Second Edition

MEDICAL-SURGICAL NURSING AND RELATED PHYSIOLOGY

JEANNETTE E. WATSON, R.N., M.Sc.N.

Professor Emeritus, Faculty of Nursing,
University of Toronto, Toronto, Canada

1979

W. B. SAUNDERS COMPANY

Philadelphia/ London/ Toronto

W. B. Saunders Company: West Washington Square
Philadelphia, PA   19105

1 St. Anne's Road
Eastbourne, East Sussex BN21 3UN, England

1 Goldthorne Avenue
Toronto, Ontario M8Z 5T9, Canada

Library of Congress Cataloging in Publication Data

Watson, Jeannette E

Medical-surgical nursing and related physiology.

Includes bibliographies and index.

1. Nursing.   2. Surgical nursing.   3. Physiology,
   Pathological.   I. Title. [DNLM: 1. Medicine – Nursing
   texts.   2. Nursing care.   3. Physiology–Nursing
   texts. WY150 W342m]

RT41.W37 1979   610.73   78–64732

ISBN 0–7216–9136–6

Medical-Surgical Nursing and Related Physiology   ISBN   0-7216-9136-6

Last digit is the print number: 9   8   7   6   5   4   3   2   1

CONTRIBUTORS AND CONSULTANTS TO THIS EDITION

KAREN WOODS CHAPMAN, R.N., M.Sc.N., Head Nurse, Hospital for Sick Children, Toronto, Canada

JOHN IAZETTA, Pharm.D., Clinical Coordinator, Drug Information Services, Sunnybrook Medical Center, University of Toronto; Assistant Professor, Faculty of Pharmacy, University of Toronto.

PATRICIA M. KEARNS, R.N., M.Sc.N., Clinical Nurse Specialist, Department of Cardiology, Sunnybrook Medical Center, University of Toronto; Clinical Associate, Faculty of Nursing, University of Toronto.

MARYLEA KENLY, R.N., Nursing Co-ordinator, Department of Neurology and Neurosurgery, Toronto General Hospital, Toronto, Canada.

S. L. NAQUI, B.Sc., M.D., F.R.C.P.(C), Department of Medicine, Sunnybrook Medical Center, University of Toronto; Assistant Professor, Faculty of Medicine, University of Toronto.

DONNA SHIELDS, R.N., C.N.M., M.Sc.N., Former Assistant Professor, Faculty of Nursing, University of Toronto.

ENID WILSON, R.N., B.Sc.N., Nurse Clinician and Enterostomal Therapist, Sunnybrook Medical Center, University of Toronto.

PREFACE
TO THE
SECOND
EDITION

The planning and writing of this edition began with consideration of the suggestions provided by readers of the previous edition. The author was grateful for the comments, and when the suggestions were consistent with the aims and scope of this textbook, an effort was made to make the changes.

The objective of this edition has been to have the content reflect many of the changes that have taken place in nursing since the previous edition was published. It is hoped that the information presented will contribute to effective patient care by providing knowledge and understanding for nursing students and practicing nurses.

The general format of the first edition has been retained. A brief review of structure and function relevant to understanding pathophysiologic changes appears at the beginning of each chapter when applicable. Frequently, when clinical nursing topics are presented alone, the physiology, which usually has been studied separately, may not be appropriately applied.

The sequence of topics is the same in this edition. However, most of the chapters have been substantially revised to include new information and current concepts. Chapters that have undergone extensive revision include Chapter 1 on patient-centered care, the chapters on the respiratory and gastrointestinal systems, and the chapter on burns and skin disorders. In Chapter 19 on the urinary system, additional emphasis has been placed on care of the patient with renal failure. Additional detail on joint disorders, especially arthritis, has been added to Chapter 25 on joint and collagen diseases. Chapters on the eye and the ear also have been expanded considerably.

The material on shock is much more extensive in this edition and now makes up a separate chapter. The material on cardiovascular nursing has been reorganized and expanded by a clinical nurse specialist in cardiovascular nursing.

v

Today's increasing emphasis on the nursing assessment of the patient has been taken into account in this revision. There is also additional material concerned with the psychological support of the patient and his family recognizing the nurse's concern with the whole patient and his problems.

Numerous new illustrations and tables are included, among them a number of new drawings by Mr. John Parker. References have been carefully selected and brought fully up-to-date. They have been chosen to provide information not included because of space limitations and for their ready availability to nurses.

The author is deeply grateful to Mrs. Joan Phillips, R.N., B.Sc.N., who typed the manuscript and provided assistance and support that made completion of the second edition possible.

The guidance and assistance received from the publisher throughout the preparation of the second edition are greatly appreciated. Special thanks are due to Miss Helen Dietz, Nursing Editor, for her guidance and patience, Mrs. Louise Robinson for her work as copy editor, Mrs. Laura Tarves for her assistance as production manager, and Mr. John Parker for many of the illustrations.

JEANNETTE E. WATSON

CONTENTS

Pain Perception 116
Pain Reactions... 116
Types of Pain.. 117

Chapter 8
THE PATIENT WITH CANCER 125

Neoplasms... 125
Cancer 126
Incidence and Trends 126
Etiologic Factors.. 128
Manifestations and Effects of Cancer...................... 131
Prevention and Early Detection............................... 132
Treatment 135
Nursing Problems Common to Patients with Cancer
and the Nurse's Role.. 150

Chapter 9
THE UNCONSCIOUS PATIENT...................................... 156
Karen Woods Chapman and Jeannette E. Watson, R.N., M.Sc.N.

Consciousness 156
Sleep... 157
Unconsciousness 157

Chapter 10
THE SURGICAL PATIENT 164

Preparation of the Patient for Surgery 164
Postoperative Nursing... 176
Postoperative Complications 184

Chapter 11
AGE—IMPLICATIONS FOR NURSING 190

Introduction 190
Nursing the Younger Patient 190
Nursing the Senescent (Significant Factors in Nursing the
Older Patient).. 201

PART II

Chapter 12
NURSING IN BLOOD DYSCRASIAS................................ 215

Composition and Physiology of Blood............................ 215
Functions of the Blood.. 215
Blood Components.. 215
Blood Groups 224
Hemostasis and Blood Coagulation........................... 227

Chapter 13
NURSING IN CARDIOVASCULAR DISEASE 269
Patricia M. Kearns, R.N., M.Sc.N.

Chapter 14
NURSING IN SHOCK 371

Chapter 15
NURSING IN RESPIRATORY DISORDERS 381

PART I

1

Comprehensive Care and the Nursing Process

KAREN WOODS CHAPMAN
JEANNETTE E. WATSON

Nursing demonstrated a remarkable preoccupation for many decades with illness and disease processes, without sufficient concern for the factors that contributed to the individual's illness. Little or no consideration was given to how the disease might have been prevented, and to what would happen to the person following discharge from the health care agency. In recent years nursing has endeavored to broaden its goals and provide services that are preventive, therapeutic, supportive and restorative in order to assist individuals and families with the promotion and maintenance of their health. Current nursing is patient-centered rather than disease-centered. It has also expanded to include consideration of the health needs of families, as well as those of the person who becomes ill. Each individual's physical, emotional, and psychological well-being is influenced markedly by the relationships, conditions and health practices within the family unit.

The provision of care is directed toward meeting the total health needs of individuals. The patient is a human being in a social setting — he has psychological and social as well as physical needs. Those of one category do not operate independently of the others; the interaction of psychological and physiological factors and their effect on health are well documented. For example, a patient's rapid pulse, diarrhea, or urinary frequency may result from the effect of his fear and anxiety on his autonomic nervous system and its control of body activities.

The breadth of current nursing practice requires much more than the technical competence and manual skills involved in the provision of physical comfort and prescribed treatment. These skills, although not less important, are only a fraction of total nursing care and may not be effective if the patient's psychological and social needs are ignored. The service expected of the nurse is patient- and family-centered comprehensive nursing — a process that attempts to recognize and meet the physical, psychological and social needs of patients and their families. Immediate and long-term goals are directed toward having patients achieve and maintain optimum physical and mental well-being.

3

Setting long-term goals implies that the nurse assumes some responsibility for the continuity of care even after the patient is discharged from the direct health service.

Included in comprehensive care are such activities as:

1. Assessment of patient's and family's health status and needs.

2. Planning and implementation of an individualized plan of care.

3. Provision of supportive, protective and comfort measures.

4. Assistance with diagnostic investigation and the prescribed therapeutic medical care.

5. Interpretation and explanation of the illness and care to the patient and family.

6. Counseling and teaching the patient and family about their health needs and how they may be met.

7. Working cooperatively with other health team members and coordinating the multidisciplinary contributions.

8. Making referrals to appropriate health and welfare personnel and agencies to ensure continuity of care and rehabilitation.

Nursing is no longer confined to the bedside; nurses assist in the delivery of health care in a variety of settings, and make contributions as consultants at all governmental levels. They, along with members of several disciplines, comprise a health team which has a common goal — the patient's and family's welfare. The composition of this team depends upon the needs and problems to be resolved; it may include one or more physicians, a dietitian, physiotherapist, social service worker, religious adviser, rehabilitation officer and community health and welfare personnel, as well as the nurses involved in providing the required care. Nurses require some knowledge and understanding of the services contributed by other health disciplines and agencies; cooperation and united efforts are necessary for the best interest of the patient.

SKILLS FOR NURSING PRACTICE

In order to provide comprehensive nursing care, the nurse must possess skills that are basic to high quality practice. These skills are interdependent and fall into three major categories: cognitive, technical and interpersonal.

Cognitive Skills

These pertain to the knowledge that the nurse has, and its application in carrying out the nursing process in providing comprehensive care. An appreciation of health that is characteristic of the various age groups (infants, children, adolescents, mature persons, senescents), the recognition of physiological and psychological disturbances and responses, and providing the required assistance demand a body of knowledge. The component activities of the nursing process (assessment, planning, implementation and evaluation) require the application of knowledge from the biological, physical and social sciences, and medicine. The profession has identified principles from related sciences and has established nursing theories and concepts as a basis for the application of the nursing process.

Recognition of influences that may be impinging upon the patient at any given time requires knowledge and skilled thought processes. For example, anorexia may be due to a physiological disturbance, or it may have a subtle psychological origin such as fear and suspicion of a malignant diagnosis, or a disturbed interpersonal relationship, or it may exist because the food is unfamiliar to the individual's ethnic dietary customs.

Technical Skills

Such skills are learned through education and practice. They are based on knowledge and have a specific role in patient care, but in actuality frequently require modification and adaptation to the condition and responses of the individual patient. The monitoring of vital signs, administration of medications, provision of fluid, nutrients, hygienic care and comfort, and doing surgical dressings are only a few of the many manual skills performed by the nurse.

Interpersonal Skills

These important skills are developed from knowledge derived principally from the psychological and sociological disciplines. An understanding of human behavior, adaptation mechanisms, an individual's values, belief systems and attitudes, and cultural influences is basic to the interpersonal process and to the establishment of satisfactory relationships.

The nurse-patient relationship is of great importance in all phases of nursing. The relationship that is established influences all that the nurse does with and for the patient, and can profoundly affect the quality and effectiveness of the service.

Mutual acceptance is basic to the achievement of a satisfactory relationship. The nurse must accept the patient without bias or prejudice. If the patient's behavior manifests stress, emotional disturbance or unacceptance, his set of circumstances and the situation should be examined carefully to determine why he reacts as he does, and if his behavior is actually an expression of some need. It is also important for the nurse to be aware of behavior responses characteristically associated with persons of different cultural backgrounds and of different age groups. As the nurse conveys an appreciation of the patient's concerns and what he is experiencing, he will accept the nurse and develop trust and confidence. A sincere interest and willingness in helping the patient may be demonstrated by acceptance, thoughtfulness, anticipation of needs, a patient, kindly, nonjudgmental manner, and a readiness to listen to the patient and answer questions. Frequently, the light touch of the nurse's hand conveys understanding, interest and caring. The patient's impressions and reactions may be influenced by the way the nurse speaks, listens and acts. Recognition of identity by addressing him by name, respect for personal preferences, and being as flexible as possible show acceptance and contribute to a satisfactory relationship. Orienting the patient to the environment, indicating how accustomed needs will be met, and explaining what is to occur and what is expected of the patient help to relieve some concern and tension.

Appreciation of the family's concerns and their need for an interpretation of what is happening to the patient conveys an understanding and warmth that instills confidence. The patient and family who develop confidence in those responsible for patient care will talk more freely about their feelings and problems. Expressing and sharing such in-

formation may prove therapeutic as well as reveal the need for appropriate nursing action.

If the patient is tense, uncommunicative, complaining or uncooperative, the nurse should analyze her own reactions and feelings about the patient. It may be that the nurse is not really accepting the patient and is being judgmental. Lack of sufficient knowledge and skills may be causing the nurse to be insecure. It may be that irritation and distraction resulting from a personal experience are responsible for the nurse's reaction in a particular situation.

During any nursing function it is evident that the three skills (cognitive, technical and interpersonal) are essential for safe, effective care and treatment. They are interdependent, interacting and overlapping. All are necessary for the provision of high quality patient care, but one may take precedence over the others in certain situations or at certain stages of the patient's illness. For example, emergency care when a person has suffered a myocardial infarction will probably necessitate the immediate application of the technical skills of resuscitation. Later, the same patient and his family require the support that can only be provided through good nurse-patient relationships.

THE PATIENT

IMPLICATIONS OF ILLNESS FOR PATIENT AND FAMILY

Patients are human individuals, not just bodies with interesting disease processes. Each has a distinctive identity as an individual, as well as a member of a family and community. Identity does not change when the role of patient is assumed. Every patient has a unique background, life style, set of values, capabilities and interests. All these factors may influence the meaning illness has for him.

A patient's concerns, responses and needs are more readily identified and interpreted if the nurse appreciates the possible implications that illness may have for the individual and his family. Illness is a stressor. It interferes with the patient's accustomed pattern of life and is likely to cause frustration, fear and anxiety. The health problem may be a threat to the individual's body integrity.

Loss of function of a body organ or part, whether temporary or permanent, may present many problems for the patient, who may fear the experience of pain, mutilation, therapeutic procedures or surgery. The health problem may be viewed as a threat to life or independence. Hospitalization is likely to initiate feelings of insecurity because the environment is strange; it lacks familiar objects and persons and an accustomed way of life.

PATIENT'S RESPONSES

The type and intensity of behavioral responses vary with each person and are influenced by such factors as:

1. The nature and severity of the patient's illness.

2. Past experiences and the patterns of behavior laid down in those experiences.

3. The resources the patient has at hand for coping and adapting to the illness.

4. The socioeconomic problems imposed or heightened by the illness.

5. The interference with plans and/or goals.

The patient's emotions may be expressed verbally or nonverbally. Verbal communication may take the form of direct statements or requests, or may hint indirectly of the patient's concern or problem. Nonverbal responses may be communicated by such manifestations as a distraught appearance, facial expressions, inability to express himself, inattention, withdrawal, depression, hostility, lack of cooperation and/or overdependency. Fear and anxiety may also account for physiological changes due to increased autonomic nervous system innervation; there may be a reduction in salivary secretion, loss of appetite, decreased gastrointestinal activity, urinary frequency, superficial vasoconstriction with resulting pallor, and cold, moist hands and feet.

PATIENT'S RIGHTS

During any illness, the patient still maintains the rights accorded to all humans and which must be respected by all health care personnel. Because of the illness the individual may not be able to maintain or establish his rights; the nurse, aware of his due privileges, assumes a protective role so that deprivation and disrespect are not suffered. Every patient has the right to:

1. High quality health care. The nurse has an obligation to endeavor conscientiously to promote high quality health care, which is a right of every citizen. A contribution can be made by every nurse by recognizing the individual's and family's health needs, maintaining high standards in her personal practice of nursing, active participation in professional organizations and research projects to promote high standards in nursing practice, cooperation in and coordination of multidisciplinary care, and assuming the professional responsibility of continuing self-education.

2. Respect and dignity as a human being. No matter how physically, psychologically or socially impaired, it must always be remembered that the patient is, first and foremost, a human being who deserves respect, kindness and understanding.

3. Life. Every person has the right to life. Conscientious endeavor to do everything that is humanly possible is required of every member of the health team. Therapeutic measures are carried out in a way that ensures safety and maximum benefit for the patient.

4. His own identity. The patient is an individual and not just a body, disease process or category of illness. Categorization or stereotyping physically or according to behavior (e.g., "the fracture or cardiac" or "the crank or complainer") does not belong in nursing.

5. Information. It is every patient's due privilege to be informed about his condition, its implications and the plan of treatment and care. By being informed, he can make appropriate decisions about his life and care, and maintain control and self-respect. Few patients prefer not to know about their illness because it may appear threatening, or because they fear the worst. The patient's responses to and feelings about illness are carefully analyzed to determine the amount of information desired.

6. The privilege of making decisions and controlling the situation. Making decisions and controlling the situation that involves self are important to the individual's security and sense of worth. If the patient is capable of good judgment, his rights of control must not be usurped. If he is incapable due to the illness or adverse intellectual, psychological

or social factors, then control must be assumed by health care personnel for the necessary length of time. If the patient is capable and informed, decisions about his care and treatment are respected.

7. Freedom of expression. The patient has the right to freedom of expression of concerns and anxieties, which should be accepted by nonjudgmental, understanding personnel.

8. Privacy. Patients have the right to claim physical and psychological privacy. Physical privacy may be protected by the use of curtains, screens, covers and closed doors, and the avoidance of abrupt, inappropriate intrusion. The right to psychological privacy is upheld by respect for the patient's wish not to discuss a subject. Repeated requests and badgering of a patient into expressing himself or reluctantly revealing some information is unwarranted. Probing into the patient's experiences or a situation for facts not relevant to the patient's health problem is unethical.

9. The presence of family and friends. The patient has the right to have others, such as family members and friends, nearby when need of their support is felt. Such persons usually have a therapeutic role that contributes to favorable progress.

BASIC HUMAN NEEDS

A large part of nursing care consists of meeting essential basic needs which are common to all persons, sick and well. Needs are ordered in terms of priority, as some are more essential for survival than others. The nurse identifies the needs according to the physical, mental and socioeconomic status of the patient and assists him in meeting those needs by the use of self and others.

Basic *biological needs* include oxygen, fluids, food, elimination of body wastes, rest and sleep, some activity and change of position, and maintenance of body temperature within a definite range.

Significant *psychosocial needs* of each person include: (1) a sense of security, or the need to feel safe and unthreatened; (2) the maintenance of identity as an individual; (3) acceptance and a sense of being wanted and belonging; (4) the opportunity for socialization; (5) independence and, at times, dependence and interdependence; (6) the freedom to make decisions; (7) the opportunity to develop and use his own potential; (8) interests and goals; (9) self-respect and usefulness; and (10) a sense of achievement. For elaboration of these points, the reader is referred to the bibliography at the end of this chapter.

The patient may or may not need assistance in meeting his requirements. When assistance is necessary, the method used must be adapted to the individual. For example, the selection of foods in meeting the fundamental need for nourishment differs, in the case of an infant or young child, from that of an adult. Modifications and special assistance may be necessary because of the patient's pathological problem. The patient with a respiratory condition may require special care in order to maintain an adequate supply of oxygen; such kinds of assistance as special positioning, suctioning to clear the airway, humidification of the air and mechanical ventilation may be necessary.

THE NURSING PROCESS

The framework for a systematic approach to identifying and meeting a patient's needs is the nursing process. It involves an ordered sequence of intellectual and physical activities directed toward a specific goal. The process consists of five logical steps:

1. Assessment of the patient and identification of his needs.

2. Establishment of priorities and planning for the necessary care.

3. Implementation of the care plan.

4. Recording.

5. Evaluation of the intervention.

Each step is part of an ongoing process and, as such, requires change, necessitating frequent reassessments. Revisions, deletions, additions and new approaches are necessary because of changes in the patient's condition and responses and the prescribed treatment from day to day. New information and more understanding of the patient and family may reveal factors that demand attention. In many instances, new needs develop when initial ones have been met; for example, a patient in the acute stage of illness has different needs when he enters the convalescent stage.

Assessment of the Patient

Patient assessment is an organized method of collecting and analyzing data about the individual's physiological, psychological and socioeconomic status. It is the first step in providing comprehensive, patient-centered care. What the nurse learns about the patient not only guides her activities for care but may be very helpful to the physician and other members of the health team in fulfilling their specific roles.

The primary sources of information about the patient are the patient, family and friends. Talking directly with the patient and family provides the nurse with more accurate information upon which to base decisions about the individual's needs and concerns. Important secondary sources include the admission record, medical history, other personnel who have cared for or are caring for the patient and the nurse's knowledge of the patient's disease.

Two major skills are associated with assessment — observation and interviewing. Accurate, objective *observation* of the patient and his family is a skilled process requiring the use of sight, hearing, touch and smell, as well as considerable thought and practice. One must learn what to observe and then make a decision as to its relevance. For example, noting the patient's general appearance, mannerisms, reactions to the environment and methods of communication reveal valuable information needed in communicating with him and planning his care. Facial expressions may provide clues to the individual's emotions, as well as comprehension. Similarly, gestures and posture may indicate anxiety, tension, pain, interest or disinterest, or other reactions. Observing attitudes and reactions when other family members are with the patient may reveal information about existing relationships and possibly point to a source of the patient's concern.

Interviewing is also a skilled endeavor used by the nurse to assess the patient's needs. The interview is designed so as to pertain only to data needed for comprehensive care and is conducted in a private setting; sitting in a crowded noisy hallway is not conducive to establishing rapport and free discussion of personal details. If the interview is to be a valuable tool, the nurse must make an effort to put the patient at ease and reduce anxiety and possible embarrassment. Tactfully, and without appearing to probe, the patient is encouraged to talk about himself and his family, interests and activities. His knowledge of his illness and his feelings and concerns about it are elicited. The interviewer should listen attentively and periodically comment briefly to assure the patient of attention and interest. It may be appropriate to say something that will channel the conversation so that the type of information being sought will be revealed. In some instances the interviewer may find it necessary to use a nonstructured format for the interview so that the patient will converse freely without sensing he is being interviewed.

It may or may not be useful to have the patient's family present at the interview. They may provide support and increase the amount of information given but, in some instances, the family may inhibit the patient, particularly if there is an emotional problem or discordant relationship between them. If the family is not present during the patient interview, arrangements are made to interview them at some other time. They can often provide helpful information about the patient, and they may have needs and concerns of their own for which the nurse can provide assistance.

Many helath agencies have nursing history forms which are used in obtaining and recording information that is pertinent to planning and implementing patient care. Information obtained in the interview and recorded on the nursing history is selected on the basis of its value for effective planning and implementing of nursing care. It is important that it not be a repetition of data recorded in the admission record and medical history. Frequently, the type of information found on the nursing history will indicate such items as family occupation, education, interests, social activities, personal hygiene habits, food likes and dislikes, elimination habits, patterns of sleep, rest and exercise, and sensitivities and allergies.

Physical assessment may or may not be the responsibility of the nurse in a particular work situation. This is usually carried out by a physician, but if required of the nurse she will have acquired the knowledge and technical skills essential for a competent physical examination. The skills used are inspection, palpation, percussion and auscultation. The reader is referred to the bibliography at the end of this chapter for references dealing with physical assessment.

Through analysis and interpretation of the data obtained in the assessment of the patient, the nurse identifies the patient's needs. Priorities and immediate and long-term goals are established. Advice and further information may be obtained from other health care personnel when clarification of a problem is required.

Planning Care for the Patient

Once needs have been identified consideration is then given to the course of action. There are several advantages to using a deliberate, systematic approach in the planning of care for each patient. Planning leads to decisions that are patient-centered and on an individualized basis, as well as to doing things in an orderly and least time-consuming manner. It necessitates more thoughtful analysis of the information pertaining to the patient which is likely to result in more effective implementation and evaluation of nursing action. Modifications are more likely to be made in accord with the individual's preferences, accustomed activities and particular situation. The written plan is made available to all who are nursing the patient to exclude the need for repetition on the part of the patient as to his preferences and needed adaptations. Systematic planning also allows for more satisfactory use of personnel and time.

Planning is more effective when it can be done by all those who will participate in the patient's care and, when his condition and the situation permits, it is important that the patient also be involved to some extent in the planning. Increased cooperation and realization of his potential often result if the patient is a respected participant in the planning of his own care.

How the patient's needs are to be met is influenced by such factors as:

1. The patient's condition and the severity of the illness.
2. The acuteness of the need.
3. Whether the patient is ambulatory or not.
4. The amount of assistance required (i.e., the extent of independence or dependence).
5. The available facilities, resources, time and staff.

There is a tendency in hospitals to follow established routines rather than to make adjustments for meeting the individual patient's needs. *The patient, and not the hospital routine, is the focus of good nursing care.* For example, if a patient is resting after having had a sleepless night due to pain, it is far more important to let him rest than to carry out the morning routine of bed bath and bed making. Such chores can always be done later when it is more convenient for the patient. When it is desirable for the patient to participate in self-care the benefit of such activity is explained to him, since many patients expect to have everything done for them. Self-care helps to increase the patient's autonomy, plays a role in the prevention of complications, and allows him some independence and mastery of his illness.

Implementation of the Care Plan

Implementation is the actual carrying out of the care plan. In the performance of direct nursing activities, the patient is advised about what is to be done, the purpose, what may be expected, and what is expected of him. The nurse avoids rigidity and is prepared to make adaptations to accommodate the patient as long as the principles of the treatment are observed and the patient derives maximum benefits. Awareness of factors that contribute to his comfort and safety, and observation of his reactions, are necessary in all that is done with or for the patient.

Recording

The nurse's notes are an account of significant patient reactions, behavior and verbal expressions, as well as treatments and care given. Statements should be current, accurate, objective, clearly legible and concise. They keep the physician and others participating in the care of the patient informed about the patient's condition, and may contribute to the diagnosis and decisions regarding necessary treatment. The record is a confidential document; it is only available to others than those participating in the care by special permission from the patient and the health agency. The notes may also be used to assess the effectiveness of care and the patient's progress, and may provide data for research.

Evaluation of the Intervention

Evaluation of the intervention is the comparison of the expected outcome to the actual outcome. For example, if a patient is expected to learn self-administration of insulin in the treatment of diabetes mellitus within 5 days, then at the end of that period the nurse determines if the patient is capable of giving the injections. If the patient is considered capable by the nurse, then the goal of the care plan has been achieved. If the patient is unable to administer his injections satisfactorily, then the care plan will be revised and the reasons for the difficulties assessed. The practice of evaluation is not only useful in improving patient care, but it can also be an educational process for the nurse; it may reveal that there are several approaches and methods that can be applied to a single problem.

During a prolonged hospital stay, continuous evaluation is made of the patient's care. A conference of the nursing personnel involved may be used to assess the situation and consider whether the patient's needs being recognized, whether the goals are listic and are being met, whether the best methods are being used, what new goals should be set and what new approaches should be used. The evaluation process includes the comments and criticisms of the patient and family; often, it is only the patient who can truly state the effectiveness of the intervention.

Self-evaluation of one's practices is just as important as an appraisal of the intervention. Each individual nurse should reflect on and evaluate her role and performance at regular intervals. The relationship established with the patient and his family and the completeness and effectiveness of her nursing are analyzed. Decisions are made regarding necessary revisions in professional practice so that a maximum contribution to high quality nursing care can be made. Self-assessment is very much a part of the nursing process and should be encouraged. Peer review or a head nurse's appraisal may be helpful if the nurse finds self-evaluation difficult.

CONTINUITY OF CARE

In comprehensive nursing, concern for the patient extends beyond the nurse's direct care and contact with him. It is necessary to consider what happens to this person after discharge from the hospital or nursing agency. He may require continued care, adjustments in his future way of life in order to live within his functional capacity, and instruction as to specific treatments and health measures. Advice and suggestions may be indicated for the patient and family in the interest of promoting their health and preventing illness.

This part of the patient's care should not be left until the last day or two before discharge but should receive attention throughout the illness, and early plans should be made for necessary discussions, instruction and referrals so that they may be complete and effective. Some knowledge of the situation to which the patient will return is important. This may be obtained from the family and patient, or the home situation may be assessed by a district health nurse or social service worker who may indicate the necessary adjustments. Plans for discharge are made in conjunction with other members of the health team. Any suggestions for assistance are discussed with and approved by the patient and the family before a referral is made. Contact with the resource agency is accompanied by relevant information about the patient's condition and regimen of care. The patient and family are also advised of indications of the need for contacting the physician or clinic.

Some teaching of the patient and family may be incidental, but much of it involves planning and organization. Motivation and readiness for learning, as well as the setting of objectives, are important factors. The content of the teaching required to meet the needs may be related to the patient's present illness, the general health habits of the patient and family or to some specific health problem of a family member. What is taught should be authentic, expressed in terms understandable to the patient, and adapted to his age, education, socioeconomic status and culture. Content related to therapeutic measures should be approved by the physician.

Teaching may be shared by the physician, dietitian or physiotherapist. It is helpful if the nurse is familiar with their instructions so she may reinforce them and be able to answer the patient's related questions.

Incidental teaching can frequently be given while administering treatments and care, and may relate to what is actually being done. For some instruction, definite uninterrupted periods are arranged at a time when the patient is comfortable and rested. These periods should be relatively short; offering too much at one time may defeat the purpose and only leave the patient confused and discouraged. When the family is to be included, times are determined as to when they can be present. Demonstrations of procedures such as colostomy care or the giving of insulin may be broken down into several steps, and followed by opportunities for the patient or family member to carry them out under the supervision of the nurse. In some instances, group teaching may be possible if there are several patients requiring similar instruction. This is of value, as it may be followed by discussions among the patients. Discovering that there are others with similar problems does much to reduce the patient's anxiety.

Time and opportunities are made available for the patient and family to ask questions, and for repetition and reinforcement of instructions. Appropriate literature, illustrations, clear simple outlines of directions and examples of improvised equipment may serve as valuable teaching aids to clarify and reinforce the content presented to the patient and family. When teaching needs are recognized they are recorded on the nursing care plan and checked off when satisfactorily achieved.

The guidance and course of action taken to ensure continuity of care are evaluated, if possible, through some follow-up or by contacting the assisting agency or the patient himself. Getting in touch with the patient and family after discharge can be a very significant contribution to continuity of care.

References

Books

Aronson, E.: The Social Animal. San Francisco, Reddman, 1972.
Beland, I. L., and Passos, J.: Clinical Nursing, 3rd ed. New York, Macmillan, 1975. Chapter 1.
Byrne, M., and Thompson, L.: Key Concepts for the Study and Practice of Nursing. St. Louis, C. V. Mosby, 1972.
Carlson, C. (Ed.): Behavioural Concepts and Nursing Intervention. Philadelphia, J. B. Lippincott, 1970.
Carter, F.: Psychosocial Nursing: Theory and Practice in Hospital and Community Health, 2nd ed. New York, Macmillan, 1976.
DeGowin, E., and DeGowin, R.: Bedside Diagnostic Examination. 3rd ed. New York, Macmillan, 1975.
Delp, M., and Manning, R. (Ed.): Major's Physical Diagnosis, 8th ed. Philadelphia, W. B. Saunders, 1975.
Duval, E.: Family Development, 4th ed. Philadelphia, J. B. Lippincott, 1971.
Fawkes, William C., Jr., and Hunn, Virginia, K.: Clinical Assessment for the Nurse Practitioner. St. Louis, C. V. Mosby, 1973.
Jourard, S.: The Transparent Self. New York, Van Nostrand Reinhold, 1971.
King, I.: Toward a Theory for Nursing. New York, John Wiley and Sons, 1971.
Kintzel, K. (Ed.): Advanced Concepts in Clinical Nursing. Philadelphia, J. B. Lippincott, 1971.
MacBryde, C. M., and Blacklow, R. (Eds.): Signs and Symptoms, 5th ed. Philadelphia, J. B. Lippincott, 1970. Chapter 31.
Maslow, A.: Motivation and Personality, 2nd ed. New York, Harper and Row, 1970.
Rogers, M.: An Introduction to the Theoretical Basis of Nursing. Philadelphia, F. A. Davis, 1970.
Sundeen, S., Stuart, G., Rankin, E., and Cohen, S.: Nurse-Client Interaction. St. Louis, C. V. Mosby, 1976.
Toffler, A.: Future Shock. New York, Bantam Books, 1970.
Towle, C.: Common Human Needs. New York, National Association of Social Workers, 1952.

Periodicals

Arpin, K., and Parker, N.: "Developing a Conceptual Framework." Nurs. Papers (Canada), Vol. 7, No. 4 (Winter 1975–1976), pp. 28–34.
Bates, B., and Lynaugh, J.: "Laying the Foundations for Medical Surgical Practice." Am. J. Nurs., Vol. 73, No. 8 (Aug. 1973), pp. 1375–1379.

Beletz, E.: "Is Nursing's Public Image Up to Date?" Nurs. Outlook, Vol. 22, No. 7 (July 1974), pp. 432–435.

Beyers, M., and Philips, C.: "Keys to Successful Leadership." Nurs. '74, Vol. 4, No. 7 (July 1974), pp. 51–58.

Carrieri, V., and Sitzman, J.: "Components of the Nursing Process." Nurs. Clin. North Am., Vol. 6, No. 1 (Mar. 1971), pp. 115–124.

Craven, R., and Sharp, B.: "The Effects of Illness on Family Functions." Nurs. Forum, Vol. 11, No. 2 (1972), pp. 186–193.

Eggland, Eileen Thomas: "How to Take a Meaningful History." Nurs. '77, Vol. 7, No. 7 (July 1977), pp. 22–30.

Foley, J.: "Wanted: A Theory of Nursing." Can. Nurs., Vol. 67, No. 1 (Nov. 1971), pp. 28–32.

Fredette, Sheila: "The Art of Applying Theory to Practice." Am. J. Nurs., Vol. 74, No. 5 (May 1974), pp. 856–859.

Fry, J., and Majumdai, B.: "Basic Physical Assessment." Can. Nurs., Vol. 70, No. 5 (May 1974), pp. 17–22.

Fuller, D., and Rosenaur, J.: "A Patient Assessment Guide." Nurs. Outlook, Vol. 22, No. 7 (July 1974), pp. 460–462.

Grant, Carol: "A Basis for Care." Am. J. Nurs., Vol. 72, No. 4 (Apr. 1972), pp. 699–701.

Hein, Eleanor, and Leavitt, Maribelle: "Providing Emotional Support to Patients." Nurs. '77, Vol. 7, No. 5 (May 1977), pp. 38–41.

Kalisch, B.: "Strategies for Developing Nursing Empathy." Nurs. Outlook, Vol. 19, No. 11 (Nov. 1971). pp. 714–718.

———: "What is Empathy?" Am. J. Nurs., Vol. 73, No. 9 (Sept. 1973), pp. 1548–1552.

Kelly, L.: "The Patient's Right to Know." Nurs. Outlook, Vol. 24, No. 1 (Jan. 1976), pp. 26–32.

Levine, M.: "The Intransigent Patient." Am. J. Nurs., Vol. 70, No. 10 (Oct. 1970), pp. 2106–2111.

Loesch, L., and Loesch, N.: "What Do You Say After You Say Mm-Hmm?" Am. J. Nurs., Vol. 75, No. 5 (May 1975), pp. 807–809.

Mundinger, M., and Jauron, G.: "Developing a Nursing Diagnosis." Nurs. Outlook, Vol. 23, No. 2 (Feb. 1975), pp. 94–98.

Nichols, M.: "Quality Control in Patient Care." Am. J. Nurs., Vol. 74, No. 3 (Mar. 1974), pp. 456–459.

Porter, Anne Lynn: "Patient Needs on Admission." Am. J. Nurs., Vol. 77, No. 1 (Jan. 1977), pp. 112–113.

Redman, B.: "Guidelines for Quality of Care in Patient Education." Can. Nurs., Vol. 71, No. 2 (Feb. 1975), pp. 19–21.

Redmond, Barbara: "Patient Education as a Function of Nursing Practice." Nurs. Clin. North Am., Vol. 6, No. 4 (Dec. 1971), pp. 573–580.

Reilly, D.: "Why a Conceptual Framework?" Nurs. Outlook, Vol. 23, No. 9 (Sept. 1975), pp. 566–569.

Reinkeymeyer, A.: "Nursing Need: Commitment to an Ideology of Change." Nurs. Forum, Vol. 9, No. 4 (1970), pp. 340–355.

Rickles, N., and Finkle, B.: "Anxiety: Yours and Your Patient's." Nurs. '73, Vol. 3, No. 3 (Mar. 1973), pp. 23–26.

Schaefer, J.: "The Interrelatedness of Decision-Making and the Nursing Process." Am. J. Nurs., Vol. 74, No. 10 (Oct. 1974), pp. 1852–1855.

Schlotfeldt, R.: "This I Believe . . . Nursing is Health Care." Nurs. Outlook, Vol. 20, No. 4 (April 1972), pp. 245–246.

Seigel, H.: "To Your Health — Whatever that May Mean." Nurs. Forum, Vol. 12, No. 3 (1973), pp. 280–289.

Sloboda, Sharon: "Understanding Patient Behavior." Nurs. '77, Vol. 7, No. 9 (Sept. 1977), pp. 74–77.

Spicer, M.: "What About the Patient?" Nurs. Clin. North Am., Vol. 7, No. 2 (June 1972), pp. 313–322.

Standover, M.: "The Relevant Who of Problem Solving." Nurs. Forum, Vol. 10, No. 2 (1971), pp. 166–175.

Thomstad, B., Cunningham, N., and Kaplan, B.: "Changing the Rules of The Doctor-Nurse Game." Nurs. Outlook, Vol. 23, No. 7 (July 1975), pp. 422–427.

Vincent, P.: "The Sick Role in Patient Care." Am. J. Nurs., Vol. 75, No. 7 (July 1975), pp. 1172–1173.

White, M.: "Importance of Selected Nursing Activities." Nurs. Res., Vol. 21, No. 1 (Jan./Feb. 1972), pp. 4–14.

2

Rehabilitation of the Disabled

INTRODUCTION

Rehabilitation is the process whereby a disabled person is assisted to regain, and utilize fully, his physical, mental, social and vocational potential insofar as the disability permits. The individual is directed toward establishing a pattern of life that provides a sense of worth, independence and satisfaction.

In recent years there has been increasing recognition of the potential of disabled persons; given assistance, many can become self-reliant, be gainfully employed, and take their rightful place in society. Rehabilitation takes time, effort, money, personnel and facilities, but such expenditures can scarcely be questioned when one considers what rehabilitation means to the individual who is faced with remaining useless and dependent unless given assistance.

The rehabilitation process may be brief and simple for some patients, involving only a few instructions and minor adjustments that will help to cope with the environment. For others, it may require a long period and the special techniques of a multidisciplinary team to help them develop an entirely new pattern of life. Various combinations of personnel may be necessary, depending on the type of disability and the type of person. The rehabilitation program must be individualized; two patients with a similar disability do not necessarily have the same degree of handicap, and certainly they do not have the same remaining capabilities and interests. The team concerned with a single patient may include the physician, nurse, physiotherapist, speech therapist, psychologist, social worker, vocational counselor, educator, employment officer and recreational director. In other instances the team may be made up of the physician, nurse and physiotherapist. Each team member has a contribution to make, but these efforts have to be coordinated. Cooperative planning and an exchange of information between the workers are necessary for maximal effectiveness. Frequently, one team member has the opportunity to reinforce another's work, but this can be done only if each is familiar with the total rehabilitation plan.

DISABILITIES

All illnesses cause disability to some extent, but when the term is used in the context of rehabilitation it implies a prolonged or permanent impairment or the loss of some bodily function. The disability may be congenital, or may be acquired suddenly or gradually as a result of injury or disease of any system of the body and it may be static or progressive. A disability may be secondary to or a complication of a long illness in which there was prolonged inacti-

13

vity or improper positioning. According to Hirschberg, et al., the commonest prolonged and permanent disabilities that necessitate special rehabilitative considerations are "caused by involvement of the nervous system, the musculoskeletal system and the cardiopulmonary system."[1] Handicapped persons are frequently classified according to the nature of their disability. They may be referred to as physically handicapped because their mobility is restricted, or as mentally handicapped because of mental illness or a subnormal level of intelligence which results in difficulty in the management of personal affairs or adjustment in society. The visually handicapped are those with partial or total loss of vision and those with auditory handicaps have a partial or total loss of hearing.

Potential Effects

Many disabilities foster prolonged inactivity. Unless preventive measures are instituted at the onset of a physical disability, complications and secondary disabilities may develop rapidly as the result of inactivity, improper positioning, pressure, injury or misuse. Immobilization and inactivity lead to *muscle wasting* and *contracture* and to *stiffening of joints* which limits the range of joint movement. Prolonged bed rest or confinement to a wheel-chair prevents normal weight-bearing and muscle pull on the bones; this may cause a *loss of calcium from the bones* (osteoporosis), resulting in increased urinary excretion of calcium that predisposes to the formation of renal or bladder calculi.

Inactivity for long periods causes *venous stasis,* which predisposes to phlebothrombosis and pulmonary embolism. The individual experiences *impaired pulmonary function* that involves a reduction in lung expansion and total lung and tidal volumes. Atelectasis and the retention of secretions are prone to develop, leading to pneumonia. Loss of strength in the respiratory muscles and the use of sedatives or narcotics contribute to shallow breathing and depression of the cough reflex.

Prolonged inactivity may also cause *orthostatic hypotension,* making it difficult for the patient to assume a sitting or upright position. Immobility *reduces energy demands* and *metabolism;* the patient may complain of being chilly in a room in which the temperature is comfortable to others. He may become apathetic and less alert.

Prolonged pressure on an area of the body compresses the blood vessels in the tissues and inhibits a normal blood flow through the area. The tissue becomes necrotic and sloughs away, leaving a *pressure sore* (decubitus ulcer). The most vulnerable areas are those over bony prominences, such as the sacral region, lateral area of the hip over the femoral trochanter, ischial region, heels, back of the head, and shoulder and scapular regions.

Constipation and fecal impaction occur frequently as a result of inactivity and the concomitant change in the patient's diet.

Occasionally, the handicapped individual may attempt to do something beyond the limitations imposed by his initial disability; as a result, he may *sustain an injury* that adds to his problems. For example, the patient may try to walk without the necessary assistance and fall, or a joint may be overextended, injuring ligaments or the joint capsule and cause pain, weakness and instability of the joint. Similarly, use or overexercise of a limb when a joint is acutely inflamed or when insufficient healing has taken place may cause *joint damage or instability* that may increase his disability and prove a hindrance to satisfactory rehabilitation.

A disability or prolonged inactivity is certain to have some *psychological effect* on the person. The implications of a disability vary with each individual according to the nature and severity of the handicap and according to personality, values, goals and responsibilities. The loss of the capacity to function as a normal, independent, productive being strikes a severe blow. It may mean dependence on others for ordinary, personal day-to-day care. A career in which a great deal of time, effort and money have been invested may be interrupted. The individual's self-image is changed, and he may see himself as different, abnormal, worthless and a burden to his family and to society.

---

[1]Gerald G. Hirschberg, Leon Lewis and Dorothy Thomas: Rehabilitation. Philadelphia, J.B. Lippincott, 1964, p. 12.

The patient experiences bewilderment, fear, and feelings of insecurity and loneliness. The dominant emotional responses and behavior which each individual manifests are determined by his previous experiences and conditioning. The process of acceptance and adjustment will be a greater struggle for some than for others. Persons who previously possessed the capacity to meet the stresses of life successfully are usually more able to cope with this new problem; others may develop emotional and personality problems. In the initial state of conflict and turmoil, acute depression accompanied by a lack of desire to live, denial of the existence of disability, anger, hostility and a lack of cooperation are frequent reactions seen in disabled persons. The period in which the patient overcomes the initial impact of disability, faces reality and accepts the situation may be much longer for some than for others. A change in personality may become apparent; the patient may lose interest in everything beyond himself and may tend to withdraw from the world around him, or he may become resentful and hostile.

When a member of the family becomes disabled, a *change in the way of life for the whole family* may be necessary. Responsibilities are shifted, financial hardships may be experienced, and plans and goals may be shattered. Their responses to the situation are also conditioned by their life circumstances, personalities and previous experiences.

THE REHABILITATIVE PROCESS

The rehabilitative part of the disabled person's care starts when he first comes under treatment in the hospital, clinic or home and should be continued until he has learned to live and work with his remaining abilities. In many instances, some aspects of rehabilitation care are required continuously (e.g., exercises, special skin care) in order to maintain the restorative status and to prevent deterioration and debility.

During the *acute phase* of the illness, treatment and care are directed toward having the patient recover from the disabling disease or injury with a minimum of dysfunction. The prevention of complications and secondary disabilities and the provision of psychological support are equally important. The acute illness is followed by the *restorative and retraining phase* of rehabilitation. This phase includes: (1) evaluation of the patient's functional status, potentials and persisting deficits; (2) the setting of realistic goals; and (3) the planning and implementing of a program of activities for realizing these goals. Who will be involved and what activities will be necessary will depend on the nature of the handicap, the extent to which the patient is damaged, the previous pattern of life, and remaining abilities and interests.

The rehabilitation program may include: (1) measures to improve and maintain the individual's general physical condition; (2) correction of deformities that restrict rehabilitation, passive movements and active exercises; (3) helping the patient to resume self-care; (4) psychological support and therapy; (5) special techniques for specific disabilities (e.g., speech therapy or new methods of mobility through the use of mechanical devices, such as braces, crutches, or prostheses); (6) education or vocational training; (7) employment placement; (8) arranging for participation in safe, appropriate, social and recreational activities; (9) assisting the family in accepting the patient and adjusting to the enforced changes in their life; (10) teaching the family how they may best help the patient and at the same time conserve their own energy; and, if necessary, (11) helping the family to procure welfare assistance.

In *evaluation of the individual's rehabilitation potential,* a history of his background is important. His education, previous interests, occupation and achievements, and role in the family and community are ascertained. His physical and mental capacity, personality and aptitudes are then assessed. An appraisal is made which should include assessment of the patient's strength, capacity for self-care, motor functions, including the ability to move from one place to another, and communication skills. Psychological and aptitude tests may be necessary to determine his intellectual capacity and the type of vocation for which he might be prepared. Knowledge of his home, family, and the social and physical environments in which he will live is also necessary.

An interpretation of what the patient may and may not do should be made to him and his family. Then, insofar as is possible, it is very important that plans for his future should respect his interests; he should be encouraged to express what he would like most to achieve within his limitations and capacity and to participate in the decisions. He is more likely to mobilize personal resources and make progress in retraining if he is working toward a goal of personal interest. If the initial rehabilitative plans and techniques are not successful, this does not preclude attempting other methods which may yield more success. Optimism, patience and persistence are necessary in those working with the patient.

There are few disabled persons who cannot be helped to some extent by rehabilitative measures. It is important to divide the program into small, workable sequential pieces compatible with the patient's ability to succeed. Achievement is rewarding as well as motivating; with success, the individual begins to focus on and attach value to the things he can do. If the patient is seriously damaged and rehabilitation is not possible, care is designed to prevent further disability and regression, to reduce suffering to a minimum and to make life as tolerable as possible for the individual and his family.

REHABILITATION NURSING

The Nurse's Role

Although the general use of the term rehabilitation is directed toward individuals with residual limitations, rehabilitation is really a part of the nursing care of all patients, for the primary objective with any patient is to restore him to optimal health and to have him return to his home and community as an independent, productive person. In this context, rehabilitation nursing is simply a part of the comprehensive care required by a patient whose illness or injury imposes some residual disability or limitations upon him.

Through early and continuing contact with the patient, the nurse has the opportunity to contribute greatly to the patient's rehabilitation. Attitude may have a significant influence on the patient's progress. It is important to appreciate the impact of disability on the patient and to develop a positive, motivating approach which reflects an underlying belief that the situation is not hopelesss — that the patient can and will be restored to a worthwhile life. Tradition and the teaching of nursing have generally emphasized doing to and for the patient, rather than encouraging, teaching and permitting self-care. As the disabled patient's condition warrants it, he is encouraged to assume more responsibility for his own care. Overprotection and doing things for him which he can do for himself only increase his dependence, passivity and feelings of inadequacy.

Nursing the disabled person should be structured from the onset to meet rehabilitative goals. Such goals include: (1) the strengthening and maintenance of the patient's functional capacities; (2) the prevention of further impairment and secondary disabilities; (3) assisting the patient and his family in dealing with the psychological impact of disability; (4) the motivation of the patient to realize his potentials, encouraging and teaching self-care; (5) knowing and using available resources that can be of assistance in rehabilitating the patient; and (6) helping the family to adjust to the situation and to obtain necessary assistance.

Rehabilitation measures related to disabilities associated with specific conditions are presented with the nursing care in the respective ensuing chapters. The following sections include a discussion of nursing factors that are common to the care of many disabled persons, particularly in cases involving prolonged inactivity.

ASSESSMENT

An ongoing evaluation from day to day is an important part of the nurse's responsibility in caring for the patient. The disabled person's physical status and emotional reaction rarely remain completely stable; they tend to fluctuate, and the program may have to be adjusted occasionally so as to be in accord with the patient's current reactions.

The nurse listens and observes to learn about the *individual's reactions* to his disability. In working with the patient, an assessment is made as to *what is the most the patient can do today* and *what his potential is for the future*.

The *skin* is examined carefully each time care is given and at frequent regular intervals when the patient assumes self-care.

The patient's *nutritional status* is followed closely; the physical demands being made on him by the exercise program and the necessary resistance to possible infections require a well-balanced diet. Obesity is avoided as it may prove a handicap in achieving mobility and independence.

An evaluation is made of the *range of joint movement, voluntary movements,* and *self-care capacity.* Involuntary muscle movements and contractures are noted and recorded.

Positioning.

The patient's position is changed every 1 to 2 hours to prevent circulatory stasis and prolonged pressure on any one part of the body, to promote expansion of the lungs and drainage of pulmonary secretions, and to contribute to his comfort. The general principles of good body alignment are observed; overextension or strain of any joint is avoided, and a minimum of flexion used. A firm mattress is used to prevent sagging under the patient's weight and if necessary, a bed board may be added.

In the dorsal position, the body should be in a straight line. A foot board is necessary to support the feet at near-right angles to the legs with the heels resting in the space between the foot board and the mattress or on some resilient material, such as sponge rubber, to avoid pressure (see Figure 2–1). The space under the popliteal region may be filled in to prevent strain on the knee joint, and a firm trochanter roll (see Fig. 2–2) or sandbag is placed against the lateral surface of the thigh, extending from above the hip joint to below the knee to prevent outward rotation of the lower limb. If there is paralysis of an arm, it is abducted and a pillow is placed between the trunk and the arm to prevent adduction contracture. The forearm is slightly flexed and the wrist is supported with the fingers and thumb in ex-

tension. The thickness of the pillow under the head should be sufficient to maintain the head in line with the spine so that flexion and extension are avoided.

In the lateral position, the lower limbs are slightly flexed; the one that is uppermost is flexed to a greater degree than the other, and it is supported on a pillow to prevent strain on the hip joint. The uppermost arm is flexed and supported on a pillow in front of the patient (see Fig. 2–1).

When the prone position is used, the head pillow is removed, and the head is turned to one side. A flat pillow or support is placed under the patient's abdomen well below the lower border of the rib cage to prevent strain on the back. The arms are abducted and flexed at the elbows, or one may be left down alongside the trunk. The feet may be supported by a small pillow under the ankles to keep the toes free of the bed, or the forepart of the foot may be suspended over the end of the mattress. (See Fig. 2–1.)

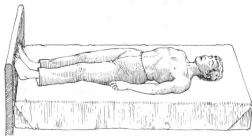

DORSAL RECUMBENT BED POSITION

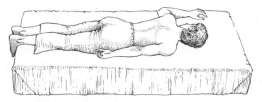

LATERAL BED POSITION

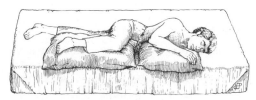

PRONE BED POSITION

FIGURE 2–1 Positioning the patient in bed.

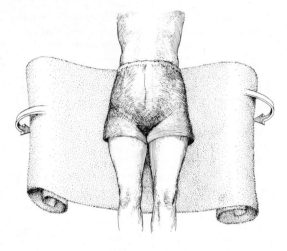

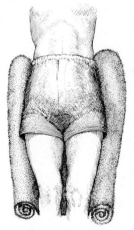

FIGURE 2–2 Trochanter roll, used to prevent external rotation of lower limb.

Skin Care

A decubitus ulcer or pressure sore will develop with startling rapidity in an area subjected to continuous pressure, but it may take weeks or months to heal. Preventive measures must be instituted promptly with all patients whose movement is restricted, who cannot shift their body weight from one area to another, and who have impaired sensory function that inhibits their awareness of the discomfort of prolonged pressure on a part. The patient's position is changed every 1 to 2 hours, and gentle massage is used to stimulate circulation in the parts subjected to pressure. Vulnerable areas may also be protected by the use of resilient surfaces, such as foam rubber, an alternating air pressure mattress and pieces of "sheepskin." The patient's skin is kept clean and dry to prevent irritation and maceration. The undersheets are kept dry, soft, and free of wrinkles and any irritating particles. Areas subjected to pressure are inspected with each change of position for early signs of ischemia and tissue damage. If damaged, the area may appear blanched and cool at first; then it becomes red or bluish-red, followed by darkening and then breakdown of the skin. Underlying layers of tissue may also be destroyed, and as the dead tissue is sloughed off a deep, open lesion remains and is referred to as an ulcer.

If an ulcer develops, the area is kept clean to prevent infection and is protected from pressure. Special treatment will be prescribed by the physician; any number of preparations are used in the forms of moist compresses, powders and ointments. Some of these may be for removal of the necrotic tissue (débridement); others may be to stimulate healing or to control infection. As the necrotic tissue is sloughed off, hopefully, the area fills in with granulation tissue and eventually heals over. The area around the ulcer is gently massaged to encourage an adequate blood supply to the area. A diet high in protein and vitamins B and C contributes to healing.

If the ulcer is large and the subcutaneous tissue is destroyed, the physician may consider skin grafting advisable.

As the disabled patient learns and assumes self-care, the importance of frequent change of position is explained, and he is taught to change his position at regular and frequent intervals. If he progresses to a wheelchair, a foam rubber cushion is provided, and the patient is advised to shift his weight and raise himself at regular, frequent intervals as prolonged sitting predisposes to a pressure sore in the ischial region. When there is loss of sensation, as with the paraplegic, the individual is taught to inspect the vulnerable areas by means of a mirror at least once daily.

Psychological Support

The disabled patient's reactions of disbelief, followed by depression and probable resentment that this has happened to him, are understandable. The nurse, knowing why he is behaving as he is, accepts his reactions; her behavior helps to convey a sense of understanding and caring. The patient is insecure, lonely and afraid; he should not be left alone for long periods. Close observation of his reactions and comments will indicate to the nurse when to encourage conversation or when it is her presence alone that is preferable to the patient. At the appropriate time, the nurse may acknowledge verbally that she knows the situation looks hopeless to him and may assure him that everything possible will be done to help him regain his strength and ability to do things for himself. Offering false hope and being overcheerful are to be avoided. Assimilation of the change in body image and pattern of life associated with his disability takes time. Gradually, as the patient recognizes the nurse's understanding, he may talk about his situation and, through this, begin to see things more realistically and explore possibilities for his future. His thinking is directed to the positive, to things he can do and would like to do. He is helped to become aware of his capabilities by being allowed to do things for himself as soon as possible. Early interpretation and initiation of rehabilitation measures offer hope and motivate the patient.

Periods of depression and withdrawal are to be expected from time to time, particularly when achievement of some aspect of his rehabilitation seems slow and frustrating. Such reactions are accepted, but with an attitude of expectation that he will persevere and ultimately succeed.

Frequent visits from family members may provide support and reinforce the impression that they are not rejecting him as a cripple. A bright, cheerful room is desirable, and being with others with similar disabilities may help.

Nutrition

Nutrition plays an important role in the patient's rehabilitation; a well-balanced diet is necessary for increasing the patient's strength. Anorexia may be a problem, due to the patient's emotional responses to his disability. An inadequate diet and nutritional deficiencies may predispose to complications that delay his restoration. Factors that encourage the patient to take adequate food include an environment that is physically, socially and psychologically acceptable, having the patient clean and comfortable, serving small amounts of high-calorie foods frequently, respect for his food preferences insofar as is possible, and provision of the necessary assistance. Most patients dislike having to be fed and frequently take less because of this. It improves morale and possibly increases the amount of food taken when the patient can manage self-feeding. Ingenuity on the part of the nurse is important in making minor adjustments so the food can be easily reached by the patient whose range of arm motion may be limited.

The total caloric intake is adjusted to maintain the individual's normal weight and to meet his energy expenditure. Increasing physical exercises and activity in his retraining program require a corresponding increase in calories. Obesity should be avoided, since excess weight increases the patient's handicap and impedes rehabilitation.

A high-protein and high-vitamin diet is encouraged; the increased protein intake is necessary to maintain muscle mass and tissue resistance. The vitamins improve the patient's appetite and increase his resistance.

Calcium-containing foods may be restricted because of the predisposition to the formation of kidney and bladder calculi (see p. 653). Precipitation of the calcium occurs more readily in an alkaline urine; a diet high in foods that leave an acid metabolic waste and drugs that acidify the urine may be ordered.

Elimination

Constipation and bowel and urinary incontinence are frequently associated with disabilities, especially if the primary problem is neurological. *Constipation* is usually the result of inactivity and changes in diet and routine. For treatment and nursing care of the patient with this problem see page 538.

Incontinence can be a serious source of emotional disturbance and discouragement for the patient. Unexpected involuntary urination or defecation when the patient has just been bathed, during meals or exercise routines, or while friends and family are visiting can be very embarrassing to him. The problem is discussed realistically with the patient; he is advised that a routine and control can be established, but it will require time and patience. The proposed plan to establish control is outlined, and the patient's role described. Mentally responsible patients are usually very anxious to cooperate.

Bowel incontinence in the disabled may be due to some damage or degenerative change of the central nervous system that causes loss of sensation of the defecation stimulus and voluntary control of the external anal sphincter.

A regular time for daily evacuation of the bowel should be decided upon, taking into consideration its convenience in relation to the day's activities and the patient's schedule when he returns home. Foods and fluids which stimulate peristalsis are included in the diet while training the bowel to empty at a specific time. One or two glycerin suppositories may be inserted into the rectum ½ to 2 hours before placing the patient on the commode or toilet, or digital stimulation may be used.

It is necessary to experiment with each patient as to the type and amount of bulky foods and fluids that are most effective in bowel training. Similarly, the number of suppositories necessary and the length of time it takes for the bowel response following insertion are determined on an individual basis. Movements are likely to occur occasionally at times other than those scheduled, particularly at first. Adjustments in diet and in the use of suppositories will probably be necessary from time to time as the patient's general condition improves and his activity increases.

Bladder control is more difficult to develop than bowel control and generally requires a longer period. Incontinence due to spinal cord injury is discussed on page 874 with the care of the paraplegic patient. When it is due to degenerative disease, loss of consciousness or other illnesses an indwelling catheter may be used. The physician's instructions may be to have the catheter drain continuously at first, then to clamp it, allowing it to drain only at stated

intervals of 1 to 2 hours. The interval is gradually increased to 3 to 4 hours; allowing the bladder to collect urine for longer periods encourages a more normal capacity. The catheter is removed as soon as possible, since it predisposes to bladder infection. A schedule is established for voiding. At first the patient is placed on a bedpan or commode hourly, and then the intervals between voidings are gradually lengthened when there is no incontinency in the shorter periods. When the intervals are short, it may be necessary to place a pad under the patient or to provide some form of drainage receptacle at night to avoid too frequent interruption of his rest. As the voidings become less frequent, the schedule becomes the same throughout the 24 hours.

A fluid intake of 2500 to 3000 ml. daily facilitates training and assists in preventing infection and calculus formation. If most of this is taken before 8 P.M., the problem of incontinency during the night is reduced. The amount voided each time is recorded, and the 24-hour volume is totaled and compared with the intake volume. This provides information as to whether the bladder is emptying completely or urine is being retained. Catheterization following a voiding may be ordered to determine if there is residual urine.

If an indwelling catheter is necessary for a relatively long period, the physician may require the bladder to be irrigated two or three times daily with an antiseptic solution to prevent infection. Disposable plastic bags may be used to receive the urine drainage; when a nondisposable drainage bottle is used it must be sterilized daily along with the drainage tubing that is connected to the catheter. The catheter is usually changed every 7 to 10 days. A urine specimen is collected every 2 to 3 days and is cultured for evidence of possible bacterial invasion. Chills, elevation in temperature and decreased urinary output may indicate urinary tract infection.

Exercises

Immobility for even a brief period causes musculoskeletal deterioration and predisposes the individual to complications that may be life-threatening as well as interfere with rehabilitation. An exercise program, approved by the physician, is started early to (1) maintain and increase the strength of functional muscles; (2) maintain the normal range of joint movement; (3) stimulate circulation and respirations and thus prevent complications, cramping and fatigue; and (4) encourage the return of function in affected muscles. Exercises also give the patient something to do that helps to relieve the boredom of lying or sitting and the restlessness and apprehension common to enforced immobility.

Exercises may be classified as passive, active, resistive, range of motion, or static. *Passive* exercises consist of movements of a part or parts of the body by some external force or by some person other than the patient. They are applied to the limbs (arm, hand, fingers, thigh, leg, foot) to prevent muscle contracture and decreased range of joint movement and to keep the muscle in readiness for active functioning. Passive exercises also have a slight stimulating effect on circulation.

Active exercises are movements that are willed and performed by the individual himself. They are effective in maintaining and increasing muscle strength, joint movement and mobility, stimulating circulation and respiratory function, and promoting a sense of well-being.

Resistive exercises are actively performed by the individual against an external force or pressure. The force may be exerted by another person; movements made within water meet with the resistance of the water. This type of exercise is used to retrain or strengthen muscles.

Range of motion exercises consist of moving a part in order to maintain or promote the range of motion of the joint involved.

Static or muscle-setting (isometric) exercises involve active contraction and relaxation of muscle(s) without movements of the respective joint and part. They are used to maintain muscle tone during a period of immobility and are applied principally to the quadriceps femoris, gluteus maximus and arm muscles. The individual maintains the contraction of the muscle(s) for several seconds before relaxing.

When a set of muscles is weak, the patient may require assistance to achieve the full range of motion of the part involved. The exercise is then referred to as *active assistive*. Only help sufficient to complete the movement is used, and this is gradually withdrawn as the muscles strengthen.

Exercises may be used with bed patients or those with restricted mobility to prevent loss of strength and complications, or they may be prescribed therapeutic activities with a specific objective such as restoring muscle function or range of joint motion, or increasing the strength and activity of a particular set of muscles to compensate for a permanent impairment that results in a mobility deficit. For example, if an individual becomes dependent on crutch-walking, shoulder and arm exercises are instituted so he will be able to cope with the crutches.

General principles to be observed in all exercise programs include the following:

1. The purpose and importance of the exercises should be understood by the patient, the family and the person responsible for the program.

2. The nurse or person responsible requires knowledge of muscle physiology, and needs to know which muscles and the joint range of motion that are involved.

3. The patient should be rested and in as comfortable a position as possible.

4. In passive movements, the parts of the body are handled very gently. The portion above the part being moved is stabilized, joints are supported and pressure on the body of any muscle is avoided.

5. Movements should be made slowly and smoothly and kept within a pain-free range.

6. Short periods of exercise repeated at intervals are preferable to fewer long periods, which cause fatigue of the patient.

7. The number of times each exercise is performed is gradually increased.

Therapeutic exercises are prescribed by a physician and are specifically defined for the patient's particular disability. In rehabilitation, the retraining of muscles may require a program of physical therapy such as hydrotherapy or thermal treatments, and exercises involving special equipment such as weights. These are directed by a physiotherapist and are usually done in a physical therapy department. The nurse should be acquainted with the program, since frequently some activities may be reinforced in nursing care.

An example of a general exercise program that may be used with a patient on bed rest or restricted mobility follows. It may require modification according to the patient's condition and should be approved by the physician before being carried out (see Fig. 2–3).

HEAD. With the pillow removed, the head may be alternately flexed forward and to each side and then, in turn, rotated to the left and right.

ARMS. To maintain shoulder joint and arm movements, each arm is successively raised over the head as far as it will go, abducted, adducted across the chest, externally and internally rotated and then circumducted. Flexion and extension of the forearm with the upper arm stabilized are used to preserve elbow function and are followed by pronation (turning the palm

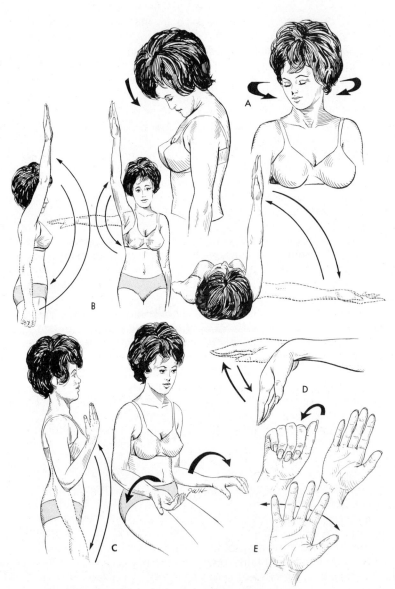

FIGURE 2–3 Series of line drawings illustrating some bed exercises. *A,* Flexion and rotation of head. *B,* Extension, abduction, adduction and rotation of arm. *C,* Flexion, extension, pronation and supination of forearm. *D,* Flexion and extension of wrist. *E,* Flexion, extension and spreading of fingers.

Illustration continued on opposite page.

downward) and supination (turning the palm upward). The hand, fingers and thumb are then moved through their normal range of movements.

LOWER LIMBS. With the lower limb, the hip joint and involved muscles are exercised by movement of the thigh with the knee flexed through flexion, extension, abduction, adduction, and internal and external rotation. Flexion and extension of the leg may be combined with similar movements of the hip. The foot is alternately dorsiflexed and plantar-flexed, then everted and inverted with the leg stabilized. Gentle raising of the toes followed by flexion will help to maintain the phalangeal joints.

If the patient is placed in the prone position, backward movement (hyperextension) of the head, arms and lower limbs may be carried out.

The series of exercises cited here may be passive movements made by the nurse to preserve range of motion. When medically permissible, the exercises become active with the patient performing them. In some instances some of the movements may be passive and the rest active exercises. For example, part of the lower limb exercises (foot and leg) may be active with the hip movements being passive.

A number of excellent references are available with detailed instructions and illustrations of active and passive exercises that the nurse may be expected to initiate

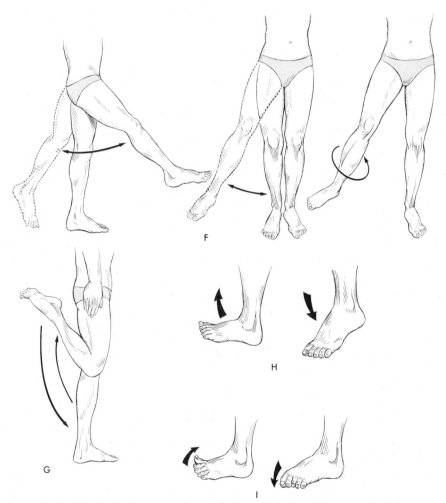

FIGURE 2–3 (*Continued.*) *F*, Flexion, extension, abduction, adduction and internal rotation of lower limbs. *G*, Flexion and extension of leg. *H*, Dorisflexion and plantar flexion of foot. *I*, Flexion and extension of toes.

and carry out. Examples of these are listed at the bottom of this page.[2-4] Others may be found in the bibliography at the end of this chapter. It is helpful if at least one or two such references are available on the hospital ward or in the visiting nurse's office. A family member or the patient himself may be instructed to carry out an exercise program at home, and he may find a booklet with illustrations of value.

Activities of Daily Living (ADL)

These activities are those normally carried out by the individual in his daily life; they contribute to independent living. Such activities include changing position (e.g., turning in bed), moving from one place to another (e.g., moving from the bed to a chair or from one room to another), feeding oneself, dressing and undressing, personal hygiene, and essential dexterous hand activities (e.g., opening doors, using the telephone, handling money, writing).

The ability to carry out self-care and to move from one place to another greatly determines the disabled person's future. A careful evaluation over a period of time will determine what he can and cannot do. Resumption of activities of daily living may simply require being given the opportunity, motivation and encouragement, or it may involve learning new ways to accomplish them.

The nurse has the first opportunity to initiate the patient's self-help measures since they begin with simple activities such as eating, washing the hands and face, combing the hair, cleaning the teeth, and cleansing oneself after going to the toilet. With the achievement of these simple initial activities the program is gradually and steadily expanded. The patient may have to learn and then practice turning in bed, rising to the sitting position, sitting on the side of the bed and transferring to a chair. Once

the latter is conquered, the next goal is locomotion; the patient learns to pull himself up to the standing position, establish his balance and then to walk. If a walker, cane or crutches are required, adjustment to the height of the patient and instruction in its use will be necessary (see p. 925). Each activity is composed of several motions, some of which may be difficult for the patient. Practice in the form of exercises is used to strengthen the muscles involved in the movement that is giving trouble.

In learning to care for himself the patient should not be rushed. Patience and restraint are required by the nurse. If the patient becomes frustrated and emotional, the nurse must guard against the sympathetic desire to take over for the patient, rather than stand by and have him struggle with and solve his own problem. Overprotection and performing his activities for him will not put the patient on the road to independence. A positive attitude of expectancy of achievement is necessary.

Eliciting from the patient what he is most interested in achieving and giving him the opportunity to participate in the setting of realistic goals and in planning his activity program will help to motivate him. When he does something successfully for himself, he will realize that he can still do things and that, although difficult, self-care is a possible and a worthwhile goal.

Rehabilitation for some patients may require *special equipment*. Disability or paralysis of the lower limbs may necessitate the use of a wheelchair. The patient is taught transferring to and from the chair and safe management in getting from one place to another. A brace may be used to stabilize the limb or assist in support of the body weight. The purpose, application and management of the brace should be taught. For self-care in patients with disability and restricted motion of the upper limbs, special devices such as a combination knife and fork, long-handled cutlery, a long drinking tube, dishes that can be stabilized and mechanical supports for a weak wrist or grasp may be necessary.

The teaching of all rehabilitation activities includes consideration of the environment in which the patient will live and work. For example, if the person dependent on a wheelchair is to be transported to

[2]Mildred J. Allgire and Ruth R. Denney: Nurses Can Give and Teach Rehabilitation. New York, Springer, 1968.

[3]Ruth Perin Stryker: Rehabilitative Aspects of Acute and Chronic Nursing Care, 2nd ed. Philadelphia, W.B. Saunders, 1977.

[4]American Heart Association: Strike Back at Stroke. New York, American Heart Association. (Available in Canada through the Canadian Heart Foundation, Toron o.)

his place of work by car, he is taught not only how to accomplish the transfer from chair to car but also the management of the collapsible type of chair and the method of getting it in and out of the car.

An *interest in personal grooming and appearance* is encouraged; some adaptations in clothing may be necessary to facilitate normal dressing, such as front openings, zippers rather than buttons or small fasteners and shoes without laces. A few illustrated texts with many suggestions and detailed instructions for improvisations and adaptations for ADL are included in the bibliography at the end of the chapter.

The Family

When a member of the family becomes disabled, it may mean a change in the way of life for the whole family. It may create financial hardships, particularly if the patient is the wage earner; responsibilities are shifted; and plans and goals may be shattered. Varied reactions on the part of the family members to the situation may be expected. Family bonds may become greater as they face the situation together; new strengths, capabilities and a determination to cope with their problems may be revealed. In other instances, the reaction of some family members may be resentment for the individual whose disability has altered their life; the patient is rejected, and his loneliness, fear and depression are increased.

An explanation of the patient's condition, the possibilities for his future, and the rehabilitative plans is made by the physician. The nurse has the responsibility of discussing with the family their role in supporting the patient. The home situation is determined, and if there is need of socioeconomic assistance, the social service worker may be asked to meet with the family and arrange for the necessary assistance. If a social worker is not available, referral to appropriate resources may be made by the nurse. This should be discussed with the family first, since they may be reluctant to accept any type of social assistance.

Marked concern for the disabled member may lead to overprotection that fosters dependence. The family is helped to realize there are things the patient can still do and others that he can learn to do if given the opportunity to use his remaining capacity. Members of the family are encouraged to talk to the nurse about their situation, express their concerns and fears, and to ask about the patient's condition and care. They are advised how they may best help him and themselves. In the initial, acute stage, having someone of his own with him who displays a realistic, optimistic attitude will provide support for the patient. This person may be taught how to assist the nurse in some aspects of the patient's care. As the patient's condition improves, it may be helpful if the family discusses their plans for their adjustments with him so he is made to feel he is still an integral part of the family.

The rehabilitative plans will include informing the family what the patient can and cannot do and what care and adaptations are necessary in his future. An assessment of the home in preparation for the patient's return is necessary. Some changes may be necessary in the environment to accommodate the patient and allow him to be as independent as possible. Appropriate reading material may be given to the family so they will have a better understanding of the disabled person's condition and necessary care. For example, an illustrated outline of the exercise routine that is to be continued or illustrations of a wall bar or raised toilet seat may prove very helpful. A referral may be made to the district visiting nurse who will give them more direct assistance in the home with the planning for the necessary adjustments and care.

When the family is being taught how to care for the patient at home, consideration should also be given to how they may conserve their energy, protect their health and live a normal life. They can be guided in the sharing of various aspects of the patient's care and can be shown that each has a part to play.

The family is advised that former associates and friends of the patient should be encouraged to visit and maintain a contact with him. They may be surprised to learn that he still has an interest in many things and may still participate in some. All too often, frequent visits are made at first and then, as weeks and months go by, tend to diminish, and the individual's life becomes needlessly narrowed to the institution or home, with limited outside contacts.

REFERENCES

BOOKS

Allgire, M. J., and Denney, R. R.: Nurses Can Give and Teach Rehabilitation, 2nd ed. New York, Springer Publishing, 1968.

American Heart Association: Strike Back at Stroke. New York, American Heart Association.[5]

———: Up and Around. New York, American Heart Association.[5]

———: Do It Yourself Again. New York, American Heart Association, 1969.[5]

Cobb, A. Beatrix: Medical and Psychological Aspects of Disability. Springfield, Ill., Charles C Thomas, , 1973.

Covalt, Nila K.: Bed Exercises for Convalescent Patients. Springfield, Ill., Charles C Thomas, 1968.

Gordon, Edward E.: A Home Program for Patients Ambulatory with Aids. New York, National Multiple Sclerosis Society, 1952.

———: A Home Program for the Care of Bed Patients. New York, National Multiple Sclerosis Society, 1952.

Hirschberg, Gerald, G., Lewis, Leon, and Thomas, Dorothy: Rehabilitation. Philadelphia, J.B. Lippincott, 1964.

Lawton, E. Buchwald: Activities of Daily Living for Physical Rehabilitation. New York, Blakiston Division, McGraw-Hill, 1963.

Licht, Sidney Herman (Ed.): Rehabilitation and Medicine. Baltimore, Waverly Press, 1968.

Robinault, Isabel P. (Ed.): Functional Aids for the Multipley Handicapped. Hagerstown, Md., Harper and Row, 1973.

Stevens, Marion Keith: Geriatric Nursing for Practical Nurses. Philadelphia, W.B. Saunders, 1975. Unit IV.

Stryker, Ruth Perin: Rehabilitative Aspects of Acute and Chronic Nursing Care, 2nd ed. Philadelphia, W.B. Saunders, 1977.

---

[5]Distributed in Canada by the Canadian Heart Foundation, Toronto

PERIODICALS

Bean, Patricia: "The Nurse: Her Role in Cardiopulmonary Rehabilitation." Heart Lung, Vol. 3, No. 4 (July–Aug. 1974), pp. 587–591.

Coogan, Joseph P. (Ed.): "Motivating the Unmotivated Patient." Nurs. '74, Vol. 4, No. 2 (Feb. 1974), pp. 31–36.

Cosin, L. Z.: "New Concepts on Rehabilitation for the Disabled and Elderly Patient." Rehabilitation, No. 95 (Oct–Dec. 1976), pp. 13–17.

Drury, John H., Jr.: "Handbook of Range-of-Motion Exercises." Nurs. '72, Vol. 2, No. 4 (April 1972), pp. 19–22.

Ford, Jack R., and Duckworth, Bridget: "Moving a Dependent Patient Safely, Comfortably." Nurs. '76, Vol. 6, No. 2 (Feb. 1976), pp. 58–65.

Griffin, Winnie, Anderson, Sara J., and Passos, Joyce Y.: "Group Exercise for Patients with Limited Motion." Am. J. Nurs., Vol. 71, No. 9 (Sept. 1971) pp. 1742–1743.

Habeeb, Marjorie, C., and Kallsstrom, Mina D.: "Bowel Program for Institutionalized Adults." Am. J. Nurs., Vol. 76, No. 4 (April 1976), pp. 606–608.

Halverston, Elizabeth Ann: "Taking Rehabilitation to the Patient." Can. Nurs., Vol. 67, No. 9 (Sept. 1971), pp. 49–51.

Hastings, J. E. F.: "Rehabilitation and Public Health." Can. J. Public Health, Vol. 53 (July 1962), pp. 279–283.

Henderson, Gloria, M.: "Teaching-Learning for Rehabilitation of the Spinal Cord-Disabled Individual." Nurs. Clin. North Am., Vol. 6, No. 4 (Dec. 1971), pp. 655–668.

Jordan, Helen S., and Kavchak, Mary Anne: "Transfer Techniques." Nurs. '73, Vol. 3, No. 3 (March 1973), pp. 19–22.

Kern, Florence C., and Poole, Laura: "Transfer Techniques." Nurs. '72, Vol. 2, No. 7 (July 1972), pp. 25–28.

Litin, Edward, M.: "Emotional Aspects of Chronic Physical Disability." Arch. Phys. Med. Rehabil., Vol. 38, No. 3 (March 1957), pp. 139–142.

Loxley, Alice Keating: "The Emotional Toll of Crippling Deformity." Am. J. Nurs., Vol. 72, No. 10 (Oct. 1972), pp. 1839–1840.

Martin, Gordon, M.: "Hazards of Inactivity." J.A.M.A., Vol. CXCVI, No. 10 (June 6, 1966), pp. 201–202.

Martin, Nancy, King, Rosemarie, and Suchinski, Joyce: "The Nurse Therapist in a Rehabilitation Setting." Am. J. Nurs., Vol. 70, No. 8 (Aug. 1970), pp. 1694–1697.

Mathews, Nancy C.: "Helping a Quadriplegic Veteran Decide to Live." Am. J. Nurs., Vol. 76, No. 3 (March 1976), pp. 441–443.

McCartney, Virginia: "Rehabilitation and Dignity for the Stroke Patient." Nurs. Clin. North Am., Vol. 9, No. 4 (Dec. 1974), pp. 693–701.

Niccoli, Arlene, and Brammell, H. L.: "A Program for Rehabilitation in Coronary Heart Disease." Nurs. Clin. North Am., Vol. 11, No. 2, (June 1976), pp. 237–250.

Norsworthy, Edith: "Nursing Rehabilitation After Severe Head Trauma." Am. J. Nurs., Vol. 74, No. 7 (July 1974), pp. 1246–1250.

Olsen, E. V., et al.: "The Hazards of Immobility." Am. J. Nurs., Vol 67, No. 4 (April 1967), pp. 779–794.

Patrick, Maxine: "Little Things Mean a Lot in Geriatric Rehabilitation." Nurs. '73, Vol. 3, No. 8 (Aug. 1973), pp. 7–9.

Perrine, George: "Needs Met and Unmet." Am. J. Nurs., Vol. 71, No. 11 (Nov. 1971), pp. 2128–2133.

Perry, Jacqueline: "The Mechanics of Walking." Phys. Ther., Vol. 67, No. 9 (Sept. 1967), pp. 778–801.

Pfaudler, Marjorie: "After Stroke Motor Skill Rehabilitation for Hemiplegic Patients." Am. J. Nurs., Vol. 73, No. 11 (Nov. 1973), pp. 1892–1896.

Rosell, Cheryl: "Pitfalls of Emotional Involvement: Sympathetic Nursing Care of a Patient with Cervical Spine Injury." Nurs. '76, Vol. 6, No. 3 (March 1976), pp. 42–47.

Rothberg, June S. (Ed.): "Symposium, Chronic Disease and Rehabilitation." Nurs. Clin. North Am., Vol. 1, No. 3 (Sept. 1966).

Smolock, Mary Ann: "The Nurse's Role in Rehabilitation of the Handicapped Child." Nurs. Clin. North Am., Vol. 5, No. 3, (Sept. 1970), pp. 411–420.

Stryker, Ruth Perin: "Every Nurse a Rehabilitation Nurse." Nurs. '72, Vol. 2, No. 1 (Jan. 1972), pp. 13–16.

Welch, Sister Regina: "Tile-Table Therapy in Rehabilitation of the Trauma Patient with Brain Damage and Spinal Injury." Nurs. Clin. North Am., Vol. 5, No. 4 (Dec. 1970), pp. 621–630.

Wolff, Ilse S.: "Acceptance." Am. J. Nurs., Vol. 72, No. 8 (Aug. 1972), pp. 1412–1415.

Zach, G. A.: "Acute Therapy and Rehabilitation of Paraplegics." Rehabilitation, No. 98 (July–Sept. 1976), pp. 13–17.

3

Disease: Causes and Tissue Responses

THE NORMAL CELL

The material of which all living matter is composed is referred to as protoplasm. It is organized in discrete microscopic units called cells. There are many different types of cells in the human body; they vary in size, shape, composition and function and are derived from preexisting cells. They all have certain common characteristics in structure and activity. All body tissues are composed of cells and cellular products.

A knowledge of the organization of the basic structural and functional unit contributes to an understanding of the structure and functions of the body and its component parts. An appreciation of the normal is necessary for recognition of the abnormal as well as for an awareness of the effects of disease and the necessary supportive measures.

STRUCTURAL FEATURES OF A CELL

All cells have three main structural parts at some time in their life cycle: a surface membrane, cytoplasm and a nucleus (see Fig. 3–1).

Cell Membrane

The cell is enveloped by a very thin membrane which gives delineation, support and protection to the cell substance, and provides the interface between the cell content and interstitial fluid. Its semipermeability, because of minute pores, allows the passage of water and small molecular solutes in and out of the cell, but it also displays an active, discriminative role in relation to what passes in and out. In addition to this transfer function, the membrane plays an important role in the constant movement of the cell surface and the entrapment of substances, and in the provision of the adhesiveness by which like cells cling together to form tissue. It is suggested that the cell membrane is also capable of differentiating between the body's own cells and alien cells (antigens).

Cytoplasm

Cytoplasm forms the bulk of the cell. Its composition varies according to the specialized function of the cell. For example, the cytoplasm of mature red blood cells features the hematin-protein compound hemoglobin for the purpose of transporting oxy-

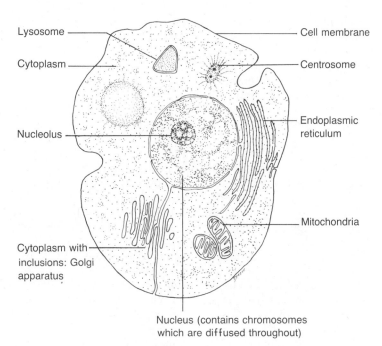

Lysosome —————————— ———————— Cell membrane

Cytoplasm ————— ———————— Centrosome

Nucleolus ————— ———— Endoplasmic reticulum

————— Mitochondria

Cytoplasm with————
inclusions: Golgi
apparatus

Nucleus (contains chromosomes
which are diffused throughout)

FIGURE 3–1 Diagram of a typical cell.

gen; muscle cell cytoplasm has compounds responsible for chemical reactions that bring about a thickening and shortening of the cell (contraction). There is a relatively high concentration of protein, potassium, magnesium, and phosphate in the cytoplasm in contrast with that of fluid outside the cell where sodium, chloride, and bicarbonate are the predominant electrolytes.

Cytoplasm is in a fluid state, consisting largely of water, and contains several functional structures or organelles — the endoplasmic reticulum, Golgi apparatus, mitochondria, lysosomes and centrosome.

The endoplasmic reticulum is a network of tubules and vesicles that are connected with the nuclear and cell membrane. The channels serve to transfer materials from one part of the cell to another. On the outer surfaces of the tubules are small granular particles called ribosomes which consist of ribonucleic acid (RNA) and protein. The ribosomes are considered to be responsible for the synthesis of protein substances characteristic of the particular type of cell. The products may be for cell use (e.g., enzymes, structural components) or for secretion.

The Golgi apparatus is a series of small vesicles associated with the endoplasmic

reticulum. It is prominent in cells which are involved with secretion, and it is suggested that secretions formed by the ribosomes are collected in these vesicles.

The mitochondria are small, oval bodies which vary in number in different cell types according to the level of cell activity. They contain oxidative enzymes to catalyze reactions that liberate energy which is needed for cellular functions. The cells that are high energy producers (e.g., muscle cells) contain more mitochondria.

Lysosomes contain hydrolytic enzymes that break down particles that are useless or harmful to the cell. Leukocytes contain an unusual number of these minute bodies in order to destroy organisms and other foreign substances taken into the cells by phagocytosis.

The centrosome consists of a pair of cylindrical bodies called centrioles and is situated close to the nucleus. This body is concerned with cell division.

Nucleus

The nucleus is a spherical or ovoid body enclosed in a membrane and, in most cells, lies centrally within the cytoplasm. This structure is the vital control center of the cell; without it the cell cannot reproduce, and its activities cease. An exception to the latter point is the erythrocyte produced by bone marrow cells; as the red blood cell matures, its nucleus is extruded, hemoglobin is formed, and the cell is released into the circulation where it functions as a transport for oxygen for approximately 120 days.

The nucleus contains the chromosomes, which determine cell characteristics and transmit the heredity of the cell and the organism from one generation to the next. All human somatic cells contain 23 pairs of chromosomes. When the cell is not in the reproductive phase the chromosomes are scattered throughout the nucleus as long, drawn-out threads. They are readily stainable and may be referred to as chromatin material. Each chromosome consists of a chain of units called genes. The gene is a large, complex molecule of a protein compound known as deoxyribonucleic acid (DNA) which is capable of self-duplication. Each gene has a specific location on a particular chromosome. The DNA of each gene has similar constituent elements, but the structural arrangement of these varies from one gene to another. The specific sequence of amino acids determines the specific genetic information. The genes contain information necessary for controlling the development and activity of the cells. They do this through directing specific protein synthesis by the cytoplasm. In other words, the DNA determines the cell properties by directing the essential cytoplasmic composition associated with the particularities of the cell's function. It is suggested that each gene is responsible for the formation and nature of one enzyme which acts as a catalyst.

A second protein found in the nucleus is ribonucleic acid (RNA). It is produced by the DNA and transmits the encoded information of the genes to the ribosomes of the cytoplasm. Within the nuclear material, minute spherical bodies called nucleoli appear. They contain RNA and other proteins, and it is thought they may be concerned with the synthesis of RNA molecules which correspond in molecular structure to the RNA derived from the chromosomes.

PHYSIOLOGICAL ACTIVITIES OF THE CELL

Metabolism

Intracellular activities are chemical reactions which are referred to collectively as metabolism. The metabolic processes are of two types. *Catabolism* refers to reactions in which there is a chemical breakdown of compounds into simpler compounds or atoms; this breakdown is accompanied by a release of energy. New compounds are synthesized from simpler substances during the anabolic process, or *anabolism*. Both types of processes occur to some extent at all times to maintain the cells and perform the functions that contribute to the overall activities and maintenance of the body as a whole. At times the rate of anabolism may exceed that of catabolism and cell substances accumulate; at times of increased body activity, catabolism proceeds more rapidly and cell substances may be markedly reduced.

A requisite to cellular health and normal functioning is the provision of adequate amounts of essential nutrients such as proteins, carbohydrates, minerals and vitamins. The substances used in metabolism are taken into the cell from the immediate extracellular fluid environment. A constant supply of oxygen is necessary for metabolism. Cellular activities cannot be sustained without the products of oxidative processes. The catabolism of many compounds to release energy results in the production of carbon dioxide, which is eliminated from the cell; this elimination of carbon dioxide and the absorption of oxygen comprise cellular respiration. In addition to carbon dioxide, various substances may be formed during metabolism which are of no use to the cell and, if retained, inhibit cellular functions. These waste products are passed out of the cell and eliminated from the body through an excretory channel. Substances called secretions are formed by some cells to serve a specific useful purpose when discharged. For example, some cells secrete mucus to protect cells from irritating materials; cells of the thyroid secrete thyroxin, which influences the rate of metabolism, particularly the oxidative process, of practically all cells in the body.

The cellular chemical reactions are catalyzed by enzymes which are produced by the ribosomes under the direction of the genes via RNA. These catalytic protein compounds are specific; that is, there is a particular enzyme for each type of chemical reaction. The reaction may be to break down a compound, transfer an atom or molecule from one compound to another or rearrange component atoms within a molecule. The breakdown of a complex compound involves a series of reactions and a specific enzyme for each reaction. If one enzyme is lacking, the normal metabolism of the substance is arrested at that level. For example, a specific enzyme is necessary to convert galactose to glucose so it can be catabolized to carbon dioxide and water and release required energy. If the gene that directs the production of the necessary enzyme is abnormal or absent, the galactose accumulates, resulting in an abnormally low blood sugar level, weakness due to the lack of energy production and mental deficiency as a result of an inadequate supply of glucose to the brain cells. The condition is known as galactosemia and is classified as an inborn error of metabolism; this implies an inherited enzyme abnormality or deficiency. Similarly, the condition known as phenylketonuria is due to a congenital deficiency of the enzyme that promotes a reaction to convert the amino acid phenylalanine (a component of many proteins) to tyrosine. Phenylalanine accumulates in the blood and spinal fluid and is damaging to the brain, resulting in mental retardation. The absence of the enzyme is detected through its excretion in the urine as phenylpyruvic acid — hence, the name phenylketonuria. If detected soon after birth, a diet low in proteins containing phenylalanine may prevent mental deficiency.

Cellular Movement

Cellular content is in fluid form. Movement of the whole or a part of a cell may occur by the flow of cytoplasm from one part to another in a manner similar to that observed in the amoeba. Leukocytes move in this way in their migration out of the blood stream into extracellular spaces and when they surround and engulf an organism or particle. The movement of a muscle cell (contraction) is achieved by shortening of the cell with a corresponding increase in the thickness; this action is the result of a series of chemical reactions within the cytoplasm. Some cells have cilia, which are fine, hair-like processes of the cytoplasm which quickly swing in one direction and then slowly resume their former position. They move particles along a surface in the direction of their initial lashing motion. Organized movement of definite parts of the cell occurs as the cell proceeds through the reproductive process.

Irritability

Cells are sensitive and will react to changes in their immediate environment. A change which will initiate a cellular response is referred to as a stimulus. The type of reaction or response of the cell will vary with the type of stimulus and the characteristics of the particular type of cell. Cells may be more irritable to a specific type of stimulus than to others.

Reproduction

New cells are necessary for growth of the organism and for replacement of worn-out cells. They are produced by a cell dividing into two cells, each having a nucleus with 23 pairs of chromosomes as well as cytoplasm with the same properties as those of the parent cell. This process of cell division is referred to as mitosis, and it involves a series of changes in which there is a rearrangement of the centrioles and chromosomes and a subsequent division of the nucleus and the whole cell.

The interval between the end of one mitosis and the beginning of the next is referred to as the interphase, or the amitotic or intermitotic phase. The changes characteristic of reproduction are described as they occur in the following four phases (Fig.3–2):

1. *Prophase*. Preceding this initial phase, cell substance is increased, and the DNA duplicates itself. Each chromosome divides longitudinally into two chromatids which remain attached by a centromere. The chromosomes coil spirally, becoming

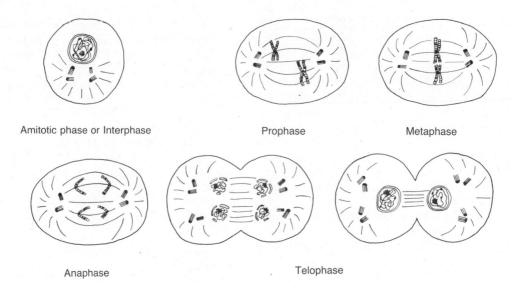

Amitotic phase or Interphase   Prophase   Metaphase

Anaphase   Telophase

FIGURE 3–2   Phases of mitosis.

shorter and thicker, and appear as distinct entities. The two centrioles move away from each other to opposite poles of the cell and develop fibrils stretching out between them. The nucleoli and nuclear membrane disappear.

2. *Metaphase.* The fibrils of the centrioles grow into the nuclear region to become attached to the centromeres of the chromosomes, which arrange themselves in a line between the two centrioles.

3. *Anaphase.* The two chromatids of each chromosome separate at their centromere; one is attracted by a fibril toward one centriole. This results in an equal number of chromatids — corresponding to the original number of chromosomes (46) — being located in either half of the cell.

4. *Telophase.* The final phase involves nuclear reformation in order to enclose each group of chromatids and constriction of the cytoplasm by indentation of the cell membrane through the center. The spindle formed by the fibrils disappears, a typical nucleus forms in each half of the cell, and the chromatids lengthen (uncoil) and diffuse irregularly throughout the nucleus. Each centriole divides to form a centrosome, and final division of the cytoplasm produces two separate cells which are identical in structure to the original parent cell.

Normally, cell reproduction is controlled to meet the tissue needs of the organism; during the growth period and as cells wear out or are destroyed they are produced in a number sufficient to produce or maintain normal tissue mass. Unfortunately, the substance or mechanism by which the rate of cell reproduction is controlled has not yet been identified. In certain disease conditions, such as cancer, this control is lost by some cells and they are produced in excess.

Meiosis (Reduction Division)

A new organism is conceived by the union of a female gamete (ovum) and a male gamete (sperm). The union forms a single cell from which all the cells of the body are derived. Obviously, the characteristic number of chromosomes (46) must be established in the initial single cell.

Initially, when both the female and male germ cells are produced by the sex glands they contain 23 pairs of chromosomes. During a maturation process, a special type of cell division takes place in which the number of chromosomes is reduced to half. This cell division process is referred to as meiosis, or reduction division. In meiotic cell division, one of each pair of chromosomes passes to an opposite end of the cell. When the two halves of the cell separate, each daughter cell contains only 23 single chromosomes (haploid chromosomes). At conception, the union of the sperm with haploid chromosomes and an ovum with a corresponding number establishes the distinctive 23 pairs of chromosomes. The resulting cell rapidly reproduces by mitosis, which continues in order to form the new organism.

HOMEOSTASIS

For normal functioning, cells require the maintenance of relatively constant conditions in the internal environment. This is referred to as homeostasis. Each cell in order to preserve its normalcy, must be surrounded constantly by a fluid with certain definite physical and chemical properties.

Homeostasis is not an absolute constancy but is rather a dynamic balance that varies within narrow limits. Derangements beyond these limits are not compatible with normal cell functioning. The extracellular environment must be within a definite temperature range; it must be capable of supplying the cells with oxygen and other essential materials, as well as removing their secretions and waste products. Cellular activities tend to produce changes, but under normal conditions body mechanisms operate continuously to restore and maintain a suitable environment. To quote Guyton: "Essentially all the organs and tissues of the body perform functions that help to maintain these constant conditions."[1]

Movement of Substances Across the Cell Membrane

There is a continuous passing of substances in and out of the cells by physical passive processes and by cellular action. The membrane, being semipermeable, permits water and small molecular substances, such as potassium and sodium, to pass through by physical processes. Active transportation by the cell involves energy — i.e., a force must be produced by the cell and applied to the substance. Various substances are transferred across the cell membrane in this way against a greater concentration or pressure gradient. The lat-

ter is an important mechanism in maintaining normal cell composition. For example, a much higher concentration of potassium is required within the cells than in the extracellular fluid; however, the reverse is true of sodium. In order to maintain these conditions, the cells actively transport potassium in and sodium out. The active movement of sodium out of the cell is referred to in physiology as the sodium pump. A method of active transportation used with large molecular substances such as protein and fat is pinocytosis. This process involves invagination of the cell membrane at the site of contact with the particle. The molecule sinks into the invaginated area and is surrounded by the membrane. A vesicle is formed which separates from the membrane and is moved into the cytoplasm where it disappears, releasing its contents.

The physical processes concerned with the movement of substances in and out of the cell are diffusion and osmosis.

Diffusion is the continual, spontaneous movement and intermingling of molecules or ions in liquids or gases. The tendency is for the particles to disperse throughout the space in which the solution or gas is contained so as to produce a uniform concentration. Random movement continues when uniformity is achieved. Water, gases and some solutes diffuse readily through a semipermeable membrane; if the distribution is equal on both sides, the constant random motion of particles results in the movement of as many particles in one direction as the other. The diffusion of more molecules of a substance in one direction than in the opposite is dependent upon a concentration gradient. Large particles diffuse more slowly than smaller ones.

Diffusion is responsible for the movement of gases between the alveolar air of the lungs and the blood and between the blood and the cells. Similarly, many substances absorbed from the intestine create a pressure gradient between the blood and the interstitial fluid and between the interstitial fluid and the intracellular content; this results in the diffusion of these substances from the blood to the interstitial fluid and on into the cells. In the opposite direction, products of metabolism diffuse from the cells into the interstitial fluid and then into the blood.

---

[1]Arthur C. Guyton: Textbook of Medical Physiology, 5th ed. Philadelphia, W. B. Saunders, 1976, p. 3.

Osmosis is the movement of water through a semipermeable membrane from a solution of lesser solute concentration to one of greater concentration. It occurs only when two solutions with different concentrations of solutes are separated by a semipermeable membrane through which the solutes do not readily diffuse. The volume of water that is retained by the solution of greater concentration is dependent upon the osmotic pressure exerted by the solute of that solution. Solutes in a solution tend to hold or attract water; this affinity or drawing power is referred to as osmotic pressure.

Osmosis is illustrated in Figure 3–3. Figure 3–3A represents a 5 per cent aqueous solution in compartment X and a 15 per cent aqueous solution in compartment Y, which are separated by a semipermeable membrane. The latter is permeable to the solvent and this particular solute, with the

result indicated in A_2. Diffusion of water and the solute occurs, and eventually an equal volume of a homogeneous solution is found in both X and Y compartments.

In Figure 3–3B the 5 per cent aqueous solution in compartment X is separated from the 15 per cent aqueous solution by a semipermeable membrane that permits the solvent to pass from one compartment to the other (i.e., diffuse in both directions), but is impermeable to the solute particles in both solutions. Although the membrane is permeable to the solvent on both sides, the osmotic pressure (drawing power) of the greater number of solute particles in compartment Y results in a net gain in the volume of solvent in that compartment. The water diffusing from X to Y continues to be retained in compartment Y until the hydrostatic pressure created by the solution counteracts the osmotic pressure. The fluid

A   MEMBRANE PERMEABLE TO BOTH SOLUTE AND WATER

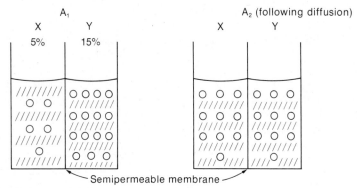

O = Solute particle
/ = Water

B   MEMBRANE PERMEABLE ONLY TO SOLVENT

O = Solute particle
/ = Water

FIGURE 3–3   Osmosis. See text for explanation.

pressure in Y reaches a point that opposes diffusion of water molecules from X to Y.

The degree of osmotic pressure of a solution is proportional to the number of particles of solute. Because the molecular weight of the molecules or ions of the solute does not influence the osmotic pressure, the unit used to quantify osmotic pressure or indicate the concentration according to the numbers of particles is the *osmol* or *milliosmol*. The *osmolality* of a solution refers to the number of solute particles in a solution per unit of solvent; the greater the number of particles, the greater the osmolality of that solution. In a solution of sodium chloride (NaCl) each molecule of the solute dissociates and forms two osmotically active particles, Na^+ and Cl^-. In a solution of glucose the molecules of the solute do not dissociate into component ions, so that one molecule of glucose represents only one osmotically active particle or one osmol.

The term *osmolarity* indicates the number of osmols or milliosmols in 1 liter of solution. A solution that has one osmol dissolved in each liter of the solution is said to have an osmolarity of 1 osmol per liter. If the solution has only 1/1000 (0.001) osmol dissolved in each liter of solution, the osmolarity is expressed as 1 milliosmol per liter.

The osmolarity of normal extracellular and intracellular fluids is approximately 300 milliosmols per liter.[2]

As stated previously, a greater concentration of potassium, phosphate, magnesium and protein exists within the cells as compared to that of the extracellular fluid. Sodium, bicarbonate and chloride are found in higher concentration outside the cell than within. Normally the osmotic pressure created by the solutes remains relatively constant on both sides of the cell membrane, and water diffuses in and out of the cell without a net loss or gain on either side of the membrane. Under such circumstances, the fluids are said to be isotonic; that is, the fluid on each side of the membrane has the same osmotic pressure.

When the osmotic pressure within the cell becomes greater than that of the interstitial fluid, osmotic equilibrium is quickly restored by the movement of water into the cell. Conversely, when the solutes of the extracellular fluid become concentrated, water passes out of the cell. This latter situation may occur in dehydration, which may be due to an excessive loss of extracellular fluid from the body or to an inadequate fluid intake. Unless the extracellular fluid volume is restored, the loss of water from the cells may interfere with normal cell functioning.

Solutions administered intravenously may be classified as isotonic, hypertonic or hypotonic (Fig. 3–4). An isotonic solution has the same osmotic pressure as the plasma.

A hypertonic solution has a greater number of solute particles than the plasma. When such a solution is given intravenously, the increased osmotic pressure of the plasma causes water to pass out of the blood cells and from the interstitial spaces across the capillary membranes. A hypertonic solution of glucose or a preparation of urea may be given to a patient with cerebral edema. The increased osmotic pressure of the blood draws fluid into the capillaries in the brain, thus reducing the edema.

A hypotonic solution has a lower osmotic pressure than the plasma. When given intravenously it reduces the plasma osmotic pressure, and water passes into the blood cells, causing them to swell and burst.

GENERAL ORGANIZATION OF THE BODY

Going from the simplest to the more complex, the structural units of the body are the cells, tissues, organs and systems.

Tissues

As cited previously, the cell is the basic structural and functional unit of the body. Those similar in structure and function are held together by an intercellular substance to form a tissue. The distinctive features of a tissue are determined by the special characteristics of the constituent cells and intercellular substance. Just as the cells of one type of tissue vary in composition, size, shape and arrangement from those of

---

[2]Ibid., p. 49.

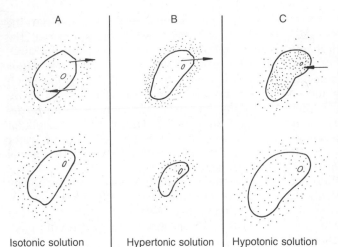

A   B   C

Isotonic solution   Hypertonic solution   Hypotonic solution

FIGURE 3–4 Isotonic, hypertonic and hypotonic solutions. *A,* Isotonic solution. Osmotic pressure of fluid introduced is same as that of the plasma and intracellular fluid. No net gain or loss to the cell. *B,* Hypertonic solution. Osmotic pressure of fluid introduced is greater than that of the plasma and intracellular fluid. Water moves out of the cell. *C,* Hypotonic solution. Osmotic pressure of fluid introduced is less than that of the plasma and intracellular fluid. Water moves into the cell, causing it to swell.

another, the intercellular substance varies in nature and amount. It may be dense and hard, fluid or gel, or may occur in the form of fibers. It may be rigid or pliable, elastic or nonextensible, and tough or fragile. In certain tissues, the intercellular substance is minimal; in these cases the cells provide the bulk and the particular function of the tissue. In other tissues there is more intercellular substance which plays a major role.

There are four major types of tissues: epithelial, connective, muscular and nervous. Variations occur in the tissues of these major categories as the cells and intercellular substance are adapted to meet the various needs of the body.

Epithelial tissues function in protection, secretion, absorption and filtration. They are found covering all external and internal surfaces as well as in secreting structures and consist mainly of cells with a minimal amount of intercellular substance. The cells reproduce readily, which is essential to the maintenance of surface and lining tissues. Examples of epithelial tissues are the skin, mucous and serous membranes, and the endothelial lining of the blood and lymph vessels and heart chambers.

Connective tissues are concerned mainly with the physical form and the mechanical activities of the body rather than with its physiological activities. They provide an internal supporting framework, protection for other structures and connections between parts of the body so they become a functional unit. The intercellular substance predominates in connective tissues and gives them their special characteristics. Examples are bones, tendons, ligaments, cartilage, fascia and adipose tissue. Blood is classified as a connective tissue; in this instance the cells have an equally significant role as that of the intercellular substance, plasma.

Muscular tissue is responsible for all movements of the body and its organs. The elongated cells (fibers) with their contractile property are important functional units; the relatively small amount of intercellular substance serves only as retaining material. The cytoplasm of muscle cells is called sarcoplasm. Muscle fibers, with the exception of those of visceral muscle, are not capable of cell reproduction; when severely damaged they degenerate and are replaced by connective tissue.

Nervous tissues form the brain, spinal cord and the network of nerve fibers throughout the body. There are two types. One consists of specialized cells (neurons) which initiate and transmit impulses to control and coordinate the physical and mental activities by which the body adapts itself to changes in its external environment. The neurons are incapable of cell division; if a cell process (nerve fiber) outside the brain or cord is injured, it may regenerate only if the cell body is uninjured (see p. 814). The other type of nervous tissue is made up of neuroglial cells and is found in the brain and spinal cord. It serves to support and protect the nervous tissue proper.

Organs

A combination of different types of tissues which are arranged to work in conjunction with one another forms an organ, such as the heart, liver, or stomach. Each organ has a definite form and location in the body and performs specialized activities which are dependent upon the functional contribution of each constituent tissue.

Systems

Several organs are arranged and correlated to form a system, which performs an overall major body function. For example, the digestion of food is dependent upon the coordinated activity of the alimentary tract and accessory organs of the digestive system. The skeletal, muscular, circulatory, respiratory, digestive, excretory, nervous, endocrine and reproductive systems compose the major complex structural units. Total body functioning is dependent upon the coordinated activities of its various systems. No system functions independently of the others.

DISEASE

INTRODUCTION

Health and disease are relative terms which are difficult to define precisely. The condition of the organism is the composite result of interaction between the cells within the body, and between the body and its environment. The organism demonstrates an amazing ability to adapt to internal and environmental changes, and to repair or compensate for stress and damage that it experiences. As long as the interaction and adaptive mechanisms can maintain normal structure and optimum functional efficiency accompanied by a sense of well-being, the individual is said to be healthy. Disease is a departure from health due to an interruption or disorder of function. There are varying degrees of departure from normal; they may be severe enough to cause incapacity of the individual, or may be less serious, allowing the individual to remain active but without a sense of well-being.

In some instances, a disturbance in function may develop without becoming apparent to the patient or to others; examples of this may be seen in the early stages of some heart diseases, cancer, tuberculosis and cirrhosis of the liver. This may be due to a sufficient number of normal cells which maintain an adequate degree of functioning, or it may be due to compensatory mechanisms, such as hypertrophy. The effects of a disturbance in the function of one part of the body is likely to be reflected in the functioning of other or all parts because of the dependence of each system on the others for its oxygen, nutrients, elimination of wastes and other essentials.

Cellular or tissue dysfunction may occur without any observable change in structure. In other instances, a disturbance in cellular activity may lead to changes in tissue structure. Structural changes resulting from disease in tissues are called lesions. The presence of lesions classifies a disease as being *organic* rather than functional; *functional disease* is characterized by a disturbance in function without demonstrable lesions. It may be associated with biochemical disturbance within the cells. The manifestations of changes in function and structure are referred to as *signs and symptoms*.

Pathology is the study of the cause (etiology), developmental process, and effects of disease. Investigation of the effects notes the characteristic signs and symptoms, the changes in physiology (pathophysiology) and mental function (psychopathology), the associated socioeconomic changes and the likely outcome (prognosis). Knowledge of these factors is useful in all aspects of nursing. An appreciation of the cause and factors that favor the development and progress of disease may be applied in preventive nursing. Some understanding of the disease process and its effects on the individual's structure, function and life style provides the basis for supportive and therapeutic measures and may alert the nurse to possible complications.

CAUSES OF DISEASE

The cause of some diseases is unknown, and continuous study goes on searching for the etiologic factor in such conditions as cancer, multiple sclerosis, rheumatoid arthritis, leukemia and psychosis. In some diseases, predisposing and perpetuating factors have been recognized even though the primary causative factor has not been identified. Such information contributes to preventive care. When the cause is unknown, care and therapy are based principally on the signs and symptoms.

Recognized causes of disease include the following:

Heredity

When an ovum is fertilized by a spermatozoon, each contributes 23 chromosomes which combine to form the nucleus of the single cell that is the origin of a new being. The chromosomes of the gametes transmit traits and characteristics from one generation to the next by their genes' influence on the biochemical activity of the cells of the new organism.

The number of abnormal conditions attributed to chromosomal aberrations seem to increase progressively as more research is carried out in this clinical area. Hereditary disease may be transmitted from one generation to another by a genetic or chromosomal disorder in one or both gametes. Abnormal cellular development and activity may result from an irregularity in chromosomal number or structure. As a result of nondisjunction in meiosis, the cells may have more or fewer than the normal number of chromosomes. Down's syndrome, a relatively common inherited disease, is characterized by an extra chromosome; the cells contain a total of 47 rather than 46. the cells in Turner's syndrome manifest a deficiency of chromosomes — one sex chromosome is missing.

Structural aberrations result from the abnormality of one or more genes of a chromosome. The patterns of these defects vary and include: (1) the separation of a chromosomal fragment or gene and its attachment to another chromosome (translocation); (2) the exchange of places by two genes from different chromosomes (reciprocal translocation); (3) omission of a gene or segment of a chromosome (deletion); or (4) breaks along the chromosome and ensuing realignment and change of gene locus.

The abnormality resulting from a change in a chromosome or gene is known as a mutation. The cause is unknown, but mutation can be induced experimentally by radiation and some chemicals. If the mutation is present in a gamete, the abnormal trait is passed on to the offspring and may be expressed as an hereditary disease, depending upon the gene dominance. The mutant gene may be carried by one of the autosomes, which are the 22 pairs of chromosomes not involved in sex determination. The mutation, then, is referred to as autosomal. If the mutation is in a chromosome of the twenty-third pair, which is concerned with sex determination, it is known as a sex-linked mutation. Mutant genes in sex-linked inherited disease are carried by the X chromosomes. If the mutant gene is recessive in penetrance, the disease will not be expressed in a female who has two X chromosomes unless both genes for that particular trait are mutant. In the case of a male the disease will be expressed, since the twenty-third pair of chromosomes is X and Y. There is no gene on the Y chromosome corresponding to the mutant gene on the X chromosome, so the mutation is fully expressed whether or not the mutant gene is dominant or recessive.

The expression or actual development of some diseases classified as hereditary is dependent upon predisposing factors. An individual may carry a mutant gene which predisposes him to a particular disorder that does not develop unless the cells are subjected to certain circumstances. Diabetes is an example of such a disorder; obesity provides the circumstance favorable for expression of the disease.

A gene for each trait is received from each parent; in some instances, the new organism may receive only one defective gene, and the manifestation of disturbance will depend on whether the gene is dominant or recessive. If it is dominant, the abnormality will be expressed, but if it is recessive the normal gene will dominate, resulting in normal structure and functioning. If each parent contributes a defective recessive gene for a particular trait, the abnormality is expressed as an hereditary disease.

Developmental Defects

Some abnormal structural and functional defects that are present at birth are due to a failure or an abnormality in the developmental process during the embryonic or fetal stage. The cause in most cases is unknown. Developmental defects are seen in some infants born to mothers who have had a viral infection during the first trimester of pregnancy. It is suggested that the virus may pass through the placenta and into the developing tissues of the embryo, thus interfering with normal tissue development. Toxic chemicals taken during pregnancy, such as the drug thalidomide, may disturb normal fetal development. Lysergic acid diethylamide (LSD) and radiation are also suspects.

Biological Agents

One of the commonest causes of disease is the invasion of the body by bacteria, viruses, fungi or parasites. They harm or destroy the tissues by their direct action on the cells or by the toxins they produce. The disease is referred to as an infection, which is discussed in the next chapter.

Physical Agents

Tissues may suffer injury or destruction as a result of external forces in the environment. These include pressure, blows, falls, lacerations and the entry of foreign bodies, such as bullets.

Cells may be destroyed when subjected to extreme heat or cold. Exposure to excessive sun rays and to radiation from x-rays or radioactive material may alter cell structure and activity or may actually cause destruction of the cells.

Chemicals

When some chemicals are introduced into the body they have an injurious effect on tissue cells. The chemical may disrupt normal cellular chemical reactions either by forming incompatible compounds or by interfering with normal enzymatic action within the cells.

Deficiencies and Excesses

An inadequate supply of materials essential to normal tissue structure and activity may cause a variety of diseases. The deficiency may be due to an insufficient intake of nutritional substances or a specific element, lack of absorption from the intestine, or an interference in the delivery of the essential substances to the cells by the circulatory system.

The lack of a normal oxygen supply to any tissue seriously impairs its function. If the supply is completely cut off, the cells quickly die. The deficiency may be local or general; local hypoxia may be due to a blockage of the vessels supplying the affected area. General oxygen deprivation may be due to respiratory insufficiency or a disturbance in the oxygen-carrying or delivery mechanisms.

An excess of nutrients may also create problems, such as increased demands on body function and the storage of excess fat. Morbidity statistics indicate a higher incidence of hypertension, cardiovascular diseases and diabetes in obese persons.

Emotions

Psychological reactions to stressful situations may influence a person's autonomic nervous system and alter its control of visceral activities. Changes in autonomic innervation may increase or decrease the function of certain structures; this may have marked effects on total body functioning.

Tissue Responses

Illness may be caused by the responses or reaction of tissues to an injury or irritation. Examples of this are inflammation and allergic reaction, both of which are discussed in ensuing sections of this chapter.

BODY RESPONSES TO DISEASE AGENTS

Body responses and manifestation patterns are frequently similar for different disease agents. Examples of reactions common to many primary causative factors include changes in body temperature, pulse, respirations, physical ability, body comfort and food tolerance. Pathologic agents initiate nonspecific as well as specific reactions. In many instances the reaction is produced as a defense mechanism but may be more damaging and stressful than the primary disease agent. The effects of disease vary not only with the type of primary agent but also with the particular individual and his responses. Defensive and adaptive capacities vary among persons; they are influenced by the individual's inherited constitution, environmental circumstances, total life style and sum total of past experiences.

When tissue cells are subjected to adverse conditions they may exhibit one or more of the following: inflammation, regeneration and repair, degeneration, necrosis, atrophy, hypertrophy, hyperplasia, metaplasia, neoplasia or the immunologic response.

INFLAMMATION

The process of inflammation is a local tissue reaction to injury or irritation. It is designed to remove or destroy the injurious agent (inflammant), keep the injury localized and repair the damage.

The causes of inflammation are many, but they may be broadly classified as: physical (e.g., mechanical agents, extreme heat and cold, radiant energy), chemical (e.g., strong acids and alkalies, irritating gases, poisons, products of necrotic tissue, products of altered metabolism), biological (e.g., microorganisms) and immunologic (e.g., antigen-antibody and autoimmune reactions). The intensity of the reaction depends on the nature and severity of the causative factor and on the reactive capacity of the individual.

The process of inflammation consists of three phases: (1) the cellular and vascular responses: (2) the formation of the inflammatory exudate; (3) systemic responses; and (4) the repair of tissues.

Cellular and Vascular Responses

In the initial phase there is a momentary constriction of the blood vessels at the site of injury. This is immediately followed by their dilation, an increased local blood supply (hyperemia) and a marked increase in vascular permeability (Fig. 3–5). These changes are attributed to the action of histamine and other chemicals that are released by the injured tissue cells. The increased filtration pressure created by hyperemia and the greater vascular permeability result in the escape of relatively large amounts of plasma and some blood cells into the interstitial spaces. As the intravascular volume is reduced the rate of blood flow decreases in the dilated vessels and the blood cells, especially the leukocytes, move out of the central portion of the stream and collect along the vessel walls; this process is referred to as margination or pavementing. The leukocytes, along with macrophages,[3] migrate through the capillary walls to the inflammatory site, where they attack the offending agent and assist in disposing of the cellular debris by phagocytosis. The leukocytes, which at this stage are principally neutrophils, and macrophages are attracted to the site of injury by chemicals released from the damaged cells. The number of neutrophils available for migration may be increased rapidly. The reacting tissues may release a globulin substance referred to as the leukocytosis-promoting factor which is carried from the area and eventually reaches the bone marrow via the blood. It stimulates the release of white blood cells, especially neutrophils, by the marrow. If the initiating factor involves an antigen, antibodies are brought to the site in the escaping plasma, which make the offending agent more susceptible to phagocytosis or which may neutralize toxins liberated by the agent.

Fibrinogen, a normal protein component of blood, is delivered to the site with the plasma. Here it is converted to fine insoluble fibers called fibrin by a cellular substance. The fibers form an interlacing network that walls off the affected area, retards or blocks the escape of the fluid and blood elements from the area via the lymphatics, and forms a framework for reparative tissue.

If the causative agent is not checked in these early responses, an increased number of macrophages are produced through the release of increased numbers of lympho-

---

[3]*Macrophages* are large wandering phagocytic cells capable of engulfing large particles. Monocytes comprise the majority of these cells.

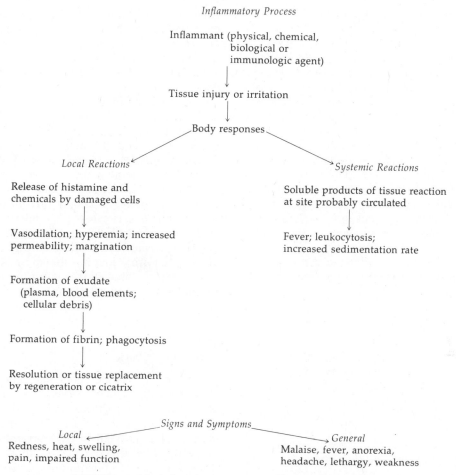

Inflammatory Process

Inflammant (physical, chemical,
biological or
immunologic agent)

↓

Tissue injury or irritation

↓

Body responses

Local Reactions

Release of histamine and
chemicals by damaged cells

↓

Vasodilation; hyperemia; increased
permeability; margination

↓

Formation of exudate
(plasma, blood elements;
cellular debris)

↓

Formation of fibrin; phagocytosis

↓

Resolution or tissue replacement
by regeneration or cicatrix

Systemic Reactions

Soluble products of tissue reaction
at site probably circulated

↓

Fever; leukocytosis;
increased sedimentation rate

Signs and Symptoms

Local
Redness, heat, swelling,
pain, impaired function

General
Malaise, fever, anorexia,
headache, lethargy, weakness

FIGURE 3–5 The inflammatory process and signs and symptoms.

cytes and monocytes by reticuloendothelial tissues (e.g., lymph glands, spleen). These leukocytes become larger, more motile and more capable of phagocytosis as they are attracted to the affected tissues by chemotaxis.

The Inflammatory Exudate

The fluid and blood elements that escape from the intravascular compartment, the products released by the injured and dead tissue cells, and the causative agent, if it is invasive or endogenous, comprise the inflammatory exudate. The nature and amount of the exudate depend upon the intensity and nature of the cause and the tissues involved.

A *serous exudate* consists chiefly of fluid with few cells and little or no fibrin. It is seen in the early stages of inflammation or when the injury is mild. An example is the fluid in a blister or that which accumulates when a serous membrane, such as the pleura or the peritoneum, is irritated. In the last two examples cited, much of the fluid is an increased secretion of serum by the affected membrane.

Purulent exudate, or pus, is a thick fluid made up of leukocytes, dead and living microorganisms which caused the injury, liquefied dead tissue cells, and the fluid and blood elements that escaped from the vessels. The formation of pus may be referred to as suppuration, and organisms that cause it are classified as pyogenic. A localized collection of purulent exudate is called an abscess. The localization is maintained by surrounding the area with leukocytes and fibrin. If the organisms migrate through the barrier to surrounding tissues, the infection spreads and is called cellulitis.

Fibrinous exudate indicates a vascular permeability that allows a greater amount of fibrinogen to leak into the interstitial area. The protein is precipitated by tissue extract (thromboplastin), which is released by injured cells and blood platelets and forms fibrin. An excessive amount of fibrin may form a membranous coating over a tissue surface, and its stickiness may cause the surfaces to adhere. The fibrin may be replaced by fibrous tissue, and bands of fibrous adhesions may form between two surfaces. Adhesions develop most frequently on serous surfaces such as the pleura, pericardium and the intestines.

A *hemorrhagic exudate* contains a large number of erythrocytes and may be described as sanguineous.

Systemic Responses

In many inflammatory conditions, especially in those caused by invasive microorganisms, an examination of the blood reveals a greater than normal number of leukocytes. This is referred to as leukocytosis. The mechanism by which this is initiated was mentioned earlier. An increase in the blood sedimentation rate also occurs. (This is the rate at which the erythrocytes settle out of blood in 1 hour.) If the cause is microorganisms, a serum titer may demonstrate a significant increase in antibodies.

Soluble products of the tissue reaction may diffuse into the blood stream or be delivered via the lymph stream to be circulated throughout the body, causing general body irritation and responses. These produce nonspecific responses which are manifested as the general signs and symptoms (see below). The severity of general responses depends upon the amount and toxicity of the absorbed inflammatory products, which in turn are determined by the nature and intensity of the offending agent.

Signs and Symptoms of Inflammation

The local manifestations include: (1) redness and heat of the affected area as a result of the hyperemia; (2) swelling and firmness due to the accumulation of the exudate in the interstitial spaces; and (3) pain caused by the pressure of the exudate on nerve endings and by chemical irritation due to substances released from the damaged cells. Impaired function of the area may be manifested, depending upon the part of the body involved.

General manifestations as well as local vary with the intensity of inflammation, the site involved and the nature of the agent. The individual may complain of "not feeling well" (general malaise), loss of appetite, headache, lethargy and weakness. Fever is common, especially if the inflammatory process is caused by invasive microorganisms or by considerable destruction of tissue cells. If the process is associated with a low nutritional intake, tissue protein catabolism takes place and the patient may demonstrate severe debilitation.

Reparative Phase

Once the causative agent has been overcome and the debris cleared away by the leukocytes, macrophages and lymph drainage, the affected area returns to normal or, if necessary, is filled in by regeneration of the respective tissue cells or fibrous scar tissue, or by a combination of the two.

When the injury is slight, cell changes may be reversible, and a complete recovery occurs. If the irritant caused the inflammatory response without cellular necrosis, the exudate is removed and the area returns to normal; this result is called *resolution*.

In the case of a more severe injury, the damage to some cells may be irreversible and they die. The area is healed by replacement of the destroyed tissue with living cells. The healing is by *regeneration* if the new cells produced by the surrounding cells are similar in structure and function to the cells being replaced. The ability to reproduce cells varies greatly from one type of tissue to another. Nervous, muscular and elastic tissues have very little or no regenerative capacity after structural growth is completed. Epithelial, fibrous, osseous, lymphoid and bone marrow tissues exhibit a much greater ability to reproduce like cells.

When regeneration is not possible, repair

occurs by replacing the lost tissue with fibrous tissue. The fibrin of the inflammatory exudate, which was formed in response to the injury, provides a framework in which granulation tissue develops. The latter is formed by the ingrowth of capillaries from surrounding vessels and by fibroblasts from marginal connective tissue. The formation of granulation tissue in an injured area is sometimes referred to as "organization." At this stage, the tissue appears as a very soft, gelatinous-like red mass because of its many newly-formed capillaries and large immature fibroblasts around which collagen fibers develop. As the fibroblasts and collagen fibers mature, the tissue shrinks, many capillaries are constricted and obliterated, and an area of firm fibrous tissue remains, known as a *cicatrix,* or *scar.* Marginal surface epithelium (e.g., skin) proliferates to form a surface covering.

The fibrous tissue substitution for the original specialized cells may reduce the functional capacity of the affected structure or may cause mechanical interference because of its firm, constricting nature, such as is seen in pyloric obstruction when a peptic ulcer heals. Factors which delay healing include:

1. *Tissue trauma and a reduced blood supply.* The more serious the tissue injury and the greater the interference with the blood supply to the affected area, the longer will be the period required to replace the destroyed tissue.

2. *Infection.* Invasion of the wound by microorganisms may increase tissue destruction and impede the formation of granulation tissue.

3. *Nutritional deficiencies.* A deficient intake of protein results in a lack of the essential amino acids from which new tissue is constructed. An insufficient supply of vitamin C (ascorbic acid) prevents the formation of collagen fibers that support the developing fibrous tissue.

4. *Mechanical factors.* Friction on a wound destroys the soft granulation tissue. The presence of a foreign body that prevents the apposition of wound edges retards healing.

5. *Adrenocortical hormones.* An excess of these hormones inhibits inflammation and, as a result, retards the formation of granulation tissue.

Classification of Inflammation

Inflammation may be classified in a variety of ways:

1. ACCORDING TO THE DURATION OF THE REACTION. It may be termed *acute* if it has a sudden onset and progresses quickly to recovery, permanent injury or death. *Chronic* inflammation usually has an insidious onset and persists over a period of months to years. A *subacute* inflammatory process is usually considered intermediary to the foregoing types in both severity and duration.

2. ACCORDING TO THE STRUCTURE AFFECTED. The suffix *-itis* is used to denote inflammation of the particular tissue or structure indicated by the preceding part of the word. For example: myocarditis implies inflammation of the muscle fibers of the heart; pneumonitis, inflammation of the lung tissue; laryngitis, inflammation of the larynx; peritonitis, inflammation of the peritoneum; and so on.

3. ACCORDING TO THE NATURE OF THE EXUDATE. Fibrinous inflammation indicates that a relatively large amount of fibrin is formed. Purulent inflammation implies suppuration.

4. ACCORDING TO THE ETIOLOGIC AGENT. Another basis of classification that may be used occasionally relates to the nature of the inflammant. The terms traumatic, chemical, bacterial or allergic may be used as descriptive terms.

Nursing in Inflammation

Much of the care of the patient with an area of inflammation is determined by the site of the process, the function which is disturbed and the nature of the inflammant. The following general principles apply:

The affected part is placed at rest and, when this is not possible, demands upon it should be reduced to a minimum.

If a limb is involved, the patient may receive some relief from pain by elevation of the part. This encourages venous and lymphatic drainage which may reduce the swelling, and it also increases the flow of a fresh supply of blood into the area with more elements to combat the offending agent and restore the tissue to normal.

Hot or cold applications to the affected

area may be ordered. Heat favors an increased blood supply to the part and relaxation of muscle tissue, which may be in spasm because of the injured cells. Cold applications cause constriction of the vessels and thus reduce the volume of exudate and diminish the swelling which is responsible for the pain. Cold also reduces the sensitivity of the inflamed nerve endings, and when bacteria are the causative agent their activity and multiplication may be delayed.

If the inflammant is known to be microorganisms, antimicrobial drugs such as antibiotics, sulfonamide, antitoxin or specific preparations are prescribed. A corticoid preparation (e.g., prednisone) may be prescribed in some chronic inflammatory conditions (e.g., colitis, Crohn's disease) because of its anti-inflammatory effect. The nurse should be familiar with the possible side effects of these drugs and should report their early manifestations. In the case of corticoid preparations side effects include acne, moon face, hirsutism, hypertension, decreased resistance to infection and osteoporosis.

General rest is beneficial in increasing the patient's ability to combat the disease, particularly if constitutional symptoms are manifested. The patient is encouraged to take plenty of fluids to promote dilution and elimination of absorbed toxic products. The caloric intake must be considered, and an effort made to prevent a negative nitrogen balance.

DEGENERATIVE CHANGES

Degeneration of cells is characterized by changes in the chemical reactions and composition of the cytoplasm, as well as a corresponding decrease in cell function. It may be due to a diminished blood supply, inadequate oxygen or nutrients, trauma, infection, toxic substances, or an alteration in the enzyme systems within the cells. The cells may contain an accumulation of an abnormal substance or an excess of normal materials which they cannot metabolize or extrude.

Descriptive terms such as fatty, cloudy, swelling, hyaline (translucent), amyloid (waxy, starch-like) and mucoid may be applied to degeneration according to the changes observed in the composition and the appearance of the cells.

NECROSIS

Necrosis is the death of cells or tissue within a living organism. It may be caused by a lack of essential materials for cell activity, mechanical injury, extreme heat or cold, chemical or bacterial poisons or radiation. The dead cells may be liquefied by their contained enzymes. They may disintegrate and coagulate to form a relatively firm dry mass or may disintegrate to form a mass of caseous material which is grayish-white and soft and cheesy in consistency. The latter is characteristic of cells destroyed by tuberculous infection.

Gangrene is the death of a relatively large area of tissue; it may involve a part or the whole of an organ or limb. *Infarction* is a term used to denote necrosis of an area of tissue caused by ischemia (inadequate blood supply to the part).

ATROPHY

A decrease in the size of a structure may be due to a reduction in the size of the individual tissue cells or a decrease in the number of constituent cells. The latter is due to a failure of the replacement of cells to keep pace with cells destroyed or worn out; this is commonly seen in the later years of life. The cause of atrophy may be nutritional deficiency, a reduced blood supply, excessive functional demands on the tissue, disuse, interruption of the nerve supply to the part, toxic substances or physiological aging mechanisms (e.g., atrophy of the uterus and breasts after menopause due to a change in the concentration of sex hormones).

HYPERTROPHY AND HYPERPLASIA

A frequent response of a tissue to increased demands placed upon it is hypertrophy, which is achieved by an increase in the size of the individual cells. It may be observed in the enlargement of skeletal muscles with increased work and exercise.

An increase in the volume of tissue due to an increased number of cells is called hyperplasia.

Hypertrophy and hyperplasia are beneficial in cases in which an increase in function is necessary. The heart, for example, may compensate for increased resistance to the flow of blood from a chamber by the hypertrophy of the myocardial fibers of the walls of that chamber. Hyperplasia of the bone marrow and lymphoid tissues increases the number of leukocytes and is helpful in severe infection. In other instances, an increase in the size of a structure may be harmful. Hypertrophy of the heart muscle may require a greater blood supply than the coronary arteries can supply. An enlarged organ may cause pressure or obstruction in some situations. A frequent example of this is hyperplasia of the prostate gland; the enlarged gland imposes upon the urethra, causing retention of urine.

METAPLASIA

This tissue response to adverse conditions is the replacement of tissue by cells that are different from their predecessors. For example, following repeated injury and irritation, the normal, ciliated, mucus-secreting epithelial lining of the respiratory tract may be replaced by a thicker, nonsecreting squamous epithelium. This substitution reduces the normal, protective cleansing mechanisms and predisposes to infection.

NEOPLASIA

This term means new formation or growth. Normally, the production of cells is a regulated process allowing for growth of the organism in early life and for replacement of worn-out or damaged cells throughout the total life span. Occasionally the control of cell reproduction is lost in some tissue and an excessive production occurs. The cells are usually atypical, serve no useful purpose, develop at the expense of surrounding tissues and continue their characteristics through successive generations of cells. The resulting mass is referred to as a *new growth* or *neoplasm*.

When the neoplasm produces an evident swelling, it may be called a tumor. If it is confined by a capsule, remains localized and the rate of growth of the cells is relatively slow, the new growth is said to be *benign. Malignant neoplasms* (cancers) grow more rapidly, are not encapsulated and spread into surrounding tissues. Some of their cells may be carried from the site of their origin and may set up colonies of the malignant cells (metastases) in other areas of the body. The proliferative growth of malignant cells with their invasion and destruction of normal tissue may end in death of the patient. Cancer is discussed in Chapter 8.

THE IMMUNE RESPONSE

The immune response is a physiological reaction of the body to factors that it considers threatening and foreign to it. A factor which evokes the immune response is referred to as an *antigen* and may be foreign protein or polysaccharide in the form of bacteria, viruses, toxins, or tissue cells from another organism. The response involves: *first,* the body's ability to recognize what is foreign to it, what is self and nonself and what is threatening; and *second,* a sequence of events that results in the production of special, sensitized cells (immune bodies), which are capable of inhibiting and overcoming the offending agent and providing protection for the individual against the antigen. This type of protection against pathogens (disease-producing agents) is called *immunity.* The immune bodies may be antibodies or special lymphocytes.

Antigens are usually exogenous (from outside the body). Occasionally the body may object to and react with some of its own cellular products, which are then referred to as *endogenous antigens* or *autoantigens.* The immune response to the latter antigens is known as an *autoimmune reaction.*

Two mechanisms are involved in the immune response; one is referred to as humoral immunity and the other as cell-mediated immunity. The *humoral immune response* entails the development and circulation of molecules of gamma globulin when antigens invade the body. These globulin molecules are known as immunoglobulins or antibodies, and are formed by plasma cells.[4] Guyton indicates that these particular plasma cells are dormant until exposed to an antigen. They then multiply rapidly and produce immunoglobulins.[5]

Immunoglobulins or antibodies have been classified and may be designated as belonging to one of the following groups: IgG, IgA, IgM, IgD or IgE. The IgG type is found to be in greatest concentration, normally composing about 75 per cent of the total. IgD and IgE normally occur in very small serum concentrations. In identifying the class to which the various antibodies belong, information has been determined about their molecular structure, concentration and distribution, movement through capillary walls, movement across the placenta into fetal circulation, and reaction with antigens.

The *cellular immune reaction* is mediated by sensitized lymphocytes, sometimes referred to as T lymphocytes because of their original association with and conditioning by the thymus gland.[6] It is suggested that these lymphocytes develop antibodies within, or "antibody-like receptors" on their surfaces. The original lymphocytes capable of becoming sensitized are considered to be produced or processed within the thymus gland very early in life and distributed to lymphoid tissues throughout the body.[7]

Antigen-Antibody Reaction

Immune bodies, whether antibodies or T lymphocytes, are specific for each antigen — that is, they are capable of opposing only the antigen which initiated their formation. For example, diphtheria antibodies will not be effective if the invaders are typhoid bacilli.

Antibodies react with antigens in a variety of ways and, in some instances, more than one type of antibody will react with the same antigen, differing in the type of reaction pro-

duced. The reactions that may occur, by which antibodies may be classified, include: (1) precipitation of the antigens from their fluid medium (precipitins); (2) lysis, which results in dissolution of the antigens (lysins); (3) agglutination, in which the antigens are clumped together, thus rendering them ineffective (agglutinins); (4) opsonization, a process which facilitates phagocytosis of the antigens (opsonins); and (5) neutralization, in which the antibody neutralizes the toxic products of the antigens (antitoxins).

A group of at least nine serum protein substances have been recognized as playing an important role in some antigen-antibody reactions. They are referred to collectively as the complement system; individually, they are numbered according to the order in which they enter the reaction (C1, C2, C3, ... C9). The complement components do not act directly on the antigen but combine with the antibody after it attaches to the antigen. This interaction activates the complement, which then initiates a sequence of enzymic reactions that cause disruptions of areas of cell membranes and eventual irreversible destruction of the cells.

When an antigen is present for the first time, the antibody concentration (titer) is not significant until about the sixth or seventh day, when the immune bodies rapidly increase. As a result of the lag, the host develops the disease. When the antigen is eliminated, the immune bodies gradually decline over a period of several weeks. The period of immunity developed following the invasion by some antigens may be brief and transient, such as that which occurs with the common cold and pneumonia. With other diseases the immunity lasts for long periods, even for life (e.g., measles and diphtheria). In the latter case a phenomenon referred to as "memory" by immunologists remains in the dormant plasma cells and lymphoblasts in lymphoid tissues. On reexposure to the same antigen production of the special immune bodies promptly occurs; the number increases rapidly enough to overcome the antigens before the disease develops, thus providing the individual with immunity. This recognition of the antigen by the body, and the effective response, is the basis of the single booster doses of immune-producing preparations. Initially, in artificially induced immunization, administration of a series of antigen doses is

---

[4]*Plasma cells* are produced chiefly by reticulum cells in the lymphoid tissue in lymph nodes, spleen and gastrointestinal tract.

[5]Guyton, op. cit., p. 119.

[6]The *thymus* is a bilobed lymphoid gland situated in the thoracic cavity, posterior to the upper part of the sternum. It is larger and more active during the first few weeks of life, gradually declining and becoming less active during childhood.

[7]Guyton, op. cit., pp. 78–79.

necessary to evoke immune body production and establish the "memory" by which the tissues recognize the antigen. After that only a small amount of the antigen is necessary to maintain effective protection.

Natural Immunity

Immunity to some diseases occurs naturally and congenitally, and is dependent upon certain substances occurring normally in the blood. Those substances which react with antigens include phagocytic cells (e.g., leukocytes), lysozyme, which breaks down microorganisms, and some polypeptides, which react with certain types of bacteria.

Natural immunity varies with species, races and individuals. A species of animal may be very susceptible to a certain antigen which is incapable of producing disease in humans. An example is the high susceptibility of cats and dogs to distemper and the natural immunity to the causative agent possessed by humans. Persons of the Negro race exhibit a poor resistance to tuberculosis as compared with that of Caucasians, but the exact reverse is apparent in relation to malaria. Natural resistance or immunity to certain antigenic microorganisms may be present in some individuals but absent in others; this is evident when a family or group is exposed equally for the first time to a specific antigen and all but one or two become ill. In addition to the protective substances normally present in the blood, age is considered to be a factor in natural immunity; certain infections have a higher incidence in children and rarely occur in adults.

Acquired Immunity

This type of immunity may be active or passive. Actively acquired immunity develops when the host forms his own antibodies in response to an antigen. An individual may acquire this immunity by having had the disease, or it may be produced artificially by a series of injections of the antigen. The length of time active immunity lasts varies; it may be very brief for some antigens, while for others it may be lifelong because of the established ability of the tissues to recognize the antigen promptly and produce the appropriate immune bodies rapidly.

Passive acquired immunity may be natural or artificially induced. Natural passive immunity occurs in the newborn infant. This type is passive because the antibodies were developed by the mother and passed through the placenta to the fetus. These maternal antibodies provide a temporary immunity, protecting the infant only through the first few months of life.

Artificial passive immunity is conferred by injecting serum taken from another organism, usually an animal, which has actively produced immune bodies. This type of immunity is rapidly established but is of short duration. The antibodies are foreign to the recipient and are destroyed in a relatively short period. As previously indicated, it takes time to produce antibodies upon first exposure; serum that contains specific immune bodies is administered only to those who already have the disease or who are known to have been exposed to the antigen. The foreign antibodies provide an immediate defense during the period in which the recipient is forming his own antibodies.

Since the immune response has such a significant defensive role in specific infections, further discussion of immunization appears in the next chapter.

Disorders of the Immune Response

"More than ever it has become apparent that dependent as man is for his survival on the immune system, so vulnerable is he to the wide-ranging disorders in its function."[8] Normally, the immune response is a physiological defense mechanism, but it may fail as such as a result of a deficiency in the necessary elements, or because of an exaggerated, altered or inappropriate reaction, referred to as hypersensitivity or allergy. The severity of the disorders varies greatly, ranging from slightly to totally incapacitating and life-threatening.

Immunologic Deficiency Disease

An immunologic deficiency state may be the result of dysfunction within the humoral-mediated immune system, the cell-mediated (T cell) immune system, or both.

---

[8]Stanley L. Robbins and Marcia Angell: Basic Pathology, 2nd ed. Philadelphia, W. B. Saunders, 1976.

HYPOGAMMAGLOBULINEMIA. Deficiency in the humoral immune system is manifested by susceptibility to infections, especially those of bacterial origin. Inadequate amounts of the gamma fraction of serum globulin results in a failure in antibody formation. Hypo- or agammaglobulinemia may be primary or secondary. Primary deficiency in immunoglobulins is congenital and is thought to have a sex-linked (X chromosome) recessive hereditary basis. The congenital deficit may not show up in the first few months of life because of the infant's passive immunity acquired from the mother in utero. Immunologists indicate that a selective deficiency may occur within the immunoglobulins — that is, that only one of the classes (IgG, IgM, IgA, IgD, IgE) of antibodies may be lacking. IgA is cited as the one most frequently decreased or absent. Individuals with hypogammaglobulinemia experience recurrent upper respiratory infections and also show a higher incidence of autoimmune diseases.[9, 10]

Acquired hypogammaglobulinemia may be secondary to disease affecting the reticuloendothelial tissues (e.g., Hodgkin's disease, leukemia). It may also develop as a result of an excessive loss of blood protein as found with the nephrotic syndrome and some intestinal disturbances.

An *abnormal antibody formation* may result from a malignant proliferation of the plasma cells responsible for synthesizing one of the classes of immunoglobulins (antibodies). For example, the plasma cells undergo transformation to malignant tumors within the bone marrow, causing *multiple myeloma*. The immunologic reactions are impaired because normal plasma cells involved in antibody production are displaced by the abnormal tumor cells. The individual experiences recurrent infections, as well as weakness and severe bone pain. Weakening of the bone structure may cause spontaneous pathologic fractures. Blood investigation shows anemia, elevated sedimentation rate and increased serum globulin level. The urine is likely to contain an abnormal serum

protein produced by the cells of the tumors, referred to as Bence Jones protein.

CELL-MEDIATED IMMUNE DEFICIENCY. Individuals with this type of deficiency are particularly susceptible to viral infections. There is a diminished production of the special, sensitized small lymphocytes (T cells). Primary deficiency in the cell-mediated immune mechanism is usually accounted for by failure in the development of the thymus (thymic aplasia or dysplasia). The diminished protection shows up early in life; individuals do not usually survive beyond the first two or three years of life. Cell-mediated immune deficiency may be secondary to Hodgkin's disease, leukopenia, severe stress incurred by trauma or acute infection, or excessive corticoid blood levels.[11]

CARE IN IMMUNE DEFICIENCY. The individual with primary immunoglobulin deficiency receives regular monthly intramuscular injections of human serum gamma globulin. If the deficit is secondary, treatment is directed towards the primary disorder.

An explanation of the deficiency and its implications is made to the patient and family. The importance of avoiding persons with infections and the practice of medical asepsis are discussed with them in detail. It is not sufficient to say merely that the affected person should avoid others with infections. The necessary precautionary measures can be emphasized by citing those that are necessary when a family member has a minor infection such as a cold or sore throat. Explanations include: (1) the ways in which organisms may be transmitted; (2) disinfection of the infected person's dishes and linens, the telephone, etc.; (3) the importance of frequent washing of the hands under running water, the covering of the mouth during coughing and sneezing, and the disposal of contaminated articles such as tissues; and (4) the avoidance of crowds and close personal contact with infected persons. They are advised of the importance of a well-balanced nutritious diet, adequate rest and warmth and avoidance of fatigue in maintaining resistance.

The patient is instructed to report the earli-

[9]G. W. Thorn, et al. (Eds.): Harrison's Principles of Internal Medicine, 8th ed. New York, McGraw-Hill, 1977.

[10]Paul B. Beeson and Walsh McDermott (Eds.): Textbook of Medicine, 15th ed. Philadelphia, W. B. Saunders, 1979.

[11]*Adrenocortical secretions* depress lymphoid tissue activity and the production of lymphocytes.

est signs of a disorder immediately; antibiotic therapy is instituted promptly. If the patient with immune deficiency requires hospitalization, it is important to provide protection by reverse isolation (reverse barrier technique). The patient is cared for in a single room and only sterile linen and equipment are used. Personnel contacting or caring for the patient are screened for possible infection and are required to wash their hands thoroughly under running water before attending the patient. A clean coverall type of gown and a mask are worn at the bedside. In some situations a cap and shoe covers may also have to be worn. Visitors are restricted to one or two immediate family members who are free of infection. They also are required to wear a gown, mask, cap and shoe covers and are requested not to go within 3 to 4 feet of the bedside. The floor is wet-mopped and the furniture is washed frequently to reduce possible contaminated dust particles. More effective isolation may be achieved in a unit which protects the patient against airborne organisms by means of a special mechanical ventilator which filters the air entering the unit. A plastic curtain or barrier with portholes may be placed along one side of the bed; care and treatments are administered through the portholes.

Efforts have been made to improve some immune-deficient victims by the transfer of immunologically competent cells from other individuals. The experimental donor tissue may come from the spleen, a lymph node, bone marrow, or the thymus of a newborn. Obviously, immunosuppressive drugs cannot be administered to those transplant recipients who are already very susceptible to pathogens. Unless the deficiency is in both immune systems, rejection occurs.

Hypersensitivity (Allergy)

The term hypersensitivity or allergy implies an altered state of tissue reactivity. Some persons have an unusual sensitivity to certain substances and, upon contact with them, manifest an adverse reaction not seen in most people. The substance may be referred to as an *allergen* or an *antigen* since it causes an immunologic response.

The allergen is usually a protein. In the few exceptions in which it is nonprotein, it becomes linked to a protein in the body and forms a compound to which the tissues are sensitive. The reaction-producing substance is specific to the individual and may be a food, an animal or plant emanation (e.g., horse dander, pollen), a chemical (e.g., dye) or a drug. It may reach the tissues by inhalation, ingestion, parenteral injection, or by direct contact with the skin. In the case of ingestion, the allergen may have a local effect upon the gastrointestinal tissues, or may be absorbed unchanged and carried by the blood to sensitive tissues.

Immune responses are usually beneficial, but in hypersensitive persons they become adverse and harmful in response to certain antigens. The first contact with the allergen may not produce manifestations of hypersensitivity, but subsequent contacts produce an inappropriate and exaggerated response that injures tissue cells and may result in the release of harmful chemical substances which are circulated, producing adverse effects on other tissues. The inflammatory process may develop at the site of the injured cells.

Common immunologic disorders attributed to exogenous allergens include hay fever, asthma, eczema, urticaria, dermatitis, specific drug sensitivity (e.g., penicillin, sulfonamide preparations, aspirin, foreign serum) and specific food sensitivity (e.g., milk, wheat, eggs, shellfish, mushrooms). There is an increasing awareness of the possibility that hypersensitivity to unknown foreign or endogenous materials may account for a wide variety of pathologic conditions. A hypersensitive reaction is considered to be the causative factor in rheumatic fever and glomerulonephritis. Currently there are an increasing number of references suggesting a similar etiologic basis for rheumatoid arthritis and collagen diseases such as lupus erythematosus, polyarteritis and scleroderma.

Cells in which a sensitivity is most frequently manifested appear to be those of the epithelial, connective and smooth muscle tissues. Areas of the body most frequently involved are the respiratory tract, skin and gastrointestinal tract. Reactions may take the form of: (1) itching, excessive secretion and edema of the nasal pharyngeal mucous membrane (hay fever); (2) spasmodic constriction of the muscle tissue of the bronchial tubes and swelling and edema of their mucosa (asthma); (3) erythematous, vesicular and inflammatory eruptions of the skin (urticaria, eczema, dermatitis); (4) vomiting and diarrhea (food sensitivity); (5) increased permeability of blood vessels and generalized edema (angioneurotic) or (6) vasodilation leading to circulatory failure, manifested by a weak pulse, sharp fall in blood pressure and collapse (anaphylaxis). Combinations of these may occur in the same patient. One allergen may cause a reaction in more than one area of the body. For example, a person with hypersensitivity to a particular food may develop both gastrointestinal and skin reactions, or may develop asthma and a gastrointestinal reaction. The reaction varies in different persons, depending upon their tissue sensitivity.

Genetic factors are of significance in allergic reactions; it is thought that the capacity to develop a hypersensitivity can be inherited. Abnormal immune reactions tend to occur in families. The disorder may differ from one family member to another — one may exhibit a skin reaction; another may suffer from asthma. At the same time, siblings or offspring of the affected person may not manifest any hypersensitivity. When there is a history of an allergy on both the maternal and paternal sides, a greater number of the offspring becomes affected and reactions appear at an earlier age.

TYPES OF HYPERSENSITIVITY

Abnormal and harmful immunologic reactions to antigens may be classified as immediate or delayed, and according to the mechanism or nature of the response.

Immediate hypersensitive states develop as the result of antigen-antibody interaction. This classification includes those abnormal immune reactions characterized by the rapid appearance of manifestations, usually within 5 to 15 minutes of antigen-antibody contact.

Delayed hypersensitive reaction is brought about by the interaction of an antigen and immunologic lymphocytes (T cells). The first signs and symptoms appear within approximately 12 hours and become progressively more intense, reaching a peak in 2 to 4 days.

The most widely accepted categorization of hypersensitivity reactions, that of Gell and Coombs,[12] indicates three immediate reactions; anaphylactic or type 1 reaction, cytotoxic or type 2 reaction, and immune complex or type 3. The delayed reaction is referred to as the T cell-mediated hypersensitivity or type 4. Irvine cites two other reactions, *stimulating antibody reaction, type 5* and *lymphoid (K) cell-dependent antibody-mediated cytotoxicity, type 6.*[13]

ANAPHYLACTIC IMMEDIATE HYPERSENSITIVITY (TYPE 1)

Until recently, anaphylaxis always implied a very severe life-threatening allergic reaction which caused severe shock. Currently, it has a broader concept and refers to a particular immune mechanism rather than to the severity of the response.

This type of reactivity results from the reaction of an antigen with IgE antibodies. The antigen and antibodies become "fixed" to the surface of mast cells.[14] The individual who manifests this type of immune response has formed more IgE antibodies than are found in those who are not hypersensitive. The antigen-antibody interaction with the cells leads to the release of certain chemicals, which cause an increase in capillary permeability and the contraction of smooth muscle in some structures. The chemically active mediators that are released include histamine, serotonin and "slow-reacting substance of anaphylaxis." These chemicals, along with plasma kinins (bradykinin and kallidin), are responsible for the various manifestations of anaphylaxis. The plasma kinins are peptides formed from plasma globulins by enzymes of the complement system. The severity of the hypersensitive response is dependent upon the concentration of chemical mediators and the tissues and structures they affect.

---

[12]P. G. H. Gell and R. R. A. Coombs (Eds.): Clinical Aspects of Immunology, 2nd ed. Philadelphia, F. A. Davis, 1968.

[13]W. J. Irvine: "Immunologic Factors in Disease." *In* J. Macleod, Ed.: Davidson's Principles and Practice of Medicine, 11th ed. Edinburgh, Churchill Livingstone, 1974, p. 28.

[14]*Mast cells* are wandering cells that are found in most tissues and are especially abundant in connective tissues.

The anaphylactic reaction may be local or systemic, depending upon the portal of entry of the antigen. *Local reactions* occur when the antigen-antibody reaction is on cells in the mucosa of the respiratory tract. The commonest allergens in this hypersensitivity are airborne particles of dust, pollen, molds and animal dander. The individual experiences the sneezing, nasal congestion, and increased secretion, and itching and "watering" of the eyes characteristic of allergic rhinitis (hay fever). If the antigen is inhaled, bronchospasm (asthma) and/or laryngeal edema may cause respiratory distress. The intestinal mucosa in a sensitized person may react locally to the antigen causing crampy pain, vomiting and diarrhea. If the antigen is absorbed, a combined systemic and local reaction may develop. The *systemic form* of anaphylaxis is likely to be severe and potentially fatal, and may be called *anaphylactic shock*. It nearly always develops very rapidly following parenteral injection of the antigen, but may occur rarely after the ingestion of food or drug allergens. The commonest antigens in anaphylactic shock are foreign serum (e.g., tetanus antitoxin), some drugs such as penicillin and streptomycin, contrast medium used in intravenous pyelograms, and bee venom from a sting.

The signs and symptoms of systemic anaphylaxis appear rapidly. The first may be a diffuse erythema and urticaria, sneezing and coughing. The patient may complain of diffuse pruritus and/or tightness in the chest which is followed by sneezing, dyspnea and cyanosis. The condition rapidly worsens. Gastrointestinal disturbance may be manifested by nausea, vomiting, colicky pain and diarrhea. There is a sharp decrease in blood pressure as vascular collapse develops; the pulse is rapid and weak and may quickly become imperceptible. The skin becomes pale and cold, pupils dilate and the patient may lose consciousness. The picture is one of cardiorespiratory failure and severe shock.

Care in Anaphylactic Shock. Urgent treatment is necessary to prevent the reaction from proving fatal.

1. Application of tourniquet. If the injection of the antigen has been made in a limb, a tourniquet is applied above the site to decrease circulation of the drug. The tourniquet must be released every 15 minutes for 3 to 5 minutes.

2. Position. The patient is placed in the recumbent position, with the neck extended and head turned to promote a clear airway. The lower extremities are elevated and constricting clothing is loosened or removed.

3. Drug therapy. Epinephrine hydrochloride (aqueous solution 1:1000) 0.1 to 0.4 ml. is prescribed to be given immediately subcutaneously or intramuscularly, or 0.1 to 0.2 ml. in 10 ml. of normal saline is administered slowly by intravenous infusion. The epinephrine is given to relax bronchial and laryngeal spasm and may be repeated if respiratory distress persists. An injection of 0.1 to 0.3 ml. may also be made at the site of injection.

Diphenhydramine hydrochloride (Benadryl) 25 to 50 mg. may be given slowly by intravenous infusion.

An antihypotensive drug such as levarterenol bitartrate (Levophed), 8 to 16 mg., or metaraminol bitartrate (Aramine), 100 to 200 mg., may be administered in 500 ml. of 5 per cent glucose in water intravenously. The rate of flow is prescribed according to blood pressure, which is monitored every 15 minutes.

If the patient experiences severe bronchospasm (asthma) without vascular collapse and shock, aminophylline, 250 to 500 mg., may be given very slowly over 15 to 30 minutes intravenously to promote bronchial dilation.

A corticosteroid preparation such as hydrocortisone sodium succinate (Solu-Cortef) or methylprednisolone (Solu-Medrol) may be given intravenously to reduce tissue sensitivity. A corticosteroid preparation (e.g., prednisone) is usually administered orally for several days following recovery from the critical phase of the reaction.

4. Maintenance of an airway. It may be necessary to introduce an oropharyngeal airway if the patient loses consciousness and the tongue and jaw are blocking passage of air. Suction is used to remove secretions and fluid. If the respiratory distress is unrelieved, and laryngeal spasm and edema are suspected, an endotracheal tube is passed or a tracheostomy may be necessary to establish an airway.

Oxygen 40 per cent is administered to decrease the hypoxia resulting from respiratory insufficiency. The method of administration used will depend on whether the patient is intubated or has a tracheostomy.

Vascular collapse leading to cardiorespiratory failure necessitates cardiopulmonary resuscitation (see p. 332).

5. Observation. A nurse remains in constant attendance on the patient. Vital signs are checked and recorded at intervals of 10 to 15 minutes; the intervals are gradually lengthened as the patient shows improvement.

Close observation is necessary for several days in the event of a recurrence of reactions and irreversible damage from the anaphylactic shock.

6. Psychological support. Systemic anaphylactic reaction is a frightening experience. The seriousness of the situation is readily sensed by the patient and some explanation of what is occurring is necessary, as is reassurance that everything possible is being done. It is helpful if someone is available to devote his full attention to reducing the patient's fears and providing the much needed support, and to meet requests such as notification of a family member. This arrangement prevents possible interruption and delay of the therapeutic team.

CYTOLYTIC IMMEDIATE HYPERSENSITIVITY (TYPE 2)

This type of reaction, which may also be called cytotoxic, is destructive to the sensitized tissue cells that are attacked by antibodies. The cells have an antigenic component, which may be an integral part of the cells, or an exogenous substance such as a drug that has become firmly attached to the cells. The interaction with the antibodies, which are usually of the IgG class or occasionally the IgM class, may produce agglutination, lysis and cell destruction. Factors in the complement system facilitate the adverse antigen-antibody reactions and subsequent dissolution of the cell.

Examples of the cytotoxic hypersensitive response include incompatible blood transfusion reaction, hemolytic anemia, drug-induced leukopenia and glomerulonephritis.

IMMUNE COMPLEX IMMEDIATE HYPERSENSITIVITY (TYPE 3)

Two types of disorders fall into this category of hypersensitivity: the *Arthus reaction,* which produces localized lesions, and *serum sickness,* which is more systemic and diffuse. The offending immunoglobulin is most often of the IgG group, but in some instances similar reactions occur if the individual has a high level of circulating IgE antibodies. The antigen-antibody precipitates and holds complement-forming complexes that are deposited in certain tissues. The complement initiates a sequence of reactions and polymorphonuclear leukocytes are attracted to the sites. Inflammation is induced in the tissues by the interactions and release of enzymes.

The Arthus reaction occurs at the site of injection of the antigen. The complex formed in this type of hypersensitivity has a predilection for the small blood vessels; vasculitis develops and may progress to irreversible vascular damage or occlusion of the vessels, leading to interference with the blood supply to some tissues and ensuing necrosis.

Serum sickness may follow the administration of a foreign serum, such as diphtheria antitoxin and tetanus antitoxin, or the giving of some drugs such as sulfonamide, penicillin or streptomycin. The area affected by the antigen-antibody complex is not confined to the site of injection. Deposition of the antigen-antibodies and subsequent inflammatory reaction may be in: (1) the joints, causing swelling, reduced mobility and pain; (2) the kidneys, resulting in glomerulonephritis; or (3) the respiratory system, giving rise to laryngeal edema, bronchospasm or interstitial pneumonitis. Involvement of diffuse skin areas may be manifested by rashes or urticaria.

CELL-MEDIATED DELAYED HYPERSENSITIVITY (TYPE 4)

This type of hypersensitivity is most commonly induced by infectious agents such as the viruses that cause measles, herpes, smallpox, mumps, and bacteria, such as the tubercle bacilli, *Treponema pallidum,* streptococcus and salmonellae. The reaction may also occur in the form of contact dermatitis in individuals who become allergic to chromium, nickel, primula plants and poison ivy. These substances become antigenic by combining with proteins in the skin. The dermatitis is manifested by redness, swelling, vesicles (blisters), exudation ("weeping") and scaling. The cell-mediated allergic response is also involved in the rejection process that may follow tissue or organ transplantation (see p. 641).

The example most often used to illustrate

this delayed immunologic response is the reaction to an intradermal injection of tuberculin[15] which is used as a test for sensitivity to tubercle bacilli. The individual who has been sensitized by previous entry of the tubercle bacilli into the body produces an inflamed, indurated area at the site of the injection gradually over 18 to 48 hours. The delayed hypersensitive reaction is not brought about by circulating immunoglobulins but by specially sensitized lymphocytes (T cells). The site of "attack" by the antigen becomes infiltrated with a large number of reticuloendothelial cells, mainly lymphocytes. In interacting with the antigen, the lymphocytes release substances currently referred to as lymphokines, which have varied effects — some have a chemotactic effect, which attracts still more lymphocytes to the site, and others are toxic to tissue cells. One is said to suppress the migration of macrophages, and is referred to as the migration inhibitor factor (MIF). Immunologists indicate that there still is much to be determined concerning the mechanism of cell-mediated hypersensitivity.

STIMULATING ANTIBODY REACTION (TYPE 5)

It is suggested that in this type of allergic reaction, certain IgG immunoglobulins have the ability to stimulate the tissue cells involved in the reaction rather than damage them. Some cases of thyrotoxicosis, and especially neonatal hyperthyroidism, are attributed to this class of hypersensitivity.[16]

LYMPHOID (K) CELL-DEPENDENT ANTIBODY-MEDIATED CYTOTOXICITY REACTION (TYPE 6)

Irvine attributes this hypersensitivity to lymphocytes which are not of the type usually involved in immune responses. These cells react with an immunoglobulin-antigen "fixed" by complement on the surface of the sensitive tissue cells. As a result of the interaction, the lymphocytes have a toxic effect on the tissue cells, causing inflammation or degenerative changes. It is suggested that

these cells are active in autoimmune thyroid disease (Hashimoto's thyroiditis).[17]

AUTOIMMUNE DISEASE

The body differentiates between its own body constituents and exogenous or foreign protein. Generally, immune bodies are formed only in response to an exogenous antigen. Occasionally, an antigen may be developed within a person (autoantigen) which stimulates the formation of antibodies (autoantibodies). The antigen may be produced by the entrance of a foreign nonantigenic substance which combines with an endogenous protein, altering it and making it antigenic. The formation of immune bodies by the body against its own protein is known as autoimmunization. The antigen-antibody combination may cause a reaction, and the resulting disease is classified as autoimmune.

IDENTIFICATION OF ALLERGENS

The most important factor in the care of the hypersensitive person is avoidance of the allergen (antigen). Identification of the offending factor becomes paramount.

HISTORY. An effort is made to learn of any allergic disorders in the family and a detailed history is taken of the patient's past illnesses, current complaint(s), personal activities, occupation and environment. The allergen may be recognized readily by the patient, family or nurse when repeated reactions are associated with the inhalation, ingestion or injection of a certain substance. For example, the individual may become ill each time he eats a particular food or may develop a rash following the wearing of a particular article of clothing, or the nurse may note that certain signs or symptoms are manifested whenever he receives a certain drug.

Physicians and institutions concerned with the investigation of hypersensitivity usually have an especially constructed history form on which relevant information is recorded. Detailed questions are presented under major headings such as: Present illness and presenting symptoms; Past illnesses; Family allergic disorders; Drugs; Immunization; Occupation; Recreation; Responses to weather;

---

[15]The solution used is a purified protein extract from cultures of tubercle bacilli. It is administered in a 1:1000 dilution.

[16]Irvine, op. cit., p. 36.

[17]Ibid., p. 36.

Foods; Skin applications; Contact with animals; Contact with plants; Environments (home, occupation, others); Patient's observations and comments (suspected allergen).

SENSITIVITY TESTS. Sensitivity to a substance may be detected by an intradermal or scratch skin test in which extracts of common allergens (dust, molds, feathers, animal danders, pollens, cosmetics, dyes, wool, synthetic clothing material and various foods and drugs) are used. The intradermal method involves the injection of a minute dose of each extract into the superficial layers of the skin. A small amount of normal saline is injected and used as a control or comparison. In the scratch test, a drop of each allergen is applied at areas along a superficial scratch. A small mark is made at the exact site of the allergen injection or application so that the size of the local response can be measured.

The arm or the upper back may be the site used for the test; the former is preferable so that at early signs of a reaction a tourniquet can be applied to slow absorption and prevent anaphylaxis. Emergency equipment and drugs that are used in the treatment of anaphylactic shock (see p. 51) should be readily available for immediate use.

The sites are observed 15 to 30 minutes after the administration of the allergens. A positive reaction is indicated by itching and the appearance of erythema and a wheal (a blanched elevation surrounded by redness). The area of reaction is measured and recorded in centimeters, which the physician then interprets as positive — 1+, 2+, 3+, etc. The patient may be very apprehensive about the many injections or scratch areas and evident positive reactions. Before the allergens are administered he should be given an explanation of the nature and purpose of the tests.

During investigation of an immunologic disorder, blood serum studies may be performed to determine the concentration of gamma globulin, antibodies and the various immunoglobulin classes. Tests may also be made to detect autoimmune antibodies, as well as complement fixations in antigen-antibody reactions (complement fixation test). A differential leukocyte count may be done, since eosinophils and lymphocytes may be increased in certain allergic disorders.

NURSING IN HYPERSENSITIVITY[18]

Factors to be considered in the care of the patient with an immunologic disorder include avoidance of the allergen, drug therapy, hyposensitization, the necessary instruction and assistance in self-care, and psychological support.

AVOIDANCE OF THE ALLERGEN. Avoidance of the allergen may involve such things as moving to another geographical area, a change of occupation, air conditioning to reduce pollen and dust inhalation, the elimination of a particular food from the diet, the use of foam rubber pillows instead of those filled with feathers, the use of nonallergenic cosmetics, avoidance of clothing of certain synthetic material, or the removal of certain pets from the environment.

DRUG THERAPY. Drugs commonly used in immunologic disorders include the following:

1. Antihistamine preparations, such as chlorpheniramine maleate (Chlor-Tripolon, Chlorphenamine), diphenhydramine hydrochloride (Benadryl), and tripelennamine hydrochloride (Pyribenzamine).

2. Cortisone (prednisolone, prednisone).

3. Epinephrine hydrochloride (Adrenalin) used in severe reactions, especially bronchospasm.

4. Isoproterenol (Isuprel) may be nebulized and inhaled to promote bronchial dilation. Phenylephrine hydrochloride (Neo-Synephrine) may be used locally in spray form to relieve nasal congestion in allergic rhinitis (hay fever).

5. In skin reactions, examples of topical applications that may be prescribed are adrenocorticoid cream or ointment (hydrocortisone ointment, 0.5 per cent) and calamine lotion. If the skin allergic response is generalized, oatmeal or hydrolyzed starch baths may reduce pruritus.

HYPOSENSITIZATION. This consists of a series of subcutaneous injections of the specific allergens to which the patient showed a positive reaction in sensitivity tests. The first few doses are very small, and are then progressively increased over an extended period of time. The exact mechanism by which this procedure reduces the patient's hypersensi-

---

[18]For care in anaphylactic shock see p. 51.

tivity is not understood clearly. It is suggested that with the resulting increase in antibodies, a larger amount of the allergen is required to elicit a reaction, or that the antibodies are so increased that they block the access of the allergen to the sensitive tissue cells.

It must be remembered that with the administration of any allergen there is the possibility of an immediate anaphylactic reaction. Equipment and medications used in anaphylaxis should be at hand in the event of such an emergency (see p. 56). If the antigen injection is given in an outpatient clinic or physician's office, the patient is asked to remain for 20 to 30 minutes for observation.

INSTRUCTION AND ASSISTANCE. The nurse may play an important role in helping the patient and family to understand and accept the condition, imposed limitations and necessary adjustments and treatment. Considerable planning, teaching and direction are necessary to prepare the patient for self-care and the prevention of hypersensitive reactions.

If the antigen is a food, the patient is advised as to what should be eliminated from the diet and what substitutions may be made in order to meet nutritional requirements.

When the excitant substance is an inhalant, efforts are made to control the individual's environment as much as possible. Procedures are used to reduce pollens, molds, feathers and dander to a minimum. The ideal solution is, of course, a mechanical system of air filtration and conditioning in the home and place of work, but this may not be economically feasible. Practical procedures include the removal of pets, damp dusting and vacuum cleaning, the replacement of feather pillows and cushions with foam rubber or a synthetic, the enclosure of mattresses in plastic, and the removal of rugs, drapes and other "dust catchers."

The patient and family are made familiar with the early signs and symptoms of a reaction and instructed as to the appropriate action. Prescribed medications are discussed with them; the purpose, dosage, times at which they should be taken and possible side effects are outlined. For example, in relation to side effects, if the patient is taking an antihistamine he is alerted to the possibility of drowsiness and the associated risk in driv-

ing; timing of taking the drug may require adjustment in accord with his activities. Corticosteroids used to reduce sensitivity may result in the development of moon face, acne and lowered resistance to infection. The avoidance of self-medication and nonprescribed drugs is stressed.

The importance of maintaining resistance to prevent recurrence of the allergic disorder is cited; adequate nutrition and rest, avoidance of chilling and physical and mental exhaustion, appropriate recreation and personal habits are reviewed. Allergic responses may be readily aggravated by emotional stress. The immunologic disorder may create emotional stress which in turn exacerbates the disorder, setting up a vicious circle. If the patient is known to be allergic to insect bites (e.g., bee sting) he is warned that he should avoid areas where he may be exposed and that he should always carry a tourniquet and emergency drugs.

The need to carry a card that indicates the allergy and to register with Medic Alert are explained. Medic Alert is an organization that registers the individual and provides an identification pendant or bracelet that immediately alerts contacts to the fact that he has a hypersensitivity.

PSYCHOLOGICAL SUPPORT. The imposed limitations and essential adjustments may entail sacrifice on the part of the patient and family. A change of residence, occupation, and forms of recreation, and the giving up of a pet, certain foods, cosmetics and/or other things may be necessary. The proposed therapeutic change in the individual's accustomed way of life is likely to cause some emotional disturbance. The patient may become depressed and angry, and signify nonacceptance of the restriction. Family members may show some resentment, blaming him for adjustments required of them.

The nurse, realizing that the patient and family require time to work through the prescribed therapeutic regime, conveys an appreciation of the demands. They are encouraged to verbalize their feelings and, by being an understanding listener, the nurse is helping. Efforts are made to explore possible solutions with them. The need for various types of assistance (e.g., socioeconomic, educational) may be recognized, and a referral made to a social service agency.

PREVENTION OF SERIOUS ALLERGIC REAC-

TIONS. Observation of the following precautions may avert a serious reaction in some instances. Patients should be questioned as to allergy and drug and food sensitivity upon admission to hospital and clinic, and also when an initial home visit is made. If any such sensitivity is indicated, it should be reported to the doctor and clearly and conspicuously marked on the front of the patient's chart and nursing care plan. Reactions may be prevented if the patient carries a notice of his allergic problem in his wallet or pocket, or if he wears a Medic Alert tag.

Before administering the first dose of a drug that is known to be a common allergen, it is advisable to ask the person if he has ever taken it before; this may elicit a history of a previous reaction. The patient is observed closely after the first two or three doses of any of these drugs for signs of an untoward reaction. Common offenders include penicillin, streptomycin, animal serum (e.g., tetanus antitoxin), acetylsalicylic acid and iodide preparations used as contrast media in x-rays. Penicillin, radiopaque contrast media and serums are responsible for the greatest incidence of anaphylaxis. Before giving the initial dose of either of these, a small test dose should be given intradermally. A sensitivity is manifested by the appearance of itching, erythema and a wheal at the site of administration within 15 to 20 minutes. When the initial dose of a drug known to cause adverse reactions is given in a clinic or doctor's office, the patient is asked to remain for 20 to 30 minutes.

An emergency tray or cart should be kept fully equipped and quickly available. It should be familiar to all staff in the event of a serious reaction. Minimal equipment on such a tray would be tourniquets, nasopharyngeal airway, endotracheal tube and laryngoscope, sterile syringes and needles, alcohol sponges, and a drug box containing ampules of epinephrine 1:1000 (aqueous), normal saline, and diphenhydramine hydrochloride (Benadryl).

Early signs of anaphylaxis are redness and itching at the site of injection, repeated sneezing, pallor, and complaints of a peculiar sensation in the throat, a tightness of the chest or faintness.

Tissue Transplantation

The transplantation of tissue or an organ from one person to the body of another has recently received a great deal of attention. Some degree of success has been achieved in the transplantation of a kidney from one person to another, but homograft rejection still poses a serious problem. Rejection of the graft by the recipient is an immunologic response. Laboratory research and experimentation continue to search for a means whereby the rejection process can be controlled so that a healthy organ may be transplanted from one person to another and be accepted.

Foreign tissue is treated as antigenic and the body rejects it by producing immune bodies which attack it. All tissue cells contain antigens which differ from one individual to another except identical twins, in which case there is histocompatibility because they are genetically identical. Although there are many tissue antigens, some are stronger than others and are more likely to be effective in causing the immunologic response that comprises rejection. The stronger antigens have been designated as belonging to the HL-A system.

In selecting donor tissue the search is for tissue that has similar strong antigenic components, or one that has at least very few differences. In other words, it is the extent of the "strong" antigenic differences between the donor and the recipient that determines the fate of the graft. The strong antigens of the HL-A system occur in almost all tissue cells except red blood cells. Erythrocytes contain antigens which belong to the blood grouping (ABO) system. Leukocytes contain all the antigens of the HL-A system and are used in tissue typing and in identifying a histocompatible graft. The tissue donor must also be of the same blood type as the recipient. The closer the relationship between the donor and recipient, the greater is the chance for success.

The rejection process is considered to be a cell-mediated delayed immunologic (type 4) reaction (see p. 641). In an effort to prevent rejection following an allograft[19] several different measures may be used to suppress the immune response. These include the administration of immunosuppressive drugs such

---

[19]An *allograft* or *homotransplant* is the transfer of tissue or an organ from one person to another with a different genetic constitution. An *isologous graft* or *isotransplant* is the transfer of tissue or an organ from one person to another who is genetically the same; the donor and recipient are identical twins.

as azathioprine (Imuran), corticosteroid preparations (e.g., prednisone), and antilymphocytic globulin and, rarely, body irradiation. Unfortunately, the side effects of these "preventive" measures not infrequently prove fatal as a result of their toxicity or their effect of decreasing resistance to infection.

Further reference is made to organ transplant (kidney, cornea) in the respective ensuing chapters.

References

Books

Anderson, W. A. D., and Scotti, T. M.: Synopsis of Pathology, 8th ed. St. Louis, C. V. Mosby, 1972.

Beeson, P. B., and McDermott, W. (Eds.): Textbook of Medicine. 15th ed. Philadelphia, W. B. Saunders, 1979.

Gell, P. G. H., and Coombs, R. R. A. (Eds.): Clinical Aspects of Immunology, 3rd ed. Philadelphia, J. B. Lippincott, 1975.

Guyton, A. C.: Textbook of Medical Physiology, 5th ed. Philadelphia, W. B. Saunders, 1976. Chapter 10.

Humphrey, J. H., and White, R. G.: Immunology for Students of Medicine, 3rd ed. Oxford, Blackwell Scientific Publications, 1970.

Macleod, J. (Ed.): Davidson's Principles and Practice of Medicine, 11th ed. Edinburgh, Churchill Livingstone, 1974, pp. 15–42.

Robbins, S. L., and Angell, M.: Basic Pathology, 2nd ed. Philadelphia, W. B. Saunders, 1976.

Schottelius, B. A., and Schottelius, D. D.: Physiology, 17th ed. St. Louis, C. V. Mosby, 1973. Chapters 2–4.

Smith, A. L.: Microbiology and Pathology, 11th ed., St. Louis, C. V. Mosby, 1976. Chapters 11, 12, 14, 39 and 40.

Sodeman, Wm. A., Jr., and Sodeman, Wm. A.: Pathologic Physiology, 5th ed. Philadelphia, W. B. Saunders, 1974. Chapters 4 and 18.

Thorn, G. W., et al. (Eds.): Harrison's Principles of Internal Medicine, 8th ed. New York, McGraw-Hill, 1977.

Walter, J. B., and Israel, M. S.: General Pathology, 4th ed. Edinburgh, Churchill Livingstone, 1974.

Weir, D. M.: Immunology for Undergraduates, 3rd ed. New York, Longmans, 1973.

Weiss, L.: The Cells and Tissues of the Immune System. Englewood Cliffs, N. J., Prentice-Hall, 1972.

Periodicals

Craven, R. F.: "Anaphylactic Shock." Am. J. Nurs., Vol. 72, No. 4 (April 1972), pp. 718–720.

Fox, C. F.: "The Structure of Cell Membranes." Sci. Am., Vol. 226, No. 2 (Feb. 1972), pp. 31–38.

Lister, J.: "Nursing Intervention in Anaphylactic Shock." Am. J. Nurs., Vol. 72, No. 4 (April 1972), pp. 720–721.

O'Loughlin, J. M.: "Immunologic Deficiency States." Med. Clin. North Am., Vol. 56, No. 3 (May 1972), pp. 747–757.

Samter, M. (Ed.): "Symposium on Allergy in Adults." Med. Clin. North Am., Vol. 58, No. 1 (Jan. 1974).

Scheffer, A. L.: "Treatment of Anaphylaxis." Postgrad. Med., Vol. 53, No. 4 (April 1973), pp. 62–66.

Taylor, H. E.: "The Clinical Application of Antilymphocyte Globulin." Med. Clin. North Am., Vol. 56, No. 2 (March 1972), p. 419.

4

Infection

The term infection implies entrance into the body of pathogenic (disease-producing) organisms. The invasion may not always produce a disease state; it depends on the particular organism, its virulence and the host's resistance.

Much progress has been made in recent decades in the fields of microbiology and epidemiology,[1] which has resulted in a marked decrease in the incidence of many infectious diseases (e.g., diphtheria, typhoid fever, smallpox, poliomyelitis). Knowledge of the sources, modes of transmission, nature and tissue predilection of many pathogenic organisms has led to more effective preventive measures such as immunization, health education and improved sanitation. Although the discovery of many new antimicrobial drugs has contributed to a reduction in deaths as a result of invasion by microorganisms, much absenteeism and illness can still be attributed to infections.

Infection affecting specific body systems is discussed in the ensuing respective chapters. This chapter presents some information relevant to infection in general.

INFECTIOUS AGENTS

The organisms capable of producing infection include bacteria, viruses, fungi, protozoa and parasitic worms.

Bacteria are forms of plant life which are microscopically visible and are broadly classified according to their shape as cocci (spherical), bacilli (rod-shaped) or spirochetes (spiral). They may be found almost anywhere. They are present in the soil, air, water, food and refuse and are also found in some body cavities and on the body surface.

Bacteria are a major cause of disease. Examples of bacterial diseases are diphtheria, streptococcal infection, staphylococcal in-fection, typhoid fever and tetanus. Many types are nonpathogenic, some species normally inhabit a particular area of the body without causing disease and are referred to as the normal bacterial flora of that area or commensals. For example, the skin is a normal habitat of staphylococci, colon bacilli are always present in the intestine, and lactobacilli inhabit the vagina. Commensals may play an essential role in the body; for instance, a main source of vitamin K, which is necessary for bloodclotting, is the bacterial action in the intestine. The bacterial flora may be potential pathogens if they gain access to other areas of the body.

Viruses are the smallest pathogenic organisms and may only be seen under electron-microscopic magnification. They produce disease by entering the host's cells and may cause proliferation, degeneration or destruction. When viruses invade the body cells they may be destroyed by the host's defense mechanisms, or may survive and become established indefinitely. The initial clinical effect of the invasion may disappear but the virus may remain dormant within the host's cells, only to cause further trouble later as a result of some stimulus. When the entrance of a virus into tissue cells stimulates cell reproduction (proliferation) the new cells contain the virus. There are many varieties or strains, and their intracellular location within the hosts has made effective therapy and control more difficult. Examples of viral diseases are the common cold, influenza, measles, mumps and smallpox. There is also accumulating evidence that viruses are associated with the development of some malignant diseases.

Fungi are multicellular, mold-like organisms which produce interlacing filaments or chains. A disease caused by a fungus is called a mycosis, or it may be indicated by the suffix *-osis* preceded by the name of the causative fungus. Thrush, ringworm and histoplasmosis are examples of mycotic disease.

---

[1]*Epidemiology* is the study of the occurrence and distribution of a disease.

Protozoa are single-celled organisms that belong to the animal kingdom and are more complex in structure and activity than bacteria. Diseases that are caused by protozoa include malaria, sleeping sickness, amoebic dysentery and trichomoniasis.

Infection may be caused by *parasitic worms,* which may be referred to as helminths. The helminthic infections most commonly seen are those caused by the roundworm, pinworm, tapeworm and *Trichinella spiralis.* The latter causes trichinosis. The filarial worm (fluke) that causes filariasis or elephantiasis and the hookworm are more prevalent in tropical areas.

SOURCES AND TRANSMISSION OF PATHOGENIC ORGANISMS

The sources of pathogenic organisms may be humans, animals, insects or inanimate objects. The most common source is a human who may be in the incubation period, acute stage or convalescence of the disease, or may be a carrier (vector). The latter may appear healthy but harbor pathogenic organisms which can be transmitted to others.

Tuberculosis and brucellosis (undulant fever) are examples of infections that may be contracted from cows. Animals infested with parasites may be a source of disease if they are used as meat. Rabies is acquired from rabid dogs, cats or other infected animals. The source of psittacosis in man is usually a parrot, and the mosquito is the source of sleeping sickness.

The most common inanimate sources are soil and decaying animal and vegetable matter. Tetanus usually develops as a result of soil contamination of a wound. Soil may also be a source of some pathogenic fungi.

Pathogenic agents may be transmitted from their source by direct or indirect contact. In direct spread the infecting agent is transferred directly from the source to the person. Indirect contact implies an intermediary-contaminated conveyor or object. Conveyors frequently support the life and growth of the organisms. Transmission of the disease-producing organism by indirect contact occurs in airborne infections (e.g., respiratory diseases) and water and food infections (e.g., food poisoning, typhoid fever). *Fomites* is a term applied to inanimate objects that spread infection; examples are bedding, towels, dishes, instruments and furniture.

The infecting agents may enter the host through the respiratory tract, the alimentary tract, a break in the skin or the genitourinary tract. A fetus may become infected by transplacental transmission. Normally the placenta is an effective barrier, but certain organisms, such as the spirochete that causes syphilis and viruses if present in the mother, are likely to cross into the fetus.

Many microorganisms have an affinity for certain tissues and organs. For example, the virus that causes mumps has a predilection for the parotid glands. Similarly, the pneumococcus readily affects the lungs, and the meningococcus prefers the meninges.

THE INFECTION PROCESS

The pathogenic organisms must enter an area of tissue before infection occurs. Disease may or may not develop when pathogenic organisms invade body tissues. This depends on the virulence of the organisms and the host's resistance. *Virulence* refers to the capacity of the organisms to survive, multiply and injure the host's tissues. It is greater in some types and in certain strains of the same type. A serious influenza epidemic occurs because the prevalent organism is so virulent that practically everyone whom it invades becomes ill. An organism of weaker virulence may be quickly destroyed by the host's defense mechanisms, or in some instances the organism may remain alive within the host but is unable to multiply to the number necessary to overcome the defenses and injure tissues sufficiently to produce disease. In the latter situation, the host may become a carrier who is capable of transmitting the organism to others whose defenses may be weaker.

If the organisms survive the body's defense mechanisms, they multiply. The period between invasion and the clinical manifestations of an infection, during which the organisms are multiplying, is referred to as the *incubation period.* Its length varies with different organisms; for example, the incubation period for streptococcal infection is about 2 to 4 days, and for measles about 10 to 14 days.

Progressive multiplication of the pathogens leads to inflammation, tissue damage, impaired function of the part and the release of toxins which are absorbed into the blood. If the defenses cannot confine the organisms they may be disseminated throughout the body, giving rise to other areas of infection and/or septicemia. If the defense mechanisms confine the infection and overcome the organisms, the exudate and dead pathogens and cells are cleared away by phagocytes and in the lymph drainage. Resolution takes place. If the infection is more destructive, pus may be formed, which, if confined locally, results in an *abscess*.

The major way in which infecting agents cause disease is by their production of harmful chemical substances called toxins. The toxin may be liberated by the organism while it is alive (exotoxin), or it may be released with its disintegration (endotoxin). Toxins may injure the cells at the site of their release and may also be absorbed into the blood and affect other structures throughout the body. In most instances, a toxin is specific as to the tissues it affects; for example, the exotoxin produced by diphtheria bacilli injures cardiac muscle cells and may cause myocarditis.

HOST DEFENSES

Defenses against pathogens are natural (innate) or acquired.

Innate Defenses

Normal body structure and activities provide the individual with considerable protection against infection. Externally, the skin is an effective barrier against the entry of organisms as long as it remains intact. The acidity and fatty acid content of its glandular secretions tend to destroy or inhibit the growth of many pathogens. Microorganisms are ever present on the skin; they penetrate the hair follicles and the ducts of the sweat and sebaceous glands. Thorough washing and scrubbing under running water reduce their number but do not produce a sterile surface. This makes the use of sterile gloves necessary when handling sterile equipment if asepsis is to be maintained.

The mucous membrane of the respiratory tract plays an important protective role. Its secretion traps and carries away organisms; the cilia filter the air and sweep out offenders. The mucus may also induce coughing, which forcefully expels material bearing organisms from the tract. Drying of the membrane, destruction of the cilia and loss of the cough reflex reduce the protective mechanism.

The mucus secreted in the gastrointestinal tract protects the mucous membrane lining from the hydrochloric acid and digestive enzymes. Absence of the mucus could result in ulceration that would permit the entrance of pathogens. The acidity of the gastric secretion destroys many organisms that are ingested.

The microorganisms that are normal inhabitants of some areas of the body may play a defensive role. For example, the reaction of the natural flora of the secretions of the vaginal mucosa produces an acidity that creates a resistance to infective agents.

Another important natural defense mechanism is phagocytosis; pathogens that invade the body may be engulfed and destroyed by leukocytes and macrophages. In many infections the number of leukocytes in circulation is rapidly increased, and they migrate to the site of invasion. Changes in the proportion of different types of leukocytes are characteristic of infection by certain types of organisms. Lymph nodes are strategically situated along the course of the lymphatics and filter out bacteria to be destroyed by phagocytosis.

The inflammatory process is a protective mechanism and is described on page 40.

Body fluids contain some substances that are antibacterial. One of these is an enzyme (lysozyme) that destroys bacteria by breaking down their cell walls. Plasma contains gamma globulin which forms antibodies in response to infective agents or their toxins.

Good health habits such as optimal nutrition and hydration, adequate rest and exercise, and the avoidance of fatigue and stress promote the body's natural resistance to infection.

Some persons have what is referred to as a natural immunity to certain diseases. Immunity may be defined as the resistance of the body to pathogenic organisms. Natural immunity to certain pathogens varies with species, races and individuals. A species of animal may be very susceptible to infection by a certain type of organism which is incapable of producing disease in humans. Persons of the Negro race exhibit a poor resistance to tuberculosis as compared with Caucasians, but the exact reverse is apparent in relation to malaria. A natural resistance to certain infections may be present in some individuals; this is evident when a family or group is equally exposed to an infectious disease and all but one become ill. Age is considered to be a factor in natural immunity; certain infections have a higher incidence in children and rarely occur in the elderly, and infections characteristic of the later years of life have a lesser incidence in younger persons.

Acquired Defenses

Immunity to an infection may be acquired by an individual as a result of contact with the infecting agent or its products. The host develops an immunity by forming antibodies or special conditioned lymphocytes. Immunity is discussed in the preceding chapter under "The Immune Response."

Artificially induced active immunity for certain diseases is recommended for every child. The mother of a newborn infant is advised of the recommended immunization program, which may be started in the second or third month. The program may vary from one province or state to another, but the nurse urges the mother to consult her physician or inquire at a clinic as to when the infant should receive the immunizing agents.

Currently, the initial immunizing preparation that is used is a combination of diphtheria toxoid, tetanus toxoid, pertussis vaccine and poliomyelitis vaccine.[2] Three 1.0-ml. doses of the combined immunizing agents are administered subcutaneously in the third, fourth and fifth months, *or* in the second, fourth and sixth months. At 12 months the child receives the trivalent immunizing agent for measles, mumps and rubella. Smallpox vaccination is not given as early as it used to be; the child is not vaccinated before his

second year and some physicians prefer to delay it until the child has reached school age.

Artificially induced immunity becomes weaker over a period of months to years; it varies in relation to the different diseases. As a result, reinforcing doses of some immunizing agents are necessary. Presently, the child receives a booster dose of the quadrivalent immunizing agent for diphtheria, pertussis, tetanus and poliomyelitis at 18 months and 5 to 6 years. A booster dose for diphtheria, tetanus and poliomyelitis is given at 10 to 12 years and again at the age of 16 to 18 years.

The combined vaccine is not used for adults since there is a greater possibility of a sensitivity reaction. Immunization for each disease is done separately. A record of the immunization received and the date is issued for each individual and should be kept safe for future reference. A pamphlet with information about the vaccine and directions for administration and storage accompanies each vial and should be carefully read by the nurse. See Table 4–1 for a sample immunization program.

There is always the possibility that the person may be hypersensitive to a vaccine and will develop a serious reaction. For this reason, he may be asked to remain for 20 to 30 minutes for observation. Epinephrine hydrochloride (1:1000) and sterile equipment for its administration should always be readily available in the event of an undesirable reaction.

See Table 4–2 for information relating to common communicable diseases.

Text continued on p. 68

[2]In some countries, a preparation of poliomyelitis vaccine is given orally in preference to parenteral administration.

TABLE 4–1   SAMPLE IMMUNIZATION PROGRAM

Immunizing Agent	Age	Doses
Combination of diphtheria toxoid, tetanus toxoid, pertussis vaccine and poliomyelitis vaccine	Commencing at 3 months *or* Commencing at 2 months	Three doses at monthly intervals Three doses at intervals of 2 months
	18 months	Single booster dose
	5 to 6 years	Single booster dose
Combination of measles, mumps and rubella vaccines	12 months	Single dose
Combination of diphtheria toxoid, tetanus toxoid and poliomyelitis vaccine	10–12 years	Single booster dose
	16–18 years	Single booster dose
Smallpox vaccine	2–6 years	—

TABLE 4–2 COMMON COMMUNICABLE DISEASES*

Communicable Disease	Causative Agent	Source(s) and Transmission	Portal of Entry
Chickenpox (varicella)	Virus (varicella-zoster virus)	Infected persons; articles contaminated by discharge from vesicles and mucous membranes Transmitted by direct contact with infected person—respiratory droplets, crusts of lesions; indirect via articles contaminated with respiratory discharge or discharge of lesions	Nasopharynx suggested
Common Cold	Numerous viruses	Respiratory droplets of infected persons Transmitted by direct contact with infected person.	Nasopharynx
Diphtheria	Diphtheria bacillus (*Corynebacterium diphtheriae*)	Respiratory secretions and saliva of infected persons or carriers; food Transmitted by direct or indirect contact	Nasopharynx
Encephalitis	Viruses	Bite from infected mosquito	Skin
Gas gangrene	Clostridia (anaerobic spore forms)	Soil and human intestinal tract Transmitted by soil or soil-contaminated articles, feces	Deep wounds
Gonorrhea	Gonococcus (*Neisseria gonorrhoeae*)	Urethral or vaginal secretions of infected persons Transmitted by sexual intercourse	Urethral or vaginal mucosa; eyes, anal canal and throat may also be portals of entry
Hepatitis (infectious type A)	Hepatitis A virus	Feces and blood of infected persons Transmitted by contaminated food and water	Gastrointestinal tract
Hepatitis (serum type B)	Hepatitis B virus	Blood from infected persons or carriers Transmitted by parenteral injection	Skin and blood vessel
Infectious mononucleosis	Virus	Saliva and respiratory secretions of infected person Transmitted by direct oral contact with infected person	Mouth

*Information compiled from: Lynda Cranston: "Communicable Diseases and Immunizations." Can. Nurs., Vol. 72, No. 1 (Jan. 1976), pp. 34–40; S. Katz (Chairman): Report of the Committee on Infectious Diseases, 17th ed. Illinois, American Academy of Pediatrics, 1974; M. Krupp, N. Sweet, E. Jaweta, et al.: Physician's Handbook, 18th ed. Los Altos, Calif., Lange Medical Publications, 1976.

Incubation Period	Isolation	Immunization	Comments
10–21 days	Patient isolated until all lesions have crusted	Active by disease; passive by human hyperimmune globulin	Virus can infect adults and cause herpes zoster (shingles)
1–4 days	Precautions to prevent spread of respiratory droplets and secretions of infected persons	None.	
2–6 days	Strict isolation until several (usually six) successive, daily negative throat and nasal cultures are obtained	Active: 1. By disease 2. Toxoid Passive: Diphtheria antitoxin, which is rarely used because of possible severe reactions; an antibiotic is usually given in preference	Schick test may be made to determine the presence or absence of specific antibodies; immunized persons can become carriers of the infective organism
4–21 days	None; not transmitted from man to man	Formalinized virus vaccines for high-risk persons	Prophylactic measures are directed toward eradication of the mosquito
1–4 days	Modified; strict precautionary measures to prevent spread by wound drainage	Polyvalent antitoxin	Early extensive débridement of deep macerated wounds; patient receives antibiotics and a high concentration of oxygen; the latter is administered in a hyperbaric oxygen chamber
3–8 days	Careful handling and disposal of articles contaminated by discharge	None	Treatment is administration of penicillin; efforts are made to identify and treat contacts
15–50 days	Modified; use of gown when giving direct patient care; careful handling and disposal of emesis and fecal discharge	Passive: Gamma globulin	
6 weeks to 6 months	Modified; careful handling and disposal of blood, wound discharges and excreta		Prophylactic measures include careful selection of blood donors and adequate sterilization of equipment used in parenteral injections
2–6 weeks	None	None	

Table continued on following page

TABLE 4–2 COMMON COMMUNICABLE DISEASES—*Continued*

Communicable Disease	Causative Agent		Portal of Entry
Influenza	Numerous viruses (types A, B, C)	Respiratory secretions of infected persons	Nose or mouth
		Transmitted by direct contact; respiratory droplets possibly airborne	
Malaria	*Plasmodium* virus	Mosquitoes and blood of infected persons	Skin
		Transmitted by bite from infected mosquito	
Measles (rubeola)	Virus	Nose and throat secretions, blood and urine of infected persons	Respiratory tract
		Transmitted usually by droplet spread	
Meningitis	Meningococcus, numerous viruses and other organisms such as streptococcus, tubercle bacillus	Respiratory secretions from infected persons or carriers	Nose and mouth
		Transmitted by respiratory droplets	
Mumps (epidemic parotitis)	Virus	Saliva of infected persons	Nose and mouth
		Transmitted by direct contact with infected persons, respiratory droplets and oral secretions	
Paratyphoid fevers	*Salmonella* species of organisms	Urine and feces of infected persons	Gastrointestinal tract
		Transmitted by ingestion of contaminated water and food	
Pertussis (whooping cough)	Pertussis bacilli	Respiratory secretions of infected persons	Respiratory tract
		Transmitted by droplet spread	
Poliomyelitis	Viruses	Gastrointestinal tract of infected persons and carriers	Gastrointestinal tract
		Transmitted by direct contact with nasopharyngeal secretions of infected persons, vomitus	
Rabies	Virus	Saliva of infected animals and persons	Skin
		Transmitted by bite from rabid animal	
Rubella (German measles)	Rubella virus	Infected persons	Respiratory tract
		Transmission by direct contact or droplet spread of nasopharyngeal secretions	

Incubation Period	Isolation	Immunization	Comments
1–4 days	Avoid direct contact during acute symptoms	Vaccines vary as to viruses	
6–37 days	Careful handling and disposal of articles contaminated by blood of infected persons	None	Prophylactic measures include antimalarial drugs for persons exposed to infected mosquitoes and programs to eradicate mosquitoes

10–15 days	Isolate from 7 days after exposure to 5 days after rash appears	Active: 1. By disease
		2. Vaccine
		    a) Live attenuated measles virus vaccine
		    b) Inactive measles virus vaccine
		Passive: Serum gamma globulin	

Varies with causative agent	Strict isolation with meningococcal meningitis; careful handling and disposal of articles contaminated by respiratory secretions		
14–21 days	Isolation for 9 days from onset of swelling	Active: 1. By disease; 2. Live attenuated mumps vaccine	
1–14 days	Modified; use of gown when giving direct patient care; thorough disinfection of articles contaminated with urine and feces.	Paratyphoid A and B vaccine (combined with typhoid vaccine)	An important prophylactic measure is strict sanitary precautions in the handling of food and water
10–21 days	Modified; measures to prevent spread of respiratory secretions; disinfect soiled articles	Active: 1. By disease 2. Pertussis vaccine	
7–21 days	Strict isolation until temperature returns to normal; careful handling and disposal of respiratory secretions, emesis and feces during the acute stage	Active: 1. By disease 2. Salk vaccine or Sabin vaccine (oral)	
10 days to 6 months	Strict isolation	Rabies hyperimmune serum vaccine daily for 14 days; wound is infiltrated with hyperimmune serum	Vaccine is only given if rabies is suspected because of an animal bite; if the animal remains healthy for 10 days injections are discontinued
14–21 days	None	Active: 1. By disease 2. Live attenuated rubella virus vaccine Passive: Gamma globulin	Pregnant women should avoid any possible contact with infected person; congenital anomalies result from infection in first trimester of pregnancy

Table continued on following page

TABLE 4–2 COMMON COMMUNICABLE DISEASES—*Continued*

Communicable Disease	Causative Agent	Source(s) and Transmission	Portal of Entry
Scarlet fever	Group A hemolytic streptococcus	Infected persons or carriers Transmission by direct or indirect contact with patient or carrier by droplet spread	Pharynx
Smallpox (Variola)	Poxvirus variola	Infected persons Transmission by direct contact and droplet and crust spread	Nasopharynx
Syphilis	*Treponema pallidum*	Exudate and blood of infected persons Transmitted by sexual intercourse; contact with open lesions; blood transfusion	External genitalia, mucosal surfaces, blood stream
Tetanus (lockjaw)	Tetanus bacillus (*Clostridium tetani*)	Animal feces and soil	Deep macerated wounds
Tuberculosis	Tubercle bacillus	Sputum from infected persons; milk from infected cows Transmission by droplet spread; ingestion of contaminated milk	Respiratory or gastrointestinal tract
Typhoid fever	*Salmonella typhi* (*typhosa*)	Excreta of infected persons and carriers Transmitted by contaminated food and water	Gastrointestinal tract

Incubation Period	Isolation	Immunization	Comments
1–5 days	Strict isolation for 7 days	None	
7–14 days	Strict isolation until lesions have healed	Active: 1. By disease 2. By vaccination	
10–90 days	Careful handling and disposal of articles contaminated by discharge from lesions	None	Careful screening of donor blood before use
3–21 days	None	Active: Tetanus toxoid Passive: Human immunoglobulin; tetanus antitoxin	If a patient has not received tetanus toxoid and receives an injury, an injection of tetanus antitoxin or tetanus immune globulin may be prescribed as a prophylactic measure
Varies	Careful handling and disposal of articles contaminated by secretions	Active: 1. Infection not absolute immunity, but individual is less likely to develop disease on subsequent exposure to disease 2. BCG vaccine given to persons showing negative tuberculin tests provides some protection	Chemoprophylactic drugs may be administered to persons who are known to be infected; these preparations arrest progress of the infection and development of the disease; they include streptomycin, isoniazid (INH) and para-aminosalicylic acid (PAS)
7–21 days	Strict isolation until stool tests are repeatedly negative	Active: 1. By disease 2. Typhoid vaccine	

FACTORS PREDISPOSING TO INFECTION

Factors that influence the host's resistance and susceptibility to infection include the following:

Nutrition

Poorly nourished persons have an increased susceptibility to infection, particularly if their diet has been deficient in protein and vitamins. Their natural tissue resistance and ability to form antibodies are reduced.

Age

Infants, children and elderly persons are less able to resist infection.

Occupation

Certain occupations provide increased exposure to infecting agents or may reduce the efficiency of one's protective mechanisms. For example, persons working with cattle may be exposed to undulant fever; those working in mines are more susceptible to tuberculosis.

Exposure to Cold

A lowering of the body temperature below normal is thought to decrease the ciliary movement in the respiratory tract, reduce the blood supply to superficial tissues and suppress antibody formation, all of which are natural defense mechanisms.

Metabolic Disturbances and Other Diseases

The person who already has some abnormality in function within the body is less able to resist or cope with an infection. For instance, the diabetic is prone to infection.

Corticoid Medication

The patient receiving corticoid therapy exhibits a marked susceptibility to infection. The steroids suppress the protective inflammatory response and the production of lymphocytes and antibodies.

Radiation

Exposure to large doses of radiation, particularly total body irradiation, reduces the patient's defense mechanisms. Leukocyte and antibody production are suppressed.

TYPES OF INFECTIONS

Certain terms may be used to describe infection. *Local* or *focal* means the infection remains confined to one area. A *generalized* or *systemic* infection is one in which the organisms are disseminated throughout the body. A *mixed* infection is due to more than one type of pathogen. If a person becomes infected by another type of organism during the course of an infection, it is termed a *secondary* infection, and the initial one is referred to as *primary*. An infection may be *acute* or *chronic*.

The presence of bacteria in the blood produces *bacteremia*. *Septicemia* means organisms have entered the blood stream and are actively multiplying and producing toxins. *Toxemia* implies a concentration of bacterial toxins in the blood. *Pyemia* is a type of septicemia in which the organisms are clumped together or incorporated into small thrombi (blood clots). The clumps, or thrombi, may become deposited at various sites throughout the body and may cause small, scattered abscesses.

MANIFESTATIONS OF INFECTION

Manifestations common to many infections include the following systemic and local symptoms: fever, which may be preceded by chills; an increase in the pulse and respiratory rates; anorexia; nausea and vomiting; headache; apathy and fatigue; joint and muscle pain; and general malaise. The patient may appear hot and flushed, and the tongue is frequently furred and dry. There may be enlargement and tenderness of the lymph nodes that receive the lymph from the site of infection. If the infection is local, the area becomes red, swollen, hot and painful. In addition to these common signs and symptoms, specific features characteristic of a specific infection may be present and may play an important role in the diagnosis. For example, certain infections cause a rash, while others may give rise to a marked increase in a particular type of leukocyte.

DIAGNOSTIC PROCEDURES USED IN INFECTIONS

Leukocyte Count and Differential

Some infections cause an increase in the white blood cells well above the normal, while in others there may be a decrease below the normal. An increase in a particular type of leukocyte is recognized as characteristic of certain infections.

Normal:
  7000 to 9000 per cu. mm.
Normal differential:
  neutrophils — 54 to 62 per cent of all leukocytes
  eosinophils — 1 to 3 per cent of all leukocytes
  basophils — 0.5 per cent of all leukocytes
  monocytes — 3 to 7 per cent of all leukocytes
  lymphocytes — 25 to 35 per cent of all leukocytes

Erythrocyte Sedimentation Rate

The rate at which the red blood cells settle in a specimen of blood is increased in infection.

Normal:
  Westergren — male, 0 to 15 mm. in 1 hour; female, 0 to 20 mm. in 1 hour
  Wintrobe — male, 0 to 9 mm. in 1 hour; female, 0 to 15 mm. in 1 hour
  Cutter — male, 0 to 8 mm. in 1 hour; female, 0 to 10 mm. in 1 hour

Antibody Tests

A specimen of blood may be examined to determine the concentration of antibodies present; this is referred to as an antibody titer. Tests may also be done to detect the presence of certain antigens or antibodies; a known antibody may be used to determine the presence of an antigen, or a known antigen may be used to detect antibodies.

Identification of the Causative Organism

The infective agent may be identified by direct microscopic examination, culture or animal inoculation.

In *direct examination* a specimen of sputum, blood, spinal fluid, urine, feces, or the discharge or scrapings from a lesion may be stained and examined under the microscope for organisms. Appearance, shape, and certain staining characteristics assist in identifying different organisms.

A *culture* involves the sterile collection of suspect material from the patient and the introduction of the material to cultural media (food materials). The media are observed for a period of time for the growth of organisms. The material to be cultured may be sputum, nasal or throat secretions, blood, urine, feces, wound discharge or spinal fluid.

Animal inoculation may be used for the identification of the organism of a few diseases such as tuberculosis and mycotic infections. Appropriate material from the patient is injected into a laboratory animal. The animal is killed after a certain period and examined for evidence of the suspected disease.

All specimens collected to determine the presence and type of pathogenic organism must be collected with sterile equipment and placed in a sterile container. Special sterile containers are usually provided by the laboratory for particular specimen materials, along with directions as to the necessary precautions to be observed in the collection. The specimen should be delivered promptly to the laboratory to avoid drying; if this is not possible, it is recommended that it be stored in the refrigerator until it can be cultured or examined.

Some anti-infective drugs are only effective in infection caused by certain organisms, while others can be used for a much greater variety of infections. In order to select an antimicrobial drug, the physician may ask for an *organism sensitivity test.* When the infecting organism is identified, a culture of it is tested with several antimicrobial drugs, such as different antibiotics, to identify which drug is most effective in destroying the organism.

Skin Tests

Two commonly used skin tests are the tuberculin (Mantoux) and Schick tests. In the tuberculin test, a small dose of old tuberculin or purified protein derivative tuberculin is injected intradermally on the flexor surface of the forearm. A positive reaction is indicated by swelling and edema at the site of injection and a surrounding redness in 2 to 3 days; this result means the individual has or has had an infection by tubercle bacilli. The test is considered negative if there is no reaction. If the first test is negative, the test may be repeated with a larger dose of tuberculin.

The Schick test is used to determine susceptibility to diphtheria. A small dose of diphtheria toxin is administered intradermally into a forearm, and a dose of inactivated toxin is given intradermally in the opposite arm. The latter is used as the comparative control. In a positive reaction, the site of the active toxin injection manifests redness in 48 hours which persists for 1 to 2 weeks. The control shows no reaction. A positive reaction indicates that the recipient of the toxin does not have antibodies to neutralize the toxin and is considered susceptible. A negative Schick test shows no reaction on either arm and indicates the person has sufficient antitoxin antibodies to protect him.

NURSING IN INFECTION

Care of the patient with an infection is directed toward: (1) improving and supporting the host's defenses; (2) destruction of the organism; (3) provision of symptomatic relief and comfort; and (4) prevention of the transmission of the infecting agent to others.

Increasing the Patient's Resistance

The patient's fluid intake is increased to a minimum of 2500 to 3000 ml. unless contraindicated by cardiovascular impairment or fluid retention. Fluids promote the dilution and excretion of toxins and are also necessary because of the fever that is a characteristic of many infections.

A diet high in protein and vitamins plays an important role in the formation of antibodies and the support of natural tissue resistance. Anorexia may be a problem; frequent small amounts of concentrated nourishing foods may be necessary.

Increased rest is planned for the patient in order to minimize the demand on body struc-

tures. Treatments and care activities are planned so that uninterrupted periods are possible. For example, when the patient must be disturbed for the administration of an anti-infective drug, other therapeutic and supportive measures are carried out at that time if at all possible.

In the case of a localized infection warm, moist applications (compresses, soaks or poultices) may be ordered by the physician. Precautions must be observed to avoid burns. The area may have to be incised to provide drainage if suppuration develops. The wound receives aseptic care to prevent a secondary infection. If local application of an antimicrobial preparation is prescribed, the wound should be cleansed of pus and tissue debris before the application to insure contact of the drug with the living infective agents.

Vital signs are recorded at frequent intervals and the patient observed closely and examined for changes that might indicate spread of the infection or complications. For example, if there is infection in a foot, the complete limb is examined for redness, tenderness, and swelling, and the lymph nodes in the groin are checked for tenderness and swelling.

Destruction of the Causative Organism

Anti-infective drugs are prescribed. It is very important that these drugs be given promptly at the times specified by the physician in order to maintain an effective blood concentration. The patient is questioned about any known allergies or drug reactions before the first dose is administered. The nurse must be familiar with the possible side effects of the drug being used and must be alert for very early signs of untoward reactions.

Provision of Comfort

Various nursing measures may be necessary to provide symptomatic relief. In the early stages of the infection, the patient may complain of chilliness; extra covers and warmth should be provided. When the patient develops a fever, cool or tepid sponges may be given to reduce the temperature, the bed covers are reduced to a minimum, and efforts are made to maintain a cool environment. Cold compresses or an ice bag may provide some relief for the headache that often is experienced during infection. Frequent changes of position, massage of the back and turning of the pillows, etc., often help the patient to rest.

The dry mouth, coated tongue and sordes that frequently accompany infectious disease and fever are a source of discomfort. Regular cleaning of the teeth, frequent mouth rinses and the application of a cream or oil to the lips as well as increased fluid intake are used to promote comfort.

The patient may experience pain in the infected area; a cradle over the area to take the weight of the bedding may help. An analgesic for the relief of pain will be prescribed by the physician.

An important nursing measure that contributes to the patient's comfort is the needed relief of anxiety and apprehension that are common in any illness. The patient is advised of his condition, the treatment and care plan and his role in this, and his progress. Opportunities are provided for the patient and family members to ask questions and receive answers. Some evidence of sincere interest, consideration of personal preferences and a willingness to keep the patient informed can be very reassuring to the patient and family.

Prevention of the Transmission of Infection to Others

The nurse caring for a patient with an infection requires knowledge of the means by which his infective agents may leave his body and be transmitted. With this understanding, appropriate precautionary measures are used to prevent transmission of the organisms to other persons and to guard against reinfection of the patient.

Pathogenic organisms leave the body of an infected person via respiratory tract exhalations and secretions, bladder and bowel excreta, and wound discharge. Transmission may be direct (from one person to another) or indirect (via contaminated persons and articles). For example, the infected patient may cough out organisms, which become airborne and are inhaled by others. Obviously, a precautionary measure that one would institute here would be to teach the patient that, when coughing, he should cover his

nose and mouth with a tissue, which is then disposed of in a paper bag.

Infective excreta or wound discharge may be deposited on the patient's clothing and bedding or may be transferred from his hands to articles handled by him. Organisms may be picked up from these possible sources by a nurse, family member or other personnel, who may become infected or may transfer the pathogens to another person. A constant awareness of the source of infection and of what is likely to be contaminated as well as the observance of precautionary measures to avoid the spread of infection are necessary.

Since medical asepsis, surgical asepsis and isolation techniques are topics introduced early in the nursing student's preparation, details are not presented here. If a review is necessary, the reader is referred to texts that present the introduction to basic principles and practice of nursing.

THE NURSE'S ROLE IN THE PREVENTION OF INFECTION

The nurse should be cognizant of the fact that the hospital carries a high risk of infection. Many patients with different infections are potential sources. Unless precautions are taken and strict medical asepsis is observed, infection may be transmitted from one patient to another. Hospital personnel may harbor organisms without manifesting illness themselves. But, unfortunately, if these infective agents are transmitted to patients, whose defense mechanisms are less effective because of their illness, the infection can be a serious complication and may be life-threatening.

The nurse has a responsibility in any situation where infection is known to exist, or where there is the possibility to practice and promote measures that will confine the organisms and prevent their spread to other persons.

The nurse also has an important role in urging those suspected of having an infection to seek treatment, as well as assuming personal responsibility to prevent infecting others.

Prevention of infection involves: (1) education of the public as to the importance of immunization and how it may be obtained; (2) sanitary practices in the handling and storage of foods; (3) awareness of factors which promote and assist in maintaining resistance to infective agents (appropriate foods, rest, etc.); (4) knowledge of how disease organisms may be conveyed from one person to another and practical measures to prevent this occurring; and (5) the role of health departments.

References

Books

Anderson, W. A. D., and Scotti, T. M.: Synopsis of Pathology, 8th ed. St. Louis, C. V. Mosby, 1972.

Dubay, E. C., and Grubb, R. D.: Infection: Prevention and Control. St. Louis, C. V. Mosby, 1973.

Hopps, H. C.: Principles of Pathology, 2nd ed. New York. Appleton-Century-Crofts, 1976.

Krupp, M., Sweet, N., and Jaweta, E., et al.: Physician's Handbook, 18th ed. Los Altos, Cal., Lange Medical Publications, 1976.

Macleod, J. (Ed.): Davidson's Principles and Practice of Medicine, 11th ed. Edinburgh, Churchill Livingstone, 1974, pp. 43–110.

Smith, A. L.: Microbiology and Pathology. 11th ed. St. Louis, C. V. Mosby, 1976.

Sodeman, William A., Jr., and Sodeman, William A.: Pathologic Physiology, 5th ed. Philadelphia, W. B. Saunders, 1974. Chapter 20.

Thorn, G. W., et al.: Harrison's Principles of Internal Medicine, 8th ed. New York, McGraw-Hill, 1977.

Periodicals

Brown, M. S.: "What You Should Know about Communicable Diseases." Nurs. '75; Part 1, Vol. 5, No. 9 (Sept. 1975), pp. 70–72; Part 2, Vol. 5, No. 10 (Oct. 1975), pp. 56–60; Part 3, Vol. 5, No. 11 (Nov. 1975), pp. 55–60.

Cranston, L.: "Communicable Diseases and Immunizations." Can. Nurse, Vol. 72, No. 1 (Jan. 1976), pp. 34–40.

Frances, B. J.: "Current Concepts in Immunization." Am. J. Nurs., Vol. 73, No. 4 (April 1973), pp. 646–649.

Katz, S. (Chairman): Report of the Committee on Infectious Diseases, 17th ed. Illinois, American Academy of Pediatrics, 1974.

5

Fluid and Electrolyte Balance; Acid-Base Balance

FLUID AND ELECTROLYTE BALANCE

Normal body functioning demands a relatively constant volume of water and definite concentrations of certain chemical compounds known as electrolytes. The distribution of certain proportions of total body water and certain electrolytes in the various fluid compartments is also important. An electrolyte is a compound that dissociates in solution; it breaks up into separate electrically charged atoms or radicals called ions. For example, sodium chloride (NaCl) in solution forms sodium ions (Na^+) and chloride ions (Cl^-), sodium bicarbonate ($NaHCO_3$) breaks up into sodium ions (Na^+) and bicarbonate radicals (HCO_3^-), and calcium chloride ($CaCl_2$) yields calcium ions (Ca^{2+}) and two chloride ions (Cl^-) for each calcium ion because calcium is bivalent. The ions that carry a positive charge are called cations, and those that are negatively charged are anions. The number of cations in a solution equals the number of anions so that the electrical chemical balance is maintained.

The body fluid and electrolytes are balanced when water and the various electrolytes are present in normal amounts in the major fluid compartments of the body. The relative constancy or balance is maintained by a number of regulatory processes that involve the cardiovascular and urinary systems.

BODY WATER

Water is essential for all body processes; it transports substances to and from the cells, promotes necessary chemical activities, and maintains a physicochemical constancy that is important in normal cellular functions.

Approximately 60 to 65 per cent of the total body weight of an average adult is water, and represents about 40 to 45 liters. The proportion of body weight that is water varies with age and the amount of fatty tissue. In the newborn infant, water comprises about 75 per cent of the body weight but progressively decreases with age to adult levels. This level is maintained until early senescence, when a gradual decrease again begins. Since fatty tissue is practically free of water, the proportion of water to body weight is less in an obese individual.

73

Distribution of Body Water

Body water is contained within two major physiological reservoirs — the intracellular and extracellular compartments. Intracellular fluid comprises about 40 per cent of body weight. The extracellular fluid, which is about 20 per cent of the total body weight, is subdivided into the intravascular and interstitial fluids (see Table 5–1). The intravascular fluid is that contained within the blood vessels and refers to the plasma component of the blood. The interstitial fluid is that contained in the tissue spaces between the blood vessels and the cells and includes that found within the lymph vessels. The latter provides an internal environment for all cells as well as an exchange medium between the blood and the cells. These major fluid compartments are separated by semipermeable membranes.

Another compartment of fluid has recently been referred to as the transcellular fluid. This represents a much smaller proportion of total body water and is of less clinical significance in assessing the patient's hydrational status and maintaining the normal fluid balance. The transcellular fluid includes gastrointestinal secretions, cerebrospinal fluid, intraocular fluid, and pleural, peritoneal and synovial secretions.

Normally, body water is in a dynamic state; there is constant loss and replacement, and changes in location and volume. Osmotic forces are the principal controlling factors in distribution of water in the intracellular and extracellular compartments. The osmotic forces are determined by the solutes dissolved in the body water; these include inorganic and organic substances. The inorganic solutes are electrolytes and, with the hydrostatic pressure of the blood, play a major role in the movement of water between compartments and in regulating the volume of total body water.

The organic solutes are of both large and small molecular size. The smaller organic solutes (e.g., amino acids, glucose, urea) diffuse across semipermeable membranes and are less important in the distribution of water, but if present in excessive amounts they may promote the retention of water. The large molecular organic substances are the blood proteins (albumin, globulin fibrinogen), which have a major influence on the movements of fluid between the intravascular and interstitial compartments. The size of the molecules inhibits free diffusion of the blood proteins across the capillary membrane.

Electrolyte Composition of the Fluids

Although the extracellular and intracellular fluids are separated by the cellular semipermeable membrane, marked differences exist between the electrolyte concentrations in the two compartments. The difference is maintained by the cells, which actively reject certain electrolytes and retain others. For example, sodium is in much higher concentration in the extracellular fluid; the difference is maintained by cellular action referred to as the sodium pump, which ejects sodium from the cells.

The major ions of cellular fluid in order of their quantity are potassium (K^+), phosphate (PO_4^{2-}), magnesium (Mg^{2+}) and protein (Pr^-). Much lesser amounts of sodium (Na^+), sulfate (SO_4^{2-}), bicarbonate (HCO_3^-), chloride (Cl^-) and calcium (Ca^{2+}) are also present.

In the extracellular compartments, sodium (Na^+), chloride (Cl^-) and bicarbonate (HCO_3^-) are of greatest abundance; protein (Pr^-), calcium (Ca^{2+}), potassium (K^+), magnesium (Mg^{2+}) and phosphate (PO_4^{2-}) and sulfate (SO_4^{2-}) occur in much lesser amounts. A significant difference between the intravascular and interstitial fluids is the greater quantity of large molecular protein in the former. The other electrolytes diffuse readily between the two compartments, but the large particles of protein are unable to

TABLE 5–1 DISTRIBUTION OF BODY WATER
Total Body Water (60 to 65 per cent of adult body weight)

Extracellular water (approximately 20 per cent of body weight)	Intracellular water (approximately 40 per cent of body weight)
1. Intravascular fluid (approximately 5 per cent of body weight)	
2. Interstitial fluid (approximately 15 per cent of body weight)	

pass through the capillary membrane (see Table 5–2).

EXCHANGES BETWEEN COMPARTMENTS

Movement of Water Between Fluid Compartments

A continuous exchange of water takes place between the intravascular and interstitial fluids and between the cellular and interstitial fluids. Water diffuses readily through the semipermeable membranes which separate the compartments. But the net exchange of water is dependent on two principal forces: the osmotic pressure created by the electrolytes and the blood proteins, and the hydrostatic pressure of the blood. When the osmotic pressure changes in one compartment, water moves across the semipermeable membrane from the area of lesser osmotic pressure to that of the greater until an equilibrium is established (see p. 34). The hydrostatic pressure created by the volume of blood flowing through the vessels is the driving force that causes filtration of fluid through the semipermeable membranes of the capillaries.

1. EXCHANGE BETWEEN INTRAVASCULAR AND INTERSTITIAL COMPARTMENTS. The total volume of fluid that moves across the capillary membranes is enormous because of the vast number of capillaries, but the net exchange between the intravascular and interstitial compartments is very small. Fluid moves out at the arterial end of the capillary and moves back in at the venous end.

TABLE 5–2 ELECTROLYTES IN BODY FLUIDS

Intracellular	Extracellular
Potassium (K^+)	Sodium (Na^+)
Phosphate (HPO_4^{2-})	Chloride (Cl^-)
Magnesium (Mg^{2+})	Bicarbonate (HCO_3^-)
Protein (Pr^-)	Protein (Pr^-)*
Sodium (Na^+)*	Calcium (Ca^{2+})*
Bicarbonate (HCO_3^-)*	Potassium (K^+)*
Sulfate (SO_4^{2-})*	Phosphate (HPO_4^{2-})*
Chloride (Cl^-)*	Magnesium (Mg^{2+})*
Calcium (Ca^{2+})*	Sulfate (SO_4^{2-})*

*Occur in much lesser amounts.

Two opposing forces exist within the vascular compartment: the hydrostatic pressure of the blood, which forces fluid out through the semipermeable membrane, and the osmotic pressure of the blood proteins, which is a holding or pulling force. The volume and direction of movement of fluid depends on the difference between these two opposing forces. When the blood enters the arterial end of the capillaries the hydrostatic pressure is greater than the protein osmotic pressure, and fluid filters out of the vessels, taking with it diffusible solutes. The movement of fluid out is also opposed by the hydrostatic pressure exerted by the volume of interstitial fluid, which is negligible if lymphatic drainage is normal. The effective filtrative force which moves fluid from the vascular compartment to the interstitial spaces may be expressed as the following equation:

Blood hydrostatic pressure (B.H.P.) − protein osmotic pressure (Pr. O.P.) − interstitial hydrostatic pressure (Int. H.P.) = effective filtrative pressure

These pressures are approximately:

B.H.P. 34 mm. Hg − Pr. O.P. 24 mm. Hg − Int. H.P. 2 mm. Hg = filtrative pressure 8 mm. Hg

The blood hydrostatic pressure is reduced as the blood flows through the capillaries and becomes less than the protein osmotic pressure. As a result, fluid is drawn into the vascular compartment from the interstitial spaces at the venous end of the capillaries. The effective osmotic pressure (Fig. 5–1) may be expressed as follows:

Pr. O.P. 24 mm. Hg − B.H.P. 14 mm. Hg − Int. O.P.[1] 2 mm. Hg = vascular osmotic pressure 8 mm. Hg.

2. EXCHANGE BETWEEN EXTRACELLULAR AND INTRACELLULAR COMPARTMENTS. The net exchange of water between the cellular and interstitial fluids is governed by differences in the osmotic pressure in the two compartments (Fig. 5–2). In the extracellular fluid, the principal osmotic forces are exerted by the sodium and chloride ions. Potassium, magnesium and phosphate are mainly responsible for the osmotic pressure within the cells. Nor-

---

[1]A small amount of blood protein may escape in the filtrate into the interstitial spaces.

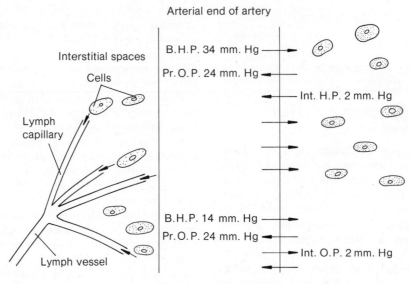

FIGURE 5-1 Exchange of water between intravascular and interstitial compartments. B.H.P. = Blood hydrostatic pressure; Pr.O.P. = protein osmotic pressure; Int.H.P. = interstitial hydrostatic pressure; Int.O.P. = interstitial osmotic pressure.

mal electrolyte concentrations maintain equal osmotic pressures in both compartments, and water diffuses freely between the compartments without net gain or loss in either. A decrease in the volume of extracellular water causes an increase in the concentration of ions and a corresponding increase in the osmotic pressure. This results in the movement of water from the cellular compartment into the interstitial space to establish an equilibrium. Conversely, if the osmotic pressure within the cells exceeds that of the interstitial fluid, water moves into the cells.

Movements of Solutes Between Fluid Compartments

The principal mechanisms responsible for the movement of solute particles across the semipermeable membranes are diffusion, filtration, solvent drag and active transport by cell membranes.

Only small molecular solutes *diffuse* through the membranes. Although their continuous random movement results in their transfer in both directions, the net movement tends to be to the compartment having the lower solute concentration. The diffusion of solutes through the membranes occurs at a much slower rate than water. Diffusion is also influenced by the electrical charges of the solute ions. When there is a difference in potential between two compartments the ions move, attempting to equilibrate the positively and negatively charged ions, positive ions move to the area that is negatively charged and negative ions move in the opposite direction.

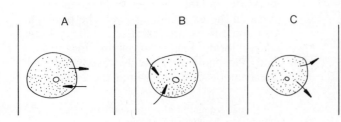

FIGURE 5-2 Exchange of water between cellular and interstitial compartments. *A,* Osmotic pressure of interstitial fluid is equal to that within the cell. Water passes freely between the compartments without net gain or loss. *B,* Osmotic pressure of interstitial fluid is less than that within the cell. Water passes into the cell. *C,* Osmotic pressure of interstitial fluid is greater than that within the cell. Water passes out of the cell.

The *filtration* process involves the forcing of water and small molecular solutes through the semipermeable membranes. The force is created by a difference in hydrostatic pressure on the two sides of a membrane. Filtration operates across the capillary walls, promoting the movement of water and small molecular solutes in the plasma into the interstitial compartment.

Solvent drag refers to the molecules of solutes that tend to flow with the water across the membranes. The amount is not great, but a small amount always moves with the solvent in such a dynamic situation.

Active transport by the cell was referred to in Chapter 3. The cell actively engages in the transport of sodium out to maintain a low sodium concentration in the intracellular compartment. At the same time it actively transports potassium into the cell and retains it to maintain a high potassium concentration within. Both sodium and potassium ions diffuse readily through the semipermeable membranes but are prevented from establishing equal concentrations within the intracellular and extracellular compartments by the sodium-potassium pump within the cells.

Active transport in the form of pinocytosis and phagocytosis also occurs. These processes take substances into the cell and are important in the movement of larger, nondiffusible molecules. Conversely many substances, such as wastes and hormones, must be moved out of cells. This process may be referred to as exocytosis, or reverse pinocytosis.

FLUID BALANCE

A minimum daily intake equal to certain obligatory fluid losses is necessary to maintain the optimum volume and distribution of body fluid. The daily obligatory losses total approximately 1300 ml., which include the water evaporated from the skin and lungs and the minimum volume required by the kidneys to excrete the solid metabolic wastes. Approximately 900 ml. are lost in perspiration and respiration, and 400 ml. is considered the minimum quantity required by normal kidneys to eliminate the metabolic wastes (see Table 5–3).

Sources of body fluid are the ingested fluid and foods and the cellular oxidation processes. The average fluid and food intake by healthy persons usually provides a volume well in excess of the obligatory losses.

A balance is maintained between the intake and output by certain mechanisms in order to preserve a constancy in fluid volume. When the intake is reduced or if there is an excessive loss, as in vomiting or diarrhea, the urinary output is decreased and one is prompted to increase the intake by the sensation of thirst that usually develops. Conversely, if there is an increase in the intake, a corresponding increase in the urinary output occurs.

When the intake volume does not equal that of the obligatory loss, body fluid is drawn upon, and the normal volume is reduced. One then develops a *negative fluid balance (dehydration)* which may seriously affect body functioning if not corrected promptly. Electrolyte concentrations and osmotic pressures are altered, resulting in abnormal fluid shifts between compartments. Faulty excretion with a continued intake may result in an excessive volume in the fluid compartments, producing a *positive fluid balance*. Electrolyte concentrations are changed, and harmful excesses and wastes are retained.

Regulation of the fluid intake and output

TABLE 5–3   AN AVERAGE DAILY WATER INTAKE AND OUTPUT

Intake		Output	
Fluid ingested	1300 ml	Urine	1500 ml.
Water content of ingested food	1000 ml.	Feces	150 ml.
Water of oxidation	250 ml.	Via lungs and skin	900 ml.
Total intake	2550 ml.	Total output	2550 ml.

to preserve constancy in the internal environment occurs through the sensation of thirst, neural and hormonal mechanisms, and renal activity.

Thirst

This is a sensation which one interprets as a need for fluid. The fluid may be needed to cover a loss or to reduce an elevated osmotic pressure of the extracellular fluid which may be due to an excessive sodium or protein intake. A group of cells in the hypothalamus is sensitive to variations in the osmotic pressure of the extracellular fluids. An increase results in impulses that evoke the sensation of thirst. Dryness of the oral and pharyngeal mucous membrane and a decrease in the intravascular volume, as in hemorrhage, also initiate the thirst sensation. Ganong suggests that the decrease in intravascular volume stimulates the kidneys to secrete renin. Renin acts on a protein in the blood; the resulting angiotensin acts on an area of the hypothalamus, causing stimulation of the cerebral area concerned with the sensation of thirst.[2]

Adjustment of Kidney Output

The kidneys perform the most important role in regulating the volume and chemical composition of body fluids. Certain factors from outside the kidneys influence them in the amount of fluid and electrolytes they should reabsorb or eliminate in the urine to preserve homeostasis.

A large amount of water and solutes is filtered out of the blood into the renal tubules. The production of the filtrate depends upon the hydrostatic pressure of the blood; if there is a fall in blood pressure, there is a corresponding decrease in the volume of filtrate. About 80 per cent of the filtrate is quickly reabsorbed in the proximal portion of the renal tubules. Absorption of water and salts in the distal portion of the tubules is adjusted to the amount necessary to maintain normal volume and osmotic pressure of the body fluids.

The tubules are governed as to how much water to reabsorb by the antidiuretic hormone (ADH). This hormone is secreted by the hypothalamus and is delivered to the posterior lobe of the pituitary gland (neurohypophysis) where it is stored and released as required. Within the hypothalamus are cells (osmoreceptors) that are sensitive to variations in the osmotic pressure of the extracellular fluid. An increase in the osmotic pressure above the normal results in impulses being delivered to the posterior pituitary lobe, which bring about the release of ADH. The increased osmotic pressure may be due to a water deficit, an increased intake of sodium chloride or an excessive amount of glucose. The hormone stimulates the tubules to reabsorb water from the filtrate. This increases the extracellular water and reduces the osmotic pressure. Conversely, a fluid intake that lowers the osmotic pressure results in ADH being withheld, and the kidneys then allow a greater loss of water.

A second hormone that indirectly influences water balance is aldosterone, which is secreted by the adrenal cortex. It stimulates the renal tubules to reabsorb sodium. Sodium is chiefly responsible for the osmotic pressure of the extracellular fluid; an increased absorption brings about the release of ADH and a resulting decrease in the water loss. The regulation of the aldosterone secretion is not clearly understood. Currently, physiologists theorize that aldosterone secretion is influenced directly by the plasma potassium and sodium concentrations, by the renin-angiotensin mechanism cited above, which is set in operation by a reduction in the blood volume and pressure in the renal arteries, and/or by the hypothalamus via the pituitary secretion of adrenocorticotropin (ACTH). The hypothalamus influences the secretion of ACTH. In stress situations (e.g., surgery, trauma, anxiety) it is suggested that the hypothalamus stimulates the pituitary to release ACTH, which in turn increases the output of aldosterone by the cortex of the adrenal glands.

Water loss via the kidneys is also affected by the load of solid wastes they are required to eliminate. There is always a certain amount of solid metabolic wastes to be excreted, but it may vary with diet and cellular activities. If there is an increased amount, the kidneys may require more

[2]William F. Ganong: Review of Medical Physiology, 7th ed. Los Altos, Cal., Lange, 1975, p. 163.

water to eliminate them. An example of this is seen when the blood sugar exceeds the normal; a greater volume of water is excreted in order to eliminate the excess sugar. This accounts for the increased urinary output and excessive thirst which are characteristic of diabetes mellitus.

ELECTROLYTES

As mentioned previously, normal body functioning requires the presence of certain electrolytes in relatively definite concentrations. Electrolytes are the principal source of the osmotic forces that control the volume and location of fluid in the body. Certain ones have a specific role in maintaining an optimum alkaline reaction (acid-base balance) and in vital cellular activities. For example, normal bone structure is dependent upon a certain ratio of calcium to phosphorus; maintenance of a particular concentration of potassium is essential to normal cardiac muscle function.

Fluid balance and electrolyte balance are interdependent; a disturbance in one is immediately reflected in the other. A loss or gain in any one of the major compartmental ions alters the osmotic pressure, with a subsequent water shift occurring. Changes in their concentration also alter cellular activities and may pose a threat to life.

Measurement of Electrolyte Concentration

In clinical investigation of the electrolyte composition of body fluids, the physician is interested in the effective chemical activity of the electrolytes. For this reason the concentration is expressed in the number of milliequivalents per liter of body fluid.

When chemicals react or combine, each does so in a certain definite unvarying proportion. An *equivalent* represents a unit of chemical activity or the combining power of a substance. It may be defined as being equal to the combining power of 1 gram of hydrogen (H^+). In clinical application the amounts in equivalents are very small, so they are expressed in milliequivalents. One milliequivalent (mEq.) is 1/1000 of an equivalent.

Information as to the number of units available for physiological chemical activity is more meaningful than a statement of the weight of the substance in mg. or Gm. per cent. A small amount of one substance may react or combine with a much larger amount of another. For instance, 1 mg. of hydrogen may replace 23 mg. of sodium and combine with 35 mg. of chlorine.

The proportion in which chemicals react or combine is related to the atomic weight of the substance and, in the case of electrolytes, to the number of electrical charges each ion carries. The latter is known as the valence of a substance. Ions which carry one charge are termed monovalent, and those with two charges are divalent or bivalent. An ion with one positive charge will combine with an ion with one negative charge (e.g., $Na^+ + HCO_3^- \rightarrow NaHCO_3$; $H^+ + Cl^- \rightarrow HCl$). An ion with two positive charges will react with two ions, each having a negative charge, or with one ion that carries two negative charges (e.g., $Ca^{2+} + Cl^- Cl^- \rightarrow CaCl_2$); $Ca^{2+} + SO_4^{2-} \rightarrow CaSO_4$). From this it may be seen that the chemical activity of an electrolyte is proportional to the total number of electrical charges carried by the ions in a given volume of fluid.

To determine the number of milliequivalents (chemical combining units) of an electrolyte, the weight in mg. in 100 ml. of blood serum is established. This figure is then divided by the atomic weight of the particular electrolyte, which yields the number of ions in 100 ml. of serum. Since the chemical activity depends on the valence, the above figure is then multiplied by the valence of the electrolyte to obtain the number of milliequivalents in 100 ml. In clinical practice it is customary to express the number of milliequivalents present in a liter (1000 ml.) of body fluid, so the number in 100 ml. must be multiplied by 10. The formula may be written as follows:

milliequivalents per liter (mEq./L.) =
$$\frac{\text{mg. per cent}}{\text{atomic weight}} \times \text{valence} \times 10$$

To illustrate:

1. A solution contains calcium 20 mg. per cent (20 mg. per 100 ml.). Calcium is divalent and has an atomic weight of 40. Using the formula:

$$\text{mEq./L. of calcium} = \frac{20}{40} \times 2 \times 10 = \frac{400}{40} = 10$$

2. A solution contains sodium 207 mg. per cent (207 mg. per 100 ml.). Sodium is monovalent and has an atomic weight of 23. Using the formula:

$$\text{mEq./L. of sodium} = \frac{207}{23} \times 1 \times 10 = \frac{2070}{23} = 90$$

See Table 5–4.

Other units of measurement relevant to chemical solutes of body fluids include moles, millimoles, osmoles and milliosmoles.

One *mole* (mol) of a substance is the molecular weight of that substance in grams (e.g., one molecule of NaCl = 58.5 Gm.).[3] One *millimole* (mM.) is 1/1000 of a mole and is expressed in milligrams (e.g., 1 mM. of glucose ($C_6H_{12}O_6$) = 180 mg.).

Osmole (Osm.) is the unit of measurement of osmotic pressure. One *milliosmole* (mOsm.) is 1/1000 of an osmole. Osmotic pressure is determined by the number of particles of solute (molecules, atoms, ions). The osmotic activity of solutions is influenced by the extent to which the solutes ionize. An increase in the number of particles from ionization of the molecules of solute increases the osmotic pressure. A solute that does not ionize, such as glucose, produces less osmotic pressure. One mole of a substance that does not dissociate into ions is equal to 1 osmole. One mole of sodium chloride which dissociates almost completely into a sodium ion and a chlorine ion equals 2 osmoles. For example, 1 liter of a solution with 60 mM. of sodium chloride dissolved in it contains 120 mOsm./liter of the solution.

Osmole concentration of the body fluids plays an important role in the exchange and distribution of water and dissolved substances. The osmotic activity is a result of the combined osmotic pressure of several solutes. Clinically, the *osmole concentration* per unit of solvent, or *osmolality*, may be determined by measuring the depression of the freezing point of a fluid compared to water rather than by calculating the concentration and ionization of the various solutes in the particular body fluid. The device used is an osmometer.[4, 5] The normal range of serum osmolality is 275 to 300 mOsm./liter.

TABLE 5–4 MILLIEQUIVALENTS PER LITER OF ELECTROLYTES IN SERUM

Electrolyte	mEq./L.
Bicarbonate (HCO_3^{2-})	25 to 27
Calcium (Ca^{2+})	4.5 to 5.5
Chlorine (Cl^-)	98 to 106
Magnesium (Mg^{2+})	1.5 to 2.5
Phosphorus (PO_4^{2-})	1.0 to 1.5
Potassium (K^+)	3.5 to 5
Sodium (Na^+)	140 to 145

DISTURBANCES IN FLUID BALANCE

Fluid Deficit

A fluid deficit is a negative fluid balance; the fluid loss exceeds the intake and there is a reduction in the normal volume of body fluid. A negative water balance not only implies changes in the water volume, but involves changes in electrolyte concentrations. The latter may exceed the normal concentration if the fluid intake is reduced or if the water loss exceeds the rate of electrolyte loss. In some instances the electrolytes may be depleted by excessive losses with the fluids; for example, a loss of gastrointestinal secretions involves losses of certain electrolytes in addition to loss of water.

Extracellular fluid is depleted first. This increases the osmolality in that compartment; the fluid becomes hypertonic and causes water to move out of the cells. Cellular dehydration alters cellular concentrations and eventually disrupts normal cellular activities. The movement of water from the intracellular compartment helps to maintain intravascular fluid within near normal limits, and blood pressure, pulse vol-

---

[3]A *mole* is the molecular weight of a substance; an equivalent is the atomic weight divided by the valence.

[4]E. Goldberger: A Primer of Water, Electrolyte and Acid-Base Syndromes, 5th ed. Philadelphia, Lea and Febiger, 1975.

[5]H.A. Harper: Review of Physiological Chemistry, 15th ed. Los Altos, Cal., Lange, 1975, p. 537.

ume, and the hematocrit may remain within normal range for a period of time. If the fluid deficit is not corrected, the intravascular fluid is eventually depleted and is reflected in a fall in blood pressure, progressive weakening of the pulse and a rise in the hematocrit. Blood flow through the kidneys is reduced and the urinary output falls below the obligatory output. This leads to the retention of metabolic wastes and acidosis.

A deficit of water is usually accompanied by a loss of potassium ions, mainly from the cells. They are excreted by the kidneys or retained in the extracellular fluid in higher than normal concentration. The loss of potassium from the cells lowers the osmotic pressure of the intracellular fluid. As a result more cellular water is lost to the extracellular fluid.

In order to offset the fluid deficit, there is an increase in the secretion of the antidiuretic hormone as a result of the hypertonicity of the extracellular fluid. The increased reabsorption of water by the renal tubules minimizes the loss of body water.

Causes of Fluid Deficit

A negative fluid balance may be caused by: (1) an excessive loss of fluid from the body; (2) an insufficient intake of fluid; or (3) a deficiency of electrolytes.

1. EXCESSIVE LOSS OF FLUID. Excessive loss of body water can occur in the following ways:

a. Loss of fluid from the gastrointestinal tract by vomiting, diarrhea, suction drainage, fistula or ileostomy drainage.

b. Excessive perspiration in fever or exposure to a high environmental temperature.

c. A rapid respiratory rate, which may deplete body water as a result of the increased evaporation that accompanies the increased respirations.

d. A deficit of body fluid, which may develop rapidly as the result of hemorrhage or the loss of plasma in severe burns.

e. If a deficiency occurs in the secretion of the antidiuretic hormone (ADH), as in diabetes insipidus or following the ingestion of alcohol, the kidney tubules fail to reabsorb the normal amount of water, thus increasing the volume of the urinary output.

f. An excess of solute or increased load of solid wastes, which demands more water for elimination by the kidneys. For example, the accumulation of glucose in the blood in diabetes mellitus results in polyuria (excessive output of urine), causing too great a loss of water.

g. Chronic kidney disease, which may impair the renal ability to concentrate wastes. The kidneys use a greater volume of water to dilute the wastes for excretion and the individual may develop dehydration unless the fluid intake compensates for the increased loss.

h. Wounds with profuse drainage, which can result in marked fluid loss.

2. INSUFFICIENT FLUID INTAKE. An inadequate intake of fluid may be due to:

a. The inability to swallow. This may occur with esophageal disease (e.g., stricture, newgrowth), or in comatose or seriously debilitated patients.

b. A lack of available fluid. This occurs rarely and mainly with persons lost or trapped by injury in a desert or woods. Fluid may not be available to infants and young children because of their dependence on others who do not provide an adequate amount for them.

c. Lack of thirst or failure to recognize need. Patients whose sense of thirst is impaired by cerebral injury or disease and elderly persons are likely to be deficient in fluid intake for this reason.

3. DEFICIENCY OF ELECTROLYTES. A reduction in body fluid may develop with a concentration of electrolytes below normal. Body mechanisms operate to restore the normal osmotic pressure by eliminating water.

a. This is seen in Addison's disease, in which a deficiency of aldosterone secretion by the adrenal cortices results in an inadequate reabsorption of sodium by the renal tubules. The osmotic pressure of the extracellular fluid is reduced; this in turn prompts a decrease in the secretion of the antidiuretic hormone (ADH) and causes a reduction in reabsorption of water by the renal tubules.

b. A relative deficit of electrolytes may develop when an excessive amount of water is ingested or a nonelectrolyte solution is administered intravenously. The concentration of the body electrolytes is lowered; also, as the excessive water is eliminated, some electrolytes may be washed out with it.

Effects of Fluid Depletion

The effects of dehydration depend on the volume of the fluid deficit and the rate at which it develops. Effects are more acute when it develops rapidly, when the patient is an infant, a young child or an elderly person, and if the patient is debilitated.

Interstitial fluid is depleted first, resulting in an increase in the osmotic pressure that causes water to move out of the cells. Cellular dehydration alters cellular concentrations and eventually disrupts normal cellular metabolism.

Signs and Symptoms

The manifestations depend on the severity of the fluid deficit. The sensation of thirst is usually the first symptom. It is suggested that this occurs when water loss is equal to about 2 per cent of body weight (approximately a loss of 2 to 3 pounds). There is a loss of weight proportional to the degree of the fluid deficit.

The skin becomes dry as perspiration secretion decreases, and loses its turgor. Salivary secretion is reduced; the mouth, pharynx and tongue become dry and a source of discomfort to the patient. Swallowing of solid food is difficult and the dryness of the mucous membranes may interfere with clarity of speech. The eyes appear sunken and the eyeballs become soft as intraocular fluid is reduced.

Blood pressure and pulse volume remain normal in the early stage of dehydration as the intracellular water moves out to replace the extracellular loss. However, if the fluid deficit is not corrected, the intravascular volume is eventually depleted; the blood pressure falls, the pulse becomes progressively weaker and the patient presents a picture of shock.

Urinary output is decreased (oliguria), which leads to the retention of metabolic wastes and acidosis. The patient is constipated and the hard, dry stool may cause impaction and considerable discomfort.

An elevation of temperature develops as a result of the decreased evaporation of fluid from the body surface, which normally is an important temperature control mechanism.

Laboratory data reveal changes, dependent upon the extent of the fluid loss. Reduction in the plasma volume and the resulting hemoconcentration is reflected in elevated hemoglobin (normal: women 12 to 16 Gm/100 ml., men 14 to 18 Gm./100 ml.) and hematocrit, which is the volume percentage of red blood cells (normal: women 37 to 47 per cent, men 45 to 52 per cent). Serum electrolyte levels are determined, as concentration and osmolality changes are likely to occur, and serve as a guide in fluid replacement. Urinalysis shows an increased concentration of solid wastes by an increase in specific gravity (normal range: 1.003 to 1.030). Estimations of the excretion of particular solids may also be made; for example, a high sodium loss may be incurred in an effort to reduce the osmolality of the extracellular fluid.

At the onset of dehydration, the patient experiences a loss of strength and manifests apathy. With a persisting and increasing negative fluid balance, the individual progressively becomes weaker and disoriented, and may eventually lapse into coma. Death may ensue.

Implications for Nursing

It is important that the nurse realize the significance of normal amounts of water and electrolytes in body functioning and the need for recognition of early deficits.

1. OBSERVATIONS. The patient's daily fluid intake and output volumes should be known to the nurse. If the output exceeds the intake, there is an immediate need for an increased fluid intake unless the patient previously has had a positive fluid balance and edema. A form is usually available for accurate recording and tabulation of the fluid intake and output volumes for each 24-hour period. Headings under intake include the various routes by which fluids may be introduced, such as oral, intravenous, interstitial and rectal. The time and character of the fluid administered are noted, as is the volume. Output columns provide for the recording of losses of urine, emesis, suction drainage, wound drainage, blood, perspiration and stool. Some of these can

be measured accurately but estimates have to be made with perspiration, respiratory evaporation and wound drainage.

The patient is weighed daily, if possible, as losses or gains serve in assessing the deficit as well as provide a guide for fluid replacement. The individual is weighed at the same time each day on the same scale and with the same weight of clothing. The weight may be recorded on the fluid balance sheet. A urinary specific gravity in excess of 1.030 should be noted also as a need for an increased fluid intake unless contraindicated.

The condition of the patient's mouth and skin is also a good source of information as to the patient's hydrational status.

When a fluid deficit is known to exist a frequent check should be made of the patient's vital signs (temperature, pulse and blood pressure), general appearance and responses.

2. FLUID REPLACEMENT. The necessity to restore normal hydration and electrolyte concentrations is urgent in order to restore normal metabolism, circulation and renal function. The method used for the administration of replacement fluids will depend on the patient's condition. Intravenous infusion is used to reestablish a satisfactory balance quickly. When ordering the quantity and type of solution to be given the physician considers the cause, source and volume of the losses and excesses as well as the general condition of the patient. Blood chemistry studies are done to determine possible electrolyte and acid-base imbalances. The choice of solution is an individual matter based on each patient's needs.

Before the intravenous infusion is started, the nurse explains the purpose and the procedure to the patient and advises him of his role. It may be necessary to splint the limb that is used or provide some form of restraint in order to prevent dislocation of the needle and maintain the flow of solution into the vein. Displacement of the needle by withdrawal from the vein or secondary puncture results in solution running into the interstitial spaces. This causes swelling and discomfort at the site of injection.

Once the intravenous infusion is started, the nurse is responsible for maintaining the desired rate of flow, detecting any difficul-

ties and noting the patient's reactions. If the patient is an infant, young child, an elderly person or a patient with a cardiac or pulmonary condition, the rate of flow must be carefully controlled. Too rapid infusion may overload the circulatory system and lead to pulmonary edema and cardiac dilatation.

If no specific rate of flow is ordered, the clamp is usually adjusted to deliver 60 to 80 drops (gtt.) per minute. If the fluid depletion is severe, the solution may be administered more rapidly (100 to 120 gtt./min.) for the first 1000 ml., then run more slowly. The flow is monitored frequently, since the rate may change as the volume in the solution container lessens or if the needle shifts or is partially or totally plugged. Because the size of the drop delivered may vary with different makes of intravenous equipment, the nurse should note the time taken to deliver 50 to 100 ml. and adjust the rate of flow accordingly.

The site of injection and the vein pathway are examined for possible interstitial infusion and irritation of the vein by the solution. The patient's pulse and respirations are also assessed frequently; dyspnea and unfavorable changes in the pulse are reported promptly. The usual procedure when untoward reactions are suspected is to slow the rate of flow and consult the physician immediately.

Frequently, medications are added to the intravenous solution; this is usually done by a physician or by nurses with special training. A safeguard is to have a second nurse check the preparation and dosage. Strict aseptic technique is observed and the medication is thoroughly mixed with the intravenous solution so that it is adequately diluted. A label is placed conspicuously on the container indicating the drug, amount and the time it was added. The rate of flow is usually slower if a drug is added, and the patient is observed closely for possible unfavorable reactions. The purpose, expected effect, and possible side effects must be familiar to the nurse responsible for the care of the patient.

Intravenous infusion need not interfere with care of the patient if the needle and distal portion of the tube are anchored securely with adhesive. The patient may be turned at regular intervals or encouraged to move about himself if he is able.

Reevaluation of the serum electrolytes and reassessment of the individual's hydrational status are necessary. Volume and electrolyte composition of the solution are adjusted according to the findings. For example, if the sodium level was initially elevated above normal, the solution administered would probably be glucose 5 per cent in distilled water; later, when the serum sodium level returns to normal, an isotonic solution is used.

If the patient is permitted oral fluids, some persuasion and resourcefulness may be necessary on the part of the nurse. The patient's cooperation is sought by advising him of the importance and role of fluids in his recovery and in health. Small amounts are given at frequent intervals. Preferences for certain fluids should be ascertained and respected if possible, and the necessary assistance in taking a drink is provided. The patient may be too sick or too weak to reach out and take the fluid himself; holding the glass and elevating his head will prove more effective than simply placing the fluid at the bedside with instructions to the patient to take it.

3. MOUTH CARE. The mouth requires frequent cleansing and rinsing. Oil, petroleum jelly or cold cream may be applied to the lips to relieve the dryness and prevent cracking.

4. SKIN CARE. Frequent bathing or temperature sponges may help to reduce the fever that may develop, as well as provide comfort for the patient. The amount of bedding and the room temperature should be adjusted to the patient's temperature.

5. HEADACHE. Cold compresses to the forehead and a quiet environment with subdued lighting may relieve the patient's headache to some extent.

6. REST. The patient is encouraged to rest as much as possible in order to lessen the demand on cellular activities. Nursing care is planned so that there will be a minimum of disturbance for the patient.

7. SAFETY PRECAUTIONS. Bed sides or rails and close observation are necessary to protect the patient if there are indications of confusion and disorientation.

Fluid Excess

Edema is the accumulation of an excessive amount of fluid in the interstitial spaces locally or generally. If it occurs generally, it implies a positive fluid balance in which the fluid intake has exceeded the output, and there is an increase in total body water and sodium.

Causes of Fluid Excess

The mechanisms of formation of edema include the following:

1. INCREASED VENOUS PRESSURE. If for any reason there is an increase in the hydrostatic pressure of the blood in the venous end of the capillaries in excess of the blood protein osmotic pressure, the return of interstitial fluid into the capillaries is inhibited. This mechanism contributes to the formation of edema in cardiac failure; the impaired heart contractions cannot forward an adequate volume of blood. As a result of the incomplete emptying of the chambers, the heart cannot receive all the blood being brought to it in the large veins. This causes an increase in venous volume and a consequent increase in venous pressure. Increased venous pressure may also be caused by an obstruction to the flow of blood in a large vein, possibly as the result of thrombosis or extrinsic pressure on the vein.

2. OBSTRUCTION TO LYMPHATIC DRAINAGE. Interference with the drainage of interstitial fluid that is normally carried away in the lymphatic vessels results in edema. This produces a localized edema and may be seen in the arm of a patient who has had a radical mastectomy which involves resection of the axillary lymphatics and lymph nodes that drain the arm. This type of edema is also seen in elephantiasis, in which filarial worms cause an obstruction in the lymphatics.

3. DEFICIENCY OF BLOOD PROTEINS. A decrease in the amount of blood proteins (albumin, globulin and fibrinogen) reduces the osmotic pressure of the intravascular fluid. Much of the fluid that is filtered out of the arterial end of the capillaries remains in the interstitial spaces because the protein osmotic pressure is not sufficient to return it at the venous end. This may be seen in nephrosis, a kidney disease in which serum albumin escapes from the glomeruli into the renal tubules and is lost to the body in urine. It may also occur in malnutrition, in which a lack of protein results in decreased formation of blood proteins.

4. INCREASED CAPILLARY PERMEABILITY. An excessive amount of fluid in the

interstitial spaces may be due to permeable capillaries. An example of this type of edema is that seen in inflammation, hypersensitivity reactions and burns.

5. RENAL INSUFFICIENCY. Diminished kidney filtration may cause an insufficient output of water, resulting in an accumulation in the interstitial compartment. This may be due to disease in the kidneys (e.g., acute nephritis) or to a decreased blood flow through the kidneys (e.g., heart failure, shock).

6. EXCESSIVE HORMONES. An excessive secretion of adrenocortical secretions, particularly aldosterone, increases the reabsorption of sodium by the renal tubules. In turn, the excess of sodium and the corresponding increase in extracellular osmotic pressure causes an increased release of ADH. More water is reclaimed in the kidney tubules and eventually accumulates in the interstitial spaces.

If for any reason there is an abnormal release of ADH, an excess of water is conserved and forms edema.

Manifestations of Edema

Indications of the presence of edema include weight gain, swollen tissues which pit on finger pressure, weakness, apathy, slowness or absence of responses, anorexia and a decreased urinary output. The patient may experience dyspnea and there may be moist gurgling sounds with respirations, indicating fluid accumulation in the airways (pulmonary edema) as a result of circulatory overload.

A gain in weight is one of the earliest symptoms of fluid retention. A person may accumulate approximately 5 to 10 pounds of water before it becomes apparent on the surface. There is a gain of approximately 2 to 2.5 pounds for each liter of fluid retained. If the person is ambulatory, edema may be observed first in swelling of the feet and ankles. The bed patient usually exhibits signs of fluid accumulation first in the sacral region. Localized edema according to the patient's position is referred to as dependent edema. Later, as the total interstitial compartment becomes overloaded, a generalized edema is evident.

Implications for Nursing

The treatment and nursing care of the patient depends on the cause of edema. Only general principles as related to the edema are cited here.

An accurate record is made of the fluid intake and loss. The patient is weighed daily or every other day if possible. This should be done at the same time each day, with the patient wearing the same amount of clothing, and on the same scale each time.

Specific orders should be received from the physician as to the patient's fluid and salt intake. Salt is usually restricted except in localized edema. Fluid restrictions are governed by the patient's circulatory status and urinary output.

The skin requires special attention since edematous tissue is poorly nourished and breaks down readily. The patient's position is changed frequently. Vulnerable pressure areas are examined, bathed and gently massaged every 2 to 3 hours. The skin may also be protected by placing the patient on a resilient surface; an alternating pressure air mattress, foam rubber or a sheepskin may be used. Gentle handling is also very important.

The excess of fluid in generalized edema may cause mental confusion and disorientation. Safety precautions such as bed sides and closer attendance to the patient may be necessary.

If a diuretic is ordered, an accurate record is made of the volume of urine excreted. If the patient is ambulatory, he should be close to a bathroom. Frequent use of a urinal or commode will be necessary for the bed patient. He should not be kept waiting or receive an impression that his demands are excessive. The frequent voiding can be quite exhausting for the patient; necessary assistance in getting on and off the pan and allowing the patient to rest undisturbed between voidings help to conserve his energy. Serum electrolyte levels are determined, as an excessive loss may be incurred with the diuresis.

In the case of pulmonary edema, the patient is usually placed in the semirecumbent position. This helps to decrease the venous return to the heart and lungs and may reduce the pulmonary edema.

Water Intoxication

This is a fluid imbalance in which there is an increase in body water without a comparable increase in body sodium. The osmotic pressure of the extracellular fluid is less than that of the intracellular fluid. As a result, water leaves the interstitial spaces and enters the cells, disturbing their normal concentrations and activities. The amount the cells will hold is limited, so an excess may also remain in the interstitial spaces.

The cause of water intoxication is a decreased urinary output with a continuing intake of water, or an excessive intake of water without salt.

The signs and symptoms are similar to those seen in the person with a sodium deficiency. The patient experiences headache, muscle cramps, nausea and vomiting, and excessive perspiration. Cerebral disturbances are manifested in drowsiness, confusion and loss of coordination. Convulsions and coma may develop if the condition is not corrected in the early stages.

Water intoxication is treated by restriction of the fluid intake and the administration of a diuretic. If the serum sodium level is below normal, a small volume of hypertonic solution of sodium chloride may be given intravenously. This increases extracellular osmolarity and promotes the movement of excess water out of the cells.

SPECIFIC ELECTROLYTES AND IMBALANCES

Sodium (Na+)

Sodium is the major cation found in the extracellular fluids. Its concentration is maintained relatively constant within a narrow range (140 to 145 mEq./L, or 320 to 340 mg./100 ml.), although the amount ingested varies greatly from day to day.

FUNCTIONS. Sodium plays an important role in fluid balance by maintaining the normal osmolality of the extracellular fluids. The osmotic pressure created by sodium is the principal factor in the movement and volume of body water. A normal concentration of sodium in the interstitial and intravascular fluids prevents excessive fluid retention or fluid loss.

Sodium contributes to normal muscular irritability or excitability. It is essential in the transmission of electrochemical impulses along nerve and muscle cellular membranes.

Cell permeability is affected by the sodium concentration; it is considered essential in the

movement of some substances across the cell membrane.

Sodium ions are also important in conjunction with chlorine and bicarbonate in acid-base regulation.

REQUIREMENT, SOURCES, METABOLISM. The average diet contains sodium well in excess of the suggested body requirement of 2 grams (5 grams of sodium chloride). The individual with a family history of hypertension is advised to restrict sodium chloride intake to 1 to 2 grams per day. Sodium occurs naturally in unprocessed foods, and much is added in the form of sodium chloride in the preparation and preservation of foods.

Ninety-five per cent of the sodium removed from the body is excreted in the urine, with the remainder leaving the body in perspiration and feces. The adrenocortical secretions, especially aldosterone, influence the metabolism of sodium. The steroid secretions promote reabsorption of sodium by the renal tubules. A deficiency of the cortical secretions (Addison's disease) causes an increase in sodium excretion in the urine and a lower serum sodium level.

HYPONATREMIA (SODIUM DEPLETION). Since normal kidneys are very efficient in conserving sodium when the intake is reduced, an adequate concentration for normal body functioning is usually maintained. Depletion of sodium ions in the extracellular fluid most often results from an excessive loss rather than a deficient intake. A low serum level may also occur because of fluid retention; excessive fluid volume causes dilution of the sodium. This is referred to as dilutional hyponatremia.

The *causes* of hyponatremia include: (1) diaphoresis (profuse perspiration) in fever or high environmental temperature; (2) loss of gastrointestinal fluids by vomiting, suction, diarrhea or fistula; (3) a deficiency of adrenocortical secretions, which results in failure of the renal tubules to reabsorb sodium; and (4) renal disease that impairs tubular function. It is also suggested that a loss of sodium ions from the extracellular fluid to the cells (the intracellular compartment) may occur when the cells are deficient in potassium.

Dilutional hyponatremia may occur, in which a low serum sodium level develops because of dilution of the sodium by a disproportionate increase in extracellular fluid. This may follow the ingestion of a large volume of water, an abnormally high secretion of the antidiuretic hormone (ADH), a loss of sodium without a corresponding loss of water, or an intravenous infusion of a nonelectrolyte solution. The increase in ADH may occur with a cerebral injury, disease or tumor. Rarely, a decreased intake of sodium may account for a deficit as a result of a prolonged low sodium therapeutic diet.

Normally, a lowered concentration of extracellular sodium initiates a decrease in the release of ADH and an ensuing increase in the volume of water excreted in the urine. This response is made in an effort to restore normal osmolality of the extracellular compartments, but it sacrifices fluid volume. Some extracellular fluid also moves into the cells; the cells become swollen, normal cellular electrolyte concentrations are altered and cell activities may be impaired. If the sodium deficit is severe, depletion of the extracellular fluid results in the development of dehydration and its manifestations.

The movement of water into cells and the excessive loss of water are considered responsible for the *symptoms* of sodium deficit. The individual experiences apprehension, lethargy, headache, muscle and abdominal cramps and weakness. Nausea and vomiting and diarrhea may accompany the abdominal distress. The muscular disturbance may progress to twitching and convulsions. Urinary output is increased in the early stages but, as the extracellular total fluid volume is reduced, oliguria develops. The patient may develop all the signs and symptoms of dehydration (p. 82). If the sodium deficiency persists, complicated by a marked reduction in total extracellular fluid, the individual lapses into unconsciousness and manifests circulatory failure and shock.

A sodium deficit is not uncommon in those working in a high environmental temperature in industry, or for prolonged periods in the hot sun. The increased sweating causes an excessive loss of water and sodium; the individual experiences thirst and may drink large amounts of water without replacing the salt lost. In such situations the problem should be anticipated and sodium chloride tablets provided, which the workers are advised to take to prevent sodium deficiency.

Treatment of hyponatremia consists of the ingestion of a salt-containing solution or, if necessary, an intravenous infusion of an iso-

tonic sodium chloride solution (0.9 per cent). The volume and additional electrolytes that may be needed are determined by the presenting symptoms, pulse rate and volume, blood pressure, urinary output, and laboratory reports of serum electrolytes. While receiving the intravenous infusion of sodium chloride, the patient is observed closely for the disappearance of the symptoms manifested and the appearance of other changes. The rate of administration of the infusion is usually reduced after the first liter is given. A rapid increase in extracellular sodium and osmolality may induce the movement of an excessive amount of water from within the cells to the interstitial compartment. If the low serum sodium level is due to dilution, the intake of water is restricted and diuresis may be initiated by the administration of a diuretic, such as furosemide (Lasix).

HYPERNATREMIA (EXCESS SODIUM). An excess of sodium in extracellular fluid and consequent hyperosmolality may develop as a result of an excessive ingestion of sodium chloride, an inadequate water intake, or water loss without a corresponding excretion of sodium. Hypernatremia may be associated with intracranial injury or disease that causes disturbance in the hypothalamic response to changes in the osmolality of extracellular fluid; the disorder may incur a deficiency of ADH (e.g., diabetes insipidus). Decreased excretion of sodium by the kidneys may be caused by hyperactivity of the adrenal cortices, as in Cushing's disease, or by the administration of corticoid preparations which may promote reabsorption of sodium ions by the renal tubules. Retention of sodium may also occur in renal insufficiency, especially if the sodium intake is not reduced.

Normally, the responses to an increase in the osmolality of the extracellular fluids above normal include an increased release of ADH, thirst, decrease in perspiration and movement of water out of the cells.

The *signs and symptoms* of an elevated serum sodium include dry, sticky mucous membranes, rough dry tongue, thirst, and flushed dry skin.

The disorder is *treated* by giving water orally and/or by the administration of glucose 5 per cent in water by intravenous infusion. The underlying cause must also be investigated and treated. A low sodium diet is prescribed; depending on the cause of the hypernatremia, the restriction may vary from "No added salt" (2 to 3 Gm.) to the more severe restriction of being permitted only 500 mg. per day.

Potassium (K⁺)

Potassium is the major cation found in the intracellular fluids and, to maintain homeostasis, the amount in the body is kept relatively constant within a range of 3.5 to 5 mEq. per liter of blood serum. The amount of total body potassium is about twice that of sodium. It is present only in small amounts in the extracellular fluids but is especially abundant and active within the cells.

FUNCTIONS. Within the cells, potassium plays a significant role in creating the osmotic pressure that is important in preserving normal cellular fluid content. Normal volume of water, in turn, contributes to the maintenance of normal electrolyte concentrations. Potassium also influences the acid-base balance.

Potassium ions in the extracellular fluids are essential for the normal functioning of all muscle tissue, and are especially important in cardiac muscle activity. In conjunction with sodium and calcium, potassium regulates neuromuscular excitability and stimulation and is necessary for the transmission of the nerve impulses that prompt contraction of muscle fibers.

Potassium is also active in carbohydrate metabolism. It is required in the conversion of glucose to glycogen and in its subsequent storage. This element is also used in fairly large amounts in the synthesis of muscle protein.

REQUIREMENT, SOURCES, METABOLISM. Potassium is widely distributed in foods; a deficiency is unlikely if there is an adequate intake of food, since the average daily diet contains 2 to 4 Gm. Meats, whole grains, bananas, oranges, apricots, prunes, tomatoes, squash, legumes and broccoli have a high potassium content. Potassium is readily absorbed from the small intestine. The digestive secretions contain potassium but this portion, as well as much of that found in digested foods, is reabsorbed.

Kidney activity is the chief regulatory mechanism for potassium; reabsorption, secretion and excretion of potassium ions by the tubular cells operate to maintain an optimum serum concentration. The kidneys can readily increase the excretion of potassium if the intake is high. The excretion of the ions is influenced by changes in the acid-base balance; the serum potassium level is higher in acidosis and lower in alkalosis. The serum level may also be influenced by the adrenocortical secretion, aldosterone. The latter promotes renal excretion of potassium ions in exchange for sodium.

ABNORMAL LEVELS. Even small variations outside the narrow normal range should receive prompt attention because of possible serious effects on cardiac activity. Slight variations in extracellular fluids are readily reflected in electrocardiographic changes.

HYPOKALEMIA (POTASSIUM DEPLETION). The causes of a potassium deficit include: (1) excessive urinary loss that may be caused by some renal tubular disease, uncontrolled diabetes, diuretic (especially thiazide) or corticoid medications, or increased adrenocortical secretion; (2) gastrointestinal loss incurred by diarrhea, intestinal fistula, enterostomy, vomiting or gastric suctioning; (3) increased movement of potassium ions into the cells as a result of excessive alkali administration or parental administration of glucose and insulin; or (4) a deficient intake of potassium if the individual is unable to eat or has been deprived of food for a period of time and has not received parenteral potassium. Some potassium continues to be excreted in the urine, progressively establishing a deficit.

When the potassium concentration of the extracellular fluid is depleted, potassium tends to move out of the cells, creating an intracellular deficit. The cells retain more sodium and hydrogen ions in an effort to establish an ionic balance. These ionic shifts seriously affect normal cell functioning, and the normal alkalinity of the extracellular fluid is altered because of its loss of hydrogen and sodium ions.

Signs and symptoms of hypokalemia are neuromuscular disturbances manifested by skeletal muscle weakness and loss of tone, numbness, and loss of reflexes. Cardiac muscle disturbance is manifested by arrhythmias, electrocardiographic changes and increased sensitivity to digitalis that may lead to digitalis toxicity if the medication is continued. ECG changes include a flattening of T waves and depressed S T segments. The disturbance in myocardial functioning may progress to cardiac arrest. If the potassium deficiency becomes progressively greater, paralysis of the arms, legs and respiratory muscles may develop. Smooth muscle disturbance is manifested by diminished peristalsis in the gastrointestinal tract, leading to abdominal distention, nausea and vomiting and an absence of bowel sounds and elimination (paralytic ileus). Alkalosis may develop; the kidney tubules secrete hydrogen ions in excess and reabsorb bicarbonate. Less water is reabsorbed, so the patient experiences polyuria.

Hypokalemia may be *prevented* in patients known to be predisposed to it because of receiving diuretic or corticosteroid medication by increasing foods high in potassium in their diet, and by taking a supplemental preparation. Patients receiving digitalis are followed closely and observed for early symptoms of potassium depletion. Even a slightly below normal serum level may precipitate digitalis toxicity, manifested by bradycardia (slow pulse), irregular pulse, anorexia, vomiting and/or diarrhea.

Treatment of hypokalemia involves the administration of potassium orally or by intravenous infusion. If the patient's condition permits, oral administration is preferred because the low normal concentration can readily be exceeded and the problem may become one of hyperkalemia. Potassium-rich foods are given, and potassium chloride may be prescribed in liquid or tablet form. If a liquid preparation (usually 10 per cent) is prescribed, each dose is diluted in orange or grape juice and given immediately following a meal to avoid nausea and gastric irritation. The tablet preparation (e.g., Kaochlor or Slow-K) is enteric-coated to prevent gastric distress.

Considerable caution is necessary if the patient is receiving potassium by intravenous infusion. It is necessary to note what the patient's urinary output has been and to keep a close record of it during and following the infusion. Potassium is not usually prescribed if the patient has oliguria or if there is any question about the adequacy of renal function, since it is the major channel by which excess is eliminated. The nurse requires a specific order as to the rate at which the solution is to be administered. It is generally kept within the range of 8 to 20 mEq. per hour, depending upon the severity of the deficit, and is usually given in normal saline rather than glucose 5 per cent since the latter may result in still further decrease in the serum level.

Close observation is made of the individual receiving potassium by infusion. The pulse is checked at 15- to 30-minute intervals or may be continuously monitored by electrocardiogram. It is necessary to be familiar with the changes that may indicate hyperkalemia. Laboratory assessment of the serum potassium level is made at frequent intervals. The patient's responses and skeletal muscle strength are noted.

HYPERKALEMIA (EXCESS SERUM POTASSIUM). An excessive concentration of serum potassium may be the result of decreased renal excretion, increased catabolism or the administration of excessive amounts. Inadequate renal excretion is usually associated with renal failure, severe oliguria caused by dehydration, or adrenocortical insufficiency. The destruction of tissue such as occurs in crushing injuries, extensive burns, and severe infection causes the release of intracellular potassium into the extracellular fluid. Metabolic acidosis also causes hyperkalemia as potassium shifts from the cells. The disorder rarely occurs as a result of an excessive intake if renal function is normal.

Manifestations of high serum potassium levels resemble those of low levels in many respects. Neuromuscular disturbances include muscular weakness, which may progress to paralysis. The patient is lethargic, may become confused and may experience intestinal disturbance and abdominal distention. Myocardial contractions and the conduction of cardiac impulses are impaired. The electrocardiogram shows tall peaked T waves and depressed S T segments. Disordered cardiac function may progress to ventricular fibrillation (rapid, irregular, weak and ineffective contractions) and cardiac arrest.

It is important to recognize the possibility of hyperkalemia developing in patients with impaired kidney function and oliguria. The serum level is checked, the intake controlled and observations made of early indications of increased extracellular potassium.

Treatment of hyperkalemia involves measures to restrict the intake of potassium, antagonize the effects of the high concentration of potassium, move potassium into the cells and increase the excretion of potassium.

Medication containing potassium and foods high in potassium are restricted. Intravenous therapy should not include any potassium-containing solution.

A slow intravenous injection of a calcium solution (calcium gluconate or chloride) may be given by the physician to counteract the effects of the potassium on the heart. Boedeker and Dauber suggest that a calcium preparation must not be given if the patient is receiving digitalis.[6]

Glucose and regular insulin may be given intravenously to promote the movement of potassium ions into the cells. If there is no edema or cardiovascular overload, a solution of sodium bicarbonate may be added to the glucose or administered separately intravenously to enhance the shift of potassium into the cells, especially if the electrocardiogram reflects serious cardiac disturbance.

Potassium ions may be removed from the body by giving a cation-exchange resin such as sodium polystyrene sulfonate (Kayexalate). It may be prescribed to be given orally (20 to 50 Gm.) or by rectum (50 Gm. dissolved in 200 ml. of water and given as a retention enema). When oliguria is present, hemodialysis or peritoneal dialysis (see p. 63) may be used to reduce extracellular potassium ions.

Calcium (Ca²⁺)

Calcium is present in the body in a greater amount than any other mineral. It comprises about 2 per cent of the body weight and most of it (approximately 99 per cent) is in the bones and teeth in the form of calcium phosphate. A relatively small amount is present and essential in the body fluids. Normal total serum calcium is within the range of 4.5 to 5.5 mEq./L., or 9 to 11 mg./100 ml. About half of this calcium is free diffusible calcium ions (2.3 to 2.8 mEq./L., 4.5 to 5.6 mg. per 100 ml.), and the remainder is bound with plasma proteins or occurs as part of other compounds.

FUNCTIONS. In addition to being the major inorganic constituent of bone tissue, calcium also has an essential role in the blood clotting process, normal muscle contraction and relaxation, and nerve impulse transmission. It influences cellular permeability and is necessary for the activation of some enzymes; for example, it activates adenosine-triphosphatase in the release of energy for muscle fiber contraction.

REQUIREMENT, SOURCES, METABOLISM. The minimum daily requirement of an adult is estimated to be 600 to 800 mg.; the latter is equivalent to about three 224-ml. glasses of milk. Demands are greater during the growth period and during pregnancy and lactation.

Dairy products are the richest source of calcium. Other sources, although they contribute much less, include egg yolks, nuts, green leafy vegetables, legumes, and whole grains.

Absorption of calcium from the intestine is largely dependent upon the presence of vitamin D. It is also influenced by contents of the diet; a high phosphate concentration tends to reduce absorption, and free fatty acids may cause the formation of insoluble, nonabsorbable calcium salts. An increased pH (increased alkalinity) of intestinal fluid reduces absorption. Serum calcium ion concentration also affects absorption; even a slight decrease promotes increased absorption.

The principal regulator of calcium concentration in the body fluids is the hormone parathyrin, which is secreted by the parathyroid glands. A decrease in serum calcium stimulates the secretion of parathyrin, which causes a withdrawal from the stores of calcium within bone tissue, decreased excretion by the kidneys and probably increased absorption of the mineral from the intestine. When the serum level of calcium is increased above normal, parathyrin is not released, less calcium is added to the body fluids and more is excreted by the kidneys. Urinary excretion is the principal mechanism by which excess calcium is eliminated from the body. A small amount is also excreted with the intestinal digestive secretions, especially bile.

A reciprocal relationship exists between phosphorus and calcium levels in the extracellular fluids. An elevation in one accompanies a decrease in the other, but their functions are not comparable.

HYPOCALCEMIA (CALCIUM DEFICIT). A deficiency of calcium may occur as a result of a dietary deficiency, decreased intestinal absorption, hypoparathyroidism, or impaired kidney function.

Calcium is the mineral most likely to be

---

[6]E. C. Boedeker and J. H. Dauber (Eds.): Manual of Medical Therapeutics, 21st ed. Boston, Little, Brown, 1974, p. 45.

deficient in the human diet because of its limited sources. Decreased intestinal absorption may result from a deficiency of vitamin D, increased alkaline or fatty acid intestinal content, or disease of the intestine. Absorption may also be reduced if the content is hurried through the small intestine and eliminated, as in diarrhea, or if it is lost in the drainage of an intestinal fistula.

A decrease in parathyrin secretion produces an abnormally low concentration of calcium. This may occur as a result of a new growth in the parathyroid glands or of trauma during a surgical procedure, such as thyroidectomy.

Calcium depletion may also develop in chronic renal disease because of impaired reabsorption of the ions from the filtrate or because abnormal amounts of phosphate are being retained, resulting in a compensatory decrease in calcium.

Lowered serum calcium produces *manifestations* of disturbed neuromuscular function, resulting in hyperirritability and tetany. The patient complains of "pins and needles" and numbness in the extremities and twitching of the facial muscles. In more severe deficits, painful tonic spasms of skeletal muscles occur beginning in the hands, and may be followed by convulsions. Spasm of the larynx and respiratory muscles may interfere with breathing. The individual may also experience diplopia, abdominal cramps and urinary frequency. Hypocalcemia may also inhibit blood coagulation; bleeding from the mucous membranes or into the tissues, or excessive bleeding of a wound may result. Calcium ions are necessary in the conversion of prothrombin to thrombin in the blood clotting process.

Treatment depends on the cause; the deficiency, especially the acute form which is quickly and recently developed, may be rapidly corrected by the intravenous administration of a calcium solution (e.g., calcium gluconate 10 per cent; calcium chloride 5 per cent). The solution is given slowly. Following the initial administration of 10 to 30 ml. a continuous infusion of a weaker solution may be given to maintain a satisfactory calcium concentration. Laboratory assessment of serum level is made at intervals and the individual observed for positive changes or increasing severity of symptoms. Oral calcium supplements are given if the condition per-

mits. If the patient is allowed foods, those with high phosphorus content are omitted to promote maximum calcium absorption. Vitamin D, 100,000 to 200,000 units per day for 3 to 4 days, may be prescribed if the deficit is severe; the dosage is reduced in 2 to 3 days since the drug is accumulative.

If the cause is hypoparathyroidism and is not readily corrected by intravenous calcium, parathyroid extract in doses of 100 to 200 units may be prescribed.

HYPERCALCEMIA (EXCESS SERUM CALCIUM). An excess of calcium in the extracellular fluid may be caused by overadministration of vitamin D, hyperparathyroidism, thyrotoxicosis, prolonged immobilization, the breakdown of bone tissue by malignant disease, the prolonged ingestion of large amounts of milk, or impaired renal function.

Manifestations of hypercalcemia include anorexia, nausea, vomiting, loss of muscle tone, weakness, constipation, increased urinary output with resulting thirst and dehydration, and dullness and confusion which may progress to coma. The high urinary content of calcium may lead to the formation of kidney or bladder calculi. The individual may also experience pain in bones as their structure is weakened by the withdrawal of calcium.

Treatment is directed to the primary cause, and to prompt lowering of the serum calcium level because of the serious, adverse effects on neuromuscular functions. Since renal sodium excretion is accompanied by calcium excretion, an intravenous infusion of saline is given. A diuretic such as furosemide (Lasix) may also be prescribed to promote sodium excretion. Serum levels of the electrolytes sodium, potassium and calcium are determined at intervals to ascertain progress and to determine whether serum sodium and potassium are being depleted by the diuresis.

If the hypercalcemia is secondary to sarcoidosis (a collagen disease) or newgrowth a corticosteroid preparation such as prednisone may be given, which is thought to decrease intestinal absorption and renal tubular reabsorption from the glomerular filtrate. The level of serum sodium is observed in case hypernatremia develops.

If the increased serum calcium is the result of malignant neoplasm in bone tissue mithramycin, a cytotoxic chemotherapeutic agent used in malignant disease, is very occasionally administered intravenously because of its side effect of hypocalcemia. If given, the nurse observes the patient for other possible side effects, which include bleeding as a result of a decrease in thrombocytes and impaired renal function.

Dietary intake of foods with high calcium content is restricted. Care of the patient involves precautions against falls and heavy lifting because of the weakened bone structure and the predisposition to fractures.

Other disorders associated with calcium metabolism include osteoporosis, osteomalacia and rickets, discussed in Chapter 24.

Phosphorus (Phosphate; PO_4^{2-})

Phosphorus is closely associated with calcium in the body and occurs mainly in the form of phosphate. About 80 to 85 per cent of the total is combined with calcium in the bones and teeth. The remainder is combined with protein, lipid and carbohydrate compounds, and with enzymes and other substances throughout all body cells. The normal serum level is 1 to 1.5 mEq./L., or 3 to 4.5 mg./100 ml.

FUNCTIONS. Phosphate functions as a component in the structure of bone tissue and teeth. It is essential in the metabolism of almost all cells and is especially important in the absorption process of glucose and glycerol in the intestine, and in the formation of many enzymes essential to the intracellular oxidation process and production of energy. As part of the buffer system, it is active in maintaining acid-base balance. Through its combination with fatty acids and the formation of phospholipids it prevents an excess of free fatty acids.

REQUIREMENT, SOURCES, METABOLISM. The requirement is comparable to that of calcium and, since phosphorus is present in nearly all foods, a dietary deficiency is not likely to occur. Dairy products and lean meats have a high phosphate content.

The metabolism is closely associated with that of calcium as mentioned in the previous discussion. Vitamin D promotes the absorption of phosphorus from the intestine but is not actually essential for its transfer. The kidneys regulate the serum phosphorus level by their tubular excretion and reabsorption mechanisms. This regulation is influenced by the parathyrin hormone secreted by the para-

thyroid glands. With an increase above normal in the serum phosphate level, parathyrin is released to block renal tubular reabsorption of phosphorus from the glomerular filtrate, with an ensuing increase in the amount excreted in the urine. Conversely, a decrease below the normal serum level results in increased reabsorption in the renal tubules.

HYPOPHOSPHATEMIA (PHOSPHATE DEFICIT). Phosphorus may be depleted as a result of impaired intestinal absorption because of a disease such as celiac disease or sprue. It may also be low in hyperparathyroidism and in osteomalacia, in which there is an imbalance of calcium and phosphorus. The main *symptoms* of phosphorus deficit are lethargy and muscle weakness as a result of decreased energy production caused by defective enzyme systems and metabolism. The primary disease that leads to the phosphorus deficit is treated.

HYPERPHOSPHATEMIA (EXCESS PHOSPHATE). A serum phosphate level above normal may occur because of renal failure or hypoparathyroidism. Serum calcium falls and the patient may manifest the effects of hypocalcemia (see p. 90). Treatment is aimed at the primary causative condition.

Magnesium (Mg^{2-})

The adult contains about 20 to 21 Gm. of magnesium; 50 to 70 per cent is insoluble and in combination with calcium and phosphorus in bone tissue. The remainder is found in soft tissues and in body fluids. The normal serum level of magnesium is within the range of 1.5 to 2.5 mEq./L., or 2 to 3 mg./100 ml.

Magnesium is essential in the function of many enzyme systems, and also influences neuromuscular activities.

REQUIREMENT, SOURCES, METABOLISM. The suggested daily requirement for an adult is 250 to 300 mg. The main food sources are whole grains, legumes, seafood, soybeans, cocoa and milk. The metabolism of magnesium is similar to that of calcium.

HYPOMAGNESEMIA (MAGNESIUM DEFICIT). A serum magnesium level below normal may be associated with vomiting, diarrhea, prolonged gastric suctioning, starvation or hypoparathyroidism. The magnesium level may be depleted in a patient who is sustained by intravenous infusion for a long period of time without magnesium being supplied in some form. The deficiency may also occur with alcoholism or with excessive urinary losses.

Signs and symptoms of a magnesium deficit are frequently difficult to identify as such because the deficiency is likely to be compounded by other electrolyte deficiencies. The manifestations are predominantly neuromuscular disturbances evidenced by muscle weakness, twitching and tremors, which may progress to convulsions. Nystagmus (rhythmic lateral, vertical or rolling movement of the eyes) may be observed. The patient may be restless and disoriented. Hypertension and cardiac arrhythmias may develop.

The serum level is determined and the deficit corrected by intravenous administration of a magnesium sulfate or chloride preparation (e.g., 50 mEq. of $MgSO_4$ in glucose 5 per cent or in normal saline). The solution is given very slowly over 12 to 24 hours because it is a strong central nervous system depressant. This may be repeated daily until the serum concentration returns to nearly normal levels.

HYPERMAGNESEMIA (EXCESS SERUM MAGNESIUM). An excessive concentration of serum magnesium is usually associated with renal insufficiency. Treatment is directed toward promoting urinary output; hemodialysis or peritoneal dialysis may be used.

Chlorine (Cl⁻)

Chlorine is a vital electrolyte for the maintenance of homeostasis, and occurs in the body as the chloride ion. It is found in greatest concentration in extracellular fluids; it is the major anion in the extracellular compartment.

FUNCTIONS. Chloride ions, along with sodium, help to maintain normal extracellular osmotic pressure and regulate water balance. Chloride is important in the chloride shift that occurs between red blood cells and plasma (see p. 96). In this latter function it contributes to acid-base equilibrium. Chloride ions are also essential for the production of hydrochloric acid by gastric mucosal cells to provide the necessary acid medium for normal gastric digestion.

REQUIREMENT, SOURCES, METABOLISM. No actual requirement for chlorine has been established. The intake is satisfactory if the sodium intake is adequate. Both intake and output are inseparable from those of sodium. Chloride is almost completely absorbed from the intestine; only an insignificant amount is lost in feces. It is excreted by the kidneys according to the need to maintain acid-base balance. The reabsorption of chloride ions, as with sodium, is promoted by adrenocorticoid secretion, especially aldosterone.

Disorders of chloride metabolism generally are associated with disorders of sodium; excessive sodium losses, as in Addison's disease (adrenocortical insufficiency), diaphoresis, and diarrhea, are accompanied by chloride depletion.

A loss of chloride ions in excess of sodium may occur with the loss of gastric secretions incurred by prolonged vomiting, gastric suctioning, or pyloric or duodenal obstruction, causing hypochloremia. As a result of the chloride deficit there is an increase in bicarbonate ions, and alkalosis develops.

ACID-BASE BALANCE

Normal cellular activities require that the concentration of hydrogen ions (H^+) in body fluids be maintained within a very limited range.

The acidity or alkalinity of a solution depends upon the concentration of hydrogen ions (H^+). When these are in excess of those contained in a neutral solution, the chemical reaction is *acid;* if fewer, it is *alkaline.* Normally body fluids are slightly alkaline; slight deviations in hydrogen ion concentration results in an imbalance that is disturbing and threatening to body metabolism.

Acids are substances which contain hydrogen ions that can be freed or donated by chemical reaction to other substances. Conversely, *bases* are chemical substances that can combine with hydrogen ions in a chemical reaction. A compound that completely dissociates its hydrogen ions is referred to as a strong acid; for example, hydrochloric acid, which completely dissociates when placed in water, is a strong acid ($HCl \rightarrow H^+$ Cl^-). One that only partially frees its hydrogen ions is referred to as a weak acid; for example, a molecule of carbonic acid dissociates into one hydrogen ion and a bicarbonate ion ($H_2CO_3 \rightarrow H^+ HCO_3^-$), and therefore is termed a weak acid.

The symbol pH is used to express the hydrogen ion concentration, or the degree to which a solution is acidic or alkaline. It represents the negative logarithm of the hydrogen ion concentration. For example, a neutral solution, such as water, with a pH of 7 contains 10^{-7} or $\frac{1}{10,000,000}$ or 0.0000001 gram of hydrogen ions per liter. A solution with a pH of 6 contains 10^{-6} or $\frac{1}{1,000,000}$ or 0.000001 gram of hydrogen ions per liter; it contains 10 times as many hydrogen ions as a solution with a pH of 7. A pH of 8 indicates a hydrogen ion concentration per liter of 10^{-8} or $\frac{1}{100,000,000}$ or 0.00000001 gram. Since a solution of pH 7 is neutral, as the pH decreases below 7, the hydrogen ion concentration increases, and the solution becomes acidic. Conversely, as the pH increases above 7 and the hydrogen ion concentration decreases, the solution becomes alkaline. In other words, a pH of 7 denotes neutrality. A pH of less than 7 indicates acidity, and the smaller the figure, the greater the degree of acidity; a pH greater than 7 denotes alkalinity, and the greater the figure, the greater the degree of alkalinity.

Obviously the use of the symbol pH is less cumbersome than the expression of the hydrogen ion concentration by fraction or decimal.

ACID-BASE REGULATION

Body fluids normally have a pH of 7.35 to 7.45. Certain mechanisms operate to maintain the normal pH within this very narrow range; a variation of a few tenths in either direction is incompatible with normal cellular activity and life.

An arterial blood pH of below 6.8 or over 7.8 is considered incompatible with life. Cellular chemical processes produce relatively large amounts of acids, but the body is equipped with control mechanisms that maintain the required normal alkalinity.

The chief acid resulting from metabolism is carbonic acid, which is formed by the chemical combination of water and carbon dioxide ($H_2O + CO_2 \rightarrow H_2CO_3$). The combination is promoted by the enzyme carbonic anhydrase within the cells. In addition to carbonic acid, cellular activity produces a substantial quantity of stronger acids such as sulfuric, phosphoric, lactic, uric, acetoacetic, β-hydroxybutyric and hydrochloric acid. The acids must be rapidly neutralized or weakened by chemical reactions and, since their production is continuous, there must be a constant elimination of them from the body. The volatile carbonic acid is removed by the lungs by eliminating carbon dioxide; the nonvolatile acids are excreted by the kidneys.

Control Mechanisms

The optimum pH of body fluids is maintained by acid-base buffer systems in the body fluids, respiratory excretion of carbon dioxide, and selective excretion of hydrogen ions or bases by the kidneys.

BUFFER SYSTEMS. Buffers are substances which tend to stabilize or maintain the constancy of the pH of a solution when an acid or a base is added to it. They do this by rapidly converting a strong acid or base to a weaker one which does not dissociate as rapidly.

A buffer system consists of two substances — a weak acid and a salt of that acid. The buffer systems of body fluids include the following pairs:

$\dfrac{\text{carbonic acid}}{\text{sodium (or potassium) bicarbonate}}$	$\dfrac{H_2CO_3}{NaHCO_3 \text{ (or } KHCO_3)}$
$\dfrac{\text{acid phosphate}}{\text{alkaline phosphate}}$	$\dfrac{NaH_2PO_4}{Na_2HPO_4}$
$\dfrac{\text{acid plasma protein}}{\text{proteinate}}$	$\dfrac{HPr}{Na \text{ proteinate}}$
$\dfrac{\text{hemoglobin}}{\text{potassium hemoglobinate}}$	$\dfrac{Hb}{KHb}$
$\dfrac{\text{oxyhemoglobin}}{\text{potassium oxyhemoglobinate}}$	$\dfrac{H \cdot HbO_2}{KHbO_2}$

The principal buffer pair of the plasma is the carbonic acid–sodium bicarbonate system. Maintenance of a normal pH is greatly dependent upon the ratio of carbonic acid concentration to that of bicarbonate, which normally occurs as 1:20. *As long as there are 20 bicarbonate ions to one carbonic acid molecule, the pH will remain within normal range regardless of the actual amounts of the two substances.*

When a strong acid is added to a fluid that contains the carbonic acid–bicarbonate system, it combines with the bicarbonate ion to form carbonic acid. Thus, the strong acid which dissociates readily to yield many hydrogen ions is replaced by a weaker acid which frees fewer hydrogen ions. This reaction may be illustrated by the following equations: hydrochloric acid + sodium bicarbonate yields carbonic acid + sodium chloride $(HCL + NaHCO_3 \rightarrow H_2CO_3 + NaCl)$; lactic acid + sodium bicarbonate yields carbonic acid + sodium lactate $(HLa + NaHCO_3 \rightarrow H_2CO_3 + NaLa)$. If a strong base is added to a fluid containing this buffer system, the base combines with the carbonic acid to form bicarbonate (weaker base) and water as shown in the following: sodium hydroxide + carbonic acid yields sodium bicarbonate + water $(NaOH + H_2CO_3 \rightarrow NaHCO_3 + HOH)$.

When an acid is added to a solution with the acid phosphate–alkaline phosphate system, it combines with the alkaline phosphate to form acid phosphate. To illustrate, hydrochloric acid + sodium alkaline phosphate yields sodium acid phosphate and sodium chloride $(HCl + Na_2HPO_4 \rightarrow NaH_2PO_4 + NaCl)$; and carbonic acid + sodium alkaline phosphate yields sodium acid phosphate and sodium bicarbonate $(H_2CO_3 + Na_2HPO_4 \rightarrow NaH_2PO_4 + NaHCO_3)$. The phosphate system is especially active in the kidneys where the acid phosphate that has been formed is eliminated.

Oxyhemoglobin and reduced hemoglobin act as the acids of buffer pairs in the erythrocytes, and the potassium salt of the hemoglobin forms the other part of the systems. Oxyhemoglobin is a stronger acid (i.e., it dissociates its hydrogen ions more freely) than reduced hemoglobin and carbonic acid, and the latter is a stronger acid than reduced hemoglobin. When carbon dioxide diffuses into the red blood cells carbonic acid is formed:

$$CO_2 + H_2O \xrightarrow{\text{carbonic anhydrase}} H_2CO_3$$

This is also a reversible reaction. The carbonic acid is buffered by potassium hemoglobinate to form the weak acid hemoglobin and potassium bicarbonate $(H_2CO_3 + KHb \rightarrow HHb + KHCO_3)$. When the acid hemoglobin is oxygenated to oxyhemoglobin in the lungs it becomes a stronger acid and is rapidly buffered by potassium bicarbonate to form potassium oxyhemoglobinate and carbonic acid $(HHbO_2 + KHCO_3 \rightarrow KHbO_2 + H_2CO_3)$. Carbonic anhydrase reverses its action and the carbonic acid is broken down into carbon dioxide and water; the carbon dioxide diffuses out of the cells into the blood and into the alveoli of the lungs (see Fig. 5–3).

RESPIRATORY REGULATION. A second important factor in the maintenance of the normal pH of body fluids is the elimination of carbon dioxide in respiration. Carbon dioxide is constantly produced in cellular metabolism and diffuses from the cells into the blood and erythrocytes. As a result, carbon dioxide is in greater concentration in the blood when it enters the pulmonary capillaries than in the air in the alveoli of the lungs. The pressure gradient results in some carbon dioxide diffusing from the blood into the alveoli from which it is exhaled. This reduces the amount available to form carbonic acid in the body fluids.

The neurons of the respiratory control center in the medulla are extremely sensitive to the concentration of carbon dioxide and hydrogen ions in body fluids. An increase in either stimulates the center to increase the rate and volume of respirations so more carbon dioxide may be eliminated. Conversely, a decrease in the concentration of carbon dioxide or hydrogen ions below the normal results in slower shallow respirations so that carbon dioxide is retained to form carbonic acid.

Obviously any condition that impairs the capacity of the lungs to eliminate carbon dioxide from the body predisposes to an increase in the carbonic acid level and a decrease in the pH of body fluids; on the other hand, increased pulmonary ventilation may increase the pH of the body fluids by the excessive loss of carbon dioxide.

KIDNEY REGULATION. The kidneys play an important role in maintaining the acid-base balance by excreting hydrogen ions and forming bicarbonate in amounts as indicated by the pH of the blood. The cells of the distal portion of the renal tubules are sensitive to changes in the pH; when there is a decrease below the normal, hydrogen ions are excreted and bicarbonate is formed and retained. Conversely, when there is an increased alkalinity above the normal, hydro-

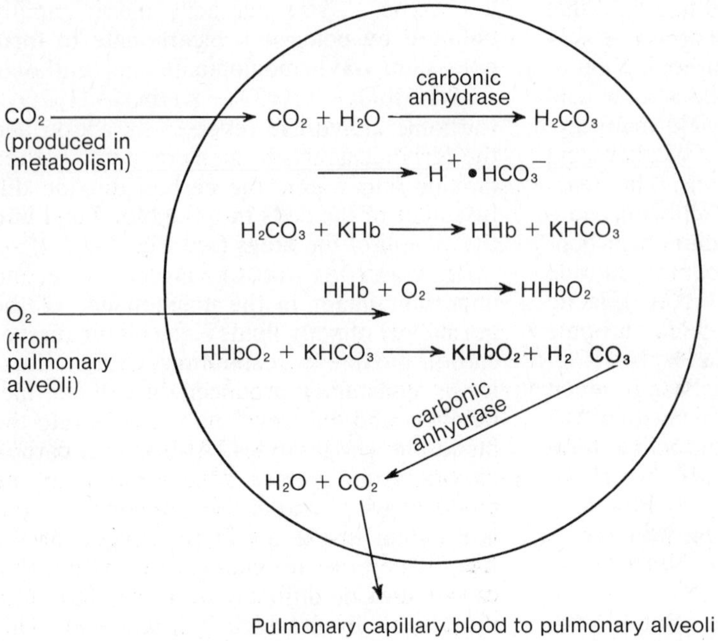

FIGURE 5–3 Role of the red blood cell in pH regulation.

gen ions are conserved and base-forming ions are excreted. In other words, the kidneys may excrete many or few hydrogen ions and form more or less bicarbonate according to the need.

The elimination of acid ions and the formation of bicarbonate involve the following processes:

1. Within the renal tubular cells, carbon dioxide and water form carbonic acid

$$(CO_2 + H_2O \xrightarrow{\text{carbonic anhydrase}} H_2CO_3)$$

which ionizes to release hydrogen and bicarbonate ions (H^+ HCO_3^-). The hydrogen ion moves out into the renal tubule.

2. The alkaline sodium phosphate (Na_2HPO_4) in the tubular fluid is converted to acid sodium phosphate (NaH_2PO_4) by accepting a hydrogen ion and releasing a sodium ion (Na^+). The acid sodium phosphate is excreted in the urine.

3. The sodium ion passes into the tubular cell in exchange for the hydrogen ion that moved out. There it combines with the bicarbonate ion to form sodium bicarbonate ($NaHCO_3$), which diffuses into the blood.

4. Additional hydrogen ions may be eliminated by the kidneys to form ammonia and eliminate it as an acid salt. Within the tubular cells, the amino acid glutamine is broken down and ammonia (NH_3) is released into the tubule. Sodium chloride in the tubular fluid ionizes ($NaCl \rightarrow Na^+ Cl^-$); the ammonia combines with a hydrogen ion and a chlorine ion to form ammonium chloride ($NH_3 + H^+ + Cl^- \rightarrow NH_4Cl$), which is eliminated in the urine. The sodium ion passes into the tubular cell to form sodium bicarbonate, which passes into the blood.

In summary, to preserve the normal pH, the kidneys secrete hydrogen ions into the renal tubules in exchange for sodium ions, acidify alkaline phosphate, form and retain sodium bicarbonate and form an ammonium acid salt (see Fig. 5–4).

ACID-BASE IMBALANCE

Normally the pH of body fluids is maintained within the narrow range of 7.35 to 7.45. When the alkalinity falls below 7.35 the condition is known as acidosis or acidemia; when it is above 7.45 the condition is referred to as alkalosis or alkalemia.

Tests for Acid-Base Imbalance

Significant blood tests used in determining an acid-base imbalance include the following:

1. BLOOD GASES. An estimation is made of the carbon dioxide and oxygen concentrations of the blood. These may be expressed in volumes per cent, or as mm. Hg partial pressure. The normal values for the oxygen in arterial blood is 17 to 21 volumes per cent, or a tension of 80 to 100 mm. Hg. The latter is recorded as paO_2 80 to 100 mm. Hg. If a sample of venous blood is used, the normal value is 10 to 16 volumes per cent (pO_2 10 to 16 vol. %).

The normal value for carbon dioxide in arterial blood is in the range of 35 to 45 mm. Hg. Plasma normally contains 21 to 30 mEq./L., or 50 to 70 volumes per cent of carbon dioxide. This represents the carbon dioxide in the blood as carbonic acid and bicarbonate, as well as that free in solution.

Arterial blood values for blood gases are used clinically more often than venous estimations. The collection of arterial blood samples for the evaluation of blood gases involves certain measures to prevent exposure of the specimen to the air. True values cannot be obtained if air contacts the blood sample.

A readily accessible artery, such as the brachial at the antecubital space, the radial or femoral, is used. The site is cleansed with an antiseptic. A solution of heparin is drawn up into the syringe to be used to rinse the

inner surface, and is then discarded. All air must be excluded from the syringe and needle.

When the needle is passed through the arterial wall, the patient is likely to experience deep sharp pain; the patient is advised of this during the preparation for the procedure and asked not to move the limb. Anticipating this possibility, the assisting nurse provides the necessary restraint.

Blood flows readily into the syringe because of the arterial blood pressure and pulsations. When the needle is withdrawn it is quickly inserted into a rubber stopper or capped to prevent the entry of air. The syringe is placed in a container of crushed ice, labeled and, with the requisition, is delivered immediately to the laboratory. If the analysis is delayed, true values are altered.

Pressure is applied to the arterial puncture site for at least 5 minutes. When the nurse is assured that there is no bleeding, a sterile dressing is applied. The area is checked and re-dressed at frequent intervals.

2. CARBON DIOXIDE COMBINING POWER. This provides information as to the amount of carbon dioxide carried in the blood in the form of bicarbonate. The normal is expressed as 50 to 65 volumes per cent, or 21 to 28 mEq./L.

3. pH. The hydrogen ion concentration

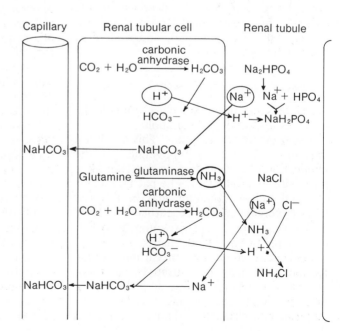

FIGURE 5–4 The role of the kidneys in pH control.

is determined by an estimation of the pH. The normal value is 7.35 to 7.45.

4. SERUM ELECTROLYTES. It is necessary to determine the serum concentration of various electrolytes, especially sodium, bicarbonate and potassium. See p. 80 for normal levels.

5. URINALYSIS. Analysis of the urine may also provide useful information. Significant factors are: a. The pH of the urine. The normal range is 5 to 8, depending upon the diet and drug therapy.

b. Total volume. Normally a minimum of 1000 to 1500 ml. are excreted in 24 hours.

c. Amounts of various solids, ammonia, bicarbonate, calcium, chloride, ketones and potassium.

Acidosis

When the hydrogen ion concentration is increased in body fluids, the three control mechanisms (buffer systems, respiration, and kidney activity) endeavor to reestablish a normal pH. If the carbonic acid–bicarbonate ratio can be kept normal by increased respiratory elimination of carbon dioxide and by increased kidney elimination of hydrogen ions and formation of sodium bicarbonate, the pH is kept within normal range. The condition is then said to be *compensated acidosis*. If the mechanisms cannot compensate adequately, a decrease in the carbonic acid–bicarbonate ratio develops, the pH falls below normal, and a state of uncompensated acidosis exists.

Types of Acidosis

Acidosis may be classified according to the cause as respiratory or metabolic.

RESPIRATORY ACIDOSIS. This condition develops as a result of hypoventilation; the elimination of carbon dioxide does not keep pace with its production. The $paCO_2$ level is elevated and the condition may be referred to as hypercapnia or hypercarbia. The level of serum carbonic acid rises above normal and the pH of body fluids decreases.

Inadequate elimination of carbon dioxide by the lungs may be caused by acute or chronic respiratory disease (e.g., pneumonia, chronic obstructive lung disease such as emphysema), circulatory failure or impaired perfusion of the alveoli, depression of the respiratory center by drugs or cerebral disease, or weakness of the respiratory muscles. Impaired carbon dioxide excretion is usually accompanied by reduced paO_2 (hypoxia) because of the decreased alveolar gas exchange.

The kidneys respond to the increased level of carbon dioxide by secreting more hydrogen ions into the tubules for excretion in exchange for sodium ions. The latter combine with the bicarbonate ions left behind by the hydrogen ions, forming sodium bicarbonate. *The serum bicarbonate level becomes elevated.* The kidneys also increase their formation and excretion of ammonia, which uses more hydrogen ions. These renal compensatory responses require one or more days to be effective and can do so only if there is adequate blood circulation. The compensation is of greater value in acidosis associated with chronic respiratory disease such as emphysema and bronchiectasis.

MANIFESTATIONS. The retention of carbon dioxide and the decreased pH cause a depression of the central nervous system. The patient is restless and apprehensive and may complain of headache at the onset, but gradually his mental responses become slow and dulled. If ventilation does not improve he may be disoriented and eventually lapse into coma. Peripheral vasodilation and a rapid pulse may be associated with acute respiratory acidosis. If the acidosis is caused by chronic respiratory disease, the individual's respirations are labored and the expiratory phase is prolonged.

TREATMENT. Treatment is directed toward relieving the respiratory insufficiency. Tracheal intubation or a tracheostomy with the use of a mechanical ventilator may be necessary. If the respiratory center has been depressed by a drug, the appropriate antidote is prescribed. For further details of the care required in respiratory insufficiency see p 431.

METABOLIC ACIDOSIS. This occurs as a result of an excessive production or ingestion of acid, the retention of nonvolatile acid or depletion of the bicarbonate base.

An excessive production may be seen in uncontrolled diabetes mellitus and starvation in which there is an excessive catabolism of fat by the cells as a source of energy. Ketone bodies, e.g., acetoacetic acid, βhydroxybutyric acid, and acetone, are produced in abnormally large amounts and at a greater rate than that at which the cells can complete their oxidation to energy, carbon dioxide and water. The acids deplete the bicarbonate buffer, and the pH of the body fluid falls.

Overdosage or prolonged administration of ammonium chloride, acetylsalicylic acid (aspirin) or acetazolamide (Diamox) may give rise to acidosis. With ammonium chloride, the ammonium radical is converted to urea, leaving hydrochloric acid, which uses up bicarbonate in buffering. Acetazolamide may depress the ability of the renal tubular cells to form sodium bicarbonate and secrete hydrogen ions to acidify urine.

A decreased urinary output, whether due to renal disease or a condition such as severe dehydration or shock, will obviously result in the retention of nonvolatile acids which are constantly produced in metabolism. Respirations and the buffers can compensate for a period of time, but eventually the bicarbonate is depleted as the acids accumulate and no bicarbonate is being formed by the renal tubular cells. In chronic kidney disease, the tubular cells may be damaged and their ability to secrete hydrogen ions and form sodium bicarbonate and ammonia is impaired. As a result, acidification of the urine is diminished and excessive amounts of hydrogen ions are retained.

A frequent cause of metabolic acidosis is an abnormal loss of alkaline secretions that are normally reabsorbed. The secretions that comprise the intestinal juice have a high sodium and potassium bicarbonate concentration; diarrhea, an intestinal fistula, vomiting or suction of fluids from the intestine may deplete the body's bicarbonate.

In an effort to decrease the carbonic acid level, respirations are increased in rate and volume to promote carbon dioxide elimination. The serum bicarbonate concentration is reduced and insufficient to buffer the increased nonvolatile acids. The kidneys increase hydrogen ion secretion into the distal portion of the tubules for elimination in the urine.

MANIFESTATIONS. The patient complains of headache, fatigue and drowsiness. The decreased pH causes a depression of the central nervous system; mental responses are slow and dulled and, if the acidosis is not corrected, the patient may become disoriented and eventually comatose. Anorexia, nausea and vomiting are common. Respirations increase in rate and volume (hyperpnea). The urinary output is increased; dehydration develops rapidly as a result of the vomiting, diuresis and decreased intake. The serum bicarbonate level is reduced and disturbances in the concentration of other electrolytes develop. Buffering of the increased fixed (nonvolatile) acids results in the movement of potassium out of the cells; the serum potassium level rises. This may necessitate treatment for hyperkalemia (see p. 89). The elimination of potassium in the urine will be increased. Later, when the acidosis is corrected, potassium ions move back into the cells and may cause a potassium deficit (see p. 89).

TREATMENT. The primary cause is treated and, if renal function is not impaired, fluid and the indicated electrolyte deficits are replaced by intravenous infusion. If acidosis has developed as a result of renal insufficiency, hemodialysis or peritoneal dialysis may be necessary.

Implications for Nursing

OBSERVATIONS. The patient with acidosis is critically ill and requires close observation of vital signs, fluid balance, orientation and level of consciousness. Frequent collection of urine specimens may be required and may necessitate the use of a retention catheter. Blood specimens are taken at frequent intervals for pH and electrolyte assessment. The required equipment is kept readily available and the necessary assistance is provided in the collection of the blood. The nurse is alert for signs and symptoms of specific electrolyte deficits or excesses, especially potassium.

FLUIDS. If the patient is conscious, oral fluids are encouraged. The fluids permitted may vary with the cause of the acidosis. For example, salted broth, orange juice and milk may be given in diabetic acidosis, but in the case of acidosis associated with renal failure these may be contraindicated because of the potassium and sodium content. Parenteral fluids are administered; the solutions given are based on the blood chemistry reports and kidney function. The rate of flow should be defined by the physician; frequently a limited amount is given fairly rapidly if the patient is dehydrated, and then the rate is slowed.

MOUTH CARE. Frequent mouth care is especially important because of the hyperpnea, mouth breathing, vomiting and dehydration that commonly accompany acidosis.

PRECAUTIONS. Safety precautions are necessary if the patient manifests disorientation. If comatose, all the points applicable to the care of an unconscious patient will require consideration (see p. 159).

PSYCHOLOGICAL SUPPORT. The patient and family require support and reassurance that everything possible is being done. They are kept informed as to the progress and advised of treatment procedures. Time is taken to listen to their concerns and to answer their questions.

Alkalosis

This is an acid-base imbalance in which there is an increase in the pH in excess of 7.45 due to a carbonic acid deficit or an excessive amount of bicarbonate. It may be classified as respiratory or metabolic.

Types of Alkalosis

RESPIRATORY ALKALOSIS. This disorder is due to an excessive loss of carbonic acid by hyperventilation. Carbon dioxide is being excreted by the lungs in excess of its production. The rapid deep breathing may be caused by an anxiety state, hysteria or central nervous system disease that is producing overstimulation of the respiratory center, high fever or hypoxia.

EFFECTS AND MANIFESTATIONS. The pH of the blood and the ratio of carbonic acid to bicarbonate are increased. If the condition is prolonged, large amounts of base are excreted by the kidneys, resulting in increased losses of sodium and potassium. There is a corresponding decrease in the excretion of chloride and hydrogen ions.

The patient frequently complains of dizziness. Tetany may develop as a result of increased neuromuscular irritability; signs and symptoms of this are tingling in the distal portions of the extremities, cramps, and tonic spasms of muscles which may progress to convulsions.

IMPLICATIONS FOR NURSING. If the condition is of psychological origin, an explanation of the overbreathing and its effects may lead to voluntary correction. An effort is also made to help the patient resolve his concerns. He is encouraged to verbalize his fears or problems. The prescription of a tranquilizing drug may be necessary to reduce the anxiety.

Having the patient rebreathe his own carbon dioxide by breathing into a paper bag is helpful. Inhalation of 5 per cent carbon dioxide in oxygen may be ordered.

Oxygen inhalation may be ordered if the respiratory alkalosis is caused by hypoxia and, if the latter is due to anemia, a transfusion of whole blood or packed cells may be administered (see p. 264).

METABOLIC ALKALOSIS. This increase in pH may develop as the result of an abnormal loss of hydrochloric acid from the stomach in vomiting or gastric suctioning, excessive ingestion of alkaline substances (e.g., sodium bicarbonate) or a potassium deficit. The plasma concentration of bicarbonate is elevated with a corresponding increase in the pH and carbonic acid–bicarbonate ratio.

EFFECTS AND MANIFESTATIONS. Respirations become slow and shallow in an effort to increase the carbonic acid content of the blood. If the hypopnea is prolonged, it may produce an oxygen deficiency and the patient become cyanotic.

Kidney compensation is by conservation of hydrogen and chloride ions and by increased excretion of bicarbonate. If the alkalosis is caused by vomiting, there is likely to be an associated dehydration which leads to decreased urinary output and reduced renal compensation.

The patient is restless and apprehensive; tremors and twitching may be observed and tetany may ensue. Nausea, vomiting and diarrhea may be present.

IMPLICATIONS FOR NURSING. An intravenous infusion of normal saline is usually ordered immediately in the treatment of metabolic alkalosis. The plasma concentration of potassium is determined and, if there is a deficit, potassium in some form is prescribed. It may be administered orally or intravenously; if the latter method is used, the rate of flow is specified by the physician. It is usually given very slowly and limited to a definite amount in a certain number of hours.

The patient receiving a potassium solution intravenously is observed closely for signs of hyperkalemia, which include a slow, weak pulse, restlessness and muscular weakness. Ammonium chloride may be prescribed intravenously or by mouth, especially if the alkalosis is due to vomiting, which depletes the chloride ions. Precautions similar to those mentioned above in relation to parenteral potassium administration are necessary if ammonium chloride is given intravenously.

Close observations are made of the vital signs. The intake and output are recorded accurately to serve as a basis for fluid administration. Signs and symptoms of a deficit or excess of potassium are noted.

Early signs of disturbed neuromuscular functioning and tetany should be noted and reported promptly. These include muscle twitching and spasms. Trousseau's sign, which is characteristic of the onset of tetany, may be positive. It involves carpal spasm, which can be elicited by compression of the upper arm.

Frequent blood specimens are collected to determine the pH, serum electrolyte levels and blood gases. The necessary equipment and assistance should be readily available to prevent delays. The laboratory data are carefully followed as a basis for care and therapy.

Safety precautions are taken in the event of the patient becoming confused.

References

Books

Beeson, Paul B., and McDermott, Walsh (Eds.): Textbook of Medicine, 15th ed. Philadelphia, W. B. Saunders, 1979.

Black, D. A. K.: Essentials of Fluid Balance, 4th ed. Oxford, Blackwell, 1967.

Boedecker, E. C., and Dauber, J. H. (Eds.): Manual of Medical Therapeutics, 21st ed. Boston, Little, Brown, 1974. Chapter 2.

Chapman, W. H., et al.: The Urinary System: An Integrated Approach. Philadelphia, W. B. Saunders, 1973. Chapters 1, 4.

Davenport, H. W.: The ABC of Acid-Base Chemistry, 6th ed. Chicago, University of Chicago Press, 1974.

Ganong, William F.: Review of Medical Physiology, 7th ed. Los Altos, Cal., Lange, 1975. Chapters 1, 40.

Goldberger, E.: A Primer of Water, Electrolyte and Acid-Base Syndromes, 5th ed. Philadelphia, Lea and Febiger, 1975.

Guyton, Arthur C.: Textbook of Medical Physiology, 5th ed. Philadelphia, W. B. Saunders, 1976. Chapters 20, 33, 37.

Harper, H. A.: Review of Physiological Chemistry, 15th ed. Los Altos, Cal., Lange, 1975. Chapters 1[1], 19, Appendix.

Harrington, Joan, and Brener, Etta Rae: Patient Care in Renal Failure. Philadelphia, W. B. Saunders, 1973. Chapter 3.

Krupp, M. A., and Chatton, M. J.: Current Medical Diagnosis and Treatment. Los Altos, Cal., Lange, 1975. Chapter 2.

Masoro, Edward J., and Siegel, Paul D.: Acid-Base Regulation: Its Physiology, Pathophysiology, and the Interpretation of Blood-Gas Analysis. Philadelphia, W. B. Saunders, 1971.

Nave, Carl R., and Nave, Brenda C.: Physics for the Health Sciences. Philadelphia, W. B. Saunders, 1975. Chapter 9.

Pitts, R. F.: Physiology of the Kidney and Body Fluids, 3rd ed. Chicago, Year Book Medical Publishers, 1974.

Robinson, J. R.: Fundamentals of Acid-Base Regulation, 4th ed. London, Blackwell, 1972.

Thorn, G. W., et al. (Eds.): Harrison's Principles of Internal Medicine, 8th ed. New York, McGraw-Hill, 1977.

Periodicals

Boyd, D. R., and Baker, R. J.: "Osmometry: A New Bedside Laboratory Aid for the Management of Surgical Patients." Surg. Clin. North Am., Vol. 51, No. 1 (Feb. 1971), pp. 241–250.

DeVeber, George A.: "Fluid and Electrolyte Problems in the Postoperative Period." Nurs. Clin. North Am., Vol. 1, No. 2 (June 1966), pp. 275–284.

Gentry, W. D., et al.: "Anxiety and Urinary Sodium and Potassium as Stress Indicators on Admission to a Coronary Care Unit." Heart Lung, Vol. 2, No. 6 (Nov.–Dec. 1973), pp. 875–877.

Grant, M. M., and Kubo, W. M.: "Assessing a Patient's Hydration Status." Am. J. Nurs., Vol. 75, No. 8 (Aug. 1975), pp. 1306–1311.

Kee, J. L.: "The Critically Ill Patient and Possible Fluid and Electrolyte Imbalances." Nurs. '72, Vol. 2, No. 3 (March 1972), pp. 6–11.

———, and Gregory, A. P.: "The ABC (and mEq's) of Fluid Balance in Children." Nurs. '74, Vol. 4, No. 6 (June 1974), pp. 28–36.

Lee, C. A., et al.: "Extracellular Volume Imbalance." Am. J. Nurs., Vol. 74, No. 5 (May 1974), pp. 888–891.

———, "What to do When Acid-Base Problems Hang in the Balance." Nurs. '75, Vol. 5, No. 8 (Aug. 1975), pp. 32–37.

Levenstein, B. P.: "Intravenous Therapy: A Nursing Specialty." Nurs. Clin. North Am., Vol. 1, No. 2 (June 1966), pp. 259–267.

Metheny, N. A.: "Water and Electrolyte Balance in the Postoperative Patient." Nurs. Clin. North Am., Vol. 10, No. 1 (March 1975), pp. 49–57.

Reed, G. M.: "Confused About Potassium? Here's a Clear Concise Guide." Nurs. '74, Vol. 3, No. 3 (March 1974), pp. 21–27.

Sharer, J. E.: "Reviewing Acid-Base Balance." Am. J. Nurs., Vol. 75, No. 6 (June 1975), pp. 980–983.

Trunkey, D. D.: "Review of Current Concepts in Fluid and Electrolyte Management." Heart Lung, Vol. 4, No. 1 (Jan.–Feb. 1975), pp. 115–121.

Voda, A. M.: "Body Water Dynamics." Am. J. Nurs., Vol. 70, No. 12 (Dec. 1970), pp. 2594–2601.

Wareham, Darryl V., and Deliganis, Sam G.: "Rational Fluid and Electrolyte Therapy Utilization Review." Drug Intell. Clin. Pharm., Vol. 11, No. 9 (Sept. 1977), pp. 549–553.

Wilson, J. A.: "Infection Control in Intravenous Therapy." Heart Lung, Vol. 5, No. 3 (May-June 1976), pp. 430–436.

6

Body Temperature

INTRODUCTION

Accurate monitoring of body temperature is an important nursing measure. Temperature reflects the heat content of the body, and may provide information during an illness or following an injury that contributes to making the diagnosis and decisions as to the necessary therapeutic care. It may signal a change in the patient's condition that indicates the need for immediate action.

Body temperature is the balance between the heat produced and acquired by the body and the amount lost. Normally, the body maintains a relatively constant temperature within the range of 36° to 37° C. (97° to 98.6° F.) regardless of the environmental temperature (Fig. 6–1). For this reason, man is classified as homoiothermic or warm-blooded as opposed to the poikilothermic or cold-blooded species whose body temperature fluctuates with variations in the environmental temperature.

HEAT PRODUCTION AND DISSIPATION

Constancy of a temperature of 36° to 37° C., which favors normal cellular activity, is maintained by physiological processes that preserve a balance between heat production and heat dissipation. An increased production of heat is compensated by increasing the loss; conversely, a decrease below normal body temperature initiates a decrease in the heat loss as well as an increase in the production of heat.

Heat is generated in the body by chemical reactions within the cells. The more active the tissue, the greater is its production of heat; as a result, especially large amounts of heat are produced by the muscles and liver. A small amount may be acquired from external sources by radiation and conduction. Heat production is dependent upon cellular activity, and biochemical reactions (metabolism) increase as body temperature increases. A decrease in body temperature slows the rate of cellular activity, decreasing heat production. Body temperature may also be increased by the hormones thyroxine, epinephrine, norepinephrine and progesterone.

Normally, an excess of heat is produced within the body and must be eliminated to maintain a normal temperature. The excess is dissipated by the physical processes of radiation, conduction, convection and vaporization. Most of it is lost through the skin by evaporation and the remainder is eliminated in respirations and excreta.

Radiation is the process by which radiant energy is transmitted from one object to another without direct contact. Conduction is the transfer of heat between two objects that are in contact. Convection is the process by which heat is carried away from a surface by air currents passing over it, such as occurs when a fan is used. Evaporation of 1 gram of water from the surface of the skin and respiratory tract utilizes about 0.58 calorie. The sweat glands pour their secretion onto the skin surface; the heat of the blood in peripheral vessels is utilized in

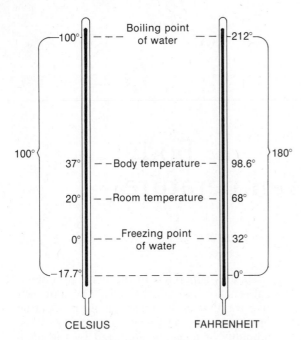

FIGURE 6-1 Two temperature scales, F. and C.

evaporating the secretion. Some vaporization takes place constantly, but the amount taking place on the skin varies. If there is a need to increase the heat loss, the sweat glands increase their secretion and peripheral vasodilation occurs, resulting in increased vaporization. If there is a need to conserve body heat, less moisture is released onto the skin surface and vasoconstriction reduces circulation to the periphery.

Heat loss by radiation, conduction and convection depends on a temperature gradient. If the environmental temperature is equal to or greater than that of the body, these processes are ineffective and heat dissipation becomes completely dependent on the evaporation process.

TEMPERATURE REGULATION

Temperature-regulating mechanisms are essential to prevent the damaging effects on body tissues by extremes of heat and cold.

Responses to changes in body temperature are evoked by sensory nerve impulses that originate in temperature receptors in the skin and by the direct effect of the blood temperature on the hypothalamus. Guyton suggests that it is likely that there are also temperature receptors in some internal organs.[1]

Receptor cells that are sensitive to heat and cold are located in the skin. When changes in the cutaneous temperature occur, the receptors give rise to nerve impulses that are delivered to the cerebral cortex and hypothalamus of the brain. Those that reach the cerebral cortex make the individual conscious of the temperature change. He may then produce voluntary responses to aid in correcting the change. For example, if he experiences the sensation of cold, he may voluntarily increase muscle activity to generate more heat, seek a warmer environment and add clothing to reduce the heat loss. In a hot environment, the voluntary responses might be to decrease activity in order to lower the heat production and to change to lighter clothing to permit more radiation.

In the anterior portion of the hypothalamus is a group of neurons that is referred to as the thermostatic or heat-regulating center. This center responds to cutaneous temperature impulses and to changes in the temperature of the blood. When the body temperature rises above normal, impulses

---

[1] Arthur C. Guyton: Textbook of Medical Physiology, 5th ed. Philadelphia, W. B. Saunders, 1976, p. 961.

are discharged that cause dilation of the cutaneous blood vessels and stimulation of the sweat glands. Heat loss is increased by evaporation of the additional sweat as well as by radiation from the larger volume of blood brought to the surface.

If the normal body temperature is threatened by a reduction in body heat, the center initiates impulses which reduce heat loss and increase the production of heat. Superficial blood vessels constrict, secretion by the sweat glands is inhibited, and shivering occurs.

MONITORING BODY TEMPERATURE

The thermometers for measuring body temperature may be scaled in Fahrenheit (F.) or Celsius (C. centigrade) and it may be necessary at times to know the equivalent of one in the other system.

The difference between the freezing point (0° C.) and the boiling point (100° C.) on the Celsius scale is 100 degrees; on the Fahrenheit scale the difference is 180 degrees (32° F. = freezing point; 212° F. = boiling point). This indicates that 100 Celsius degrees equal 180 Fahrenheit degrees, or one Fahrenheit degree equals 5/9 of a Celsius degree. The freezing point on the Fahrenheit scale is 32 degrees, but on the Celsius scale it is 0 degrees; therefore, when converting to Celsius the 32 must first be subtracted in order to find the number of degrees to be converted. When converting to Fahrenheit the 32 must be added to the product so that the result will be adjusted for the Fahrenheit scale. The following formulas may be used when conversion from one system to the other is necessary.

The formula to convert Fahrenheit degrees to Celsius is

$$(\text{F. degrees} - 32) \times \frac{5}{9} = \text{C. degrees}$$

Example: The conversion of 100° F. to C. degrees.

$$(100° \text{ F.} - 32) \times \frac{5}{9} = 37.7° \text{ C.}$$

The formula to convert Celsius degrees to Fahrenheit is:

$$\left(\text{C. degrees} \times \frac{9}{5}\right) + 32 = \text{F. degrees}$$

Example: The conversion of 39° C. to F. degrees.

$$\left(39° \text{ C.} \times \frac{9}{5}\right) + 32 = 102.2° \text{ F.}$$

Body temperature may be measured by placing a clinical thermometer in the sublingual area of the oral cavity, the rectum or the axilla. The site used depends upon the patient's rationality, age, and local conditions which would preclude accuracy (e.g., recent food or fluid ingestion or smoking, inflammatory disease in the site). The results of several studies indicate that "for ordinary, regular assessment, the most accurate reflection of the body's core temperature is obtained by using the sublingual pocket."[2] In oral monitoring, the proximity of the thermometer to the lingual and sublingual arteries provides for greater accuracy. A period of 15 minutes should elapse following the ingestion of hot or cold fluids, or smoking before taking the oral temperature.

Studies have also suggested the optimum period of time that the thermometer should remain in each of the sites in order to have the maximum temperature recording.[3] These are: for oral recording, 7 minutes; for rectal recording, 3 minutes; and when the axilla is used, 10-minute placement is suggested.

If the body temperature shows a progressive increase towards dangerously high levels, or if a patient's condition is likely to produce fluctuations, establishing a system of continuous recording is preferable to very frequent monitoring by the usual method. It is less anxiety-producing and less disturbing for the patient, as well as more convenient for the nursing staff.

Continuous monitoring is possible with

[2]Carol Gohrke Blainey: "Site Selection in Taking Body Temperature." Am. J. Nurs., Vol. 74, No. 10 (Oct. 1974), p. 1861.

[3]G. A. Nichols and P. J. Verhonick: "Time and Temperature." Am. J. Nurs., Vol. 67, No. 11 (Nov. 1967), pp. 2304–2306.

an electric thermometer, which operates on the principle that heat alters the resistance of a conductor to the flow of an electric current. Depending upon the material used as the conductor, the resistance may be increased or decreased. In continuous recording of body temperature, a temperature sensor (probe) in which a conductive material is encased may be placed in the esophagus or rectum. A small electrical current of constant voltage is directed through the conductor. The resistance is proportional to temperature, and the voltage of the current conducted through the probe is calibrated in terms of temperature. The temperature may be determined from the position of the pointer on a Fahrenheit or Celsius scale, or the model being used may be equipped with an automatic chart recorder.[4, 5]

VARIABLES WITHIN THE NORMAL

The body temperature shows slight variations within the normal range from one individual to another and under certain circumstances. Variations within the normal may have several causes.

Time of Day

The temperature is higher in the late afternoon and evening following an individual's activities during the day. It decreases during the night with the reduced activity, being lowest from about 4 to 6 A.M. If the individual is active during the night and sleeps during the day, the times of higher and lower temperatures are usually inverted.

Age

Infants and young children have a higher normal temperature. Their heat production is greater owing to the higher metabolic rate associated with their growth and activity. Also, the ability to regulate heat loss and production is not sufficiently developed in the early years to regulate a constancy of temperature efficiently.

Older people have a somewhat lower normal temperature because of their slower metabolic rate and reduced muscular activity. Their mechanisms of heat production, conservation and dissipation are less efficient.

Exercise

Strenuous exercise may cause an elevation of 0.5° to 1° C. in temperature, but it quickly returns to normal when the activity ceases. Women in labor frequently show an increase in temperature, attributed to their increased muscular activity.

Menstrual Cycle

A variation in temperature is characteristic of certain phases of the menstrual cycle. There is an increase of 0.3° to 0.5° C. when ovulation occurs, which is usually about the middle of the cycle. This is attributed to the increased activities of the endometrial cells, initiated by the secretion of progesterone. The slight increase is maintained until a day or two before the onset of menstruation, when it falls to the previous normal level.

Pregnancy

A slight increase in temperature occurs in the first 3 to 4 months of pregnancy and is followed by a gradual fall of 0.5° to 1° C. The lower temperature continues to full term and returns to the individual's normal level after parturition.

ABNORMAL BODY TEMPERATURE

FEVER

Fever, or pyrexia, is an elevation of the body temperature above normal. It is a manifestation of tissue injury or a disorder that results in an increase in heat production in excess of the rate of dissipation, or in an impairment of the heat-dissipating or control mechanisms.

[4]Carl R. Nave and Brenda C. Nave: Physics for the Health Sciences. Philadelphia, W. B. Saunders, 1975. Chapter 15.

[5]Charles W. Hagerman, Jr.: "Electronic Thermometers." Nurs. '71, Vol. 1, No. 1 (Nov. 1971), pp. 21–26.

Causes of Fever

The imbalance in body heat content may be caused by malfunction of the temperature-regulating center, the response of the center to a pyrogen, exposure to a very high environmental temperature, or impaired dissipation.

Disturbance in regulation by the center may be the result of the direct action of brain disease or increased intracranial pressure, or by the action of a substance that is released into the blood at the site of tissue injury or disintegration anywhere in the body. The substance, which may be referred to as a pyrogen, is thought to be the product of the injured or disintegrating cells or of leukocytes which invade the area. On the basis of experimental work, there is increasing support for the theory that the pyrogen is released by the leukocytes.[6]

Stimulation of the hypothalamic heat center by the pyrogen is analogous to the setting of the thermostat of an automatic heating system to a higher level; heat is produced until the set level of temperature is achieved. The higher temperature is maintained as long as the pyrogen is present. As the concentration of the pyrogen is reduced, the level of the thermostat is lowered, and there is a corresponding decrease in the fever by activation of the heat-dissipating responses, peripheral vasodilation and sweating.

In the case of fever due to exposure to a high temperature, the body cannot dissipate heat as fast as it is being received from the exterior.

Fever occurring because of the inefficient heat-dissipating mechanisms is seen most often when severe dehydration develops. The secretion of sweat is reduced, resulting in a marked decrease in heat loss by evaporation.

Manifestations and Effects of Fever

The onset of fever may be sudden and rapid, or the rise in body heat may develop gradually without the individual being aware of it. The initial manifestations of fever vary with the degree of disturbance in the thermostatic center. If the elevation is moderate and gradual, the patient may experience slight chilliness for a brief period, general malaise, headache and anorexia. With a sudden and greater degree of stimulation of the center, the patient has a chill in which he shivers and feels very cold, even though his temperature may already be above normal. Epinephrine is released which accelerates metabolism, increasing heat production. In turn, the rise in temperature further accelerates the metabolic rate and heat production. The skin becomes pale and is cold to the touch because of peripheral vasoconstriction. The shivering is increased muscular activity for the purpose of producing heat; it may be severe enough to cause chattering of the teeth and shaking of the whole body. Small elevations of skin (gooseflesh) appear and the small fine hairs become erect owing to the contraction of small muscles attached to the hair follicles. The chill lasts until the temperature reaches the level set by the stimulated thermostatic center in the hypothalamus. Then, as long as the pyrogen is effective, a balance between the heat production and dissipation maintains the temperature at approximately this higher level.

Frequently the onset of fever in infants and young children is accompanied by a convulsion which is due to the immaturity and instability of their nervous systems.

With subsidence of the chill, the patient's skin becomes hot and flushed, and he complains of being hot. Disorientation and delirium are not uncommon when the fever is high, especially in older persons.

The basal metabolic rate is increased in proportion to the elevation of temperature. With a fever of 40.5° C. (105° F.) there is an increase in metabolism of approximately 50 per cent. A negative nitrogen balance develops with the increased destruction of body protein in metabolism, and there is a loss of weight. Respirations and the heart rate are accelerated. There is a greater loss of fluid by evaporation from the hot skin and in the increased respirations.

If the temperature rises above approximately 40.5° C. (105° F.), there is danger of cellular damage. The hypothalamus may lose its capacity for temperature regulation, resulting in a progressive increase in fever until death occurs. The limit to which the

---

[6]A. C. Guyton: Medical Physiology, 5th ed. Philadelphia, W. B. Saunders Co., 1976, p. 966.

temperature may rise before causing death is about 43.3° to 44.4° C. (110° to 112° F.).

When the pyrogenic factor is suddenly removed, the mechanisms that contribute to heat loss are set in operation. There is marked peripheral vasodilation and profuse sweating (diaphoresis); heat is lost rapidly by radiation and vaporization. This sudden lowering of the temperature is referred to as the *crisis of fever*. If the temperature returns to normal gradually over a period of several days, the process is known as *lysis*.

Fever is thought to serve a useful purpose in some infections. A high temperature will destroy a large number of causative organisms in gonorrhea and neurosyphilis. Other pathogenic organisms may be made less virulent by a high fever. It is also suggested that the increased metabolism supports an increased production of antibodies, since patients who fail to develop a marked febrile response in a severe infection usually do less well.

Types of Fever

Fever may be classified according to its variation within 24 hours or 2 to 3 days. An intermittent fever is one in which the temperature falls to normal and rises again within the 24-hour period; a remittent fever manifests a variation of 1 or 2 degrees, but does not reach normal within the 24 hours. A relapsing fever occurs when there are alternating periods of one or several days of normal and elevated temperature.

Heat Stroke

A heat stroke occurs with relatively long exposure to extreme heat. At first the individual may experience headache, visual disturbances, nausea and vomiting. Weakness, flaccidity of the muscles, a rapid bounding pulse and rapid respirations are manifested. The individual becomes delirious, collapses, and lapses into coma. The skin is hot and dry, and there is an absence of sweating due to dehydration and central nervous system damage. The temperature progressively rises to 40.6° to 43.3° C. (105° to 110° F.).

Unless the condition is discovered in the early stages and the body is rapidly cooled, circulatory failure develops and the patient dies. The patient may be immersed in a cold bath, or given a cold sponge bath followed by the application of ice bags, or a cooling blanket that is used to induce hypothermia may be applied.

Nursing in Fever

The care of the fever patient depends largely on the causative condition, but the following points require consideration.

REST. Fever produces an increased metabolic rate, so the patient is advised to decrease his activity. With an elevation of 37.7° C. (100° F.) or higher, bed rest is usually recommended. Anticipation of the patient's needs is important in order to avoid activity on his part and unnecessary expenditure of energy. Information about his condition and treatment is given to reduce the patient's apprehension and level of anxiety. Concern and fear may stimulate the release of epinephrine, which accelerates cellular metabolism and heat production.

OBSERVATIONS. The temperature, pulse and respirations are usually noted every 4 hours; they may be checked oftener in high fever and when these vital signs may indicate complications. For example, when caring for a patient with brain disease or trauma, it may be necessary to record the temperature, pulse and respirations at least hourly. An increase in temperature and a decrease in pulse and respirations may indicate an elevation in intracranial pressure. Frequent monitoring may create anxiety. A judicious explanation with reassurance will be necessary. The degree of concern aroused by the repeated checking may necessitate continuous recording using an electric thermometer.

Observations are made of the individual's nutritional status and state of hydration, since fever tends to be very debilitating and dehydrating. There is generally a corresponding increasing weakness with increasing fever. Notation is made of the color of the skin and whether it is moist or dry. If the skin is pale rather than flushed and dry, heat dissipation is inefficient. Patient responses and orientation should be noted, especially if the temperature rises to the levels of hyperpyrexia.[7] Cerebral disturb-

---

[7]*Hyperpyrexia* and *hyperthermia* are terms used to indicate fever when the temperature is over 40° C. (104° F.)

ance may develop as less oxygen becomes available to the brain cells.

If the fever is of unknown origin, the nurse observes the patient closely for the development of signs and symptoms which may be helpful to the physician in making a diagnosis.

CARE DURING A CHILL. If the patient experiences a chill at the onset of the fever, several light covers are used and tucked in closely to the body to prevent heat loss. If heat applications in the form of hot water bottles or an electric blanket or heating pad are employed, extreme precautions are necessary to avoid burning the patient. As soon as the chill is over, heat applications are removed and covers reduced to prevent loss of body fluid and sodium by excessive sweating.

FLUIDS AND FOOD. Unless contraindicated by the patient's disease, the fluid intake in fever is increased to a minimum of 2500 to 3000 ml. for an adult because more fluid is lost by evaporation from the skin and in the increased respirations. The inclusion of broths and soups is recommended for their salt content. A record is made of the fluid intake and output.

Since fever is accompanied by an increase in metabolism and in destruction of body protein, an increase in the caloric and protein intake is necessary. This may be difficult during the acute stage owing to the anorexia and the patient's condition, but it should be effected as soon as possible. When the patient's intake consists mainly of fluids, calories and protein may be increased by giving milk drinks, eggnogs, and gruel, and by adding cream, glucose, or lactose to a commercial nutritional supplement.

COOLING PROCEDURES. Care of the fever patient may include cooling measures to prevent the temperature reaching the level at which tissue damage may occur. The various procedures used may be classified as external surface cooling, internal surface cooling, or extracorporeal cooling.

External surface cooling is the method most often employed and may be achieved by a variety of measures. An increase in the loss of body heat by radiation and convection may be promoted by reducing the covers to a minimum, lowering room temperature, and directing air currents from electric fans over the patient. Cooling may be induced by sponging the body with cool water or a cool solution of approximately 35 per cent alcohol in water. The alcohol solution is not used with infants and children, as they may be affected by the intoxicating fumes. If the skin remains pale and cool to the touch after sponging, gentle rubbing of the skin is used to stimulate superficial circulation; the increased volume of blood brought to the surface promotes heat radiation and conduction. An alternative to the sponge may be the placing of a cold, wet sheet over the patient. Currents of air from fans are then directed over the sheet. This method facilitates heat loss by evaporation and convection. In some instances, an effort is made to reduce fever by the application of ice bags to the head, axillae, groins and sides of the trunk.

Internal surface cooling is occasionally used to lower body temperature. Repeated enemas or a colonic irrigation of ice water may be prescribed.

The use of extracorporeal cooling is generally reserved for reducing body temperature during cardiac, vascular and brain surgery that necessitates interference with normal circulation, resulting in a reduced oxygen supply to the tissues. This cooling procedure involves diversion of the blood from a large vessel to outside the body where it is pumped through the heart-lung machine. While passing through the machine, the blood is cooled to a "set" temperature and then returned to the body. The cooled blood lowers body temperature, which in turn reduces the metabolic rate and cellular requirements. The latter decreases the oxygen need, reducing possible tissue damage as a result of oxygen deficiency.

In all cooling procedures shivering is to be avoided, since it is muscular activity that increases heat production. If the patient develops shivering, the physician is consulted as to the necessary action. A drug to depress the heat-regulating center and prevent the shivering response may be prescribed.

MEDICATIONS. If the temperature approaches dangerous levels, a drug that lowers the sensitivity of the heat-regulating center and produces diaphoresis may be ordered. The antipyretic drug most commonly used is acetylsalicylic acid (aspirin) in doses of 0.3 to 0.6 Gm. for an adult every 3 or 4 hours.

COMFORT MEASURES. The mouth becomes very dry and a source of discomfort to the fever patient. Sordes, an offensive accumulation of secretions, epithelial cells and organisms, tends to collect on the lips and teeth. The mouth should be cleansed and rinsed with a mild antiseptic solution every 2 hours. Petroleum jelly, oil or cold cream may be applied to the lips to prevent cracking.

Herpes simplex (fever blister, cold sore) may develop about the mouth. The lesion appears first as a sore, burning papule; then a vesicle forms, followed by encrustation and scab formation. It is due to a virus which has probably been latent in the cells and becomes activated by the higher body temperature. An ointment may be prescribed to inhibit the spread and soften the encrustation. If the lesions occur within the mouth, they may discourage the taking of fluids and nourishment; a mouthwash containing a topical anesthetic may be ordered.

Frequent back rubs, changes of position and changes of linen may help to reduce the patient's discomfort. Frequent bathing is necessary because of the increased perspiration.

An enema may be necessary to relieve constipation, which is frequently associated with fever as a result of the dehydration.

HYPOTHERMIA

Hypothermia means a subnormal body temperature and is encountered much less frequently than fever. The cause may be prolonged exposure to cold, reduced metabolism as occurs in hypothyroidism (myxedema) or depression of body activities by alcohol intoxication, heavy sedation or circulatory failure. Clinically, the term hypothermia is used most often to indicate deliberate cooling of a patient for therapeutic purposes.

Prolonged Exposure to Cold

When an individual is accidentally exposed to extreme climatic cold, the first physiological responses are peripheral vasoconstriction, increased heat production by shivering and accelerated metabolism, and an increase in the pulse and respiratory rates. With continued exposure, the internal body temperature is gradually lowered. The cooling of the brain results in a depression of the heat-regulating center in the hypothalamus, and the ability to protect the body temperature is lost. There is a progressive depression of metabolism and a slowing of mental and muscular responses. The individual becomes drowsy, eventually lapses into coma, and may develop respiratory and circulatory failure.

The patient suffering cold exposure is treated by immersion in a warm bath of 42° to 43° C. (107° to 110° F.) for 10 to 20 minutes; this warms the peripheral blood and tissues. It is not prolonged since superficial vasodilation would reduce the blood supply to the vital centers. Rewarming is then continued at normal room temperature. Some instability in body temperature control is likely for 7 to 10 days, so the patient is usually kept at rest and under observation during that period.

Induced Hypothermia

PURPOSE AND EFFECTS. Hypothermia may be intentionally produced to decrease the rate of metabolism and oxygen utilization. The low temperature may be maintained for an hour to several days, depending on the purpose and the patient's condition. It may be employed during surgery on the heart, large blood vessels or brain which necessitates a temporary interruption of the blood flow in the area. It may also be used following cerebral surgery or severe head injuries in order to prevent or reduce severe cerebral edema or hyperthermia. Cooling of the cells reduces their activity and prevents the damage that would normally ensue with a decreased oxygen supply.

The temperature most frequently used in induced hypothermia is within the range of 32° to 26° C. (89.6° to 78.8° F.). The decrease in cellular activity and oxygen requirement is proportional to the decrease in temperature. A decline to 30° to 28° C. reduces metabolism by approximately 50 per cent. The pulse and respiratory rates are slowed and are accompanied by a fall in blood pressure. The patient becomes stuporous and may lose consciousness with lower hypothermic levels. There is a loss of the gag reflex and corneal and pupillary reactions, and the response to pain is diminished. The viscosity of the blood increases. The urinary output may not be markedly reduced at first, but it progressively decreases and has a low specific gravity.

METHODS OF INDUCTION. Hypothermia may be produced by the application of cold to the surface of the body or by extracorporeal cooling of the blood.

Surface cooling methods include immersion in an ice water bath, enclosure of the patient in large plastic sheets filled with crushed ice, placing the patient between electrically controlled blankets with coils through which a cold fluid is circulated, and the application of ice bags over the body surface. The latter may be combined with the circulation of cool air over the body by fans.

The blanket method is the most satisfactory and the one in current use; it is simpler and provides better control. The temperature of the fluid flowing through the coils is maintained at the level at which the gauge on the accompanying refrigerating unit is set. The blankets may also be used to rewarm the patient following hypothermia by adjusting the temperature controls on the machine.

The extracorporeal method of cooling is used during surgery. The blood is diverted from a large vessel, circulated through a cooling coil outside the body, and returned to another blood vessel. The heart-lung machine (pump-oxygenator), which is used in cardiac and vascular surgery as a mechanical pump to maintain circulation and to add oxygen to the blood, is also equipped with a heat exchanger that may be used to either cool or warm the blood. The extracorporeal circulation of the blood through a heat exchanger has certain advantages; the patient may be cooled more quickly, better control of the body temperature is provided, and the patient may be quickly rewarmed on completion of the surgical procedure.

Reduction of the body temperature can only take place when heat production does not compensate for heat loss. Before hypothermia induction is commenced, the pa-

tient receives a drug that depresses the heat-regulating center and prevents the shivering response. Shivering must be avoided because of the associated heat production and the marked increase in the utilization of oxygen. The sedative effect of the drug also reduces the unpleasantness of the cooling for the conscious patient. Examples of the drugs used are chlorpromazine (Thorazine), promethazine hydrochloride (Phenergan), and meperidine hydrochloride (Demerol), all of which may be administered intramuscularly or intravenously.

The internal body temperature is monitored continuously during hypothermia by special electric thermometers. Probes which record the temperature are placed in the esophagus or rectum. These are connected to a transducer that converts the heat energy to electrical energy, which is registered on a scale. When the temperature is within 1 or 2 degrees of the desired level, the cooling procedure is discontinued or reduced, and a downward drift of 1 or 2 degrees will continue. Obese persons cool more slowly and manifest a greater tendency to drift.

REWARMING. Following surgery, the patient may be rewarmed before leaving the operating room. As cited above, if extracorporeal cooling is used, the heat exchanger of the heart-lung machine may be used to rewarm the patient. If the blanket method is used, warm water may be circulated through the coils. In many instances, the patient is simply covered with blankets and allowed to rewarm at his own rate.

Nursing Responsibilities in Hypothermia

PREPARATION. The conscious patient and the patient's family may have considerable apprehension when advised that hypothermia is to be used. The purpose and method to be used should be explained, and their questions answered to reduce their anxiety.

If surface cooling is to be used, the skin should be clean and inspected for discolored areas and lesions. If the hypothermia is to be prolonged, a light protective application of oil or lanolin is usually made to the entire body surface.

Collapse of the peripheral veins occurs with the cooling; for this reason, an intravenous infusion is started prior to induction so fluid, electrolytes and medications may be administered during the treatment. An indwelling catheter is inserted so that renal function and the fluid output may be assessed.

The preinduction medication is given as ordered, and the patient's blood pressure, pulse, respiratory rate, level of consciousness and responses are noted for a comparative baseline later. An electric thermometer is inserted in the esophagus or rectum for continuous temperature recording.

Emergency equipment that should be assembled and readily available includes an intermittent positive pressure respirator, oxygen, tracheostomy set and an emergency drug tray with vasopressors and cardiac and respiratory stimulants.

CARE DURING HYPOTHERMIA. A nurse remains in constant attendance. Frequent observations and recording (usually at 15 to 30-minute intervals) are made of the pulse rate and rhythm, respirations and blood pressure. Cardiac irritability may increase with cooling, and fibrillation may develop. Changes in the color of the skin, lips or nail beds are noted. A continuous monitoring of the temperature is necessary; any change in the level or indication of shivering is reported promptly to the physician. There is danger of cardiac arrest and permanent tissue damage if the temperature falls too low.

The patient is turned or moved hourly to prevent frostbite and fat necrosis, especially in areas where skin over bony prominences may be in prolonged contact with the hypothermia blanket. The skin is carefully inspected every 1 to 2 hours; discolored or firm immovable areas may indicate fat necrosis or frostbite, in which there is a crystallization of the tissue fluid. If pillows are used, the nurse makes sure they are placed under the lower blanket. In prolonged hypothermia, the light application of oil or lanolin is repeated to protect the skin. Good body alignment is kept in mind when positioning the patient in order to prevent contractures and hyperextensions; if his condition permits, passive range of motion exercises are used during prolonged hypothermia to preserve normal joint movement and prevent circulatory stasis.

The fluid intake and output are accurately recorded; the fluid intake is determined by the 24-hour output. The hourly urinary output is noted, and frequent specimens are collected for analysis.

The conscious patient is encouraged and given the necessary support to breathe deeply and cough hourly. This is done at the same time the position is changed in order to keep the essential disturbances to a minimum. Since the cough and gag reflex are usually depressed, he may not be successful in coughing.

The mouth is cleansed and moistened every 2 to 3 hours, and the nasal passages are kept clear of secretions. Precautions are necessary when cleansing the mouth to avoid fluid aspiration because of the associated depression of reflexes.

Since the corneal reflex may be absent and normal secretions are diminished, moist normal saline patches may be applied to the eyes for protection or an artificial tear solution (methyl cellulose) instilled.

REWARMING. During the rewarming period, constant observation of the patient is just as important as during the hypothermic phase. As the temperature approaches normal, the extra blankets used in rewarming are gradually removed to prevent it from rising above the normal level. Frequent checking of the pulse, respirations and blood pressure is still necessary. If medications were administered during hypothermia or the rewarming period, the nurse must be alert for possible accumulative effects of the drug(s).

After the patient is rewarmed, the special thermometer probes are removed, but recording of the temperature every 3 or 4 hours continues for 2 or 3 days, as there may be some instability of the hypothalamic heat-regulating center, especially in the young and aged. Frequent checking of the pulse continues for the first 24 to 48 hours since the patient may still develop cardiac irregularity or fibrillation.

The indwelling catheter is removed when a normal urinary output is established. Oral fluids are administered in small amounts and progressively increased as tolerated.

References

Books

Anthony, C. P., and Kolthoff, N. J.: Textbook of Anatomy and Physiology, 9th ed. S. Louis, C. V. Mosby, 1975.

DuGas, Beverly Witter: Introduction to Patient Care: A Comprehensive Approach to Nursing, 3rd ed. Philadelphia, W. B. Saunders, 1977. Chapter 25.

Guyton, Arthur C.: Textbook of Medical Physiology, 5th ed. Philadelphia, W. B. Saunders, 1976. Chapter 72.

Nave, Carl R., and Nave, Brenda C.: Physics for the Health Sciences. Philadelphia, W. B. Saunders, 1975. Chapter 15.

Sabiston, David C., Jr. (Ed.): Davis-Christopher Textbook of Surgery, 11th ed. Philadelphia, W. B. Saunders, 1977. Chapter 9.

Sodeman, W. A., and Sodeman, W. A., Jr.: Pathologic Physiology: Mechanisms of Disease, 5th ed. Philadelphia, W. B. Saunders, 1974.

Periodicals

Atkins, Elisha, and Bodel, Phyllis: "Fever." N. Engl. J. Med., Vol. 286 (Jan. 6, 1972), pp. 27–34.

Beaumont, Estelle: "Hypo/Hyperthermia Equipment." Nurs. '74, Vol. 4, No. 4 (April 1974), pp. 34–41.

Blainey, Carol Gohrke: "Site Selection in Taking Body Temperature." Am. J. Nurs., Vol. 74, No. 10 (Oct. 1974), pp. 1859–1861.

Denney, Ann Marie, and Kingsbury, Barbara A.: "Hypothermia in Fact and Fantasy." Am. J. Nurs., Vol. 72, No. 8 (Aug. 1972), pp. 1424–1425.

Erickson, Roberta, and Storlie, Frances: "Taking Temperatures: Oral or Rectal, and When." Nurs. '73, Vol. 3, No. 4 (April 1973), pp. 51–53.

Grass, Suzanne: "Thermometer Sites and Oxygen." Am. J. Nurs., Vol. 74, No. 10 (Oct. 1974), pp. 1862–1863.

Hagerman, Charles W., Jr.: "Electronic Thermometers." Nurs. '71, Vol. 1, No. 1 (Nov. 1971), pp. 21–26.

Nichols, G. A., and Kucha, D. H.: "Taking Adult Temperatures: Oral Measurements." Nurs. Res., Vol. 22 (Jan.-Feb. 1973), p. 93.

Nichols, G. A., and Verhonick, P. J.: "Time and Temperature." Am. J. Nurs., Vol. 67, No. 11 (Nov. 1967), pp. 2304–2306.

Verhonick, P. J., and Nichols, G. A.: "Temperature Measurement in Nursing Practice and Research." Can. Nurse, Vol. 64, No. 6 (June 1968), pp. 41–43.

7

The Patient with Pain

PAIN

Pain is a distressing sensation generated when pain receptors in the skin or viscera produce impulses that are carried by an afferent nerve pathway to the brain. It plays an important protective role; one progressively learns from early childhood to avoid and correct the situations which cause pain. When the sensation is lost in an area of the body as it is in spinal cord injury or leprosy, the lack of awareness of injury and the absence of normal protective responses may lead to extensive tissue damage. Pain is one of the most impelling symptoms that prompt a person to seek medical advice. It also provides information that aids the physician in making a diagnosis. It should be remembered, however, that there are serious diseases, such as cancer and heart disease, which may be painless at the onset; as a result, persons may delay seeing a physician until the disease is in an advanced stage.

PAIN MECHANISM

The structures essential for the pain sensation are receptors that are sensitive to pain stimuli, an impulse pathway to and within the central nervous system (brain and spinal cord), and areas within the brain for perception, interpretation and the initiation of responses.

Pain Receptors

Stimuli that cause pain sensation are received by freely branching bare nerve endings which form a diffuse network in the tissue. The concentration of these receptors varies throughout the body; they are abundant in the skin and on joint surfaces, but there are relatively fewer in the deeper tissues and viscera.

Pain Stimuli

A wide variety of stimuli evoke pain; these stimuli include mechanical agents (e.g., cutting, blow, friction, distention), thermal agents (extremes of heat and cold), chemicals (e.g., chemicals released by injured cells or microorganisms), electric current, ischemia and sustained muscle contraction. Many are nonspecific but elicit pain through their intensity. For instance, light pressure produces an awareness of touch, but increasing the intensity of the pressure causes pain. Similarly, heat and cold must reach a certain intensity to stimulate pain receptors.

Pain Impulse Pathways

The sensory, or afferent,[1] nerve fibers, whose bare terminal branches form the

---

[1]*Sensory,* or *afferent,* nerve fibers carry impulses toward the central nervous system (brain and spinal cord). *Motor,* or *efferent,* nerve fibers transmit impulses away from the central nervous system to peripheral structures.

pain receptors, provide a peripheral pathway to conduct the impulses into the spinal cord or brain stem. These sensory nerve fibers are of two types: some are larger, have a fatty insulating sheath (myelin) and are classified as A delta fibers; the others are smaller, nonmyelinated and designated C fibers. The myelinated fibers transmit the impulses very rapidly. A sudden, pain-producing stimulus causes two pain sensations. The impulses transmitted by the myelinated fibers produce the sharp pain that is felt immediately when the injury occurs. The nonmyelinated fibers conduct more slowly and are responsible for the more diffuse, throbbing pain or ache that follows the immediate sharp pain associated with the initial injury.

Various theories have been presented to explain the physiology of pain, none of which has proved entirely satisfactory. Currently, the specificity theory and the gate control theory are favored.

The *specificity theory of pain* proposes that there are specific structures (afferent nerve fibers and central nervous system pathways and neurons) concerned with the pain sensation. Pain impulses are transmitted by specific sensory nerve fibers from the stimulus site and enter the spinal cord via the dorsal root ganglia to neurons within the dorsal column or horn of gray matter. Some impulses may be passed to motor neurons to initiate impulses that are carried out of the cord along motor or efferent nerve fibers to skeletal muscles (see Fig. 7–1). These motor impulses produce a reflex response, such as withdrawal of the injured part from the object producing the pain stimulus (as seen in the withdrawal of the finger that receives a pin prick or touches a very hot object). The other pain impulses cross to the other side of the cord and ascend the lateral spinothalamic tract to the thalamus in the brain. From here they are relayed via a thalamocortical pathway to the appropriate sensory area of the cerebral cortex.

It is suggested that the individual becomes aware of the pain when the impulses reach the thalamus. Interpretation of the site of the stimulus and the quality and intensity of pain is made at the cortical level. In addition to interpretation, impulses are initiated which activate the physical and psychological responses to pain.

Recognition of the specific pain pathways inherent in the specificity theory provides the basis for surgical intervention in intractable pain. The procedure interrupts the pain pathway and impulses do not reach conscious level.

Siegele explains that the *gate control theory* advanced by Melzack and Wall proposes that pain impulses can be regulated, modified or blocked by certain cells within the central nervous system. It is thought that impulses can be prevented from reaching the transmission cells of the dorsal column by the action of the substantia gelatinosa[2] cells, which are said to "close the gate." Whether or not the gate is open to permit the conduction of impulses through the dorsal horn cells and hence to higher levels is dependent upon the nature of the impulses delivered to the substantia gelatinosa. Siegele indicates that when cutaneous impulses aroused by such stimuli as vibration, scratching, cold and heat are transmitted by large fibers in the afferent nerve they can negate the input of the fibers of smaller di-

---

[2]The *substantia gelatinosa* is an area of special neurons located close to each dorsal column of gray matter and extending the length of the spinal cord.

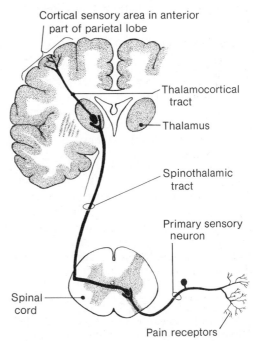

FIGURE 7–1 Diagram illustrating pathway of pain impulses.

ameter. That is, they close the gate. It remains open to impulses transmitted by small fibers if there is "relatively little activity in the large fibers."[3] The activity of the gating mechanism may also be affected by emotion and impulses in descending tracts from areas of the brain (brain stem, thalamus and cerebral cortex).[4]

The gate control theory establishes a basis for the following procedures in lessening pain and suffering: (1) distraction; (2) reducing fear and lowering the level of anxiety; (3) analysis of the pain and reactions by the individual, and participation in the planning to cope; (4) local counterirritants, massage and heat applications; (5) electrical stimulation; and (6) probably acupuncture.

The pain sensation has two components: perception and reactions.

PAIN PERCEPTION

Perception is the awareness or feeling of pain. The severity of the pain perceived depends upon the intensity and frequency of the pain impulses. Qualifying the type of pain and relating it to various stimuli are learned experiences. The child gradually learns to associate the unpleasant feeling with objects and situations that cause pain.

Pain Threshold

The point at which a stimulus first elicits the awareness of pain is referred to as the pain threshold. The threshold is considered fairly constant and uniform for all persons and differences occur mainly in the responses.[5] The threshold may be elevated by such things as distraction, strong stimuli in other parts of the body (e.g., pain in one part of the body raises the threshold in other parts) and pathologic conditions which involve the pain receptors, impulse pathways or cortical sensory areas. Depressed activity of the cerebral cortex due to certain drugs, alcohol, shock or debilitation may also raise the threshold.

A lowering of the pain threshold (hyperalgesia) may occur with inflammation or injury of structures concerned with the pain sensation or of neighboring tissues to such structures. The pain threshold may also be lowered by a reduction of other stimuli. The latter accounts for a patient's increased pain during the night when ordinary stimuli are at a minimum.

PAIN REACTIONS

The reaction component of pain is composed of all the psychological, physical, voluntary and involuntary responses that are made when pain is perceived.

The physical reactions include those of skeletal muscles and the involuntary physiological responses implemented through the release of adrenalin and stimulation of the autonomic nervous system.

Muscle Responses

Skeletal muscle reaction may be the immediate withdrawal reflex (cited previously), involuntary contraction, or increased tone in an attempt to splint or immobilize the affected part (e.g., rigidity of the abdomen). The individual may support or rub the part, assume a position that he thinks may provide relief, clench his fists, rock or pace back and forth or toss about. Voluntary muscle activity may also be involved in correcting the situation when the individual removes the offending object, treats the site or seeks assistance.

Autonomic Nervous System Responses

The physiological responses seen most commonly are mediated by sympathetic innervation and the secretion of adrenalin. Superficial vasoconstriction occurs; the blood supply to the skeletal muscles and brain is increased as a defense mechanism; the blood pressure, pulse and respirations increase; salivary secretion and gastrointestinal activity decrease; perspiration increases, and the pupils dilate. The individual manifests pallor, cold clammy skin and dry lips and mouth.

If the pain is deep, severe and prolonged, the above reactions may not develop and

---

[3]D. S. Siegele: "The Gate Control Theory." Am. J. Nurs., Vol. 74, No. 3 (March 1974), pp. 449–450.

[4]William F. Ganong: Review of Medical Physiology, 7th ed. Los Altos, Cal., Lange, 1975, p. 73.

[5]A. C. Guyton: Textbook of Medical Physiology, 5th ed. Philadelphia, Saunders, 1976, p. 667.

the patient may exhibit shock and extreme weakness; the blood pressure falls, the pulse weakens and nausea and vomiting may occur.

Psychological Responses

Even when the intensity and the nature of the pain stimulus are the same for several persons, the type and degree of reactions are likely to vary considerably because of individual differences in psychological makeup. The nature of a person's psychological reactions is determined, to a large extent, by his past experiences and the degree of threat and frustration inherent in the pain for him. Some may audibly complain by moaning, crying or verbal expression of suffering and fear and may further indicate their distress by restlessness and purposeless movements. Others may be very stoical, remain still and suffer in silence.

Factors which may influence patients' responses include the following:

1. SOCIOCULTURAL BACKGROUND An individual's responses become conditioned by social and cultural attitudes to pain. Some learn from those around them that pain is to be endured without obvious emotional reactions. If others have been accustomed to persons in pain exhibiting outward responses which are accepted and which receive attention, they consciously or unconsciously develop a similar pattern of response.

2. EMOTIONAL STATE. If the patient is in an emotional state to begin with, his evaluation of pain is likely to be exaggerated. If the illness has disrupted plans or created financial or home problems, or the origin of the pain is the heart or a common site of cancer, the patient is threatened to a greater degree and is more fearful.

3. PHYSICAL CONDITION. Psychological reactions are usually greater in weak and fatigued persons. For instance, the obstetrical patient whose labor is prolonged may be quite calm and uncomplaining at first, but as she becomes fatigued and fearful that something is wrong, her pain becomes less tolerable.

4. PREVIOUS PAIN EXPERIENCE. Responses may be either increased or decreased by the memory of previous pain.

Fear of a repetition of former severe suffering may produce marked outward reactions. With some a greater tolerance and resignation may develop.

5. SIGNIFICANCE OF THE PAIN. Apprehension is always greater when a situation is not understood or when one does not know what to expect. The patient who fears he has cancer may manifest greater pain reaction until he learns that the biopsy report is negative for malignancy.

To children, pain is a new, unpleasant and frightening experience which they cannot understand; overt expressions may be expected. The labor patient who has been prepared during her pregnancy by explanations of the source and purpose of the labor pains is less anxious and calmer than the unprepared patient.

6. DISTRACTION. Reactions as well as perception are influenced by the amount of the patient's attention that is focused on the pain. If a situation commands considerable concentration on the part of the individual or creates pleasurable emotion, pain responses are minimized. The person actively engaged in competitive sport may not even be aware of the pain of an injury he receives. But if the patient focuses his whole attention on his discomfort, reactions are more pronounced.

7. INTENSITY AND DURATION OF PAIN. If the pain stimulus is very intense, the individual feels more threatened. He may find it difficult to control his emotional responses and may even become quite disorganized. Similarly, pain of long duration is wearying and may initiate more overt reactions; on the other hand, the patient may become more resigned to the pain and take the attitude that he has to live with it.

TYPES OF PAIN

Some of the more common terms used to classify pain are as follows:

Superficial pain occurs when the receptors in surface tissues are stimulated. Conversely, *deep pain* arises from deeper tissues, such as muscle, periosteum and viscera.

Localized pain arises directly from the site of the disturbance. *Referred pain* is that which is felt in a part of the body which is remote from the actual point of stimulation. The impulses usually arise in an organ, but the pain is projected to a surface area of the body. A classic example of referred pain is that associated with angina pectoris; the pain originates in the heart muscle as a result of ischemia, but it may be experienced in the midsternal region, the base of the neck and down the left arm. Pain arising in the gallbladder or bile ducts may be referred to the epigastrium and the right scapular region. (See Figure 7–2.)

The mechanism of *referred pain* is not clearly understood. Several explanations have been offered. The one most commonly accepted appears to be one which states that the area of stimulation and that in which the pain is felt are both innervated by nerve fibers that arise from the same segment of the spinal cord. Each spinal nerve contains sensory fibers that are distributed to certain viscera, skeletal muscles and an area of superfical tissues. The pain impulses from all of these areas are delivered to the same segment of the spinal cord from which they ascend via a common spinothalamic tract to the thalamus and then relayed to the cerebral cortex. It is suggested that the faulty localization in the brain may be attributed to the infrequency of visceral pain impulses as compared with the frequency of impulses arising in cutaneous areas.

Another theory suggests that the fibers carrying the pain impulses from the viscera and those from peripheral tissues converge upon the same neuron at some point in the pain pathway within the central nervous system. The impulses are then interpreted as coming from the superficial area because of previous experience.

Referred pain may also be explained by the fact that it is usually perceived as being in a structure that has had the same segmental embryonic origin as the part in which the pain stimulus occurs. For example, the heart and the arm deveop from the same embryonic segment.

Projected pain occurs when impulses are set up at some point along the pain pathway beyond the peripheral pain receptors. The pain is perceived as arising at the site of the pain receptors served by the pathway in which the pain originated. A person who has had an amputation may experience what is referred to as *phantom limb pain*.

Stimuli arising from the stump may be localized on the basis of the previously established body image, and as a result the pain is projected to the portion of the limb that was removed.

Persistent, severe pain that cannot be effectively controlled by the usual medications is referred to as *intractable pain*.

Headache is a frequent discomfort experienced by many persons, and applies to the pain sensation that is perceived as being in the cranial vault (i.e., facial pain, toothache and earache are excluded). Headache is a common complaint in many illnesses in which the primary disturbance is quite remote from the head.

The pain receptors within the cranium occur in the walls of the arteries and in the meninges. The actual brain tissue is devoid of pain receptors. Headache may originate with tension or spasm of associated muscles at the back of the neck. Extracranial pain is usually well localized to the area where superficial pain receptors are being stimulated.

Psychogenic pain is that experienced when there is no detectable organic lesion or peripheral stimulation. It is thought that the pain is the conversion and physical expression of a distressing psychic disturbance or problem. It must be remembered that the discomfort is very real to the individual and that efforts must be made to provide relief.

Care of the Patient with Pain

The nurse plays an important role in the relief and support of a patient who is experiencing pain and may also make a significant contribution to the diagnosis and treatment through accurate observations.

A person may mention to a nurse that he has a pain but doesn't consider it severe enough to consult a doctor. The nurse, without alarming the patient, should urge him to see his physician, since pain is an indication of some disturbance which, if recognized early, may be corrected before causing more severe suffering and inconvenience.

Important considerations in the care of a patient with pain are:

1. ATTITUDE OF THE NURSE. When acceptance, gentleness and a desire to pro-

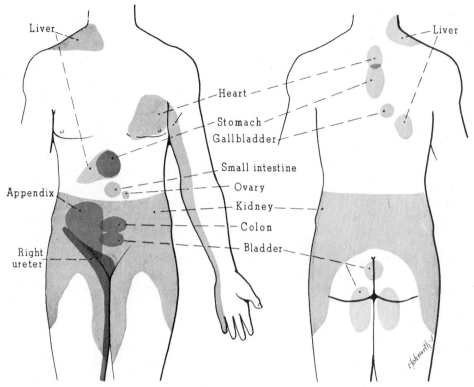

Liver
Liver
Heart
Stomach
Gallbladder
Small intestine
Appendix
Ovary
Kidney
Colon
Right ureter
Bladder

FIGURE 7–2 Common areas of referred pain. (From Jacob et al.: Structure and Function in Man, 4th Ed. W. B. Saunders Co.)

vide relief are evident in the nurse's response to his suffering, the patient senses an emotional warmth and understanding that allay much of his fear and make the pain more tolerable.

The nurse guards against forming personal opinions as to whether the patient really has pain of the intensity expressed. Criticism of the patient's behavior is avoided; it is extremely important for the nurse to have an appreciation that cultural background, past experience and circumstances condition each person's emotional responses. Whether or not the intensity of the pain is due entirely to the physical disturbance or is aggravated because of anxiety or sociocultural factors, it is real to the patient and requires attention.

2. **OBSERVATION.** Assessment and observation of the patient with pain is an important nursing responsibility. Certain information about the pain is obtained from the patient and his family and is objectively recorded. Alert observations are made of the patient for associated symptoms and the effect of the pain on the individual. Failure to recognize a patient's pain and its characteristics could lead to a delay in diagnosis and necessary treatment.

Pain is wholly subjective; only the person experiencing the pain knows the nature, intensity and location of it. Information that should be elicited from the patient includes:

LOCATION. This should be as specific as possible. For example, abdominal pain may be localized to the lower or upper right or left quadrant, epigastrium or mid-abdomen. The site may be well defined or diffuse or the path may radiate, involving a widespread area.

TYPE. Crampy; stabbing; sharp; dull; throbbing; burning; aching; boring.

INTENSITY. Mild; severe; excruciating.

ONSET. Sudden or gradual. The time it began is noted.

DURATION. Persistent; intermittent. What the patient thinks would provide relief or help him is considered as well.

The nurse also takes note of:

CHANGES IN THE SITE. Tenderness; swelling; discoloration; firmness; rigidity.

POSITION ASSUMED OR MOVEMENTS. Knees drawn up; resting on his knees; sitting up; refuses to change position; clasping or holding a part; pacing the floor; thrashing about.

EMOTIONAL RESPONSES. Crying; screaming; restless; thrashing about; anxious.

GENERAL APPEARANCE. Color (flushed, pale, gray, cyanosed); distressed; pinched facies; weak; prostrated.

VITAL SIGNS. Pulse, respirations, blood pressure and temperature.

ANY PROVOKING OR RELIEVING FACTORS. Is the occurrence or relief of pain related to meals, medication, activity, a certain position, treatment, or coughing? Does it occur or become worse at any particular time of the day?

ASSOCIATED SYMPTOMS. Nausea and vomiting; profuse perspiration; fainting; inability to perform usual functions; dulling of senses; apathy; clouding of consciousness; disorientation; inability to rest and sleep.

PATIENT'S HISTORY AND CIRCUMSTANCES. Is the patient worried about the diagnosis and outcome of his illness or about a family or financial problem? Is he lonely and fearful in the strange new environment?

3. POSITIONING. A change of position may provide some relief for the patient by reducing the pressure and tension on the affected area. Venous and lymphatic drainage are promoted in order to decrease the accumulation of fluid in the tissue and thereby relieve pain. Adequate assistance and extreme gentleness are necessary when turning or moving the patient. It is done slowly, and support is provided for the painful area. It is often helpful to ask the patient how the movement can be made least distressing for him. Good body alignment contributes to comfort by eliminating tension and hyperextension. Support and elevation of a painful limb on a pillow may be helpful. Immobilization and support by mechanical devices may ease the patient's pain and lessen the discomfort associated with moving. Examples of such devices are a fracture board and firm mattress, a splint applied to a limb, an abdominal or chest binder, and a Stryker or Foster bed.

4. REST AND RELAXATION. Care is planned so that the patient is disturbed as little as possible. Consideration should be given to his location in the ward. Noise in the environment should be kept to a minimum; the more the patient is alerted, the more acutely he is aware of his pain.

Efforts are made to promote relaxation; tension of muscles predisposes to pain and discomfort by the ischemia and accumulation of metabolites that are likely to develop. Simple nursing measures that may help include frequent change of position, support to the affected part, passive or active movements of limbs, bathing, massage of back and limbs (unless contraindicated by varicosities or phlebitis) and instructions to the patient to relax — to consciously "let go and become limp."

5. REDUCE FEAR AND ANXIETY. Relief of worry may substantially contribute to the relief of pain. If the patient is overly anxious about his illness and its outcome, it may be helpful to encourage him to talk about it. His concern could be brought to the attention of the doctor, who will then talk with the patient about his condition. An understanding of the cause of the pain and its probable duration may reduce the patient's anxiety. Pain may become less severe if the patient knows that the nurse has taken care of a worrisome home problem by arranging for assistance from a social worker or visiting nurse.

The person in pain should not be left alone and unattended for long periods. Visits at frequent intervals by the nurse to see how he is getting along are reassuring; he knows someone is aware and concerned about him and is available if he needs assistance.

The patient who is advised ahead of time that he is likely to experience some pain (e.g., the surgical patient) may suffer less if he knows it is expected and is not an indication that he is not progressing favorably. When explaining the pain, the nurse assures the patient that everything possible will be done to provide relief and minimize his discomfort.

6. DIVERSION. In some instances, de-

pending on the nature of the illness and on the particular individual, some diversion which is acceptable to the patient provides distraction that may reduce his concentration on the pain or "close the gate." A brief visit and chat with someone, a few moments with his religious adviser, reading or listening to a radio may prove beneficial.

7. **LOCAL APPLICATIONS.** The application of moist or dry heat or cold (subject to the approval of the physician) may produce relief of pain. The effects of heat are the relaxation of muscle tension or spasm and the increased rate of blood flow through the area. Precautions against burning are necessary, since the patient in pain may be less sensitive to excessive heat.

Cold applications stimulate constriction of the local blood vessels and reduce the amount of blood in the area and the accumulation of tissue fluid (lymph). This diminishes the painful swelling and congestion in the affected area. Cold also reduces the sensitivity of the pain receptors.

Applications which cause irritation of the skin (counterirritants) may provide relief (see discussion of gate control theory). Examples of applications used are menthol and methyl salicylate ointment preparations and mustard plasters.

8. **SUPPORTIVE CARE.** Remaining with the patient, holding his hand or placing a hand on his arm or shoulder, and making an occasional comment that acknowledges his suffering or offers encouragement all convey to the patient that someone understands and cares. Such support may make the pain more tolerable. Simple nursing measures such as bathing the face and hands with cool water, rinsing of the mouth or offering sips of fluid, gentle massage of the back or tense muscles and change of position may contribute to relief. Simple nursing measures may not seem significant to the nurse, but the patient feels something is being done for him.

9. **ANALGESICS.** The drugs used to relieve pain include those that depress pain perception, reduce the patient's response to pain or relax muscle spasm.

It is important that the nurse be familiar with the action of the prescribed drug, the usual dosage, factors that influence the dosage and effectiveness, the frequency with which it may be given and the possible side effects. A knowledge of the condition of the patient who is to receive the analgesic is also necessary. Frequently the administration is left to the discretion of the nurse since the order may be "give when required" (P.R.N.). The prescribed analgesic should be used judiciously and under conditions that will contribute to maximum benefit for the patient. Treatments and nursing measures are carried out before or immediately following the administration of the drug so the patient may remain undisturbed as much as possible. The administration of the drug should not be withheld unnecessarily since pain may initiate harmful physiological responses and may contribute to shock. Also, the longer the patient suffers, the more fearful and apprehensive he becomes, making it more difficult to achieve relief. In other words, pain is easier to control if it can be relieved soon after the onset. When persistent, severe pain, such as that often associated with terminal malignancy, is being experienced, the patient is observed closely to determine the duration of the effect of an analgesic; the nurse's observations are then discussed with the doctor. Administration at more frequent and regular intervals may be ordered to prevent the pain from reaching severe intensity.

At no time should an analgesic replace nursing measures that, in many instances of less severe pain, may provide relief.

A great variety of drugs are used as analgesics; they range from mild acetylsalicylic acid (aspirin) to strong opiates and synthetic preparations. Examples of nonnarcotic analgesics are aspirin, aspirin compound (aspirin, phenacetin and caffeine), acetaminophen, and propoxyphen (Darvon). Narcotics used as stronger analgesics include morphine, codeine, meperidine hydrochloride (Demerol), and pantopium hydrochloride (Pantopon).

If the patient is apprehensive, a sedative, such as sodium amytal phenobarbital or flurazepam (Dalmane), or a tranquilizer, such as diazepam (Valium), may be ordered as an adjunct to an analgesic in order to decrease the patient's fear and tension and reduce his pain responses. A sedative or tranquilizer may enhance the effectiveness of a smaller dose of an analgesic.

When the cause of pain is known to be

muscle spasm, a preparation that produces relaxation of the muscle tissue may be prescribed. For example, spasm of the smooth muscle tissue of the gastrointestinal tract, the urinary tract and biliary tract may be relieved by antispasmodic preparations, such as tincture of belladonna, atropine sulfate, methantheline bromide (Banthine) and propantheline bromide (Pro-Banthine). These drugs are effective by reducing the parasympathetic impulses to the visceral muscle.

The analgesic drugs may produce side effects, the incidence and nature of which vary from one patient to another. Nausea and vomiting are two of the most common reactions. The time relationship between the administration of the drug and the onset of the nausea or vomiting should be noted and brought to the physician's attention. Frequently, patients who are upset by morphine and codeine may tolerate meperidine.

The more potent analgesics, such as opiates and meperidine, cause some depression of the respiratory center. The rate and volume of respirations should be noted following the administration of these drugs, particularly in the cases of older patients and those known to have respiratory dysfunction.

One must be always alert to the possibility of addiction when a patient is receiving repeated doses of analgesics or sedatives. It is not likely to become a problem if given over a period of a few days when the patient's condition is such that pain may be expected. If the patient requests the drug for relief beyond this period, it is brought to the physician's attention. If a patient is experiencing intractable pain, he may develop a decreasing response to the prescribed dose. The rate at which the patient increases his tolerance for an analgesic may be slowed by giving him a tranquilizer or sedative as well as regular doses of an analgesic.

Constipation, dry mouth, impaired ability to make decisions and occasionally disorientation are also side effects of analgesics that may occur and for which the nurse must be alert.

Neurosurgery to Relieve Pain

In some instances, *intractable pain* which cannot be effectively controlled by analgesics is relieved by surgical interruption of the pain impulse pathway either outside or within the central nervous system. The procedure is usually reserved for patients with an incurable disease or cancer and those who suffer the excruciating pain of tic douloureux (trigeminal neuralgia).

When the source of the pain is localized to a relatively small area of the body a neurectomy may be done. This involves severing or crushing the peripheral sensory nerve fibers to the affected area.

A second neurosurgical procedure used is a rhizotomy, in which the sensory pathway which carries impulses from the affected area is interrupted just before it enters the spinal cord. (The area of fibers that is severed or crushed lies between the associated dorsal ganglion and the cord.) The disadvantage of a rhizotomy is that it causes the loss of the sense of touch and position in the area, so it is used principally to relieve pain in the upper part of the trunk.

When intractable pain is in the lower part of the trunk and the lower limbs or if it involves a large part of the body which is supplied by several spinal nerves, the pain pathways in the spinal cord and, rarely, in the brain stem or thalamus are interrupted. The procedure currently in use is *percutaneous cordotomy*. The surgeon inserts a needle into the spinothalamic tracts of the spinal cord. An electrode is passed through the needle into the area, followed by an electrical current which damages the tissue. A *tractotomy* may be done by severing the pain impulse–conducting pathway in the cord. This operative procedure is used less often because it involves "open" surgery and a laminectomy to expose the cord.

Interruption of these pathways causes permanent loss of the temperature sensation, as well as that of pain below the level of the interruption. Loss of these sensations eliminates natural body defenses. Precautions are necessary to avoid burns, ischemic sores from pressure, and injury. An explanation is made to the patient and instructions given as to how to avoid prolonged periods of pressure and injuries.

Electrical Stimulation to Relieve Pain

Based on the theory of the gating mechanism, electrical stimulation of peripheral nerves is being used for the relief of phantom pain and the pain associated with degenerative spinal conditions and arthritis. Electrodes are applied to the surface of the skin or implanted in an area of contact with a major sensory pathway. An electric current is discharged into the electrode and produces stimulation of large afferent nerve fibers. When these impulses reach the dorsal column of the spinal cord, the substantia gelatinosa cells are activated and the "gate is closed," blocking impulses to the spinothalamic tract.

Electrical stimulation may be used for relief of chronic pain by implanting the electrode in the spine so that the impulses enter the dorsal column directly. The operative procedure for implanting the electrode of the dorsal column stimulator involves open surgery and a laminectomy.

Acupuncture to Relieve Pain

Acupuncture, a very old Chinese medical procedure, has received considerable attention in North America recently. It is currently being used as an analgesic in some pain clinics with patients experiencing chronic and intractable pain.

The procedure involves the insertion of several long fine probes to varying depths at selected points. The sites for insertion depend upon the patient's particular problem. The probes are rotated as they are introduced and after they are in place; this enhances the stimulation. The practice sometimes involves applying electrical stimulation through them following their insertion.

The physiology of acupuncture, and the reason for its effectiveness in relieving pain are not clearly understood. Currently its effectiveness is explained on the basis of the gate control theory of pain. Pain impulses arising from the insertion of the needles and electrical stimulation activate the blocking system in the central nervous system.

References

Books

Beeson, Paul B., and McDermott, Walsh (Eds.): Textbook of Medicine, 15th ed. Philadelphia, W. B. Saunders, 1979.

Ganong, William F.: Review of Medical Physiology, 7th ed. Los Altos, Cal., Lange, 1975. Chapter 7.

Guyton, Arthur C.: Textbook of Medical Physiology, 5th ed. Philadelphia, W. B. Saunders, 1976. Chapter 50.

MacBryde, C. M., and Blacklow, R. (Eds.): Signs and Symptoms, 5th ed. Philadelphia, J. B. Lippincott, 1970.

Roddie, I. C., and Wallace, William F. M.: The Physiology of Disease, London, Lloyd-Luke, 1975. Section 7, p. 275.

Thorn, G. W., et al. (Eds.): Principles of Internal Medicine, 8th ed. New York, McGraw-Hill, 1977.

Periodicals

Armstrong, M.: "Acupuncture." Am. J. Nurs., Vol. 72, No. 9 (Sept. 1972), pp. 1582–1588.

Billars, K. S.: "You Have Pain? I Think This Will Help." Am. J. Nurs., Vol. 70, No. 10 (Oct. 1970), pp. 2143–2145.

Cashatt, B.: "Pain: A Patient's View." Am. J. Nurs., Vol. 72, No. 2 (Feb. 1972), p. 281.

Clark, M. C.: "Chest Pain." Heart Lung, Vol. 4, No. 6 (Nov.-Dec. 1975), pp. 956–962.

Collins, S.: "Intractable Pain: How Nursing Care Can Help." Nurs. '74, Vol. 4, No. 9 (Sept. 1974), pp. 55–59.

Copp, L. A.: "The Spectrum of Suffering." Am. J. Nurs., Vol. 74, No. 3 (March 1974), pp. 491–495.

Drakontides, A. B.: "Drugs to Treat Pain." Am. J. Nurs., Vol. 74, No. 3 (March, 1974), pp. 508–513.

Gaumer, William R.: "Electrical Stimulation in Chronic Pain." Am. J. Nurs., Vol. 74, No. 3 (March 1974), pp. 504–505.

Goloskov, J., and LeRoy, P.: "Use of the Dorsal Column Stimulator." Am. J. Nurs., Vol. 74, No. 3 (March 1974), pp. 506–507.

Harmon, V.: "Doing it Better." Nurs. '74, Vol. 4, No. 9 (Sept. 1974), pp. 91–92.

Johnson, J. E., and Rice, V. H.: "Sensory and Distress Components of Pain." Nurs. Res., Vol. 23, No. 3 (May-June 1974), pp. 203–209.

Mastrovito, R. C.: "Psychogenic Pain." Amer. J. Nurs., Vol. 74, No. 3 (March 1974), pp. 514–519.

McCaffery, M.: "Patients in pain." Nurs. '73, Vol. 3, No. 6 (June 1973), pp. 41–50.

———: "Intelligent Approach to Intractable Pain." Nurs. '73, Vol. 3, No. 11 (Nov. 1973), pp. 27–32.

McLachlan, E.: "Recognizing Pain." Am. J. Nurs., Vol. 74, No. 3 (March 1974), pp. 496–497.

Munley, M. Joan, and Keane, Mary C. (Eds.): "Symposium on Impressions of Pain: A Nursing Diagnosis." Nurs. Clin. North Am., Vol. 12, No. 4 (Dec. 1977), pp. 609–668.

Murphy, T. M.: "Cancer Pain." Postgrad. Med., Vol. 53, No. 5 (May 1973), pp. 187–194.

Pace, J. Blair: "Helping Patients Overcome the Disabling Effects of Chronic Pain." Nurs. '77, Vol. 7, No. 7 (July 1977), pp. 38–43.

Siegele, D. S.: "The Gate Control Theory." Am. J. Nurs., Vol. 74, No. 3 (March 1974), pp. 498–502.

Storlie, F.: "Pain: Describing it More Accurately." Nurs. '72, Vol. 2, No. 6 (June 1972), pp. 15–16.

Wise, Thomas N.: "The Complaint of Pain." Primary Care, Vol. 2, No. 1 (March 1975), pp. 1–7.

The Patient with Cancer

NEOPLASMS

Normally, the production of cells is a regulated process which allows for growth in early life and for the replacement of wornout or damaged cells throughout life. The mechanisms for the initiation of cell reproduction when tissue cells increase or replacement is needed and the control of that reproduction so that it does not exceed the needs of the organism are not understood. Occasionally the control of cell reproduction is lost in some cells in a particular area of the body and an excessive production occurs, forming an abnormal mass that is referred to as a *newgrowth* or *neoplasm*. The cells of the neoplasm serve no useful purpose and use nutrients and oxygen, causing deprivation in the host's normal tissues. The newgrowth may be benign or malignant.

Benign Neoplasms

A benign newgrowth is considered much less of a threat to the host's life because it does not spread to other sites. It is usually possible to cure benign neoplastic disease by surgical removal of the mass.

Growth of a benign neoplasm is slow and tends to be expansive rather than invasive; the mass remains localized, frequently is encapsulated, and the cells may show little abnormality compared with those of the normal tissue from which they originated. When excised, it rarely recurs. Since a benign newgrowth is a space-occupying lesion, it may cause serious effects on neighboring structures, depending on its size and location. In some instances it may obstruct blood vessels or a passageway or may cause pressure on vital tissues leading to serious malfunction. Some benign lesions tend to become malignant if left untreated; examples are polyps in the stomach and intestine, papillomas of the bladder and larynx, and pigmented moles.

Malignant Neoplasms

A malignant newgrowth is a distinct threat to life by virtue of its ability to proliferate destructively into surrounding tissue and to other parts of the body. Some of the cells become detached form the primary mass and are carried via the blood or lymph to a distant area of the body, where they set up colonies of the malignant cells (metastasis). The neoplastic cells tend to grow and reproduce rapidly and change in structure and activity in varying degrees. They lack normal cellular differentiation and are atypical in size, shape and staining properties (see Table 8–1).

In addition to being classified as malignant or benign, a neoplasm is also named according to the type of tissue involved. Classification of the more common neoplasms is found in Table 8–2.

Neoplastic disease is discussed as it relates to specific organs in the respective ensuing chapters. In this chapter, certain features and problems common to malignant newgrowths are presented to give this major health problem special emphasis.

125

TABLE 8–1   DIFFERENCES IN BENIGN AND MALIGNANT NEOPLASMS

	Benign	Malignant
Cells	Relatively normal and mature.	Little resemblance to normal; poorly differentiated, atypical in size and shape, nonuniform, and immature.
Growth	Slow and restricted. Noninvasive of surrounding tissue; expansive, pushing aside normal tissue.	Usually rapid and unrestricted. Invasive of surrounding tissue.
Spread	Remains localized. Usually encapsulated.	Metastasizes via blood and lymph streams.
Recurrence	Rarely recurs.	Frequently recurs.
Threat to host	Prognosis favorable. The effect depends on size and location. May cause pressure on vital organs or obstruct a passageway, which is usually corrected by surgical excision of neoplasm.	Threatens life by reason of its local destructive proliferation and formation of secondary neoplasms in other structures. Prognosis more favorable with early diagnosis and treatment, when cells show less departure from the normal and there is no metastasis.

CANCER

Cancer is a term commonly used to designate any disease that is a malignant neoplasm; it is not one specific disease but a group of diseases. As cited previously, malignant neoplasms have certain common characteristics, but there are also marked differences from one type to another because of the type of tissue involved, the location, and the degree of departure from normal of the cells of the newgrowth. They differ as to signs and symptoms, effects on the host, rate of growth, metastasis, form of treatment used and their response to treatment.

Cancer begins as a localized disease, known as *carcinoma in situ* (cancer in its original site). When the cells commence invasion of surrounding tissues it may be referred to as *invasive cancer*. In the more advanced stages of the disease, cells become detached from the neoplasm and are carried by lymph or blood vessels to other parts of the body, where more cancer develops. This process, as mentioned earlier, is described as *metastasis*. The cells carried in the lymph may be trapped in lymph nodes near the original site, producing disease in the nodes and causing what is known as *regional involvement*. Eventually these areas of disease disseminate cancer cells to other parts.

Certain areas are known to be the most frequent sites of metastases from certain organs. For example, in breast cancer when the disease is advanced beyond regional involvement, frequent sites are the lungs, brain and bones. In cancer of the stomach, the most common site of metastasis is the liver.

INCIDENCE AND TRENDS

Cancer diseases account for a large number of deaths each year. They are second only to heart disease as a killer in the United States and Canada, and it is estimated that one out of every four persons develops cancer. In 1977, 690,000 new cases of cancer were reported in the United States.[1] In Canada in 1974, it claimed 150.4 lives per 100,000 of the population.[2] Statistics indicate that in recent years cancer has accounted for an increasing number of deaths. Factors which have probably contributed to the increase include: (1) a greater number of persons living to an older age, which increases cancer susceptibility; (2) the increased risk of developing

---

[1]Lisa Begg Marino, "Helping Cancer Patients—Effectively." Horsham, Pa., 1977, pp. 17–22.

[2]Report compiled by the Canadian Cancer Society, Toronto, 1976.

TABLE 8–2 CLASSIFICATION OF MALIGNANT AND BENIGN NEOPLASMS

Tissue of Origin	Benign Neoplasms	Malignant Neoplasms
Epithelium Surface epithelium	Papilloma	Carcinoma Epithelioma (squamous or basal cell carcinoma)
Glandular epithelium	Adenoma Papilloma Polyp	Adenocarcinoma Papillary carcinoma Papillary adenocarcinoma
Melanocytes (cells that synthesize the pigment melanin)	Nevus Melanoma	Malignant melanoma
Connective Tissue Fibrous tissue Embryonic fibrous tissue Bone Cartilage Fatty tissue	Fibroma Myxoma Osteoma Chondroma Lipoma	Sarcoma Fibrosarcoma Myxosarcoma Osteosarcoma Chondrosarcoma Liposarcoma
Muscle Tissue Smooth muscle Skeletal muscle	Leiomyoma Rhabdomyoma	Leiomyosarcoma Rhabdomyosarcoma
Endothelial Tissue Blood vessels Lymph vessels	Hemangioma Lymphangioma	Hemangiosarcoma (angiosarcoma) Hemangioendothelioma Lymphangiosarcoma Lymphangioendotheliosarcoma
Hematopoietic and Reticuloendothelial *Tissues* Bone marrow		Myelogenous leukemia Multiple myeloma Ewing's sarcoma (endotheliosarcoma)
Lymphoid Tissue		Hodgkin's disease Lymphocytic leukemia Lymphosarcoma Lymphoma
Nerve Tissue Nerve Ganglion Brain	Neuroma Neurofibroma Ganglioneuroma Glioma	Neurogenic sarcoma Neuroblastoma Glioblastoma Astrocytoma Medulloblastoma
Meninges	Meningioma	Malignant meningioma
Placental Tissue	Hydatid mole	Choriocarcinoma
Adrenal Medulla	Pheochromocytoma	Malignant pheochromocytoma
More than One Tissue (Mixed) Gonads	Teratoma (e.g., dermoid cyst of ovary)	Malignant teratoma (e.g., Wilms' tumor or embryonal carcinosarcoma)

certain cancers because of greater exposure to specific carcinogens (e.g., cigarette smoking); (3) new and improved diagnostic procedures; and (4) a decrease in deaths from diseases such as pneumonia, scarlet fever and other acute infections.

Statistics also show a significant change in the incidence of cancer between the two sexes over the past two decades. The mortality rate for females has decreased, owing mainly to a lesser incidence of uterine, gastric and intestinal malignant neoplasia. The death rate for males has increased, which may be attributed mainly to the greater occurrence of cancer of the lung and prostate.

Other important trends reported are changes in the occurrence of certain types of cancer. The incidence of gastric and uterine cancer has decreased but the mortality rates for leukemia and cancer of the lung, breast and male urinary system have increased.[3] Figure 8–1 shows the distribution of different types of cancer.

Such changes in incidence may provide clues to predisposing factors and causes in relation to environment, occupations, health habits and customs, and may also indicate the value of preventive and early detection programs. For instance, the decrease in uterine cancer may be correlated with the increasing practice of an annual Papanicolaou vaginal smear (Pap test). The increase in cancer of the respiratory tract, particularly the lungs, is attributed to increased cigarette smoking in both sexes.

The incidence of cancer varies with age. It occurs in infants and children as well as adults but increases with advancing age. Leukemia and neoplasms of the central nervous system account for many of the malignancies occurring in children up to 5 years of age. Between the ages of 5 and 15 years there is a lesser incidence, but from 15 on there is a steady increase.

ETIOLOGIC FACTORS

A great deal of effort on the part of microbiologists and medical research scientists has been directed toward identification of a specific cause and treatment of cancer.

Much information has been obtained about cancerous diseases, and new and improved therapeutic measures have resulted in an increase in survival rates. Intensive study of cancer cells has led to the conclusion that the uncontrolled multiplication of atypical cells characteristic of cancer is due to a change in the structure of the deoxyribonucleic acid (DNA) in the nucleus of a cell. Once these atypical cells develop, the abnormal characteristics are continued in the cells that result from their mitosis. Certain chemical and physical agents have been recognized as being active in causing some cancers, but a common specific etiologic factor that initiates and promotes the transformation of a normal cell into malignant cells remains obscure.

It has become apparent that a number of factors, both intrinsic and extrinsic, play a role in the development of the disease. Agents that incite malignant changes in cells are referred to as *carcinogens*.

Intrinsic Factors

Contributory or controlling factors within the individual are considered to be heredity, hormonal balance and immunologic response.

The *genetic make-up* of the cells is thought to be responsible for a predisposition to develop one of the malignant diseases. Hopps states that "the incidence of cancer in siblings born of parents both of whom have (or get) cancer is approximately four times greater than that of siblings, neither of whose parents have (or get) cancer."[4] Familial occurrence of some neoplasms such as retinoblastoma, multiple polyposis of the colon, neurofibromatosis (von Recklinghausen's disease) and multiple endocrine adenomas has been recognized, but a hereditary relationship has not been established for all neoplastic diseases.

An *excessive concentration of certain hormones* appears to influence the change of some normal cells to malignant ones, with subsequent uncontrolled growth. Such cancers are said to be hormone-dependent and manifest changes in growth activity when the concentration of certain hor-

[3]Canadian Cancer Society: Cancer Can Be Beaten. The Facts. Toronto, 1976.

[4]H. C. Hopps: Principles of Pathology, 2nd ed. New York, Appleton-Century-Crofts, 1976, p. 34.

DISTRIBUTION IN 100 MALES

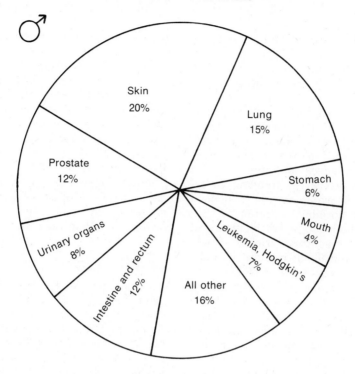

DISTRIBUTION IN 100 FEMALES

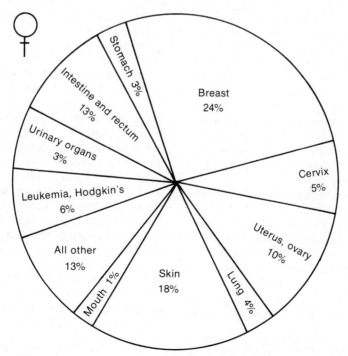

FIGURE 8–1   Distribution of cancer. (Courtesy of the Canadian Cancer Society.)

mones is altered. For instance, estrone and estradiol (ovarian estrogenic hormones) favor the growth of some breast cancers, while androgens (male hormones) tend to suppress their progress. Cancer has been produced experimentally in mice by the injection of estrogen. Whether the hormone is the primary incitant in hormone-supported cancer in humans or whether it simply produces a tissue susceptibility to a primary factor is not known. There are striking differences in the incidence of some cancers in males and females. The fact that breast cancer is frequent in females and rare in males may be explained on the basis of hormonal differences. But the reason for the much higher incidence of cancer of the stomach and urinary system in males than in females is not understood.

In the last decade there has been renewed interest in *cancer immunology*. Considerable attention and support are being given to the concept that the abnormal cells of the newgrowth contain substances that are foreign to the host's normal body cells and are therefore antigenic. The neoplastic antigens prompt an immune response in the host that controls the development, growth and spread of the disease. There is evidence that spontaneous regression and disappearance of the neoplasm have occurred; on the basis of the immunologic concept, the host's immune mechanisms have destroyed the neoplastic cells. If the host's immune response is deficient the abnormal cells multiply rapidly, invade surrounding tissues and spread to distant areas. It has been observed that there is a higher incidence of cancer in persons with an inadequate immune response, which may be due to primary immunodeficiency disease, immunosuppressive drugs, radiation exposure, or the aging process.[5, 6]

Frei and Bodey suggest that the immunologic response is primarily cell-mediated (see p. 46), but that in some instances "humoral 'enhancing' or blocking substances" are produced which favor and accelerate neoplastic growth. These sub-stances may block lymphocytic action (cell-mediated immune response).[7]

Investigation of immunologic factors in cancer continues with the hope of determining why the patient's defense mechanisms fail. Researchers also hope to find a safe antigenic preparation that will stimulate immune mechanisms specific to cancer cells (active immunity), or a serum that will transfer immunity (passive immunity) to destroy the neoplastic cells or confine them locally.

An attenuated solution of the bacillus Calmette-Guerin (BCG) is currently being used as a form of active nonspecific immunotherapy in acute myeloid leukemia and malignant melanoma.

Extrinsic Factors

It has been well established that the development of most cancer diseases is due to or enhanced by some factors in the environment. These include certain chemicals, physical agents and viruses. Certain *chemical and physical agents* are recognized as having an etiologic role. Many chemicals in the environment are being studied as possible carcinogens and a number have been determined to be offenders. The latter include asbestos, hydrocarbons (coal tar products), aniline dyes, chromates, nickel and arsenic. Many of these have been recognized through the high incidence of cancer associated with occupational exposure to the specific chemical. For example, persons working with an aniline dye, which may be absorbed through the skin and excreted in the urine, show a high incidence of urinary bladder cancer. An etiologic relationship has also been established between asbestos and lung cancer. Insecticides and herbicides are highly suspect, and animal growth-stimulating hormones and some food additives are being investigated as potential carcinogens. Cigarette smoking as a cause of cancer of the respiratory tract and the bladder has been well documented. Air pollutants are also of concern, especially in lung cancer. Research has indicated that there is usually a relatively long latent period between exposure to chemical carcinogens and cancer development.

[5]J. Macleod (Ed.): Davidson's Principles and Practice of Medicine, 11th ed. Edinburgh, Churchill Livingstone, 1974, p. 42.

[6]David C. Sabiston, Jr. (Ed.): Davis-Christopher: Textbook of Surgery, 11th ed. Philadelphia, W. B. Saunders, 1977, p. 550.

[7]G. W. Thorn, et al. (Eds.): Principles of Internal Medicine, 8th ed. New York, McGraw-Hill, 1977.

Significant physical carcinogens include excessive exposure to the sun's rays, radiation and chronic irritation. A large percentage of skin cancers are attributed to excessive exposure to the sun's rays. Fair-skinned individuals with less natural pigmentation of the skin, and those whose occupation keeps them outdoors (e.g., farmers), appear to be more susceptible to neoplastic changes in the dermal cells as a result of excessive sun exposure. X-rays and radioactive substances have proved beneficial in the diagnosis and treatment of some diseases, but repeated and heavy radiation may lead to malignant neoplasia. The adverse effects may not be seen for quite a long period following irradiation, since the effects can be cumulative. Repeated exposures to an amount that is considered harmless may eventually be of pathologic significance. This was unfortunately found to be the case with personnel working with x-ray equipment before the need for more adequate shielding was recognized; many developed leukemia or cancer of the skin.

Chronic irritation of an area and repeated tissue destruction and repair are thought to be contributory factors in the development of cancer. For example, the incidence of cancer of the lip is greater in pipe smokers; similarly, cancer of the cervix is more prevalent in women with unrepaired cervical lacerations.

Scientists have established that various types of *viruses* produce some forms of malignant neoplasia in experimental animals. As a result, intensive research is being conducted in an effort to identify viruses as a cause of cancer in man. Viral etiology is particularly suspect in leukemia and lymphomas.

MANIFESTATIONS AND EFFECTS OF CANCER

The manifestations and effects of cancer depend upon the location of the neoplasm, its stage, and whether there are secondary conditions such as ulceration, hemorrhage, infection and metastases. With few exceptions, cancer is a space-occupying lesion. It may obstruct a passageway, compress blood vessels, neighboring tissue or organs,

exert pressure on regional nerves, causing pain or even paralysis, or it may produce malfunctioning by its invasion and replacement of normal tissue.

Unfortunately, in the early stage of some cancers, signs or symptoms are not evident to the host. Important early symptoms that should be stressed in public education are: (1) *unusual bleeding or discharge from any body orifice;* (2) *a lump or thickening in the breast or elsewhere;* (3) *a sore that does not heal;* (4) *a persistent change in bowel or bladder habits;* (5) *a persistent cough or hoarseness;* (6) *indigestion or difficulty in swallowing;* and (7) *an obvious change in a wart or mole.* The presence of any one of these disturbances does not necessarily mean that cancer has developed, but early recognition followed by prompt treatment increases the chances for cure and survival. It should be known that frequently at the onset, cancer does not cause pain.

As the lesion grows, there is an insufficient blood supply and inadequate nutrition to maintain it and the normal tissue. Necrosis of a portion of the normal tissue results, with subsequent ulceration. Vessels may be eroded, leading to *chronic hemorrhage* and *anemia.* If the bone marrow is involved, as well as anemia, the individual will also experience deficient leukocyte and thrombocyte production.

Frequently there is a marked loss of weight and strength as the rapidly growing cells compete with normal cells for nutrients, and *disturbances develop in the normal metabolic and physiological processes* throughout the body.

Disfigurement and amputations associated with the involvement of superficial tissues and limbs handicap the individual and cause a disturbing loss of body image.

Infection can be a serious problem as a result of decreased efficiency in immunologic responses and defense mechanisms and the patient's general debility.

Pain usually develops following the initial stage of the cancer, but may be associated with early development if the new-growth is close to a sensory nerve or within bone tissue. The pain of cancer generally becomes progressively more severe as the disease infiltrates more and more tissue, causes obstruction, and/or metastasizes.

If the patient's disease is not arrested, he develops increasing general debility and malnutrition, his color is poor, and he appears emaciated, very sick and weak. This syndrome may be referred to as *cachexia*.

An important effect of malignant disease is the *emotional disturbance* it creates. All ill persons usually experience some psychological as well as physical stress, but it is especially true of those who are advised or even suspect that they have cancer. The individual's anxiety may be concerned with a belief that all cancer is incurable, fear of a prolonged painful illness and death, unfulfilled goals, or the distress that his illness or death will create for the family. The behavioral response will vary from one person to another, depending upon each one's circumstances and previous attitude and pattern of responses to stressful situations. Some patients become very depressed and give up; others may withdraw and avoid any discussion or mention of the problem but may manifest their anxiety in other ways, such as restlessness, inability to sleep and loss of interest in everything and everyone. Certain patients may be resentful that this should happen to them and show anger, and a few become completely disorganized.

Some of the disturbances and discomfort manifested by the patient with cancer may be the effects of the treatment being used (surgery, radiation, and chemotherapy). In some instances, the signs and symptoms of the disease become more severe for a period as a result of the treatment; such effects may be classified as *iatrogenic*.

PREVENTION AND EARLY DETECTION

At present it is not possible to prevent all types of cancer, but some types can be prevented by avoidance of recognized carcinogens. The public needs to understand the cancer problem more thoroughly, and every nurse has an obligation to participate in disseminating the necessary knowledge. Every opportunity should be taken to advise uninformed persons of the importance of avoiding exposure to carcinogenic agents and of the role of early detection and treatment. Many persons need more hopeful and con-

structive attitudes because of their abnormal fear and fatalistic point of view of cancer. Many do not realize that several types of cancer can be detected in an asymptomatic phase by certain examinations (e.g., cervical Pap test), and that some cancers can be cured if treated in the early stage. Cure is directly related to early detection. Statistics indicate that one out of two patients is cured.[8] A person with an early sign may delay a visit to the physician or clinic because of fear of being told that he has cancer. Malignant neoplasm begins as a localized disease; if all the cancer cells are confined to their source of origin, most cancers may be successfully treated. Delay in detection and treatment diminishes chances of cure and survival, since it permits the growing neoplasm to invade surrounding tissues, with cells becoming detached and carried to other body areas (metastases). In many instances, on investigation of early symptoms, the findings are negative and the individual who has put off the visit to the doctor because of fear has experienced much needless anxiety.

The National Cancer Society has instituted intensive campaigns to alert the public to potential causes of cancer, high risk factors, early detection and the fact that "cancer can be beaten." When more people are informed, a more positive, hopeful attitude to the disease will develop. As part of its public education, the Canadian Cancer society advocates the following "Seven Steps to Health":

1. Have a medical and dental checkup.

2. Watch for any change in your normal state of health.

3. Find out about any lump or sore that does not heal.

4. Protect yourself against too much sunlight.

5. Do not smoke.

6. Have a Pap test.

7. Do a monthly breast self-examination.[9]

---

[8]C. Gordon Zubrod: "Successes in Cancer Treatment." Cancer, Vol. 36, No. 1 (Suppl.; July 1975), p. 267.

[9]Canadian Cancer Society, op. cit.

Emphasis is placed on the role of regular periodic examinations. The nurse has many opportunities to discuss with her patients and friends the importance of regular self-examination of the breasts and the annual Pap smear (see section in this chapter on Exfoliative Cytologic Tests). The breast self-examination procedure should be explained and the excellent pamphlet, published by the National Cancer Society, which clearly outlines and illustrates the examination steps, should be made available. Many persons also require information regarding the significance of avoiding excessive exposure of the skin to the sun's rays.

The nurse also should inform people that cigarette smoking causes lung cancer and help them to break the habit. The nurse who continues to smoke is setting a very poor example and is contributing to defeat in the battle against smoking.

In some instances, a person delays seeking medical consultation because he does not have a private physician or because he cannot afford it. The nurse can help in advising him of a cancer detection clinic or an outpatient department to which he may go for assistance. If these are not available, a referral may be made to a local health department or local branch of the National Cancer Society, where arrangements will be made for him to see a physician.

In some occupations the employees may be brought in direct contact with a carcinogenic substance in the work situation. Industrial regulations are necessary to protect employees and communities from carcinogenic hazards. In addition to protective measures for those in a high-risk work situation, the workers require an understanding of the risk and the significance of conscientious respect for the precautions. They should be advised of early symptoms that must be reported promptly, and should receive frequent regular examinations. Some industries may disseminate offending substances that could affect many citizens in the community. Governments are becoming more aware of such hazards and are requiring protective measures.

All industries, as well as those cited above, should be encouraged in their employee health program to provide cancer education. An attempt should be made to identify high-risk individuals such as heavy smokers and those with a family history of the disease, and appropriate measures for early detection established.

In order to assume the expected role in cancer prevention and an early detection program, the nurse must keep informed as to the trends in the incidence of cancer and current advances being made. The work and the publications of the National Cancer Society should be familiar to the nurse. An important contribution can be made by advising the public of the organization and work of the National Cancer Society and its local branches. Support of organizations such as these makes possible continuous cancer research, education and treatment, as well as a variety of services to cancer patients and their families. Films, pamphlets and speakers are available for cancer education for both professional and lay groups.

Radiologic Examination

Internal parts of the body may be examined for form and density by x-ray. A radiopaque substance may have to be administered before the examination to provide a contrast medium when soft tissues are to be viewed. For instance, the patient may receive barium by mouth if the esophagus, stomach or intestine is to be viewed (see p. 495); for kidney and ureter x-ray a radiopaque dye (an iodide preparation) is given intravenously (see p. 620).

Radiology has become increasingly useful in the diagnosis and treatment of disease, but it is also potentially harmful unless it is carefully controlled and certain precautions are observed. As is the case with most drugs, an excessive amount can be very damaging and may prove fatal. Even an x-ray for diagnostic purposes involves the absorption of a small amount of x-radiation by the patient. Most of the exposed cells recover, but there is a small residual injury which is irreversible — so small that it is insignificant. With many such exposures, however, the irreversible damage adds up, or is cumulative. For this reason x-rays are to be used judiciously and with precautions.

Radioactive Isotopes

Radioactive isotopes and compounds are also used in diagnosing some cancers. A specific isotope or radioactive tagged compound is given according to the tissue being investigated; some tissues are known to absorb and concentrate a certain chemical. If a radioactive substance is administered, special instruments may then be used to detect and record the localization, distribution and concentration of the substance in the body. This process of detecting radiation within the body is known as *scanning*. The first radioactive isotope used for this purpose was iodine[131] to detect disease of the thyroid. Since then a number of radioactive isotopes have been introduced for both diagnostic and therapeutic purposes. Scanning may be used to detect both primary and secondary cancerous lesions.

Examples of some radioactive chemicals used in diagnosis are iodine[131] (I^{131}) in thyroid disease, iodine[131] rose bengal in liver disease, gold[198] (Au^{198}) in liver disease, radioiodinated serum albumin (RISA) in brain disease and for tracing circulation in the lung, chromium[51] (Cr^{51}) in red blood cell studies, iron[59] (Fe^{59}) in iron absorption and hemoglobin studies, calcium[47] (Ca^{47}) in bone disease, and strontium[85] (Sr^{85}) in bone disease. For a discussion of the nature of radioisotopes and the nursing care of patients who receive a radioactive isotope, please see the section on Internal Radiotherapy in this chapter.

Exfoliative Cytologic Tests

These tests involve the microscopic examination of smears of secretion or fluid taken from a body cavity. Cells are continuously shed from the epithelial surface tissue of the body cavities; this process is referred to as exfoliation or desquamation. Normally, cell replacement by the basal layer of epithelium parallels the exfoliation. Cancer may attack the epithelial lining of organs or body cavities, and some of the neoplastic cells become separated from the tissue and appear in the secretions found on the internal surface of the cavity. Cancer may be detected through recognition of these malignant cells before there are any other recognizable signs or symptoms, resulting in early successful treatment. Specimens may be taken from the cervix, vagina, respiratory tract, mouth, esophagus, stomach, urinary tract, prostate and the pleural and peritoneal cavities. The examination generally may be referred to as a Pap smear; "Pap" is derived from Papanicolaou, the name of the physician who introduced the use of smears for cytologic examination. "Pap smear" in clinical practice refers to a vaginal smear. An annual vaginal or cervical Pap smear on all women over 30 years of age is recommended by the National Cancer Society. The increase in this practice has led to early recognition and treatment of cancer of the uterus in many women and may be correlated to the recent decline of deaths due to uterine cancer.

Pathologists grade the degree of their findings in examination of a specimen of tissue or tissue cells by the following classification:

Class I. Normal

Class II. Very slightly atypical — probably normal

Class III. Doubtful — more atypical characteristics, possibly malignant

Class IV. Moderately atypical — probably malignant

Class V. Definitely cancer — markedly atypical and showing very little differentiation

Endoscopy

This is the introduction of a lighted tube (endoscope) into a body passage or organ for direct inspection of the area. At the same time a biopsy may be obtained by means of a biting forceps passed through the endoscope. This method of examination may be used in the larynx (laryngoscopy), bronchi (bronchoscopy), esophagus (esophagoscopy), stomach (gastroscopy), colon (colonoscopy), sigmoid (sigmoidoscopy) and rectum (proctoscopy). These are discussed in Part II of this book in connection with the specific sites.

Hematologic and Serological Tests

Some serologic tests are used for certain types of malignant neoplasia. For example, the serum acid phosphatase level is used in investigation for carcinoma of the prostate; it is elevated when the disease is present. Blood and plasma cell evaluations are important in diagnosis and assessment of malignant disease of the bone marrow and reticuloendothelial system.

TREATMENT

Cancer may be treated by surgery, ionizing radiation, drugs, immunotherapy or a combination of these.

A. Surgery

Surgical excision is considered the most effective therapy, provided the disease is still localized. The operation may be simple, as in the case of a basal cell cancer of the skin, or it may be quite radical and probably disfiguring. The lymphatics and lymph nodes which drain the area are also removed if there is evidence of regional involvement.

In some breast cancers, surgery may involve the removal of unaffected glands which secrete hormones that are supportive of the so-called hormone-dependent neoplasm; the ovaries and adrenal glands may be removed.

B. Radiotherapy

Radiation may be used alone or in conjunction with surgery or chemotherapy to treat cancer. It may be derived from an external source, or from a radioactive substance placed within the body or applied to the surface.

Radiation is composed of electromagnetic waves, or streams of nuclear particles from atoms of a radioactive substance. The sources of diagnostic and therapeutic radiation are the x-ray machine and radioactive isotopes.

Units of Measurement of Radiation

Several units are used in referring to amounts of radiation.[10, 11]

The *curie* (Ci) was the first unit to be introduced but is not satisfactory for use in medicine. It is used to measure the strength of a radiation source — that is, the amount of radioactivity. Since the ionizing effect may be altered with increasing distance from the source, the measurement in curies of the radioactivity of the source does not indicate the amount that is actually absorbed.

The units commonly used to express therapeutic and diagnostic dosage are the roentgen (R), rad and rem. The *roentgen* may be used to indicate the intensity of the radiation exposure received from x-rays or gamma rays.

The *rad* is a unit of measurement of the absorbed ionizing radiation and is defined as an "absorbed dose of 100 ergs of energy per gram of tissue."

The *rem* (roentgen-equivalent-man) may be defined as the amount of radiation that has the same biologic effectiveness as 1 rad of x-ray.

Different types of radiation (x-rays, gamma rays, alpha particles, beta particles) have different degrees of biologic effectiveness. The effect of 1 rad, 1 roentgen and 1 rem of x-rays and gamma rays is equivalent, but it differs with the radiation by alpha and beta particles. For example 1 rad of alpha particle radiation is equivalent to 20 rems.

Smaller units of the curie and roentgen that may be used are: the *millicurie* (mCi), which is 1/1000 of a curie; the *microcurie* (μCi), which is 1/1,000,000 of a curie; and the *milliroentgen* (mR), which is 1/1000 of a roentgen.

Types of Radiation Used

X-RAY RADIATION. X-rays are electromagnetic waves which are produced in a special vacuum tube. An electric current of high voltage is passed into an electron source at one end of the tube. Freed electrons rapidly bombard a metal plate (tungsten or molybdenum) at the opposite end of the tube, resulting in the emission of electromagnetic waves (x-rays). Wavelengths can be varied; the higher the voltage of the electrical current applied to the tube, the more penetrating are the x-rays produced. As a result, high or super voltage machines are used in the treatment of cancer in deep-lying structures. Lower voltage machines which produce low-energy rays are used in diagnostic procedures and in the treatment of superficial neoplasms. Heavy dense substances, such as bone tissue, barium, iodides and lead absorb x-rays; soft

[10] Benjamin F. Miller and Claire B. Keane: Encyclopedia and Dictionary of Medicine and Nursing. 2nd ed. Philadelphia, W. B. Saunders, 1978.

[11] Carl R. Nave and Brenda C. Nave: Physics for the Health Sciences. Philadelphia, W. B. Saunders, 1975, p. 280.

tissues and less dense elements do not absorb these electromagnetic waves, which is why barium or iodide preparations are used in radiologic examination of certain body areas.

RADIOACTIVE ISOTOPES. The second source of radiation used in diagnosis and therapy is radioactive isotopes. The radiation emitted by these elements is due to instability in their nuclei. Before discussing radioisotopic therapy, a brief explanation of the nature of radioactive isotopes may be necessary.

Varying forms of the same element may occur as the result of differences in atomic weights, and are referred to as *isotopes*. The isotopes of an element have a constant number of protons in the nuclei, identical atomic numbers and similar chemical properties, but they differ in the number of neutrons in the nuclei; this results in the variance in atomic weights.[12] To illustrate, there are two isotopes of hydrogen (H) — deuterium (H^2) and tritium (H^3). They each have an atomic number of 1, which is the same as hydrogen. The nucleus of the regular hydrogen atom contains one proton and no neutrons. The deuterium nucleus has one proton and one neutron, making the atomic weight 2, and the atomic weight of tritium is 3 because its atomic nucleus contains one proton and two neutrons. Uranium is another example of an isotope; some of its atoms may have an atomic weight of 235 (U^{235}) and others occur with an atomic weight of 238 (U^{238}).

Those elements which have an atomic weight greater than 209 tend to be unstable.[13] For example, radium, an unstable element

with an atomic weight of 226, has 88 protons and 138 neutrons in its atomic nucleus. The atoms of unstable elements constantly undergo some disintegration or decay until stability is established. This disintegration gives rise to the emission of particles and high-energy electromagnetic waves, and the element or isotope is said to be radioactive. The period of time in which the radioactivity (instability) of an isotope is reduced by half is referred to as the *half-life* of the isotope; this varies from seconds to years with different isotopes.

The particles emitted by the isotope are of two types, alpha (α) and beta (β). The alpha particles are capable of penetrating only a few centimeters of air and a fraction of a millimeter of tissue and are therefore of little therapeutic value. The beta particles are capable of penetrating surface tissue. The waves of energy released in radioactivity are known as gamma (γ) rays, which are similar to x-rays. These are highly penetrating and are capable of passing through concrete several feet thick. A dense metal such as lead is required for shielding from gamma radiation.

Types of Radiotherapy

EXTERNAL RADIOTHERAPY. This may be provided by an x-ray machine or by a radioactive substance such as cobalt[60] or cesium[137] which emits gamma rays. External radiotherapy may be referred to as teletherapy. Patients undergoing external radiation treatment receive a series of exposures (fractionated doses) rather than one massive dose, which would produce excessive damage to normal tissue that might cause death. The number and spacing of the treatments are determined for each individual by the radiologist.

Gamma rays emitted by a radioisotope may be used in external irradiation. Radioactive cobalt[60] (or cesium[137]) is encased in a large lead container which only allows the escape of gamma rays through a controlled aperture. The patient is placed at a considerable distance from the source in order to reduce skin damage. Mechanical devices permit rotation of the radiation beam or of the table on which the patient is placed. The beam is directed at an angle that results in continuous penetration of the affected area

[12]*Atomic Structure*. The atom of an element consists of electrons (negatively charged particles), protons (positively charged particles) and neutrons (neutral particles). The protons and neutrons form a dense core, or nucleus, around which the electrons revolve in rings or orbits.

Example: One atom of oxygen consists of eight electrons, eight protons and eight neutrons.

Atomic Number. The atomic number of an element is equal to the number of protons or the number of electrons, since both are the same.

Atomic Weight or Mass. Protons and neutrons are the heavy particles of the atom. The atomic weight, or mass, of an element is equal to the sum of the protons and neutrons in an atom. The mass of an electron is equal to roughly 1/2000 of that of a proton.

[13]Hessel H. Flitter: An Introduction to Physics in Nursing, 7th ed. St. Louis, C. V. Mosby, 1976.

but that reduces the amount of exposure of any one area of the skin.

This type of unit differs from the x-ray machine in that the latter does not give off rays once the electricity is turned off. Radioactive cobalt[60] emits rays continuously, and the opening through which the rays exit must be closed by heavy shielding shutters when the unit is not being used for treatment. Both the x-ray machine and the cobalt[60] unit are housed in rooms with specially constructed walls through which x-rays and gamma rays cannot pass. While treatment by either is in progress only the patient remains in the room. A means of communication between the patient and the radiologist or technician is provided, and a window is available through which the patient may be observed.

The objective is to deliver sufficient radiation to destroy the malignant tissue, with a minimum of damage to normal tissue. The x- or gamma rays are directed to a circumscribed area of the body. The parts of the patient's body not being treated are usually protected by lead sheets. Particular attention is given to the protection of the patient's gonads to prevent sterility and genetic mutations. The patient is positioned by the radiologist and asked to remain immobile during the treatment. Patients who cannot be relied upon to maintain the desired position may receive a sedative before going to the treatment unit, and straps or sand bags may also be necessary.

INTERNAL RADIOTHERAPY. Radioisotopes may be introduced into the body or applied topically to deliver radiation to an affected part. The radioactive element may be encased or sealed within a nonradioactive metal that screens out alpha and beta waves, or the isotope may be unsealed and in liquid form. The radiation may be delivered by administering the radioisotope orally or intravenously, placing it within a body cavity, or implanting it interstitially in the affected area.

The selection of a radioisotope which is to be administered orally or intravenously is based on the affinity of the affected tissue or organ for a particular element. The uptake and concentration of the radioisotope is comparable to that of the nonradioactive form of the element. For instance, radioactive phosphorus (P^{32}) is administered orally or intravenously, and is concentrated in bone tissue from which its radiation readily penetrates to the bone marrow. This accounts for its use in treating polycythemia vera and myelogenous leukemia. Radioactive iodine (I^{131}) is taken up by the thyroid tissue and is concentrated in the thyroid gland. It may be used in the diagnosis and treatment of thyroid disease.

Colloidal radioactive gold[198] (Au^{198}), which emits both beta and gamma radiation, is used principally in the treatment of pleural or peritoneal effusion due to cancer of the lung or cancer within the abdomen. The gold suspension is injected into the pleural or peritoneal cavity and the patient is turned every 15 minutes (side, prone, opposite side, back, and sitting positions) for 2 hours, then every half hour for 2 hours and hourly for 3 hours to provide even distribution within the cavity. The gold preparation that is injected is purple; as a result, leakage at the site of injection is readily detected and special precautions are taken in the changing and disposal of the dressing and linens to protect the handler from radiation. A patient who receives radioactive gold is usually very ill; should death occur, the body is conspicuously tagged as having had the radioisotope, and the mortician is advised as to the necessary precautions.

Radioisotopes sealed in a metal case are used therapeutically. The encasement containing the radioactive element may be in the form of needles, seeds, tubes, wires or molds. They are placed within the tissue or a body cavity for a prescribed period of time and then removed unless the radioisotope used has a short half-life. Seeds which generally contain radon[222] (Rn^{222}) are frequently permanently implanted; radon is an inert gas that is formed by the disintegration of radium and is radioactive. Its half-life is short (approximately 3.8 days).

Molds are designed specially for specific areas of the body and may be applied directly to a mucous membrane lining or to the skin.

The implantation of these sealed forms is done under aseptic conditions in an operating room. Radioisotopes commonly used in the sealed form in therapy include:

Radium[226] (Ra^{226}) Half-life 1,580 years
Radon[222] (Rn^{222})   "   3.8 days
Cobalt[60] (Co^{60})   "   5.3 years

Gold[198] (Au^{198})	"	2.7 days
Iodine[131] (I^{131})	"	8.0 days
Phosphorus[32] (P^{32})	"	14.3 days

Radioisotopes which are not sealed within metal are used in liquid form. They may be given orally or intravenously and are selected on the basis of the specific affinity of the affected tissue for a particular element. The liquid radioisotope may be introduced directly into a body cavity to treat a malignant effusion or may be placed in a nonmetal capsule or balloon for irradiation within a body cavity such as the urinary bladder. Examples of radioisotopes used unsealed in therapy include:

Iodine[131] (I^{131})
Phosphorus[32] (P^{32})
Gold[198] (Au^{198})
Bromine[82] (Br^{82})
Sodium[20] (Na^{20})

Effects of Radiation

In radiation, the rays and particles that are emitted damage or destroy the cells which they enter by the ionizing (molecular dissociation) effect produced. The injury may result in mutations by disrupting chromosomes, or in the inability of the cells to reproduce. If not destroyed, much of the tissue recovers but some permanent residual damage occurs. Subsequent exposures result in increasing accumulations of permanent cellular damage.

Uncontrolled radiation causes serious disturbances in hematopoietic tissues (bone marrow and lymphoid tissue), skin, mucous membranes and the reproductive system. Genetic mutations, sterility and malignant disease, especially skin cancer and leukemia, can develop. Exposure to intense radiation over a short period of time produces death or a serious illness, as was observed in the victims of the Hiroshima and Nagasaki atomic bomb blasts. The reaction or illness following a large dose is referred to as the "acute radiation syndrome or sickness." This critical condition has a gradual onset, with the person developing lassitude, anorexia, nausea and vomiting. There may be a remission and then, later, these manifestations become more severe and serious blood disorders and gastrointestinal and central nervous system disturbances are manifested. Anemia, leuko-penia and thrombocytopenia develop as a result of the depression of the bone marrow, predisposing the individual to infection and hemorrhage. The damage to the mucous membrane lining of the gastrointestinal tract results in ulceration, diarrhea and bleeding. Rapid weight loss, dehydration and slow and disturbed responses become manifest. The individual may die or make a long slow recovery. Those who recover are predisposed to the development of cancer in later years.

This brief discussion of exposure to intensive and uncontrolled radiation has been included to emphasize the need for extreme caution and the use of protective measures when there is any possibility of nontherapeutic exposure to sources of ionizing radiation.

The effects of a *prescribed dose* of radiation are influenced by the following:

1. The rate at which the dose is administered. If it is fractionated and spread over a long period of time, it will produce less damage than if given in one dose.

2. The size of body area being irradiated. The larger the area is, the greater the effects.

3. The particular tissue cells receiving radiation. Some types of cells are more susceptible to ionizing radiation than others. Hematopoietic cells of the bone marrow, lymphocytes, gonadal cells and those of the mucous membrane of the mouth and gastrointestinal tract are the most sensitive. These are cells which divide and reproduce rapidly. Malignant neoplastic cells which also reproduce rapidly and are poorly differentiated are more susceptible than normal cells.

4. Individual variability in response. Some individuals have greater reactions than others to similar dosage.

Fortunately, severe reactions are not often seen; increased knowledge and improved therapeutic techniques have reduced radiation side effects. Reactions that may occur may be local and/or systemic, and all patients manifest some emotional response. Some patients experience only feelings of tiredness for 2 or 3 days following each treatment, while others develop disturbances of varying degrees of severity.

Local reactions occur in the area being treated; the therapeutic rays are directed to the cancer but overlying and surrounding healthy tissues also receive some radiation. Usually no reactions are evident for several days or weeks after the treatments are commenced.

Some local skin reaction may be expected with external radiation, since the therapeutic rays are directed through the skin overlying the cancer site. The severity of the skin reaction may be described as mild, moderate or severe. The manifestations of each stage are:

1. Mild reaction. The skin exhibits a slight redness for a brief period, with transitory epilation (loss of hair).

2. Moderate reaction. The skin is erythematous and dry, and some desquamation may occur. A temporary suppression of sweat gland activity develops, as well as some loss of hair.

3. Severe reaction. With larger doses and more sensitive skin, more severe responses are likely to occur. Marked erythema may be followed by purple discoloration, blister formation and moist desquamation. Ulcerated areas may appear and the patient experiences considerable discomfort. Healing is slow and leaves the skin dark, atrophied, thin, and very sensitive to heat, cold and trauma. There is also permanent epilation and destruction of sweat glands in the area.

The reactions of irradiated mucous membrane are similar to those of the skin. Dryness due to suppression of mucous secretion, ulceration and bleeding may follow. If the mouth, throat or gastrointestinal tract is involved, the irritation and damage to the mucous membrane lining frequently interfere with the intake of food and fluids, leading to malnutrition and dehydration; diarrhea may also contribute to these complications.

If the larynx is treated, the patient is observed for possible edema and occlusion of the airway which would necessitate prompt intubation or a tracheostomy.

Irradiation of the bladder or neighboring structures may cause urinary frequency and pain. Radiotherapy of uterine cancer may result in some sloughing of the endometrium and vaginal mucosa. Vaginal discharge or bleeding may be troublesome.

Systemic reactions also occur in varying degrees of severity. Many patients experience *anorexia* and a sense of fatigue following a treatment. Some are nauseated and vomit, particularly if thoracic or abdominal viscera have been exposed. With large doses, the hematopoietic tissue may be depressed; anemia, leukopenia and thrombocytopenia may develop.

As cited previously, most patients receiving radiation treatments experience some *psychological reaction*, especially when first advised of the need for therapy, and then with the initial treatment. This probably accentuates the nature of the disease, as many lay persons are familiar with the use of "x-ray treatment" for cancer. Many persons may fear radiotherapy because of knowing or having heard of someone who had severe reactions to treatments before the present improved techniques were introduced. A third factor that causes an emotional reaction is fear of the radiation equipment, which at first appears rather ominous. If internal radiation is used, the patient may react to the precautions that are used to protect those in his environment.

Radiation Safety Factors

No one would dispute the value of radiation in medicine but, as cited previously, it can be biologically harmful. Like many other things in our environment it has both positive and negative potentials. The negative aspects depend mainly upon whether certain precautions are observed to protect the patient and attendant personnel. When using either external or internal diagnostic or therapeutic radiation three basic principles regarding protection should be kept in mind and respected in practice. These involve *time, distance* and *shielding*.

The first principle to be observed is that the shorter the period of time one spends in an area where x-rays or gamma rays are being emitted, the less hazardous is the exposure. When caring for a patient who contains a radioactive substance, necessary treatments and care should be well planned and expedited to minimize the time spent at the bedside. A monitoring badge is worn so that the amount of exposure can be estimated. If this approaches what is considered the maximum level for safety, a reassignment of personnel is made.

The second basic fact important in radiation protection is that the greater the distance from the source, the less radiation will be received. When the distance is doubled, the intensity decreases by a factor of 4. For instance, at 4 feet from the source there is only 1/16 of the exposure that there would be at 1 foot from the source.

Thirdly, effective shielding materials are available for protection. Ionizing rays lose energy when they come in contact with solid matter. The denser and thicker the matter, the fewer are the rays that will pass through it. Because of its density, lead is used extensively for shielding. One-eighth of an inch of lead will provide as much protection as several feet of concrete.

Nursing Responsibilities in Radiotherapy

The nurse caring for the patient whose treatment plan includes radiotherapy requires some understanding of radiation, its sources, how it is administered and its effects on body tissues. This is necessary for the nurse's role in reducing the patient's apprehension, providing the needed psychological support, preparing the patient for therapy and providing adequate postirradiation care. The nurse also requires an appreciation of the radiation hazards that may be experienced by those working in an environment of possible radiation exposure. Protective principles and measures must be familiar to and respected by all personnel working with radiotherapy.

1. PSYCHOLOGICAL PREPARATION. Many lay persons have erroneous ideas of radiation treatments. Some patients have the misconception that this type of treatment means that the disease is advanced, that the surgery that was performed was not successful, and that this is a last resort. It is important for the patient to be advised of the purpose of the treatment and of the curative role of radiation in cancer.

Before the initial treatment, an explanation is made to the patient as to what he may expect and what is expected of him; understanding is a defense against fear. If external radiotherapy is to be used, a brief description of the machine, which may appear rather ominous, will help to reduce anxiety. He is advised that although he will be alone in the room he will be under constant observation by the radiologist or technician, with whom he may communicate. He is also told that the treatment period will be brief. He should be informed that no pain or sensation will be felt as the rays penetrate, and that it is important for him to maintain the position in which he is placed by the radiologist. Time should be taken to talk with the patient and family, answer questions, and reassure them that the treatments are well controlled and adequate protection is used. They should know that the individual will not be radioactive following the treatment.

If the patient is to receive internal radiotherapy, it is necessary that the plan of treatment and aftercare be outlined to the patient and family; otherwise, the isolation and protective precautions that may have to be observed for a time are likely to cause great concern. Emphasis is given to the fact that such measures are temporary as well as necessary for the protection of family and friends who might visit, and for hospital staff.

2. PHYSICAL PREPARATION. The skin of the area to be treated is gently cleansed with water only and dried. It should be intact and free of any lesions or infection. Blood cell counts (erythrocytes, leukocytes and thrombocytes), hemoglobin concentration, and blood urea and uric acid concentrations are usually determined and may be used as a base line for comparison when assessing radiation reactions later. Special preparation for internal radiotherapy may be necessary, depending upon the site. For example, preparation for internal radiation therapy of uterine cancer usually includes perineal cleansing and shaving, cleansing enemas and a cleansing antiseptic vaginal douche. The patient will likely receive a general anesthetic, so food and fluid are withheld for the 6 to 8 hours preceding the insertion of the applicator with the radioactive isotope.

3. POSTEXTERNAL RADIOTHERAPY CARE. OBSERVATIONS. Following the treatment, the skin of the area irradiated is examined daily for reaction; if the mouth was involved, it is checked for dryness and ulceration; the patient is observed for fatigue, weakness and anorexia. Blood studies are repeated and are noted for possible depression of the hematopoietic tissues (anemia, leukopenia, thrombocytopenia). The temperature is recorded four times daily for 2

to 3 days for possible elevation, and any observed, or complained of, disturbance or change in body function, such as nausea and vomiting, is reported.

Reactions, their symptoms and severity, and the length of time they last will vary considerably with the site being treated and the amount of tissue irradiated.

PSYCHOLOGICAL SUPPORT. The occurrence of reactions may alarm the patient; he may interpret them as unfavorable progression of his disease. The nurse, recognizing his discouragement, provides the necessary reassurance and explains that the reactions are not unexpected, are temporary and are not an indication of a worsening of the cancer.

SKIN CARE. Some local skin reaction may be expected. Instructions as to the care are given by the radiologist. The area is cleansed with tepid water and patted dry. Soap is not used and brisk rubbing is avoided. The radiologist usually outlines the area to which the radiation beam is to be directed; these markings circumscribing the area should remain until the series of treatments is completed. Alcohol, powders, oils, lotions, creams and ointments are not used unless prescribed by the physician. If the axillae have been irradiated, deodorants must not be applied. The site is kept dry and may be covered lightly with smooth cotton. Adhesive tape is never applied. Pressure is prevented by avoiding any restricting clothing and prolonged periods of lying on the area. No hot or cold applications are used on the site, which must also be protected from exposure to direct sunlight. In the case of the male patient, if the face or neck has received radiation, shaving may be permitted after a few days. If itching and irritation accompany the erythema, the radiologist is consulted. Applications of plain calamine lotion (i.e., without phenol) or cornstarch may be suggested if the area is dry. Later, when the erythema has disappeared, and if the skin is dry and desquamating, a light application of lanolin or an oil may be permitted.

DIET AND FLUIDS. Maintaining an adequate nutritional and fluid intake may be a problem because of anorexia and lethargy. A high-protein, high-calorie diet is necessary to promote the patient's resistance, healing and replacement of the tissue destroyed by radiation. An explanation of the importance of food and fluids should be made to the patient. Small amounts of those foods preferred by him, offered in small amounts at frequent intervals through the day, may be more acceptable than fewer, larger quantities. An increased fluid intake is encouraged to promote elimination of the products of tissue breakdown (e.g., creatinine).

An antiemetic (antinauseant) preparation such as dimenhydrinate (Dramamine, Gravol) may be prescribed for oral or parenteral administration to control nausea.

MOUTH CARE. If the mucous membrane of the mouth or pharynx has been irradiated, frequent rinsing of the mouth with a mild alkaline mouthwash may provide some relief for the dryness and discomfort. If the patient is experiencing considerable discomfort the doctor is consulted, especially if there is evidence of ulceration. The teeth are cleansed with absorbent cotton rather than the usual brush to avoid injury to the soft tissues. If the esophagus is involved, the diet may be modified to bland, soft or liquid foods to lessen the dysphagia.

REST. Extra rest is necessary during the first few days after the treatment, but the patient is encouraged to move about and have some activity. Rest periods are planned with the patient.

PREVENTION OF INFECTION. Contact with persons having an infection is avoided, especially those with any respiratory infection, because of the patient's lowered resistance and possible reduced immune responses. If the leukocyte count is low, it may be necessary to use reverse isolation.

TEACHING. In the case of an outpatient receiving external radiotherapy, possible minor reactions are discussed and the patient and family advised that any other disorders should be reported promptly to the physician. Written instructions concerning skin care, the need for additional rest, nutritional and fluid intake and the importance of avoiding contact with infection are given. These instructions are reviewed with the patient and a family member, and time is taken to listen to and answer their questions. They are informed of someone to contact if a question or concern arises at home. Emphasis is placed on the importance of keeping the appointment for the next treatment; if the patient is not well enough, the physician or radiologist should be contacted.

4. CARE DURING INTERNAL RADIO-THERAPY. When radioisotopes are implanted or injected for therapeutic purposes, the patient becomes a temporary source of radioactivity. In addition to being concerned with the patient's reactions and psychological and physical needs, the nurse is concerned with the precautions necessary to protect herself and others from radiation that may be emitted from the patient and his body discharges in some instances.

The radioisotope laboratory is consulted as to the precautions to be used with each patient who receives internal radiation; care and precautions vary with different radioisotopes.

PRECAUTIONARY MEASURES. The nurse caring for a patient receiving internal radiotherapy should know the half-life of the radioisotope used and, when it is a liquid, it is also necessary to know how it is excreted from the body. The three safety factors that apply to protection from external radiation sources — time, distance and shielding — must also be kept in mind and respected (see p. 139).

The patient is usually placed in isolation in a single room for a period of time equal to the half-life of the radioisotope used. A notice is placed on the door that indicates radioactivity, and warns that no visitors are permitted to enter. Preferably the room should have both a window through which the patient can be observed and an intercommunication system, so that the time spent in the room by staff is minimized. A card or sheet is placed on the front of the patient's chart with appropriate information, and a wristband indicating radioactivity is placed on the patient.

The patient is likely to be apprehensive or resent his isolation unless he is oriented to the plan of treatment, and understands that it is temporary as well as necessary for the protection of others.

The nurse's time in the room is restricted to a minimum and, when doing anything for the patient that brings her in close contact, she should wear a gown and rubber gloves. She works quickly and remains only long enough to give the necessary care, having thoughtfully anticipated the patient's needs and planned ahead of time as to what observations should be made, as well as the details of care to be carried out. All nurses participating in the patient's care are required to wear a monitoring badge which records the amount of radiation received by the patient.

Specific directions are necessary regarding the disposal of excreta and contaminated dressings. For instance, radioactive iodine is eliminated in the urine, so it is collected in a lead-encased container and taken to the laboratory, where it is stored until the radioactivity has decayed. In addition to wearing gloves, the nurse should wash her hands very thoroughly with soap and running water after any contact with the patient or handling of bedding, bedpan, dressings, syringes, needles and other equipment. If an area of the nurse's skin becomes contaminated, it is washed with soap and water and monitored for radioactivity. If contamination is still indicated, the washing and monitoring are repeated. Linen is usually placed in metal containers and stored until monitoring indicates it is safe. Dishes may have to be washed and kept in the room. Nondisposable syringes, needles and other treatment equipment are thoroughly washed with soap and water and kept in the room until monitoring indicates safety, before being returned to general stock.

Any displacement or loss of radioactive implant(s) is promptly reported to the physician or radioisotope laboratory. Any radioactive implant is handled with a long forceps, never with the hands. All dressings and bedding are checked before disposal in case they contain dislodged implants. This is important because they could be a source of danger to others; also, most of these implants are very costly and are reusable.

The nurse should know the time at which the temporary implant is to be removed. The patient may be returned to the radiology department for this procedure or it may be done in the patient's room. The equipment should be ready in advance and, if necessary, the person responsible for the removal reminded. If the procedure is carried out in the patient's room, the nurse should be familiar with the disposition of the implant.

If the implantations are permanent (e.g., radon seeds), precautions are observed for the half-life of the radioisotope. A permanent type of implant may be used in the treatment of cancer of the urinary bladder. In this case all urine is collected and checked for radioactivity during the half-life of the implant.

When the isolation is terminated, the room and remaining equipment are monitored, cleansed by persons who are adequately protected with gloves, gown and shoe covers, and then monitored again. The room is left until safety is indicated.

The patient is advised as to the elimination of the isotope so he will not think he is a continuing source of danger to his family and others.

PSYCHOLOGICAL SUPPORT. The isolation and precautionary measures may be frightening to the patient even if it was explained before the radioisotope was implanted or administered. It is helpful if there is a telephone available during the period of restrictions so he can talk with his family and friends. A radio or television and reading material may also help to relieve the boredom and anxiety. Long periods of total isolation are avoided; brief visits from the doorway or frequent contact via the communication system will let the patient know he has not been forgotten.

OBSERVATIONS. The patient's temperature is taken every 4 hours; an elevation over 38°C. (100°F) is reported. As with external radiotherapy, any complaint or observed change in body function is reported to the physician. Blood tests may be done to detect possible changes that might indicate some depression of hematopoietic tissues.

PHYSICAL CARE. Nutritional and fluid intake require the same attention as that suggested for the patient who has received external radiation. The usual hygienic care is provided; the nurse works quickly when caring for the patient, keeping the time spent at the patient's bedside to a minimum without making the patient feel at all neglected.

In the case of mouth, lip or tongue therapy specific orders are received as to mouth care. Following a mouthwash, the solution is examined before it is disposed of to make sure no implants have been dislodged.

When the patient has had a uterine implantation, the patient may be required to remain in the dorsal recumbent position. Back rubs and a small pillow to fill in the space in the "small of the back" may relieve some discomfort. An indwelling catheter is usually passed at the time the implantation is made, since the patient will not likely be able to use the bedpan because of the applicator which protrudes from the vagina. A low-residue diet may be ordered so that the patient will be less likely to have a bowel movement.

If a liquid isotope has been given, the patient may be ambulatory but is requested to remain in his room during the precautionary period.

C. Chemotherapy

Drug therapy has assumed increasing importance in recent years in the treatment of some cancers, particularly those which are too widespread to be treated by surgery or radiation (e.g., leukemia, lymphoma, metastatic cancer). It may be used alone or in conjunction with surgery or radiation. Unfortunately, the drugs used are nonspecific in action, and many are highly toxic and damaging to normal cells as well as to neoplastic cells. As in radiation, the cells that proliferate rapidly are those most susceptible to the toxicity, and patients may experience irritation and ulceration of the mouth and gastrointestinal tract and suppression of the hematopoietic tissues.

The drugs used may be classified as polyfunctional alkylating agents, antimetabolites, plant alkaloids, antibiotics, hormones or steroids, and miscellaneous (a few that are used which do not fit into any of the above categories).

The *polyfunctional alkylating agents,* also known as antimitotic drugs, act within the nucleus of the cell and alter the deoxyribonucleic acid (DNA) molecules, resulting in inhibition of cell growth and reproduction.

The *antimetabolites* resemble substances that are essential to cellular activities, and which are therefore taken up by the cells. These preparations are sufficiently different from normal metabolites so as to alter metabolism and inhibit growth and reproduction. They include folic acid and purine antagonists and pyrimidine analogues.

The *plant alkaloids* currently in use are derived from periwinkle plants. They block cell reproduction during metaphase (second stage of division of the cell nucleus).

Certain *antibiotics* have been found to be of value in inhibiting some types of neoplastic cells. They act by interfering with DNA and/or RNA synthesis of the cells.

The *hormones* used in the treatment of malignant disease change the chemical environment of the cancer cells and counteract the hormone which may be favoring their

Text continued on page 148

TABLE 8-3 DRUGS USED IN CANCER THERAPY*

Chemotherapeutic Agent	Method(s) of Administration	Uses in Cancer	Toxic Effects
1. Alkylating Agents			
Mechlorethamine (nitrogen mustard; Mustargen)	Intravenous Intracavity	Lymphomas (e.g., Hodgkin's disease) Bronchogenic cancer Malignant effusion	Nausea and vomiting Anorexia Bone marrow suppression
Chlorambucil (Leukeran)	Oral	Lymphomas Lymphocytic leukemia Ovarian cancer	Anorexia Bone marrow suppression
Cyclophosphamide (Cytoxan)	Oral Intravenous	Lymphomas Multiple myeloma Lymphocytic leukemia Breast, ovarian and bronchogenic cancer Neuroblastoma	Anorexia, nausea and vomiting, diarrhea Stomatitis Bone marrow suppression Alopecia Hemorrhagic cystitis
Busulfan (Myleran)	Oral	Chronic myelogenous leukemia Polycythemia vera	Anorexia Bone marrow suppression
Melphalan (Alkeran)	Oral	Multiple myeloma Breast, ovarian and testicular cancer	Anorexia Bone marrow suppression
Triethylenethiophosphoramide (thio-Tepa)	Intravenous Intracavity Intra-arterial Oral	Lymphomas Breast and ovarian cancer Effusions	Anorexia Headache Fever and allergic reactions Bone marrow suppression
2. Antimetabolites			
6-Mercaptopurine (Purinethol; 6MP)	Oral	Leukemia	Nausea and vomiting Anorexia Bone marrow suppression Diarrhea and intestinal ulceration
5-Fluorouracil (5-FU; 5-fluorodioxyuracil)	Oral Intravenous	Cancer of breast, ovary, stomach, colon and pancreas	Anorexia Nausea and vomiting Bone marrow suppression Stomatitis Gastrointestinal ulceration Diarrhea

Drug	Route	Indications	Side Effects
Cytosine arabinoside (cytarabine; Cytosar; Ara-C)	Intravenous	Acute myelogenous leukemia Lymphomas	Nausea and vomiting Diarrhea Anorexia Stomatitis Bone marrow suppression
Methotrexate (A-Methopterin; MTX)	Oral Intravenous Intra-arterial	Acute leukemia Choriocarcinoma Cancer of head, neck, breast and testicle	Nausea, vomiting, diarrhea Stomatitis Gastrointestinal ulceration Bone marrow suppression Alopecia
Thioguanine (6-TG)	Oral	Acute myelogenous leukemia	Bone marrow suppression Stomatitis Diarrhea Skin rash Jaundice Photosensitivity
3. *Plant Alkaloids* Vinblastine (Velban)	Intravenous	Lymphomas Choriocarcinoma	Nausea and vomiting Diarrhea Bone marrow suppression Alopecia Neurotoxic effects (paresthesias, urinary retention, constipation, loss of reflexes and coordination)
Vincristine (Oncovin)	Intravenous	Acute lymphoblastic leukemia Lymphomas Wilms' tumor Neuroblastoma	Nausea and vomiting Stomatitis Neurotoxic effects (as above)
4. *Antibiotics* Actinomycin D (Dactinomycin; Cosmegen)	Intravenous	Wilms' tumor Neuroblastoma Rhabdomyosarcoma Choriocarcinoma Testicular carcinoma Ewing's sarcoma	Nausea and vomiting Stomatitis Diarrhea Bone marrow suppression Mental depression
Adriamycin (Doxorubicin)	Intravenous	Leukemia Wilms' tumor Neuroblastoma Lymphomas Ewing's sarcoma Breast, ovarian, lung, and bladder cancer	Stomatitis Bone marrow suppression Alopecia Cardiac function disturbance

Table continued on following page

TABLE 8–3 DRUGS USED IN CANCER THERAPY* (*Continued*)

Chemotherapeutic Agent	Method(s) of Administration	Uses in Cancer	Toxic Effects
Bleomycin (Blenoxane)	Intravenous Intramuscular	Cancer of skin, head, neck, cervix and testicle Lymphomas	Nausea and vomiting Stomatitis Alopecia Anaphylactic reaction Fever
Mithramycin (Mithracin)	Intravenous	Testicular cancer	Nausea and vomiting Fever Hypocalcemia and hypokalemia Stomatitis Headache and drowsiness
Daunorubicin (daunomycin; rubidomycin)	Intravenous	Leukemia	Bone marrow suppression Disturbed cardiac function Stomatitis Alopecia
Mitomycin (Mutamycin; Mitomycin C)	Intravenous	Cancer of pancreas, stomach, breast and bronchus Melanoma	Nausea and vomiting Fever Stomatitis Pruritus Alopecia Paresthesias
Streptozotocin (streptozocin)	Intravenous	Cancer of pancreas Carcinoid	Nausea and vomiting Impaired renal function Stomatitis Hypoglycemia Abdominal cramps
5. *Hormones* Estrogens (diethylstilbestrol; estradiol; Premarin; estrone; Estinyl)	Oral Intramuscular	Cancer of prostate and breast	Fluid retention Feminization of male Uterine bleeding Hypercalcemia
Progestins (hydroxyprogesterone; Delalutin; Provera)	Intramuscular	Cancer of endometrium and breast	Thrombophlebitis Impaired liver function } Rarely Hypercalcemia
Androgens (testosterone propionate; methyltestosterone; testolactone; fluoxymesterone; calusterone)	Intramuscular Oral	Breast carcinoma	Fluid retention Masculinization Hypercalcemia

Drug	Route	Indications	Side Effects
Corticosteroids (prednisone; prednisolone; dexamethasone)	Oral Intramuscular	Leukemia Lymphomas Multiple myeloma Cancer of breast	Increased appetite Euphoria Sodium and fluid retention Hypokalemia Hypertension Moon face and trunk obesity Peptic ulcer Osteoporosis Predisposition to infection
6. Miscellaneous			
L-Asparaginase (an enzyme; Elspar; L-ASP)	Intravenous	Acute lymphoblastic leukemia	Nausea and vomiting Fever Anaphylaxis Impaired liver function Hyperglycemia
Hydroxyuria (Hydrea)	Oral	Chronic leukemia Melanoma	Nausea, vomiting, anorexia Bone marrow suppression Pruritus Alopecia Stomatitis with ulceration
Procarbazine hydrochloride (Matulane; Natulan)	Oral	Lymphomas Bronchogenic cancer	Leukopenia and thrombocytopenia Joint and muscle pains Drowsiness
Bischloroethyl nitrosourea (alkylating agent; BCNU; Carmustine)	Intravenous	Neoplasia of central nervous system Multiple myeloma Melanoma	Nausea and vomiting Bone marrow suppression Impaired liver function
Lomustine (alkylating agent; CCNU)	Oral	Lymphomas Neoplasia of central nervous system Gastrointestinal, bronchogenic and renal cancer	Nausea and vomiting Bone marrow suppression Impaired liver function
Methyl-CCNU (alkylating agent; Semustine)	Oral	Neoplasia of central nervous system Melanoma Gastrointestinal, pancreatic and bronchogenic cancer	Nausea and vomiting Bone marrow suppression

*Compiled from the following sources:
M. J. Cline and C. M. Haskell: Cancer Chemotherapy, 2nd ed. Philadelphia, W. B. Saunders, 1975.
Mary W. Falconer et al.: The Drug, the Nurse, the Patient, 6th ed. Philadelphia, W. B. Saunders, 1978, pp. 353–358.
Elizabeth Begg Marino and Dona Harris LeBlanc: "Cancer Chemotherapy." Nurs. '75, Vol. 5, No. 11 (Nov. 1975), pp. 22–33.

growth. Adrenal corticosteroids are commonly used because they suppress cell reproduction through inhibition of cellular protein synthesis.

Table 8–3 lists some drugs used in cancer therapy and indicates the method(s) by which they may be administered, the cancer disease in which they may be used, and the possible toxic effects. New drugs are introduced frequently, and the search continues for a drug that will be selective and prove toxic to malignant cells without damaging normal tissue.

Methods of Administration

The channels by which anticancer drugs are administered are intravenous, oral, intramuscular, intracavity and intra-arterial. The latter method of administration may be intra-arterial infusion or perfusion.

In intra-arterial infusion, the drug is introduced directly into the artery that supplies the malignant area. The drug circulates through the affected part in high concentration before it becomes diluted in the general circulation. An arterial catheter is introduced into the appropriate artery under fluoroscopy. For instance, in liver cancer, the organ may be infused with the drug of choice via a small catheter introduced into the hepatic artery. Since it is intra-arterial, pressure is required to overcome the arterial blood pressure. A small mechanical pump may be used which delivers a certain amount of the drug at a prescribed rate.

Intra-arterial perfusion is a more complex procedure, involving an extracorporeal circulation. It is carried out in an operating room and requires the use of a pump-oxygenator (heart-lung machine). The venous blood from the affected part is diverted into the tube of the pump where the anticancer drug is added. The blood is returned to the artery that supplies the structure to be treated. The isolated circuit is maintained for ½ to 1 hour. This method of treatment prevents the circulation of the toxic drug through the total body and maintains a higher concentration in the malignant tissue for a longer period. In some instances, on completion of the perfusion, the blood may be replaced by transfusion blood to prevent the toxic drug from entering the general circulation. Since some blood containing the drug may escape into the systemic circulation, the patient must still be observed for possible toxic reactions.

Nursing Care of the Patient Receiving Chemotherapy

Anticancer drugs generally cause side effects that may be quite serious and distressing for some patients. The toxic reactions most commonly associated with the chemotherapeutic agents include bone marrow depression leading to anemia, leukopenia and thrombocytopenia, stomatitis, nausea and vomiting, diarrhea or constipation, and fluid retention. Since the side effects vary with different drugs, it is essential that the nurse know the chemotherapeutic agent given, the possible toxic reactions of that particular drug, their significance and how they are manifested.

The routine for administration varies with the drug used and with the patient's reactions to it. In some instances, a "course" of the anticancer drug is given over several days and then a period of time elapses before it is administered again. Some drugs are given in larger doses for a few days, and then in smaller maintenance doses. The dosage also is a very individual matter, being influenced by the patient's size and weight, whether one anticancer drug or a combination of two is being used, radiotherapy the patient may also have received, and reactions to the initial dose of the drug.

PREPARATION OF THE PATIENT AND FAMILY. The patient and family are informed as to what to expect; otherwise, the side effects of the drugs may engender alarm and hopelessness. When explaining the treatment plan and drug action, the potential benefits of the drug must be emphasized. The patient and family are advised that persons vary in their reactions to drugs, and the patient should tell the nurse or doctor if he feels different or observes any change in body function after he has received the drug.

The erythrocyte, leukocyte and thrombocyte counts and hemoglobin concentration are determined before the therapeutic regimen is commenced.

SIDE EFFECTS. When a patient has been given an anticancer drug he is observed closely for manifestations of possible side effects.

Leukopenia makes the patient very susceptible to infection; the avoidance of contact with persons with infection, frequent antiseptic mouthwash, and good skin care to keep it intact and free of lesions are preventive measures to be observed. The temperature is taken regularly; an elevation above normal may indicate the onset of infection. Antibiotic therapy may be instituted with even a slight elevation of temperature or any other indication of infection. Blood cell counts are usually repeated daily or every other day; if the white cells are reduced to 2000 per cu. mm., the patient will probably be cared for with reverse isolation procedures (barrier nursing; see p. 49). A marked decrease in the white blood cells is promptly brought to the physician's attention; the dosage of the therapeutic agent will likely be decreased, or the administration may be discontinued until the bone marrow recovers and leukocyte production improves.

Anemia may be manifested by weakness, complaints of constant tiredness, pallor, and shortness of breath with even slight energy expenditure.

Depression of the bone marrow may also result in a deficiency of thrombocytes, and ensuing impairment of the blood clotting process. The patient is observed for signs of hemorrhage which could be ecchymoses, blood in the stool or urine, bleeding into the sclera, or vaginal bleeding. When thrombocytopenia develops parenteral injections are avoided, if possible. Blood transfusions may be given to support the patient while his bone marrow recovers.

Many patients on chemotherapy experience nausea and vomiting which may be relieved by the use of an antiemetic. Anorexia is also a problem; every effort is made to encourage the patient to take nourishment and adequate fluids. Small amounts of high-calorie foods which may appeal to him, attractively served at frequent intervals rather than larger amounts served less often, are likely to be more acceptable. If the oral mucosa is irritated and sore, bland nonirritating foods are selected. A mouthwash just before and after each meal may help.

Diarrhea may be troublesome with the administration of an antimetabolite or antibiotic chemotherapeutic agent. An antidiarrheic preparation may be prescribed; foods that seem to initiate stools should be identified and eliminated. Bulky foods that absorb fluid (such as bran) may be added to the patient's diet and prove helpful. If the diarrhea persists dehydration may further complicate the patient's condition, and necessitate the administration of parenteral fluids.

Stomatitis (inflammation of the oral mucosa) is not uncommon in patients receiving some anticancer drugs. The mucosa becomes inflamed and tender and may ulcerate, causing considerable discomfort and interference with the ingestion of food and fluids. The mucosa readily becomes infected. Frequent oral irrigations with a mild antiseptic or alkaline solution are used, and the teeth are cleaned with a very soft brush or absorbent. An application of a mild topical anesthetic (e.g., Xylocaine preparation) may be prescribed, especially before meals.

Retention of fluid commonly occurs in patients receiving steroid drugs. The patient's fluid intake, output and weight are recorded daily. Observations are made for dependent edema. Indications of a positive fluid balance are promptly reported to the physician.

Sensory and motor innervation may be impaired in a patient receiving one of the plant alkaloid preparations. He may experience some loss of sensation, coordination and reflexes, and severe constipation. Precautions are taken to prevent possible falls. The patient is encouraged to move and prevent long periods of pressure on any one area. Bulky foods and increased fluids are given, as well as a stool softener to promote normal bowel elimination.

Many patients receiving chemotherapy suffer a temporary loss of hair (alopecia). Although the patient was informed of the possibility before receiving his drug, he may have a severe emotional reaction when it occurs. Loss of hair from the head may be reduced by using a scalp tourniquet during intravenous administration of the chemotherapeutic agent; this decreases the concentration of the drug reaching the hair follicles. The tourniquet is left in place 10 to 15 minutes after the administration. The use of scarves, turbans and wigs is discussed, and the fact that the hair will grow in again when the drug is discontinued is emphasized.

PSYCHOLOGICAL SUPPORT. The patient may become very discouraged with the discomfort and the illness experienced following the administration of an anticancer drug.

The patient presents such a distressing picture that his family members may consider "his suffering is not worth it." The nurse indicates that she understands what the patient is experiencing and appreciates the family's reaction, and again emphasizes that the effects are temporary and stresses the potential benefits. The treatment may mean less suffering, a resumption of activities and years of life.

D. Immunotherapy

Considerable attention is being directed to cancer immunology. It is suggested that probably the host's immune response is deficient, which permits the abnormal antigenic cells (neoplastic cells) to multiply rapidly. Based on this suggested etiologic factor, the administration of an immunostimulant is being used with some cancers (acute and chronic leukemia, lymphomas, melanoma, and bronchogenic cancer).

The immunostimulant currently in use is a solution of the bacillus Calmette-Guerin (BCG). It is nonspecific but stimulates both cellular and humoral immune mechanisms. The administration may be intradermal, intratumor or intravenous. Local reactions at the site of injection include inflammation, necrosis and scarring. General systemic reactions that may occur are anaphylaxis, fever and tuberculosis. The latter is treated with antituberculosis drugs (e.g., isoniazid, streptomycin, aminosalicylic acid, rifampin).

NURSING PROBLEMS COMMON TO PATIENTS WITH CANCER AND THE NURSE'S ROLE

The nursing related to cancer of specific sites is considered in the appropriate sections in Part II. Only some general problems that are common to many cancer patients are discussed here.

Psychological Impact

Cancer has become one of the most dreaded diseases, and the majority of persons believe that once a diagnosis of the disease has been made, a death warrant has been issued.

Certainly not every patient with cancer can be cured, but neither can all patients with heart conditions. Something can be done for almost every cancer patient; some can be cured, and the survival rate has shown a steady improvement (one in two[14]). Many patients whose disease is not cured live normal useful lives, symptom-free for long periods following treatment. It is necessary for the nurse to see the disease in its proper perspective and to develop a hopeful, positive attitude if she is to help the patient and his family with the emotional burden imposed by cancer.

The decision as to whether or not the patient is told he has cancer rests with the physician and the patient's family. It is influenced by the patient's circumstances, his responsibilities and obligations, the anticipated course of the disease, and by knowledge of the patient's philosophy of life and death and how he has accepted or coped with crises in the past. It may be necessary to tell the patient so he can deal with business affairs and make arrangements to prevent difficulties and hardships for the family.

At present, with the prevalence of cancer and the amount of publicity given to it, it is difficult for a patient not to suspect the possibility. In many instances, evasion of answers and deception on the part of those around him only reinforce the patient's suspicions. The uncertainty of not knowing may cause more continuous anxiety and agitation than actually knowing the diagnosis. On the other hand, some patients do not ask because they do not want their suspicion verified.

Emotional reactions to cancer are not specific. They are the same as for other serious illnesses, but cancer tends to evoke a greater degree of anxiety than other diseases. Reactions vary greatly with each individual, influenced by past and present life experiences and the hopes and goals that were held for the future. The nurse respects the patient's responses and endeavors to gain insight into some of his fears and concerns; the same illness can hold different meanings for different individuals. The patient may believe that cancer is incurable, or he may fear death, loss of usefulness and independence; his concern may be mutilation by surgery and loss of body image, with ensuing rejec-

---

[14]Canadian Cancer Society, op. cit.

tion by family and friends. The patient and family are faced with a jarring and difficult experience. There are many psychosocial factors associated with cancer. By identifying and understanding the fears and concerns of both the patient and family, the nurse is better prepared to provide assistance and support, correct misconceptions, and discourage hopelessness; tension is reduced and the patient is more likely to achieve maximum benefit from care and treatment.

The nurse must know what the doctor has told the patient and the family in order to be prepared for their questions and discussions. When she knows that the patient has been told, his reactions are observed, and if he wishes to talk about the problem, the nurse should listen and not try to avoid the situation. At times, the nurse will probably need the assistance of the physician or the patient's spiritual adviser to reinforce the support she is endeavoring to give the patient and his family. His religious faith frequently proves a source of comfort and peace that helps him to accept the situation.

The nursing student or recent graduate may need assistance from the head nurse or clinical supervisor in these difficult situations. She may have had little or no experience with death and may not yet have developed a philosophy or acceptance that it must come to all at some time. It may be helpful if she is given an opportunity to talk about the situation and her feelings and explore how she can be supportive to the patient and family. A continued, sincere interest in his welfare and attention to the details of his physical, mental and social needs assure the patient of support and confidence that help to reduce his despair and keep hope and faith alive.

Nutrition and Fluids

The fluid intake for cancer patients may have to be increased by 1000 to 1500 ml. above the normal, particularly if they are receiving radiotherapy. The products of the rapid cellular breakdown place additional demands on the kidneys. For example, the uric acid concentration increases, and unless it is well diluted and eliminated it may crystallize in the kidney tubules, leading to renal insufficiency or shutdown. The patient's cooperation is sought by advising him that plenty of fluids are important, and a supply is kept at the bedside. For the person who is weak and finds even taking a drink an effort, the necessary assistance is provided. If sufficient fluids cannot be taken by mouth, intravenous infusions are administered.

Anorexia, impaired digestion and absorption, and severe weight loss are common problems with many cancer patients. Every effort and considerable ingenuity may be necessary on the part of the nurse to tempt the patient and to help him maintain a satisfactory nutritional intake. The form of food given will depend on the location of the neoplasm. If the patient is unable to eat, tube feeding or parenteral alimentation (see p. 504) may be necessary. For the patient who can take food in the regular form, preferences and ethnic customs (consistent with his condition) are considered, the family is encouraged to bring in his favored dishes, protein supplements are used in drinks, and small amounts of high-calorie foods are offered at frequent intervals rather than three regular full meals. The surroundings should be clean, tidy and free of odors. Vitamin supplements may be ordered to meet deficiencies and to improve the patient's appetite.

Pain

The patient may be free of pain in the early stages of his disease, but later as the neoplasm invades surrounding tissues and metastasizes it causes pressure and involves sensory nerves. Nursing measures such as a change of position, a back rub, the use of pillows to provide support to a part, and a little time spent at the bedside listening and talking to the patient should be used to reduce the amount of analgesic needed and to enhance the effectiveness of that given. Initially, the patient's pain may be relieved by mild analgesics such as aspirin and propoxyphene (Darvon). Later a more potent drug, in progressively larger doses, may be necessary as the patient develops a tolerance for the analgesic and the pain becomes more severe. Prompt response to the complaint of pain means a great deal to the patient. Knowing that relief of pain is quickly available reduces his apprehension and may even lessen the amount of drug needed. If a patient is kept waiting while in pain, he may develop the habit of registering his complaint well before the hour he knows the drug may be repeated.

Skin Care

Frequently, the cancer patient becomes emaciated and his tissue has less vitality and resistance. Pressure sores readily develop unless preventive measures are used. Frequent turning, gentle massage, cleanliness and dryness are very necessary. An air or alternating pressure mattress and a sheepskin placed under the areas subjected to pressure are helpful. The vulnerable areas are inspected frequently; any discoloration is brought to the physician's attention, and pressure on the site is avoided as much as possible.

Infection

Infection is a common problem with cancer patients, and is often a terminating factor. The high incidence may be attributed to general debility and lowered resistance. The patient is susceptible as a result of impaired immune reactions and failing defense mechanisms. Those who receive radiation and chemotherapy are predisposed because these forms of treatment have an immunosuppressive effect. Many patients' disease (e.g., leukemia) involves hematopoietic and/or lymphoid tissues which play an important role in protection against infection. Another factor that probably contributes to the incidence of infection is that the greater number of cancer patients are in the older age group, and normally the aging process reduces the effectiveness of immune responses.

The nurse must be constantly aware of the problem and observe the necessary preventive measures. If the patient is in bed, a regimen of deep breathing, coughing and turning is established. Contact with persons with any type of infection is to be avoided, and the nurse practices strict medical asepsis to avoid cross infection. Nutrition plays a role in maintaining the patient's resistance; protein is essential for keeping the blood proteins at a level at which they can produce antibodies. Any breaks in the skin are treated aseptically until healed. Good hygienic care of the skin and mouth is important. If the patient's leukocyte count falls markedly, it may be necessary to protect the patient by reverse isolation.

Esthetic Factors

The sloughing of tissue in cancer and secondary infection is likely to cause an offensive odor which may produce considerable embarrassment for the patient and family. Dressings must be changed frequently, and the patient and bedding must be kept scrupulously clean. Irrigations or dressings of potassium permanganate 1:10,000 to 1:5000 may be helpful, and a number of commercial deodorants are available. Some cancers are disfiguring and the patient is likely to be very sensitive. He will be less embarrassed if he is in a private room. The room should be cheerful and attractive and have soft lighting.

Activity

Just as with other patients, those with cancer are encouraged to resume their normal pattern of life if they are able. Going back to work is good for the patient's and his family's morale, and being occupied prevents concentration on his disease. Independence within his physical limitations is encouraged and guidance as to the care required will be necessary. If the patient has a colostomy or tracheostomy or requires a prosthesis, the necessary instruction for care and adaptation to daily living is given. (Specific problems such as these are discussed in the related sections in Part II.)

The patient who cannot return to work may still be well enough to go home. As well as receiving instruction as to the necessary care at home, the patient and his family are advised of the available resources for assistance. A referral may be made to the visiting nurse association, welfare department or local branch of the National Cancer Society according to the need. When necessary, local branches of the National Cancer Society will provide dressings, colostomy equipment and drugs, loan certain equipment such as a wheelchair or hospital bed, and arrange for nursing and housekeeping services. The National Cancer Society may also have volunteer workers who make home visits and transport patients to the clinic or physician's office.

The patient is kept active and independent as long as possible; inactivity and prolonged bed rest only add to the problems by promoting circulatory stasis, muscular atrophy and weakness, pressure sores and elimination difficulties. Judgment is needed; activity should not be unduly urged beyond the patient's actual physical capacity. Details in good grooming, such as shaving, a shampoo, and a haircut or hairdo, are encouraged and arranged. This type of attention conveys a sense of worth and hope to the patient. Some form of diversion which may interest the patient is made available. Visitors, association with others and participation in social activities are advocated as long as the patient is well enough. Oversolicitous family members may need suggestions as to how to spare themselves and protect their own physical and mental health.

If the patient is in the advanced stage of his disease, the goal may simply be to keep the patient as comfortable as possible and to provide emotional support for the family. Thoughtful attention to small details which may appear rather insignificant to the nurse may assume great importance to the dependent patient.

The Role of the Visiting Nurse in Cancer

The visiting nurse has a responsible role to play in disseminating factual knowledge that will help the public develop a more optimistic attitude toward cancer. More people need to learn that many kinds of cancer are preventable, and by what means, and that many persons with cancer are cured. They should be alerted to the "seven danger signals" and the importance of diagnosis and treatment while the disease is still localized.

During her home visits and health discussions in clinics, the nurse has the opportunity to stress regular periodic examinations and monthly breast self-examination. National Cancer Society pamphlets which explain the hazards of cigarette smoking and excessive exposure to sun rays and certain chemicals may be distributed and discussed. An early sign or symptom which a person ignores or considers insignificant may be recognized and prompt investigation urged. In some instances, it may be necessary for the visiting nurse to make an appointment with the doctor or clinic for the patient. A follow-up visit is made to see if the patient kept the appointment and if further assistance is required. Should the patient be scheduled for hospital admission for further investigation or treatment, an explanation is made as to what may be expected. There may be questions to answer which could help to allay unrealistic fears on the part of the patient and his family. The home situation may be such that the patient feels that he or she cannot leave to go to the hospital. The nurse explains that any delay should be avoided, and she may be able to make suggestions or arrange for assistance that will solve the immediate home problems.

The cancer patient and his family frequently require the assistance of the visiting nurse after discharge from the hospital. There may be some residual functional interference; it is important to explain the meaning of the defect to the individual and the attendant needs. Contributions which the visiting nurse may make include recognition of the needs of the patient and his family, the actual giving of care, instruction as to treatment and activity, provision of emotional support, and arrangements for necessary socioeconomic help.

References

Books

Boedeker, Edgar C., and Dauber, James H. (Eds.): Manual of Medical Therapeutics, 21st ed. Boston, Little, Brown, 1975. Chapter 16.

Bouchard, Rosemary, and Owens, Norma F.: Nursing Care of the Cancer Patient, 3rd ed. St. Louis, C. V. Mosby, 1976.

Canadian Cancer Society: Cancer Can Be Beaten. The Facts. Toronto, Canadian Cancer Society, 1976.

Cline, Martin J., and Haskell, Charles M.: Cancer Chemotherapy, 2nd ed. Philadelphia, W. B. Saunders, 1975.

Donovan, M. I., and Pierce, S. G.: Cancer Care Nursing. New York, Appleton-Century-Crofts, 1976.

Flitter, Hessell H.: An Introduction to Physics in Nursing, 7th ed. St. Louis, C. V. Mosby, 1976.

Garner, H. H.: Psychosomatic Management of the Patient with Malignancy. Springfield, Ill., Charles C Thomas, 1966.

Krupp, Marcus A., and Chatton, Milton J.: Current Medical Diagnosis and Treatment. Los Altos, Cal., Lange, 1975. Chapter 32 and pp. 911–912.

Nave, Carl R., and Nave, Brenda C.: Physics for the Health Sciences. Philadelphia, W. B. Saunders, 1975. Chapter 21 and pp. 258–259.

Sabiston, David C.: Davis-Christopher: Textbook of Surgery, 11th ed. Philadelphia, W. B. Saunders, 1977, Chapter 23.

Schottenfeld, David: Cancer Epidemiology and Prevention. Current Concepts. Springfield, Ill., Charles C Thomas, 1975.

Periodicals

Berlin, N. I.: "Current Status of Research in Detection and Diagnosis." Cancer, Vol. 37, No. 1 (Jan. 1976), pp. 417–420.

Bingham: Carol Ann: "The Cell Cycle and Cancer Chemotherapy." Am. J. Nurs., Vol. 78, No. 7 (July 1978), pp. 1200–1205.

Boeker, Elisabeth H. (Ed.): "Symposium on Radiation Uses and Hazards." Nurs. Clin. North Am., Vol. 2, No. 1 (March 1967).

Breeding, Mary A., and Wollin, Myron: "Working Safely Around Implanted Radiation Sources." Nurs. '76, Vol. 6, No. 5 (May 1976), pp. 58–63.

Chaney, Patricia (Ed.): "Surviving." Nurs. '76, Vol. 6, No. 4 (April 1976), pp. 40–50.

Clarkson, B., and Lawrence, W.: "Perfusion and Infusion Techniques in Cancer Chemotherapy." Med. Clin. North Am., Vol. 45, No. 3 (May 1961), pp. 689–708.

Craytor, Josephine K.: "Talking with Persons Who Have Cancer." Cancer, Vol. 69, No. 4 (April 1969), pp. 744–748.

Gatti, R. A., and Good, R. A.: "Occurrence of Malignancy in Immunodeficiency Diseases." Cancer, Vol. 28, No. 1 (July 1971), pp. 89–95.

Golden, Susan: "Cancer Chemotherapy and Management of Patient Problems." Nurs. Forum, Vol. XIV, No. 3 (1975), pp. 278–303.

Harper, B. C.: "Social Aspects of Cancer Recovery." Cancer, Vol. 36, No. 1 (Suppl.; July 1975), pp. 274–276.

Hess, Cynthia M.: "Intra-arterial Chemotherapy: Making It Safer and More Successful." Nurs. '74, Vol. 4, No. 5 (May 1974), pp. 30–34.

Holland, James F.: "Prospectus for Cancer Treatment," Cancer, Vol. 36, No. 1 (Suppl.: July 1975), pp. 299–303.

Hubbard, Susan, and Devita, Vincent: "The Patient's Perspective on Cancer." Cancer, Vol. 36, No. 1 (Suppl. July 1975), pp. 279–280.

————: "Chemotherapy Research Nurse." Am. J. Nurs., Vol. 76, No. 4 (April 1976), pp. 560–565.

Jackson, Bettie S., and Armenaki, Doris W.: "A Tumor Classification System." Am. J. Nurs., Vol. 67, No. 8 (Aug. 1976), pp. 1320–1322.

Johnson, Philip C.: "Benefits and Risks in Nuclear Medicine." Am. J. Public Health, Vol. 62, No. 7 (July 1972), pp. 909–916.

Halman, Marc, and Suttinger, John: "Family-Centered Care for Cancer Patients." Nurs. '78, Vol. 8, No. 3 (March 1978), pp. 42–43.

Kelleher, Anne, et al.: "Drug Therapy by Indwelling Arterial Catheter." Am. J. Nurs., Vol. 75, No. 11 (Nov. 1975), pp. 1990–1992.

Levine, Myra E.: "Cancer Chemotherapy — A Nursing Model." Nurs. Clin. North Am., Vol. 13, No. 2 (June 1978), pp. 271–280.

Marino, Elizabeth B., and LeBlanc, Dona H.: "Cancer Chemotherapy." Nurs. '75, Vol. 5, No. 11 (Nov. 1975), pp. 22–33.

McCorkle, Margaret R.: "Coping with Physical Symptoms in Metastatic Breast Cancer." Am. J. Nurs., Vol. 73, No. 6 (June 1973), pp. 1034–1038.

McMullen, Kathleen: "When the Patient Is on Bleomycin Therapy." Am. J. Nurs., Vol. 75, No. 6 (June 1975), pp. 964–966.

Miller, Daniel G.: "What Is Early Diagnosis Doing?" Cancer, Vol. 37, No. 1 (Jan. 1976), pp. 426–432.

Miller, Suzanne: "Oncology Nurse and Chemotherapy." Am. J. Nurs., Vol. 77, No. 6 (June 1977), pp. 989–993.

O'Neill, Marcella P.: "Psychological Aspects of Cancer Recovery." Cancer, Vol. 36, No. 1 (Suppl.; July 1975), pp. 271–273.

Parsell, Sue, and Tagliareni, Elaine M.: "Cancer Patients Help Each Other." Am. J. Nurs., Vol. 74, No. 4 (April 1974), pp. 650–651.

Parsons, Joanne (Ed.): "Symposium—Needs of the Cancer Patient." Nurs. Digest, Vol. V, No. 2 (Summer 1977).

Ringer, Lynn D.: "A Cancer Patient's Message to Physician." Med. Times, Vol. 106, No. 3 (March 1978), pp. 64–67.

Schein, Phillip S.: "Current Concepts in the Drug Treatment of Cancer." Med. Times, Vol. 106, No. 3 (March 1978), pp. 26–27.

Schreier, Ann McBride, and Lavenia, Jamie: "The Nurse's Role in Nutritional Management of Radiotherapy Patients." Nurs. Clin. North Am., Vol. 12, No. 1 (March 1977), pp. 171–182.

Shubin, Seymour: "Cancer Widows: A Special Challenge." Nurs. '78, Vol. 8, No. 4 (April 1978), pp. 56–60.

Silverstein, Melvin J., and Morton, Donald L.: "Cancer Immunotherapy." Am. J. Nurs., Vol. 73, No. 7 (July 1973), pp. 1178–1181.

Theologides, A.: "Why Cancer Patients Have Anorexia." Geriatrics, Vol. 31, No. 6 (June 1976), pp. 69–71.

Tiedt, Eileen: "The Psychodynamic Process of the Oncological Experience." Nurs. Forum, Vol. XIV, No. 3 (1975), pp. 264–277.

Trowbridge, Janet E.: "Oral Care of the Patient Having Head and Neck Irradiation." Am. J. Nurs., Vol. 75, No. 12 (Dec. 1975), pp. 2146–2149.

Winters, Wendell: "Viruses and Cancer." Am. J. Nurs., Vol. 78, No. 2 (Feb. 1978), pp. 249–253.

Zubrod, C. Gordon: "Successes in Cancer Treatment." Cancer, Vol. 36, No. 1 (Suppl.; July 1975), pp. 267–270.

9

The Unconscious Patient

KAREN WOODS CHAPMAN
JEANNETTE E. WATSON

Unconsciousness is the result of impaired function of one or more areas of the brain, and is a common nursing problem that may be associated with a variety of disorders in any clinical field. Regardless of the location or nature of the primary disease process that led to the loss of consciousness, certain nursing principles and measures are common to the care of all unconscious patients.

CONSCIOUSNESS

Consciousness may be defined as the complete awareness of self and environment, with appropriate responsiveness to stimuli. The waking state and full consciousness depends upon interaction between the cerebral cortex and the central reticular formation. The central reticular formation, more often referred to as the reticular activating system, is a subcortical mass of relatively undifferentiated neurons located throughout the central portion of the brain stem. The ascending tracts of the central reticular formation receive branches from all sensory pathways that enter the brain via the spinal cord and the cranial nerves. Impulses are transmitted from the central reticular formation to the thalami, and from there to the cortex. The cortical neurons are then activated, producing a state of alertness.

It has been postulated that the reticular activating system may influence consciousness by discriminatory receptor neurons.[1] These receptors act as a "gate," selecting the input that is to continue to the cortical level, and inhibiting or rejecting extraneous incoming information (see Fig. 9–1). If the discriminatory receptors were not present, the cortex would be bombarded with numerous streams of signals or information that it is not prepared to process, and confusion would result. Rapid, precise selection and discrimination of the incoming information is the most important function of the reticular activating system and its receptors.

Once excited, the cerebral cortex gives rise to impulses which are conducted back to the reticular formation, which in turn initiates further stimuli to the cortex. A cycle is thus established between the reticular activating system and the cerebral cortex that maintains wakefulness and cerebral alertness. This continuous circuitry of arousal prepares the cortex for the reception and interpretation of ingoing sensory impulses.

Consciousness depends not only upon the normal neural circuitry with the central reticular activating system, as described above, but also upon a second factor. This second

---

[1]P. Milner: Physiological Psychology. New York, Holt, Rhinehart and Winston, 1970, p. 282.

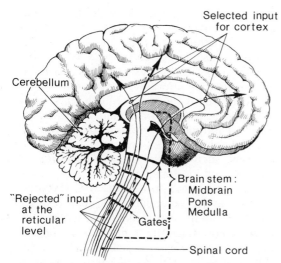

Selected input for cortex

Cerebellum

"Rejected" input at the reticular level

"Gates"

Brain stem:
Midbrain
Pons
Medulla

Spinal cord

FIGURE 9-1 Impulses transmitted to the reticular activating system may be blocked and not carried to the cerebral cortex.

factor is the normal metabolic functioning of the human body which ensures that adequate oxygen is available to the brain along with sufficient nutrients, especially glucose. In addition, the rate and volume of the cerebral blood flow, normal oxyhemoglobin dissociation and the permeability of the blood brain barrier are important factors.

SLEEP

Normal sleep is physical and mental inactivity from which a person can be roused to consciousness. It is a reversible suppression of the reticular activating system that creates a depression in the activity of the cerebral cortex. Sleep is believed to result from the eventual fatigue of the neurons and a decrease of impulses being sent through the "gates" of the reticular formation. With sleep, consciousness is lost and changes in an individual's physiological functions occur. For example, there is a decrease in the respiratory and pulse rates and blood pressure, the pupils contract and react more slowly than during wakeful periods, and the eyes deviate upwards. The electroencephalogram also shows decreased brain activity. The cerebral cortex is still capable of some mental activity, as indicated by dreams.

During sleep a person may be easily aroused to wakefulness or consciousness by cerebral arousal through stimuli such as pain or unaccustomed noise. The return to wakefulness shows that the reticular activating system is still functioning and capable of screening and discrimination.

UNCONSCIOUSNESS

Interruption of impulses from the reticular activating system, or failure of the cerebral cortical neurons to respond to incoming impulses, produces a loss of consciousness. Other than destruction of the cortical or cortical activating cells (reticular formation) by trauma, the basic factors contributing to unconsciousness are considered to be oxygen and glucose deprivation. Neurons require a constant supply of both of these substances for cellular activity. A deficiency of oxygen for even a few seconds decreases neuronal metabolism to a point at which unconsciousness ensues.

Levels of Impaired Consciousness

Impaired consciousness may be described in several different ways. It may be classified according to the responses to various stimuli, or it may be graded according to the perceptual ability and degree of responsiveness. It may be described in such terms as confusion, obtundation, stupor, light or semicoma, or deep or profound coma.

Confusion is an inappropriate reaction to the environment. For example, the patient may be unable to orient himself in time or place. *Obtundation* is a state of dullness or drowsiness, in which the patient's mental acuteness is inhibited. A patient who has reached the *stuporous* level requires vigorous and often continuous stimulation from external sources to maintain arousal. His answers to questions are likely to be incoherent. *Light or semicoma* is the state of unconsciousness in which the patient cannot be aroused but in which the peripheral reflexes (e.g., corneal, plantar, withdrawal from pain) are present. Incontinence of urine and feces occurs, and some restlessness may be manifested by the patient at the semicomatose level. *Deep or profound coma* is the level at which there is no arousal, the peripheral reflex responses of the body are lost, and incontinence of both urine and feces occurs.

Deep coma may progress to involve the vital centers (respiratory, cardiovascular) in the medulla, resulting in death from respiratory and/or circulatory failure.

The level of consciousness may be denoted by indicating the stimulus used and the response made. This method provides a more definite evaluation that can be used for comparison when the stimulus is repeated. Examples of such an assessment are:

1. Responds when spoken to; is alert, oriented and cooperative.

2. Responds when spoken to and obeys simple commands but is confused as to day, date and place.

3. No response to auditory stimuli; withdraws limb on painful stimulus (needle prick or pressure).

4. No response to painful stimuli. Gag reflex absent.

5. No response to any external stimuli.

In some clinical situations, the practice in indicating the level of response in a patient may be to use something similar to the following:

4+ indicates: normal.
3+ indicates: responsive to spoken word but confused and disoriented; reflexes normal.
2+ indicates: responsive to painful stimuli only.
1+ indicates: deep coma.

Loss of consciousness may be preceded by a period of progressive apathy or excited confusion. Recurring sudden, brief periods of unconsciousness followed by full recovery are characteristic of syncope, epilepsy and the Adam-Stokes cardiac disorder.

Causes of Impaired Consciousness

Impaired consciousness may result from a variety of intracranial or systemic disorders.

INTRACRANIAL CAUSES. Disorders within the cranium that may cause loss of consciousness include: (1) head injuries that involve concussion, depressed skull fracture, hemorrhage or a penetrating wound; (2) cerebral vascular disease, such as hemorrhage (stroke), aneurysm, thrombosis and embolism; (3) compression of brain tissue by a space-occupying lesion which may be a newgrowth, abscess or hematoma, or by an elevated intracranial pressure due to an increased volume of cerebrospinal fluid; (4) infections, such as meningitis and viral encephalitis; and (5) epilepsy.

EXTRACRANIAL OR SYSTEMIC CAUSES. Coma may be secondary to a disorder that has its origin in an area that is extracranial or quite remote from the brain. Such disorders include: (1) metabolic diseases that may result in a deficiency of glucose that is very essential to neurons of the brain (hypoglycemia, diabetic ketoacidosis), or that lead to an accumulation of metabolic wastes that are harmful to the brain (renal and hepatic failure); (2) diseases that interfere with the delivery of an adequate oxygen supply to the brain (cardiac failure, severe loss of blood, anemia, shock, respiratory insufficiency); (3) overwhelming infection in which the toxins are depressive and harmful to brain cells; (4) intoxication and poisoning (alcohol, overdoses of drugs such as barbiturates, narcotics and carbon monoxide); and (5) hypothermia.

Effects of Unconsciousness

The normal person has a variety of sensory and response mechanisms which enable him to be aware of his environment and to protect himself. Even during sleep many of these are preserved; for example, discomfort prompts one to change his position, and pain awakens him. With loss of consciousness, the mechanisms for awareness and responses essential to comfort, protection and self-preservation no longer operate. Protection and preservation become the responsibility of those caring for the patient.

Loss of skin sensation and immobility may lead to pressure sores or to burns if heat applications are used. The absence of certain reflexes poses a threat. Loss of the corneal reflex and depression of lacrimal secretion may result in prolonged exposure, drying and injury of the cornea, which may lead to ulceration. Respiration is threatened by the absence of the pharyngeal and laryngeal reflexes that normally prevent the aspiration of mucus, food and vomitus. Secretions and foreign material are retained in the respiratory tract when the cough reflex is depressed. Obstruction of the airway may occur as a result of relaxation of the lower jaw and tongue, and respirations may be infrequent and weak because of depression of the respiratory center.

Immobility and the loss of skeletal muscle tone predispose to circulatory stasis and thrombosis. Metabolic activity is usually depressed throughout the body, resulting in reduced heat production unless there is an infection or involvement of the heat-regulating center in the hypothalamus.

Normal controlled bowel and bladder elimination do not occur; the individual is usually incontinent or there may be urinary retention and constipation.

Nursing Management of the Comatose Patient

ESTABLISHMENT AND MAINTENANCE OF AN AIRWAY. The first priority in caring for an unconscious patient is the establishment of a patent airway. The comatose patient is placed in a lateral or semiprone position (unless contraindicated by a chest or spinal injury), with the neck aligned with the spine. Either position facilitates the drainage of mucus and vomitus and prevents obstruction of the airway by the relaxed tongue and jaw. If mucus collects in the oropharyngeal cavity, frequent suctioning with a flexible catheter will be necessary. The catheter should have several holes at its tip for adequate collection of the mucus during suctioning. The catheter is moistened with water prior to its insertion and is handled gently with intermittent suctioning to avoid trauma of the mucous membranes.

If the patient is restricted to the dorsal position because of his condition (e.g., a patient who is unconscious due to a motor vehicle accident may also require traction), or his breathing is hindered in the semiprone position, an artificial airway may be needed. An oropharyngeal airway or an endotracheal or a tracheostomy tube may be inserted to maintain the airway and facilitate the removal of secretions by suctioning. (See pp. 416–421 for a discussion of intubation and tracheostomy.)

ASSESSMENT. The unconscious patient requires constant, close observation. Skilled observations and recording of the patient's manifestations are important in assessing progress and in some cases in detecting the cause of unconsciousness.

The nursing assessment of any unconscious patient includes the following:

1. The vital signs (i.e., temperature, pulse, respirations and blood pressure) are recorded frequently, with the frequency depending upon the patient's condition. For example, if the coma is due to a head injury or intracranial disorder, the nurse may be required to record the pulse and blood pressure every 15 or 30 minutes and the temperature every 1 or 2 hours. In addition to observing the rate, rhythm and depth of the respirations, the equality of the chest excursion on both sides and any sounds associated with inspiration or expiration are noted. The chest is auscultated for possible retention of secretions and inadequate ventilation of some lung areas.

2. Observation is made for any change in the level of consciousness that may be manifested by a response to an external stimulus or by spontaneous behavior, such as movement of the limbs.

3. The reaction, size and equality of the pupils are noted and the eyes are examined for retracted lids ("open eyes"), discharge and edema. The nurse may also be expected to test the corneal reflex occasionally. This involves touching the cornea lightly with a wisp of cotton to determine if the normal reflex response of closing the eye is present. It is obvious that judgment is necessary when testing this reflex; too frequent use of it by other than knowledgeable, experienced persons could result in damage to the cornea.

4. The skin is checked for discoloration, temperature, and dryness or moisture. If the skin is cold and moist it may indicate unfavorable progress or shock and is brought to the physician's attention. If it is very dry, the patient may require fluids. Discoloration of pressure areas signifies possible tissue damage and the need for more intense skin care

of these vulnerable areas. Blueness or cyanosis of the extremities indicates a lack of adequate oxygen delivery which may be due to interference with the circulation to the part, or to cardiac or respiratory insufficiency.

5. Skeletal muscles are examined for increased spasticity or flaccidity which may point to central nervous system involvement. Rigidity of the neck and hyperextension of the head are important manifestations.

6. The nurse may be expected to assess the patient's responses and reflexes. Simple tests for responses include speaking to the patient, making verbal commands, gentle squeezing of a hand, and exerting finger pressure to the supraorbital area or on a finger, elbow, knee or ankle joint. Patellar and biceps tendon reflexes are commonly tested; normally the leg extends quickly when the patellar tendon is tapped and the arm flexes when the biceps tendon is used. If a blunt object is moved along the lateral portion of the sole of the foot, it normally elicits the response of flexion of the toes. Dorsiflexion of the toes (especially the great toe) reflects some central nervous system involvement (contralateral corticospinal tract).

The gag reflex may be tested when mouth care is being given. If it is absent, it indicates deep coma and emphasizes the need for efficient drainage and removal of oropharyngeal secretions to prevent aspiration and ensuing respiratory complications.

7. The fluid intake and output are measured and the fluid balance determined.

8. Various laboratory tests and investigational procedures may be carried out to determine the cause of the patient's unconsciousness, or to assess the disorder that is known to be the etiologic factor. The nurse provides the necessary protection and support for the unconscious person during procedures that involve moving, special positioning or body invasion. The family may be concerned about the patient being subjected to some of the investigative procedures (e.g., x-rays, lumbar puncture, electroencephalogram, taking of blood specimens); the nurse takes time to advise them of the procedure and its purpose and that she will be with the patient.

POSITIONING. When the patient is placed in the lateral or semiprone position (as cited above), attention is given to good body alignment and to the prevention of contractures, foot and wrist drop, muscle strain, joint injury, and interference with circulation and chest expansion. The head is positioned so that the neck is aligned with the spine. The arm that is uppermost is flexed at the elbow and rests on a pillow to prevent a drag on the shoulder and wrist drop. The arm that is down is drawn slightly forward, flexed at the elbow, and lies on the bed parallel with the neck and head. The lower limb that is uppermost is flexed at the hip and knee, and supported on a firm, plastic-covered pillow; the other lower limb is slightly flexed. Dorsiflexion of the feet is maintained by the use of firm pillows, sandbags or a footboard (see Fig. 9–2).

The patient is turned hourly to promote circulation and to prevent the accumulation of pulmonary secretions and the development of pressure sores. A minimum of two or three persons is necessary to turn the unconscious patient in such a manner that hyperextension and joint and muscle strain are avoided.

In some conditions (e.g., cerebral injury and following some brain operations), the patient may have to remain on his back. The arms are slightly adducted and supported on pillows. Trochanter rolls are used to prevent outward rotation of the lower extremities, and the space under the knees may be filled in by a folded towel or small pillow. The feet are supported in the dorsiflexion position.

The extremities are passively moved through their normal range of motion at least twice daily to preserve joint function and prevent circulatory stasis.

PROTECTION FROM INJURY. The side rails of the bed are always maintained in the up position unless someone is in constant attendance on the patient. He could suddenly regain consciousness, be confused and fall out of bed if the side rails are not up. It may be necessary to pad the sides of the bed if the patient is restless and thrashing about. Placing mittens on the hands may be necessary if the patient is restless, scratches himself, or pulls on the nasogastric or intravenous tube,

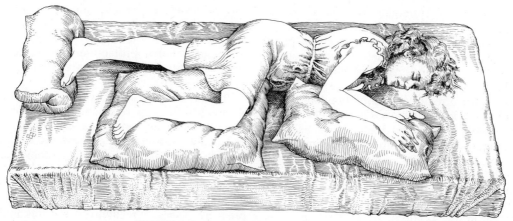

FIGURE 9–2   Position of the unconscious patient.

or the urethral catheter. The mittens are removed twice daily; the hands are bathed, the nails are kept clean and short, and the fingers put through their normal range of motion by passive exercise.

The use of restraints is avoided if possible. The patient often becomes more restless if restrained when he is in the confused or obtunded state or when he arouses from the comatose state. The nurse does not attempt to force resisting extremities (such as in decorticate or decerebrate rigidity) to assume a different position. Forcing a rigid extremity into a different position could result in a fracture of that limb.

FLUIDS AND NUTRITION. At no time should the unconscious patient be given food or fluid by mouth; a poor or absent swallowing reflex could lead to the aspiration of either into the respiratory tract. The patient's nutrition may be sustained by intravenous infusion, feedings given via a nasogastric tube or hyperalimentation (see p. 504). The

liquid tube feeding contains the essential food elements and may provide 1500 to 2500 calories per day. A feeding of 100 to 200 ml. may be given every 2 to 3 hours. If there is any regurgitation (fluid welling up around the tube into the mouth), the volume given at one time is decreased, and the frequency of the feedings is increased. If the patient's condition permits, it is helpful to elevate the head of the bed slightly during the feeding. The tube is rinsed with 30 to 45 ml. of water after each feeding.

The presence of the tube in a nostril tends to irritate the mucous membrane and stimulate mucus secretion. The area is cleansed twice daily with applicators which have been moistened with normal saline, and is then also lubricated lightly. The tube is secured loosely enough so that it does not continuously press on any one area of the nostril.

When a patient is unconscious for a prolonged period nourishment may be provided by parenteral alimentation. This procedure is a means of supplying the individual's complete nutritional needs by intravenous infusion of solutions of amino acids or protein hydrolysates, glucose, lipids, electrolytes, and vitamins. An indwelling venous catheter is introduced into the subclavian vein (either directly or via the brachial vein) or the superior vena cava (via the subclavian and innominate veins) under rigid aseptic technique, and the solution is administered slowly at a prescribed, constant rate. A very fine filter (millipore) is incorporated into the intravenous line to remove any possible organisms and solid particles that might be present in the solution.

Infection is a hazard to which the nurse must be constantly alert; the solutions used provide an excellent medium and the direct open line into the blood stream predisposes the patient to septicemia unless asepsis is strictly observed. Specific directions are received from the physician as to the care of the catheter and the site at which it is introduced. For further details about hyperalimentation see p. 504.

ELIMINATION. The comatose patient has urinary incontinence or may have retention with incontinent overflow. An indwelling catheter is passed to assess output and prevent skin irritation. The catheter may be clamped for specified intervals to maintain normal bladder tone and capacity. It is taped to the thigh or secured to the bed to prevent undue traction. The indwelling catheter used may be a triple lumen tube; one lumen is to inflate the "balloon" that holds the catheter in the bladder, another is to provide for an inflow of an irrigating solution, usually an antibacterial preparation, and the third lumen allows bladder drainage (urine and irrigating solution). The complete set of tubes and drainage receptacle constitutes a closed sterile system. The urethral meatus and surrounding area are cleansed with an antiseptic solution two or three times daily. A gauze dressing moistened with the antiseptic may be placed around the catheter at the meatus.

If a retention catheter is not used, frequent attention is necessary to protect the skin. Pads are used to absorb the urine and are changed promptly after voiding. The bed may be protected by a square of absorbent material with an undersurface of plastic. The skin is washed after each voiding, dried thoroughly and a protective powder (e.g., zinc stearate) or a moisture-repellant ointment is applied.

The patient may have involuntary stools, particularly if he is receiving tube feedings. Prompt cleansing and changing of soiled pads and bedding are necessary. If the bowels do not move, a cleansing enema may be ordered every second day.

SKIN CARE. The unconscious patient is predisposed to the rapid development of pressure sores. Precautions are taken to keep the skin clean and dry and the bedding free of wrinkles. In addition to a complete daily bath, pressure areas are bathed and gently massaged frequently to stimulate the circulation and prevent a breakdown of the skin. Powder, lanolin or a light, oily preparation may be used on the skin during massage. A resilient, soft material, such as sponge rubber or sheepskin, is placed under the pressure areas, or an alternating air pressure (ripple) mattress may be used. If a pressure sore develops it is treated aseptically, just as any wound, and as little pressure as possible is placed on the area.

CARE OF THE EYES. If the corneal reflex is absent and the eyelids are retracted, eyeshields or eyepads are applied to protect the cornea from possible injury and continuous exposure. Daily irrigations with sterile normal saline and the instillation of a drop of an ophthalmic solution are essential care measures to provide moisture and protection.

CARE OF THE MOUTH AND NOSE. Dentures are removed in case they become displaced and interfere with breathing. The mouth and tongue tend to become dry and coated, necessitating cleansing every 2 hours with swabs which have been moistened in an antiseptic mouthwash. An application of mineral oil to the tongue and of oil, petroleum jelly or cold cream to the lips helps to prevent drying and encrustations.

The nostrils are examined daily for accumulated secretions, which are removed by cotton applicators moistened with water.

PSYCHOLOGICAL CONSIDERATION. Conversation should be guarded in the presence of the patient; nothing is said that would not ordinarily be said if the individual were conscious. Occasionally things that have been said are recalled with startling accuracy when the patient regains consciousness.

The individual's right to dignity and respect is observed. The hair is combed and kept tidy, the fingernails are kept clean and short, and the male patient is shaved if his condition permits. At all times the patient is protected from unnecessary body exposure.

The patient cannot indicate needs and discomforts; it is the nurse's responsibility to make every effort to recognize these and to do everything possible to provide high quality care. For example, the temperature of the environment and the number of covers are controlled according to the patient's temperature and the warmth of his skin.

The family and their concern for the patient requires consideration. Time should be taken to talk with them, answer their questions and reassure them that everything that can be done is being done. It may be helpful to them if a family member is allowed to remain at the bedside and participate in some aspects of the care. For example, the relative might assist with the turning and positioning of the patient. Family socioeconomic problems may have resulted from the illness; a referral to the appropriate social or welfare service may provide the necessary assistance.

RECOVERY OF CONSCIOUSNESS. When a patient recovers consciousness he is likely to experience a period of confusion and bewilderment. He may be unable to appreciate what has happened and where he is. The presence of a familiar face and voice will mean much to the patient at this time. A family member or friend is encouraged to be with him. He is reoriented and advised as to what has occurred.

There may be some residual disability that necessitates the planning and initiation of a rehabilitation program.

References

Books

Beeson, Paul B., and McDermott, Walsh (Eds.): Textbook of Medicine, 15th ed. Philadelphia, W. B. Saunders, 1979.

Beland, Irene L., and Passoo, Joyce Y.: Clinical Nursing, 3rd ed. New York, MacMillan, 1975, pp. 261–263.

Boedeker, Edgar C., and Dauber, James H. (Eds.): Manual of Medical Therapeutics, 21st ed. Boston, Little, Brown, 1974. Chapter 21.

Brain, L., and Walton, J.: Brain's Diseases of the Nervous System, 7th ed. London, Oxford Press, 1969.

Carini, Esta, and Owens, Guy: Neurological and Neurosurgical Nursing, 6th ed. St. Louis, C. V. Mosby, 1974.

Ganong, William F.: Medical Physiology, 7th ed. Los Altos, Cal., Lange, 1975. Chapter 11.

Krupp, Marcus A., and Chatton, Milton J.: Medical Diagnosis and Treatment. Los Altos, Cal., Lange, 1975, pp. 550–551.

Milner, P.: Physiological Psychology. New York, Holt, Rinehart and Winston, 1970.

Thorn, G. W., et al. (Eds.): Principles of Internal Medicine. 8th ed. New York, McGraw-Hill, 1977.

Periodicals

Brooks, H. L.: "The Golden Rule for the Unconscious Patient." Nurs. Forum, Vol. 4, No. 3 (1965), pp. 12–18.

———: "Evaluation of the Unconscious Patient." Med. Clin. North Am., Vol. 57, No. 6 (Nov. 1973), pp. 1363–1372.

———: "Coma." (Panel discussion). Nurs. '74, Vol. 4, No. 5 (May 1974), pp. 24–29.

Gardner, M. Arlene: "Responsiveness as a Measure of Consciousness." Am. J. Nurs., Vol. 68, No. 5 (May 1968), pp. 1034–1038.

Locke, S.: "The Neurological Aspects of Coma." Surg. Clin. North Am., Vol. 48, No. 2 (April 1968), pp. 251–256.

Luessenhop, A.: "Care of the Unconscious Patient." Nurs. Forum, Vol. 4, No. 3 (1965), pp. 6–11.

Olmstead, R. W., and Murtagh, F.: "The Unconscious Patient." Pediatr. Clin. North Am., Vol. 9, No. 1 (Feb. 1962), pp. 3–16.

Tate, G.: "Assessment and Direction of Nursing Care for Patients with Acute Central Nervous System Insult." Nurs. Clin. North Am., Vol. 6, No. 1 (March 1971), pp. 165–171.

10

The
Surgical
Patient

Surgery is defined as the treatment of disease, injury or deformity by manual or instrumental procedure.[1] This indicates the special feature that categorizes the patient as being surgical, but the care that contributes to the restoration and maintenance of optimum physiological status before and after the operation comprises a large portion of the total surgical treatment and is extremely important in determining the patient's progress and recovery.

Surgical operations may be classified as elective, essential or emergency. An *elective operation* is not necessary for the patient's survival but is expected to improve the patient's comfort and health. *Essential surgery* is considered necessary to remove or to prevent a threat to the patient's life. An *emergency operation* is one which must be done with a minimum of delay in the interest of the patient's survival.

Operative procedures vary greatly. They range from one that is quite simple and uncomplicated, taking only a brief period, to a prolonged, complex, major procedure that has severe traumatic effects. Many necessary considerations and nursing measures are common to the care of all surgical patients, regardless of their particular type of surgery. The basic components of the plan of care

may require modification and/or additional specific details according to the particular operative procedure, the individual's psychological or physiological status, and the type of anesthetic used.

PREPARATION OF THE PATIENT FOR SURGERY

The preoperative period, which begins with the decision that surgery is to be performed, may extend over an hour to several days or weeks. Whenever the patient's condition permits, sufficient time is taken to assess and treat the patient so that he goes to the operation in the best condition possible. Intelligent, conscientious preoperative nursing may contribute much to having the patient achieve an optimum condition that favors a satisfactory postoperative progress and minimizes the possibility of complications. When the surgery is elective or essential, there is usually a period of several days or weeks that the patient is at home awaiting admission to the hospital. A visiting nurse may contribute to the patient's physical and psychological preparation during this time. Some of the patient's and family's questions may be answered, psychological support provided and advice given on such matters as nutrition and rest. Possible solutions to social and economic problems that are precipitated by the impending surgery may also be suggested by the visiting nurse.

---

[1]Benjamin F. Miller and Claire Brackman Keane: Encyclopedia and Dictionary of Medicine, Nursing and Allied Health, 2nd ed. Philadelphia, W. B. Saunders Co., 1978, p. 969.

Psychological Preparation

PATIENTS' FEARS. Few patients face surgery without some degree of anxiety. The concerns and fears vary from one person to another; some may be anxious about the pain and discomfort, others fear possible disfigurement and incapacity, loss of control of self, or death. They may be worried because of the expense being incurred, absence from work, lack of support for dependents, lack of care for the family or disruption of plans. Many are disturbed because they simply don't know what to expect; the unknown tends to be more threatening than the known.

The patient's emotional state and physical condition should receive equal consideration. Psychic stress evokes physiological responses that may impair health; fear initiates adrenal medullary responses (release of epinephrine and norepinephrine) which may have an unfavorable effect, especially if prolonged. The emotionally disturbed patient may experience a greater problem with vomiting, urinary retention, pain and restlessness during the postoperative period.

PSYCHOLOGICAL SUPPORT. Through more prolonged and intimate contact with the patient, the nurse has the opportunity to assess his perception of the situation and identify his attitudes and concerns. Many of his and his family's fears may be unrealistic, based on misinformation and misconceptions about the surgery. The surgeon, in a limited time, will have discussed the operation with the patient and family: what it involves, why it is necessary and the expected results. Frequently, the patient and his family are so emotionally overcome at the time that they do not grasp all that has been said. Later, they want clarification and usually have a number of questions. The nurse should determine what information was given them by the doctor and, in simple understandable terms, answer their questions. Tact is necessary in order to avoid increasing their anxiety.

The patient is encouraged to reveal his fears and concerns, which are accepted by the nurse as reasonable and to be expected. The problems are explored and, through verbalizing them and receiving some explanation or available assistance, some of the apprehension may be allayed. The fact that someone expects him to have some qualms and is sufficiently interested to listen to him is in itself a comfort to the patient. Some patients may be reluctant to express their fears because they think of them as a personal weakness within themselves, but they may be manifesting their insecurity in other ways such as tenseness, restlessness or withdrawal. The nurse, recognizing the problem, may initiate a discussion by saying, "I am sure you are concerned about your operation; there may be something I could clarify for you if you would like to talk about it." There may be the occasional patient who displays a total lack of concern; this person may have considerable deep underlying concern which for some reason he is denying. His reaction is brought to the surgeon's attention.

The patient receives an explanation of why several days of hospitalization are necessary before the actual operation. He is kept informed as to the purpose and what is involved in the investigative and preparatory procedures. What he may expect on the day of operation and in the postoperative period is discussed. Ignorance of what is going to happen usually causes more fear and mental suffering than being advised of the facts.

Any anticipated permanent change in body function or appearance is explored, and the patient is advised as to the available assistance and how he may manage his life; emphasis is placed on the positive aspects. For instance, a woman who is to have a mastectomy may be concerned about her appearance but is relieved when she learns that special prosthetic brassieres are available. A patient who is being prepared for a permanent colostomy may be encouraged to see and talk with a person who has had the same operation and is living a relatively normal, active life.

It is an established practice in some institutions to have an operating room nurse who will be involved with the patient's surgery visit him 2 or 3 days before the day of operation. This has distinct advantages for the patient. It tends to lessen "the fear of the unknown" for the patient. The visit means that when he is received in the operating room, the nurses will not all be complete strangers. It also indicates an interest on the part of the staff, which is reassuring to the patient. The nurse reviews the patient's history, talks with his ward nurse and advises the patient of the purpose of this visit. The discussion includes such matters as transportation to the operating room, the type of room he will be in, any preanesthetic checks, why staff are gowned and masked, the anesthetic, and the postoperative return to the recovery room or the surgical ward. The patient is encouraged to ask questions. The visit to the ward and patient provides the operating room nurse with information about the patient that enables the operating room staff to be prepared more fully for this particular patient. For example, the patient may have a disability that necessitates preparation for placing him in a different position than that normally used.

Consideration is given to placement on the ward by selecting a unit that is quiet and nearer to those less likely to increase anxiety in the patient. Long periods in which the patient is entirely alone should be avoided; relatives are encouraged to visit and the nurse should "drop in" at frequent intervals. Some form of diversion in which he is interested may be provided. The patient may find his religious adviser a source of strength and courage, but one must be cautious about suggesting such a visit. The patient may request it, or the nurse might tactfully suggest it to the family without increasing their anxiety. In some instances help beyond that which the nurse can provide is needed to reduce the patient's fear. It may be necessary to consult the surgeon or anesthetist and have one of them talk further with the patient.

If the patient is ambulatory and hospitalized for several days before surgery, he is encouraged to spend some time in the ward lounge to meet and mix with other patients. Most patients tend to talk readily to each other about their problems and share their preoperative fears. The fact that many of the same concerns are experienced by others seems to put them in proper perspective and make them less ominous to the patient.

Family members are kept informed, and time is taken to talk with them, answer their questions, and advise them as to how they can offer support to the patient.

Physical Preparation

PHYSICAL ASSESSMENT. Common concerns with all surgical patients are cardiac, pulmonary and renal function, blood volume and composition, nutritional status, and fluid and electrolyte balance. Basic laboratory tests for all preoperative patients include urinalysis, hematocrit, hemoglobin, leukocyte count, and bleeding or clotting time. An electrocardiogram is usually done, and the chest is examined by auscultation and probably x-ray. Other laboratory tests, functional studies and x-rays may be done, as well as specific investigative procedures relevant to the patient's particular disorder and physiological status. These studies should be understood by the nurse so that the necessary explanation, support for the patient and the appropriate adaptations in nursing care plan can be made.

The patient's history and physical examination records are reviewed for significant information that may influence both preoperative and postoperative care. For example, if an incident of an allergic reaction is recorded, further questioning of the patient and family may be necessary to elicit sufficient information. The nurse makes sure the physician is aware of this so that possible allergens are avoided, which might be certain drugs. If the health history reveals that the patient has had several episodes of pneumonia, the nurse looks for early signs of a respiratory complication and takes extra precautions to protect the individual from possible contact with infection.

The nurse is constantly alert for signs and symptoms that might indicate a condition or change in the patient which could interfere with the patient's progress and predispose to complications. Such factors as the following are promptly reported to the physician: an elevated temperature; a significant change in pulse, respirations or blood pressure; a rash; a cough, complaint of sore throat or nasal discharge that might point to a respiratory infection; bleeding gums, which may indicate a vitamin C deficiency; onset of menstruation; diarrhea; nausea and vomiting; and a deficient food or fluid intake.

NUTRITION. The patient who is malnourished tolerates surgery less well. Protein deficiency delays healing and decreases the resistance to infection because of a slower response in antibody formation. Vitamin C also plays an important role in healing since it is necessary for the laying down of collagen fibers. It also contributes to capillary integrity. Optimum amounts of the vitamin B complex are necessary for normal glucose metabolism and for the maintenance of cellular enzymes. A deficient intake of carbohydrate depletes the liver glycogen, leaving the body without a reserve source of glucose during the period when food intake is decreased, which leads to catabolism of the body tissues.

If the patient is not obese and can tolerate it, he is given a high-calorie (3000 to 4000 calories), high-carbohydrate diet and vitamin supplements. The patient is more likely to cooperate if he is advised of the significant role nutrition plays in his postoperative progress. Feeding the patient or providing some assistance may be necessary if he is weak or uncomfortable. Frequent small feedings may prove more successful than three large meals. When possible, the patient is consulted as to foods that he would prefer.

If the patient's condition is such that the ordinary solid food cannot be taken, fluids containing commercial protein concentrates and glucose may be tolerated. When oral intake is insufficient or not possible, intravenous solutions of glucose, protein preparations, plasma or whole blood may be administered.

There is a considerable increase in the risk in surgery on obese persons. They have a greater tendency to develop cardiovascular, pulmonary and wound complications. The excessive fat tissue frequently makes the operative procedures more difficult. The patient who is overweight is advised of the need to lose weight before his operation and may be placed on a diet of 800 to 1200 calories.

FLUIDS AND ELECTROLYTES. A normal fluid balance is extremely important in the surgical patient; dehydration predisposes to shock, a retention of metabolic wastes, and disturbances in electrolyte concentrations. The patient who has been ill for some time particularly if his disorder is gastrointestinal, frequently has a fluid and electrolyte deficit. A record of the fluid intake and output is kept, and the patient is observed for signs of dehydration (see p. 82). A minimum intake of 2500 to 3000 ml. is encouraged unless contraindicated. Blood chemistry studies are done to determine electrolyte concentrations, and any deficiencies are corrected by oral or parenteral preparations.

REST AND EXERCISE. The patient awaiting an operation may find it difficult to rest and sleep because of anxiety and decreased activity. It is brought to the doctor's attention, and regular small doses of a mild sedative may be prescribed to provide relaxation and the necessary rest. The patient is encouraged to read or pursue an appropriate hobby which will occupy his mind and prevent constant, intense concentration on his condition and impending surgery.

When the patient is well enough, he is usually kept ambulatory and encouraged to get some exercise. This prevents general weakness, contributes to normal fatigue and rest, and diminishes the probability of circulatory complications later.

INFORMATION AND INSTRUCTION. The patient is informed where he will be following the operation — that is, whether he will be taken to a recovery room or a surgical ward or returned to his present unit. If the recovery room is used, the nurse describes that unit and what occurs there, and indicates how long he will be cared for in that department.

Deep breathing and coughing at frequent intervals will be necessary after the operation. These are to prevent pulmonary complications by fully expanding the lungs and removing secretions. The purpose is explained to the patient, and he is taught how they are done and encouraged to practice. Assurance is given that the necessary assistance and support will be provided. The patient is requested not to smoke; any irritation of the respiratory tract predisposes to pulmonary complications.

Postoperative lower limb exercises to prevent circulatory stasis and thrombosis are described and demonstrated. The patient is also advised that he will be assisted in getting out of bed for brief periods in the early postoperative period, as this promotes normal body processes and reduces problems such as vomiting, gas pains and difficulty with voiding. He is also told that he need not be alarmed by the nurse's frequent checking of his pulse and blood pressure; they are checked on all patients to provide information as to their condition. If the use of drainage tubes (e.g., chest or gastric) or special equipment such as a respirator is anticipated, these are also discussed so that he won't think his condition is worse than had been expected.

SPECIFIC THERAPY. Certain treatments to correct secondary physiological disturbances or coexistent disease may comprise a large part of the preoperative preparation. The patient who has developed anemia because of a loss of blood or nutritional deficiency may receive one or more blood transfusions (see p. 263). A course of an antimicrobial drug may be necessary to clear up some infection. A diabetic patient may require dietary and insulin therapy to bring his disease under control, lower the blood sugar, and have the urine free of sugar and ketone acids. The purpose of any such treatments and their significance to the surgery are explained to the patient and his family.

Operative Consent

Before any operation, it is necessary to obtain the patient's signature to a statement which gives consent for the anesthetic and operation.[2] The purpose is to protect the hospital, surgeon and anesthetist against claims of unauthorized anesthesia and surgery. The statement indicates that the nature of the anesthetic and operation have been explained and that consent is given. A clause is usually included that permits further or alternative procedures that are deemed necessary during the operation. Exceptions may be added at the patient's request. When asked to sign the consent, the patient must be rational, alert and not under the influence of any drug that might impair comprehension and judgment. Preferably, the signing is done a day or two before the day of operation, not just before bedtime the night before the operation or the morning of operation, as it is likely to increase the patient's anxiety at such a time.

The signing of an operative consent must be witnessed by a person authorized to do so by the hospital; in some institutions only a doctor is permitted to act as a witness, while in others it may be either a doctor or a nurse. The witness attests to the fact that in his or her presence the statement has been read and explained to the signatory, who stated that he or she understood and then signed the consent.

If the patient is a minor, the permit must be signed by a parent or legal guardian. If he is a minor but is married or earning his own living, he may sign the consent. When a relative of a minor is not close by, consent by telephone, letter or telegram may be accepted. In the case of an emergency involving a minor or an unconscious patient, consent may have to be obtained by telephone. If a relative cannot be reached and immediate surgery is necessary in the interest of the patient's life, a brief statement explaining the circumstances may be signed by two physicians.

For operations that are likely to alter the patient's functional ability or appearance permanently, the signature of a close relative is required as well as the patient's. For instance, when a hysterectomy is to be done, the husband's consent may also be necessary. Other examples of cases in which two signatures may be required are operations on the brain and amputations. It is advisable for the nurse working in a new or unfamiliar situation to determine the policies pertaining to informed consents in that particular hospital.

Immediate Preoperative Preparation

The following preparatory measures receive consideration the day before and on the day of operation.

FOOD AND FLUIDS. The patient's stomach should be empty when he goes to the operating room to prevent the possibility of aspiration of vomitus. No solid food is given after a light evening meal on the day before operation. Clear fluids are permitted and encouraged up to 6 hours before the scheduled hour for the surgery. An explanation is given to the patient as to why food and fluid are withheld. If the patient's mouth becomes dry and uncomfortable, he is given a mouthwash. Parenteral fluids may be ordered the morning of operation, particularly if the surgery is scheduled for late in the day. When a patient inadvertently takes food or fluid, the surgeon or anesthetist is promptly notified. It will probably necessitate a postponement of the operation or the passing of a gastric tube to evacuate the stomach content.

When the patient is a child, the doctor may stress the giving of clear sweetened fluids for 24 hours up to 4 to 6 hours before operation. This is to promote an optimum glycogen reserve in the liver since it is normally proportionately less than in the adult and will be depleted quickly.

---

[2]A consent signed by the patient is also necessary for some major diagnostic procedures.

If the patient is to receive a local anesthetic, a light breakfast may be permitted by the physician.

ELIMINATION. The physician's orders may or may not include a cleansing enema. If the patient has had a normal bowel movement the day before operation, it may not be considered necessary. Some surgeons prefer all patients having major surgery to have a cleansing enema the evening before surgery to prevent constipation following the operation when diet and activity are restricted.

The bladder should be empty when the patient goes to the operating room in order to prevent incontinence during the anesthetic induction and operation. In the case of low abdominal or pelvic surgery, a full bladder may interfere with the surgical procedure by making the site less accessible, and it may also increase the risk of accidental injury to the bladder wall. The patient is asked to void just before the preoperative sedative takes effect. If the patient is unable to void, or to be certain that the bladder is empty, catheterization may be ordered. The doctor may want an indwelling catheter passed and attached to a drainage system if the patient is receiving continuous intravenous infusion or if he wants the bladder to remain collapsed throughout the operation.

LOCAL PREPARATION. Although the details of the preparation of the site of the operation vary according to the area and the surgeon's preference, the principles are the same. The site is treated to have it as free as possible of dirt particles, hair, desquamated cells, secretions and organisms.

When the skin is to be prepared, the site of the incision and a generous surrounding area are carefully shaved and thoroughly cleansed with water and a detergent-germicide the afternoon or evening before operation (see Fig. 10–1 for areas). In some instances, the cleansing is followed by an application of an antiseptic such as benzalkonium chloride (Zephiran Chloride) 1:1000. Further cleansing and the application of an antiseptic are carried out in the operating room.

If a patient is discovered to have acne or infected lesions, the operation may be delayed until the condition is corrected. Daily antiseptic baths or the application of an antimicrobial preparation may be prescribed.

Special preparation extending over several days may be ordered by the surgeon for some operations such as skin grafts and orthopedic procedures. Specific instructions for local preparation are received for any surgery on the head, face and eye.

When vaginal surgery is to be done, in addition to shaving and cleansing the area surrounding the vaginal orifice, a cleansing antiseptic douche may be ordered.

For rectal and lower bowel surgery, the patient may be required to have water or saline enemas until the return is clear. These are given high and slowly, and the patient is allowed to rest following each one. They should also be given early enough to make sure all fluid is expelled before the patient is taken to the operating room. The perineum and surrounding area are thoroughly cleansed with water and detergent following the final evacuation.

In the case of operations on the mouth or throat, unless specific preparatory instructions are given, the teeth are cleaned and the mouth rinsed well with an antiseptic mouthwash the night before and the morning of the day of operation.

PERSONAL CARE. Depending on the patient's condition, he has a tub bath, shower, or bed bath on the morning of operation. If the surgeon approves, the patient who is able is encouraged to do this for himself, since the ambulation and activity stimulate circulation and deeper respirations. If the operation is scheduled for an early hour, the bath is taken the night before so the patient is disturbed as little as possible in the morning. A clean hospital gown is provided.

The teeth are cleansed and an antiseptic mouthwash is used the night before and the morning of the day of operation to make sure all food particles are removed. Dentures are removed because they may become displaced and interfere with respirations. They are placed in an appropriate container in the patient's locker. Occasionally, the anesthetist may ask to have the dentures left in place so the anesthetic mask will fit more closely to the face. Any prosthesis, such as an artificial eye or limb, is removed and safely stored.

The hair is combed, neatly braided if long enough, left free of hairpins, and secured under a turban so that it does not become soiled or interfere with the anesthetic. Colored nail polish and make-up are removed since checking of the color of the lips and nail beds for cyanosis is necessary. All jewelry is removed for safekeeping. If the patient does not wish to remove a wedding ring, it is

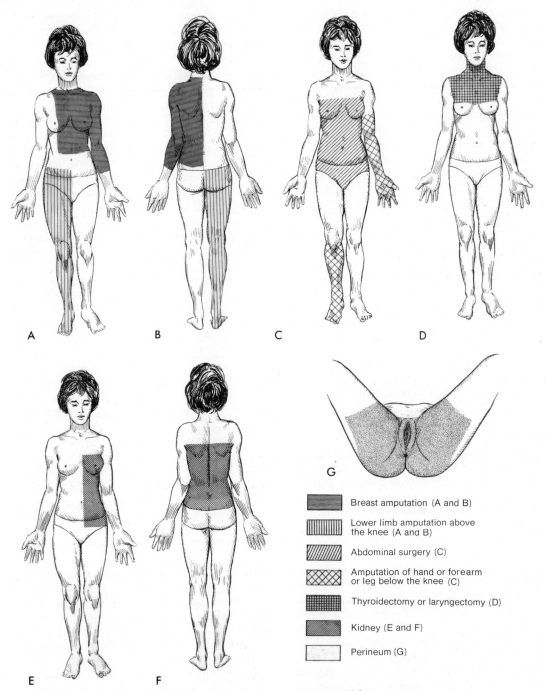

FIGURE 10–1 Areas of the skin prepared for surgery.

A   B   C   D

E   F   G

▓ (dark)	Breast amputation (A and B)
‖ (vertical)	Lower limb amputation above the knee (A and B)
⫽ (diagonal)	Abdominal surgery (C)
⊠ (crosshatch)	Amputation of hand or forearm or leg below the knee (C)
▦ (grid)	Thyroidectomy or laryngectomy (D)
▒ (gray)	Kidney (E and F)
░ (light)	Perineum (G)

securely taped or tied to the hand. The identification wristlet is checked to make sure it is clearly legible and secure.

SPECIAL PROCEDURES. Some special procedures may be ordered preceding certain operations. A nasogastric or duodenal tube may have to be passed, an intravenous infusion started, or an intravenous cutdown done and a cannula inserted for the administration of intravenous solution or whole blood. The nurse sees that the necessary equipment is available at the bedside so that the procedure may be completed by the time the patient receives the preoperative sedation.

MEDICATION. When the immediate preoperative orders are written, it should be clarified as to whether there are any preceding orders for medications; if so, it should be cleared with the physician whether these preparations are to be withheld or given. The patient may have been receiving digitalis, insulin or other important drugs and the omission of such could have serious effects.

A sedative is usually given the night before operation to ensure a good night's sleep for the patient. A barbiturate such as phenobarbital, amytal sodium, pentobarbital sodium or flurazepam (Dalmane) is commonly used. The patient is advised not to get up after taking the drug but to signal for the nurse if he wishes something or is unable to sleep. Frequently, simple nursing measures such as a back rub, change of position, turning the pillow or staying with the patient briefly may reduce tension and apprehension and promote sleep. Since an older person sometimes becomes confused after receiving a barbiturate, side rails are placed on his bed.

Approximately 45 to 90 minutes before operation, the patient usually receives an injection of a drug such as meperidine hydrochloride (Demerol) to produce relaxation and allay anxiety. The physician's choice of drugs is based mainly on the patient's condition and age. For example, if the patient is known to develop respiratory problems readily, morphine is not used because of its depressing effect on the respiratory center. Milder sedatives such as phenobarbital are used for children.

If a general anesthetic is to be given, the patient may also receive atropine or hyoscine hydrobromide (scopolamine) to reduce salivary and respiratory secretions. Scopolamine tends to make the respiratory secretion less tenacious than atropine. It may be administered alone without a sedative to young children since it depresses mental activity as well as secretions.

All preparatory procedures should be completed before the preoperative sedative is given. The patient is then left undisturbed, and silence is maintained. A relative may remain in the room to provide comfort and security for the patient.

A final check and recording are made of the pulse, respirations and blood pressure about ½ hour after the preoperative drug has been given.

PATIENT'S CHART. Treatments and any pertinent reactions of the patient are recorded, and the complete chart including the nurses' notes, diagnostic reports, progress notes, patient's history and the operative consent are put together and taken to the operating room with the patient. A sheet on the front of the chart should list any factors that may be considered particularly important for the anesthetist, surgeon and operating room staff to note. Examples are allergies, drug sensitivity, coexistent disease and limitation of joint movement in a limb. The latter may be significant in relation to positioning the patient on the operating room table. The patient's blood type is also noted.

PATIENT'S FAMILY. The family is notified when the operation is to take place and usually one or two members come to the hospital before the operation. They are allowed to visit the patient briefly before the preoperative sedation is given. As cited previously, one may remain quietly in the room as long as the patient is not disturbed.

After the patient is taken to the operating room, the relatives are directed to a place where they may wait and are advised that they will be notified as soon as the patient returns. The nurse stops to speak to them occasionally and may provide a cup of coffee or suggest where they may go to get refreshments. During a long operation, the surgeon may send someone from the operating room to advise them of the progress. He usually sees them as soon as the operation is completed to inform them of the patient's condition.

Emergency Preoperative Preparation

Preoperative preparation in emergency surgery is limited to basic essentials. When the patient is in shock or is bleeding, the hemoglobin is checked and the blood typed immediately. An intravenous infusion is started using normal saline or a plasma expander (dextran 6 per cent) until compatible whole blood is available.

If the patient is to have an inhalation anesthetic and has most likely taken food and fluid within the last 6 to 8 hours, a gastric tube is passed to evacuate the stomach content. In the case of hemorrhage from a peptic ulcer, perforation of an ulcer or intestinal obstruction, a nasogastric or duodenal tube is passed and intermittent suction-siphonage started in order to keep the stomach or duodenum free of fluid and gas.

As soon as possible, the patient is asked to void to obtain a specimen for urinalysis and to have the bladder empty for the surgery. If the patient is unable to void, catheterization is usually ordered, as it is important to know before operation whether the urine contains sugar, or abnormal constituents that might indicate diabetes mellitus or impaired renal function.

The skin at the site of operation is shaved and thoroughly cleansed, the permit for operation is signed, and preoperative medication is given. Any dentures or prostheses and jewelry are removed, and the hair is covered with a turban.

If the patient has just been admitted and is not accompanied by a relative, the nurse makes sure she obtains the name and telephone number of a family member and notifies the person as soon as possible.

Transportation of the Patient to the Operating Room

At the appropriate time, the patient is taken to the operating room either in his bed or on a stretcher. If the bed is used, the woolen blanket is replaced with a flannelette sheet to prevent the possibility of creating static electricity in the operating room since many of the anesthetic drugs are explosive and inflammable. The bedding is tucked in along the sides, and a name tag is attached to the bed so the patient will be returned to his own bed postoperatively. When a stretcher is used, sufficient covers are used to protect the patient from exposure and drafts. The covers are tucked in and either side rails or straps used to guard against the patient falling off the stretcher.

Two nurses or a nurse and an orderly accompany the patient. A nurse remains with the patient until a member of the operating room staff takes over. If the patient is awake, the ward nurse leaves him with a cheerful reassuring word that indicates a genuine interest in his welfare. He should not be left alone or exposed to the commotion and conversations that are frequently common to an operating room corridor. Such experiences only arouse the patient's anxiety. If he has to wait for a period of time, it should be in a quiet room.

Anesthesia

Anesthesia implies loss of sensation. The term is applied most commonly to the partial or total loss of sensation deliberately induced to prevent pain perception and promote relaxation during a surgical procedure. All sensation requires a stimulus to excite a receptor; this initiates nerve impulses which are transmitted along nerve fibers into the central nervous system. There, they are conducted through neurons and along impulse pathways to the brain, resulting in sensory perception — that is, awareness of the stimulus. If the impulse is blocked, the pathway interrupted, or the neurons responsible for the awareness inactivated, anesthesia occurs.

TYPES OF ANESTHESIA. Anesthesia may be general or regional (see Table 10–1). *General anesthesia* produces unconsciousness; the agent used acts on the brain, causing reversible inactivation of the cerebral neurons that are responsible for awareness and responses. In *regional anesthesia*, the agent used temporarily blocks the sensory receptors in the surgical area or in some area of the sensory impulse conduction pathway without loss of consciousness.

METHODS OF ANESTHETIC ADMINISTRATION. A *general anesthetic* agent may be administered intravenously or by inhalation. Often the practice is to start with an agent that is given intravenously and takes effect quickly, and then to continue with one or more inhalation agents.

Regional anesthetic agents are administered by a variety of methods.

1. *Local infiltration* entails the injection of the anesthetic agent into the surgical area. This makes the receptors unresponsive to stimuli.

2. *Topical or surface anesthesia* is produced by the application of the agent to the skin or mucous membrane. This method also blocks the sensory receptors.

3. *Peripheral nerve block* involves the injection of an anesthetic agent into the area of a large nerve trunk or a nerve plexus. This procedure interrupts the conduction of nerve impulses.

4. *Field block anesthesia* is produced by the injection of an anesthetic agent all around the operative site.

TABLE 10–1 TYPES OF ANESTHESIA

Type of Anesthesia	Method of Administration	Anesthetic Agents	Comments
General anesthesia	A. Inhalation	1. Nitrous oxide (gas)	Nonflammable. Always given with oxygen. In high concentration causes hypoxia.
		2. Cyclopropane (gas)	Flammable. Given with oxygen. May cause cardiac arrhythmia and postanesthetic nausea and vomiting.
		3. Halothane (Fluothane) (volatile liquid)	Nonflammable. Usually given with nitrous oxide and oxygen. Rare incidence of postanesthetic nausea and vomiting. Depresses respirations, which may lead to respiratory acidosis. Cardiovascular depressant; may cause reduced cardiac output and hypotension. Postanesthetic liver dysfunction may occur.
		4. Ether (volatile liquid)	Flammable. Irritating to respiratory tract membrane. Causes postanesthetic nausea and vomiting. Prolonged and restless induction and recovery periods.
		5. Methoxyflurane (volatile liquid)	Nonflammable. Postanesthetic nausea and vomiting rarely occurs. Slow recovery of consciousness. Possible renal tubular damage with large dosage.
		6. Enflurane (volatile liquid)	Nonflammable. May depress cardiovascular and respiratory function.
	B. Intravenous	1. Thiopental sodium (sodium pentothal)	Fast-acting. Used for induction before inhalation anesthetic. Danger of respiratory depression with large dose.
		2. Innovar (a combination of fentanyl, an analgesic, and the tranquilizer droperidol)	May cause some respiratory depression. Used as an adjunct to inhalation anesthetic or to regional anesthesia.
		3. Ketamine	Produces a "state of dissociative anesthesia." Patient may appear to be awake but is insensitive to nonvisceral pain. Used for changing burn dressings or brief orthopedic manipulative procedures. Not used if patient is hypertensive.
Regional	A. Local infiltration	1. Procaine hydrochloride (Novocain) 2. Lidocaine (Xylocaine) 3. Tetracaine (Pontocaine)	The preparations used in regional anesthesia are synthetic preparations with the exception of cocaine. All these preparations are toxic drugs, especially cocaine; it is used only for topical anesthesia.

Table continued on following page

TABLE 10–1 TYPES OF ANESTHESIA (*Continued*)

Type of Anesthesia	Method of Administration	Anesthetic Agents	Comments
Regional (*Continued*)	B. Topical or surface	1. Cocaine 2. Lidocaine (Xylocaine) 3. Benzocaine 4. Tetracaine (Pontocaine) 5. Butacaine 6. Nupercaine	Patients are observed for possible reaction. Epinephrine is added to many of the preparations. Epinephrine causes vasoconstriction which slows the absorption of the anesthetic agent. This prolongs duration of the anesthesia and minimizes the dose required.
	C. Peripheral nerve block	1. Lidocaine (Xylocaine) 2. Tetracaine (Pontocaine) 3. Mepivacaine	
	D. Field block	(As for local infiltration)	
	E. Spinal anesthesia	1. Procaine hydrochloride (Novocain) 2. Lidocaine (Xylocaine) 3. Tetracaine (Pontocaine) 4. Amylocaine hydrochloride	
	F. Epidural	1. Procaine hydrochloride 2. Lidocaine (Xylocaine) 3. Mepivacaine 4. Tetracaine (Pontocaine)	

5. *Spinal anesthesia* entails the injection of an anesthetic agent into the cerebrospinal fluid in the subarachnoid space, usually in the lumbar region (between the second and fourth lumbar vertebrae). The agent blocks impulses at the origin of the peripheral nerves. The area anesthetized is determined by the level to which the drug rises in the spinal canal as well as by the amount of the drug used. This type of anesthesia is used principally in low abdominal and lower limb operations. Chest and high abdominal surgery would require that the agent be carried to higher levels, which could cause the blocking of impulses to the respiratory muscles, with ensuing respiratory failure.

6. *Epidural or caudal anesthesia* is induced by the injection of an anesthetic agent into the extradural space of the lower part of the vertebral canal (sacrococcygeal region). The drug blocks impulses along the fibers of the cauda equina. This type of anesthesia is mostly used in obstetrics during labor and delivery and occasionally in rectal and perineal operative procedures.

Hypothermia is used very occasionally as a supplement to anesthesia in some prolonged operative procedures, especially in cardiac surgery (see p. 110).

ANESTHETIC AGENTS. A wide variety of drugs are used as anesthetic agents. The choice depends mainly upon the method of administration used, the surgery to be performed and the physical and psychological conditions of the patient. In addition to producing anesthesia, some agents produce more relaxation of the muscles in the operative area than others; this may also be a factor in the choice of the agent. Preparations of muscle relaxants are available and frequently are given intravenously during surgery (e.g., tubocurarine chloride). The resulting relaxation facilitates surgery and decreases the amount of anesthetic required.

IMPLICATIONS FOR NURSING. It is not the intention here to mention the responsibilities of the nurse assisting with the administration of various types of anesthetics. For details of such a role the reader is referred to an operating room procedure text or a book on anesthesia. The nursing care for the surgical patient does require some information about the anesthetic agents commonly used. A compilation of pertinent information is presented in Table 10–1.

Some *significant factors in relation to anesthesia* generally are as follows:

1. Anesthetics are toxic drugs and have

potentially dangerous side effects. They produce physiological changes, especially those used to produce general and spinal anesthesia. Complications develop most often in respiratory, cardiovascular and central nervous system functioning. The patient's physiological and phychological status should be carefully assessed before he receives an anesthetic; any deficiency, sensitivity or impairment noted by the nurse is brought to the physician's attention and corrected, if possible, before anesthesia. The choice of anesthetic may be influenced by such findings and serious complications prevented.

Many inhalation anesthetics are flammable; special precautions are necessary to prevent the possibility of static electricity igniting the flammable substances. The responsibility for the control of hazards usually rests with the anesthesia and operating room staffs of the hospital, but every nurse entering the department should be aware of such hazards. Unless wearing appropriate shoes and clothing (that is, conductive shoes and clothing such as cotton that does not produce static electricity), personnel are not permitted in rooms where flammable anesthetic agents are stored or in use.

2. In *general anesthesia,* the degree of anesthesia is described as light, moderate and deep. Light anesthesia requires less anesthetic and may produce loss of consciousness but only slight muscle relaxation. This "depth" may be adequate for a superficial operation of short duration, but greater depth is necessary for surgical procedures that are longer in duration and require muscle relaxation. The amount required also varies with individuals; a large robust man requires more than a slight frail person. Deep general anesthesia is more hazardous; shock, cardiac dysfunction and postoperative complications are more likely to develop. Fortunately, the introduction of muscle relaxants into surgery has greatly reduced the depth of anesthesia required and has made anesthesia much safer. The anesthetist makes a continuous assessment of the depth and the patient's responses. Cardiovascular and respiratory functions are monitored, certain reflexes are tested frequently (e.g., pupillary and corneal reflexes) and muscle relaxation, especially in the operative site, is observed. Manifestations of an excessive and dangerous level of anesthesia are fixed full dilation of the pupils,

absence of reflex responses, muscular flaccidity, cyanosis or grayish pallor, hypotension, weak pulse, cardiac arrest and respiratory insufficiency or failure.

Inhalation anesthetics are administered by an open, closed, or semiclosed system, and in nearly all instances more than one drug is used. The open method is seldom used except for some very brief operative procedures or in an emergency. It involves placing a gauze mask over the nose and mouth and dropping a volatile anesthetic agent on the mask.

The closed and semiclosed methods require more complex equipment, which provides sources for anesthetic agents and oxygen, and a mixing chamber. Flow meters for gauging the amount of anesthetic agent and oxygen delivered to the patient are also necessary. In the closed system, the equipment allows for rebreathing of the exhaled anesthetic agent and removal of carbon dioxide within the circuit. In the semiclosed system, a valve operates to direct the patient's expired "air" into the atmosphere. The anesthetic and oxygen mixture may be inhaled from a mask placed over the patient's mouth and nose or, in prolonged surgery, it may be delivered with each inspiration via an endotracheal tube. Intubation ensures a patent airway, provides better control of respiration, facilitates the removal of secretions and lessens the dead space (the area in the respiratory tract in which no gas exchange occurs). The intubation method accounts for some "throat" irritation and temporary loss of voice above a whisper that some patients may experience in the immediate postoperative period.

The patient who is to receive general anesthesia is often more apprehensive and concerned about this phase of the impending surgery than about the actual operation. He may fear loss of consciousness and the complete loss of self-control. An explanation is given of what to expect and what occurs. Reassurance may be given by advising the patient and family of the tremendous progress that has been made in recent decades with the introduction of the safer, new agents and methods of administration. They are also made aware of the constant monitoring that will take place. If fear and apprehension persist it should be brought to the attention of the physician or anesthetist before the day of surgery.

3. As mentioned previously, the patient remains conscious when regional anesthesia is used. This may be of concern to the patient during the preoperative period; he may fear that he will experience pain. During the operative phase the individual's anxiety may be increased by the very strange and awesome environment. He may hear disturbing remarks unless staff conversation is carefully guarded. He is advised before the operation that he will be able to express pain or "hurt," which will alert the surgeon to the need for more anesthesia or a longer period of waiting for it to take effect.

The use of regional anesthesia must not be taken lightly by the nurse. The patient can develop unfavorable reactions to the regional anesthetic agent. The pulse, blood pressure, respirations and color are noted throughout the operative phase and postoperatively. Some patients find surgery under regional anesthesia extremely anxiety-producing and may experience reactions to that stress for several hours after the surgery is completed.

Spinal regional anesthesia is not usually used if the patient has a history of frequent severe headaches. When it is used, the drug injected into the subarachnoid space may block autonomic innervation as well as incoming sensory impulses. The interference with sympathetic impulses may cause widespread vasodilation and, as a result, decreased venous return to the heart and ensuing reduced cardiac output and hypotension. The patient is usually given a sympathetic stimulant such as ephedrine or epinephrine hydrochloride (Adrenalin) as a prophylactic measure, just before the spinal anesthetic is given. Continuous monitoring of the patient's vital signs is necessary until he recovers from the anesthesia. If hypotension occurs, a vasopressor drug such as norepinephrine (Levophed or levarterenol) may be administered intravenously. With spinal anesthesia the patient loses sensation and motor ability from the upper abdominal region down. He cannot move his lower limbs and lower trunk. This may be very frightening for the patient even though it was explained preoperatively. He requires reassurance that it is a reversible condition.

Following the surgery, the patient is kept in a supine position, and is usually not permitted to sit up or get up for at least 8 hours. Some patients complain of headache after a spinal anesthetic and are more likely to develop it if they assume the erect position within the first 6 to 8 hours postoperatively. The headache is thought to be due to loss of cerebrospinal fluid through the membrane puncture or to chemical irritation of the meninges. Loss of the fluid results in a lack of fluid support and protection for the structures within the cranium, especially when the patient assumes the upright position. If the patient does experience headache, he is kept quiet and subjected to a minimum of stimuli and movement. An ice bag is applied and an analgesic given. The giving of fluids is important so that the volume of cerebrospinal fluid may return to normal.

POSTOPERATIVE NURSING

All surgery has certain common effects that vary in extent and intensity with each particular individual and each specific operation. It produces tissue trauma, pain, psychological reactions and loss of blood. There is an increased possibility of invasion of body tissues by pathogenic organisms through a break in the continuity of the skin, or by the introduction of foreign objects into the body. In addition, there are disturbances in body functions which are due directly to the surgical procedure or indirectly to the responses of the autonomic nervous system and the adrenal glands to the associated psychic and physical stresses.

The nurse who is caring for a patient following an operation must possess knowledge and understanding of the implications of the particular surgery for the patient, its possible effects on the patient's body functions, and the care and support required to assist in his return to normalcy with a minimum of discomfort and pain. A constant watchfulness of the patient's clinical progress is necessary. Adverse changes and their possible significance must be recognized promptly and the surgeon alerted. If it is possible, the nurse who is to care for the patient in the postoperative period has had an opportunity to become acquainted with the patient and learn something of his condition before the operation. The patient may be more confident with a nurse who is not a complete stranger, and the nurse, knowing something of the patient, is better able to evaluate his reactions and condition.

Preparation to Receive the Patient

Most hospitals have a recovery room, either within the operating room department or adjacent to it, to which the patient is taken on completion of the surgery. In a few instances, the patient may be returned directly to his ward unit. The recovery room has several distinct advantages: constant surveillance is provided by a staff experienced in immediate postoperative care and whose attention is undivided; proximity to the operating room reduces the distance the patient is transported in this critical period; equipment necessary for emergencies is concentrated in the area and is in immediate readiness; and one nurse may care for two or three patients — a situation which would not be possible on the ward, where each patient is in a different location. The patient remains in the recovery room until he fully regains consciousness and his vital signs are stabilized.

Most hospitals have intensive care units apart from the recovery room in which critically ill patients and patients with a special problem, such as respiratory insufficiency, receive care. The patient who has had major surgery or who has developed serious complications may be transferred directly from the operating room to the intensive care unit, where the type of care given in the recovery room may be extended for several days or weeks. The advantages of such a unit are similar to those of the recovery room, but the latter provides a briefer period of care. In a few situations, the two units may be combined, using the same staff and equipment.

In the unit to which the operative patient is to go, certain basic preparations are made to receive the patient. The bed is made up with two flannelette sheets to provide warmth and absorption of skin moisture. The top bedding is fan-folded to one side to facilitate the transfer of the patient. A piece of waterproof material is placed at the head of the bed over the bottom flannelette sheet and covered with a towel or draw sheet; if it becomes soiled with vomitus it can be changed with a minimum of disturbance to the patient. If drainage from any area of the body is anticipated, the same precaution is taken. Side rails are attached to the bed and are ready for use in the event that the patient becomes restless and confused during recovery from the anesthesia.

Basic equipment to be assembled at the bedside includes a sphygmomanometer, stethoscope, oropharyngeal airway, tongue depressor, tongue forceps, two emesis basins, tissues, face towel, recording sheets and infusion pole. A suction apparatus, a portable emergency respirator (Ambu bag with oxygen), and an emergency tray with cardiac and respiratory stimulants, sterile syringes and needles, tourniquet and alcohol swabs should be quickly available.

Equipment most likely to be needed because of the nature of the surgery is also assembled in readiness for prompt use. For instance, if the patient is having gastric surgery, equipment for gastric suction-siphonage drainage will be necessary; if the operation is an amputation, tourniquets must be at the bedside.

The room or unit is ventilated and tidied; unnecessary equipment and objects are removed, and daily cleaning is done in order to prevent disturbance of the patient later. The light signal is tested to make sure it is in order should assistance be required.

Transportation of the Patient from the Operating Room

On completion of the operation, the patient is dried if the skin is moist with perspiration, and a clean gown and flannelette sheet are applied. He is then lifted gently and without unnecessary exposure by a mechanical lifting device or by a sufficient number of persons to provide adequate support and prevent strain on any part, particularly the operative area. When the bed is used the patient is placed in the lateral or semiprone position, and the side rails are raised. If the transfer is to a stretcher, the dorsal recumbent position is more likely to be used, and straps may be placed over the patient (one above the elbows, the second just above the knees) and secured for safety. Side rails are also used. Sufficient covers are used to ensure warmth and protection from drafts. The head is extended and an oropharyngeal airway is probably in place to facilitate breathing. If the patient is on his back and an airway is not used, the lower jaw must be held up and forward to prevent the tongue from obstructing breathing. The anesthetist and a nurse accompany the patient to the recovery room or the ward. Along with immediate treatment orders, the nurse taking over receives a report on what was done, the patient's condition and anything special for which she should be alert.

Postoperative Care

The discussion presented here deals with general postoperative considerations applicable to most surgical patients. Modifications and additional care as related to specific surgery are included in the respective sections in Part II.

A nurse remains in constant attendance until the patient fully regains consciousness, is oriented to his surroundings and his vital signs are stabilized.

ASSESSMENT. When the patient is received, an immediate check is made of the respirations, pulse, blood pressure, color of the skin and mucous membranes, condition of the skin (warm or cold, dry or moist) and the level of consciousness. The wound area is examined for bleeding and drainage. If there is a catheter or other type of drainage tube, it is checked for patency. These initial observations and the patient's preoperative vital signs serve as a comparative base line which assists the nurse later in recognizing favorable and unfavorable changes and in making decisions as to actions. Cardiac arrhythmia, weak pulse, a decrease or fluctuations in the systolic blood pressure, abnormal respiratory rate and volume, and bleeding in the wound area are reported promptly to the physician.

The vital signs are recorded every 15 minutes for 2 hours; if they are satisfactory, the intervals are then progressively extended to every half hour, every hour and then every 2 hours over the next 12 to 24 hours; then they are recorded every 4 hours.

Observation of the patient's color, skin condition, and operative site for any untoward signs continues, and the patient's responses are noted. The fluid intake and output are accurately recorded until normal fluid and food intake and normal urinary elimination have been resumed.

MAINTENANCE OF ADEQUATE VENTILATION. Inadequate ventilation (hypoventilation) is a common problem in the immediate postoperative period for the patient who has had a general anesthetic, and it may lead to serious respiratory complications. Hypoventilation implies that the volume of air being moved in and out of the alveoli (air sacs of the lungs) with each respiration is below normal. It leads to hypoxemia (deficiency of oxygen in the blood) and the retention of carbon dioxide (hypercarbia) and pulmonary secretions. If the latter are retained a bronchial tube may become plugged, resulting in the collapse of a segment of the lung (atelectasis). Bronchitis or pneumonia may develop, since retained secretions provide an excellent medium for the growth of pathogenic organisms. Postoperative hypoventilation may result from: (1) central nervous system depression by the anesthetic agent(s); (2) the depression of respiratory muscle activity by a muscle relaxant; or (3) partial airway obstruction caused by the tongue or lower jaw blocking the pharyngeal area, excessive mucus secretions or laryngeal edema. Laryngeal edema may develop if endotracheal intubation was used by the anesthetist.

Hypoventilation may be recognized by: (1) abnormally slow or shallow respirations; (2) audible, moist, gurgling respirations, indicating excessive secretions; (3) wheezing, or "crowing" respirations (stridor); (4) rales or nonentry of air into an area detected by auscultation; or (5) restlessness, cyanosis and rapid pulse rate that are characteristic of hypoxemia.

Measures to promote adequate ventilation include the following:

1. During unconsciousness, unless contraindicated by the nature of the surgery, the patient is placed in a lateral or semiprone position without a pillow under the head. This position lessens the danger of aspiration of mucus and vomitus, and of the relaxed tongue and lower jaw "falling back" to block the pharynx. The head is hyperextended to facilitate free entry of air and expiration. A firm pillow may be placed at the patient's front and back, if necessary, to maintain the desired position. The knees are flexed to reduce strain, and the uppermost limb is flexed to a greater degree than the lower one. The arm that is uppermost is supported on a pillow so that chest expansion is not restricted. If the patient must be kept on his back, an oropharyngeal airway may be necessary during the unconscious period to prevent occlusion of the airway.

2. Excessive secretions may be removed by pharyngeal suctioning. A Y connecting tube is attached to the tube leading from the source of negative pressure. The suction catheter is

attached to the one arm of the Y connecting tube, moistened, and directed into the pharyngeal area. The other area of the Y tube is then occluded by the thumb and suction established. The catheter is rotated and withdrawn slowly. If the secretions are beyond pharyngeal suctioning, intratracheal suctioning may have to be undertaken. (See p. 413 for details of deep suctioning).

Increased humidification of the air may be necessary if the secretions are tenacious, thick and difficult to remove.

3. Oxygen may be administered as a supportive measure and to prevent hypoxemia. It may be given by nasal cannulae or a mask (see p. 408).

4. As soon as the patient regains consciousness, he is encouraged to do deep breathing and voluntary forced coughing every 1 to 2 hours to expand the lungs fully and remove tracheobronchial secretions. Even though the patient has received instruction and practiced these procedures before the operation, he may be very reluctant to carry them out because of the fear of pain. He must be assisted to the sitting position and given the necessary encouragement and support. One hand is placed at the patient's back and the other may be placed over the wound site to provide support during the coughing. The deep breathing and coughing are repeated eight to ten times every 2 hours. If the patient is very weak or complains of dizziness, it may be necessary to start with fewer deep breaths and then increase them progressively as the patient's tolerance improves. Physical therapy may be indicated to promote removal of secretions and normal ventilation (see p. 414).

5. The patient is turned from side to side frequently to allow full expansion of both lungs. When consciousness has been regained the patient may be turned side to side to back to side. If any one position is restricted, it will be indicated by the surgeon. For example, a patient who has had a pneumonectomy (removal of a lung) is not usually permitted to lie on the nonoperative side since it diminishes the expansion of the remaining lung. Specific orders for positioning are necessary following cerebral surgery.

Two nurses are necessary for turning the patient until he is alert and responsive. During the first 24 to 48 hours changes of position are made slowly, since the vascular reflexes which adjust the distribution of blood with postural changes may be dulled and slower.

6. If hypoventilation persists the concentration of blood gases is determined. Mechanical ventilatory assistance may be necessary (see p. 424 for details).

FOLLOWING SPINAL ANESTHESIA. When the patient has had a spinal anesthetic the foot of the bed is elevated. The patient will be conscious but is not permitted a pillow and is advised to keep his head down. This is necessary because there is usually an associated decrease in blood pressure due to the effect of the anesthetic on the vasomotor nerves which cause vasodilation. The position is maintained until sensation and motor ability have returned to the lower limbs and the systolic blood pressure is over 90 mm. Hg.

TREATMENTS. The physician's orders are noted immediately for specific treatments. For instance, oxygen, intravenous infusion, appropriate drainage system, special positioning and observations, and drug therapy may be indicated by the doctor's orders.

Any drainage tubes that are to be connected to appropriate bottles or a suction-siphonage system must receive prompt attention, as they are usually clamped during transit from the operating room. If drainage is not quickly established, the tube may become plugged, or sufficient pressure may be built up within the body cavity to cause serious effects. For example, if a gastrointestinal tube remains clamped following gastric or duodenal surgery, distention may cause a leakage of secretions into the peritoneal cavity and may result in peritonitis.

RECOVERY FROM ANESTHESIA. While the patient is emerging from anesthesia, he may be restless. Other than side rails and a splint to the arm that has a needle in a vein for intravenous infusion, restraints are not used. The nurse protects the patient from injuring himself and prevents the tubes from being dislodged. As the patient regains consciousness, he is reassured that someone is with him.

Should the patient not respond within 2 to 3 hours, the physician is notified of the delay. It may be because of slow elimination or metabolism of the drugs and anesthetic agents, or it may be due to shock or depressed brain activity due to a lack of oxygen.

When consciousness is regained, a few simple nursing measures may lessen the patient's discomfort. The flannelette sheets are removed if the body temperature is within normal range; excessive perspiration is avoided since it may deplete body fluids. The face and hands are bathed, the mouth rinsed with a cool mouthwash, the back rubbed, and the position changed. The environment should be quiet and ventilated without exposing the patient to drafts. The direct shining of light in the patient's eyes is avoided by lowering the window shade or adjusting the lamp.

COMMON POSTOPERATIVE DISCOM-FORTS. Discomforts common to many postoperative patients include pain, nausea, and vomiting, gas pains and apprehension.

PAIN. Complaints of pain in the operative area are to be expected because of the unavoidable tissue trauma in surgery. Inadequate control of postoperative pain may cause restlessness and contribute to shock and injury to the operative site. The surgeon usually orders an analgesic such as meperidine hydrochloride (Demerol), Pantopon or codeine to be given every 4 hours if required (p. r. n.) for the first 24 to 48 hours. The patient should be kept relatively free of pain, but excessive use of the drug is to be avoided. Careful judgment is required of the nurse, since narcotics tend to depress respirations. Respirations are checked before and after the administration of each dose. If the respirations are only 12 or less per minute, the analgesic is not given until the physician is consulted. The use of analgesics is more hazardous with older persons, patients with some respiratory insufficiency (e.g., patients with chronic bronchitis or emphysema) and with young children.

The patient's position is changed, and deep breathing, coughing and necessary treatments are done just before or immediately following the drug injection so that the patient may derive maximum benefit. After the first day or two, the dose of the analgesic is usually reduced or a milder drug is substituted. When the doctor has not specified a time limit on the drug, the question is raised by the nurse after 48 hours.

Prevention of strain on the operative site by good positioning and support with a pillow contributes to the prevention and relief of pain. For instance, a patient with a pendulous abdomen who has had abdominal surgery may suffer less discomfort if the strain on the wound is relieved.

Occasionally, a patient may complain of a backache or pain in a shoulder which may have been caused by prolonged immobilization during surgery. Gentle massage may provide relaxation and relief. If the lower limbs are causing discomfort, the patient is encouraged to do a few simple movements such as flexion of toes, feet and legs. Massage is never used, but a change of position and support under the full length of the limbs may be helpful. Massage of the lower limbs is discouraged because of the danger of dislodging a thrombus that may have formed because of venous stasis.

NAUSEA AND VOMITING. Surgical patients may experience some nausea and vomiting immediately after the operation as a result of the toxic effects of the anesthetic and the handling of viscera in abdominal surgery. Assistance is provided by having the basin available, holding the patient's head, providing a mouthwash and wiping the patient's mouth. If the patient is still under the influence of the anesthetic or drugs, precautions are taken to prevent aspiration by turning the patient's head to the side and if necessary using suction to make sure the vomitus is removed from the mouth and pharynx. Oral fluids are usually withheld, and the patient is kept quiet and is disturbed as little as possible. Emesis basins are emptied promptly, soiled linen is changed, and the room is ventilated. Vomiting that persists beyond 24-hours after operation is reported, as it may indicate a complication or intolerance to the analgesic being used. (For a fuller discussion of nausea and vomiting see p. 489.)

FLATULENCE. Patients who have had abdominal surgery may experience some pain and distention which are caused by an accumulation of gas in the gastrointestinal tract. Most of the gas is air that is swallowed during nausea or when the patient is tense and fearful. The depressing effects of anesthetics and drugs, handling of the intestine during surgery, and the lack of food intake in the tract may contribute to a reduction in peristalsis. The discomfort may be relieved by the insertion of a rectal tube for a brief period or by an enema. When the distention is high, a nasogastric tube may be passed and suction-decompression used (see p. 500). If the distention persists, it may indicate a serious complication such as paralytic ileus, bowel obstruction or peritonitis (pp. 544 and 563). Frequent turning, early ambulation, and normal fluid and food intake are helpful in reestablishing normal peristalsis and preventing distention and gas pains.

APPREHENSION. The postoperative patient may be apprehensive and concerned about his condition; this anxiety is likely to cause restlessness and aggravate discomfort and pain. An explanation of what has taken place and what he may expect may relieve some of his concern. He is also told that the nurse is close by and will be in and out frequently to check on him. Having a family member visit or remain quietly in the room may be helpful. It may be necessary for the nurse to remain at the bedisde until the patient regains sufficient confidence and control. If he is worried about the findings at operation, it may be helpful to have the surgeon advise him as to his condition and the prognosis.

FLUIDS AND NUTRITION. A blood transfusion will probably be given during a major operation or immediately after to replace the blood loss or to combat shock if the blood pressure falls below 90 mm. Hg. Before the transfusion is started, the blood is checked by two persons to be certain that the label bears the patient's name. The blood bank labels the blood with the patient's name after making sure it is the right type and is compatible. The blood should be at room temperature or cooler when given. The patient is observed for signs or symptoms of untoward reactions, which may be a chill, fever, dyspnea, pain in the lumbar region or chest, or a fall in blood pressure. Later, the urine may contain hemoglobin and hematin crystals because of hemolysis of red blood cells. The rate of flow is set by the doctor; initially, it may be introduced very slowly (2 to 3 ml. per minute): symptoms of a reaction are usually manifested during the infusion of the first 50 to 100 ml. of each unit of blood. After 100 ml., the rate may be increased to 4 to 10 ml. per minute. The rate of flow will depend on the reduction in the patient's vascular volume, blood pressure and cardiac function. It is usually considerably slower in an elderly person.

If a reaction is manifested, the transfusion is stopped and the doctor is notified immediately. In some situations, the blood and equipment are then returned to the blood bank for examination to determine the cause of the reaction.

Oral fluid and food are restricted during the period of nausea and vomiting and following abdominal operations. Intravenous infusions of electrolyte and glucose solutions are given to meet the patient's daily requirements and maintain normal fluid and electrolyte balance. Frequent rinsing of the mouth and cool, moist compresses laid over the lips will help with the patient's discomfort of thirst.

As soon as fluids are permitted, sips of water are given and gradually increased in amount. The intake is then progressively increased as can be tolerated through fluids and soft diet to general diet. The resumption of a normal diet as soon as possible promotes normal gastrointestinal functioning. The patient is less likely to experience abdominal distention, gas pains and constipation. Normal nutrition also favors wound healing, maintenance of strength and a sense of wellbeing.

In the case of a patient who has had surgery on the alimentary tract (gastric or intestinal), all oral intake is withheld until specifically ordered by the physician.

The postoperative patient may be rather indifferent to food, but he may be encouraged to take more by the offering of small amounts of those foods for which the patient has indicated a preference. Frequently food and fluids are not taken simply because the patient is weak and finds the effort expended in reaching and feeding himself too exhausting. The necessary assistance should be provided until the patient regains sufficient strength. The amounts of food and fluid taken are recorded until a normal diet is resumed.

ELIMINATION. The postoperative patient may have a temporary inability to void because of a depression of the bladder sensitivity to distention; the impulses that produce the desire to void and the reflex emptying are not initiated. The inhibition may be due to the anesthetic, drugs or trauma in the region of the bladder. The recumbent position, nervous tension and fear of pain may also contribute to urinary retention. The patient may have the desire to void but is unable to do so because of spasm of the external sphincter. When the bladder becomes distended, a small amount may be voided frequently, but the bladder is not emptied; this is referred to as retention with overflow. Restlessness, complaints of pain or of a feeling of pressure in the pelvic area, and a palpable fullness above the symphysis pubis are associated with retention.

Distention and stagnation of urine predispose to inflammation and infection of the bladder. If the patient has not voided for 10 to

12 hours, efforts are made to induce voiding by leaving the patient alone on the bedpan or with the urinal, opening taps to produce the sound of running water, pouring warm water over the vulva of the female, and by elevating the head of the bed, unless contraindicated. The unnatural position of being in bed is one of the common problems; the surgeon may allow the patient to get out of bed and use a commode or a bedpan placed on a chair. The male patient may be permitted to stand at the side of the bed to use a urinal. If the patient is permitted to get up, someone must remain with him in case he becomes faint.

Difficulty in voiding may have been anticipated by the physician and an order left to catheterize the patient if necessary in 10 to 12 hours. If there is no order and the patient has not passed urine for 12 hours, a report is given to the doctor. The amount of fluid the patient has had since last voiding should be noted. Strict asepsis and gentleness are necessary in the passing of a catheter to avoid trauma of the mucous membrane and the introduction of infection.

In major abdominal and pelvic surgery, an indwelling catheter may be passed and left in place for 2 or 3 days to avoid repeated catheterization as well as pressure from a full bladder on the internal operative site. An indwelling catheter may also be used to determine hourly secretion of urine if the patient is in shock or has some renal insufficiency due to disease. There is concern if the output is less than 30 ml. per hour.

Since the bowel is usually empty at the time of surgery and food intake is restricted for 2 or 3 days, bowel elimination is not an immediate postoperative concern. The patient, probably accustomed to a daily bowel movement, may be worried unless he is advised that the delay is to be expected and will not be harmful.

If a normal diet is quickly reestablished, a laxative or enema may not be necessary. Some doctors order a mild laxative, glycerine suppository, or a small enema 2 days after operation. Early ambulation and being allowed to go to the toilet or use a commode help in reestablishing normal bowel elimination.

ACTIVITY AND POSITIONING. Bed rest and inactivity predispose to problems of flatulence and abdominal distention, retention of urine, loss of strength, joint stiffness, and respiratory and vascular complications. Gastrointestinal peristalsis is sluggish, venous stasis occurs, and respirations are shallow.

To minimize these potential difficulties, some activity and frequent change of position are promoted. Venous stasis and the resultant danger of thrombus formation, particularly in the lower limbs, may be prevented by stimulating the circulation with foot and leg exercises. These are usually commenced 8 to 10 hours after the operation and done every 2 to 3 hours until the patient is up and walking. Alternating active flexion and extension of the toes, dorsal and plantar flexion of the feet, and flexion and extension of the legs and thighs are carried out under the direction of the nurse.

If early ambulation is not possible and the surgeon approves, self-care and the following exercises are included as soon as the patient's condition permits: (1) flexion and extension of the head; (2) flexion and extension of the fingers, hands, forearms and arms; (3) abduction, adduction and external rotation of the arms at the shoulders; and (4) contraction of the abdominal muscles. The purpose of self-care and the exercises are explained to the patient; otherwise, he may feel resentful and consider he is not receiving due care. The proposed activities stimulate circulation and respirations and prevent contractures and loss of strength (see Fig. 10–2).

EARLY AMBULATION. Within 24 to 48 hours after surgery, if the vital signs are stable and the general condition satisfactory, the patient is assisted out of bed and encouraged to walk about. At first the patient may take only a few steps, but movement can be progressively increased as the patient feels stronger and more secure. This early ambulation promotes the return of normal physiological activities such as gastrointestinal peristalsis, reduces the incidence of respiratory and circulatory complications, prevents the loss of muscle tone, improves the patient's morale, and shortens the period of hospitalization and convalescence.

The patient is likely to be very fearful and helpless the first time he gets out of bed and will need assistance and support. The head of the bed is lowered, and he is turned to a lateral position near the edge of the bed with his legs and thighs flexed. The patient is then slowly assisted to the sitting position and his legs are put over the side of the bed. After a brief rest in this position while the nurse puts his slip-

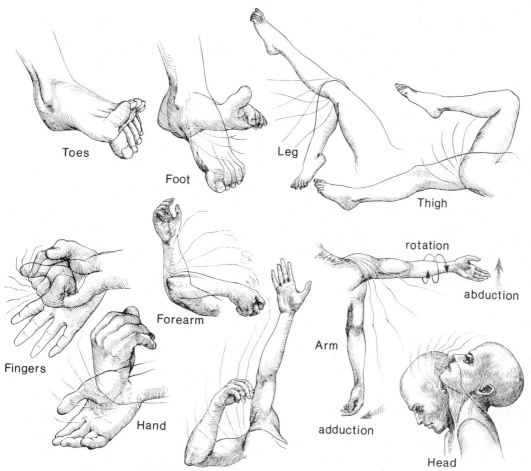

FIGURE 10–2 Bed exercises for postoperative patients.

pers and dressing gown on him and notes his reactions, the erect position is assumed. Then, with help, he is encouraged to take a few steps. This is repeated two or three times each day and the walking is increased. Sitting in a chair for prolonged periods is discouraged since it favors venous stasis in the lower limbs and lower abdomen.

The patient is encouraged to use a commode or go to the toilet while up to promote normal bladder and bowel elimination. Precautions against overactivity are necessary when the patient is up more frequently for longer periods because the reparative processes are still going on within the body.

Early ambulation is contraindicated or delayed when there is shock, hemorrhage, infection, or cardiac insufficiency, and in the case of feeble, elderly persons.

WOUND CARE. The objectives in wound care are to have it remain uninfected and heal firmly with a minimum of scar tissue. On completion of the surgery, the incision is cov-

ered with a sterile gauze dressing and the area is inspected frequently during the immediate postoperative period for signs of drainage or bleeding. If the dressing becomes moist with serous drainage, it is reinforced by the application of sterile pads without disturbing the initial dressing. Should bright blood be evident, the doctor is notified promptly. In 2 or 3 days, the surgeon may order the dressing removed and the wound left exposed or covered with a thin layer of gauze. This is to eliminate warmth and moisture which favor infection and maceration of the wound edges, and the use of adhesive which can be irritating to the skin. The sutures are removed in 5 to 7 days.

A drain may have been inserted at the time of surgery to allow the escape of serum, pus or a body fluid such as bile. The tube may pass through the incision or a separate small stab wound. Specific orders are given as to the required care and when the tube is to be removed. Precautions are necessary when moving or bathing the patient in order to prevent dislodgement of the tube, particularly when it is attached to a drainage system.

PREPARATION FOR DISCHARGE FROM HOSPITAL. Surgical patients remain in the hospital for a much shorter period now than they did a few years ago. Early ambulation, self-care, and early resumption of a normal diet hasten recovery and help to maintain the patient's strength, making a shorter period of hospitalization possible.

Since the reparative processes continue, the patient and his family receive instructions as to the amount of activity permitted and the necessary rest. If dressings or treatments are required, the patient and a family member are taught how these are carried out, or a referral may be made to a visiting nurse organization. The nurse discusses with the doctor when he wants to see the patient for an examination and arranges a clinic or office appointment. The doctor may give the patient some idea of when he may return to work before he leaves the hospital, or it may not be decided until he has his initial follow-up examination.

POSTOPERATIVE COMPLICATIONS

It is important that the nurse caring for the postoperative patient appreciate the complications that may develop following surgery. Only the more common complications are presented here; specific complications that may be associated with particular operations are presented in the respective chapters in Part II.

Shock

This is a circulatory failure that results in an inadequate perfusion of tissues and organs. This failure at the microcirculatory level reduces the delivery of oxygen and other essentials to a level below that required for normal cellular activities. It may develop during or immediately following the surgery, or it may develop more slowly and become evident several hours after operation. It may be secondary to a severe infection or respiratory complication that occurs later.

Early manifestations are a decrease in blood pressure, restlessness, inappropriate anxiety, ashen pallor, cold moist skin, rapid weak pulse and decreased pulse pressure.

Shock is serious and immediately life-threatening; prompt recognition and action are necessary to prevent the condition from becoming irreversible. For details see Chapter 14.

Hemorrhage

Postoperative bleeding may occur as a result of a slipped ligature or from an increase in the blood pressure opening up previously collapsed vessels or dislodging the clot that plugged a severed vessel.

The hemorrhage may become evident externally at the site of operation, or it may be concealed internally and only manifested and recognized by changes in the vital signs and the patient's general appearance and complaint of weakness. Loss of blood causes: a fall in blood pressure; a rapid, thready pulse; deep, rapid respirations which are referred to as air hunger; pallor; apprehension; restlessness; and weakness.

Any suspicion of hemorrhage must be immediately reported. The patient is kept as quiet and undisturbed as possible; Pantopon or meperidine hydrochloride (Demerol) is usually ordered to allay apprehension and reduce restlessness. The head is lowered to prevent cerebral ischemia. The dressing is reinforced as required. If the bleeding is from a limb, a tourniquet and pressure dressings are applied, and the part is elevated. An intravenous infusion of a plasma expander (e.g., Dextran 6 per cent) may be given while blood is being obtained for a transfusion. The patient may have to be returned to the operating room to have the blood vessel ligated.

Secondary hemorrhage may occur several days or weeks after the operation because of the erosion of a blood vessel by infection or malignant disease.

Respiratory Complications

The respiratory complications seen most often postoperatively are hypoventilation, atelectasis, pneumonia and pulmonary embolism. Whatever the disorder that develops, the common denominator is hypoxia and hypercarbia. An oxygen deficiency affects the entire body. Hypoxia may be manifested by headache, restlessness and irritability, and then apathy, dullness and clouded sensorium. The pulse rate increases and arrhythmias may develop. The respiratory rate increases as the carbon dioxide level rises.

As noted earlier in this chapter, *hypoventilation* occurs frequently in the immediate postoperative period as a result of respiratory center depression by drugs or the anesthetic agent. Suggestions for improving ventilation were presented in the earlier discussion.

Obstruction of a bronchial tube by aspirated material or a plug of mucus results in *atelectasis*, the collapse of the portion of the lung distal to the obstruction. If the collapsed area is large, the patient becomes dyspneic and cyanosed; his respirations are rapid and shallow, chest expansion is decreased on the affected side and intercostal retraction may be evident. The pulse rate and temperature are elevated. On examination there is percussion dullness and an absence of breath sounds in the area. Trapped secretions tend to harbor organisms, leading to infection (pneumonia) in the collapsed area.

A chest x-ray may be ordered to determine the extent of the area involved. Frequent deep breathing, coughing and turning are required. Percussion of the chest by a physiotherapist to dislodge the mucus is done several times daily. An expectorant may be ordered, and an increased fluid intake and humidification of the air are used to promote liquefaction of the secretions so they can be raised. Endotracheal (deep) suctioning may be used, depending upon the location of the collapsed area and the amount of secretions in the tracheobronchial tree. If the mucus plug cannot be dislodged, bronchoscopic aspiration may be necessary. An antimicrobial preparation is prescribed to combat infection

Pneumonia may develop independently of atelectasis. Any secretions retained in the alveoli and bronchial tubes readily become infected. The patient usually develops a cough and may complain of chest pain. The temperature, pulse and respirations are elevated, and the sputum becomes purulent and blood streaked. (See p. 449 for a detailed discussion of pneumonia.)

Prevention of postoperative respiratory complications begins with the preoperative preparation. Recognition of even a very mild respiratory infection is important and should be reported. Unless the surgery is an emergency, the operation is deferred until the infection is cleared up. A good nutritional status contributes to the patient's resistance, and smoking should be discouraged. It is extremely important that the patient's stomach be empty when receiving an anesthetic to decrease the danger of aspiration of vomitus.

Postoperative nursing measures that contribute to the prevention of respiratory complications include the following: (1) lateral or semiprone positioning of the patient during recovery from general anesthesia to prevent obstruction of the airway and promote drainage of secretions and vomitus to prevent aspiration; (2) use of suction when necessary to remove secretions from the pharynx and mouth; (3) frequent deep breathing, coughing and change of position; (4) protection of the patient from chilling and exposure to persons with a respiratory infection; (5) ambulation as soon as ordered; and (6) prompt recognition and reporting of adverse signs and symptoms.

Cardiovascular Complications

Cardiac and vascular complications that may develop postoperatively include cardiac arrest, phlebothrombosis, thrombophlebitis and embolism.

CARDIAC ARREST. Rarely, sudden heart failure occurs in the postoperative patient and demands rapid emergency treatment. External cardiac massage and artificial respirations by the mouth-to-mouth method are initiated immediately. The cardiac arrest is due to failure of the heart muscle to contract or to ventricular fibrillation. In the latter, the normal synchronized contractions of the muscle fibers of the ventricles are replaced with rapid, irregular, uncoordinated contractions that result in incomplete filling and emptying of the chambers and insufficient blood being pumped into the systemic circulation. A defibrillator may be used by which one or two electric shocks are delivered to the heart.

Drug therapy may include an antiarrhythmic drug given by intravenous infusion (see p. 328), epinephrine hydrochloride (Adrenalin) 1:1000, calcium chloride 10 per cent for direct intracardiac injection to stimulate contractions, and sodium bicarbonate (44.6 mEq. per ampule) intravenously to combat the metabolic acidosis that develops rapidly with the oxygen deficiency in the tissues. (For details of cardiopulmonary resuscitation see p. 331.)

PHLEBOTHROMBOSIS AND THROMBO-PHLEBITIS. *Phlebothrombosis* is the formation of a clot in the veins due to a stasis of the blood. It develops most often in the lower limbs. Pressure on the calves of the legs and prolonged flexion of the legs should be avoided. Although the patient may find a pillow under the knees or the elevation of the Gatch frame at the knees very comfortable, these are hazardous since they promote venous stasis. Frequent foot and leg exercises play an important role in the prevention of phlebothrombosis in the bed patient.

The thrombus formation is a "silent" process; there may be some tenderness in the calf of the leg that is accidentally discovered on pressure, but generally there are no evident signs or symptoms. If phlebothrombosis is suspected or recognized, the patient is placed at rest with the foot of the bed elevated. An anticoagulant (e.g., heparin) may be prescribed to prevent enlargement of the thrombus. The condition is very dangerous because the clot may be carried along in the blood stream and eventually may block a vital blood vessel, causing what is called an embolism, which may be fatal. Since venous stasis is more likely to occur in varicosed veins, as a precautionary measure the surgeon may order an elastic type of stocking or the application of elastic bandages to the lower limbs from the foot to the thigh before surgery. These usually remain until just before the patient is discharged or resumes a normal amount of activity. The nurse removes and reapplies them twice daily to give the necessary skin care.

Thrombophlebitis is due to trauma, infection or chemical irritation of the wall of a vein, initiating a local inflammatory reaction and clot formation. In this instance the clot is fairly firmly attached to the wall of the vein. The condition is quickly recognized because the surrounding tissue becomes edematous, reddened and painful, and there is an elevation of temperature and pulse.

The patient may be kept on bed rest with the affected limb elevated. External heat may help to relieve the pain caused by vasospasm, and an anticoagulant may be ordered to prevent enlargement of the thrombus. The affected limb is handled very gently and is never massaged, in order to avoid dislodging the clot and the possibility of an embolism.

PULMONARY EMBOLISM. This is a serious vascular postoperative complication that compromises the individual's gas exchange and the volume of blood returned to the left side of the heart. Embolism involves the transport by the blood stream of a detached blood clot (thrombus) or mass of "foreign" material (tissue, fat globules, air) to a site remote from its origin or point of entry into the vascular system. It is most often a thrombus which eventually lodges in a vessel, obstructing the flow of blood and causing an infarction in the area.

A frequent site of embolism is a pulmonary artery, and the size of the artery occluded determines what happens to the patient. If it is a large pulmonary artery, the patient may experience sudden severe chest pain and respiratory distress and collapse and die immediately. If a smaller pulmonary artery is blocked, the patient experiences chest pain, dyspnea, coughing and elevation in temperature, pulse rate and respirations. He may expectorate blood-streaked mucus. If it is a relatively large infarction, shock develops rapidly. In a few hours an area of dullness may be detected by percussion, and auscultation may reveal an area in which there are no breath sounds, as the alveoli in the infarct gradually collapse. A chest x-ray is done and the blood pH and gas (oxygen and carbon dioxide) concentrations are determined frequently.

Oxygen is administered by nasal cannulae or a mask, and an analgesic such as meperidine hydrochloride (Demerol) may be ordered to relieve the patient's pain and anxiety. An anticoagulant (heparin) is given by intravenous infusion.

Postoperative embolism occurs more often following pelvic surgery, prolonged bed rest, fractures, and orthopedic surgery. It develops more readily in elderly persons and in those with varicosities or a history of a recent leg injury. It is also suggested that women who have been using an oral contraceptive (anovulatory drug) are predisposed to embolism.[3, 4]

Frequent foot and leg exercises and early mobilization are important measures in the prevention of embolism. (For a more detailed discussion of pulmonary embolism and nursing intervention see p. 467.)

---

[3]G. W. Thorn, et al. (Eds.): Harrison's Principles of Internal Medicine, 8th ed. New York, McGraw-Hill, 1977.

[4]Edgar C. Boedeker and James H. Dauber (Eds.): Manual of Medical Therapeutics, 21st ed. Boston, Little, Brown, 1974, p. 178

Wound Complications

INFECTION. In the operative site, infection is manifested by fever, increased pulse rate, general malaise and redness, swelling and tenderness of the wound area. Spontaneous purulent drainage occurs unless the infection is deep, in which case the surgeon may remove a suture and probe the area to facilitate drainage. A swab of the first discharge is taken for culture to determine the causative organism. An antimicrobial drug (antibiotic or sulfonamide) is administered and frequent application of hot, moist dressings may be ordered to increase the blood supply to the area and to promote drainage of the exudate. Even though the wound is infected, strict aseptic dressing technique is used to prevent the introduction of a secondary infection. When the soiled dressings are removed they are immediately placed in a paper bag for disposal, and precautions are taken to avoid contamination of the bedding and other objects in the environment to prevent the transmission of the infection to others.

DEHISCENCE. Excessive strain on a wound, such as occurs in prolonged abdominal distention or severe coughing, wound infection, malnutrition, and general debilitation, may cause separation of the edges of the incision; this separation is called *dehiscence*. Resuturing or the application of adhesive straps may be used to pull the edges together.

EVISCERATION. If there is some separation of all the tissue layers (skin, fascia and peritoneum) in an abdominal wound, protrusion of a loop of intestine onto the surface of the abdomen may occur. This is referred to as *evisceration*. It is usually sudden, and the patient experiences "something giving way" and a warm sensation on the skin surface due to the escape of peritoneal fluid and viscera. The surgeon is notified and sterile dressings moistened with sterile normal saline are applied to the exposed intestine. If a large portion of the bowel is eviscerated, a sterile towel moistened with the saline will provide better protection. A binder may be applied for support. The patient is requested to lie very still and the head and shoulders and the lower limbs are slightly elevated to reduce the strain on the abdominal wall. Someone remains with the patient to provide reassurance, and a sedative may be ordered to allay fear. Since the patient will most likely be returned to the operating room, an anesthetic and operative consent is signed after the surgeon has explained what is necessary, and the family is notified. The anesthetist or surgeon is advised as to when the patient last took food and fluid so that necessary precautions are taken to prevent aspiration. Lavage or induced vomiting are contraindicated since intra-abdominal pressure would be increased and more intestine eviscerated.

Gastrointestinal Complications

Persistent vomiting beyond 24 hours after operation causes concern. It may be due to the patient's sensitivity to the drugs which have been given, or it may be caused by *acute dilatation of the stomach* which can occur after almost any surgery if there is shock. Gastric dilatation is characterized by frequent vomiting of small amounts without effort, and upper abdominal distention which imposes on the diaphragm, causing dyspnea. A nasogastric tube is passed and suction-decompression established (see p. 501).

Mechanical intestinal obstruction, paralytic ileus and *peritonitis* are serious complications and may develop following abdominal surgery. These conditions are discussed in Chapter 16.

HICCUPS (SINGULTUS). Hiccups may occur as a troublesome, exhausting, postoperative complication, particularly after abdominal operations. They are paroxysmal, intermittent contractions of the diaphragm with the glottis closed. The cause is mechanical or chemical irritation of the diaphragm, a phrenic nerve, or the respiratory center of the brain. They may be associated with gastric dilatation, abdominal distention, peritonitis, pleurisy, pneumonia, uremia or the ingestion of very hot or cold fluids.

The hiccups may cease spontaneously as the cause is corrected. If persistent, a tranquilizing drug such as chlorpromazine hydrochloride (Thorazine) may be prescribed. The inhalation of carbogen (carbon dioxide 5 per cent in oxygen) for 5 minutes at frequent intervals to stimulate deep regular respirations may provide relief. Rebreathing the air in a paper bag held closely over the mouth and nose may be used. Suction-decompression via a nasogastric tube is established if the hiccups are associated with gastric dilatation or abdominal distention.

PAROTITIS. Dehydration, lack of oral intake and the omission of frequent hygienic mouth care predispose the patient to infection of the parotid gland. Normally, parotid salivary secretion is stimulated with fluid and food intake; this secretion washes out any organisms that may have found their way into the parotid ducts (Stensen's ducts). In the absence of secretion and adequate mouth care, organisms multiply in the mouth and have access to the glands. A painful swelling appears at the angle of the jaw on the side of the infected gland, and the patient develops a fever and systemic signs of infection. Older persons seem to have a greater predisposition to parotitis, and it may prove fatal when secondary to surgery or other illnesses.

Prevention involves keeping the mouth clean and moist and encouraging the patient to take adequate fluids and food as soon as permitted. Chewing gum or sucking a sour fruit candy may be helpful in stimulating salivary secretion if the ingestion of fluids and food is restricted.

Treatment involves local heat applications and antimicrobial drug administration. If suppuration develops, surgical drainage may be necessary.

References

Books

American College of Surgeons, Committee on Pre- and Postoperative Care: Manual of Preoperative and Postoperative Care, 2nd ed. Philadelphia, W. B. Saunders, 1971. Part 1.
Beland, Irene L., and Passos, Joyce Y.: Clinical Nursing, 3rd ed. New York, Macmillan, 1975. Chapter 17.
Falconer, Mary W., et al.: The Drug, The Nurse, The Patient, 6th ed. Philadelphia, W. B. Saunders, 1978. Chapter 15.
Sabiston, David C., Jr. (Ed.): Davis-Christopher: Textbook of Surgery, 11th ed. Philadelphia, W. B. Saunders, 1977. Chapter 5.
Schwartz, Seymour I., et al. (Eds.): Principles of Surgery, 2nd ed. New York, McGraw-Hill, 1974. Chapters 1–12 (inclusive).

Periodicals

Preoperative

Derksen, Wendy S., and Shewchuk, Muriel G.: "Preop Visits Expand the O.R. Nurse's Role." Can. Nurs., Vol. 71, No. 6 (June 1975), pp. 27–30.
Egbert, L. D., et al.: "Reduction of Postoperative Pain by Encouragement and Instruction of Patients." N. Engl. J. Med., Vol. 270, No. 16 (April 16, 1964), pp. 825–827.
Laird, Mona: "Techniques for Teaching Pre- and Postoperative Patients." Am. J. Nurs., Vol. 75, No. 8 (Aug. 1975), pp. 1338–1340.
Lindeman, Carol A., and Van Aernam, B.: "Nursing Intervention with the Presurgical Patient: The Effects of Structured and Unstructured Preoperative Teaching." Nurs. Res., Vol. 20, No. 4 (July/Aug. 1971), pp. 319–332.
Lyons, Mary Lou: "What Priority Do You Give Preop Teaching?" Nurs. '77, Vol. 7, No. 1 (Jan. 1977), pp. 11–12.
Merkatz, Ruth, et al.: "Preoperative Teaching for Gynecologic Patients." Am. J. Nurs., Vol. 74, No. 6 (June 1974), pp. 1072–1074.
Prasla, Helena: "Admission Unit Dispels Fear of Surgery." Can. Nurs., Vol. 70, No. 12 (Dec. 1974), pp. 24–26.
Winslow, Elizabeth Hahn, and Fuhs, Margaret Frances: "Preoperative Assessment for Postoperative Evaluation." Am. J. Nurs., Vol. 73, No. 8 (Aug. 1973), pp. 1372–1374.

Postoperative

Blackwell, Ardith K., and Blackwell, William: "Relieving Gas Pains." Am. J. Nurs., Vol. 75, No. 1 (Jan. 1975), pp. 66–67.

Burgess, Miriam G.: "A Nursing Care Plan for the Postoperative Patient in the Recovery Room and the Intensive Care Unit." Nurs. Clin. North Am., Vol. 3, No. 3 (Sept. 1968), pp. 499–502.

Campbell, Robert M.: "Fluid and Electrolyte Management in the Postoperative Surgical Patient." Nurs. Clin. North Am., Vol. 3, No. 3 (Sept. 1968), pp. 492–494.

Codd, John, and Grohar, Mary E.: "Postoperative Pulmonary Complications." Nurs. Clin. North Am., Vol. 10, No. 1 (March 1975), pp. 5–15.

Collart, Marie E., and Brenneman, Janice K.: "Preventing Postoperative Atelectasis." (Report of a study.) Am. J. Nurs., Vol. 71, No. 10 (Oct. 1971), pp. 1982–1987.

Friedman, Barbara: "Cardiac Surgery: Skilled Nursing During the Critical Postoperative Period." Nurs. '74, Vol. 4, No. 12 (Dec. 1974), pp. 37–40.

Gardhill, Norma, Campbell, Robert M., et al.: "Postoperative Management of the Surgical Patient." (Panel discussion.) Nurs. Clin. North Am., Vol. 3, No. 3 (Sept. 1968), pp. 491–505.

Garrett, John J.: "Oliguria in Postoperative Patients." Nurs. Clin. North Am., Vol. 10, No. 1 (March 1975), pp. 59–67.

Hamilton, William P.: "Common Cardiovascular Problems in the Postoperative Period." Nurs. Clin. North Am., Vol. 10, No. 1 (March 1975), pp. 27–41.

Heironimus, Terring W.: "Postoperative Respiratory Problems of the Surgical Patient." Nurs. Clin. North Am., Vol. 3, No. 3 (Sept. 1968), pp. 495–496.

Libman, Robert H., and Keithley, Joyce: "Relieving Airway Obstruction in the Recovery Room." Am J. Nurs., Vol. 75, No. 4 (April 1975), pp. 603–605.

Maykoski, Kathleen, and Fabre, Diane: "Nursing Assessment of the Surgical Intensive Care Patient." Nurs. Clin. North Am., Vol. 10, No. 1 (March 1975), pp. 83–106.

Metheny, Norma A.: "Water and Electrolyte Balance in the Postoperative Patient." Nurs. Clin. North Amer., Vol. 10, No. 1 (March 1975), pp. 49–57.

Murray, Ruth L. E.: "Assessment of Psychologic Status in the Surgical ICU Patient." Nurs. Clin. North Am., Vol. 10, No. 1 (March 1975), pp. 69–81.

Parsons, Mickey C., and Stephens, Gwen J.: "Postoperative Complications: Assessment and Intervention." Am. J. Nurs., Vol. 74, No. 2 (Feb. 1974), pp. 240–244.

Smith, Betty J.: "After Anesthesia." Nurs. '74, Vol. 4, No. 12 (Dec. 1974), pp. 28–32.

Smith, R. Brian, et al.: "In a Recovery Room." Am. J. Nurs., Vol. 73, No. 1 (Jan. 1973), pp. 70–73.

Walker, Betty J.: "Nursing Care to Assess and Prevent Common Cardiovascular Problems." Nurs. Clin. North Am., Vol. 10, No. 1 (March 1975), pp. 43–48.

Wyper, Mary: "Pulmonary Embolism." Nurs. '75, Vol. 5, No. 10 (Oct. 1975), pp. 30–38.

11

Age—
Implications
for Nursing

INTRODUCTION

Significant structural, physiological, intellectual and behavioral differences exist between individuals in different stages of the life cycle. Every nurse should appreciate the growth and developmental processes and the physical and psychological norms characteristic of the various age groups. The chronological and developmental ages of a person greatly influence health care needs, how they are expressed and the ways in which they should be met. It must be recognized that an individual can be an adult chronologically, but may be younger than an adult physically, intellectually and/or behaviorally.

Medical-surgical nursing references generally relate to the mature individual who falls within the physical and psychological norms, but many disorders that are discussed may also occur in children and elderly persons. Adaptations in the care cited are necessary because of existing variants due to age.

NURSING THE YOUNGER PATIENT

Factors in Adapting Care to Children

Nursing a child differs from caring for an adult in several ways, and the nurse's re-

sponsibilities for assessment, decisions, protection and fostering development are greater. Adults have the right and responsibility to make decisions about and participate in their own care; they may be dependent because of physical impairment but, if conscious, are able to communicate feelings and needs.

The following paragraphs include some important considerations in the care of the sick child. They are certainly not all-inclusive, but they may serve to indicate that differences do exist and to prompt the reader to refer to pediatric nursing texts for details. Although children may experience many of the illnesses to which adults are subject, infections, dysfunctions associated with congenital defects, nutritional problems and accidents have a much higher incidence. Neoplastic, metabolic and degenerative diseases occur less frequently in the earlier years of life.

ILLNESS AND HOSPITALIZATION. Illness and pain are new and frightening experiences to a young child and he has no understanding of them. If hospitalization is necessary, it imposes separation from the parents, strangeness and loneliness, which may have adverse effects on the child. Anything that is strange and unknown is potentially threatening; in addition to physical care he requires attention that will develop a sense of trust and security.

If the child is old enough, it is helpful if

190

the parents prepare him for hospitalization. A simple truthful explanation is made as to what a hospital is, why boys and girls are there, and why he must go. If he is not prepared, hospitalization may be interpreted as desertion or punishment. It is helpful if the child receives a general description of his hospital bed, how he will receive his meals, what he will wear, the use of the bedpan, and the personnel who will care for him. A number of picture and story books are available that are useful in preparing the child for hospitalization.[1] A copy of one of these may be obtained from the local children's hospital or the library. It is comforting if one or two favorite toys are taken along so that he will have something familiar close to him. When possible, the child is placed in a room or ward with children of his own age.

Individual differences in responses to frightening situations occur and depend largely on previous experiences and training. For example, although some preparation is still necessary, hospitalization for the child of school age is less difficult. He has had the experience of separation from his mother and home for part of each day and has usually developed some degree of independence. Some children may fight and resist the nurse, while others may withdraw and become listless, probably because of feelings of being forsaken by their parents. Understanding and accepting the child's fears and insecurity, the nurse provides the attention and care that hopefully leads to his recognition of her as a source of affection and security.

The child needs the mother's support in adjusting to the strange environment and situation. She is encouraged to remain close to the child, to undress him and to participate in the admission procedure. The nurse takes over gradually, and the child, seeing the mother's approval of this, becomes more accepting of the nurse. When the child is old enough to understand, the parents should tell him that they are leaving but will return and will take him home as soon as he is better. The nurse accepts

the child's concern and behavior when they leave, gives him attention and tries to introduce new interests. Although an occasional child may be inconsolable, the nurse patiently persists in her efforts to provide comfort and emotional support and establish a relationship that provides security. To give up and leave him alone only adds to his despair and insecurity.

PARENTS. The young child is totally dependent upon his parents, particularly his mother. His security and source of satisfaction in relation to his physical and emotional needs are vested chiefly in her or the person who mothers him. The mother as well as the child usually experiences considerable emotional disturbance on separation, and needs the understanding support of the nurse. She may fear the outcome of the illness or be concerned about the child suffering. She may develop feelings of inadequacy and guilt and may attribute the situation to some neglect on her part. Some of the parents' anxiety may be due to the expenses being incurred by the illness; a referral to the social or welfare service may be necessary for the provision of assistance.

The nurse assesses the parents' reactions and, on recognizing anxiety, makes an effort to avoid giving the impression that she is taking over the child. The mother is encouraged to talk about the child, remain with him as much as possible, especially at first, and to participate in his care. Her participation reassures the child, provides an outlet for the mother and establishes a better nurse-parent relationship in that it acknowledges the normal mother-child relationship. The nurse inquires as to whether there is anything special she should know about the child's accustomed care, such as food likes and dislikes, how he communicates his need to go to the toilet, his sleeping habits (his usual bedtime and whether he has a nap during the day), patterns of play, and what independent behavior he has developed. As well as providing information to be used in nursing, this manifests an interest in the child and respect for the care he has received from his parents.

Free visiting is permitted by many pediatric units now. The mother is usually anxious to spend a good deal of time with her sick child but may require guidance in the interest of the care of other children at

---

[1]Examples: Margaret and H. A. Rey: Curious George Goes to the Hospital. Boston, Houghton-Mifflin, 1966.

The Hospital for Sick Children, Toronto: Billy Goes to Hospital. Toronto, Women's Auxiliary of the Hospital for Sick Children.

home. In participating in the child's care, she should not be required to do more than she desires or she may think the nurse does not want to care for him. The nurse is still responsible for his total care and must know what takes place. Working with the mother provides an excellent opportunity for teaching and improving health practices which are favorable to the child's health and development. The mother may learn much simply by observing the care given.

GROWTH AND DEVELOPMENT. An important factor that influences the nursing of children is that the patients are in a period of physical growth and psychological and social development. It is necessary for the nurse to be familiar with the norms for the age of the child in her care. She has a responsibility to foster normal growth and developmental processes and recognize abnormalities and regression, as well as to meet the needs incurred by the child's illness. The amount of attention related to this aspect of nursing will vary with the age of the child, the nature and length of his illness, and the parents' understanding of his needs.

Until one has had considerable experience with children and the application of knowledge of growth and development, it may be necessary to refer to texts to determine the norms for the age of the child for whom care is being planned and implemented. It is not the intention to present a review of the characteristics of normal development here since there is an abundance of literature in this field. Several suitable textbooks are included in the references at the end of this chapter.

Illness frequently produces some regression in young children, particularly those in the preschool age group. Earlier patterns of behavior and greater dependency may be manifested; for example, the child may not indicate a need to go to the toilet and may revert to bedwetting, or he may make no attempt to feed himself. Information as to the child's independent and self-care activities is obtained from the parents, and opportunities are provided for their continuance within the limits imposed by his illness. If the need to learn and "to do for himself" is ignored, overdependence develops, motor skills regress, and the child is less able to cope with the situation.

The child requires opportunities to play, explore, learn, express himself, and achieve in association with his peers if he is to develop. This cannot be left to chance but takes planning, patience and time on the part of the nurse. A variety of toys and amusements are necessary and are selected according to the child's age, condition, interests and level of development. A play room or section of the ward is made available for ambulatory and wheelchair patients and is staffed by trained workers. For the children confined to bed, games may be organized that will involve several patients. Toys or games may be selected from carts which are taken through the wards, or as part of nursing care a story may be read to the bed patient. It should be remembered that a child has a short attention span; new interests and stimulation are needed. Most pediatric nursing texts include a chapter on play in which specific suggestions are made for play and amusement suitable for the various age groups. Play activities which promote motor coordination and dexterity, perception, and self-expression are also indicated.

A person tends to develop responses that are satisfying to him, but these may not always be acceptable to society. It is important that the child develop patterns of behavior that are acceptable to those around him. Group play provides opportunities for socialization and the learning of appropriate approved behavior.

If the school child is in the hospital or is confined to bed at home for a prolonged period, his school work is continued by a visiting teacher provided by the local school board. His diet will probably require periodic adjustment to meet his growth requirements.

SIGNS, SYMPTOMS AND OBSERVATION. Signs and symptoms of illness in an infant and child differ somewhat from those in a mature patient because of the effect of the disorder on immature developing tissues and organs. The onset of an illness is frequently more abrupt and acute. An evident change in behavior, fussiness, refusal of food, vomiting, diarrhea and fever are common to many conditions in children and do not point to the specific nature or site of the problem. A convulsion is common at the onset of a fever, and the temperature rises to higher levels than in an adult. Serious dehydration leading to shock may develop as a result of vomiting, diarrhea, fever and reduced intake. The child loses weight and becomes debilitated quickly because of the lack of nutritional reserves. The provision of fluids and nourishment becomes an immediate concern with any sick child.

Observation is an important part of all nursing, but it plays an even more significant role in the care of children. The infant and the young child are unable to verbalize and describe their discomforts and needs; the physician and nurse are dependent on objective signs. Many nonverbal communications in the form of behavioral manifestations have meanings that are just as important as the vital signs. The diagnosis and treatment may be greatly influenced by the nurse's accurate, objective description of the child's physical, mental and emotional responses.

Pertinent factors that should be noted and recorded include the following:

1. *Crying* — whether it is the normal strong vigorous cry or is shrill and piercing, feeble, or a whimper.

2. *Body movements and position*— whether restless, making purposeless movements, abnormally still and favoring one position, cries and protests when a particular part or area is moved or touched or when he is picked up.

3. *Abnormal loss or increase in muscle tension* (e.g., rigidity and hyperextension of the neck).

4. *Frequent brushing or rubbing of a part* (e.g., face or ear).

5. *Apathy* — passive, withdrawn, indifferent to environment.

6. *Increased dependence* — appears fearful and bewildered, clings to the nurse or parent.

7. *Failure to eat and drink.*

8. *Change in the number and character of stools.*

9. *Change in the volume and character of urine.*

10. *Skin eruptions.*

11. *Facial expression and color* — drawn, aged appearance, pallor, eyes sunken, shadows under the eyes, mottling or cyanosis.

12. *Any behavior that differs from that expected for the age and level of development* or from that which was previously exhibited.

13. *Excessive sweating* is not normal and is brought to the physician's attention since it may indicate some autonomic nervous system dysfunction.

Continuity of care by the same nurses is important so that physical and behavioral changes will be recognized promptly. It is also better for the child as he becomes accustomed to the same nurses to whom he can relate; lack of a continuing warm relationship causes anxiety in the child and later a cold indifference to everyone.

RESISTANCE. Children are more susceptible to infection and, the younger the child, the greater the susceptibility. As he becomes older, he develops antibodies and some immunity following repeated infections. The infant is born with a natural passive immunity to some infections through having received antibodies from the mother's blood. Measles, diphtheria, poliomyelitis, smallpox, and streptococcal and pneumococcal infections are relatively rare in infants up to 6 months of age. The antibodies which diffused across the placenta from the mother's blood into the fetus gradually diminish over the first 5 to 6 months of life, and the child begins to manufacture his own antibodies after repeated exposures to invading pathogenic organisms (antigens). The principal defense mechanisms and the reticuloendothelial tissues concerned with antibody formation are immature and slower to respond in the child, contributing to the high incidence of childhood infections.

Parents should be urged to consult their physician as to the recommended schedule for active immunization for their infant (see p. 61). When it is learned that a hospitalized child has had no inoculations, it is brought to the doctor's attention.

Because of their lower resistance, children should be protected from contact with known and suspected sources of infection. The child with an infection requires prompt attention and treatment; his immaturity and lack of antibodies and reserves may lead rapidly to an overwhelming infection.

FLUIDS. There is a proportionately greater volume of water in the body of the child than in the adult; approximately 70 to 80 per cent of body weight is water, as compared to approximately 60 per cent of the adult's weight. The water in the young is used more rapidly; the increased heat production results in a greater amount being vaporized and the urinary output is proportionately greater since the immature kidneys are less efficient in conserving water and concentrating wastes.

Serious dehydration, acid-base imbalance and shock can develop with startling rapidity when there is a reduced fluid intake or an increased loss of fluid as in vomiting, diarrhea and fever. Unfortunately all of these latter factors commonly occur together in childhood illnesses. An early assessment of the ill child's state of hydration is necessary. Vomiting, diarrhea, high fever and failure to take fluids should be reported promptly so that body fluids may be brought up to the optimal level. Signs of dehydration are dry mouth with thick stringy saliva, loss of tissue turgor, sunken eyes, depressed fontanelles in the infant, apathy and loss of weight. If it is allowed to progress to greater fluid depletion, the reduced intravascular volume causes shock, which is manifested by pallor, cold skin, rapid weak pulse and an abnormally low blood pressure.

Resourcefulness and patience are necessary on the part of the nurse in getting the child to take an adequate amount of fluid by mouth. A pleasant positive approach, assuming the child is going to take the fluid, rather than a demanding, urgent manner is helpful. Overurging may only result in the child's vomiting. Allowing the young child to choose between two or three fluids and to select a colored straw may capture the child's cooperation. An accurate record of the intake and output is necessary.

When sufficient fluid cannot be given orally, parenteral fluids are administered by intravenous or interstitial infusion (hypodermoclysis). Sites used for intravenous infusion in the young include a vein on the medial side of an ankle and a scalp vein. If the latter is used, the area is shaved in preparation. A cutdown may be necessary; if so a local anesthetic is injected into the skin at the site and a small incision is made to expose the vein. A cannula or needle is then introduced into the vein and secured by suture material. The area is protected by a sterile dressing. Adequate restraint is necessary during the starting of an intravenous infusion and later to prevent dislodgement of the needle or cannula. The mummy restraint which encloses the arms, trunk and lower limbs, and immobilization of the head with sandbags are used if the scalp vein is the site of the infusion. When a limb is used, clove hitch restraints and a splint on the particular arm or leg may be applied. The volume and rate of flow of the intravenous fluid are indicated by the physician and carefully controlled. If the fluid is given more rapidly than it can pass from the intravascular compartment into the tissues, the cardiovascular system may become overloaded, leading to serious and even fatal results.

In interstitial infusion (hypodermoclysis) a quantity of fluid is introduced slowly into the subcutaneous tissues. Sites which may be used are the anterior aspects of the thighs and the scapular and pectoral areas. The rate at which the solution is administered is regulated according to the rate of absorption. If it is allowed to run too rapidly it will cause considerable local swelling and discomfort. Hyaluronidase, an enzyme, may be added to the fluid to promote absorption.

NUTRITION. Infants and children require more calories in proportion to size and weight than adults in order to support their growth process, higher metabolic rate and physical activity. The daily requirement is approximately 110 to 120 calories per kilogram of body weight during the first 2 years of life and gradually declines to 40 to 60 calories per kilogram at maturity. Malnutrition is manifested quickly in a child with an inadequate caloric intake, as his reserves are very limited.

The sick child frequently presents nutritional problems; food may be refused because of a loss of appetite, the strange environment, despair at being separated from his parents, or because the food is not what he is accustomed to at home. The nurse needs to know the nutritional requirements of the child according to his age, the necessary restrictions because of his disorder, how much he is actually taking and changes in his weight. As with the giving of fluids, resourcefulness and patience are frequently necessary to have the patient receive sufficient nourishment. The following suggestions may be helpful:

1. A positive approach should be used, assuming the child is going to take the food.

2. He should not be hurried or bribed and is commended when he eats what is offered.

3. Milk may be withheld until later if he is inclined to drink it all and then refuse the solid foods.

4. Similarly, only the more important food principles (eggs, meat, vegetables) may be offered and carbohydrates, such as bread and desserts, withheld so he doesn't satisfy his appetite on those first. Giving him a choice when possible may add some enticement. Self-feeding is permitted and encouraged unless it is contraindicated by his illness. When the condition permits, the child usually eats better when at a table with others.

In some instances it may be beneficial to have the mother visit at mealtime, provided she does not become overanxious and aggravate the problem. Her presence may provide a situation with which the child is familiar. Normally, parents are discouraged from bringing in home-cooked food, but occasionally it may be of value to permit them to bring the child some food which he likes and is accustomed to receiving at home, and which is compatible with his condition.

If the child is obese, fats and starches are reduced. In long-term illness, it is important that adjustments be made from time to time in the caloric intake and diet according to the child's age and progressive growth requirement.

NAUSEA AND VOMITING. Vomiting commonly occurs with any illness in a child. Nausea may precede the vomiting but cannot be verbalized by the young. In some instances it may be suspected and vomiting anticipated when the child manifests pallor, increased salivation, restlessness and sweating.

Regurgitation, which is nonforceful, effortless vomiting that occurs without abdominal muscle contraction, is common in infants because of the incomplete development of the cardiac sphincter. The cause of this type of vomiting is more often the swallowing of air or gastric distention due to overfeeding.

The immaturity of the neuromuscular system, which results in less efficient reflexes, increases the possibility of aspiration or vomitus; the infant or child must be quickly turned to the prone position to promote drainage from the pharynx and mouth. The nursing observations and responsibilities cited in the care of the patient who is vomiting (p. 489) will also apply to the child. It must be remembered, though, that the child lacks the reserve which the adult is likely to have and, in vomiting, will develop serious dehydration and malnutrition more rapidly.

ELIMINATION. The normal infant has an average of two stools per day; after the age of 1 year, bowel elimination is usually decreased to one stool per day. Stools are examined for changes in volume, color, composition and consistency. The characteristics of the stool normally are determined by the food; changes from the normal may indicate a necessary dietary adjustment, particularly in infants.

Elimination which is too frequent or is absent, excessive straining at stool, and abnormality of the stool are reported and recorded. An abnormal stool is saved for the physician's inspection and for possible laboratory examination. An enema or laxative is only administered when ordered by the physician since either causes loss of fluid.

REST AND SLEEP. The increased activity, higher metabolic rate and lesser reserve of the young result in their need for more rest and sleep than mature persons. Nursing includes plans for regular rest periods and naps during the day as well as a regular early bedtime hour at night. Special bedtime rituals are determined from the parents and followed as much as possible; for example, the child may be accustomed to saying his prayers to someone or to having a certain toy or blanket to cuddle.

VITAL SIGNS. The young child's temperature-regulating mechanism is not fully developed, and as a result fever rises to higher levels than in adolescents or adults. He tolerates exposure to cold less well because his ability to conserve body heat by vascular constriction is less efficient.

The temperature is taken rectally up to the age of 7 to 8 years. The thermometer is held and the other hand is placed on the child during the recording to prevent sudden movement and possible breaking of the thermometer in the rectum. For a fever over 38.8° C. (102° F.), temperature-reducing measures such as a tepid sponge bath and the administration of antipyretic drugs (e.g., acetylsalicylic acid) may be ordered. The tepid sponge bath is discontinued if cyanosis, weak pulse or a slow respiratory rate is manifested.

The pulse and respirations vary with age, activity, emotions and crying. The volume and rhythm of the pulse are more significant than the rate. More accurate information may be obtained if they are checked when the child is sleeping and before the temperature is taken, since the insertion of the rectal thermometer may disturb the child and cause variation. The pulse rate gradually decreases, reaching adult levels by adolescence. The average normal range for different age groups is as follows:

Infant	140 to 120 per minute
1 to 5 years	120 to 90 per minute
5 to 10 years	90 to 80 per minute
10 to 16 years	90 to 74 per minute

The respirations are more rapid and shallow in the infant and preschooler than in the older child and adult. They vary from 30 to 50 per minute in infancy and gradually decrease to adult levels of 16 to 20 per minute by the age of 10 to 12 years.

The blood pressure is considerably lower in infancy and childhood than in maturity; it gradually increases with weight. The width of the cuff used in determining the blood pressure varies with the size of the child. If the cuff is too narrow, the blood pressure recorded will be higher than it actually is; if it is too wide, a lower reading is obtained. The cuff used should be approximately two-thirds the length of the upper arm. Cuffs usually appropriate for different ages are as follows:

Infants	cuff of 1 to 2 inches
2 to 8 years	cuff of 3 inches
8 to 12 years	cuff of 4 inches
12 to 14 years	cuff of 5 inches

The child should be at rest for an accurate recording of blood pressure; fear, restlessness and excitement are likely to produce an erroneously high systolic pressure. The average normal blood pressures according to age are found below.

	Systolic pressure
Infancy	85 mm. Hg
1 to 6 years	85 to 90 mm. Hg
6 to 10 years	90 to 100 mm. Hg
10 to 16 years	100 to 118 mm. Hg

	Diastolic pressure
Infancy	50 mm. Hg
1 to 6 years	50 to 60 mm. Hg
6 to 10 years	60 to 65 mm. Hg
10 to 16 years	65 to 70 mm. Hg

URINARY SYSTEM. The urinary output in infants and young children is proportionately larger than in children over 8 or 9 years and adults. The immature kidneys have less discriminatory ability; they are unable to conserve water and regulate the output according to the intake and to concentrate wastes to the same extent.

Pyelonephritis (infection of the kidney pelvis and tissue) due to colon bacillus is relatively common in young females because of the short urethra. Prevention necessitates prompt changing of soiled diapers or underclothing and thorough cleansing following defecation. In cleansing, precautions are taken to avoid the possibility of transmitting contamination toward the urethral meatus.

RESPIRATORY SYSTEM. In the early years, on inspiration the chest cavity is enlarged mainly by the contraction and lowering of the diaphragm. The infant's and young child's ribs are horizontal and the intercostal muscles have a lesser role in respiration. As a result, the rise and fall of the chest wall during respiration is less noticeable than in the older child and adult, and movement of the abdomen is more evident.

The lumen of the respiratory tract is smaller and so is more readily occluded in inflammatory conditions and aspiration. The larynx is sensitive, and irritation or inflammation may quickly cause spasmodic contraction, making breathing difficult. The nasal passages, being small, obstruct easily in respiratory infections, making sucking difficult. The cough reflex is absent in the infant and less efficient while developing in the young child; as a result, they do not get rid of secretions or a foreign body as readily as older children and adults. Because of these several differences, infants and children with respiratory infection require prompt treatment and close observation for respiratory insufficiency. Sternal and intercostal retraction and flaring of the nostrils frequently accompany severe respiratory difficulty and must be reported promptly to the physician. Prolonged, rapid respirations exhaust a young child more rapidly than an older child or adult. Mucus should be wiped away quickly or removed by nasopharyngeal suctioning to prevent aspiration. The patient is kept on his side or in the semiprone position as much as possible to promote drainage of secretions. Cool moist air and increased fluid intake are provided to liquefy the mucus and facilitate its removal.

If oxygen or air is administered directly under pressure into the child's respiratory tract, the pressure must be kept low for a child up to 12 years so that the lungs are not damaged by overdistention. Similarly, caution is also necessary if mouth-to-mouth resuscitation is used.

Middle ear infection (otitis media) is a common complication of respiratory infection in children. The incompletely developed eustachian tube is straighter and wider, making it a more accessible pathway by which organisms may enter the middle ear from the pharynx.

NERVOUS SYSTEM. The child's developing nervous system is unstable. As a result, convulsions frequently accompany illness in children up to 4 or 5 years of age, especially if there is a fever. A nurse should remain with the child during the seizure to protect him from injury. Suction is quickly made available to remove excess oral secretions when the child relaxes. The seizure is reported promptly and the following observations recorded:

1. Child's condition and activity immediately preceding the seizure.

2. The parts of the body involved.

3. Whether the movements are jerky (clonic) or whether the body or involved parts remain contracted and rigid (tonic).

4. The patient's color, secretions, eye movements and pupillary changes.

5. The length of the seizure and period of unconsciousness.

6. Incontinence.

7. Temperature, pulse, and respirations, as well as any changes in behavior and awareness following the seizure. It must be remembered that convulsions may not always be due to the immaturity of the central nervous system; they may be associated with metabolic or central nervous system disorders.

Immature reflexes and lack of complete muscular coordination predispose the developing child to falls and accidents, necessitating greater protective measures on the part of those responsible for him. Blows to the infant's head are more serious because of the open fontanelles and incompletely developed suture lines in the skull.

BLOOD VALUES. Normal blood values for the infant and the child up to 12 years differ from those for adults. Erythrocytes (red blood cells) are more numerous at birth and gradually decrease to a lower level over the first 2 or 3 months; adult levels are usually reached by the age of 12 years. The leukocyte count is higher in the infant and in the child up to about 12 years with a higher percentage of lymphocytes. In Table 11–1 the normal blood values for various ages are presented.

SAFETY MEASURES. The child's normal curiosity, desire to explore, and lack of experience and understanding necessitate special precautions and constant alertness on the part of the nurse to reduce the possibility of injury from falls, the swallowing or aspiration of foreign bodies, burns, suffocation and poisoning. Essential protective measures include the following: crib sides must be kept up and securely fastened unless the nurse or a parent is right at the bedside, facing the child. If the nurse must turn from the child to get something during direct care or if the child is on a treatment table, she keeps a hand on the child. The sides should also be kept up on empty cribs to discourage ambulant children from climbing. Young children, whether in bed or up, are not left unattended for long periods.

TABLE 11–1 HEMATOLOGIC VALUES DURING INFANCY AND CHILDHOOD

Age	Hemoglobin gm./100 ml. %		Hematocrit %		Reticulocytes %	WBC/MM.³		Neutrophils %		Lymphocytes % Mean (Relatively Wide Range)	Eosinophils % Mean	Monocytes % Mean	Nucleated Red Cells /100 wbc
	Mean	Range	Mean	Range	Mean	Mean	Range	Mean	Range				
Cord blood	16.8	13.7-20.1	55	45-65	5.0	18,000	(9-30,000)	61	(40-80)	31	2	6	7.0 (3-10)
2 weeks	16.5	13.0-20.0	50	42-66	1.0	12,000	(5-21,000)	40		48	3	9	0
3 months	12.0	9.5-14.5	36	31-41	1.0	12,000	(6-18,000)	30		63	2	5	0
6 mos.-6 yrs.	12.0	10.5-14.0	37	33-42	1.0	10,000	(6-15,000)	45		48	2	5	0
7-12 yrs.	13.0	11.0-16.0	38	34-40	1.0	8,000	(4500-13,500)	55		38	2	5	0
Adult Female	14	12.0-16.0	42	37-47	1.6	7,500	(5-10,000)	55	(35-70)	35	3	7	0
Male	16	14.0-18.0	47	42-52									

All values represent compromises between a number of standard sources and published reports. Greatest variations in "normal" are seen in infancy and early childhood. (From V. C. Vaughan and R. J. McKay: *Nelson Textbook of Pediatrics.* 10th ed. Philadelphia, W. B. Saunders Company, 1975, p. 1110.)

If a restraint is necessary, that applied to the trunk must fit closely enough to remain in position and prevent the child from wriggling out of it. When restraints are applied to the limbs, precautions are necessary to avoid interference with the circulation.

The use of soft pillows and plastic sheeting is avoided; if either is used, it must be secured to the bed to prevent the possibility of the child pulling it over his face and smothering. All of the windows should have screens firmly secured in position. Radiators, electrical outlets and fans are covered, and doorways and the entrances to stairways are guarded by gates if children are ambulatory. Sharp-edged toys and those with loose or detachable small parts that might be swallowed or aspirated are removed. Safety pins are kept closed and out of reach.

Medications are kept in a locked cupboard and never left at the bedside or within reach of a child. During administration, the nurse must not turn her back on a medicine tray or cart that has medication on it. The term "candy" should not be used as a means of persuasion when giving the child a pill, as it may lead to his taking an overdose of available pills at a later date.

A positive identification of the child by checking the necklace or bracelet and the bassinette or crib card is necessary before administering a treatment and medication, since the infant or child is not capable of questioning or advising the nurse that he is the wrong patient.

Medications, fluids and foods are not forced because of the possibility of causing aspiration as well as fear and resentment in the child. Infants' feeding bottles must not be propped because of the danger of aspiration.

Extreme caution is necessary with the use of steam inhalations and applications of heat. With the former, the steam outlet is screened and kept out of reach. Hot water bottles must not be more than 44° to 46° C. (110° to 115° F.) and must be tightly stoppered and covered. Taps must be turned off tightly; bath water is tested with a thermometer before placing a child in it.

Sufficient assistance should be available during treatments to provide adequate restraint to ensure safety.

Whenever the opportunity presents, the child who is old enough to understand is taught what is safe and unsafe. The nurse also has a responsibility for educating parents and others as to their role in the prevention of accidents.

MEDICATION. Drug dosage for children is based on their weight and age, and must be very accurate. Children and particularly infants are observed closely for the effects of drugs given since their immature enzyme systems, liver and kidneys may not completely metabolize and excrete the drugs. Although the doctor prescribes the dose of the drug to be given, the nurse should be familiar with how a dosage is determined. If not familiar with the drug or if there is reason to question the dosage, the nurse makes a quick check before administering the drug. In many instances, the label or brochure accompanying the drug will indicate the dosage or the amount to be given per kilogram of body weight. Or the dosage may be checked by using Clark's rule, which is:

Infant's or child's dose =

$$\frac{\text{weight of child in pounds} \times \text{adult dose}}{150 \text{ (which is the average adult weight)}}$$

Occasionally for older children, Young's rule may be used:

Child's dose =

$$\frac{\text{age of child in years} \times \text{adult dose}}{\text{age of child in years} + 12}$$

When administering drugs to children, a positive, firm approach is used. The nurse's attitude and comment reflect no doubt about the child's cooperation. The child's questions are answered honestly. For infants and children up to 5 or 6 years, tablets and pills are crushed and put into solution. Medications should not be disguised in food, as this may cause future refusal of that particular food. Many medications are placed in fruit-flavored syrups which disguise any disagreeable taste. As cited under safety measures, special precautions are taken by the nurse to be sure of the right child. Care is taken to avoid force in administering oral medication. The head and shoulders are elevated during the taking of oral medicine to avoid possible aspiration.

Infants and children tolerate opiates

poorly, and a smaller dose than might be expected according to the previously mentioned rules is always prescribed.

When children are to receive hypodermic or intramuscular injections, if they are old enough to be frightened and resist, they should receive some preparation. Sufficient assistance should be available to hold the child securely and provide support. Needles are selected according to the child's size and should be sharp and in good condition. Afterwards, the child's crying and protestations are accepted; the nurse acknowledges his hurt and tries to comfort the child by picking him up or in the case of an older child by staying with him.

NURSING PROCEDURES. The child's size must always be considered, since it dictates variations in certain procedures. Oversized equipment such as tubes or needles can be traumatizing to the child's tissues and interfere with effectiveness of the treatment.

Procedures are described in simple terms to the child who is old enough to understand even part of what is being said. Sometimes it is possible and helpful to let the child explore the equipment, see illustrations, or in some instances demonstrate to some extent on the child's doll or toy animal. Resourcefulness is needed to devise approaches and methods. The child is approached with a patient, positive attitude rather than a domineering, demanding manner that threatens him. It is helpful if the child is involved and is asked to do something that contributes. Whenever possible, the same nurse gives the treatment. Sufficient assistance must be available to provide the restraint necessary to make the treatment safe. The temperature of treatment solutions is tested by a thermometer and should not be used if over 40.5° C. (105° F.) unless specified by the physician.

When positioning an infant or young child it should be remembered that prolonged pressure from remaining in one position for a long period may alter the shape of young developing bones. It is particularly significant in relation to the skull because of the fontanelles and developing suture lines. Freedom of movement is necessary to promote muscular development and coordination.

When possible, the infant and young child are held during feeding and some nursing care procedures; physical contact is reassuring and tends to make the situation less frightening.

The Adolescent

Adolescence is the period of transition from childhood to adulthood and extends roughly from the thirteenth to the nineteenth year. It is characterized by marked structural, physiological, emotional and social behavioral changes. The individual is seeking independence and a new set of values and standards, and struggling with identity conflict and developing sexuality.

PHYSIOLOGICAL AND STRUCTURAL FACTORS. There is an increased secretion of the sex and somatotropic (growth) hormones, producing structural and physiological changes which include a spurt in physical growth (an increase in both height and weight), the appearance of secondary sex characteristics, the onset of menstruation in girls and the production of sperms in boys. The physical growth occurs more rapidly than nervous control can be established, resulting in some awkwardness or ungainliness in the young adolescent. The secondary sex characteristics evident in the female are:

1. An enlargement of the breasts and hips.

2. A broadening of the pelvis.

3. The growth of pubic and axillary hair.

4. The onset of menstruation, which indicates increased concentrations of sex hormones, ovulation and the ability to reproduce.

In boys, the secondary sex developments include:
1. Enlargement of the genitals.

2. The growth of hair on the pubis, axillae, chest and face.

3. A general increase in skeletal muscle mass.

4. An increase in the size of the larynx, which produces voice changes.

The activity of the sebaceous and sweat glands is increased in both sexes, giving rise to the common adolescent problem of acne.

PSYCHOSOCIAL FACTORS. Adolescents are faced with the body changes, new feelings and reactions that puberty brings. They become very self-conscious and sensitive and frequently display mood shifts and emotional instability. Their responses to situations are unpredictable; interests, moods and attitudes may vacillate between extreme opposites. For example, teen-agers tend to be ambivalent, alternately displaying acceptance and resistance to authority, content and discontent, and independence and dependence. They frequently go through a phase of rebelling against adult opinions and conventional society in general; on the other hand, they place tremendous importance on identification and conformity with their peers. They want to make their own decisions but are generally not sufficiently experienced to sever dependence and parental control entirely. Adults often make the problem more difficult by telling an adolescent he is old enough to know that or to do that and in the next breath tell him he is too young to know or to decide what is best. In this period of life, the decision must also be made as to a vocation or career for the future. Adolescents facing the changes, problems and necessary adjustments characteristic of this period of life require understanding and ubobtrusive guidance from adults.

ILLNESS. Illness is disturbing to the adolescent for different reasons than for the child; he resents the interference with his freedom and school and social activities and feels threatened by the imposed dependence. He becomes the focus of his parents' attention at a time when he has been trying to be independent of them. If hospitalization is necessary, the adolescent is likely to be humiliated if placed in a children's ward. If no adolescent ward is available, careful consideration is given to placement in an adult ward because the impressionable teen-ager is readily influenced by the conversation and behavior of the adults.

In many instances a student nurse may be assigned to care for the patient and, being an adolescent herself, has problems similar to those of the patient. She may find the situation difficult and require the guidance and support of a mature, understanding instructor or head nurse. The patient's ever-changing moods and attitudes must be accepted, and the nurse's approach adapted to elicit cooperation.

The nurse should be prepared to listen to the adolescent's opinions and concerns, treat them confidentially, and give advice or explanations when the opportunity presents but avoid an authoritarian manner. For example, adolescents usually have great concern about their bodies and welcome assistance in understanding the changes they are experiencing and reassurance that these are normal developments.

Because the adolescent is very sensitive and easily humiliated, it is important that precautions be taken to avoid any unnecessary exposure and to provide adequate privacy. It is helpful to include him as much as possible in planning his care. Procedures are carefully explained, as he is likely to show more interest in detail than either younger or more mature patients. This approach and manifested interest and concern on the part of the nurse mean much to the adolescent; it promotes acceptance and trust. If restrictions on certain activities or foods are necessary, the reason(s) for these are presented in a way that reflects no doubt about the adolescent's cooperation. Given responsibility for assuming self-discipline and self-care activities, or being asked to assist with other patients or a ward chore, furthers his self-esteem.

The nutritional and energy requirements of the teen-ager are markedly increased; the daily intake to meet these needs may vary from 2200 to 3000 calories depending on his activities and rate of growth. Protein content should be kept high — 80 to 100 grams per day. Emphasis is placed on the inclusion of meat, fish, eggs, cheese, fresh vegetables and fruits, whole grain cereal and milk. When planning the diet during illness, it is important to consider the growth needs of the adolescent as well as the cause of his illness.

NURSING THE SENESCENT (Significant Factors in Nursing the Older Patient)

Aging and life's stresses result in structural and functional changes which appear throughout the later years of the life span. The changes are regressive and degenerative in nature, and the age at which they appear and their rate of progression are individual factors. Chronological age and the degree of change do not necessarily correspond for all persons; stereotyping of the elderly according to their number of years is often erroneous and misleading. It is important for the nurse to know that although there is marked individual variation, there are certain changes which may be expected in the advanced years and that elderly people are structurally and functionally different persons than they were in their youth and maturity. Their needs, the ways in which these are expressed and should be met, and their responses to illness differ.

Illness and Hospitalization

Illness is usually more threatening to the older person simply because of his age and his recognition of a difference in his body efficiency. If hospitalization is necessary, he may be very apprehensive and pessimistic in regard to the outcome of his illness. In some instances, the older person becomes resentful at being transferred to a hospital or nursing home because it is interpreted by him as an indication that the family does not want to look after him. Adjustment to the hospital is likely to be difficult; the unfamiliar environment and personnel and the change in the patient's accustomed routine and way of life produce insecurity. The stress may bring about confusion and marked behavioral changes, necessitating special precautions to protect him. Frequently, the older person has experienced the loss of his spouse and a number of his contemporaries, and illness and hospitalization seem to further emphasize his aloneness. He is accustomed to having familiar personal possessions around him, and to have all of these except a few toilet articles removed suddenly may be very distressing and frequently initiates protests and restlessness.

If the illness necessitates confinement to bed, the enforced inactivity is very hazardous and must be kept to a minimum with senescents. Circulatory stasis, hypostatic pneumonia, decubitus ulcers and loss of strength become immediate concerns. The slowing up of the circulation to the brain predisposes to disorientation and confusion. Many older citizens have an income inadequate for the present cost of living. Expenses incurred by illness and dependence may only add to their financial worries.

Repeated orientations to the situation are needed because the senescent forgets quickly. Explanations are necessary about such things as to why he is in bed and in the hospital, how his regular needs (e.g., meals, toilet) will be met, the whereabouts of his family members and when they will come, and the location of his personal belongings. A clock and a calendar in the room or unit may help to reduce the confusion that some experience and their possible concern about day and time. The figures on them should be large so they can be seen by the senescent, whose visual acuity may be reduced. Rigid adherence to routines may be very disturbing to the elderly. In many instances, the practice of some hospital customs could be delayed and introduced gradually.

Consideration in regard to the placement of the older person in the hospital ward is necessary; proximity to patients with infections is avoided because of his lowered resistance. If ambulatory, being near the bathroom is important. He should not be left unobserved or alone for long periods.

Structural and Functional Changes — Implications for Nursing

GENERAL CHANGES. Some basic cellular changes develop gradually as part of the aging process. The rate of cell division (reproduction), growth and repair becomes slower. In some areas, regeneration becomes less than the rate of cell destruction, resulting in tissue atrophy and, in the case of injury or disease, diminished recovery and healing ability. There is also less specialization in the cells being produced; in many instances, cells are replaced by those of a less specialized order, such as fibrous or fatty tissue cells. These less specialized cells require less oxygen and nutrients but are incapable of the specialized activities of the cells replaced.

There is a reduction in the fluid maintained within the cells and their environment. An inadequate fluid intake or an excessive loss of fluid may quickly lead to serious dehydration. The rate of metabolism decreases with advancing years and reduces the amount of energy and heat produced. The homeostatic mechanisms become less efficient in maintaining the normal constancy of the internal environment (e.g., chemical concentrations, fluid volume, pH, temperature). The reduced efficiency in regulation leaves a decrease in the body's reserves and a lesser margin of safety.

Such general changes obviously influence the functional ability of various organs and systems and must be kept in mind when caring for the elderly.

CARDIOVASCULAR SYSTEM. The heart is one of the few organs that do not atrophy. More often, it is found to hypertrophy because of the increased demands on it created by vascular changes and hypertension. It no longer has as great a capacity for increasing the rate and strength of contractions to meet increased demands as incurred by physical exercise. The endocardium tends to thicken and patchy sclerosing occurs; the valves become thicker and less pliable, making their closing and opening less efficient. The myocardium gradually becomes slower in recovering irritability and contractility in the cardiac cycle.

The walls of the arteries become less distensible because of a loss of elastic tissue and the development of patchy areas of fatty and calcium deposits in the walls. The intima becomes thicker, and the lumen of the vessels narrows. Resistance is offered to the flow of blood, the blood pressure (both systolic and diastolic) is elevated and there is a diminished blood supply to organs and tissues, lowering their level of function.

The walls of veins are thinner and weaker, predisposing to the slowing of venous drainage and the pooling of blood.

The blood itself has greater constancy than most other tissues in the body. Unless an actual blood dyscrasia develops or dietary deficiencies are experienced, the plasma volume and blood composition show little change. The serum albumin level shows some decrease but the other blood proteins do not usually show any change.

IMPLICATIONS FOR NURSING. Changes in the cardiovascular system necessitate a reduction in the physical demands on the patient. He is cautioned to move more slowly to avoid sudden increases in cardiac demands and output. A large part of the animal fat in the diet should be replaced by vegetable fat, which may reduce the blood cholesterol and the formation of atherosclerotic plaques in the walls of the arteries.

If an intravenous infusion is to be administered, the rate of flow is slower than that used with a younger person. The less elastic arteries and weaker heart may not be capable of accommodating a rapidly increasing intravascular volume. The rate of flow and the volume to be given in 24 hours are usually stated by the physician.

Immobility and prolonged bed rest are avoided, since they predispose to circulatory stasis and thrombosis. When bed rest is necessary, a change of position every 1 to 2 hours and passive and active exercises, particularly of the limbs, are important to promote venous drainage and circulation.

RESPIRATORY SYSTEM. In later years, the respiratory system is likely to be less efficient and less resistant to infection. The bronchial walls become thinner. The cough reflex is less responsive and less effective in clearing the tract owing to loss of muscle tone and strength and reduced sensitivity of the tract, resulting in retained secretions which favor infection. The elasticity of the lungs and the compliance of the chest wall are reduced, which results in a reduction in the vital capacity and maximum breathing capacity and an increase in residual air in the alveoli. Underventilation of alveoli, especially in the bases of the lungs, reduces the exchange volumes of carbon dioxide and oxygen between the blood and alveolar air. Oxygen concentration of the blood may be reduced, which encourages degenerative changes throughout the body. When the older patient is at rest, shallow breathing and slower pulmonary circulation predispose to the escape of fluid into the alveoli and ensuing coughing, dyspnea and hypostatic pneumonia. The cilia are fewer and less efficient in "sweeping out" mucus and foreign particles as a result of atrophy and dryness of the epithelial lining of the tract.

IMPLICATIONS FOR NURSING. In order to encourage better oxygenation and prevent respiratory complications, it is necessary to have the patient breathe deeply five to ten times, cough and change position every 1 to 2 hours. One should be sure that the position assumed allows for free chest expansion for better ventilation. Frequent auscultation of the chest will reveal retention of secretions and areas that are not being ventilated. Early ambulation and activity within the limitations imposed by the illness are encouraged. Protection of the elderly patient from exposure to persons with an infection is necessary because of the lowered resistance. Respiratory infection in the older person should receive prompt attention; otherwise, it may become serious very quickly.

DIGESTIVE SYSTEM, NUTRITION AND FLUIDS. The stomach of the elderly person loses muscular strength and tone and takes longer to empty. There is usually some decrease in secretions and acidity; some persons may have a reduced tolerance to certain foods, such as fats. Fewer active taste buds combined with decreased activity contribute to a decrease in appetite. The loss or neglect of teeth may interfere with the taking of essential foods.

Loss of muscular tone in the intestine reduces peristalsis; the content is moved along more slowly, which may cause constipation.

The metabolic rate as well as physical activity is reduced, so that fewer calories are necessary than in previous years. If the person continues the same caloric intake, obesity is likely to develop; this should be avoided since it increases the demands on the cardiovascular system and on the weight-bearing joints.

IMPLICATIONS FOR NURSING. Nutritional deficiencies are frequently found in older persons and may be due to living alone or a reduced interest in and desire for food. In others, the malnutrition may be attributed to an inadequate income, limited cooking facilities and refrigeration, ill health or the lack of dentures.

In order to keep tissue destruction to a minimum, emphasis is placed on high-protein foods, fresh fruits and vegetables in the older person's diet. Vitamin supplements, especially A, B complex and C, may be prescribed to correct deficiencies, improve appetite and the condition and resistance of mucous membranes, correct anemia and promote a feeling of well-being. A protein concentrate preparation (e.g., dried skim milk) added to liquids may be helpful to make up calories and meet the daily requirements. The nurse may have to combat anorexia with frequent small servings, by determining and respecting the patient's food choices if possible, and by feeding the patient. If he is ambulatory, the meals may be more appealing and pleasant if arrangements are made to have him eat with others. If dentures are posing a problem, the dietary department is advised so that the meat

is minced and other foods are appropriately prepared. A referral may be made to a dentist when the patient's condition permits.

As cited previously, the elderly person may develop dehydration very quickly. An explanation of the importance of fluids, the frequent offering of small amounts and giving the patient his choice may be helpful in having him take an adequate amount. The older person will often take twice as much water if it is not ice cold. An accurate record of the intake and output is made until a normal fluid balance is well established. A negative or positive balance is brought promptly to the physician's attention.

The inadequate fluid intake which is common in illness and the somewhat decreased salivary secretion in the aged readily lead to dryness of the mouth and tongue and an accumulation of tenacious offensive matter (sordes). Frequent care is necessary to keep the mouth moist and clean and to prevent parotitis. Infection and inflammation of a parotid gland is a complication that may occur, particularly in older persons, if good oral hygiene is not maintained.

In preparation for the patient's discharge from the hospital, he should receive counseling as to his nutritional needs and the selection, purchase and preparation of foods in accordance with his circumstances. The reasons for needed dietary changes are explained. Since it is difficult for an older person to remember, written suggestions and pamphlets on recommended dietary allowances should be provided. A referral may be made to the local welfare department or Visiting Nursing Association so that some guidance may be provided when he goes home.

BOWEL ELIMINATION. Loss of intestinal muscle tone, inactivity and lack of a well balanced diet and adequate fluids contribute to constipation in an individual in later years. Frequently the older person is overconcerned about daily bowel elimination and resorts too readily to taking nonprescribed laxatives, which may result in excessive fluid and mineral loss.

If constipation is a problem, more bulky foods such as bran, cereals, whole wheat bread, fresh fruits and vegetables, and fluids are gradually introduced into the diet to regulate bowel elimination. If a laxative is needed, the patient receives a bulk-forming laxative such as a preparation of psyllium seed (Metamucil), a stool softener or a lubricant such as mineral oil. The latter is used for only a brief period, since it may prevent the absorption of the fat-soluble vitamins. Dependence upon the continuous use of any laxative should be discouraged.

URINARY SYSTEM. Sclerosed areas in the kidneys may develop as a result of a decrease in the renal blood supply. The ability of the kidneys to concentrate wastes may be reduced, and they require solids to be well diluted for elimination. The bladder loses some of its tone and may not be completely emptied during voiding. The residual urine undergoes some decomposition which predisposes to bladder inflammation and infection; the urea releases ammonia which accounts for the ammoniacal odor characteristic of some old persons' urine. Frequency and incontinence are common problems, particularly in illness, and can be embarrassing to the patient and may lead to social withdrawal.

IMPLICATIONS FOR NURSING. The reduced ability of the kidneys to concentrate wastes indicates the need for a minimum of 1500 to 2000 ml. of fluid per day. Because of the urgency and frequency of urination, the ambulatory patient is placed near the bathroom. If incontinence develops, the patient may become very discouraged. Involuntary voiding causes embarrassment, physical discomfort and odor. The individual loses self-esteem, and tends to withdraw and decrease his social interaction.

Every effort must be made to retrain the bladder and correct the incontinence. The patient's fluid intake is increased to 2500 to 3000 ml. daily to improve bladder tone and lessen any irritation that may be contributing to the problem. A variety of fluids is used to make it easier for the patient to take the required amount. The patient goes to the toilet, or is placed on the commode or bedpan, every 2 hours. Fluid intake is discontinued at 8 P.M.; this permits longer uninterrupted periods of rest at night. The schedule and expected outcomes are carefully explained to the patient at the onset.

Understanding and patience are necessary on the part of the nurse with the patient who experiences frequency or incontinence. Manifestations of displeasure and impatience only create more anxiety for the patient, which in turn further aggravates the problem.

The use of an indwelling catheter is discouraged because it provides an entry for bacteria and promotes loss of bladder muscle tone, making reestablishment of normal voluntary control still more difficult. The hazards are emphasized with those caring for the patient who may consider the catheter the procedure of choice. If a retention catheter must be used it should be left in for as short a period as possible. Drainage is by a closed sterile system of tubing and receptacle and the fluid intake is increased to 2500 to 3000 ml. daily, unless contraindicated, to reduce the predisposition to infection and stasis of urine that may lead to the formation of urinary calculi. When the catheter is removed the retraining program described above is commenced. The intervals between the voiding events are gradually lengthened and, as the patient's general condition improves and he is more secure, the normal conditioned reflex and voluntary control are likely to be resumed.

When the patient is incontinent, the skin should be cleansed and the bedding changed promptly. The skin may be protected by the application of a protective cream or lotion or a moisture-repellant powder following each voiding and cleansing.

REPRODUCTIVE SYSTEM. The earliest senescent changes in the female occur in the reproductive organs. Ovulation and menstruation cease and there are changes in the concentrations of sex hormones. The uterus, vagina, genitals and breasts atrophy. The vaginal mucosa becomes thinner, dry and less resistant to infection and irritation.

Reproductive ability persists to a much later age in the male; atrophy of the testicles occurs at a later age than atrophy of the ovaries. There is a decline in sexual energy in both sexes, but some interest and activity in sexual relationships persists for many older persons through the late decades. The need for such intimacy and affection should be accepted and never ridiculed. The older male may experience hypertrophy of the prostate gland which leads to difficulty in voiding and incomplete emptying of the bladder.

IMPLICATIONS FOR NURSING. Careful cleansing and frequent bathing of the female perineal area provides protection against infection. Patients are urged to have a complete physical examination annually and given assistance in arranging for it if necessary.

If the male is a bed patient, he may have

difficulty in voiding unless allowed to assume the upright position. If his condition permits, he may be assisted to stand beside the bed or go to the bathroom rather than have to be catheterized.

SKIN. The older person's skin is dry, thin and wrinkled and, as a result, is easily damaged by pressure, chemicals and trauma. Loss of elastic and subcutaneous fatty tissue causes flabbiness and wrinkles. Diminished secretions due to atrophy of the sebaceous and sweat glands contribute to the dryness. Pigmented areas frequently appear on exposed areas. The superficial blood vessels are less efficient in dilating and contracting to regulate body temperature. As a result, in hot weather heat dissipation is poor and, when exposed to cold, the body is not as capable of conserving heat. Local sensation of heat, pressure and painful stimuli may be less acute and are not as reliable in initiating protective reflexes and responses.

Fingernails and toenails tend to thicken and become brittle. The hair loses its color and tends to become dry, thin and gray.

IMPLICATIONS FOR NURSING. The skin of the elderly patient requires special attention because of the changes associated with the aging process. Daily bathing may be inadvisable because of the dryness. A mild soap is used sparingly, and lanolin or a cold cream is applied after bathing. Bony prominences and pressure areas are massaged gently every 2 or 3 hours and are examined for any indication of pressure sores or trauma. Frequent changes of position, prompt changing of soiled linen and cleansing of the patient following incontinence, placement of a sheepskin pad under pressure areas, and the use of an alternating air pressure mattress (ripple mattress) contribute to keeping the skin intact and in good condition when the patient is confined to bed.

Soaking of the feet in warm water followed by an application of lanolin or oil will soften and remove much of the hard, dry scaly skin that tends to accumulate. The oil softens the nails, making it easier and safer to cut them.

If local heat applications are used, special precautions are necessary to avoid burns because of the reduced sensitivity. Exposure to extremes of temperature is avoided. In hot weather, the patient's activity is kept to a minimum, and the room temperature is controlled as much as possible. The older person is more sensitive to cold; he produces less body heat and is less able to conserve body heat. In a room temperature which others find comfortable, he may be chilly. For this reason, the older patient usually requires warm clothing and extra lightweight bed covers.

Skin wounds heal more slowly and are more easily infected in the aged because of the reduced blood supply to the area and the lower general resistance. Aseptic care of wounds and good nutrition play an important role in preventing infection and promoting healing.

MUSCULOSKELETAL SYSTEM. The bones become more brittle in the later span of life. There is a reduction in the organic material and osteocytes, and some demineralization usually takes place as a result of the changes in the concentration of some endocrine secretions (e.g., estrogen). These alterations in bone structure increase the incidence of fractures in older people. Joint action may become restricted and painful because of degeneration of the cartilage on the ends of weight-bearing bones. Osteoarthritis, the formation of adhesions, or calcium deposits in the joints interfere with joint function and frequently lead to inactivity and decreased mobility of the patient. The intervertebral discs undergo some atrophy and the vertebrae tend to flatten; as a result the older person loses height.

There is decreased strength and some slowing of response in the muscles. If the person remains active, the muscle tissue shows some atrophy but remains relatively strong. Disuse of the muscles leads to fatty infiltration and marked weakness.

IMPLICATIONS FOR NURSING. Since the elderly tend to fall more readily and their bones fracture easily, their environment and activities are controlled as much as possible to prevent accidents. The patient should be well oriented to his surroundings, which should be well lighted. A light left burning at night so that he can readily find his way to the bathroom if ambulatory or the provision of a commode at the bedside may prevent a fall. Side rails on the bed may be necessary to lessen the danger of the patient falling out of bed or getting up when his condition does not permit ambulation. Lowering of the bed and removal of the casters also contribute to the prevention of falls. The use of scatter rugs is avoided and footstools or other pieces of furniture over which the patient might trip or stumble are removed.

Overweight in the elderly is to be avoided, as cited previously. In addition to hastening degenerative changes in the joints, it can make mobility and activity practically impossible for the person.

The nurse has to be understanding and patient with the slower responses and movements of the older person and also help the family to accept this change.

Exercise and activity are encouraged within the limitations imposed by the older person's physical condition. The family and friends frequently require guidance in relation to this; with the very best intentions, they may foster inactivity and its undesirable results by waiting on the older person and discouraging self-care and participation in other forms of activity. If left to simply rest in bed or a chair, the person regresses mentally and physically. Complete bed rest is considered one of the most dangerous forms of treatment for the elderly. It predisposes to the complications of thrombosis in the legs, pulmonary embolism, hypostatic pneumonia, loss of calcium from bones, joint stiffness, loss of muscle strength and the breakdown of skin over pressure areas.

Muscle contractures, deformities and restricted joint movement will develop rapidly in the older patient unless emphasis is placed on daily exercises. Passive movement of the limbs through their normal range by the nurse may be necessary if the patient is too ill or weak to carry out the exercises. It must be remembered that in taking the joints through their range of motion the movement is not forced beyond the range of comfort. Many of these patients may have some permanent joint changes which restrict the range of motion.

When the patient is well enough to be out of bed, it is not sufficient just to have him sitting hour after hour in a chair. He should be encouraged and assisted, if necessary, to walk a few steps and exercise his limbs. If unable to walk, standing up and raising his arms and legs at intervals is encouraged; otherwise blood pools in the lower limbs and pelvis.

SPECIAL SENSES. There is a decline in the older person's special senses, reflected especially by a loss of visual and hearing acuity.

The refractive ability of the eye is reduced owing to changes in the lens which becomes cloudy, allowing less light through to the retina. This cloudiness gradually increases and eventually the lens becomes opaque to light rays. This change in the lens is referred to as cataract.

The elderly person develops farsightedness and experiences narrowing of the visual field. Adaptation in dimly lit and darkened rooms is lost and may lead to the person tripping over objects, such as stools or chairs, and injury. Similarly, a longer period of time is required for adaptation to a bright light. A white circle may appear at the periphery of the cornea in the very elderly, referred to as the arcus senilis.

Atrophy of the auditory nerve occurs in varying degrees. Acuity for higher pitched tones is lost first. As the ability to communicate is progressively impaired, the older person's interests become limited and he tends to isolate himself socially.

A dulling of temperature perception and a decrease in the speed of the withdrawal reflex may result in burns. For example, an older person may not recognize that a hot water bottle that has been applied is excessively hot. Similarly, pain perception may be decreased; for this reason, lack of the complaint of pain or the severity of pain described is not always dependable, for it may not necessarily correspond to the degree of severity of the causative pathologic process. For example, a myocardial infarction may occur in an aged person without any complaint of the chest pain which is considered practically a classical characteristic of such an episode in a middle-aged person.

IMPLICATIONS FOR NURSING. Impaired vision places further emphasis on the need for repeated and thorough orientation of the patient to his surroundings. Good lighting is necessary, particularly for any close work or reading. For suggestions as to how those with impaired vision or hearing may be helped, please see Chapters 27 and 28.

In relation to the possible decrease in perception of temperature and pain, greater precautions are necessary in the use of heat applications and baths, and it must be kept in mind that the patient's condition may be more serious than is indicated by his complaints.

PSYCHOLOGICAL CHANGES. Some degree of organic cerebral change is associated with the aging process, but any change in personality or regression in cerebral activity varies greatly from one individual to another. Most aging minds show some loss of memory for recent events, slower comprehension, slower response, and a shorter span of concentration. Learning ability may be sustained to a surprising level if the person's interest and desire to learn are high.

One sees many variants; in addition to the pleasant, alert, elderly persons who adjust readily, there are some who are unhappy, irascible, complaining and aggressive. Many of the emotional disturbances and personality differences seen are functional and are not due to organic brain changes. In many instances, they are due to the unfortunate social and economic conditions imposed on the elderly by present-day society. Forced retirement, inadequate income, the current social attitude of society which depreciates the worth of older citizens, and the loss of close family members and friends are factors that contribute to changes in the behavior of many elderly persons. They may not be consulted or allowed to make decisions in spite of the fact that many older persons have developed greater understanding, foresight and a more balanced sense of values through their experiences in years of living. Occasionally one hears an elderly person say, "No one cares what I think or how I feel. I am completely ignored and expected to passively accept others' decisions." Just as in earlier years, these persons have the need for recognition, affection, achievement and some degree of independence. Enforced dependence and loss of self-esteem often lead to introversion; the person withdraws, isolates himself and lives in the past. The individual may experience social deprivation and a lack of sensory input which contribute to a reduced sense of reality, aberrations in behavior and responses, and confusion. Most older people tend to feel more secure in their established pattern of living and resist new ideas and changes.

IMPLICATIONS FOR NURSING. Any stress in the later years of life, whether physical or psychological, is likely to cause confusion that may last for a varied length of time. Such reactions may be anticipated when an elderly person is ill and hospitalized, which should put the nurses on guard to avoid any possible accident or crisis.

Physical care alone is not adequate for the elderly; they require respect, a voice in matters which concern them and meaningful activity to contribute to an incentive for living. It is important that the nurse understand that many emotional disturbances seen in older persons are due only in part to organic aging changes.

As with all patients, each aged person is assessed carefully by the nurse; his reactions to the circumstances, interests and mental and physical capacities are noted. The psychological status, obviously, will influence the amount of protective care required and the necessary precautions for safety. An atmosphere of acceptance and respect is reassuring to the patient. When change is necessary, it is explained, discussed, and when possible introduced gradually. The older person's wishes and pattern of living are given consideration, and unnecessary rigidity in routines should be avoided. By discussing his care with him, respect for the patient's years and individuality is manifested; by showing this respect, the nurse may avoid the reaction of resentment toward the young taking over. Enforced and abrupt change threatens and antagonizes the older patient. Preparation for events and answering questions relating to what is to take place will make the situation less stressful for the patient. Encouraging family members to visit regularly and spend as much time as possible with the older patient will help him to orient to and accept the situation. Close relatives provide ties and identity that are reassuring. If possible, having some familiar personal belongings close by and readily accessible may also help. Use of the proper form of address and using the patient's name indicate respect for his identity.

When his physical condition permits, an effort is made to promote the patient's interests and to encourage activity and socialization with others. Self-care and interest and pride in personal appearance are also encouraged.

Medications and the Elderly

Reduced efficiency in metabolism, enzyme systems, renal excretion and circulation in older persons results in a decreased tolerance for many drugs, particularly when they are given in the average adult dosage. Detoxification of drugs by the liver and various enzymes may be incomplete and may occur at a much slower rate. The products may be retained in the blood for a longer period before being eliminated in the urine. A cumulative effect develops more often in the elderly, and may build up a concentration that exceeds the maximum dose. In some instances, a delayed reaction occurs as the result of impaired circulation.

Drug reaction is less predictable than with younger persons. For this reason, these patients are observed closely following the administration of drugs. Sedatives, such as barbiturates, and analgesics, such as opiates, may cause excitement and confusion in some, while others may experience respiratory depression and such sound sleep that the resulting immobility predisposes to circulatory stasis and pressure sores. Usually smaller doses of narcotics and sedatives are used for the aged. The elderly often have multiple complaints and disorders, and one frequently finds several drugs prescribed for the various ailments. The nurse must be alert for the danger of adverse drug interactions.

Older patients are frequently required to continue drug therapy at home following discharge from the hospital. Schwartz et al. found a high incidence of errors in self-administration of drugs among elderly patients. They found an average of 1.5 errors were made by each of the 178 older persons studied.[2] The errors included omission of the drug and incorrect dosage, frequency and timing. Many of the patients lack accurate knowledge as to the purpose of the drug; others may have wrong information.[3] Self-medication presents a problem among older patients; the dangers and ineffectiveness of patent and unprescribed medicines need greater emphasis. Their use usually results in a serious delay in getting proper attention. These factors have implications for hospital and visiting nurses.

Hospital patients who are to continue a medication after discharge should receive a clear, simple explanation of its purpose, the importance of taking it as prescribed, what may happen if it is omitted and how the supply may be renewed if it is to be continued. Labels and directions for dosage, frequency

and method of taking the drug should be clearly written and reviewed with the patient. Some patients responsible for self-administration of drugs require a calendar and time sheet drawn up that will be helpful in reminding them to take the medication. Encouraging the patient to record the taking of his drug immediately may avoid repetition and a toxic dose. If there are family members, one of them should also receive the instructions. A referral may be made to the Visiting Nurse Association so that the patient will receive supervision.

Convalescence and Rehabilitation

The convalescent period following an illness is usually longer for the aged than for younger persons. The patient is likely to become discouraged because it takes him longer to regain his strength. In addition to counteracting the undesirable physiological effects of bed rest, early ambulation is promoted to improve the older person's morale. Once he is allowed up he is likely to be more optimistic about his recovery.

Many elderly persons seen by nurses have been socially isolated and emotionally starved prior to their illness. As the patient's physical condition improves, nursing care is planned and implemented to promote activities and mental and physical independence within the limits imposed by aging and his health status. Interests are determined, and mobility and socialization are encouraged. Suggestions are made to the patient and family as to the activities, interests and sources of assistance that may help to make the older person's life more useful and satisfying and to counteract the apathy, depression and complete dependence so frequently seen. A few simple adjustments such as hand rails on the wall and the side of the bathtub and a seat in the tub may permit self-care.

Most communities now have organized health and social services for senior citizens, but many older persons require information about these services and assistance in making the initial contact with them. Many clubs have been formed to provide certain types of services to older persons; an example is Meals on Wheels. Home visits may be made to those whose health inhibits them from going out; for others, appropriate programs are planned for entertainment and socialization. Those who are able are encouraged to

---

[2]D. Schwartz, B. Henley, and L. Zeitz: The Elderly Ambulatory Patient — Nursing and Psychosocial Needs. New York, MacMillan, 1964, pp. 110–113.

[3]Rosella Cunningham: "An Exploratory Study of Home Visits by Public Health Nurses to Patients with Cardiac Disorders." Toronto, the University of Toronto, 1972 (unpublished).

participate in voluntary services (e.g., baby-sitting, home and hospital visiting); this fosters their self-esteem and sense of usefulness. Special publications (newspapers, bulletins) are also made available to retired persons free of charge in many localities.

Summary

The elderly compose a large segment of our population, and many nursing hours are devoted to the care of elderly persons. Following the mature years of middle life, biological changes are an inevitable component of aging. The rate and extent of these changes vary with individuals, so that biological age is not characteristic of any particular chronological age. Stereotyping must be avoided. Too often we tend to judge on the basis of age in years and at a glance by skin changes, wrinkles and gray hair. The changes result in a progressive limiting of capacity and compensatory reserve; older persons are more vulnerable to illness and stress. Their immunologic responses are less efficient, so they require protection from contact with infection and prompt treatment if they become ill. Their physiological changes may cause potentially dangerous reactions to ordinary adult doses and combinations of drugs.

Confusion and behavioral disorders are usually the result of a combination of such factors as strange environment, separation from familiar persons, demands that exceed the individual's capacity, pathologic condition (e.g., cerebral circulatory insufficiency), drugs, physical restraints and lengthy periods without sensory input.

In planning nursing care, rehabilitation must be taken into consideration; it is just as important for these patients as for younger persons. They want to be independent and useful. Each person's potential and assets are identified and fostered. The need exists to extend concern beyond physical care; psychological and social needs must not be ignored. These older persons require friendship, understanding, activity and opportunities for communication and social interaction. Otherwise, life lacks meaning, and they withdraw and lose contact with reality. They should not go unnoticed.

References

Nursing Children and Adolescents

Books

Chin, Peggy L.: Child Health Maintenance. St. Louis, C. V. Mosby, 1974.
Latham, Helen C., et al.: Pediatric Nursing, 3rd ed. St. Louis, C. V. Mosby, 1977. Part 1.
Marlow, Dorothy R.: Pediatric Nursing, 5th ed. Philadelphia, W. B. Saunders, 1977. Chapters 2–4.
Waechter, Eugenia H., and Blake, Florence G.: Nursing Care of Children, 9th ed. Philadelphia, J. B. Lippincott, 1976.

Periodicals

Abbott, Nancy C., et al.: "Dress Rehearsal for the Hospital." Am. J. Nurs., Vol. 70, No. 11 (Nov. 1970), pp. 2360–2362.
Brooks, Mary M.: "Why Play in the Hospital?" Nurs. Clin. North Am., Vol. 5, No. 3 (Sept. 1970), pp. 431–441.
Caghan, Susan B.: "The Adolescent Process and the Problem of Nutrition." Am. J. Nurs., Vol. 75, No. 10 (Oct. 1975), pp. 1728–1731.
Gallagher, J. R. (Ed.): Symposium, "The Medical Care of the Adolescent." Med. Clin. North Am., Vol. 49, No. 2 (March 1965).
Giuffra, Mary J.: "Demystifying Adolescent Behavior." Am. J. Nurs., Vol. 75, No. 10 (Oct. 1975), pp. 1724–1727.
Grant, Dorothy: "VIP Treatment Proves This Hospital Really Cares." Can. Nurs., Vol. 72, No. 7 (July 1976), pp. 24–27.
Hymovich, Debra P.: "Keeping Up with Pediatric Nursing." Nurs. '71, Vol. 1, No. 1 (Nov. 1971), pp. 14–15.
Kitzman, Harriet: "The Nature of Well Child Care." Am. J. Nurs., Vol. 75, No. 10 (Oct. 1975), pp. 1705–1708.

Leifer, Gloria (Ed.): Symposium. "The Nurse and The Ill Child." Nurs. Clin. North Am., Vol. 1, No. 1 (March 1966), pp. 73–162.

Lockeberg, L. E.: "Reaching To-morrow's Citizens." Can. Nurs., Vol. 72, No. 2 (Feb. 1976), pp. 29–30.

Lore, Ann: Adolescents: "People, Not Problems." Am. J. Nurs., Vol. 73, No. 7 (July 1973), pp. 1232–1234.

Oremland, E. K., and Oremland, J. D. (Eds.): "How to Care for the 'Between-Ager'." Nurs. '74, Vol. 4, No. 11 (Nov. 1974), pp. 42–49.

Plank, Emma N.: "Games Little People Can Play While on Bed Rest." Nurs. '71, Vol. 1, No. 1 (Nov. 1971), p. 16.

Tisdale, Barbara: "Not for Admission." Can. Nurs., Vol. 68, No. 12 (Dec. 1972), pp. 35–39.

Turcotte, Catherine: "How Children See the Nurse." Can. Nurs., Vol. 71, No. 4 (April 1975), pp. 41–42.

Nursing Elderly People

Books

Brocklehurst, J. C.: Textbook of Geriatric Medicine and Gerontology. Edinburgh, Churchill Livingstone, 1973. Chapters 1–4.

Burnside, Irene M.: Nursing and the Aged. New York, McGraw-Hill, 1976.

Morton, P.: To The Good Long Life: What We Know About Growing Old. New York, Universe Books, 1974.

Rossman, Isadore (Ed.): Clinical Geriatrics. Philadelphia, J. B. Lippincott, 1971. Chapters 1–6.

Rudd, Jacob L., and Margalin, Reuben J. (Eds.): Maintenance Therapy for the Geriatric Patient. Springfield, Ill., Charles C Thomas, 1968.

Stevens, Marion Keith: Geriatric Nursing, 2nd ed. Philadelphia, W. B. Saunders, 1975.

Periodicals

Buch, Julius, et al.: "Preventive Medicine in a Long Term Care Institution." Geriatrics, Vol. 31, No. 2 (Feb. 1976), pp. 99–108.

Beverley, E. Virginia: "The Beginning of Wisdom." Geriatrics, Vol. 30, No. 7 (July 1975), pp. 117–128.

_____: "Nursing Homes: Matching the Facilities to the Patient's Needs." Geriatrics, Vol. 31, No. 4 (April 1976), pp. 100–110.

Cahall, Jean B., and Smith, Diana: "Considerate Care of the Elderly." Nurs. '75, Vol. 5, No. 9 (Sept. 1975), pp. 38–39.

Cunningham, Rosella: "An Exploratory Study of Home Visits Made by Public Health Nurses to Patients With Cardiac Disorders." Unpublished, Toronto, University of Toronto, 1972.

Diekelman, Nancy, and Galloway, Karen: "Exercises for the Elderly." (Excerpt from Exercises for the Elderly, by Herman L. Kamenetz.) Am. J. Nurs., Vol. 72, No. 8 (Aug. 1972), p. 1401.

_____: "The Middle Years — A Time of Change." Am. J. Nurs., Vol. 75, No. 6 (June 1975), pp. 994–996.

Duffie, John: "Frankly Speaking — Aging: The Myth and the Reality." Can. Nurs., Vol. 73, No. 4 (April 1977), pp. 40–41.

Godfry, Charles M.: "The 'Old Disease'." Can. Family Physician, Vol. 24, No. 2 (Feb. 1978), pp. 131–132.

Grenby, Mike: "Making the Most of the Golden Years." Can. Nurs., Vol. 73, No. 4 (April 1977), p. 39.

_____: "Living to Eat: Nutrition for Senior Citizens." Can. Nurs., Vol. 73, No. 4 (April 1977), pp. 42–44.

Hahn, Aloyse: "It's Tough to Be Old." Am. J. Nurs., Vol. 70, No. 8 (Aug. 1970), pp. 1698–1699.

Jenny, Jean: "Nursing in the Land of the Aged." Can. Nurs., Vol. 68, No. 12 (Dec. 1972), pp. 31–34.

Johnson, Linda: "The Middle Years — Living Sensibly." Am. J. Nurs., Vol. 75, No. 6 (June 1975), pp. 1012–1016.

Kee, Joyce L.: "Fluid Imbalance in Elderly Patients." Nurs. '73, Vol. 3, No. 4 (April 1973), pp. 40–43.

Knowles, Lois N. (Ed.): Symposium. "Putting Geriatric Standards into Practice." Nurs. Clin. North Am., Vol. 7, No. 2 (June 1972), pp. 201–309.

Lane, Harriet C.: Symposium. "Care of the Elderly Patient." Nurs. Clin. North Am., Vol. 3, No. 4 (Dec. 1968), pp. 649–748.

le Riche, W. Harding: "An Epidemiologist Looks at Retirement." Can. Family Physician, Vol. 24, No. 2 (Feb. 1978), pp. 137–138.

Macdonald, Myrtle I.: "Practical Concerns for Nursing the Elderly in an Institutional Setting." Can. Nurs., Vol. 73, No. 4 (April 1977), pp. 25–30.

Modell, Walter (Ed.): Symposium. "Use of Drugs in the Elderly Patient." Geriatrics, Vol. 29, No. 6 (June 1974), pp. 49–78.

Moody, Linda, et al.: "Moving the Past into the Present." Am. J. Nurs., Vol. 70, No. 11 (Nov. 1970), pp. 2353–2356.

Patrick, Maxine: "Little Things Mean A Lot in Geriatric Rehabilitation." Nurs. '73, Vol. 3, No. 8 (Aug. 1973), p. 7–9.

Rapelje, Douglas H.: "A Home for the Aged Where People Live." Can. Nurs., Vol. 64, No. 11 (Nov. 1968), pp. 45–48.

Rosenberg, Gilbert: "Can We Slow the Aging Process?" Can. Family Physician, Vol. 24, No. 2 (Feb. 1978), pp. 139–140.

Scott, D., and Crowhurst, J.: "Reawakening Senses in the Elderly." Can. Nurs., Vol. 71, No. 10 (Oct. 1975), pp. 21–22.

Scott, M. Louise: "To Learn to Work with the Elderly." Am. J. Nurs., Vol. 73, No. 4 (April 1973), pp. 662–664.

Sibille, Sister Michael: "Geriatric Care: Let's Make it More Than Physical Care." Nurs. '75, Vol. 5, No. 7 (July 1975), pp. 54–55.

Stevens, Carolyn B.: "Breaking Through Cobwebs of Confusion." Nurs. '74, Vol. 4, No. 8 (Aug. 1974), pp. 41–48.

_____: Symposium. "Mental Health and Aging: Life Cycle Perspectives." Geriatrics, Vol. 29. No. 11 (Nov. 1974), pp. 59–186.

Thralow, Joan V., and Watson, Charles G.: "Remotivation for Geriatric Patients (A Study)." Nurs. Digest, Vol. 3, No. 4 (July–Aug. 1975), pp. 48–49.

Tobis, Jerome S. (Ed.): Symposium. "The Special Rehabilitation Needs of the Elderly." Geriatrics, Vol. 31, No. 5 (May 1976), pp. 51–103.

Wasylenki, Donald: "Coping with Change in Retirement." Can. Family Physician, Vol. 24, No. 2 (Feb. 1978), pp. 133–136.

Wilkiemeyer, Diana S.: "Affection: Key to Care for the Elderly." Am. J. Nurs., Vol. 72, No. 12 (Dec. 1972), pp. 2166–2168.

Yeaworth, Rosalee C. (Ed.): Symposium. "Gerontological Nursing." Nurs. Clin. North Am., Vol. 11, No. 1 (March 1976), pp. 115–206.

Young, Charlotte M.: "Nutritional Counseling for Better Health." Geriatrics, Vol. 29, No. 5 (May 1974), p. 83.

PART II

12

Nursing in Blood Dyscrasias

COMPOSITION AND PHYSIOLOGY OF BLOOD

Blood is a red fluid tissue that is pumped through the vascular system by the heart. It transports cellular requirements and products from one part of the body to another. There is a continuous exchange between the fluid surrounding the cells (interstitial fluid) and the blood; this exchange serves to maintain a suitable cellular environment that varies only within narrow limits.

Blood is opaque and has a viscosity about three to four times that of water. Its color is dependent on the pigment in the hemoglobin of the red blood cells and varies with the amount of oxygen combined with the hemoglobin. A higher concentration of oxygen produces a brighter red. Blood has a slightly alkaline reaction, with a pH of 7.35 to 7.40. The average volume in the adult is 5 to 6 liters, or approximately 70 to 75 ml. per kg. of body weight. The volume remains remarkably constant.

FUNCTIONS OF THE BLOOD

The blood performs several important functions:

1. Transportation of oxygen from the lungs to the cells and carbon dioxide from the tissues to the lungs for excretion.

2. Transportation of absorbed nutrients from the alimentary tract to the cells.

3. Conveyance of metabolic wastes from the cells to the organs of excretion (kidneys, lungs, liver and skin).

4. Maintenance of a normal interstitial fluid volume. The interstitial fluid is the medium of exchange between the blood and the cells. Unless its volume is kept relatively constant, the concentration of solutes may be so altered that the passage of substances in and out of the cells is affected.

5. Distribution of hormones and other endogenous chemicals that regulate many body activities.

6. Transference of heat from the site of production to the surface of the body where it can be dissipated.

7. Protection of the individual against excessive loss of blood by coagulation and against injurious agents, such as bacteria and toxins, by its leukocytes and antibodies.

BLOOD COMPONENTS

Fifty-five to 60 per cent of the blood is a straw-colored fluid called plasma in which the formed elements of the blood (blood cells and platelets) are suspended (Table 12–1).

TABLE 12–1 COMPOSITION OF BLOOD

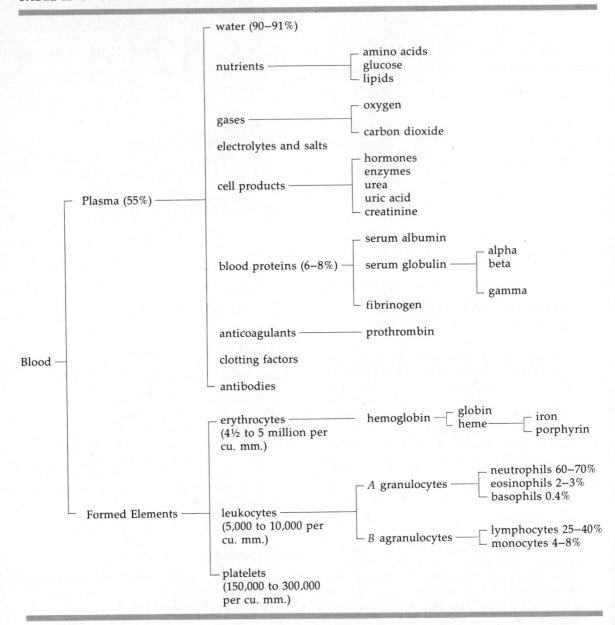

Plasma

Composition

The constituents of plasma are water (90 to 91 per cent) and a wide variety of solutes. The latter include all the substances which cells take in and use as well as many substances produced by the cells. Examples are the nutrients (amino acids, glucose and lipids), the gases (oxygen and carbon dioxide), electrolytes and salts, and cell products such as hormones, enzymes, urea, uric acid and creatinine. In addition, there are also blood proteins, anticoagulants, clotting factors and antibodies.

The concentration of the solutes remains relatively constant even though water and solutes are continually being added and removed. There are temporary variations, but, under normal conditions, certain complex interactions and mechanisms function quickly to restore the plasma to normal. A good example of a quick readjustment that is made to preserve constancy is the maintenance of the plasma concentration of glucose between 80 and 120 mg. per cent. Following a meal, the blood sugar becomes elevated, but within 1 to 2 hours the level returns to normal, owing mainly to liver cells removing excess glucose, converting it to glycogen and storing it. Conversely, much of the plasma glucose may be removed into the cells to be oxidized to produce energy, but a normal concentration in the plasma is maintained by the conversion of glycogen to glucose in the storage depots and its release into the blood.

Blood Proteins

Three types of proteins comprise the greater part of the solutes of the plasma. These are referred to as the plasma or blood proteins and are *serum albumin, serum globulin,* and *fibrinogen.* The normal concentration of the plasma proteins is about 6 to 8 Gm. per cent. They are large in molecular structure and do not readily diffuse through the capillary walls. The resulting concentration of these nondiffusible substances within the capillaries is responsible for what is referred to as the colloidal osmotic pressure of the plasma. A pressure gradient results between the tissue fluid and the blood that promotes the movement of the fluid from the interstitial spaces back into the capillaries (see p. 75). An abnormal decrease in the plasma proteins, especially albumin, reduces the colloidal osmotic pressure, resulting in an accumulation of fluid in the tissues known as edema. The proteins contribute to the viscosity of the blood, which influences circulation and blood pressure.

The plasma proteins are formed from the amino acids of ingested foods but in protein starvation they may be synthesized from tissue protein. Serum albumin and fibrinogen are formed by the liver. Albumin, because of its greater molecular weight, functions mainly in producing the colloidal osmotic pressure. Fibrinogen is concerned with the blood clotting process; its role in this is discussed on page 228.

Serum globulin is produced by reticuloendothelial cells (phagocytic cells of spleen, lymph nodes, liver and bone marrow) and may be separated into three fractions–the alpha, beta, and gamma globulins. The gamma globulin fraction contains antibodies. For this reason it may be administered to provide a temporary immunity against measles or other infections. (See Table 12–2 for normal blood protein values.)

In summary, the functions of the plasma proteins are as follows:

1. They exert an intravascular osmotic pressure that influences fluid exchange between the interstitial and intravascular compartments.

2. Fibrinogen plays a role in blood coagulation which protects the individual from an excessive loss of blood.

3. Serum globulin functions in the production of antibodies, protecting the individual against microbial agents and their toxins.

4. At the site of inflammation or injury, fibrinogen forms a medium in which the various tissues can grow and repair themselves (see Tissue Repair, p. 42).

5. Plasma proteins provide viscosity to the blood.

6. In starvation, the plasma proteins may be broken down and used as a source of amino acids for the tissues.

7. Plasma proteins will combine with both alkalis and acids and can act as buffers to maintain a normal pH of body fluids. They may accept hydrogen ions from acids or, when necessary, donate hydrogen ions to reduce excessive alkalinity.

TABLE 12–2 NORMAL VALUES OF THE PLASMA PROTEINS

	Grams Per Cent
Total plasma proteins	6–8
Albumin	4.05
Globulins	2.5
alpha globulin	0.46
beta globulin	0.86
gamma globulin	0.75
Fibrinogen	0.3

8. The proteins bind some substances such as hormones (thyroxine, adrenocorticoids, gonadal secretions), enzymes and essential ions during their transport in the blood. This prevents too rapid escape of these substances by filtration in the renal glomeruli.

Formed Elements of the Blood

The formed elements include the *red blood cells* (erythrocytes), the *white blood cells* (leukocytes) and the *blood platelets* (thrombocytes).

Erythrocytes

The normal red blood cell is an elastic biconcave disk. The blood normally contains approximately 4.5 to 5.0 million erythrocytes per cu. mm. The volume percentage of erythrocytes in whole blood is 45 to 50, and is expressed as the hematocrit.[1] Anemia is the term applied to a deficiency of red blood cells or to a lack of hemoglobin. An excessive number of red blood cells is referred to as polycythemia. Each cell has a nucleus when first formed, but the normal mature circulating erythrocyte is devoid of a nucleus.

The *function* of red blood cells, by virtue of their composition, is the transportation of oxygen and carbon dioxide between the tissue cells and the lungs. The major constituent of the cell is *hemoglobin,* which is made up of protein globin and an iron-containing pigment called heme. Heme is formed by the union of iron and the pigment porphyrin; four molecules of heme combine with one molecule of globin to form hemoglobin. Oxygen has an affinity for this compound; four molecules of oxygen combine with one molecule of hemoglobin to form *oxyhemoglobin.* Approximately 1 Gm. of hemoglobin combines with 1.3 ml. of oxygen. This is a loose combination, so when there is little or no free oxygen in the red cells' environment (plasma), oxygen is freed from the red blood cell and diffuses out of the cell into the plasma, leaving what is known as *reduced oxyhemoglobin.*

Some of the carbon dioxide in the blood (approximately 27 per cent) is carried by the red blood cells in the form of the compound carbaminohemoglobin. When the hemoglobin takes on oxygen in the lungs, the carbon dioxide is released into the plasma and then diffuses into the alveoli.

Hemoglobin is produced by the red blood cells themselves before they are released into the circulation from their source of production, the red bone marrow. Because of its pigment content, hemoglobin gives the red color to the blood. The *normal concentration of hemoglobin* is 14 to 16 Gm. per 100 ml. of blood. It is slightly higher in men than in women.

PRODUCTION OF ERYTHROCYTES (ERYTHROPOIESIS).[2] After birth, erythrocytes are produced exclusively by the red bone marrow. Prenatally, in the developing organism, they are first produced by the yolk sac and then by the liver in the second to fifth months. During the remaining months the red bone marrow develops and gradually takes over the role. During infancy and childhood most of the bones contain red bone marrow that participates in erythropoiesis. When the growth process is completed, the red blood cells are produced by the red bone marrow of the cancellous (spongy) tissue of the skull bones, vertebrae, ribs, sternum, pelvis and proximal ends of the femora and humeri.

The red blood cells, the white blood cells produced by the marrow and the thrombocytes (platelets) develop from common primitive stem cells which differentiate to become either red or white blood cells, or platelets. In erythropoiesis, the hemocytoblast forms a proerythroblast which goes through a series of nuclear and cytoplasmic changes, becoming progressively smaller. These changes are outlined in Table 12–3 and compose what is referred to as the maturation process of red blood cells.

REGULATION OF ERYTHROPOIESIS. Under normal conditions the rate of production and maturation of red blood cells approximates the rate of removal of the

---

[1]The *hematocrit* or volume percentage of erythrocytes is determined by centrifuging a blood sample, which separates the cells from the plasma. Erythrocytes normally occupy 45 to 50 per cent and the plasma 55 to 50 cent of the volume of the blood.

---

[2]*Poiesis* is the Greek word meaning formation or production.

TABLE 12–3   FORMATION OF RED BLOOD CELLS (ERYTHROPOIESIS)

Stages of Development	Description
Stem cell or → Hemocytoblast	A large, undifferentiated, nucleated cell that divides by mitosis into two proerythroblasts.
Rubriblast or → Proerythroblast	A nucleated cell with no hemoglobin that divides into two smaller nucleated cells.
Prorubricyte or → Early normoblast	A nucleated cell with no hemoglobin that divides into two cells. The nucleus is smaller than it was in the previous stage and the cytoplasm is more abundant.
Rubricyte or → Intermediate normoblast	A nucleated cell that divides. The nucleus becomes smaller and more dense, and a small amount of hemoglobin appears.
Metarubricyte or → Late normoblast	A cell in which the nucleus becomes fragmented and disintegrates as the hemoglobin content of the cytoplasm increases. No cell division.
Reticulocyte →	A nonnucleated cell with an increased amount of hemoglobin. The cytoplasm has a reticular (network of strands) appearance due to the products of the disintegrated nucleus.
Erythrocyte	The mature red blood cell from which the nuclear remnants have disappeared. It is almost completely filled with hemoglobin and is released into the blood stream.

old cells from the circulation and their destruction. The red blood cell count and the amount of hemoglobin remain relatively constant—sufficient to meet the tissues' oxygen needs but, at the same time, controlled in order to prevent a concentration of cells that would impede the blood flow.

The oxygen concentration of the blood is the essential factor in the regulation of the production of erythrocytes. If the rate of cell destruction is increased or if there is a loss of red blood cells as in hemorrhage, the concomitant decrease in the oxygen level brings about a prompt increase in erythropoiesis if the bone marrow is normal and the essential substances are available. At high altitudes where the oxygen concentration of the air is low, the body compensates by producing more red blood cells.

The red bone marrow does not respond directly to the hypoxemia (lowered concentration of oxygen in the blood). The stimulation is brought about by a hormone called *erythropoietin,* or *hemopoietin,* that is produced in response to the hypoxemia. Most of the erythropoietin is formed by the action of an enzyme (erythrogenin or renal erythropoietic factor) produced by the kidneys from a plasma globulin. The renal factor (R.E.F.) is secreted when the oxygen concentration of the blood falls below normal.[3]

Erythropoietin stimulates the bone marrow to produce hemocytoblasts and hastens the successive nuclear and cytoplasmic maturation changes. As a result of this acceleration, reticulocytes may be released into the blood stream before complete maturation and the development of a normal amount of hemoglobin.

Protein, iron, vitamin B_{12} (cyanocobalamin), folic acid (pteroylglutamic acid—a member of the vitamin B complex) and traces of copper must be available to the bone marrow to insure an adequate production of normal erythrocytes. *Protein* is a necessary element in the structure of the cell and its hemoglobin. *Iron* is essential for the formation of hemoglobin. Only a limited amount of iron is absorbed from the small intestine; it is then loosely combined with a protein (apoferritin) to form ferritin which is stored in the intestinal mucosa and liver. Ferritin is released as iron is needed by the bone marrow. Much of the iron used in the formation of hemoglobin is derived from the breakdown of worn-out erythrocytes. Only a small amount of dietary iron is necessary to maintain that required under normal circumstances. Since an excess of absorbed iron cannot be eliminated, its absorption is controlled by the small intestine; that is, the mucosa rejects or absorbs iron according to the rate of use. If erythropoiesis is increased as it is in hemorrhage, pregnancy or other conditions causing hypoxemia, more iron is absorbed. In persons who have a normal hemoglobin concentration and a normal amount of iron in storage, extra dietary iron and medicinal iron preparations do not increase the absorption; the excess iron is simply eliminated in the feces. With increased demands on the bone marrow, the iron stored in the intestinal mucosa and liver is reduced, and absorption by the intestine is increased accordingly.

Vitamin B_{12}, which is referred to as the *extrinsic factor, or antianemic factor,* is essential to normal erythropoiesis. It acts as a catalyst, promoting the synthesis of nucleic acids to form normal red blood cells. The extrinsic factor is especially abundant in liver and red meats and is only absorbed in the presence of a factor or enzyme that is secreted by the gastric mucosa. This substance, essential for the absorption of vitamin B_{12}, is known as the intrinsic factor. The vitamin is then stored in the liver and released as it is needed. In the absence of either the extrinsic factor or the intrinsic factor, the number of erythrocytes is reduced, and many that are in circulation are abnormal. Normoblasts do not divide as many times but grow larger and may contain a greater amount of hemoglobin than normal. These large cells are called macrocytes. There may also be large, primitive, nucleated cells in circulation that are known as megaloblasts.

Folic acid (pteroylglutamic acid), acting as a catalyst, also influences the production and maturation of erythroblasts and is sometimes used in the treatment of a deficiency of red blood cells. The richest dietary sources of this vitamin are liver, kidney and fresh green vegetables.

---

[3]Normal oxygen tension: arterial blood (pO$_2$), 90–100 mm. Hg. Normal oxygen content: arterial blood, 17–21 volumes per cent venous blood, 10–16 volumes per cent.

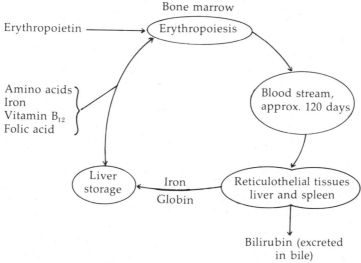

FIGURE 12–1 Life cycle of erythrocytes.

Traces of *copper* are essential to serve as a catalyst for the absorption of iron and its utilization in the formation of hemoglobin.

LIFE SPAN AND NORMAL DESTRUCTION OF ERYTHROCYTES. The average length of life of the red blood cells is 120 days. As the cell ages, the continuous friction between the blood cells and the vessel walls weakens the cell membrane, and it eventually ruptures. The cell fragments are engulfed by macrophages (large phagocytic cells of the reticuloendothelial tissues) in the liver and spleen. The hemoglobin, which composed most of the cell substance, is broken down and the globin and iron fractions are reclaimed for use. The porphyrin molecules are converted to bilirubin and excreted in bile. (Fig. 12–1).

Leukocytes

The white blood cells are less numerous and larger than the erythrocytes, and have nuclei. There are several types, which differ in structure, origin, function and staining reaction. Normally, the blood contains 5,000 to 10,000 per cu. mm. The count tends to be lower after a period of rest and increases following a meal or activity. There is a rapid increase to above normal in most infections in defense of the body. The term *leukocytosis* is applied to an increase above the normal number of white blood cells. A decrease in the white

blood cells below the normal is called *leukopenia*.

TYPES OF LEUKOCYTES. The leukocytes may be divided into two major groups on the basis of whether their cytoplasm is granular or nongranular—namely, granulocytes or agranulocytes (Table 12–4).

1. *Granulocytes.* The granulocytes are formed in the red bone marrow and have lobulated nuclei. Three types are recognized by the staining quality of their cytoplasm.

a. *Neutrophils* stain with a neutral dye, and their nuclei may have several lobes. The latter characteristic results in the neutrophils also being called *polymorphonucle-*

TABLE 12–4 TYPES AND NORMAL VALUES OF LEUKOCYTES*

Type	Per Cent of Total
Granulocytes	
Neutrophils	60–70
Eosinophils	2–3
Basophils	0.4
Agranulocytes	
Lymphocytes	25–40
Monocytes	4–8

*The total leukocyte count is normally 5,000 to 10,000 per cu. mm.

ar leukocytes. They may comprise 60 to 70 per cent of the total white blood cells.

b. *Eosinophils* stain with eosin, a red acid dye, and normally constitute about 2 to 3 per cent of the white blood cells.

c. *Basophils* stain with basic dyes and comprise about 0.4 per cent of the total leukocytes.

2. *Agranulocytes.* The white blood cells with agranular cytoplasm are of two types — lymphocytes and monocytes.

a. The *lymphocytes* are smaller than the granulocytes and have a large spherical nucleus that fills most of the cell. They are produced in the lymphoid tissue (lymph nodes, spleen, tonsils and thymus). Twenty-five to 40 per cent of the total white blood cells are lymphocytes.

b. The *monocytes* are larger than the lymphocytes and have a kidney-shaped nucleus. Differing opinions exist regarding their origin; Guyton states that they are produced by lymphoid tissue,[4] while Ganong indicates that they are produced in the red bone marrow, circulated in the blood for about 24 hours, and then enter the tissues and become macrophages.[5, 6] Monocytes make up about 4 to 8 per cent of the total number of leukocytes.

LEUKOCYTE COUNT. When a white blood cell count is requested, an estimation is made of the total number of cells per cu. mm. (as cited previously, the normal is 5000 to 10,000 per cu. mm.). Frequently, a differential white cell count is done, since it is known that certain types of cells are increased in certain disease conditions. For example, in acute infections, the neutrophils increase rapidly, in chronic infections, the lymphocytes are increased, the number of monocytes are increased in protozoal infections such as malaria, and the eosinophil count is known to rise in allergic reactions and with parasitic invasion of the body. In a differential count the percentage of the various types of leukocytes is determined.

The various types of white blood cells are produced by the stem cells in the blood cell–forming organs in three primitive

forms — the myeloblasts, monoblasts and lymphoblasts (Table 12–5). The *myeloblast,* which is produced by stem cells in the red bone marrow, is nongranular and the nucleus is not divided into lobules. Successive changes occur and are characterized by the appearance of granules in the cytoplasm; the myeloblasts become promyelocytes which change to myelocytes. The latter differentiate to form neutrophils, eosinophils and basophils. Following this, nuclear changes develop, resulting in lobulation and the release of the cell into the blood.

The *monoblast* undergoes mitotic division to form the promonocyte. The cell remains large and nongranular, but the nucleus changes, becoming oval and then kidney-shaped.

The *lymphoblast,* although produced in lymphoid tissue, goes through developmental phases comparable to the other leukocytes. The lymphoblast divides by mitosis and the cells progressively become condensed to form mature, small lymphocytes.

FACTORS IN LEUKOPOIESIS. Little is known about the physiological stimulus responsible for the production and maturation of leukocytes. It has been observed that the breakdown of white blood cells is followed by the appearance of numerous young white blood cells in the blood. This suggests that a chemical which stimulates leukopoiesis may be released from the disintegrated cells.

Increased leukopoiesis occurs in infection, hemorrhage and tissue destruction. The nutrients, protein and vitamins which are essential to all cells of the body are necessary for the production of leukocytes. Some drugs may depress the production of leukocytes; for example, sulfonamides, gold, thiouracil and cortisone preparations may result in a low white blood cell count.

CHARACTERISTICS AND FUNCTIONS OF LEUKOCYTES. The leukocytes serve as an important body defense. They destroy many injurious factors such as microorganisms and the products of degenerating tissues. This is made possible by certain special properties the cells possess — namely, diapedesis, mobility, chemotaxis and phagocytosis.

Diapedesis is the ability of the leukocytes to squeeze through the capillary walls and escape into the tissues. They are ca-

---

[4]Arthur C. Guyton: Textbook of Medical Physiology, 5th ed., Philadelphia, W. B. Saunders, 1976, p. 67.

[5]*Macrophages* are large phagocytic cells — cells that engulf and destroy microorganisms and foreign substances.

[6]William F. Ganong: Review of Medical Physiology, 7th ed. Los Altos, Cal., Lange, 1975, p. 380.

TABLE 12-5   FORMATION OF WHITE BLOOD CELLS (LEUKOPOIESIS)

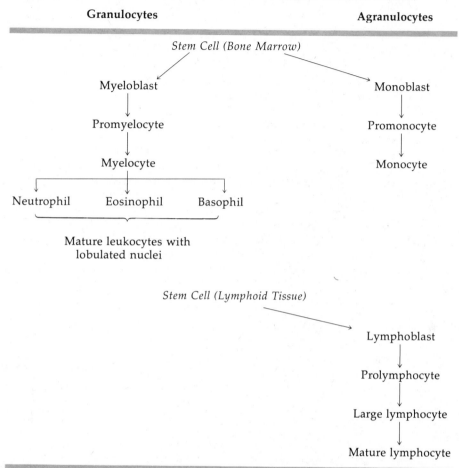

Granulocytes   Agranulocytes

Stem Cell (Bone Marrow)

Myeloblast   Monoblast

Promyelocyte   Promonocyte

Myelocyte   Monocyte

Neutrophil   Eosinophil   Basophil

Mature leukocytes with
lobulated nuclei

Stem Cell (Lymphoid Tissue)

Lymphoblast

Prolymphocyte

Large lymphocyte

Mature lymphocyte

pable of ameboid movement[7] which takes them through the tissues to the source of irritation. The neutrophils are especially mobile; they are attracted by a chemical substance which is liberated by bacteria or by the irritated tissue cells.

Phagocytosis is the engulfing and digesting of particles and is the most important function of the neutrophils and monocytes in protecting the body against microorganisms.

The lymphocytes play an important role in immunity, discussed in Chapter 3.

LIFE SPAN AND DESTRUCTION OF LEUKOCYTES. The life span of the white blood cells varies greatly with the body's protective needs and with the types of white cells,

ranging from a few hours to as long as 200 days. The granulocytes survive a shorter period than do the agranulocytes. Guyton suggests 12 hours as the average life span for granulocytes, but this may be much shorter if there is infection to combat. Many of the lymphocytes have been found to survive 100 to 300 days.[8]

It is thought that the white blood cells that are destroyed or die are disposed of by phagocytosis by the macrophages of the reticuloendothelial tissues.

Blood Platelets (Thrombocytes)

The third and smallest of the formed elements of the blood are the platelets. They are oval, nonnucleated granular structures,

---

[7]*Ameboid movement* is achieved by the cell protruding a protoplasmic extension into which the remaining cell substance streams.

[8]Guyton, op. cit., Chapter 7.

numbering 150,000 to 300,000 per cu. mm. of blood. They are produced in the red bone marrow. The stem cells form giant cells called megakaryocytes which extend bits of their membrane and cytoplasm that separate from the parent cells to form the platelets. The cell content contains important substances, including calcium, potassium, several clotting factors, serotonin, epinephrine, adenosine triphosphate (ADP) and enzymes. When an injury occurs to a vessel wall, the platelets clump and adhere to the site. Their membranes are very fragile and readily permit the escape of platelet content. It is suggested that serotonin and epinephrine are responsible for the vasoconstriction that occurs at the site of injury. The platelets become sticky, resulting in more of them adhering to the original clump and contributing to the formation of a "hemostatic plug." The clotting factors released from the thrombocytes promote coagulation.[9]

Platelet production is increased following tissue trauma and destruction and in hypoxemia. It is suggested that, as well as a reduced oxygen concentration of the blood, chemical substances liberated by degenerating or injured tissue stimulate the bone marrow to increase platelet formation.

FUNCTIONS OF BLOOD PLATELETS. The platelets initiate the blood clotting process through their disintegration and release of thromboplastin (platelet factor) which activates prothrombin (see Coagulation of the Blood, p. 228). On disintegration, they also liberate serotonin (5-hydroxytryptamine) and epinephrine which causes vasoconstriction that, in turn, contributes to reducing the loss of blood when a vessel is interrupted.

With any slight damage to the inner surface of blood vessels, the platelets clump and stick together at the site, helping to plug leaks and prevent loss of blood.

BLOOD GROUPS

Blood may differ from one individual to another according to the presence or absence of specific antigens (agglutinogens) in the red blood cells and the presence or absence of specific antibodies (agglutinins) in

the plasma. For this reason, the blood of a person taken at random cannot be used in transfusion, since the bloods might be of different types and could cause a serious reaction. The blood groups of greatest clinical significance are the ABO and Rh (Rhesus) types.

ABO Blood Groups

In the ABO system, an individual's blood is typed as A, B, AB, or O, depending on the presence or absence of agglutinogens termed A and B in his erythrocytes. If a person has A or B or both A and B naturally occurring agglutinogens, his plasma will not contain antibodies that will agglutinate his own erythrocytes.

In blood that is *typed as A,* the erythrocytes contain *agglutinogens A.* The plasma has anti-B agglutinins which only cause clumping of erythrocytes that have agglutinogens B. Blood that is *typed as B* has erythrocytes containing *agglutinogens B* and, in the plasma, *anti-A agglutinins,* which only cause clumping of red blood cells with agglutinogen A. In blood that is *typed as AB,* the erythrocytes bear both *agglutinogens A and AB.* The plasma is free of anti-A and anti-B agglutinins; otherwise, the individual's own red cells would be attacked. In blood that is typed as O, both agglutinogens are absent, but the plasma contains both anti-A and anti-B agglutinins.

The type of blood is determined by adding specially prepared serum, containing either anti-A and anti-B antibodies. The procedure is as follows:

Anti-A serum is added to a sample of the blood to be typed and, if clumping of the red blood cells occurs, the blood is type A.

Anti-B serum is added to a sample of the blood to be typed, and if clumping occurs, the blood is type B.

If clumping of the red cells occurs with the addition of anti-A and anti-B sera, the presence of both A and B agglutinogens is indicated, and the blood is type AB.

When there is no agglutination with the addition of either anti-A or anti-B serum, it indicates the absence of both A and B agglutinogens in the erythrocytes. The blood type is O.

The blood type of a person is determined genetically; a gene received from each

[8]Ganong, op. cit., p. 383.

TABLE 12–6   ABO SYSTEM

Blood Type	Agglutinogen in Erythrocytes	Agglutinins in Plasma	Plasma Agglutinates Erythrocytes of Blood Type
A	A	anti-B	B and AB
B	B	anti-A	A and AB
AB	A and B	—	—
O	—	anti-A and anti-B	A, B and AB

parent influences the type of blood of the offspring. The genes for A and B agglutinogens are equally dominant. The genotype of an individual of type A may have inherited an A agglutinogen from each parent (AA) or an A agglutinogen from one and none from the other (AO). With type B, it may be BB or BO. In the case of type AB, it is an A and B.

Blood Transfusion

When the volume of circulating blood is reduced, the clinical value of the administration of blood donated by another individual is well recognized. The blood used must be of the same type as that of the recipient. If the bloods are not of the same type, the recipient's plasma may contain agglutinins that will clump the red blood cells of the donor's blood. The agglutinated cells may block blood vessels and could prove fatal if the occluded vessels supply vital areas. In a few hours, the clumped cells are destroyed by macrophages (large phagocytic cells) of the reticuloendothelial system, releasing hemoglobin into the plasma. The disintegration of the red cells is referred to as hemolysis. The free hemoglobin in the plasma is treated as foreign protein and is excreted by the kidneys.

The important precaution to be observed in a blood transfusion is to prevent the donation of red blood cells that will be agglutinated by agglutinins in the recipient's plasma. Since type O has neither A nor B agglutinogens, this blood may be given to a recipient of any one of the four types. For this reason, the person of type O is referred to as a *universal donor*.

Conversely, since an AB type does not have either anti-A or anti-B antibodies in his plasma, the individual is considered to be a *universal recipient*.

The following table indicates possible donors for each blood type in the ABO system.

Recipient	Possible Donor
Type A	Types A and O
Type B	Types B and O
Type AB	Types AB, A, B, and O
Type O	Type O

Whenever possible, it is considered safer to use a donor with blood of the same type as that of the person requiring the transfusion. To ensure compatibility of the donor's and recipient's blood, cross matching is done. A small quantity of each of the bloods is centrifuged in separate tubes. Some of the recipient's cells are added to the donor's serum and vice versa. If no agglutination occurs in 15 minutes, the bloods are considered compatible.

Rhesus (Rh) Blood Groups

This system involves numerous antigens (agglutinogens) having varying degrees of antigenicity. The D factor is the strongest antigen and is of greatest clinical significance. Approximately 85 per cent of Caucasians possess the D factor and are classified as the Rh positive. The remaining 15 per cent are said to be Rh negative.

Plasma antibodies (agglutinins) against the D factor do not occur naturally. They only develop in the plasma of Rh(D) negative blood when the D factor is introduced. The anti-D agglutinins will clump erythrocytes containing the D factor. The formation of anti-D antibodies may be evoked

TABLE 12–7   Rh FACTOR: GENETIC POSSIBILITIES FOR AGGLUTINOGEN D*

		Rh Negative Mother X	Rh Negative Mother X	
Rh Positive Father (Homozygous)	X^D	$X^D X$	$X^D X$	**Offspring:** All heterozygous Rh positive
	Y^D	$Y^D X$	$Y^D X$	
		Rh Negative Mother X	X	
Rh Positive Father (Heterozygous)	X^D	$X^D X$	$X^D X$	**Offspring:** 50 per cent chance of Rh positive; 50 per cent chance of Rh negative
	Y	YX	YX	
		Rh Negative Mother X	X	
Rh Negative Father (Homozygous)	X	XX	XX	**Offspring:** All Rh negative (The mother will not form antibodies)
	Y	YX	YX	

*The Rh factor (agglutinogen D) is dominant. If the father is Rh positive and the mother is Rh negative, the offspring will be Rh positive and the mother will form antibodies.

within an Rh negative person receiving a transfusion of Rh(D) positive blood, or by the development of an Rh(D) positive fetus within an Rh(D) negative mother. In the case of the blood transfusion, usually no clumping of the Rh positive donor's cells in the Rh negative recipient's blood occurs with the first transfusion, because the anti-D antibodies are developed slowly and may not reach sufficient concentration before the foreign positive cells are terminated. But, if a second transfusion of Rh(D) positive blood is given, a reaction occurs, causing agglutination of the donor's cells.

When an Rh positive fetus develops within an Rh negative mother, some of the fetal red blood cells, or D factors released by worn-out erythrocytes, pass through the placenta into the maternal circulation. The mother then forms anti-D agglutinins which diffuse into the fetal circulation and cause agglutination of the fetal erythrocytes. The clumped cells are ultimately disintegrated, and the hemoglobin is broken down and converted to bilirubin, causing jaundice (yellowness of the skin and conjunctivae). This condition is known as erythroblastosis fetalis. The destruction of red blood cells may prove fatal to the fetus, depending on the concentration of antibodies that reaches

the fetal circulation. If the fetus goes to term, at birth the infant will exhibit jaundice, anemia, edema and enlargement of the spleen and liver. Prompt treatment by a series of exchange transfusions is necessary. Compatible Rh negative blood is given. The exchange is made by alternate withdrawal and injection of equal amounts of blood.

The first baby sensitizes the Rh negative mother but usually escapes the hemolytic disease. With subsequent pregnancies, the anti-D agglutinins progressively increase if the fetuses are Rh positive. Immunization of Rh negative persons seems to vary; some develop antibodies more readily than others.

The Rh blood group factors are inherited, and the gene for the D agglutinogen is always dominant (Table 12–7). One who is Rh positive may be homozygous (DD), having inherited a gene for the D factor from each parent, or may be heterozygous (D–), having inherited a gene for D from one parent only. The child of an Rh positive father who is homozygous and an Rh negative mother will always be Rh positive because of the dominance of the D factor. The child of an Rh positive father who is heterozygous and an Rh negative mother has a 50 per cent chance of being Rh positive. If the developing organism in utero is Rh negative, there is no problem.

HEMOSTASIS AND BLOOD COAGULATION

Any rupture or severance of a blood vessel is normally followed by certain responses in an effort to reduce the loss of blood. These responses are local vasoconstriction, the formation of a temporary plug, coagulation of the blood and the formation of scar tissue to close the opening in the vessel. These defense responses occur frequently in the body without the individual being aware of them. During normal day-to-day activities and in minor injuries, minute blood vessels are ruptured and the loss of blood is controlled by these mechanisms. If a large vessel, especially an artery, is interrupted, coagulation and vasoconstriction may not be adequate in checking the bleeding. Ligation, pressure or cautery may have to be used.

Vasoconstriction in Hemostasis

Local vasoconstriction reduces the blood flow to the injured site and is brought about by direct vascular muscular tissue reaction to the injury and by reflex nerve impulses that occur as a result of the trauma to the vessel. In the latter, sensory impulses arising in the injured vascular wall are transmitted into the central nervous system, causing impulses to be sent to the musculature of the vessels, and stimulating contraction. This vascular spasm is augmented by the release of serotonin (5-hydroxytryptamine) and epinephrine by the disintegrating platelets at the site of injury.

Hemostatic Plug

Injury and interruption of a vascular wall results in a clumping of thrombocytes at the site. The aggregation serves as a loose temporary plug in the opening and is the forerunner of blood coagulation and the formation of a clot.

TABLE 12–8   BLOOD CLOTTING FACTORS AND THEIR ROLES IN BLOOD COAGULATION

Factor Number	Synonym	Role in Blood Coagulation
I	Fibrinogen	Forms fibrin
II	Prothrombin	Forms thrombin which converts fibrinogen to fibrin
III	Thromboplastin	Converts prothrombin to thrombin
IV	Calcium	Serves as a catalyst in conversion of prothrombin to thrombin
V	Labile factor (accelerator globulin AcG, proaccelerin)	Necessary in the formation of active thromboplastin
VII	Proconvertin (stable factor, serum prothrombin conversion accelerator SPCA)	Accelerates the action of tissue thromboplastin
VIII	Antihemophilic factor, AHF (antihemophilic globulin, AHG)	Promotes the breakdown of thrombocytes and the formation of active platelet thromboplastin
IX	Christmas factor (plasma thromboplastin component, PTC)	Similar to Factor VIII
X	Stuart factor	Promotes the action of thromboplastin
XI	Plasma thromboplastin antecedent (PTA)	Promotes clumping and breakdown of thrombocytes and the release of thromboplastin
XII	Hageman factor	Similar to Factor XI
XIII	Fibrin-stabilizing factor (FSF), Laki-Lorand factor (LLF)	Converts the loose fibrin mesh to dense tight mass

TABLE 12–9 SCHEMA OF THE CLOTTING PROCESS

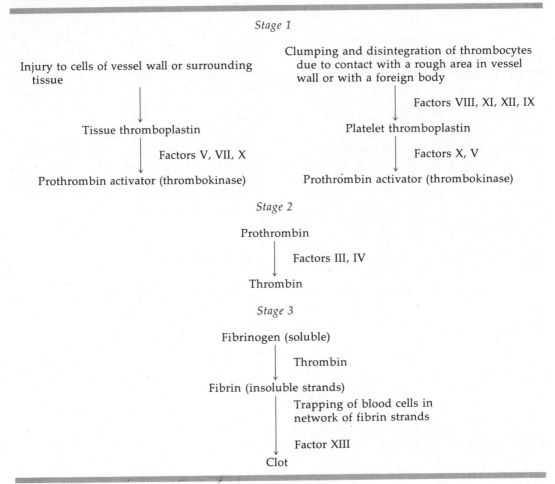

Stage 1

Injury to cells of vessel wall or surrounding tissue

Clumping and disintegration of thrombocytes due to contact with a rough area in vessel wall or with a foreign body

Factors VIII, XI, XII, IX

Tissue thromboplastin

Platelet thromboplastin

Factors V, VII, X

Factors X, V

Prothrombin activator (thrombokinase)

Prothrombin activator (thrombokinase)

Stage 2

Prothrombin

Factors III, IV

Thrombin

Stage 3

Fibrinogen (soluble)

Thrombin

Fibrin (insoluble strands)

Trapping of blood cells in network of fibrin strands

Factor XIII

Clot

Blood Coagulation

Coagulation of the blood is the formation of a jelly-like mass in the blood by the conversion of the soluble plasma protein fibrinogen to an insoluble mass of fine threads called fibrin. Blood cells are enmeshed in the fibrin to form the mass known as a clot. The conversion of fibrinogen to fibrin is dependent upon a chain of reactions between several intrinsic factors that are designated by number. Twelve factors are currently indicated; a list of these, their synonyms and their role in the blood clotting process is found in Tables 12–8 and 12–9.

The essential major steps in coagulation are:

1. The release and activation of thromboplastin by disintegrating platelets and damaged tissue cells.
2. The conversion of prothrombin to thrombin by thromboplastin (prothrombin activator) in the presence of calcium ions.
3. The conversion of fibrinogen by thrombin to fibrin.

Prothrombin is normally present in the blood and is the inactive form of thrombin. Vitamin K is essential for its production by the liver. The conversion of prothrombin to active thrombin depends upon the presence of calcium ions and thromboplastin. Information concerning the exact role of some factors is incomplete, but the absence of any one produces a bleeding tendency.

NORMAL ANTICOAGULANTS. A remarkable property of blood is its ability to remain fluid in the blood vessels; this is necessary for its circulation. Under normal circumstances, small amounts of thromboplastin are released by the disintegration of some thrombocytes and tissue cells and could initiate coagulation. In order to counteract this, coagulation inhibitors — *heparin* and *antithrombin* — are normally present in the plasma.

Large granular cells in the pericapillary connective tissue that are known as *mast cells* are the principal source of heparin. It inhibits the formation and action of thrombin. If thrombin is produced in relatively small amounts, it is neutralized by antithrombin, an alpha globulin, and the conversion of fibrinogen to fibrin does not take place. The presence of antithrombin and heparin prevents coagulation under normal conditions, but with increased tissue and platelet destruction, the greater concentration of thromboplastin is sufficient to initiate spontaneous coagulation.

Blood that is collected from one person for administration to another is prevented from clotting by the addition of sodium citrate. The citrate combines with the calcium to form insoluble citrate of calcium. Certain blood examinations require that the blood remain fluid; an oxalate which combines with the calcium is usually added.

CLOT RETRACTION AND ORGANIZATION. After a clot forms, the fibrin strands shrink (as a result of Factor XIII) and the plasma that was trapped along with the blood cells is extruded. This fluid is referred to as *serum* and differs from normal plasma because it lacks fibrinogen. The fibrin strands of the clot attach to the edges of the injured area of the blood vessel; as they shrink they pull the edges of the opening closer together, helping to check the loss of blood.

The opening in the vessel is repaired by a process called *clot organization*. Fibroblasts proliferate the clot and, as they mature, the area is filled in by fibrous tissue. Macrophages (large reticuloendothelial phagocytes) clear away the trapped blood cells. Endothelial cells of the intima proliferate to replace the vessel lining in the area.

DISORDERS OF THE BLOOD AND BLOOD-FORMING ORGANS

INTRODUCTION

Blood disorders (dyscrasias) may affect the erythrocytes, leukocytes or the coagulation process. The problem may be due to a defect originating in the blood-forming organs, the deficiency of an essential element, or the abnormal destruction of cells. The disorders may be primary or secondary to another disease.

Diseases of the blood-forming organs may involve the red bone marrow or reticuloendothelial tissue.

Investigative Procedures Used in Blood Disorders

A. Blood Tests for Assessing Erythrocytes

1. RED CELL COUNT. Normal: 4.5 to 5 million per cu. mm.

2. HEMOGLOBIN CONTENT OF ERYTHROCYTES. Normal: males, 13 to 15 Gm. per 100 ml.; females, 13 to 14 Gm. per 100 ml.; children (3 months to puberty), 10 to 14 Gm. per 100 ml.

3. HEMATOCRIT (PACKED CELL VOLUME). The volume of red blood cells in 100 ml. of blood (volume percentage of erythrocytes). Normal: males, 45 to 50 per cent; females, 40 to 45 per cent.

4. ERYTHROCYTE INDICES. Mean corpuscular volume (MCV) — average size of individual red cell. Normal: 80 to 92 cu. microns. Mean corpuscular hemoglobin (MCH) — average amount of hemoglobin per red cell. Normal: 29 to 32 micromicrograms. Mean corpuscular hemoglobin concentration (MCHC) — average Gm of hemoglobin in 100 ml. packed cells. Normal: 30 to 38 Gm. per 100 ml. packed red cells.

5. RETICULOCYTE COUNT. The percentage of circulating red blood cells that are reticulocytes. Normal: 0.5 to 1.5 per cent.

6. URINARY UROBILINOGEN. An estimation of the urobilinogen that is excreted in urine. It is increased in excessive red blood cell destruction (hemolytic anemia) and liver disease. Normal: present in very small amount (0 to 4 mg. in 24 hours).

7. FECAL UROBILINOGEN. An estimation of the amount of urobilinogen that is excreted in the feces. It is increased in excessive red blood cell destruction. Normal: 50 to 300 mg. in 24 hours.

8. SCHILLING TEST. This procedure determines the amount of vitamin B_{12} (cyanocobalamin) absorbed from the gastrointestinal tract. The test requires that the patient

fast for 8 hours; he is then given an oral dose of radioactive vitamin B_{12}. Two hours after the oral dose is given, a dose of the regular (nonradioactive) vitamin B_{12} is given intramuscularly. The urine is collected over the next 24 hours; the amount of radioactive vitamin B_{12} excreted in the urine is then determined. Normally, 15 to 40 per cent of the oral dose is excreted. The administration of the nonradioactive vitamin B_{12} saturates the blood so that the radioactive vitamin B_{12} that is absorbed is excreted in the urine.

9. BONE MARROW BIOPSY. The investigation of most blood dyscrasias includes the examination of a specimen of red bone marrow that is usually obtained by aspiration. Smears are made of the marrow specimen and the cells are examined. The number of cells in the various developmental and maturational phases and the size, shape and characteristics of cell content are noted.

The sites used most frequently for marrow aspiration are the sternum and iliac crest. Preparation of the patient involves an explanation of the procedure and its purpose, and the shaving and cleansing of the skin over the site to be used.

The area receives an application of an antiseptic and is draped with sterile towels. The physician injects a local anesthetic before introducing the aspiration needle. Considerable pressure is necessary to pass the needle through the cortex of the bone into the marrow space. The stylet is then removed from the needle, and a syringe is attached for the collection of 1 to 2 ml. of marrow. Upon completion of the procedure a small sterile dressing is applied to the puncture site.

The patient may fear the procedure and manifest considerable apprehension. In addition to explaining and describing the procedure, the nurse provides support by remaining close to the patient during the procedure.

10. OSMOTIC FRAGILITY OF ERYTHROCYTES. This test is done to determine the tendency of the red blood cells to hemolyze in increasingly hypotonic solutions. It is used in hemolytic anemias; the fragility is increased in some types of hemolytic anemia (e.g., spherocytosis) and decreased in others (e.g., sickle cell anemia).

B. Blood Tests for Assessing Leukocytes

1. LEUKOCYTE COUNT. Normal: 5,000 to 10,000 per cu. mm.

2. DIFFERENTIAL LEUKOCYTE COUNT.

An estimation of the percentage of the various types of white blood cells that constitute the leukocytes in circulation. Normal: neutrophils (polymorphonuclear leukocytes), 60 to 70 per cent; eosinophils, 2 to 3 per cent; basophils, 0.4 to 3 per cent; monocytes, 4 to 7 per cent; lymphocytes, 25 to 30 per cent.

3. BONE MARROW BIOPSY. See above.

C. Tests Used in Investigating Hemorrhagic Disorders

1. THROMBOCYTE (BLOOD PLATELET) COUNT. Normal: 150,000 to 300,000 per cu. mm.

2. BLEEDING TIME. This is the time it takes bleeding to stop naturally — that is, the period of time blood continues to escape from an "open" area. Normal: 2 to 5 minutes.

3. COAGULATION TIME. This is the time it takes blood to clot after it has been shed. Normal: 5 to 12 minutes.

4. PROTHROMBIN TIME. This is the time it takes for coagulation following the addition of thromboplastin and calcium to the specimen. Normal: 12 to 20 seconds.

5. PLASMA FIBRINOGEN. This indicates the fibrinogen concentration. Normal: 160 to 300 mg. per 100 ml. of blood.

D. Miscellaneous Tests

1. COOMBS' TEST. The erythrocytes are examined for the presence of immune bodies (agglutinins) that adhere to the red blood cells and lead to clumping and hemolysis. This is referred to as the *direct Coombs' test*. An indirect method is done on serum to test for the presence of the antibodies to the erythrocyte antigens.

The Coombs' test may be used in identifying hemolytic anemia or erythroblastosis fetalis.

2. LYMPH NODE BIOPSY. A tissue specimen of a lymph node that has undergone some change is obtained. The change may be associated with an alteration in the patient's leukocytes, especially the lymphocytes.

ERYTHROCYTE DISORDERS

Introduction

A deficiency or an excess may occur in the number of circulating red blood cells, or the cell composition may be abnormal. Variations in the size, shape and hemoglobin content may be present. Certain descriptive terms are used to denote some of these characteristics.

Erythrocytes that are larger than the normal are referred to as *macrocytes;* if they are smaller than the normal, they are *microcytes.* Cells that possess a normal amount of hemoglobin are said to be *normochromic,* but if it is deficient, they are described as *hypochromic.* Those with a volume of hemoglobin greater than the normal are *hyperchromic.* If the cells present have abnormal shapes, they are described as *poikilocytic.*

Anemia may sometimes be classified according to the characteristics of the erythrocytes. For example, in anemia which is due to an iron deficiency, the cells are hypochromic and microcytic; the disease may be referred to as hypochromic-microcytic anemia.

Anemia

The term anemia implies a reduction in the oxygen-carrying capacity of the blood as a result of fewer circulating erythrocytes than is normal or a decrease in the concentration of hemoglobin.

The abnormal reduction in the number of erythrocytes may be due to decreased erythropoiesis, excessive red blood cell destruction or hemolysis, or loss of blood. Anemia may be primary, but frequently is secondary to some other disorder, and because of this the patient may undergo extensive investigation to determine the cause. It may also be classified as acquired or hereditary. Anemia due to decreased erythropoiesis may be caused by a deficiency of factors essential for normal production or by depressed bone marrow activity. An abnormal rate of destruction of the red blood cells may be associated with intracorpuscular defects or extracorpuscular factors.

Table 12–10 outlines the principal types of anemia according to cause.

General Effects and Manifestations of Anemia

Although there are various causes and types of anemia, they present a common problem — that of a decrease in the capacity

TABLE 12–10   TYPES OF ANEMIA

A. Anemia due to decreased erythropoiesis
  1. Deficiency anemia
    a. Iron deficiency anemia
    b. Vitamin B_{12} deficiency anemia (pernicious anemia)
    c. Folic acid deficiency anemia
  2. Aplastic anemia (anemia due to depressed bone marrow activity)

B. Anemia due to excessive rate of hemolysis
  1. Hemolytic anemia due to intracorpuscular defects
    a. Congenital hemolytic jaundice (hereditary spherocytosis)
    b. Hemoglobinopathy
      Sickle cell anemia
      Thalassemia (Mediterranean anemia, or Cooley's anemia)
  2. Hemolytic anemia due to extracorpuscular factors, such as
    a. Certain infective agents
    b. Autoimmune reaction
    c. Certain drugs and chemicals

C. Anemia due to blood loss

of the blood to transport oxygen. The patients, regardless of the cause or type of their anemia, manifest signs and symptoms attributable to tissue and organ hypoxia and the ensuing reduced metabolism. The occurrence and severity of these manifestations depend on the degree of anemia present.

The person experiences general fatigue, lassitude, shortness of breath on exertion, and anorexia. Diarrhea or constipation and flatulence may be troublesome. The mucous membranes (e.g., conjunctivae) and skin become pale. Complaints of headache, dizziness, faintness, and tingling or "pins and needles" in the extremities are common. The reduced metabolic rate and consequent lowered heat production due to hypoxia frequently causes the individual to feel cold in temperatures that are comfortable for others. The pulse rate and cardiac stroke volume are increased as compensatory measures in response to the oxygen deficiency, and frequently palpitation is experienced. In severe anemia, the circulation or renal function may be sufficiently impaired to cause some edema and, probably, some fluid in the bases of the lungs. Angina pectoris due to the myocardial hypoxia may occur, especially in elderly persons. There is a general reduction in efficiency throughout the body and lowered resistance to infections.

A. Anemias Due to Decreased Erythropoiesis

1. DEFICIENCY ANEMIAS. An essential nutrient for erythrocyte production, such as iron, vitamin B_{12}, folic acid, ascorbic acid and protein, may be lacking in the diet, or there may be defective absorption of an essential factor. In some instances, there may be an increased demand within the person which the normal supply cannot meet. The deficiency anemias seen most often are those resulting from iron, vitamin B_{12} or folic acid deficiency.

a. IRON DEFICIENCY ANEMIA. Anemia due to a deficiency of iron is characterized by small red blood cells with less than the normal content of hemoglobin (microcytic-hypochromic). There is usually some slight reduction in the total number of red blood cells. The deficiency of iron may be due to: (1) an insufficient dietary intake; (2) chronic or acute blood loss; (3) impaired intestinal absorption; or (4) an increased requirement. Iron deficiency is seen frequently in children because of their increased requirements for growth. It is not uncommon in women during their reproductive years because of menstrual blood loss and because of the increased demands during pregnancy and lactation. Anemia due to an iron deficiency is uncommon in adult males unless there has been a loss of blood or the development of hypochlorhydria secondary to gastric disease or atrophy of the gastric mucosa.

In addition to the general symptoms of anemia (see p. 231), the patient with iron deficiency anemia may experience soreness and inflammation of the mouth and tongue. The tongue may be very red and may have a smooth, glazed appearance due to atrophy of the papillae. Rarely, the patient with a severe anemia complains of dysphagia (difficulty in swallowing). The combination of dysphagia, stomatitis (inflammation of the mouth) and atrophic glossitis (inflammation of the tongue with atrophy of papillae) in anemia may be referred to as the Plummer-Vinson syndrome. Changes in the fingernails are common in prolonged iron deficiency. They become brittle and concave or spoon-shaped.

A well-balanced diet containing an adequate quantity of iron-rich foods is important in the prevention of this type of anemia. A normal diet contains about 10 to 15 mg. of iron per day, of which only 5 to 10 per cent is absorbed. It is suggested that absorption is increased as the need for increased production of hemoglobin occurs. It may be necessary to supplement the dietary intake with medicinal iron during periods of increased demands, such as pregnancy and lactation. A supplement may also be necessary for the woman with an excessive menstrual flow.

Unless there is an obvious reason for an iron deficiency anemia, the patient is investigated to determine the primary cause. For example, malabsorption of iron may be the result of a reduced secretion of hydrochloric acid.

Treatment. Medicinal iron is the principal form of treatment and is usually given orally in the form of a ferrous salt. Examples of preparations commonly used are ferrous sulfate and ferrous gluconate. Oral iron medications may cause gastrointestinal irritation and crampy pain. If the patient complains of distress, the drug is administered with the meal or with a snack. The physician may recommend that it be given with a glass of orange juice, since it is suggested that vitamin C promotes iron absorption. The patient is advised that his stools will be black and tarry. He may experience some diarrhea or, with some preparations, may develop constipation, necessitating a mild laxative. Ferrous salt in a syrup or an elixir may be used for children. Any liquid product containing iron is given well diluted through a drinking tube to prevent staining of the teeth.

For patients who cannot tolerate oral preparations or if oral administration is contraindicated because of some gastrointestinal disturbance or malabsorption, iron may be given parenterally. Injections of iron dextran (Imferon) may be given intramuscularly and occasionally dextriferron (Astrofer) intravenously. When giving an iron preparation intramuscularly, the injection is made deeply into the upper outer quadrant of the buttock. The "Z" track technique[10] is used, since iron is irritating to superficial tissues. The patient

---

[10]The "Z" track technique involves pulling the skin to one side before inserting the needle. After the solution has been introduced, 10 seconds are allowed to elapse before the needle is withdrawn. The purpose of this technique is to prevent the drug leaking into the subcutaneous tissues.

is observed for toxic reactions, which are manifested by headache, dizziness, joint pains and fever. Rarely, an anaphylactic reaction may occur; the patient complains of dyspnea and chest pain, the pulse is rapid and weak and the blood pressure falls.

The patient with iron deficiency anemia is encouraged to take an adequate diet that contains iron-rich foods. These are red meats, organ meats (especially liver), eggs, fish, green leafy vegetables, enriched whole grain cereals and bread, and dried fruits.

b. VITAMIN B_{12} DEFICIENCY ANEMIA (PERNICIOUS OR ADDISONIAN ANEMIA). Vitamin B_{12} (cyanocobalamin) is essential for the production of normal red blood cells and may be referred to as the extrinsic antianemic factor. When it is not available to the red bone marrow, excessively large cells called megaloblasts are formed. The number of red blood cells produced is less than normal, and they show marked variation in size and shape. The megaloblasts contain a greater than normal amount of hemoglobin, but the deficiency in the total number of erythrocytes results in an inadequate oxygen-carrying capacity of the blood. The condition may be referred to as *megaloblastic anemia*.

The *cause* of vitamin B_{12} deficiency anemia is usually non-absorption of the vitamin. Rarely, vitamin B_{12} deficiency occurs because of an inadequate dietary intake (Table 12–11).

As cited earlier in this chapter, an intrinsic factor secreted by the gastric mucosa is essential for the absorption of vitamin B_{12}. Nonabsorption of the vitamin results from a deficiency of the intrinsic factor, which may be due to a gastric secretory defect, gastrectomy or an autoimmune mechanism. Failure of absorption of the vitamin may also occur as a result of extensive resection of the small intestine or intestinal disease such as ileitis, steatorrhea and parasitic infestation. Blind or stagnant loops in the small intestine may develop following intestinal surgery or with multiple diverticula (sacs or outpouchings in the walls) and may cause a proliferation of bacteria that use up the available vitamin B_{12} before it can be absorbed.

There appears to be some familial tendency to vitamin B_{12} deficiency anemia when the deficiency of the intrinsic factor is not secondary to partial or total gastrectomy. It is suggested that a predisposition to the dis-

TABLE 12–11 POSSIBLE CAUSES OF VITAMIN B_{12} DEFICIENCY ANEMIA

A. Nonabsorption of Vitamin B_{12}
   1. Deficiency of intrinsic factor
      a. Gastric secretory defect
      b. Gastrectomy (partial or total)
      c. Autoimmune mechanism
   2. Intestinal resection
   3. Intestinal disease (e.g., regional ileitis, steatorrhea)

B. Malnutrition
   1. Inadequate dietary intake of foods containing vitamin B_{12}
   2. Totally deficient food intake

order is inherited.[11] An autoimmune mechanism is considered to be active — that is, the individual produces antibodies to the intrinsic factor. This primary form of the disease (that due to a gastric secretory defect or autoimmune mechanism) is known as *pernicious anemia* or *Addisonian pernicious anemia*. It is more common in females, has an insidious onset, and usually develops between 35 and 65 years of age.

Manifestations. In addition to the general symptoms of anemia cited previously, the patient may experience gastrointestinal and nervous system changes. The tongue is sore and smooth. There is a loss of appetite and some intolerance for food, but the person does not always show a corresponding loss of weight. The lack of vitamin B_{12} (antianemic factor) may cause myelin and nerve fiber degeneration in the spinal cord and peripheral nerves. As a result of this degeneration, the patient may develop symmetrical tingling or "pins and needles" or coldness and numbness in the extremities. Unless the deficiency is corrected, serious motor disturbances may develop in the form of muscular weakness, ataxia (loss of coordination and staggering) and paralysis. In prolonged, severe deficiencies, degeneration of the optic nerves may occur, resulting in serious impairment of vision. When degenerative changes occur in the spinal cord, the condition is referred to as *subacute combined degeneration of the cord*.

In severe pernicious anemia, the skin may

[11]Marcus A. Krupp and Milton J. Chatton: Current Medical Diagnosis and Treatment. Los Altos, Cal., Lange, 1975, p. 273.

show some jaundice, a result of increased hemolysis. Laboratory examination of the blood reveals a deficiency of erythrocytes. The cells are unusually large with more than the normal amount of hemoglobin (macrocytic-hyperchromic). Gastric analysis demonstrates hypochlorhydria even after stimulation with histamine (see p. 498). Bone marrow aspirated by sternal puncture shows hyperplasia of the bone marrow and failure in normal erythropoiesis. The Schilling test shows that less than the normal amount of vitamin B_{12} is being absorbed.

Treatment. Pernicious anemia is treated by intramuscular injections of vitamin B_{12}. A daily dose may be prescribed for a period of time; then, the interval between injections is gradually ·increased, and the dosage is reduced to a maintenance level according to the patient's response. The patient will require regular maintenance doses of vitamin B_{12} for the rest of his life. The majority of those with pernicious anemia require 50 to 1000 micrograms monthly to maintain normal hemoglobin and erythrocyte levels. Regular red cell counts and hemoglobin estimations are necessary. Initially, the rapid regeneration of erythrocytes in response to treatment may deplete the iron stores, resulting in insufficient hemoglobin production. Ferrous sulfate may be prescribed for a period of time in addition to the vitamin B_{12}.

If the anemia is very severe, with a hemoglobin as low as 4 to 5 Gm per cent, a blood transfusion may be considered advisable. Packed cells are used to avoid a sudden increase in the blood volume which might precipitate sudden heart failure. The patient is usually kept on bed rest if the hemoglobin is less than 7 Gm. per cent. The recommended diet is light, easily digested, and rich in protein, iron and vitamins. Highly seasoned and coarse foods are avoided if the mouth is sore.

Regular medical examinations are necessary so that early and insidious regressive changes may be recognized before serious degenerative changes develop.

In contrast to pernicious anemia, the anemia associated with a dietary deficiency of vitamin B_{12} or intestinal disease does not manifest hypochlorhydria or degenerative changes of the nervous system. The dietary deficiency of vitamin B_{12} (extrinsic factor) usually occurs when the diet lacks animal protein and consists mainly of carbohydrates and vegetables. When the anemia is secondary to intestinal disease, care of the patient includes treatment of the initial cause as well as parenteral administration of vitamin B_{12}. Oral or parenteral preparations of folic acid may also be prescribed.

c. ANEMIA DUE TO DEFICIENCY OF FOLIC ACID AND VITAMIN C. A lack of folic acid or ascorbic acid may interfere with the production of normal erythrocytes. Either deficiency may result from inadequate intake or a malabsorptive problem. It is also more likely to develop during pregnancy because of the increased demand. Laboratory tests reveal the same hematologic changes as appear with vitamin B_{12} deficiency, but the patient does not manifest nervous system involvement, achlorhydria or a decreased vitamin B_{12} absorption.

Folic acid may be given orally or intramuscularly to correct the deficiency. Food sources include dark green leafy vegetables, asparagus, liver and kidney.

Vitamin C enhances the catalytic action of folic acid in erythropoiesis. If the folic acid dietary intake is satisfactory, the administration of vitamin C in anemia will assist in increasing red cell production.

2. APLASTIC ANEMIA. This type of anemia is the result of depressed bone marrow activity. There may be an actual reduction in the amount of blood-forming marrow, or the marrow may have a functional defect. Aplastic anemia usually results in a deficiency of leukocytes and thrombocytes as well as insufficient red blood cells. The disorder may involve only failure of the bone marrow to produce erythrocytes, causing anemia alone without leukopenia or thrombocytopenia. When all three formed elements of the blood are reduced, the condition is referred to as *pancytopenia.*

CAUSES. Depression of bone marrow activity may be the result of the toxic action of certain drugs or industrial chemicals, excessive exposure to radiation, chronic infection or crowding by tumors or neoplastic tissue. Drugs capable of suppressing bone marrow function include sulfonamides, antineoplastic agents (e.g., nitrogen mustard, busulfan, cyclophosphamide, methotrexate, mercaptopurine), gold salts (Myochrysine), chloramphenicol (Chloromycetin) and phenylbutazone (Butazolidin). Examples of industrial chemicals that may depress erythropoiesis include benzene, aniline dyes, lead, mercury and arsenic. Some insecticides and plant sprays may also be offenders in bone marrow failure. In relation to radiation, drugs and chemicals, there appears to be no direct correlation between the dosage and the development of the anemia. Sensitivity of the individual seems to be a contributing factor. With some patients their aplastic anemia may be idiopathic; the cause remains obscure.

SYMPTOMS AND TREATMENT. The person with aplastic anemia is critically ill and, as well as suffering severe hypoxia, he is susceptible to infection because of the deficiency of leukocytes (leukopenia). Spontaneous bleeding is also a problem due to the lack of thrombocytes. The onset of the anemia may be sudden and prostrating, or it may be insidious and gradual. The patient manifests the general symptoms of anemia (p. 231), oral and throat lesions, fever, infection and hemorrhagic areas.

Treatment includes removal of the cause, frequent transfusions of whole blood, oral antibiotic administration to control infection and a corticoid preparation such as prednisone. The latter is thought to have a stimulating effect on the bone marrow. Supportive nursing care is very important. Close observations are made for infection, hemorrhage and increasing hypoxia. Precautions are necessary to prevent infection. Reverse isolation technique is used (see p. 252). Frequent cleansing of the mouth with an antiseptic solution is important. Subcutaneous and intramuscular injections are avoided as much as possible to keep the skin intact to prevent infection.

B. Hemolytic Anemias

Excessive hemolysis (disintegration of red blood cells) causes anemia if the rate of destruction exceeds the erythropoietic ability of the red bone marrow. Premature hemolysis may result from (1) *intracorpuscular (intrinsic) defects* that reduce the ability of the cells to survive the normal life span in circulation, or it may be due to (2) an *extracorpuscular (extrinsic to the erythrocytes) factor or mechanism*.

The patient's symptoms depend on the rate, severity and duration of the cell destruction. As well as the symptoms produced by the reduced oxygen-carrying capacity of the blood, there is an increased concentra-

tion of bilirubin in the blood; this may cause jaundice, which is evident first in the sclerae. An increased amount of urobilinogen appears in the urine and feces and, rarely, free hemoglobin is detected in the plasma and urine. Laboratory examination of the blood reveals an increased number of reticulocytes in circulation (reticulocytosis) because of the constant demand for new cells, as well as a deficiency in the total number of red cells. Examination of a bone marrow specimen demonstrates hyperplasia and hyperactivity of the marrow. Acute hemolytic anemia may cause a chill followed by a high temperature, prostration, headache and pain in the back and legs.

The hemolytic anemias caused by a congenital corpuscular defect include hereditary spherocytosis, sickle cell anemia, and thalassemia. Hemolysis due to extracorpuscular factors may be caused by some infective agents, an autoimmune reaction or certain drugs.

1. HEMOLYTIC ANEMIAS DUE TO INTRACORPUSCULAR DEFECT

a. HEREDITARY SPHEROCYTOSIS. This type of hemolytic anemia is also known as congenital hemolytic jaundice, familial hemolytic anemia, and acholuric jaundice. The erythrocyte defect is an abnormal cell membrane that is excessively permeable to sodium. The influx of sodium increases the demand on the "sodium pump," adding to the total metabolic work of the cell. The high sodium content of the cells also leads to the entrance of more than the normal amount of water through osmosis, which accounts for the characteristic spherical shape of the cell rather than the normal biconcave disc. This spherical shape predisposes the cells to entrapment in the spleen and their marked fragility results in ready destruction.

The disorder is inherited from an affected parent. The gene with the abnormal trait is dominant; that is, to have the disorder expressed, one need only receive a gene for the trait from one parent. The age at which the disease is recognized varies, depending on its severity. The patient may have little difficulty and go undiagnosed until adulthood. The enlarged spleen may be discovered during a routine examination. It is usually the jaundice or the symptoms of anemia that prompt the patient to seek medical assistance. Occasionally, the increased bilirubin leads to the development of gallstones.

Treatment is removal of the spleen, which reduces the excessive destruction of the abnormal red blood cells and relieves the anemia. The abnormal erythrocytes persist, but the majority survive a normal life span in the absence of the spleen.

b. HEMOGLOBINOPATHY. The complex hemoglobin (Hb) molecule is a combination of globins (protein) and the red pigment heme (porphyrin and ferrous iron). Three forms of hemoglobin occur normally; the type is determined by slight variations in the globin fraction of the compound. The hemoglobin in the erythrocytes of the fetus is type F (Hb-F) and gradually disappears during the first few months of life. About 97 per cent of the hemoglobin that develops after birth is known as type A (Hb-A), and the remainder as type A_2 (Hb-A_2).

The term hemoglobinopathy indicates the presence of red blood cells containing an abnormal type of hemoglobin. The latter is the result of a genetic mutation which causes a disorder in hemoglobin synthesis. The abnormal hemoglobin may cause premature hemolysis of the erythrocytes. The most common hemoglobinopathies are sickle cell disease and thalassemia. The hemoglobin in the former disease is designated as Hb-S; in the latter various abnormal types may be present.

Sickle Cell Disease. This recessive, hereditary blood disorder is characterized by erythrocytes that contain Hb-S. It occurs in two forms, sickle cell trait and sickle cell anemia. *Sickle cell trait* is a heterozygous state; the individual has inherited the Hb-S gene from only one parent. Only a small amount of the individual's hemoglobin is type Hb-S. The person with sickle cell trait usually does not manifest symptoms of sickling except in some very stressful situations, especially those that cause hypoxia. He or she is a carrier, and there is a 50 per cent chance that offspring will inherit the sickle cell trait (see Table 12–12).

Sickle cell anemia occurs because the individual is homozygous for Hb-S — that is, a gene for the abnormal hemoglobin has been inherited from each parent (see Table 12–12). A large amount of hemoglobin S is present.

The disease affects both males and females and occurs almost exclusively in blacks.

Hemoglobin S is less soluble than normal hemoglobin, especially when it gives up its oxygen to become reduced oxyhemoglobin, and when the pH is below normal. Firm crystals form within the cells which are distorted and become crescent-shaped (like a sickle). The blood becomes thicker, heavier and sticky and will not flow as readily through the capillaries. Circulatory stagnation and the thrombosis that may result lead to a greater reduction of the oxyhemoglobin and ensuing local metabolic acidosis (reduced pH). Sickle cells are more fragile and hemolyze readily. Their life span is about 26 to 35 days, as compared with the 120-day life span of normal erythrocytes. These effects promote more sickling and tend to set up a vicious circle. Sickling and vascular occlusion resulting in an infarcted area may occur in any tissue or organ; the severity and site are not predictable. Frequent sites are the lower limbs, joints, kidneys, mesentery, lungs and brain.

Signs and Symptoms. The individual usually has symptom-free periods alternated with exacerbations. There is a continuous premature destruction of red blood cells, resulting in a hemoglobin level of approximately 7 to 10 Gm per cent, increased bilirubin in the blood, reticulocytosis, enlargement of the spleen and liver and hyperplasia of the red bone marrow. At intervals, an exacerbation or acute episode, referred to as sickle cell crisis, occurs. It is frequently precipitated by an infection, stress, dehydration, exposure to cold, acidosis, or any situation in which the individual experiences hypoxia. The acute episode is characterized by sickling, circulatory stagnation and thrombosis. Pain, swelling and impaired function develop in whatever area suffers the interrupted blood supply. The individual is irritable and weak and develops a fever. Jaundice is evident with the increased hemolysis. The symptoms may be quite similar to those of many diseases; for example, if the vascular occlusion occurs in the mesentery, the condition may be mistaken for appendicitis because of the acute abdominal pain and tenderness unless the individual is known to have sickle cell disease. Occlusion of kidney vessels may destroy some nephrons, resulting in renal insufficiency. Obstruction of a cerebral artery may cause some paralysis or reduced mental ability. Growth is retarded

TABLE 12–12   POSSIBILITIES OF INHERITANCE IN SICKLE CELL DISEASE*

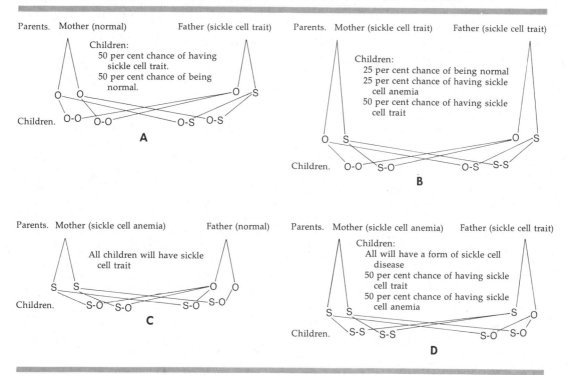

*S = gene for sickle cell trait; O = gene for normal erythrocyte.

and the individual tends to develop a thin short trunk, long extremities, narrow shoulders and hips and increased anterior-posterior diameter of the chest. Symptoms do not usually appear within the first 6 months of life because the individual is protected from sickling during this period by the hemoglobin F that is still present in the erythrocytes.

Nursing Responsibilities. During quiescent periods, care is directed toward the prevention of infection and situations that may initiate a crisis. Parents and the individual, when old enough, are advised of the nature of the disease, the importance of prophylactic care during remissions and the factors that may precipitate a crisis. The affected person is encouraged to live as normal a life as possible, but to avoid chilling, contact with infected persons, high altitude, overfatigue and stressful situations. A well-balanced, nutritious diet, adequate fluids and plenty of regular rest are important. Proper dental hygiene and immunization against infectious disease are stressed.

Regular visits to the clinic or the doctor are necessary for physical and blood examinations. In the case of the school child, the teacher should be informed of the child's problem. Identification indicating that the individual has sickle cell disease should be carried or worn at all times; as cited previously, presenting symptoms are similar to those of many other disorders. Membership may be acquired in the Medic-Alert Foundation. The member is provided with a bracelet or pendant to be worn which indicates the condition and the number of the file from which information can be obtained.

Care during a crisis includes bed rest, analgesics for the relief of pain and increased fluid intake. Clear fluids are given orally but, if they are not tolerated, intravenous infusions are used. A close check is kept on the vital signs and urinary output, and for the appearance of "new" signs and symptoms. If the anemia is severe, the patient may receive blood transfusions and oxygen. Oxygen is used only during the acute emergency period, since prolonged use and the ensuing high oxygen concentration in the blood may cause suppression of erythropoiesis.

Thalassemia. Synonyms that may be used for this type of anemia are Mediterranean anemia, Cooley's anemia and hereditary leptocytosis.

This disease occurs in two forms, major and minor, and is seen most frequently in persons of the Mediterranean countries and Southeast Asia. Both forms have the common feature of a genetically determined defect in the cellular synthesis of the globin fraction of the hemoglobin. The red blood cells are smaller than normal, fragile, irregular in shape and deficient in hemoglobin. A large percentage of the hemoglobin is of the fetal type (Hb-F). Hemoglobin A occurs in a greater amount and there is much less Hb-A than is found in normal erythrocytes.

Thalassemia major, also referred to as Cooley's anemia, is a homozygous state; a gene for the thalassemia trait has been received from each parent. The disorder is manifested in infancy or early childhood. Fortunately, this form of the disease is of lesser incidence than thalassemia minor. It produces very severe anemia and marked hyperplasia of the red bone marrow and may cause pain in the bones. Reticulocytosis occurs and immature nucleated red blood cells may appear in the circulation. The spleen and liver are enlarged as a result of the rapid hemolysis of the abnormal red blood cells, and jaundice may be apparent. The serum bilirubin level is elevated. Growth and development are retarded, and the child does not usually survive beyond early childhood. Treatment consists mainly of blood transfusions.

Thalassemia minor is a heterozygous state and is less severe. The red blood cells are smaller than normal but are less deficient in hemoglobin than those of the major type, and there is less premature hemolysis. The degree of anemia varies greatly in affected persons; some may be asymptomatic and live a normal life, with their disease only being detected by a blood cell examination. Others may be handicapped to some degree by anemia.

HEMOLYTIC ANEMIA DUE TO EXTRACORPUSCULAR FACTORS. Extrinsic mechanisms that may cause hemolysis include (a) some infections, (b) immune bodies, and (c) certain drugs and chemicals.

a. An increased rate of erythrocyte destruction may be associated with severe infections caused by the hemolytic streptococci, *Staphylococcus aureus*, pneumococcus, *Clostridium perfringens (Bacillus welchii)* and some viruses. Excessive hemolysis may also accompany malaria. The red blood cells may be damaged by the pathogenic organisms or their toxins.

b. Hemolytic anemia may be caused by antibodies which may be acquired or may be developed in response to an endogenous or exogenous antigen. Erythroblastosis fetalis (hemolytic disease of the newborn) is an example of hemolytic anemia occurring as a result of acquired antibodies (see p. 225).

When a person develops antibodies that result in the destruction of his own erythrocytes, the condition is referred to as autoimmune hemolytic anemia. Frequently, the cause of this condition is not known. In many instances, it is secondary to a collagen disease (e.g., lupus erythematosus) or to a disease involving lymphoid tissue (e.g., Hodgkin's disease). The agglutinins adhere to the red blood cells, predisposing them to entrapment and destruction, especially in the spleen and liver.

c. Hemolytic jaundice may develop in some persons receiving preparations of quinine, sulfonamide and phenacetin. Its incidence has also been reported in persons exposed to insecticides, arsenic, and coal tar products such as aniline dyes and toluene. The mechanism by which certain drugs and chemicals produce hemolysis in some persons is not known.

Treatment of autoimmune hemolytic anemia includes blood transfusions, splenectomy to reduce the trapping and destruction of the red blood cells, and the administration of a corticoid preparation such as prednisone to decrease sensitivity and antibody formation.

C. Anemia Due to Blood Loss

The loss of blood removes erythrocytes from the circulation, reducing the oxygen-carrying capacity of the blood. A blood count taken immediately after a hemorrhage does not reflect the degree of anemia since the total intravascular volume is reduced. Over a period of 24 to 48 hours, the intravascular volume is restored by the entrance of extracellular fluid into the vascular compartment and probably by intravenous infusion. The red blood cells at this time are those that remained after the blood loss and are now dispersed in a greater volume of plasma. The count (per mm.) now gives a more accurate indication of the severity of the anemia.

Normally, the bone marrow responds quickly to the tissue hypoxia, and the erythrocyte count returns to normal over a period of 4 to 5 weeks. At first, more than the normal number of reticulocytes are in circulation and some immature nucleated normoblasts may also be released. Since considerable iron is lost from the body in hemorrhage, hemoglobin production may lag behind red blood cell production. The administration of an iron preparation may be necessary to bring the hemoglobin concentration back to normal.

If the blood loss is 20 per cent or more of the total blood volume, rapid replacement by means of a blood transfusion is necessary. This quickly increases the total circulating volume as well as the number of erythrocytes to carry oxygen.

In cases of chronic blood loss in which there is a continuous loss of a relatively small amount over a long period, the bone marrow may keep the erythrocyte count close to normal. The continuous loss of iron, however, creates a deficiency of that essential element, and the erythrocytes in circulation are small and lack a full complement of hemoglobin. The anemia may be described as microcytic-hypochromic. Treatment includes correction of the cause of the bleeding and the administration of an iron preparation such as ferrous sulfate.

Nursing in Anemia

The care required by the anemia patient varies with the severity and cause of his disease. The anemia may not be severe enough to necessitate bed rest or hospitalization. It may be chronic, as in pernicious and sickle cell anemia, resulting in the patient's need for continuous treatment and supervision and modification in his way of life. With some, their anemia may be entirely cured by correction of the cause. Depending on the etiologic factor, there may be symptoms and problems in addition to those attributable to anemia. For example, in hemolytic anemia there may be the problem of jaundice; in the sickle cell type there is the serious problem of vascular obstruction. Regardless of the type of anemia, the patients have one common difficulty, namely, a decreased capacity of their blood to transport oxygen.

1. AIMS. Care is directed toward eliminating the cause, increasing the oxygen-carrying capacity of the blood, reducing the demand for oxygen, alleviating the discomforts experienced by the patient, preventing complications and, when the disease is chronic, helping the patient to live a life that is as useful and satisfying as his condition will permit.

The following considerations are not necessarily applicable to all anemia patients nor are they all-inclusive. As well as adapting the care to the individual, the severity and type of his anemia must be considered.

2. REST. Energy expenditure is reduced in order to decrease the demand for oxygen. The anemic patient fatigues quickly, may complain of lightheadedness or may faint on exertion. The ambulatory patient is encouraged to lighten his activity load and rest at intervals throughout the day. With severe anemia bed rest is necessary until the red blood cells and hemoglobin increase and there is less evidence of hypoxia. An explanation of the basis of the fatigue and weakness and the importance of rest may help the patient through this difficult period. Nursing care is planned to conserve the patient's energy; uninterrupted periods of rest, assistance in turning and feeding, and a restricted number of visitors for brief periods only are important factors. Activity short of fatigue and breathlessness is encouraged.

3. OBSERVATIONS. The patient with pernicious anemia is observed for signs of degenerative changes in his nervous system. Any complaint of tingling, numbness and sensations of "pins and needles" in distal portions of the extremities, loss of finer movements, difficulty in holding small objects, weakness of limbs, ataxia and impaired vision are immediately recorded and brought to the doctor's attention. The patient's tolerance for activity is noted.

The color of the patient's sclerae and skin is noted daily for pallor and, in the case of hemolytic anemia, for initial or increasing jaundice.

If the patient has sickle cell anemia, frequent close observation is made for swollen, tender and painful areas, and changes in body functions or the patient's mental and physical abilities that may indicate areas of thrombotic disease.

Reports of laboratory studies are followed and nursing measures adapted to indicated changes. For example, a decrease in the hemoglobin, hematocrit or erythrocyte count may be such that the patient's activity should be further reduced.

4. NUTRITION AND FLUIDS. Diet has an important role in erythropoiesis. It should be light, easily digestible and selected to provide the protein, iron, vitamins and other elements necessary for the production of red blood cells and hemoglobin. Anorexia frequently poses a problem. It is helpful to discuss with the patient the importance of foods in increasing the red cells and hemoglobin and to determine his food preferences. Small portions offered five or six times a day may be more acceptable than the usual three meals. If the patient's mouth, tongue and esophagus are sore, roughage and hot and spiced foods are avoided. Mouth care just before the food is served, remaining with the patient, provision of the necessary assistance if weakness is a problem, and a well ventilated, neat environment that is free of commotion and disturbing sights are conducive to having the patient take his food.

Extra fluids are important for the patient with hemolytic anemia, especially sickle cell, to counteract the increased blood viscosity and circulatory stagnation. The daily fluid intake is recorded. If an adequate oral intake is not tolerated, an intravenous infusion is given.

5. RESPIRATORY SUPPORT. Severe anemia may cause shortness of breath or dyspnea. The patient may be more comfortable with the head of the bed elevated and the room well ventilated. If the dyspnea is present with the patient at rest, oxygen administration may be necessary. Sufficient assistance is given the patient to avoid unnecessary expenditure of energy and increased oxygen demand. A blood transfusion of packed cells may be given to increase the oxygen-carrying capacity.

6. MOUTH CARE. In pernicious and iron deficiency anemias, a common problem is ulcerative lesions of the oral mucosa and a sore "raw" tongue. Frequent cool, mildly alkaline mouthwashes are necessary. A soft-bristled toothbrush or an absorbent applicator is used to clean the teeth. The mouth is cleansed before and after taking nourishment. As cited above, roughage and hot spicy foods are avoided.

7. SKIN CARE. The skin is more susceptible to pressure and breaks down readily because of the reduced oxygen supply in the tissues. If the patient is confined to bed, his position is changed every 1 to 2 hours; pressure areas receive frequent, gentle massage and are protected by the use of sponge rubber, sheepskin or an alternating air pressure mattress (ripple mattress).

If the anemia is hemolytic, there may be jaundice and pruritus (itching of the skin). Slightly warm or tepid water is used for bathing. Sodium bicarbonate added to the bath water, or oatmeal that is tied in a gauze bag and squeezed through the water, may help to relieve the irritation. The use of soap is avoided. Calamine lotion or caladryl may be applied for relief. The patient's fingernails are kept short and clean to prevent excoriation and infection of the skin should the patient scratch the irritated areas.

8. WARMTH. As a result of the reduced amount of oxygen available for metabolism, the anemia patient produces less body heat. He may require extra clothing and bedding and a warm, ventilated room. Local heat applications are rarely used, especially with the pernicious anemia patient, since he may have some sensory loss.

9. PAIN AND HEADACHE. Patients with anemia frequently experience severe headache as a result of the cerebral hypoxia. Symptomatic relief measures are used; the patient is encouraged to remain quiet and inactive; environmental stimuli such as bright light and noise are reduced to a minimum. Cold compresses may be helpful and an analgesic such as aspirin or acetaminophen (Tylenol) is prescribed.

Hyperplasia of the red bone marrow is associated with anemia; the increased production of marrow cells in response to the concomitant hypoxia results in pressure from the volume of tissue, which causes pain. A cradle is used to protect the site from the weight of the bedclothes. Local heat application may provide some relief and an analgesic is prescribed.

10. PREVENTION OF INFECTION. The patient with severe anemia is more susceptible to infections. Consideration is given to his placement in the hospital ward to avoid contact with a patient with infection. Visitors and personnel with any infection, such as a cold or sore throat, should not be permitted contact with the patient. The person with aplastic anemia is placed in reverse isolation since he is lacking leukocytes to provide him ordinary protection.

11. MEDICATIONS. Various medications are used in the treatment of anemia. The drug used depends on the cause and type of the anemia. These drugs have been cited in the preceding discussion of the various types of anemia. The principal antianemic drugs are preparations of iron, vitamin B_{12} and folic acid.

12. BLOOD TRANSFUSION. In severe anemia the patient may require a blood transfusion. Unless the anemia is due to blood loss, there is a danger of overloading the circulation if whole blood is given. It must be given very slowly and the patient's pulse and respirations checked frequently. In most instances, unless there has been a blood loss, packed cells are used.

13. INSTRUCTION. An explanation of the nature of the disorder is made to the patient and family; the symptoms such as weakness, fatigue, and shortness of breath are related to his anemia and the resulting deficiency of oxygen. They are advised of the importance of good nutrition. A printed outline of the important foods is provided, meal planning and foods that should be included to promote red blood cell and hemoglobin production are discussed.

If the anemia is chronic, regular visits to the doctor or clinic are stressed. The necessity of maintenance doses of vitamin B_{12} is explained to the pernicious anemia patient; even though he feels well he must not omit the prescribed vitamin B_{12}. If the disease is severe and a weekly injection is prescribed, a referral may be made to the visiting nurse organization so the patient may receive the drug at home rather than having to go to the clinic so frequently.

In the case of sickle cell anemia, the parents receive an explanation of the disease and factors that predispose to crises, and instruction is given as to the care of the affected child (see p. 237).

14. PSYCHOLOGICAL SUPPORT. The patient may be depressed and concerned about his future; the fatigue and inability to achieve prove discouraging. The nurse listens to the patient and provides reassurance that much can be done to restore his blood cells and that everything possible will be done. Patients with chronic anemia usually regain confidence and enthusiasm readily as they become aware of the improvement in the amount of energy they have and in the way they feel.

15. SPLENECTOMY. The spleen is removed in some hemolytic anemias. Preparation of the patient for surgery is similar to that for any abdominal surgery (see p. 164). The postoperative care includes that which is necessary for any patient who undergoes intra-abdominal surgery (see p. 178). The close proximity and attachment of the spleen to the diaphragm may temporarily affect diaphragmatic function and may result in reduced expansion of the left lung. Regular deep breathing, coughing and turning are important in preventing respiratory complications. Since the spleen exerts some influence on the production and liberation of cells from the marrow, there may be a marked increase in the number of thrombocytes in circulation following splenectomy, predisposing to thrombus formation. Optimal hydration to avoid hemoconcentration, frequent change of position, bed exercises and early ambulation to prevent stasis are important considerations in the postoperative nursing.

Polycythemia

An excessive number of erythrocytes and a corresponding increase in the concentration of hemoglobin is referred to as polycythemia. The red blood cell count may be 7 to 10 million per cu. mm. with a hemoglobin concentration of 18 to 25 Gm. per cent. The condition may be primary or secondary.

Secondary polycythemia is referred to as *erythrocytosis;* it is a physiological compensatory increase in the number of erythrocytes by the red bone marrow in response to a low concentration of oxygen in the blood. It occurs normally at high altitudes where the atmospheric oxygen tension is low, and in pathologic conditions in which there is inadequate oxygenation of the blood. Examples of the latter are congenital malformations of the heart which lead to blood bypassing the pulmonary-circulatory system and pulmonary conditions that interfere with normal gas exchange (e.g., emphysema).

Primary polycythemia is known as *polycythemia vera;* it is a rare proliferative disorder of the red bone marrow in which there is an uncontrolled production of an excessive number of red blood cells and hemoglobin. It may be accompanied by some overproduction of myelocytes (leukocytes produced by the marrow) and thrombocytes. The cause is unknown. The onset is usually in middle-aged persons, with a higher incidence in males and Jewish persons.

Signs and Symptoms

Polycythemia vera increases the total volume and viscosity of the blood. The blood pressure is elevated and the work load of the heart is increased. The rate of flow through the vessels is reduced and, with the increased number of thrombocytes and blood viscosity, predisposes to the development of thrombi. Occlusion of a vessel may occur, causing a cerebral vascular accident, coronary thrombosis, pulmonary infarction or gangrene of a limb. Heart failure may develop insidiously as a result of the increased cardiac demands. The spleen enlarges because of the increased number of red blood cells to be destroyed.

Symptoms vary greatly with patients; the individual may not experience any discomfort and be totally unaware of any problem until the excessive number of erythrocytes are discovered during the course of a regular physical examination. Symptoms may include headache, dizziness, a full feeling in the head, weakness and ready fatigue. The patient may complain of pruritus, especially after a hot bath, and pain in the bones as a result of hyperplasia of the red bone marrow. A high color (deep dusky red) is manifested in the lips, nose, cheeks, ears and neck. The distal parts of the limbs (especially lower) may be cyanotic at times, owing to the sluggish circulation incurred by the increased viscosity of the blood. These patients also have a tendency to develop a peptic ulcer which is attributed to an associated increase in gastric secretions.

Treatment and Care

Treatment and care of patients with polycythemia vera are aimed at decreasing the activity of the red bone marrow and at reducing the volume and viscosity of the blood. Radioactive phosphorus (P^{32}), which is taken up by the bone marrow cells, may be administered to suppress the bone marrow. Irradiation of the long bones by x-rays may be used.

Drugs such as nitrogen mustard, busulfan (Myleran) or cyclophosphamide (Cytoxan) may also be given to inhibit erythropoiesis. A phlebotomy (venesection) may be done at regular intervals to provide a temporary reduction in the blood volume. Five hundred to 1000 ml. may be withdrawn each time. The regular blood bank equipment for the collection of blood is used, and the blood is donated to the bank. Red and glandular meats and iron-containing foods are restricted in the patient's diet.

These persons are not usually hospitalized until a complication such as thrombosis, peptic ulcer or cardiac insufficiency develops. A reasonable amount of activity is encouraged to prevent circulatory stasis. They are advised of the need for regular, frequent visits to their physician or the clinic for close supervision. The family and patient are alerted to early indications of impending complications and advised of the importance of promptly getting in touch with the physician.

LEUKOCYTE DISORDERS

Alterations in the number of leukocytes may involve an increased or decreased production of the cells.

Leukocytosis

The number of leukocytes in circulation normally increases to a level in excess of the normal (7,000 to 10,000 per cu. mm.) in defense of the body in most infections and in response to necrotic tissue. This increase is referred to as leukocytosis and is usually predominant in one type of white cell. Information as to which type of leukocytes are in excess of the normal provides significant information for the physician, since some leukocytoses are known to be associated with certain pathologic conditions. For instance, neutrophil leukocytosis normally develops quickly in response to most infections (e.g., appendicitis, pneumonia) and tissue destruction (e.g., myocardial infarction); lymphocytosis is characteristic of certain infections such as measles, mumps, pertussis, and infectious hepatitis; and an increase in eosinophils (eosinophilia) accompanies many allergic conditions. The white blood cell count returns to normal when the infection is checked, the necrotic tissue is disposed of, or the initiating factor, such as an allergen, is removed.

Leukemia

Normal leukocytes progress from differentiated, proliferating blast cells (myeloblasts, lymphoblasts, monoblasts) to mature, nonproliferating, functioning white blood cells. Leukemia is a disease in which there is an excessive uncontrolled production of leukocytes in blast form. They continue to proliferate and remain immature, and consequently are unable to perform their normal functions. The cell production is comparable to the uncontrolled production of cells in malignant neoplastic disease. For this reason leukemia is sometimes referred to as cancer of the blood.

There usually is a marked increase in the number of leukocytes in circulation, and many of these are immature and abnormal. Their inability to perform their normal role in body defense makes the individual very susceptible to infection. Hyperplasia of the hemopoietic tissue and the accumulation of leukoblasts within it hamper the formation and maturation of erythrocytes and thrombocytes, leading to anemia and thrombocytopenia. The circulating leukemic cells infiltrate organs and tissues and cause dysfunction in these areas. The liver, spleen and lymph nodes enlarge. The enlargement of viscera, in addition to hyperplasia of the bone marrow, causes discomfort, pain and interference with neighboring structures.

The marked overproduction of leukocytes and the rapid rate of their destruction result in an increase in the body's metabolic rate. The use of certain substances in the proliferation of these cells deprives other cells of essential metabolic elements, and the increased amount of cell destruction increases the concentration of metabolic wastes.

Types of Leukemia

Leukemia may affect the production of granulocytes, monocytes or lymphocytes. The disease is classified according to the type of leukocyte involved and whether the process is acute or chronic. It may be *acute or chronic myelocytic* or *granulocytic leukemia,* or it may be *acute or chronic lymphocytic*

leukemia. Acute and chronic monocytic leukemia have a lesser incidence than any of the preceding types.

Acute leukemia is seen more often in children and young adults, with the lymphocytic form being the most common type in children.[13] The highest incidence of acute lymphocytic leukemia occurs in the first 5 years of life.[14] Chronic leukemia develops more often in persons over 40 years of age and there is a greater frequency of the chronic form of the disease, especially lymphocytic, in males.

While intensive research continues to search for the cause of leukemia and for a means of preventing and curing the disorder, chemotherapeutic agents used in recent years have produced remissions and prolonged the life of those with acute leukemia. The therapeutic regimen is directed toward reducing the production of leukemic cells and preventing associated complications, such as infection, anemia and hemorrhage. The chronic forms of the disease progress slowly, are less malignant and manifest more normal mature leukocytes in the blood.

Etiology

Leukemia is considered to be a fatal disease of unknown etiology in most instances. There is significant evidence that overexposure to ionizing radiation is the causative factor in some cases. This is substantiated by the high incidence of leukemia found in the survivors of the Hiroshima and Nagasaki atomic bombing, radiologists, and patients with ankylosing spondylitis (arthritis of the spine) who were treated by x-ray radiation. Viruses and absorption of the chemicals benzol, pyridine and aniline dyes have been strongly suspected of being leukemogenic. Guyton states that regardless of the initial cause, the uncontrolled production of leukocytes is the result of a cancerous mutation of a myelogenous or a lymphogenous cell.[15] Studies have shown that chromosomal abnormalities are present in the leukocytes involved.

[13]Genevieve Foley and Ann Marie McCarthy: "The Child with Leukemia — The Disease and Its Treatment." Am. J. Nurs., Vol. 76, No. 7 (July 1976), p. 1109.

[14]Krupp and Chatton, op. cit., p. 292.

[15]Guyton: op. cit., p. 75.

Manifestations

Acute leukemia usually has an abrupt onset that is frequently accompanied by weakness, general malaise and nonspecific complaints. Fever, excessive perspiration, lowered heat tolerance, tachycardia and weight loss develop because of the increased metabolic rate. Bone marrow dysfunction and the resulting anemia are manifested by pallor, shortness of breath, extreme fatigue, weakness and palpitation. External and internal bleeding may occur due to the reduced production of thrombocytes. Bleeding of the gums, nose and gastrointestinal tract is common. Petechiae or ecchymoses may appear as further evidence of the reduced ability of the blood to coagulate. The patient with myelogenous leukemia will most likely complain of tenderness and pain in the long bones and sternum from the hyperplasia and crowding in the bone marrow.

Although there is an excessive number of leukocytes, they are immature and do not provide the normal defense against infection; the patient may complain of a sore mouth and throat which exhibit infected necrotic ulcers. An acute infection such as pneumonia, septicemia or perirectal abscess may develop. The spleen and liver enlarge and, in the later stages, infiltration of the leukemic cells into the kidneys may cause renal insufficiency. Renal dysfunction also occurs as a result of the excessive blood concentration of uric acid produced by the rapid destruction of the leukocytes. Urate crystals may form and obstruct renal tubules. Sensory and motor disturbances, severe headache, convulsions or disorientation may occur, indicating central nervous system involvement. Lymph nodes enlarge and are tender, owing to infiltration by the leukemic cells. This may be readily detected in the axillary, cervical and inguinal lymph nodes.

The leukocyte count varies greatly but is usually above normal and may exceed 100,000 per cu. mm. In some instances, the count is within normal levels or may even be below normal. This is attributed to the bone marrow retaining the leukocytes because of their immature state; normally, they are not released until mature. The erythrocyte and thrombocyte counts are abnormally low. A specimen of aspirated bone marrow demonstrates the proliferation of leukemic cells.

The *chronic forms of leukemia* have an insidious onset, but are slowly progressive. They may go unrecognized for a lengthy period. The discovery is often made when the individual undergoes a regular physical checkup or is being investigated for some unrelated condition.

Chronic myelocytic (granulocytic) leukemia is manifested by a progressive development of weakness, loss of weight, anemia and thrombocytopenia. The granulocytes are in excess and upon examination reveal a deficiency of alkaline phosphatase and glycogen and an increased histamine content. An abnormality is consistently recognized in chromosome 21 or 22 (Philadelphia chromosome) of the cells produced by the bone marrow of patients with this chronic form of leukemia.[16] In the advanced stage of the disorder, the enlarged spleen may cause considerable discomfort; an infarction within it may precipitate acute, severe pain in the upper left abdomen. Large ecchymoses and other signs of bleeding appear. The temperature is elevated and the patient becomes progressively weaker because of the increased anemia. In this later stage the number of immature granulocytes (myeloblasts) in circulation shows a marked increase. Pain is experienced in the sternum and long bones owing to marrow hyperplasia.

The rate at which *chronic lymphocytic leukemia* progressively develops varies with patients. Some remain free of symptoms and in relatively good health with only mild anemia and a moderate increase in lymphocytes for several years. In others the leukemic process slowly but steadily increases in severity. The blood picture is one of an increased leukocyte count, with small atypical lymphocytes predominating. There is a decrease below normal in erythrocytes and thrombocytes. The patient experiences recurring infections because the immune and defense mechanisms are impaired; antibodies are not formed in antigenic response to organisms. The spleen, liver and lymph nodes enlarge; pressure on neighboring structures may cause impaired function, discomfort and pain. In the advanced stage many more immature lymphocytes (lymphoblasts) appear in the circulation, and the anemia and deficiency of thrombocytes become severe.

[16]John Macleod (Ed.): Davidson's Principles and Practice of Medicine, 11th ed. Edinburgh, Churchill Livingstone, 1974, p. 12.

Treatment and Nursing Care of the Patient with Leukemia

The treatment and care of the patient with leukemia are directed toward suppressing the abnormal cell production, the prevention of complications (infection and hemorrhage), and supporting the patient physiologically and psychologically.

ACUTE LEUKEMIA

1. DRUG THERAPY. The chemotherapeutic program for the patient with acute leukemia involves a variety of drugs which are given in combinations or singly. Administration usually extends over a period of 3 years. Antileukemic agents act by interfering with cell mitosis and the synthesis of the leukocyte cellular substance, and by depressing the red bone marrow. Unfortunately they affect normal cells, especially those which reproduce rapidly (e.g., mucous membrane, erythrocytes), in addition to leukemic cells, and produce serious side effects with which the nurse must be familiar as they necessitate physiological and psychological supportive measures. Drugs used in acute leukemia include vincristine sulfate (Oncovin), prednisone, L-asparaginase, methotrexate (amethopterin), 6-mercaptopurine (Purinethol), cyclophosphamide (Cytoxan), daunorubicin (daunomycin, rubidomycin), cytosine arabinoside (Ara-C, Cytosar), busulfan (Myleran), and thioguanine (6-thioguanine) (see Table 12–13). The most common side effects associated with these chemotherapeutic agents are nausea, vomiting, stomatitis and ulceration, alopecia (loss of hair), change in bowel habit (diarrhea or constipation) and bone marrow suppression that predisposes the individual to infection and hemorrhage.

An example of a therapeutic regimen that may be prescribed follows.[17-19] The patient is advised of the possible side effects or, in the case of a minor, they are discussed with the parents. A signed consent is usually required. Initially the patient receives vincristine and prednisone for 2 to 4 weeks to induce a remission, evidenced by a marked reduction or total absence of leukemic cells in the blood and bone marrow. Vincristine is given intravenously weekly and the patient is observed for possible side effects which include alopecia, abdominal cramps, constipation and neurological disturbances. Signs and symptoms of neurological disturbances are an abnormal gait, stumbling, a decrease in reflex responses, loss of coordination, paralysis and paralytic ileus. Prednisone, an adrenocorticosteroid, is given by mouth daily. Its serious side effect is the individual's increased susceptibility to infection. Gastric distress and ulceration may develop but may be prevented if the drug is given with milk or an antacid preparation such as Maalox.

When the course of vincristine and prednisone is completed, the patient is started on L-asparaginase. This is an enzyme preparation that destroys the amino acid L-asparagine, which is an important element in leukemic cell activity. L-Asparaginase is given intravenously each day to reinforce the remission. During the period in which it is being given the bone marrow recovers its ability to produce normal blood cells, since this drug does not have the side effect of bone marrow depression. When given it may produce the serious side effects of anaphylactic shock (see p. 50) and impaired liver and pancreatic function. Psychological depression may also develop. The blood glucose level is checked frequently for a possible abnormal elevation.

Infiltration of the central nervous system by leukemic cells may be referred to as "central nervous system leukemia." It usually develops late in the disease and may be manifested by headache, nausea, vomiting, exaggerated reflex responses, irritability, disorientation, papilledema[20] and head retraction with rigidity of the neck. The drugs cited above (vincristine, prednisone and L-asparaginase) are ineffective in destroying the leukemic cells which infiltrate into the brain and cervical area of the cord. This ineffectiveness is attributed to the limited amount of those drugs that crosses the blood-brain barrier, which is readily traversed by the leukemic cells. The therapeutic program usually includes prophylactic measures before central nervous system leukemia becomes evident.

[17]Paul B. Beeson and Walsh McDermott (Eds.): Textbook of Medicine, 14th ed. Philadelphia, W. B. Saunders, 1975, pp. 1490–1491.

[18]Edgar C. Boedeker and James H. Dauber (Eds.): Manual of Medical Therapeutics, 21st ed. Boston, Little, Brown, 1974, pp. 311–314.

[19]Foley and McCarthy, op. cit., pp. 1110–1113.

[20]*Papilledema*, also referred to as choked disk, is hyperemia and edema of the optic disk and is usually associated with increased intracranial pressure.

TABLE 12–13   ANTILEUKEMIC AGENTS

Agent	Classification	Administration	Potential Side Effects
Vincristine (Oncovin)	Plant alkaloid Inhibits mitosis of leukemic cells	Intravenous	Alopecia Abdominal cramps Constipation Nervous system disturbances: hyporeflexia, abnormal gait, loss of coordination, stumbling, paralysis, paralytic ileus
Prednisone	Hormone—an adreno-corticosteroid Retards leukemic cell reproduction	Oral	Gastric distress and ulceration Decreased immune responses and increased susceptibility to infection Retention of fluid
L-Asparaginase	Enzyme Deprives leukemic cells of amino acid L-asparagine	Intravenous	Anaphylactic shock Allergic reactions Impaired liver and pancreatic functions (hyperglycemia) Depression (psychological)
Methotrexate (amethopterin)	Folic acid analogue Deprives leukemic cells of folic acid	Oral Intravenous Intrathecal	Bone marrow depression Oral and gastrointestinal ulceration and bleeding Nausea, vomiting, diarrhea Dermatitis Impaired liver function Alopecia
6-Mercaptopurine	Purine analogue Deprives leukemic cells of essential purine	Oral Intravenous	Bone marrow depression Nausea and vomiting Intestinal ulceration Dermatitis
Cyclophosphamide (Cytoxan)	Alkylating agent Suppresses leukemic cell reproduction	Oral Intravenous	Bone marrow depression Hemorrhagic cystitis Alopecia
Daunorubicin (daunomycin, rubidomycin)	Antibiotic Inhibits synthesis of normal cellular substance (DIVA)	Intravenous	Nausea and vomiting Stomatitis Bone marrow depression Cardiac arrhythmia
Cytosine arabinoside (cytarabine; Ara-C, Cytosar)	Pyrimidine analogue	Intravenous Intrathecal Subcutaneous	Nausea and vomiting Bone marrow depression Stomatitis and ulceration Impaired liver function
Thioguanine	Purine analogue	Oral	Bone marrow depression Stomatitis Hepatitis
Busulfan (Myleran)	Alkylating agent Interferes with mitosis	Oral	Bone marrow depression Alopecia Nausea, vomiting, diarrhea Stomatitis Pulmonary fibrosis Hyperpigmentation of the skin
Chlorambucil	Alkylating agent Antimetabolic action	Oral	Nausea and vomiting Bone marrow depression
Hydroxyurea	Antimetabolic	Oral	Nausea and vomiting Bone marrow depression Skin changes Stomatitis Alopecia

During the first 6 to 8 weeks following diagnosis, the patient may receive methotrexate intrathecally and a series of cranial radiation treatments.

Following the course of L-asparaginase a drug or combination of drugs is administered to maintain the remission. The drugs, prescribed singly or in combination as maintenance therapy, may be methotrexate, which may be given orally or by intravenous twice weekly; 6-mercaptopurine, which may be given orally daily; and cyclophosphamide, which may be given orally daily. Reactions frequently accompany the use of these drugs, with nausea and vomiting being the most common problem. The patient receiving methotrexate is observed for anemia, hemorrhage and infection because of the potential bone marrow and antibody suppression. He may also develop oral and gastrointestinal ulceration. The latter may be manifested by abdominal discomfort and pain, vomiting, hematemesis, diarrhea and blood in the stool. Liver function may be impaired. Mercaptopurine may cause bone marrow depression and intestinal ulceration. Cyclophosphamide may depress the bone marrow and also causes alopecia. It is eliminated in the urine and may result in severe hemorrhagic cystitis unless well diluted by an adequate daily fluid intake (a minimum of 3000 ml.). In order to provide an adequate fluid intake, an antiemetic preparation such as dimenhydrinate (Gravol, Dramamine) may be ordered to counteract nausea and vomiting, or an intravenous infusion may be given.

If the patient remains free of leukemic cells, the drug therapy may be discontinued at the end of 3 years.

The drug regimen cited above (i.e., vincristine, prednisone, L-asparaginase, methotrexate, cyclophosphamide) may be prescribed for the patient with any type of acute leukemia, but its most encouraging results have been with acute lymphocytic leukemia.[21] Cytosine arabinoside (cytarabine), thioguanine, daunorubicin, and cyclophosphamide may be the chemotherapeutic agents used in the treatment of acute myelocytic leukemia.

Nursing responsibilities associated with drug therapy include the following. It is important that the nurse be familiar with the expected action, route of administration used and the potential side effects of the antileukemic agents. The patient is advised of the possible effects, that support will be provided and that those drugs now available do bring about a remission and permit the individual to leave the hospital and resume many former activities. Opportunities are provided for the patient to ask questions and discuss his feelings about his therapy and reactions to it. If the patient's need for information and assurance are not met he becomes resentful, frustrated and depressed.

A frequent assessment is made of the patient for changes and manifestations of reactions to the drug(s). Nursing measures are instituted promptly to provide necessary support and relief. For example, when the patient complains of nausea, prompt administration of an antiemetic that has been ordered "when necessary," reduction of external stimuli by dimming the light, and leaving him undisturbed may provide relief and prevent vomiting.

Allopurinol (Zyloprim) may be prescribed if the serum uric acid level is elevated to avoid renal dysfunction. It inhibits the enzyme that promotes the formation of uric acid from the products of cellular breakdown.

2. SUPPORTIVE CARE. The care plan for a patient with acute leukemia must give consideration to the following measures.

a. *Observations.* The patient's blood cell and platelet counts and hemoglobin estimation are followed closely. A deficiency of normal leukocytes, anemia and thrombocytopenia indicate necessary modifications in patient care to prevent complications. The patient is observed for regressive changes which may appear as various organs and tissues are invaded by the leukemic cells. The vital signs are checked frequently and the patient observed for indications of infection, hemorrhage, disorientation and loss of coordination. Infection may be manifested by an elevation in temperature, increased pulse and respirations, a cough or a skin lesion. Hemorrhage may be detected by blood in the urine or stools, petechiae, ecchymoses, bleeding gums, hematemesis, or rapid weak pulse and a fall in blood pressure. The patient's emotional status is assessed daily and the amount of support and attention needed in this area determined. The fluid intake and output are recorded and the balance determined.

b. *Rest.* Unless the patient is in a remission, rest and the prevention of unnecessary expenditure of energy are important because

---

[21]Boedeker and Dauber, op. cit., p. 312.

of the increased metabolic rate associated with the rapid, excessive production and destruction of leukemic cells. The individual is also experiencing some degree of hypoxia because of anemia. The acutely ill patient requires assistance in turning and moving.

c. Blood Transfusion. Transfusions of whole blood may be given if there has been bleeding. If there has been no marked loss of blood and no decrease in the circulatory volume, transfusions of packed red blood cells are used to relieve the anemia and of platelets to control and prevent bleeding. The patient is observed closely for reactions during and immediately following the transfusions. A reaction may be manifested by a chill and fever, urticaria, severe headache, lumbar pain, dyspnea, oliguria, and discoloration of the urine due to hemoglobin released by hemolysis. If a reaction occurs the transfusion is discontinued and the physician notified promptly.

d. Protection from Infection. The individual's immunosuppression and the lack of normal defensive leukocytes make him very vulnerable to serious infection. Every effort must be made to establish precautionary measures. Reverse isolation technique is used and, preferably, the patient is cared for in a room with filtered air to reduce the possibility of airborne infection. No one with an infection should be allowed to visit or care for the patient. In addition to barrier-nursing technique, preventive measures include: (1) daily examination of the skin for possible lesions; (2) regular and frequent recording of the oral or axillary temperature and prompt reporting of an elevation; (3) avoidance of taking rectal temperature to prevent mucosal damage that provides an entry for organisms; (4) the avoidance, if possible, of parenteral administration of medications but, if it is necessary, special cleansing and protection of the skin before and after; (5) antiseptic mouth care and gentle cleansing of the teeth with a soft brush to avoid mucosal damage and ensuing infection; (6) daily bathing with a mild antiseptic soap to reduce the skin flora (the patient's own body flora of the skin, mouth, nose and intestinal tract is frequently the major source of infection); (7) keeping the nails short and clean; and (8) the avoidance of constipation and the giving of an enema to prevent possible rectal mucosal trauma. The stool may be kept soft by fruit and plenty of fluids in the diet. If necessary a stool softener such as dioctyl sodium sulfosuccinate (Colace) may be given. If a local infected area develops, a culture is made immediately so that the infecting organisms can be identified and tested for antimicrobial sensitivity in order for an effective antibiotic to be prescribed.

e. Fluids. A minimal fluid intake of 2500 to 3000 ml. per 24 hours is encouraged to promote elimination of the increased serum uric acid by the kidneys. This results from the rapid leukemic cell destruction and, unless well diluted, may crystallize in renal tubules, blocking them and impairing kidney function. An adequate fluid intake is also important if the patient's temperature is elevated. Intravenous infusion is frequently necessary in order to provide optimum hydration.

f. Nutrition. Nutrition may be a problem with the acute leukemic patient; he has anorexia and his mouth may be very sore. A high-calorie, high-vitamin diet is desirable; the overproduction of cells makes an excessive demand on body nutrients. The patient's preferences and what can be tolerated are determined from day to day. Bland, nonirritating concentrated foods and nutritious fluids are used whenever possible. Cold or iced preparations are usually more acceptable and less irritating to the mouth. When there is stomatitis, rinsing the mouth with an anesthetic mouthwash just before each meal may reduce the discomfort associated with eating.

g. Oral Hygiene. Frequent special mouth care is very important because of the patient's fever, susceptibility to infection, hemorrhage, stomatitis and ulceration that are frequent side effects of several antileukemic drugs. The mouth is rinsed every 2 hours with a mildly alkaline mouthwash. A very soft-bristled toothbrush is used to gently clean the teeth. If the mouth is very sore an irrigation setup (solution container and tube) may be necessary, with the patient in the lateral position or with the head and shoulders elevated and forward to prevent aspiration. An emollient or oil may be applied to the lips to prevent "cracking" and adherence.

h. Skin Care. Because of the fever, weakness, and susceptibility to infection, the patient's skin requires special attention. Frequent bathing is necessary to remove perspiration and organisms and provide comfort. A mild antiseptic soap may be used for its antibacterial effect. The patient's position is changed frequently to prevent pressure sores and other complications. The alternating air pressure mattress (ripple mattress) is very helpful here. Extreme gentleness is required when doing anything for the patient to avoid pressure that might precipitate bleeding into the tissues. Following an injection, pressure is applied to the site for several minutes to reduce the amount of bleeding and the formation of a hematoma.

i. Relief of Pain. The patient may experience bone pain because of the marrow hyperplasia and pain in viscera that are enlarged and swollen by infiltration by leukemic cells. Severe headache accompanies infiltration of the brain. Local applications of ice packs may be used over the painful areas and a cradle will protect the parts from the pressure and weight of bedding. The administration of an analgesic may be necessary to provide relief, particularly as the disease becomes progressively more severe.

Because of the patient's fever and lowered heat tolerance (due to increased metabolic rate) and shortness of breath (due to anemia), a cooler well ventilated environment is more comfortable for him.

j. Psychological Support. The diagnosis of acute leukemia is very difficult for the patient and family to accept. There may be situations in which there is still some question as to whether the patient should be told that he has leukemia. More and more in recent years, the nature of the disease and treatment are discussed frankly with the patient as well as the family. The nurse must know what information they have received from the physician. The therapeutic program requires cooperation and participation by them. They are advised that the blood disorder is serious but that in recent years new drugs have been made available that control the problem for most patients.

When the patient has been told of his disease and the nature of the treatment that is likely to continue over a period of 3 years, he may withdraw or manifest denial or resentment. The nurse accepts his reaction, provides opportunities for him to express his feelings and conveys a willingness to listen. He needs someone to spend time with him, listen to what he has to say and answer his questions. The nurse must be prepared to fill this role as part of the care of this patient. With someone to listen to him and discuss his problems frankly, he is more likely to arrive at

acceptance. A patient with leukemia wrote that "the briefing of the patient on his progress by medical personnel trained to impart such momentous information is, over the long haul, the best instrument by which to create optimum psychological conditions for treatment, whatever the ultimate effect of that treatment."[22]

The family will be very distressed and require sympathetic understanding and emotional support from the nurse. They are encouraged to be with the patient and to participate in his care as much as possible without overtaxing themselves or neglecting other members of the family. Active assistance tends to restore their confidence, reduce their feelings of helplessness and guilt and develop a more rational perspective for them. They may find support in a visit from their religious adviser. Discussion with a family that has a member in successful remission may contribute towards acceptance and a more positive, hopeful attitude.

k. The Patient in Remission. When the patient's condition improves and a remission of the leukemic process occurs the patient goes home. The nurse plans and implements a program of discussions with him and the family to provide direction as to the necessary care and continuing health supervision. The patient is encouraged to resume as normal a pattern of life as possible. The physician will indicate if he may return to his former employment or, in the case of a child or youth, to school. The employer or the teacher is advised of the individual's limitations; for example, those concerned should know that the continuing chemotherapy and regular clinic visits are likely to necessitate some absenteeism. Some adjustments will be necessary; the demands of the treatment schedule, the side effects of the medication, the frequent regular clinic visits and the ever-present fear of a relapse impose changes in attitudes, activities and living pattern for the family as well as the patient.

The family is advised to guard against overindulgence and being oversolicitous with the patient. Promoting his independence within the limits of his ability is in his best interests as well as those of all members of the family.

Information is conveyed to the family

---

[22]Ray Hugos: "Living with Leukemia." Am. J. Nurs., Vol. 72, No. 12 (Dec. 1972), p. 2187.

about the importance of doing all they can to prevent infection, since an infection that would be a minor incident to a normal person could be very serious for the leukemic person. Early signs and symptoms of respiratory and skin infections and of gastrointestinal and urinary disturbances are reviewed. They are advised of the need to notify the physician if the oral temperature is over 38° C. (100° F.) or, in the case of a child, if it is over 38.5° C. (101° F.). Hygienic care of the mouth, teeth, skin and nails is discussed, as is the need to avoid tissue trauma. The role of frequent rinsing of the mouth, cleansing of the teeth with a soft brush, bathing and keeping the nails short and clean to prevent infection is outlined. Avoidance of exposure to or contact with persons with infection is stressed. They are advised that if a member of the family develops a cold or infection he should "keep his distance" with the patient, his dishes should be disinfected and his clothing and linen kept separate when laundered.

The chemotherapeutic schedule is reviewed and given in writing. Symptoms of potential toxic effects of the prescribed drugs are cited and the patient advised what to do if these reactions occur. Emphasis is placed on the need for the patient to continue the antileukemic drugs even though he feels good between doses. It is stressed that he should not take any drugs except those prescribed by the physician. Aspirin is not taken because of its potential to increase the bleeding tendency.

The importance of keeping clinic or medical appointments is explained; these may be necessary for the patient to receive an intravenous drug that is part of the chemotherapeutic regimen. Blood counts are done on these visits because a change in cell count is usually the first indication of the onset of a relapse. It is suggested that it is well to have a family member accompany him to the clinic; the relative learns what the patient experiences, and the physician may want to discuss the patient's progress and activities with him.

A well balanced nutritious diet is discussed, as is the need for the inclusion of fruit and vegetables to prevent constipation and the need for a laxative. A daily fluid intake of 2500 to 3000 ml. is indicated to promote normal bowel and renal function.

If the patient has experienced alopecia he will be faced with the surprise and comments of fellow workers or fellow students. Suggestions are made that a hair piece or wig might be obtained or, if the patient is a female, that a scarf or hat may be worn.

A referral may be made to a visiting nursing agency requesting home visits to provide guidance and assistance. A history of the patient's illness and the prescribed plan of therapy is given to the agency so that there can be continuity of care. Home visits also provide opportunities to assess the family's reactions to the patient at home and to see how they are handling the situation. The family is advised of the assistance available from a local cancer society.

B. Chronic leukemia

If the patient is not incapacitated by the disorder, treatment may be withheld until the leukemic process is accelerated and more severe. He is advised of his susceptibility to infection and informed of preventive measures that should be observed (see p. 249). Hospitalization is not usually necessary until the later severe stage, unless a severe infection intervenes. The patient is kept under close medical or clinic supervision. He is seen monthly or bimonthly. Leukocyte, erythrocyte and platelet counts are done and a bone marrow biopsy may be necessary periodically. Treatment and care include drug therapy, irradiation, and psychological and physiological supportive care.

1. Drug therapy. The chemotherapeutic agent most commonly used at present in the treatment of *chronic granulocytic leukemia* is busulfan (Myleran). It is given orally until the leukocytes show a decrease of about 50 per cent; this may be over a period of 4 to 6 weeks. A course of the drug may be repeated when a relapse occurs. Potential side effects of busulfan are nausea, vomiting, diarrhea, stomatitis, alopecia, bone marrow depression and, later, pulmonary fibrosis and hyperpigmentation of the skin. Hydroxyurea given orally is also used in the treatment of *chronic myelocytic leukemia*. Toxic effects may be bone marrow depression, nausea, vomiting, diarrhea, stomatitis and skin changes.

In *chronic lymphatic leukemia,* the drugs used in combination or singly may be chlorambucil (Leukeran), prednisone and cyclophosphamide (Cytoxan). Possible toxic effects of chlorambucil include nausea, vomiting, and bone marrow depression. Side effects of prednisone and cyclophosphamide have been cited previously in this chapter.

2. RADIATION THERAPY. A series of x-ray treatments may be used on the enlarged spleen and other areas (e.g., lymph nodes) where leukemic cells have invaded. This is necessary and more effective in chronic granulocytic leukemia. Radioactive phsophorus (P^{32}) given intravenously may be administered for more general irradiation.

3. SUPPORTIVE CARE. In the early stages of chronic leukemia the patient is not hospitalized but he and his family need someone to listen to them and answer their questions about the disorder, treatment and the likely course. The visiting nurse to whom the patient has been referred or the nurse in the clinic or physician's office should be prepared and take the time to meet this need.

The patient is encouraged to continue with his normal life pattern and is assured that the doctor will indicate when a change in activities is necessary. He and his family are made aware of his increased susceptibility to infection, the important preventive measures, early signs and symptoms of infection, and the prompt appropriate action that should be taken. They should be made familiar with early manifestations of a relapse in his condition that would prompt the seeking of medical attention. The importance of regular ongoing medical supervision is explained and the need for the patient to keep his clinic or doctor's appointments is stressed.

In advanced stages of the disease the problems and necessary supportive care are similar to those of the patient with acute leukemia (see pp. 245–250).

Leukopenia

Leukopenia may be defined as a reduction in the number of leukocytes below the normal lower limit of 5000 per cu. mm. It may be due to a decreased production or excessive destruction of leukocytes. The deficiency occurs most often in the granulocytes, especially in neutrophils. Lymphopenia, a deficiency of lymphocytes, occurs rarely but is seen occasionally in patients receiving an adrenocorticoid preparation or adrenocorticotropic hormone (ACTH), and in those with uremia.

Agranulocytosis (Neutropenia)

Agranulocytosis is characterized by a marked reduction in neutrophils.

Causes

In most instances, this blood disorder is the result of the toxic effects of certain drugs in persons with a sensitivity or idiosyncrasy. The drugs found most frequently to be offenders include gold salts, sulfonamides, aminopyrine (Pyramidon), phenylbutazone (Butazolidin), chlorpromazine (Thorazine) and thiouracil preparations. The condition may also be associated with typhoid fever, malaria, miliary (widespread throughout the body) tuberculosis or any severe, overwhelming infection (e.g., septicemia).

Neutropenia may be an integral part of the aplastic anemia that may develop with radiation and anticancer drug therapy, or it may be due to an excessive destruction of the neutrophils by the spleen (hypersplenism). The disease has a higher incidence in females than in males.

Manifestations

Neutrophils play an important role in defending the body against infection because of their ability to ingest and destroy organisms. Neutropenia lowers the normal resistance to infection, resulting in prompt invasion of the mucous membranes and skin by pathogenic organisms. The source of the infecting organisms may be the individual's own body flora.

The disease usually has a sudden onset and is manifested by chills, fever and prostration. The patient complains of a very sore throat and has difficulty in swallowing. Infected, ulcerated areas appear on the mucous membranes in the mouth, throat, rectum and vagina. Skin and respiratory infections may develop. Some patients complain of severe joint pain (arthralgia). The white cell count may be less than 1500 per cu. mm.

Treatment and Nursing

Treatment of neutropenia includes prompt elimination of any suspected cause. Antibiotic therapy in large doses is commenced promptly to prevent infection and check that which may be established. If the neutropenia is a part of pancytopenia, a blood transfusion may be given to relieve the anemia, but it does not alter the white blood cell count since transferred leukocytes are quickly removed from the circulation. If the infection can be controlled and supportive care provided, a gradual increase in the number of neutrophils and improvement in the patient's condition may be expected in 1 to 2 weeks.

The patient is cared for in a single room, preferably one with filtered air to reduce the possibility of airborne infection. Reverse isolation technique is used. Only sterile linen and equipment are used. Personnel contacting or caring for the patient are screened for possible infection and are required to wash their hands thoroughly under running water before attending to the patient. A clean coverall type of gown and a mask are worn at the bedside. Visitors are restricted to one or two immediate family members who are free of infection. They are also required to wear a gown and mask and are requested not to go within 3 to 4 feet of the bedside. The floor is wet-mopped, and the furniture is washed frequently to reduce the number of contaminated dust particles.

An alternative isolation method may be the use of a plastic isolator tent or "life island." This equipment completely encloses the patient and bed, creating a barrier to outside organisms. Air entering the enclosure is filtered by a mechanical ventilator. Sterile gloves are used when giving care through the sleeves or portholes in the sides of the tent. With either method of barrier nursing an explanation is made to the patient as to its protective purpose; otherwise, the procedures may be frightening.

Care of the mouth is extremely important. It is rinsed or irrigated every 1 to 2 hours with normal saline or a mild, antiseptic mouthwash. The patient should receive 2000 to 2500 ml. of fluids per day and a high-protein, high-vitamin diet. Because of the oral lesions, the patient may have difficulty taking adequate food. Nutritious fluids, soft bland foods, protein concentrates and vitamin supplements may be used.

Constipation is avoided; the hard stool may injure the intestinal mucosa, making it more vulnerable to infection.

Prevention of Neutropenia

In some instances, neutropenia might have been prevented if the affected person had understood the danger inherent in self-medication. Whenever the opportunity presents, the nurse has the responsibility of informing lay persons that drugs should only be taken under medical supervision and according to the specific directions of the physician. It is not uncommon to learn of someone who has been taking a potentially dangerous drug on his own over an abnormally long period of time. Equally dangerous is the situation in which a family member, neighbor or friend shares a drug or suggests one that has been prescribed for him and has proved helpful. They do not appreciate that a drug may affect one person quite differently from another and that it is prescribed by the doctor on an individual basis following a careful study of the patient's condition. Reactions and side effects are unpredictable; some supervision is necessary to recognize early toxic manifestations.

Multiple Myeloma (Myelomatosis)

Multiple myeloma is a malignant disease characterized by a proliferation of abnormal plasma cells in the bone marrow. Plasma cells are involved in the synthesis of the immunoglobulins that function as antibodies. In multiple myeloma the malignant plasma cells proliferate the bone marrow, forming diffuse, multiple solid tumors.

Effects and Manifestations

Diffuse areas of bone destruction develop; these areas may coalesce and leave large "punched out lesions." The breakdown in bone structure frequently results in pathologic fractures, especially in weight-bearing bones such as the vertebrae. The patient experiences pain in the areas of the bone lesions that worsens with movement, jarring and pressure. The vertebrae are a common site of involvement, and pressure on nerve roots by the tumors and/or collapsing vertebrae causes severe back and/or lower limb pain; interruption of nerve impulses may give rise to paraplegia. Changes in posture and stature become evident. The ribs and skull bones are frequently affected. As tumors and areas of bone destruction develop in the skull, soft subcutaneous masses may be palpated. As the disease progresses, the patient has more and more pain and becomes increasingly incapacitated and deformed. Skeletal x-rays show areas of bone destruction.

The excessive production of abnormal plasma cells results in a decrease in the synthesis of normal immunoglobulins. This decrease in normal antibodies predisposes the patient to infection. The patient experiences recurring infections which are usually respiratory, but bladder infection and skin lesions are not uncommon.

The production of leukocytes, erythrocytes and thrombocytes diminishes as the bone marrow is crowded and replaced by the myeloma. The reduction in white blood cells further predisposes the individual to infection. Symptoms of anemia (shortness of breath on exertion, pallor, chilliness, weakness) and a bleeding tendency (bleeding gums, petechiae, ecchymoses, melena) may be manifested.

The breakdown of bone tissue gives rise to the release of calcium and hypercalcemia develops (normal calcium: 4.5 to 5.5 mEq./L). The excretion of the serum calcium by the kidneys entails an increased loss of water. If the fluid intake is not correspondingly increased, the patient manifests dehydration, the serum calcium is retained and the urinary output falls. Nausea, loss of appetite, impaired cardiac function and disorientation may occur with hypercalcemia.

An abnormal protein, referred to as Bence Jones protein, is excreted by the kidneys. In high concentration this protein may be precipitated in the renal tubules, forming casts and damaging the tubules and possibly resulting in renal insufficiency. The high serum uric acid (normal: 3 to 7 mg. per 100 ml.) incurred by the rapid destruction of cells further contributes to impaired renal function; precipitation of the uric acid in renal tubules can obstruct and destroy them. Another factor that contributes to impaired renal function is the hypercalcemia cited above.

Laboratory blood tests reveal an elevation in erythrocyte sedimentation rate, erythrocyte, leukocyte and platelet counts below normal, and elevated serum calcium and uric acid levels. Urinalysis may record the presence of Bence Jones protein. Examination of a bone marrow specimen shows the presence of abnormal plasma cells. Serum electrophoresis demonstrates the presence of abnormal globulin.

Treatment and Nursing Care

Care of the patient with multiple myeloma involves the administration of chemotherapeutic agents, radiation therapy and supportive care.

A. DRUG THERAPY. The chemotherapeutic agents used in the treatment of multiple myeloma are melphalan (Alkeran) and cyclophosphamide (Cytoxan). Melphalan is given daily orally in combination with prednisone; it may cause nausea and bone marrow depression. Cyclophosphamide is given daily orally and may cause nausea and vomiting, bone marrow depression, alopecia and hemorrhagic cystitis. The bone marrow depression results in a decreased production of erythrocytes, platelets and leukocytes, in addition to destruction of the plasma cells. This contributes to the anemia, hemorrhagic tendency and leukopenia that are also caused by bone marrow crowding and replacement by the abnormal plasma cells. The blood cell counts are followed closely; the dosage or protocol for the drug administration may have to be readjusted.

Allopurinol (Bloxanth) may be prescribed to decrease uric acid production and prevent impaired renal function.

B. RADIATION THERAPY. A series of x-ray treatments to the local areas of involvement may be used to reduce the tumor mass and lessen the pain caused by pressure.

C. SUPPORTIVE CARE. Nursing care includes the following considerations.

1. OBSERVATIONS. Frequent assessments are necessary, as significant changes may occur in a very short period of time. Laboratory data are noted so that the nurse may make the necessary modifications in the care plan according to the findings. For example, it is important to know if the patient's anemia is worsening or improving, to be aware of the leukocyte count in order to judge susceptibility to infection, and to ascertain whether the platelet count is such that there is a predisposition to hemorrhage. The specific gravity of the urine is noted; if it is high, it may indicate an increase in serum calcium and/or uric acid and the need to increase the fluid intake.

The fluid intake and output are recorded and the balance noted.

The patient is observed frequently for signs of infection; the temperature is taken, respirations noted and the skin and mouth checked for lesions.

Posture, the degree of freedom or difficulty with which the patient moves and the amount of incapacity are evaluated constantly. Any numbness or loss of movement is promptly brought to the physician's attention. Observations are also made for the possible toxic effects of the chemotherapeutic agent(s) that the patient is receiving.

2. ACTIVITY AND POSITIONING. Ambulation and activity are promoted within the limits of the individual's capacity. Inactivity, bed rest and immobilization cause decalcification of osseous tissue, adding to the demineralization of bone tissue by the disease process and contributing to the hypercalcemia. The patient moves slowly and precautions are taken to prevent the possibility of falls.

As the disease advances and the patient becomes more incapacitated, walking with assistance and limb exercises are encouraged as long as possible. If pathologic fractures occur, bed rest and casts are used only if absolutely necessary. When the spine is involved, a brace or corset may be helpful when the patient is out of bed. Whenever assistance is provided, the nurse "handles" the patient with gentle, slow movements; support is provided for limbs and joints. Quick, jarring movements may cause a fracture or muscle spasm with severe pain.

A fracture board and firm mattress on the bed are necessary. Moving and bumping against the bed is avoided since even very slight jarring of the patient may cause muscle spasm and pain. Frequently the patient finds it difficult to find a comfortable position. The nurse must be patient as well as resourceful; soft and firm pillows of various sizes are used to provide support, and a cradle is used to take the weight of the bedding. In the advanced stages of the disease it may be easier for the patient if he is cared for on a Stryker frame.

3. RELIEF OF PAIN. Gentle supportive movement and positioning are important in reducing discomfort and providing relief of pain. If the patient is experiencing considerable muscle spasm, a muscle relaxant may be prescribed. Analgesics are used; initially, a mild preparation such as acetaminophen (Tylenol) or propoxyphene (Darvon) may provide relief. Later a stronger preparation is required. It may be helpful to give the patient an analgesic 15 to 30 minutes before bathing, getting him up or carrying out an exercise schedule.

4. FLUIDS. A daily fluid intake of at least 3000 ml. is necessary to replace the increased loss incurred by the hypercalcemia and to promote elimination of uric acid. The patient's preferences are determined and the fluids must be placed within easy reach since movement is painful. If the oral intake is inadequate, intravenous infusion is used to meet the requirement.

Because of oliguria or other renal symptoms, renal function tests or an intravenous pyelogram may be done. Fluids must not be withheld for any of these since dehydration could cause acute renal failure.

5. BLOOD TRANSFUSIONS. The patient's anemia and thrombocytopenia may necessitate blood transfusions. If the fluid balance is negative, whole blood is used. If the oral intake has been adequate, packed red blood cells and platelets are transfused to prevent overtaxing the heart by overload. The patient is observed closely for reactions during the transfusion and immediately following (see p. 265).

6. PROTECTION FROM INFECTION. The patient's susceptibility to infection necessitates special precautions.

7. PSYCHOLOGICAL SUPPORT. The nature of the disease, therapeutic program and the potential side effects of the chemotherapeutic agents are outlined to the patient and family by the physician. It is important that the nurse know that they have been told. Obviously it is a blow to them to learn that the disorder is malignant. The nurse provides opportunities and time for the patient and family to ask questions; she should be willing and prepared to listen to them and discuss the situation. The patient may be fearful of the pain he has experienced becoming more severe; he is assured that someone will be close by to provide medication for relief.

8. INSTRUCTIONS. When the initial chemotherapeutic course is completed the patient is usually permitted to go home. He and the family are advised about the following:

a. The need to keep mobile.

b. Precautions against falling. Suggestions are made to remove scatter rugs, footstools and anything that might trip him. Waxed and highly polished floors are avoided.

c. The importance of an adequate fluid intake to prevent kidney complications.

d. The need for a fracture board and firm mattress.

e. Protection against infection. Such measures as avoiding contact with those with an infection, disinfecting the infected person's dishes in the case of respiratory infection, avoiding chilling, and using good mouth and skin hygienic measures are emphasized.

f. Early recognition of respiratory infection, mouth and skin lesions, and impaired renal function, and the need for prompt contact with the clinic or the physician if these appear.

g. The need to promptly report change in posture or the contour of a limb (that might indicate a fracture), any numbness, marked weakness or loss of movement, inability to void and increased severity in pain.

h. Medications. Following the initial course of chemotherapy, the patient is continued on a maintenance dose. He will also require an analgesic preparation. Allopurinol may also be continued. The purpose of these drugs, the administration schedule and early signs of toxic reactions are reviewed. Pertinent information (dosage, frequency time and reactions that should prompt contacting the physician) should be given to the family in writing.

i. Sources of assistance. A referral should be made to the visiting nursing association. The patient and family are usually reassured by the nurse's visits. They provide frequent assessment of the patient's progress and the family situation and suggestions and guidance are provided as new problems arise.

j. The importance of keeping the frequent appointments with the clinic or physician. Frequent reassessment of the patient and blood studies are necessary. The patient's capacity is evaluated; he may be forcing himself to "keep going" to protect the family.

Infectious Mononucleosis

This is a benign infectious disease involving the lymphatic system and is seen most commonly in adolescents and young adults. The causative organism is the Epstein-Barr virus (EBV). The disease is not highly infectious, but may be transmitted by close personal contact.

Manifestations

The symptoms vary from one patient to another. Common complaints are sore throat, gingivitis, headache, tiredness, anorexia and general malaise. The patient has a fever which may be intermittent, and there is enlargement and tenderness of the superficial lymph nodes (cervical, axillary and inguinal). The spleen is usually enlarged and tender, and palpation may also reveal abdominal tenderness due to involvement of the mesenteric lymph nodes. Some patients develop an erythematous or maculopapular rash. Some patients are jaundiced as a result of the development of hepatitis.

The total leukocyte count is elevated and may range from 10,000 to 20,000 per cu. mm. A differential count reveals an increase in lymphocytes and monocytes, and many of the lymphocytes are atypical. The percentage of granulocytes may be below normal. The patient may experience anemia due to increased hemolysis. Diagnosis may be confirmed by a positive Paul-Bunnell test. Heterophile antibodies appear in the serum of patients with infectious mononucleosis; these antibodies cause the agglutination of sheep blood cells, which is the basis of the Paul-Bunnell test. The Paul-Bunnell reaction does not usually become positive until after the first week of infection. Recently a mononucleosis spot test (Monospot test) has been used; it is easier to carry out and is considered more specific.

Treatment and Care

The disease usually runs a self-limited course of 2 to 4 weeks. The treatment is symptomatic and supportive. The patient is kept in bed until the temperature is normal. Aspirin or aspirin compound (e.g., aspirin, caffeine and codeine) or propoxyphene (Darvon) is usually prescribed to relieve the headache, general body discomfort and sore throat. Warm saline throat irrigations may also help to relieve the sore throat. A high-calorie, high-protein diet is recommended to support the patient's resistance. The patient may become discouraged and depressed as the illness continues for weeks; he may even be fearful of the outcome. The nurse conveys understanding to the patient, accepts his reactions and provides reassurance that although improvement appears slow he will return to normal activities. Convalescence is usually prolonged; an effort is made to find an interest for the patient (e.g., reading, radio, television); the occupational therapy department may provide assistance. He is warned that fatigue and less than his accustomed strength and tolerance may be expected for several weeks. His previous activities should be resumed gradually and the need for extra rest is stressed.

MALIGNANT LYMPHOMAS

This is a term that may be applied to a group of neoplastic diseases that primarily affect lymphoid tissue (nodes and spleen). They are characterized by painless, progressive enlargement of lymph nodes and spleen. In some the proliferating cells invade extralymphatic tissues and organs. These diseases include Hodgkin's disease (lymphadenoma), lymphocytic lymphoma (lymphosarcoma), histiocytic lymphoma (reticulum cell sarcoma) and Burkitt's lymphoma (stem cell lymphoma). They are classified according to the cells identified with lymph node biopsy. Histologically they show marked differences, but the signs and symptoms are similar for all types. The painless enlargement of one or more lymph nodes is usually the initial presenting disturbance. The patient gradually develops general malaise, fatigue, weight loss, fever, sweating and splenic enlargement. Investigation and assessment of the extent of the disease is similar for the various types of lymphomas.

Hodgkin's Disease (Lymphadenoma)

Hodgkin's disease is a disease of unknown etiology that involves lymphoid tissue. It may develop at any age but usually occurs in adolescents and young adults. There is a higher incidence of the disorder in males. Until recently Hodgkin's disease was always considered a fatal condition. Impressive advances have been made in assessing the extent of the lymph node involvement and treating the affected areas with radiation and chemotherapeutic agents.

Signs and Symptoms

The disease has an insidious onset and is manifested by painless enlargement of one group of lymph nodes (usually cervical at the beginning). The disease spreads progressively to other lymphoid tissues throughout the body and a variety of symptoms develop, depending upon the lymphoid tissue involved. The enlarging lymph nodes may cause pressure on nerves, resulting in pain, or may impose on neighboring organs, causing dysfunction. Axillary and inguinal nodes frequently interfere with venous and lymph drainage, leading to edema in the arms and legs. Enlarged mediastinal nodes may produce a distressing cough, dyspnea or difficulty in swallowing (dysphagia). The spleen becomes enlarged, causing abdominal discomfort.

Constitutional symptoms are not prominent until the later stages. The patient gradually develops fatigue, weakness, fever, anorexia, loss of weight and pruritus. These are likely to be seriously aggravated by the treatments used (radiation, chemotherapy). Fluctuations in the symptoms and size of the nodes may occur.

The leukocyte count varies with patients; it may be increased or it may be normal or below normal. The differential count indicates a deficiency in the lymphocytes. Diagnosis is established by biopsy of an affected lymph node. Large atypical cells known as Reed-Sternberg cells are characteristic of Hodgkin's disease.

Assessment of Extent of Disease (Staging)

When the diagnosis of Hodgkin's disease has been confirmed, a series of investigative procedures are carried out to determine the extent of lymphoid tissue involvement. The treatment and prognosis depend upon the findings. A classification into four stages has been made according to the degree of involvement (Table 12–14). The classifying process may be referred to as "staging."

The assessment made to determine the stage of the disease may include chest x-rays, lymphangiography, inferior venacavography, liver, spleen and bone scans, liver function tests and laparoscopy or exploratory laparotomy.

A *lymphangiogram* involves the introduction of a radiopaque preparation into a lymphatic vessel in each foot. The "dye" is injected over 1 to 2 hours and x-rays are then taken of the lower limbs, abdomen and chest. Enlarged and diseased lymph nodes may be visualized on the films. Follow-up x-rays may be taken over a period of time to assess the

TABLE 12–14 CLASSIFICATION OF EXTENT OF INVOLVEMENT IN HODGKIN'S DISEASE (STAGING)*

Stage	Degree of Involvement
I	Disease limited to one lymph node
IE	Disease limited to an extralymphatic organ
II	Disease is confined to two or more lymph nodes on the same side of the diaphragm
IIE	Disease involves an extralymphatic organ and one or more lymph nodes on the same side of diaphragm
III	Disease involves lymph nodes on both side of the diaphragm
IIIS	Disease involves lymph nodes on both sides of the diaphragm and the spleen
IIISE	Disease involves lymph nodes on both sides of the diaphragm, the spleen and an extralymphatic site
IV	Diffuse involvement of extralymphatic organs or tissues.

*Marie E. Keaveny and Loy Wiley: "Hodgkin's Disease . . . The Curable Cancer." Nurs. '75, Vol. 5, No. 3 (March 1975), p. 53; Beeson and McDermott, op. cit., p. 1504; Boedeker and Dauber, op. cit., p. 316.

effect of the treatment without further injection of the dye, since the initial dose remains in the lymphatic nodes for many weeks.

A *venacavogram* requires the injection of a radiopaque preparation through a catheter into a femoral vein. Abdominal x-ray films are then made.

A *laparoscopy* may be done to determine extralymphatic involvement. The exploratory laparotomy provides more thorough evaluation of the extent of abdominal visceral and mesenteric lymphatic node involvement. Biopsies may be done and the spleen may be removed.

An explanation of the purpose(s) of each investigational procedure is made to the patient and what he may expect is outlined. A signed consent is required. No special preparations are required for the angiography. The laparoscopy and laparotomy require preoperative shaving and cleansing of the abdomen. A sedative is usually given ½ to 1 hour before the scheduled time, and food and fluid are withheld for the preceding 8 hours. Following the laparoscopy, the patient is observed closely for the possible complications of hemorrhage and shock. Abdominal pain, distention or rigidity is reported promptly to the physician. Laparotomy involves complete postoperative care (see p. 178).

The scans that may be done on the liver, spleen and bones require the administration of a radioisotope for which each of these structures has an affinity. A graph of the rays emitted by the radioactive substance is made, which indicates its concentration in the particular organ or structure being evaluated.

Treatment and Nursing Care

Treatment may consist of radiation therapy, chemotherapy or a combination of both. The patient requires psychological and physiological supportive care.

A. RADIATION THERAPY. This is used when the Hodgkin's disease is regionally localized. The patients in stages I and II receive a series of irradiation to all involved sites. Depending upon the extralymphatic involvement, patients in stages III and IV may also receive radiation therapy. The series of treatments, what may be expected during the x-ray treatment, the necessary care and possible reactions are discussed with the patient and family (see p. 140). When the location of the lymph nodes being irradiated is the neck, chest or abdomen, the patient is observed for coughing, dyspnea, sore throat, dysphagia, nausea and vomiting. Hemoglobin concentration and blood cell counts are determined frequently, since bone marrow depression may occur. Nausea and persisting fatigue are the most common problems. The patient is advised to plan for rest periods during the day and to retire early. Antiemetics and small, frequent, selective meals may be necessary for the nausea. The patient is reassured that it will be temporary.

B. CHEMOTHERAPY. This may be used to treat patients of stage III disease in conjunction with radiotherapy. Usually it is used alone for patients whose disease is disseminated and involves extralymphatic tissues. The drugs used include mechlorethamine (nitrogen mustard), vincristine (Oncovan), prednisone, procarbazine (Matulane), vinblastine and cyclophosphamide (Cytoxan). A combination of three or four drugs may be given over a period of 28 days. Then, after a week or so, if the blood counts are satisfactory, chemotherapy is commenced again.

Toxic reactions to the drugs include nausea, vomiting, diarrhea, stomatitis, bone marrow depression, alopecia and dermatitis. Vincristine and vinblastine are administered intravenously and precautions must be observed to avoid extravasation of the solution into the tissues because of the necrosis that may follow. These two drugs may also have some side effects on the central nervous system. The patient is observed for loss of reflexes, coordination, sensation and ability to move (see Table 12–13).

C. SUPPORTIVE CARE. The supportive care required by the patient with Hodgkin's disease is similar to that needed by the patient with leukemia (see p. 247). Following the investigational procedures and initial therapy, the patient — especially one with stage I, II or III disease — returns home and is encouraged to resume, as much as possible, his former pattern of life. The patient's care is fully discussed with him and the family; such factors as prevention of infection, the importance of regular visits to the physician or clinic for reassessment, the need for extra rest, medications and coping with therapy reactions are emphasized.

Lymphocytic Lymphoma (Lymphoma Sarcoma)

This is a neoplastic disease of lymphoid tissue characterized by a proliferation of lymphocytes. Unlike leukemia, the cells are confined within the lymphoid tissues until the later stages of the disease. It occurs more often in males and in those over 40 years of age.

The disease progresses similarly to Hodgkin's disease; usually only one area of lymphoid tissue is affected at first, but there is a gradual dissemination to other regions. The symptoms are largely dependent upon the location of the tumors. They reflect the pressure and interference imposed on neighboring structures by the enlarging lymphoid tissues. Fever and progressive debilitation accompany the extension and increasing severity of the disease. The treatment employed is the same as that used for Hodgkin's disease.

HEMORRHAGIC DISORDERS

An abnormal tendency to bleed may be due to a disorder of the clotting mechanism, an excess of anticoagulant or a vascular defect. A hemorrhagic disorder is characterized by prolonged bleeding following tissue damage; spontaneous bleeding into mucous membrane, skin and organs; and bleeding in more than one area of the body.

Failure of the clotting mechanism may result from a deficiency of any of the essential factors in the coagulation process (see p. 228). These disorders include hemophilia, hypoprothrombinemia and thrombocytopenia.

When a hemorrhagic disorder is suspected it is important to note the form in which the bleeding presents: purpural areas, hematoma, ecchymoses, oozing or free flow from wound, and whether from single or multiple sites. Wallerstein states that "Purpuric spots suggest a capillary or platelet defect; they are not characteristic of hemophilia. Hematomas, hemarthroses, or large ecchymoses at the site of trauma suggest hemophilia. Sudden, severe bleeding from multiple sites after prolonged surgery or during obstetric procedures suggests acquired fibrinogen deficiency. Massive bleeding from a single site without a history of purpura or previous bleeding suggests a surgical or anatomic defect rather than a coagulation defect."[23]

It is important to determine:

1. If the individual has a history of bleeding — that is, has this type of response been occurring since early childhood, or is this the initial incidence?

2. How long the bleeding has been taking place.

3. If there is anyone in the family with a history of a similar problem.

4. What precipitated this bleeding (e.g., trauma, visit to the dentist).

Hemophilia (A and B)

Hemophilia is a coagulation disorder that occurs in males as a result of a deficiency of Factor VIII (the antihemophilic factor) or

[23]Krupp and Chatton, op. cit., p. 306.

Factor IX (the Christmas factor). If the bleeding tendency is the result of a deficiency of Factor VIII, the disease is referred to as *hemophilia A;* if it is the result of a deficiency of Factor IX, it is known as *hemophilia B or Christmas disease.* It is inherited as a sex-linked recessive trait. The defective gene is carried on an X chromosome and is transmitted from mother to son.

The female has two X sex chromosomes, and the male has one X and one Y. If a female inherits an X chromosome bearing the hemophilic gene from her father, she becomes a carrier. The disorder is not manifested in her because the X with the abnormal gene is dominated by the normal X chromosome. If the carrier marries a nonhemophiliac, there is a 50 per cent chance her daughters will be carriers. Her male progeny have a 50 per cent chance of being hemophilic (see Table 12–15). The sons of a hemophilic father receive only a Y chromosome from him, so the disorder is not passed on to them or their descendants. All daughters of a hemophilic male carry the trait since the father's genetic contribution to each is an X chromosome, which in his case bears the defective gene (see Table 12–15).

Manifestations

Hemophilia is usually recognized within the first year or two of life. Excessive bleeding from the umbilical cord does not occur because of the transplacental transfer of the mother's clotting factors to the fetus. Occasionally, persistent bleeding when the infant is circumcised leads to early diagnosis of the disorder.

The severity varies in individuals; some bleed excessively with very slight trauma, others only with a more severe injury or during incidents such as tooth extraction or surgery. The important characteristic feature of the bleeding is its persistence rather than the amount. Most children experience some bleeding into joints, especially the knees, ankles and elbows. With some, this may be so severe that, as well as causing pain, it produces crippling deformities. As the blood clot organizes, fibrous adhesions may cause ankylosis. Hematomas and hematuria may be manifested. Early death may occur as a result of the pressure of a hematoma (collection of blood within tissue) on a vital structure or from the loss of blood. The latter is rarely fatal since blood and plasma have become so readily available.

Laboratory blood studies indicate a prolonged coagulation time (normal: 5 to 15 minutes when glass tubes are used); the bleeding time (normal: less than 7 minutes), blood platelet count (normal: 250,000 to 300,000 per cu. mm.) and prothrombin time (normal: 11 to 16 seconds) are normal. The partial thromboplastin time is prolonged (normal: 35 to 45 seconds). Quantitative assays of Factors VIII and IX are performed.

Treatment and Care

The patient (if old enough) and the family are alerted to the need for continuous ongoing care.

TABLE 12–15 GENETIC POSSIBILITIES IN HEMOPHILIA

		Normal Male		
		X	Y	XX Normal female
				XY Normal male
	X	XX	XY	X^hX Female carrier
Female Carrier				X^hY Male with hemophilia
	X^h	X^hX	X^hY	

		Male with Hemophilia		
		X^h	Y	
	X	XX^h	XY	XX^h Female carrier
Normal Female				XY Normal male
	X	XX^h	XY	

A. TREATMENT OF EPISODES OF BLEEDING. The simplest and most popular current measure used to arrest bleeding, especially in the early stages, is the administration of the factor required (commercial preparations of Factor VIII — Hemofil, Humafac, Factorate; commercial preparations of Factor IX — Konyne, Proplex). If a large volume of blood is lost, a transfusion of fresh whole blood may be given.

Cryoprecipitate of the antihemophilic factor (prepared from frozen fresh plasma) may be used when treating the patient with hemophilia A.

The advantage of the commercial concentrates and cryoprecipitate is that either can be infused in a small volume; this prevents overloading of the individual's cardiovascular system.

During an episode of bleeding the patient is confined to bed. If there is bleeding into a joint, attention is given to positioning with good alignment to reduce possible deformity. The patient may be fearful of using the joint after the bleeding has been arrested in case of further hemorrhage; he must be encouraged to resume activity as soon as possible to prevent ankylosis.

B. PROPHYLACTIC AND SUPPORTIVE MEASURES. Nursing responsibilities include planning and implementing instruction for the patient and family about the nature of the disorder, safe activities, necessary precautions, recognition of the need for factor replacement, and appropriate action when bleeding occurs. In some instances one or two members of the family may be taught the administration of the prescribed concentrate.

Patients are urged to seek prompt treatment following trauma and on the earliest symptoms of bleeding; for example, replacement of the deficient factor is recommended as soon as the patient experiences slight tightness or pressure in a joint, especially if he knows it has received a bump.

It should be emphasized that the person with hemophilia should always carry some form of identification indicating the disorder and blood type.

The patient and family are advised to carry on as normal a life as possible. The severity of the disease determines the restrictions placed on the individual's activities; they must be consistent with safety but there are nontraumatic sports, occupations and forms of recreation in which he may and should be encouraged to participate. Parents and siblings are warned against overprotection and promoting dependency. If of school age, the patient is usually able to attend a regular school. The teachers are informed of the individual's condition, the necessary restrictions and precautions and what to do if he receives an injury or bleeding commences. For the child whose disease is severe, arrangements may be made for him to pursue his education at home or to attend special classes. The problem must be kept in mind when selecting toys and sport equipment.

During the teaching sessions the patient and family are informed that patients with hemophilia must not be given aspirin because of its tendency to promote bleeding. Parenteral administrations must also be kept to a minimum; usually the introduction of a needle is restricted to the administration of the antihemophilic factor.

Good dental hygiene is stressed so that extractions may be avoided. A very soft brush to clean the teeth is recommended to prevent trauma and bleeding of the gums. The patient's dentist is advised of the disorder on the initial visit so that the necessary precautions can be taken.

A referral may be given to the visiting nursing agency so that home visits may be made to provide necessary assistance and supervision. The patient and family are acquainted with the resources of a local hemophilia society.

The genetic possibilities in offspring are reviewed with parents and young adults in the family. A referral may be made to the appropriate clinic for genetic counseling.

C. COMPLICATIONS. Some patients, after receiving several doses of a factor concentrate, develop antibodies to the factor. Precautions and activity restrictions have to be reassessed and are usually made more rigid. If a bleeding episode occurs, a much larger dose of the antihemophilic preparation may be prescribed in an effort to counteract the antibody activity.

Repeated hemarthroses (bleeding into joints) may lead to ankylosis and crippling.

Hypoprothrombinemia

Hypoprothrombinemia is a deficiency of prothrombin chiefly resulting from a deficient supply, impaired absorption or defective utilization of vitamin K. The vitamin is essential in the formation of prothrombin and Factor VII by the liver. If the diet does not supply an adequate amount, it is synthesized by the bacteria that normally inhabit the intestinal tract. The bleeding tendency in the newborn is attributed to the lack of bacterial synthesis of vitamin K during the first 2 to 3 days of life when the tract is free of organisms. Sterilization of the bowel by the oral administration of sulfonamides or antibiotics may produce a vitamin K deficiency.

Bile salts are essential in the intestine for the absorption of vitamin K. A frequent cause of a deficiency of prothrombin is obstruction to the flow of bile into the small intestine. An insufficient production of prothrombin may also occur in liver disease, such as chronic cirrhosis.

Hypoprothrombinemia due to impaired synthesis or absorption is treated with a synthetic preparation of vitamin K (menadione) which may be administered parenterally or orally. When the deficiency is due to liver disease, the patient may receive blood transfusions to supply prothrombin.

Thrombocytopenia (Thrombocytopenic Purpura)

Failure of the coagulation process may be due to a deficiency of circulating thrombocytes (blood platelets), known as thrombocytopenia. The deficiency in thrombocytes may be primary or secondary.

Primary thrombocytopenia is of unknown etiology (idiopathic thrombocytopenia). The reduced number of platelets is the result of their rapid destruction. The normal life span for platelets is approximately 8 to 10 days; in idiopathic thrombocytopenia their survival is only 1 to 3 days. An antigen-antibody reaction has been suggested in which the person develops antibodies (agglutinins) which destroy his thrombocytes.

Manifestations

The disorder is manifested by bleeding in any site. Petechiae and purpuric areas may appear in the skin or mucous membranes and bleeding from the nose or from the gastrointestinal or urinary tract may occur. Children and young adults, especially females, are more often affected. The severity of the disease varies, and alternating remissions and relapses may occur.

Treatment

The patient is kept at rest and is treated with an adrenocorticoid preparation (e.g., prednisone) and transfusions of fresh blood. If the patient does not respond favorably to these measures, splenectomy may be performed. Although the spleen does not become enlarged, it appears to be active in thrombocytopenia. It separates out and harbors the platelets and is suspected of producing some antibody.

Secondary thrombocytopenia may be the result of a number of disorders. It most frequently occurs as a result of depressed bone marrow activity which is associated with radiation exposure, anticancer drugs and drug sensitivity. Thrombocytopenia also occurs in metastatic disease in the bone marrow, leukemia and lupus erythematosus.

Excess of Anticoagulant

Hemorrhage may be a complication of excessive anticoagulant drug therapy. The products commonly used are heparin and preparations of coumarin (e.g., Dicumarol) and phenindione (Danilone). Heparin inhibits the conversion of prothrombin to thrombin. The other anticoagulants prevent the utilization of vitamin K to form prothrombin. If bleeding occurs, administration of the drug is stopped. Whole blood transfusions may be necessary and, in the case of heparin, protamine sulfate is used as an antidote. If the bleeding is due to the other two anticoagulants cited above, parenteral injections of vitamin K are administered as well as blood transfusions.

Prolonged administration of aspirin may cause bleeding in some patients. Its anticoagulant property causes reduced prothrombin formation.

Vascular Purpura

In some instances, bleeding into tissues and organs occurs because of damage to or a defect in the small blood vessels. The result may be increased permeability or inadequate vasoconstriction, predisposing to blood loss.

This type of disorder may be associated with an allergic reaction, septicemia or a vitamin C deficiency (scurvy).

A rare hereditary bleeding disorder known as *hereditary hemorrhagic telangiectasia* is characterized by dilated, thin-walled vessels (especially veins) that lack the normal amount of muscular tissue. Angiomas (tumors composed of blood vessels) appear on the skin and mucous membrane surfaces, and normal vasoconstriction does not take place in the affected vessels.

Disseminated Intravascular Coagulation (DIC) (Defibrination Syndrome)

Disseminated intravascular coagulation (DIC) is a potentially fatal condition that is a secondary development in a serious primary illness. It is characterized by two phases. In the first phase multiple diffuse microthrombi develop within the vascular system. This widespread coagulation depletes the blood of thrombocytes and several clotting factors to the extent that hemorrhage occurs. This is the second phase of the disorder. Contributing to the hemorrhagic phase is the fibrinolysis that occurs.

DIC may be seen as a complication in many disorders which include any condition associated with extensive tissue damage, shock, severe infections (especially those associated with gram-negative organisms), severe trauma, burns, extensive metastatic disease, surgery involving extracorporeal shunts, and obstetrical complications (toxemia and abruptio placentae).

The process involves diffuse traumatization of tissue cells and/or blood platelets by the primary disorder; thromboplastin is released which triggers the clotting process. The blood clots may seriously interfere with the blood supply to some tissues and organs, resulting in impaired function. Respiratory insufficiency and renal failure are common ensuing problems.

Plasminogen is activated during the pathologic clotting and forms the enzyme plasmin which breaks down the fibrin of clots and fibrinogen. The degradation products of this dissolution process inhibit the thrombin-fibrinogen reaction which yields fibrin. They cause a prolonged thrombin time and retard the production of thromboplastin. Obviously, these reactions inhibit coagulation and cause hemorrhage.[24, 25]

Manifestations

There are indications in the patient's general condition of regression. Diffuse bleeding occurs in various areas and may be evident by petechiae, ecchymoses, hematuria, gastrointestinal bleeding, vaginal bleeding, epistaxis, or persistent oozing from a surgical wound or needle puncture. The patient may complain of pain as a result of bleeding into tissues. Oliguria and respiratory distress may develop.

Laboratory blood studies indicate a marked decrease in the number of blood platelets, decreased levels of fibrinogen and Factors V and VIII, and prolonged prothrombin, thrombin and partial thromboplastin times.

Treatment and Nursing Care

Treatment is directed toward reversing the primary disorder and arresting the diffuse coagulation process.

Heparin is given intravenously to interrupt the formation of thrombi; this allows the level of blood platelets and fibrinogen to rise. Cryoprecipitate may be administered to increase other blood clotting factors. A transfusion of whole blood may be given to compensate for the loss incurred.

The patient is critically ill and the nurse is concerned with the primary condition as well as the blood disorder. Close observation is made for bleeding, and frequent assessment of the patient's vital signs and general condition is necessary. The hourly urinary output is noted. Continuous cardiac monitoring may be set up and, if respiratory insufficiency occurs, the patient may be put on a mechanical respirator (see p. 424).

Nursing Patients with a Tendency to Bleed

Specific nursing needs of patients with hemorrhagic disorders vary with each indi-

[24]Krupp and Chatton; op. cit., pp. 312–313.
[25]Gloria Gilbert Mayer: "Disseminated Intravascular Coagulation." Am. J. Nurs., Vol. 73, No. 12 (Dec. 1973), pp. 2067–2068.

vidual and with the cause, associated symptoms, and severity of the disease, but there are some common problems and general considerations applicable to all.

OBSERVATIONS. The skin and mouth are checked for the appearance of petechiae and purple patches (purpura). Excreta are examined for blood. A constant alert is necessary for symptoms of internal bleeding such as pallor, weakness, air hunger (rapid deep respirations), rapid weak pulse, fall in blood pressure and signs of disturbed organ function (e.g., cerebral dysfunction due to bleeding into the brain).

PSYCHOLOGICAL SUPPORT. The patient with a hemorrhagic disorder or tendency to bleed excessively becomes apprehensive and tense. His reactions of fear should be recognized, acknowledged and accepted by the nurse. He is advised of the treatment plan and reassured that the doctor is cognizant of his problem and that everything possible is being done. The patient is not left alone for long periods; frequent visits and assessments provide confidence and assurance. Opportunities are made to be with the patient to listen and answer his questions.

PROTECTION FROM TISSUE TRAUMA. The patient is handled gently and tissues are subjected to a minimum of pressure. If confined to bed, he is turned every 1 to 2 hours, and a soft resilient material such as sponge rubber or sheepskin is placed under the patient. As well as receiving an explanation of the importance of avoiding falls, bumps, scratches, cuts and pressure, the patient and his family receive suggestions as to how tissue trauma may be prevented during the time between bleeding episodes.

MOUTH CARE. A very soft toothbrush is used for cleaning the teeth. The mouth is rinsed frequently with a mild, cool mouthwash. Very hot, rough and highly seasoned foods are avoided in order to prevent damage to the oral and gastrointestinal mucosa.

REST. The patient is kept at rest in bed during a bleeding episode. Since he may not be experiencing any particular discomfort, he may find it difficult to remain inactive. The important role that rest plays is explained, and some suitable diversion is found for the patient.

PREVENTION OF CRIPPLING DEFORMITIES. Bleeding into joints is a common problem and causes severe pain. In many instances, bone and joint damage and contractures result. The affected joint is immobilized in óptimum alignment and protected from the weight of bedding by a cradle. When the bleeding is under control, exercises and physiotherapy are prescribed to restore function as fully as possible to the joint(s).

PARENTERAL INJECTIONS. If subcutaneous and intramuscular injections are necessary, a small gauge needle is used. Gentle pressure is applied to the site for several minutes following the administration.

IDENTIFICATION. Every person with a chronic hemorrhagic disorder should bear some form of identification (card or Medic Alert bracelet or pendant) at all times that clearly indicates his bleeding problem and blood type.

SELF-MEDICATION. Individuals with a hemorrhagic disorder are warned against taking unprescribed medicine, especially aspirin, because of its potential anticoagulant effect.

PATIENT AND FAMILY INSTRUCTION. The nature of the disease and the limitations it imposes are explained to the family and to the patient if he is old enough to understand. The restrictions and constant precautions that are necessary usually produce psychological reactions. It is very difficult for a child to refrain from participating in the activities and games of his playmates. He may become resentful and seek undesirable outlets. The nurse emphasizes positive activities and helps parents and the patient to plan for his development and education as well as for appropriate safe recreation. They are advised of the constant need to be alert to early signs of bleeding and of the necessary prompt action.

BLOOD TRANSFUSION

An infusion of blood or blood components may be given to: (1) replace blood lost during surgery or in hemorrhage; (2) replace a deficiency of specific blood components, such as erythrocytes, platelets and clotting factors; (3) increase the oxygen-carrying capacity of the blood, as in anemia; and (4) to increase the intravascular volume in shock.

When blood is taken from the donor, it is received in a special sterile container that contains anticoagulant. The anticoagulant most frequently used is a mixture of sodium citrate, citric acid and dextrose (acid citrate dextrose). The sodium citrate prevents clotting, the citric acid serves as a preservative and the dextrose prolongs the life of the erythrocytes. Heparin is used as an anticoagulant in blood that is to be transfused within 24 hours of procurement. Heparinized blood is necessary for extracorporeal shunts (as in open heart surgery). The heparin is less damaging to platelets and to the enzyme 2, 3-diphosphoglycerate (DPG) which promotes the release of oxygen from oxyhemoglobin.

The blood is labeled clearly to indicate donor number, blood type, whether Rh negative or positive, anticoagulant used, and expiration date. The blood may be given as whole blood or some of the components may be separated out for administration. Blood is stored at a temperature of 2 to 4° C. and may be used up to 21 days of having been obtained, except that which is heparinized.

Preparations used in Transfusions (Table 12–16)

1. **WHOLE BLOOD.** Whole blood is administered to replace blood loss or to increase the intravascular volume in shock. *Fresh* whole blood is needed for the patient who is on extracorporeal shunt (e.g., as in open heart surgery) or receiving an exchange transfusion or a massive transfusion (ten or more units in 24 hours). Fresh blood may also be required for patients with bone marrow depression who require platelets in addition to erythrocytes.

2. **PACKED RED CELLS.** A large portion of the plasma is removed from whole blood by centrifuging. The remaining cells are given to increase the oxygen-carrying capacity of the recipient's blood. The advantage of packed cells is that a lesser volume is added to the patient's intravascular volume, thus preventing the risk of overload. The cells may be administered in a small volume of normal saline or plasma.

3. **PLASMA.** Fresh frozen plasma may be stored for several months. It contains all the clotting factors except platelets, so it may be used to control bleeding in some patients.

4. **THROMBOCYTES.** Platelets may be concentrated and given in a small volume to avoid the administration of a large volume of fluid. This avoids the risk of overtaxing the recipient's heart and overloading the circula-

TABLE 12–16 PRODUCTS USED IN TRANSFUSION

Product	Uses
Whole blood	
Stored	Cell and intravascular volume replacement
Fresh	To provide coagulation factors
Packed red blood cells	To increase oxygen-carrying capacity in anemia
Platelet concentrate	To supply thrombocytes (thrombocytopenia)
Plasma	
Fresh	To supply coagulation factors
Stored	Volume and blood protein replacement
Cryoprecipitate (Factor VIII)	Hemophilia A (Factor VIII deficiency)
Factor IX	Hemophilia B (Factor IX deficiency, Christmas disease)
Fibrinogen	Hypofibrinogenemia (Fibrinogen deficiency)
Albumin	Deficiency of serum albumin

tory system. The platelets must be given while fresh (12 to 24 hours). Transfusion of platelets is used to control bleeding in patients with thrombocytopenia.

5. **CLOTTING FACTORS.** Concentrates of certain clotting factors (e.g., VIII, IX) are prepared from fresh frozen plasma to control bleeding in hemophilia A and B or in fibrinogen deficiency. The preparation is known as cryoprecipitate.

Patient Care

1. The patient is advised that he is to receive a transfusion; the purpose and what is involved are explained. He will likely have questions which should be answered.

2. The patient is made as comfortable as possible, as he may be less free to turn and move while the transfusion is being administered.

3. The patient's blood type has been determined and his blood crossmatched with donor blood for compatibility. Before the matched blood is given, a check is made by

two persons to insure that the blood that has been received is for this particular patient, and is of the correct type. The expiration date on the blood label should also be checked and contents examined for abnormal cloudiness and particles.

4. The rate of administration depends upon the patient's condition; if the blood volume has been markedly depleted by hemorrhage or if the patient is in severe shock, it may be delivered at a faster rate than is used if the intravascular volume is normal. A rate commonly used is 30 drops per minute or the delivery of a unit (500 ml.) over 4 hours. If the blood volume has not been depleted or if there is a risk of overtaxing the patient's heart, the rate should be reduced to 15 to 20 drops per minute. The patient is observed closely throughout the administration for signs of overloading (dyspnea, coughing, pink frothy sputum, weak pulse).

5. Precautionary measures are used. The blood is infused through a filter and is *gently* mixed at intervals to keep cells suspended throughout the plasma. A normal saline infusion is started so that the tube can be flushed before and after the blood is administered.

No medication should be given into the blood that is being administered; if a drug must be given, the blood is temporarily stopped and the normal saline infusion restarted.

The nurse remains with the patient for a period of 15 to 20 minutes following the beginning of the blood transfusion, or until at least 100 ml. has been delivered; the patient may be very apprehensive at first and most reactions usually develop within that period. The patient is assessed frequently for possible reactions and the rate of flow is checked.

Reactions

The transfer of blood or any component of it carries a risk of a reaction; "they should be viewed as potentially liquid transplants."[26] The blood or its components may act as a foreign protein or antigen that prompts an immune response or tissue reaction.

Unfavorable responses to transfusions include the following:

1. **HEMOLYTIC REACTION.** This is agglutination of the donor's red blood cells followed by their hemolysis, which occurs as a result of incompatibility. Antibodies within the recipient's blood attack the donor's erythrocytes. Hemoglobin and other products of the hemolysis are circulated throughout the body.

Early manifestations of incompatibility include chill, headache or full feeling in the head, anxiety, restlessness, pain in the lumbar region and/or chest, dyspnea, tachycardia and palpitation. Anaphylactic shock may develop; the patient's blood pressure falls, the skin becomes cold and clammy, respiratory distress is increasingly more severe, the pulse weakens and consciousness is clouded.

After several hours, even though the patient's general condition has improved markedly, hemoglobinuria and/or oliguria may appear. The hemoglobin released by the hemolyzed cells is excreted in the urine, coloring it red. The hemoglobin may be precipitated in the renal tubules by the acidity of the urine. The tubules block and are damaged, reducing the urinary output. Acute renal failure and anuria may develop if the hemolysis is extensive as a result of the patient receiving approximately 100 ml. or more of the incompatible blood.

A complication associated with a hemolytic reaction is hyperkalemia. The hemolysis of the donor's red blood cells releases potassium. The impaired renal function results in retention of the potassium, and its serum concentration exceeds the normal level. Hyperkalemia may develop when the whole blood that is being given has been stored for 5 days or more. Some red cells are broken down and the serum potassium concentration of the donor blood is increased.

TREATMENT. The administration of the blood or blood component is stopped promptly with the initial manifestation(s) of reaction. The normal saline is started again slowly to maintain an open intravenous line in case medications may have to be administered intravenously. The physician is notified immediately.

If the patient complains of shortness of breath and "tightness" in the chest, epinephrine hydrochloride 1:1000 (0.5 to 1 ml.) subcutaneously or intramuscularly may be prescribed. A marked fall in blood pressure

[26]J. Brian McSheffrey: "Effective Blood Transfusion Therapy." Can. Family Physician, Vol. 22; No. 12 (Dec. 1976), p. 36.

(hypotension) may be treated by increasing the intravascular volume with intravenous plasma or dextran.

Treatment is instituted to promote urinary output and reduce impairment of renal function by the hemoglobin released through hemolysis. The fluid intake and output must be accurately measured and recorded. An indwelling catheter may be passed so the urinary output may be measured hourly. Fluids containing potassium must be avoided. Mannitol (25 Gm.), an osmotic diuretic, may be slowly infused intravenously. If the urinary output progressively decreases, the fluid intake is limited to insensible fluid loss and losses by other channels (vomiting, bowel elimination). Anuria and renal failure may develop, necessitating hemodialysis.

2. FEBRILE REACTION. A fairly common reaction to a transfusion is fever preceded by a chill. It is attributed to the recipient's sensitivity to the donor's leukocytes, thrombocytes or plasma proteins. It may also develop as a result of a pyrogenic material in the equipment or solution used.

3. ALLERGIC REACTION. A component of the donor's blood may act as an antigen and initiate an allergic response. It is also suggested that the cause of an allergic reaction may be the response of antibodies in the donor's blood to an antigen within the recipient. The most common manifestations are urticaria and asthma. Severe bronchospasm and anaphylaxis occur less frequently. An antihistamine preparation, such as diphenhydramine hydrochloride (Benadryl), may provide relief. If the bronchospasm is severe or anaphylaxis develops, epinephrine hydrochloride 1:1000 may be administered parenterally.

4. CIRCULATORY OVERLOAD. The giving of a transfusion too rapidly, or the administration of whole blood or plasma to someone with a normal intravascular volume or who has or is predisposed to cardiac or renal insufficiency, is dangerous. The resulting increased intravascular volume places too great a demand on the heart. Heart failure and pulmonary edema ensue. The patient develops severe dyspnea, coughing, anxiety, weak pulse and cyanosis. A pink frothy sputum is expectorated.

Circulatory overload may be prevented by the slow administration of packed red cells while the central venous pressure is monitored carefully. (See p. 297 for central venous pressure monitoring.)

5. INFECTION. Hepatitis is the most common infectious problem associated with transfusions. Donors' blood is tested in blood banks for the hepatitis B antigen, but the transmission of hepatitis is still a possibility. The onset of manifestations of the infection may occur many weeks after the transfusion.

Syphilis and malaria may be transmitted by transfusion, but the possibility is minimal because of the screening of donors and the tests that are performed on all donor blood.

If a Transfusion Reaction Occurs

1. The transfusion is stopped promptly; slow infusion of normal saline is resumed to maintain an open line, and the physician is notified.

2. The remaining blood or blood component is returned in the container with the tubing to the blood bank for analysis and determination of the cause of the reaction.

3. The blood bank is notified of the nature of the reaction.

4. Blood specimens are taken from a vein other than the one that was used to administer the blood. They are sent to the laboratory for retyping, culture and estimation of free plasma hemoglobin.

5. A nurse remains with the patient; vital signs are monitored frequently and continuous assessment of the patient's condition is necessary. The patient is likely to be very apprehensive and fearful. He requires some information about what is happening and reassurance that everything possible is being done.

References

Books

Beeson, Paul B., and McDermott, Walsh (Eds.): Textbook of Medicine, 15th ed. Philadelphia, W. B. Saunders, 1979.

Ganong, William F.: Review of Medical Physiology, 7th ed. Los Altos, Cal., Lange, 1975. Chapter 27.

Guyton, Arthur C.: Textbook of Medical Physiology, 5th ed. Philadelphia, W. B. Saunders, 1977. Chapters 5, 6, 7.

Krupp, Marcus A., and Chatton, Milton J.: Current Medical Diagnoses and Treatment. Los Altos, Cal., Lange, 1975. Chapter 9.

Leavell, Byrd Stuart, and Thorup, Oscar Andreas, Jr.: Clinical Hematology, 4th ed. Philadelphia, W. B. Saunders, 1976.

MacLeod, John (Ed.): Davidson's Principles and Practice of Medicine, 11th ed. Edinburgh, Churchill Livingstone, 1974. Pp. 713–767.

Mengel, Charles E., et al. (Eds.): Hematology — Principles and Practice. Chicago, Yearbook Medical Publishers, 1972.

Schottelius, Byron A., and Schottelius, Dorothy D.: Textbook of Physiology. 17th ed. St. Louis, C. V. Mosby, 1973. Chapter 12.

Thorn, G. W., et al. (Eds.): Harrison's Principles of Internal Medicine, 8th ed. New York, McGraw-Hill, 1977.

Williams, William J., Beutler, Ernest, and Rundles, R. Wayne: Hematology. New York, McGraw-Hill, 1972.

Periodicals

Buschman, Penelope: "The Child with Leukemia — Group Support for Parents." Am. J. Nurs., Vol. 76, No. 7 (July 1976), p. 1121.

Child, Judy, Collins, Douglass, and Collins, Janis: "Blood Transfusions." Am. J. Nurs., Vol. 72, No. 9 (Sept. 1972), pp. 1602–1605.

Desotell, Susan: "A Brighter Future for Leukemia Patients." Nurs. '77, Vol. 7, No. 1 (Jan. 1977), pp. 18–23.

Doswell, Willa M.: "Sickle Cell Disease: How It Influences Preoperative and Postoperative Care." Nurs. '74, Vol. 4, No. 6 (June 1974), pp. 18–21.

———: "Sickle Cell Anemia: You Can Do Something to Help." Nurs. '78, Vol. 8, No. 4 (April 1978). pp. 65–70.

Foley, Genevieve, and McCarthy, Ann Marie: "The Child with Leukemia — The Disease and its Treatment." Am. J. Nurs., Vol. 76, No. 7 (July 1976), pp. 1108–1114.

———: "In a Special Hematology Clinic." Am. J. Nurs., Vol. 76. No. 7 (July 1976), pp. 1115–1119.

Foster, Sue: "Sickle Cell Anemia: Pathophysiologic Aspects." Heart Lung, Vol. 3, No. 6 (Nov.-Dec. 1974), pp. 955–961.

Gilbert, Marvin S., and Aledort, Louis M. (Eds.): "Symposium — Comprehensive Care in Hemophilia: A Team Approach." Mt. Sinai J. Med. N. Y., Vol. 44, No. 3 (May-June 1977).

Greene, Patricia: "The Child with Leukemia in the Classroom." Am. J. Nurs., Vol. 75, No. 1 (Jan. 1975), pp. 86–87.

———: "Acute Leukemia in Children." Am. J. Nurs., Vol. 75, No. 10 (Oct. 1975), pp. 1709–1714.

Gustavson, Lillian P., Hruby, Marilyn, and O'Brien, Richard: "When Hemophilia Heads the Problem List." Practical Family Patient Care, Vol. X, No. 18 (Oct. 1976), pp. 58–83.

Hugos, Ray: "Living with Leukemia." Am. J. Nurs., Vol. 72, No. 12 (Dec. 1972), pp. 2185–2188.

Keaveny, Marie E.: "Creative Nursing Care for Acute Leukemia." Nurs. '73, Vol. 3, No. 6 (June 1973), pp. 19–23.

———, and Wiley, Loy: "Hodgkin's Disease . . . The Curable Cancer." Nurs. '75, Vol. 5, No. 3 (March 1975), pp. 49–50.

Kikuchi, June: "How the Leukemic Child Chooses His Confidant." Can. Nurs., Vol. 71, No. 5 (May 1975), pp. 22–23.

Leventhal, Brigid G., and Hersh, Stephen: "Modern Treatment of Childhood Leukemia: The Patient and His Family." Nurs. Digest, Vol. III, No. 4 (July-Aug. 1975), pp. 12–15.

Martinson, Ida: "The Child with Leukemia — Parents Help Each Other." Am. J. Nurs., Vol. 76, No. 7 (July 1976), pp. 1121–1122.

Mayer, Gloria Gilbert: "Disseminated Intravascular Coagulation." Am. J. Nurs., Vol. 73, No. 12 (Dec. 1973), pp. 2067–2069.

McFarlane, Judith Medlin: "The Child with Sickle Cell Anemia." Nurs. '75, Vol. 5, No. 5 (May 1975), pp. 29–33.

Rogers, Jeanne: "Hodgkin's Disease: Hope Is the Key to Nursing Care." Nurs. '75, Vol. 5, No. 3 (March 1975), p. 51.

Rosen, Barbara J.: "Multiple Myeloma." Med. Clin. North Am., Vol. 59, No. 2 (March 1975), pp. 375–385.

Rossi, Ennio C. (Ed.): "Symposium on Hemorrhagic Disorders." Med. Clin. North Am., Vol. 56, No. 1 (Jan. 1972).

Rubin, Arnold D.: Symposium on Clinical Signs of Blood Disease." Med. Clin. North Am., Vol. 57, No. 2 (March 1973).

Sahakian, George J.: Management of Hodgkin's and Non-Hodgkin's Lymphomas." Med. Clin. North Am., Vol. 59, No. 2 (March 1975).

Schumann, Delores, and Patterson, Phyllis: "Multiple Myeloma." Am. J. Nurs., Vol. 75, No. 1 (Jan. 1975), pp. 78–81.

Sergis, Elaine, and Hilgartner, Margaret: "Hemophilia." Am. J. Nurs., Vol. 72, No. 11 (Nov. 1972), pp. 2011–2017.

Steinberg, David: "The Management of Acute Myelogenous Leukemia." Med. Clin. North Am., Vol. 59, No. 2 (March 1975), pp. 363–371.

Van Slyck, Ellis J.: "Supportive Care of the Leukemic Patient." Henry Ford Hosp. Med. J., Vol. 23, No. 3 (Fall 1975), pp. 117–128.

Warren, Barbara: "Maintaining the Hemophiliac At Home." Nurs. '74, Vol. 4, No. 1 (Jan. 1974), pp. 75–76.

Wilson, Patience: "Iron-Deficiency Anemia." Am. J. Nurs., Vol. 72, No. 3 (March 1972), pp. 502–504.

13

Nursing in Cardiovascular Disease

BY PATRICIA M. KEARNS, R.N., M.Sc.N.

CIRCULATION

Normal cellular activity is dependent upon a constant supply of oxygen, nutrients, and certain chemicals, as well as the removal of metabolic by-products. The unicellular organism is in direct contact with the outside environmental source of its essentials, but in complex multicellular organisms cell needs are not as simply met. Specialized organs are necessary for the processes of oxygenation, nutrition and excretion, as well as a transportation system between these organs and the cells throughout the body. This transportation of materials to and from tissue cells by the propulsion of blood through a closed system of tubes is the process referred to as circulation.

CIRCULATORY STRUCTURES

The circulatory system consists of the heart and the vascular system.

Heart

The heart is a hollow, cone-shaped, muscular organ lying obliquely in the thoracic cavity. Approximately two-thirds of it is situated to the left of the midline. The upper border (or base) lies just below the second rib; *the apex, which is directed downward, forward and to the left, lies on the dia-* *phragm at the level of the fifth intercostal space in the left midclavicular line. These boundary locations are significant in determining any abnormal enlargement and in counting the apical pulse.* The structural organization of the heart includes the pericardium, heart walls, chambers, orifices, valves and coronary system.

PERICARDIUM. The pericardium is a strong, nondistensible sac which loosely encloses the heart and attaches to the large blood vessels at the base of the heart and to the diaphragm at the apex. It consists of two layers. The outer one forms the fibrous pericardium, and the inner one, the serous pericardium, is also divided into two layers; one layer lines the sac, and the other is reflected over the surface of the heart as the epicardium, or visceral pericardium. The space formed between the sac and the heart is normally only a potential space. The surfaces are in close contact, and sufficient serum is secreted to keep them moist so that adhesion and friction between the heart and the sac are prevented. The fibrous pericardium, because of its inextensible nature, averts overdistension of the heart. It also supports the heart, preventing change of its position during postural changes. Although the pericardial sac is firm and considered nonextensible, it does extend in response to the gradual, sustained stretching imposed by enlargement of the heart (hypertrophy).

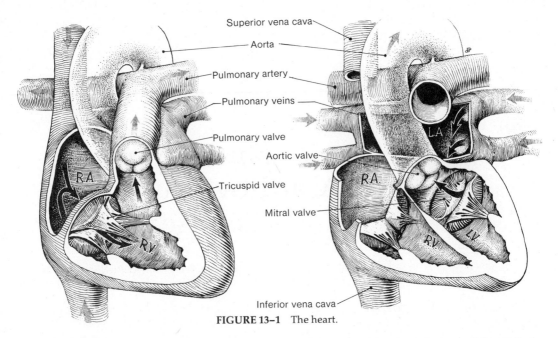

Superior vena cava

Aorta

Pulmonary artery

Pulmonary veins

Pulmonary valve

Aortic valve

Tricuspid valve

Mitral valve

Inferior vena cava

FIGURE 13–1 The heart.

HEART WALLS AND CHAMBERS. From shortly after birth, the human heart is divided longitudinally by a partition into two halves between which there is no direct communication. The cavity of each side is divided horizontally by an incomplete partition which results in two upper chambers, called the right and left atria, and two lower ones, which are the right and left ventricles (see Fig. 13–1).

The walls of the heart consist of three layers — the epicardium, myocardium and endocardium. The myocardium (heart muscle) comprises the main functional part of the heart wall; its rhythmic contractions provide the pumping force which maintains circulation. It is formed of involuntary striated muscle fibers which interlace, branch, anastomose and coalesce. This arrangement produces a very firm, closely related mass of tissue through which an excitatory impulse for contraction spreads very quickly. The muscle fibers of the atria are continuous and behave as a single mass. Similarly, those of the ventricles are also continuous and act as a single mass. Atrial muscle fibers are completely separated from those of the ventricles by fibrous tissue.

The atrial myocardium is much thinner than that of the ventricles, and the left ventricular wall is thicker than that of the right. This difference can be correlated with the force that must be given to the contained blood. The atria are receiving chambers and

are only required to deliver the blood to the ventricles, which discharge blood from the heart. The right ventricle pumps blood through the lungs to the left atrium, forming the circuit referred to as the pulmonary circulatory system. The left ventricle must provide sufficient pressure to carry blood through all parts of the body and return it to the right atrium. This latter circuit is referred to as the systemic circulatory system.

SPECIAL STRUCTURES. Two small masses of specialized tissue lie within the atrial myocardium — the sino-atrial (S-A) node and the atrioventricular (A-V) node. The S-A node is located in the upper part of the right atrium near the superior vena cava and is responsible for initiating the impulses for the rhythmic heart beats.

The A-V node lies in the lower part of the interatrial septum and is a part of the system that conducts impulses from the atria to the ventricles. A bundle of fibers called the bundle of His proceeds from junctional tissue at the A-V node into the ventricular septum where it divides into two, forming the left and right bundle branches. The left bundle branch further divides into the anterior (superior) and posterior (inferior) divisions (Fig. 13–2). As it descends, each bundle branch gives rise to a network of fine fibers which are known as the Purkinje fibers. They are distributed to the ventricular myocardial cells.

ORIFICES IN THE CHAMBERS. The right

atrium has three inlets and one outlet. Blood is received from two large veins, the superior and inferior venae cavae, and the coronary sinus. The outlet channels the blood into the right ventricle. The right ventricle has two openings — the inlet from the right atrium and an outlet into the pulmonary artery.

The left atrium has four inlets, which are the terminations of the four pulmonary veins, and one outlet into the left ventricle. The blood received from the left atrium is discharged by the left ventricle into the aorta.

ENDOCARDIUM. The endocardium is the smooth endothelial lining of the heart chambers. It covers the valves and is continuous with the lining of the blood vessels entering and leaving the heart. Its smooth surface reduces friction between the blood and the vessel.

CARDIAC VALVES. Normal circulation requires the flow of the blood in one direction only. This is maintained in the heart by a set of four valves — two atrioventricular and two semilunar.

The atrioventricular valves are formed of fibrous cusps, or leaflets, which derive from the fibrous ring that encircles each atrioventricular opening. They are covered with endothelial tissue which is continuous with the endocardium. The right atrioventricular valve has three cusps and is referred to as the tricuspid valve; the left one has two cusps and is called the mitral valve. These valves open into the ventricles but are prevented from opening into the atria by fine tendinous

cords (chordae tendineae) which insert on the free border of the leaflets and originate in small pillars of muscle projecting from the ventricular walls (papillary muscles). When the ventricles fill, the valve flaps are forced up in the direction of the atrioventricular opening. They meet, closing off the opening and, with the contraction of the papillary muscles, sufficient tension is exerted by the chordae tendineae to prevent the valves from opening into the atria (see Fig. 13–1).

The semilunar valves guard the openings from the ventricles into the pulmonary artery and aorta. Each consists of three pocket-like pouches arranged around the origin of the artery, with the free borders being distal to the ventricle (see Fig. 13–1). During the contraction of the ventricles and ejection of blood under considerable pressure into the aorta and pulmonary artery, the valve flaps lie free in the stream, offering no resistance to the flow of the blood. When the ventricles relax and there is a reversal in the direction of pressure, blood fills out the semilunar pouches, bringing their surfaces together. This closes off the aperture into each ventricle, preventing a backflow.

CARDIAC BLOOD SUPPLY (CORONARY SYSTEM). (See Fig. 13–3.) The myocardium receives its blood supply from the right or left coronary arteries, which arise from the sinuses of Valsalva in the root of the aorta. The left coronary artery divides into the anterior descending artery and the circumflex artery. The anterior descending branch is distributed to the anterior

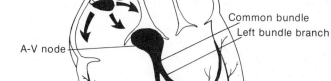

FIGURE 13–2 The impulse conduction system.

S-A node

A-V node

Common bundle
Left bundle branch

Right bundle branch

Left anterior hemibranch

Left posterior hemibranch

Purkinje fiber

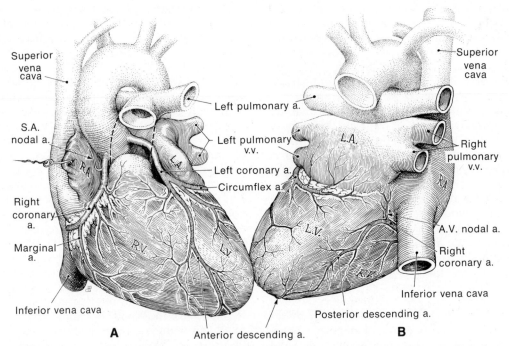

FIGURE 13–3 *A*, Circulation to the anterior surface of the heart. *B*, Circulation to the posterior surface of the heart, showing the A-V nodal artery as a branch of the right coronary artery.

part of the left ventricle and portions of the right ventricle. In addition to the anterior wall of the left ventricle, the anterior descending artery supplies the anterior papillary muscle of the left ventricle, the anterior two-thirds of the interventricular septum, and distal parts of the conduction system. The circumflex artery carries blood to the lateral and lower posterior, left ventricular walls and to the left atrium. Branches of the right coronary artery supply the remaining portions of the myocardium. The right coronary artery nourishes the sinoatrial (S-A) node in approximately 55 per cent of persons and the atrioventricular (A-V) node in 90 per cent of persons. At other times, the blood supply to these structures is provided by the left circumflex artery. The large arteries divide and subdivide to form a network of smaller arteries and capillaries throughout the heart muscle. The blood is returned to the right atrium through a system of progressively enlarging veins which terminate in the coronary sinus.

The myocardium requires a large blood supply since it must work continuously and adapt its activity to the varying needs of tissues throughout the body. The coronary ves-sels dilate to increase the supply when demands are increased. They also dilate when there is an increase in the carbon dioxide concentration of the blood and a decrease in the pH.

The flow of blood through the coronary system is dependent upon the pressure of the blood in the aorta; a reduction in blood pressure will result in a lesser volume entering the coronary arteries. The coronary volume is greater during myocardial relaxation. In systole, with the myocardium contracted, the vessels are compressed and their volume is reduced. When a person is at rest, the blood entering the coronary system is approximately 4 per cent of the total cardiac output. The coronary blood supply can be increased, but to a lesser degree than the cardiac output. That is, the work of the myocardium can be increased to a greater extent than its blood supply.

Vascular System

The blood travels from the heart successively through arteries, arterioles, capillaries and veins back to the heart (see Fig. 13–4).

The structure of each type of vessel is modified according to its function and location. One common structural characteristic of all the vessels is the smooth endothelial lining, known as the intima. The arteries and arterioles form a high-pressure distributing system; the capillaries are structured and organized for exchanging substances between the blood and interstitial fluid; the venules and veins serve as a low-pressure collecting system which returns the blood to the heart.

ARTERIES. The large arteries carry blood away from the heart and branch and subdivide many times. Their structure varies with their size, the larger ones being more elastic and less muscular. Elasticity is an important property of these vessels; with the ejection of blood from the heart, the vessel distends and on recoil exerts a slight pressure on the contained fluid, helping to force it forward. If resistance is offered to the flow of the blood, normally the arteries can stretch to accommodate the increased volume of blood, and the pressure of the blood remains within the normal range. Reduced elasticity and a thickening of the arterial walls with a narrowing of the lumen, as seen in arteriosclerosis and atherosclerosis, result in a rise in the arterial blood pressure.

ARTERIOLES. The smallest arteries emerge as arterioles which have walls composed mainly of a well developed muscular coat over the endothelium. The muscle tissue may contract or relax to decrease or increase the amount of blood through the arterioles. This feature of the arterioles gives them an important role in determining arterial blood pressure and in controlling the blood supply to tissues.

CAPILLARIES. Each arteriole channels its content into microscopic endothelial tubes, the capillaries, which anastomose with each other to form a capillary bed. These vessels are the principal functional unit of the cardiovascular system. The functions of the other structures (heart, arteries and veins) are contributory to that of the capillaries. The exchange of substances to maintain and regulate cell activity takes place as the blood passes through these minute, semipermeable vessels.

Not all the capillaries are open at all times. There are wide variations in the amount of activity in some tissues (e.g., skeletal muscle), while in others a more constant blood supply is necessary, as in brain tissue. Similarly, when an area is irritated, more blood is brought to that part in its defense (e.g. inflammation). The number of capillaries through which blood is passing at any given time is adjusted locally to meet the needs of the tissues in the area. Blood volume in the capillaries increases as tissue activity increases. Guyton states that in some resting structures only 12 to 20 per cent of the capil-

FIGURE 13–4 Artery–arteriole–capillary–vein sequence in circulation.

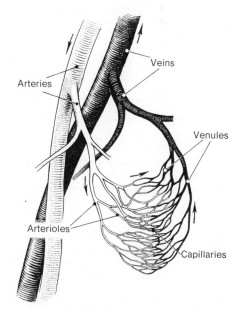

lary bed may be open to circulation. [1] This adjustment is made possible by the fact that some capillaries have at their origin a ring of plain muscular tissue which forms a precapillary sphincter.

VENULES AND VEINS. The collecting part of the vascular system originates in venules which drain the capillaries and progressively unite and enlarge to form the veins.They differ from arteries in several ways: (1) they carry blood toward the heart; (2) their walls are much thinner and less elastic with the result that they collapse when empty; (3) the contained blood is under a much lower pressure; and (4) many of the veins have valves.

The structure of veins changes as they increase in size; more muscle and fibrous tissue appear in the walls but, in comparison with arteries, the muscle fibers are sparse. Most of the pressure of the blood created by the heart is dissipated in the arterioles and capillaries and, in order to maintain the flow in one direction, valves similar in structure to the semilunar valves of the heart occur at intervals in many of the veins. They are particularly numerous in the lower extremities where the blood is flowing against gravity. The thinner walls of the veins are readily compressed by skeletal muscle contraction; this assists the blood along its course toward the heart, since backflow toward the capillaries is prevented by the valves.

PHYSIOLOGY OF CIRCULATION

Normal circulation through the cardiovascular system is dependent upon an appropriate pressure gradient throughout the system, an adequate volume of blood, a closed system of unobstructed tubes and a set of valves to ensure flow in one direction only.

Principles Applicable to the Flow of Fluids through Tubes

Since circulation is the continuous flow of blood in a pressure system composed of a pump and a series of tubes filled with the blood, it might be well at this point to consider some physical factors which govern the

flow of any liquid through tubes. The rate at which a fluid moves through a tube depends upon the pressure gradient and the resistance to flow.

PRESSURE GRADIENT. Fluids flow from an area of high pressure to one of lower pressure. The pressure of fluid at any given point in the system must be greater than that in the succeeding area into which it is to flow. This difference is referred to as the pressure gradient, or driving force. If the pressure should become the same throughout the system, no movement of fluid takes place.

The pressure gradient which maintains the normal flow of blood through the vessels is the difference between the pressure of the blood in the arterial system and that of the venous system. The main source of the driving force is the pumping action of the heart which produces a relatively high pressure in the arteries.

RESISTANCE TO FLOW. The amount of resistance offered to the flow of fluid is determined by the dimensions of the tube and the viscosity of the fluid.

The pressure of a fluid progressively decreases as it flows through a tube because of the friction between the fluid and the walls of the tube. This friction, which is referred to as peripheral resistance, causes a loss of energy. Fluid flows more slowly through a tube of smaller diameter since more friction is created between the walls and the fluid, resulting in an increase in resistance. As the blood flows through blood vessels having a lesser radius (arterioles and capillaries) resistance is increased, causing a decrease in the rate of flow and blood pressure.

Similarly, resistance is increased as the length of the tube increases, since the greater amount of surface provides more friction.

If the volume of fluid remains the same in a system of tubes, the rate of flow decreases as the tubular space (capacity) increases. This factor contributes to the marked decrease in the velocity of the blood in the capillaries. Although the radius of the capillaries is extremely small, the total cross-sectional area of the vast number of these minute tubes exceeds the total area of all the other vessels combined.

The viscosity of a fluid is an internal resistance to flow created by the friction between the molecules of fluid and their tendency to cohere. Obviously, a greater concentration

---

[1] Arthur C. Guyton: Textbook of Medical Physiology, 5th ed. Philadelphia, W. B. Saunders, 1976, p. 371.

of particles in a fluid produces an increased internal resistance. For example, an excessive number of blood cells, particularly erythrocytes, increases the viscosity of the blood and retards its rate of flow.

In summary, resistance to flow is inversely proportional to the diameter of the tube, directly proportional to the length of the tube, and directly proportional to the viscosity of the fluid. If the volume of fluid remains the same, the rate of flow decreases as the diameter of the tube increases.

The preceding principles are based on the flow of fluids through rigid tubes. Some modification is necessary in applying them to circulation. The blood vessels are not rigid tubes and their diameters are variable. Branches, division and curves occur at frequent intervals in the blood vessels. Blood is viscous and its flow is pulsatile, rather than steady, in a large part of the circulatory system.

THE ROLE OF THE HEART IN CIRCULATION

The pressure that keeps the blood in continuous movement through the circulatory system originates in the heart and is augmented slightly by the elastic recoil of the large arteries. A continuous succession of alternate myocardial contractions and relaxations, occurring rhythmically on an average of 60 to 70 times per minute, pumps the blood through the body.

Impulse Origin and Conduction in Heart Contraction

The cells of the myocardium are of two types — those which contract when stimulated and those which originate and conduct impulses. The ability to originate and conduct impulses is referred to as the electrical activity of the heart. The heart has three electrical properties: (1) automaticity, or the ability to initiate an electrical impulse; (2) excitability, or the ability to respond to an electrical impulse; and (3) conductivity, or the ability to transmit an impulse from one cell to another. The muscle fibers have an absolute and a relative refractory period. The fibers are unresponsive to any stimulus during the absolute refractory period which immediately follows a contraction. The rela-

tive refractory period is the interval in which the muscle fibers gradually recover their excitability (ability to respond to a stimulus) but will respond to a stimulus if it is stronger than the usual. The refractory period in cardiac muscle is longer than in other muscle tissue. Excitability is more slowly regained, giving the heart chambers time to fill effectively.

Contraction of the myocardium is dependent upon impulses which arise within the myocardium itself. The structures capable of generating and conducting impulses within the myocardium form the conduction system. They are the sino-atrial (S-A) node, tracts of conducting fibers originating with the S-A node, the atrioventricular (A-V) node, the bundle of His, bundle branches and the Purkinje fibers. Several areas of the conduction system are capable of the spontaneous generation of impulses — namely, the S-A node, the junctional tissue where the conducting fibers join the A-V node, the bundle of His and the Purkinje fibers. The rate at which impulses are normally fired varies in the different areas: the S-A node originates approximately 60 to 80 impulses per minute; the junctional tissue, 50 to 60 impulses per minute; the bundle of His, 40 to 50 impulses per minute; and the Purkinje fibers, 30 to 40 per minute. Since the region which is producing the highest rate of impulses sets the heart rhythm (number of contractions per minute), the S-A node is referred to as the normal pacemaker.

Impulses arising in the S-A node are quickly conducted through the atria, initiating their contraction. At the same time, impulses are transmitted to the A-V node where they are delayed; this delay allows for completion of atrial emptying and ventricular filling. From the A-V node and junctional tissue they travel through the bundle of His and along the right and left bundle branches and the widely distributed Purkinje fibers to the ventricular contractile fibers.

Electrophysiology

Electrical currents in cardiac cells are produced by ion movement across the cell membrane. There is a marked difference in the intracellular and extracellular concentrations of ions, the most important of which are sodium and potassium. The potassium concentration is approximately 30 times greater inside the cell than outside, and the sodium concentration is approximately 30 times less within the cell than outside.

During the resting state the inside of the cardiac cell is negatively charged while the outside is positively charged, and the membrane is referred to as polarized. By inserting microelectrodes inside the cardiac cell, researchers have been able to measure the potential difference in voltage across the membrane. In the resting state the potential is −90 millivolts, as shown in Figure 13–5, and is called the resting membrane potential. At this time the cell membrane is impermeable to the movement of ions through it.

During depolarization, the cell membrane becomes permeable to sodium, which rapidly shifts inside the cell. This sudden influx of sodium reverses the transmembrane potential and potassium moves out of the cell.

In Figure 13–5 the resting or polarized phase is shown as the straight line at −90 millivolts. The change in transmembrane potential is represented by the upstroke, phase 0. After excitation the action potential rapidly declines and then levels off for a short period, as represented by phases 1 and 2. This time is referred to as the absolute refractory period and further stimulation produces no response.

Repolarization, or return to the normal resting potential, occurs during phase 3, known as the relative refractory period. The inside of the cell gradually resumes its negative electrical charge. During this time a stimulus of greater than normal intensity could reactivate the cell. Phase 4 shows a period of stable resting potential which remains until the next wave of excitation.

During depolarization ions move into and out of the cell because of differences in concentration gradients on either side of the cell membrane. During repolarization, however, an active transport system is required to pump out the sodium which has entered the cell and to pump in an equivalent amount of potassium. This mechanism is known as the "sodium pump" and requires energy.

The Cardiac Cycle

The succession of events which occurs with each heartbeat is called the cardiac cycle. It consists of the relaxation and contraction of the atria and ventricles and the opening and closing of the cardiac valves in a sequence that permits the filling and emptying of the heart chambers. Contraction of the atria or ventricles is called systole; their relaxation is known as diastole. In referring to contraction or relaxation of the atria or ventricles, the terms used are atrial or ventricular systole or atrial or ventricular diastole respectively. If systole or diastole is used alone, it refers to ventricular performance only.

The sequence of events of the cardiac cycle is as follows. The atria in diastole fill with blood received from their inlet vessels. In the early part of the relaxation period, the atrioventricular (A-V) valves are closed but, as pressure builds up in the atria, it becomes greater than that in the ventricles, forcing the A-V valves open, and the blood starts to flow through into the ventricles. Atrial diastole is followed in a fraction of a second by contraction to complete the emptying of the two upper chambers, and the atria again enter their diastole.

During the filling and contraction of the ventricles the blood floats the A-V valvular flaps up, closing off the A-V openings and preventing a regurgitation of blood into the atria. In order to receive the blood from the atria, the ventricles must be in diastole and, at this time, the semilunar valves are closed. With ventricular filling the intraventricular pressure builds up until it exceeds that in the aorta and pulmonary artery, with the result that the semilunar valves open, allowing blood to flow into the arteries. The ventricular muscle contracts, and the ventricles are emptied.

During ventricular systole, the papillary muscles also contract, exerting tension on the fine tendons (chordae tendineae) inserted on the A-V valvular flaps. This prevents the flaps from opening into the atria. If this control was not placed on the A-V valves, there would be a blackflow into the atria, espe-

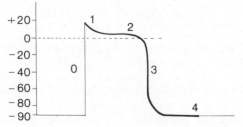

FIGURE 13–5 The electrophysiology of the cell.

cially with the ventricular contraction. The ventricles relax following their systole and emptying. This results in the pressure being greater in the arteries than in the ventricles, thus favoring the backflow of blood into the ventricles. But flow in the direction of the heart brings about the closure of the semilunar valves by the filling of the semilunar pouches; their free borders are brought together, preventing the blood from reentering the ventricles from the arteries. The cardiac cycle is now completed.

The cycle in a heart beating approximately 70 times per minute is completed in 0.7 to 0.8 of a second. The length of each phase of the cycle varies; atrial diastole lasts approximately 0.7 second, while its systole is approximately 0.1 second. Ventricular diastole is about 0.4 to 0.5 second, and its systole takes about 0.3 second. Following the ventricular contraction there is a brief period, approximately 0.4 second, in which the entire myocardium is relaxed. The ventricular diastole overlaps the atrial diastole.[2]

Heart Sounds

Two sounds are produced in quick succession in each cardiac cycle. These are followed by a brief pause before being repeated in the next cycle. Through a stethoscope the heart sounds will be heard as a lubb-dupp, and are produced by closure of the heart valves.

The first heart sound, S_1, is a prolonged low-pitched sound (lubb). It is produced by the closing of both atrioventricular valves, the mitral and the tricuspid, just before ventricular systole. Although closure of the two valves occurs almost simultaneously, the mitral valve closes slightly before the tricuspid valve. Therefore, the mitral component is heard slightly before the tricuspid and is the main component of the first heart sound.

The second sound, S_2, is briefer and higher pitched (dupp). It is produced by the closing of both semilunar valves, the aortic and the pulmonic, just before diastole. Since the aortic valve closes slightly before the pulmonic valve, the aortic component of S_2 will be heard slightly before the pulmonic. The components of the second sound are normally affected by respiration. During inspiration,

closure of the pulmonic valve is delayed because of the increased venous return to the right heart. The difference in the two components of S_2 is therefore more apparent. This is referred to as physiological splitting and disappears during expiration.

The heart sounds will differ as one listens at different locations on the chest (Fig. 13–6). The mitral component of S_1 (M_1) is best heard over the apex of the heart (the patient's fifth left intercostal space near the left midclavicular line). The tricuspid component (T_1) is softer than the mitral component and may be best heard over the patient's lower left sternal border.

The aortic component of the second heart sound (A_2) is louder than the pulmonic component and is best heard in the patient's second right intercostal space. The pulmonic valve closure (P_2) is best heard in the patient's second left intercostal space.

A third and fourth heart sound may also be heard. S_3 is a low-pitched sound produced in the ventricle by rapid filling. It may indicate ventricular decompensation and is heard in patients with congestive heart failure. An audible fourth sound (S_4), also called presystolic, is low-pitched and generated by forceful contractions of the atria. It may be present in healthy individuals but is frequent-

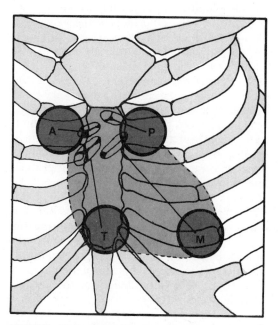

FIGURE 13–6 Auscultatory areas on the chest. Circles represent position of the stethoscope.

[2]William F. Ganong: Review of Medical Physiology, 7th ed. Los Altos, Cal., Lange, 1975, p. 413.

ly heard in patients with systemic hypertension.

Other unusual or abnormal sounds may also be heard, such as rubs, clicks, splits and murmurs, and usually indicate some pathology in the heart.

Cardiac Output

The volume of blood ejected from each ventricle in a minute is known as the cardiac output. The output of each ventricle with each contraction is called the stroke volume. In an adult, the cardiac output varies from 3000 to 5000 ml. per minute, and the stroke volume is about 60 to 70 ml. If it were 60 ml. in a person with a heart rate of 60, the cardiac output would be 3600 ml. (Stroke volume × heart rate = cardiac output per minute.)

The volume of blood that the normal heart pumps out each minute is increased in any situation that increases the body demands and activity. This is readily seen in physical exercise. In strenuous exertion the cardiac output may increase to a volume 13 times greater than the output during rest. This is achieved by an increase in the heart rate and the stroke volume. An increase in the cardiac output also occurs in high environmental temperature, emotional responses such as fear, anger or other excitement, after a heavy meal and in the later months of pregnancy.

Physiologically, the cardiac output is contingent upon the efficiency of the heart as a pump and upon the venous return. Obviously, normal heart structures, absence of disease, and an adequate supply of nutrients and oxygen are important factors in the heart's ability to produce the necessary force to eject the contained blood. If the heart is undamaged and is in a condition to respond, the strength of the heartbeat is determined mainly by the length of the muscle fibers when contraction begins. Stretching of muscle fibers, within limits, increases the strength of their contraction. The length or stretching of the myocardial fibers is dependent upon the volume of blood entering the heart. This principle is known as Starling's law of the heart and may be expressed in this manner: "the energy of contraction is proportional to the initial length of the cardiac muscle fiber."[3]

---

[3]Ibid., p. 418.

The volume of the venous return to the heart is influenced by several factors: the volume and pressure of the blood, resistance to the blood flow, physical exercise and respirations.

BLOOD VOLUME AND BLOOD PRESSURE. A decrease in the volume or pressure of the blood in the systemic circulation causes a decrease in the venous return. This is seen in hemorrhage in which the volume is reduced, and in shock, which is characterized by a fall in blood pressure. Certain areas of the body normally contain a relatively large volume of blood which may be moved out when the normal circulating volume is threatened. These areas are referred to as blood reservoirs and are the liver, spleen, large abdominal veins and venous plexuses of the skin. When necessary, the liver will increase its output into the hepatic vein, and the spleen will contract to empty as much as three-quarters of its contained blood into the circulation. Similarly, when the total circulating volume is reduced, the large abdominal veins constrict to increase their outflow. The venous plexuses of the skin, which normally contain a considerable volume of blood, will also constrict when necessary to provide a greater flow to the heart.

RESISTANCE TO BLOOD FLOW. Increased resistance to the blood flow anywhere in the circulatory system may reduce venous return to the heart and cause a corresponding decrease in cardiac output.

EXERCISE. Muscular exercise is one of the most significant factors in promoting venous return. When skeletal muscles contract, veins are compressed, and more blood is forced out of them. It must move toward the heart since the valves prevent a backward flow. Also, the increased metabolism in the muscles during exercise increases their need for oxygen and nutrients, resulting in local vasodilation of the arterioles and capillaries which reduces resistance to the flow of blood in the muscles. Since exercise usually involves a large number of muscles, this causes an appreciable decrease in the total resistance in the systemic circulation, favoring an increased venous return and cardiac output.

RESPIRATIONS. The rate and depth of respirations also have a marked effect on venous return; increased respirations increase the volume of blood entering the right atrium. On inspiration, the diaphragm descends, compressing the abdominal cavity and increasing the pressure on the veins in that area. At the same time the thoracic cavity enlarges and the pressure on regional veins is reduced. This increases the pressure gradient between the blood in the abdominal veins and that in the thoracic veins so that a greater volume flows from the abdominal veins into the thoracic vena cava and on into the heart.

The foregoing explanation of the effects of exercise and respirations on the venous return and cardiac output explains the importance of having inactive and bed patients breathe deeply at frequent intervals and do some physical exercises. These activities promote circulation and help to prevent complications that may occur with circulatory stasis.

Sympathetic nervous innervation may augment the volume of blood in circulation, and thus the venous return, by causing organs such as the liver and spleen to reduce their intrinsic volume.

The ability of the heart to increase its output commensurate with increased tissue activity and needs is referred to as cardiac reserve. The normal heart is capable of forwarding the volume of blood delivered to it and of responding to an increased demand without difficulty. It does this without causing breathlessness, tachycardia or palpitation beyond 5 to 10 minutes. It can do approximately 13 times what it does at rest if its reserve is normal.

Heart Rate

The number of heartbeats per minute varies in different persons and under different conditions. The average normal rate for an adult is 70 beats per minute, but it may range from 60 to 90. Several factors influence the heart rate. In the infant a rate of 110 to 130 is normal. It becomes progressively slower as the child grows older; by the early teens it is usually about 80. Muscular exertion will produce a marked increase, especially if one is unaccustomed to physical exercise. The rate usually increases during emotional reactions, with fever, and in the lower atmospheric pressures found at high altitudes.

Regulation of Cardiac Activity

Certain nervous, chemical and mechanical factors play an important role in the action of the heart.

NERVOUS INFLUENCE. The heart muscle is capable of generating its own impulses for contraction, but nerve impulses from the parasympathetic and sympathetic divisions of the autonomic nervous system may modify the rate and strength of the contractions. Nervous regulation is mediated by impulses which arise in the medulla oblongata in a group of neurons known as the cardiac center. Parasympathetic impulses reach the heart by way of branches of the vagus nerve (tenth cranial nerve) and are delivered to the S-A and A-V nodes and to the atrial muscle. Vagal or parasympathetic innervation has an inhibitory effect on cardiac activity; it slows the heart rate and decreases the force of the atrial contraction by reducing the excitability of the pacemaker (S-A node) and the conductivity of the A-V node and conducting system.

Sympathetic impulses enter the heart by the cardiac accelerator nerves, originating in a cervical ganglion. These impulses are transmitted to the S-A node, the conducting system, and the atrial and ventricular muscle. Sympathetic stimulation increases the heart rate and the strength of the heart contractions.

Parasympathetic innervation predominates in heart action. Normally, it exerts a fairly constant check on the heart rate, thus conserving the heart's strength.

The cardiac center may be stimulated by impulses originating in higher levels of the brain or in some part of the body which is outside the central nervous system (brain and spinal cord). One need only recall the change experienced in one's own heart action during fear, anger or other excitement. The response of increased or decreased heart activity is due to impulses being discharged by the cerebral cortical level to the cardiac center.

Sensory impulses from outside the central nervous system enter the cord or brain and may be relayed to the cardiac center, resulting in innervation of the heart. The response of the heart to peripheral sensory impulses may be referred to as a cardiac reflex. The most significant of these are the vasosensory impulses originating in the pressoreceptors and chemoreceptors. A group of sensory nerve endings in the aortic arch and in the carotid artery at its bifurcation are sensitive to changes in the blood pressure and are called pressoreceptors. In the same areas are nerve endings that are sensitive to changes in the carbon dioxide and oxygen concentration and the pH (hydrogen ion concentration) of the blood. These are known as the chemoreceptors. Impulses initiated in these receptors enter the brain or cord and are relayed to the cardiac center.

An increase in blood pressure produces a response in the cardio-inhibitory center. Vagal stimulation of the heart is increased and the heart rate decreases.[4] A decrease in the oxygen concentration, an increase in carbon dioxide concentration and a decrease in the pH of the blood result in stimulation of the cardio-accelerator center and in elevation of the heart rate.

CHEMICAL INFLUENCE. Normal, rhythmic heart contractions are greatly dependent upon an optimal concentration of potassium, sodium and calcium in the extracellular fluid.[5] These minerals play an important role in the excitability of the cardiac muscle cells and their contraction.

If the potassium level is greater than its normal concentration in the extracellular fluid, an impairment in conduction and contraction occurs. It causes a prolonged relaxation of the heart with abnormal dilation of the chambers. The pulse becomes slow. A decrease below the normal concentration of sodium results in weaker contractions. The pulse is rapid and weak, and there is a fall in blood presssure. An excess sodium concentration does not directly affect cardiac action. An excess of calcium produces a stronger and prolonged systole. Conversely, a lack of calcium prolongs the diastole.

Other chemicals of significance in heart action are oxygen and carbon dioxide. Any deficiency of oxygen is quickly reflected in a weakening of heart action. The myocardium is much more sensitive to oxygen lack than skeletal muscle; it will stand only one-fifth as much oxygen deficiency as skeletal muscle.

---

[4]Marey's law. The pulse rate is inversely related to the arterial blood pressure.

[5]Optimal serum concentrations:
K^+ 3.5–5.0 mEq./L.
Na^+ 135.0–145.0 mEq./L.
Ca^{2+} 4.5–5.5 mEq./L.

The pulse becomes rapid, weak and irregular. With an excess of carbon dioxide in the blood, as may occur in respiratory insufficiency, heart action is impaired. Conduction is slowed, the relaxation period is prolonged and the contraction is briefer than normal.

MECHANICAL INFLUENCE. The principal mechanical influence on cardiac activity is the stretching of the myocardial fibers by the volume of blood entering the chambers. As previously stated, stretching of muscle fibers increases the strength of their contraction (Starling's law of the heart, p. 278). An increase in arterial blood pressure also demands a greater force of contraction; the heart muscle must release a greater amount of energy to perform its function because of meeting greater resistance.

BLOOD PRESSURE AND PULSE

Blood Pressure

Blood pressure may be defined as the pressure exerted laterally on the walls of the blood vessels. It varies in different parts of the circulatory system, being greatest in the large arteries, with a progressive decrease as the blood continues on through the smaller arteries, arterioles, capillaries and veins. The pressure is highest in the aorta and lowest in the large caval veins which enter the heart. Blood pressure at any point in the vascular system is dependent upon the force with which the heart pumps the blood out of the ventricles, the volume of blood in the system, the elasticity of the arteries and the amount of resistance to the flow of the blood from one portion of the circulatory system to the next.

Arterial Blood Pressure

The blood pressure of greatest clinical interest is that in the arteries. The pulsatile nature of heart activity causes fluctuations in the pressure. With each contraction of the left ventricle a volume of blood is pumped into the aorta, which is already filled with blood. This causes an appreciable increase in the pressure of the blood and stretches the aortic walls. If the aorta were not elastic, the rise in pressure would be much higher and sharper. During the ventricular diastole, the elastic walls of the aorta recoil, exerting a pressure on the contained blood. If the aorta were a rigid tube which did not recoil, the pressure of the blood would fall more rapidly and to a much lower level than it does normally. The higher pressure produced by the ventricular systole is referred to as the *systolic blood pressure*. The lower pressure that occurs during the ventricular diastole is dependent upon the recoil of the large arteries and is known as the *diastolic blood pressure*. The difference between these two pressures is called the *pulse pressure*. Pulse pressure varies inversely with the elasticity of the arteries. Rigid vessels with a loss of ability to distend and recoil produce a higher systolic pressure and a lower diastolic pressure, resulting in a higher pulse pressure.

MEASUREMENT. Arterial blood pressure is most frequently measured in millimeters of mercury (mm. Hg) by means of a sphygmomanometer and a stethoscope, using the brachial artery. The rubber cuff of the blood pressure apparatus is applied to the upper arm just above the elbow and is inflated with air, which compresses the brachial artery. The pressure in the cuff is transmitted to the column of mercury of the manometer. The stethoscope is applied over the brachial artery just below the cuff.

When the cuff pressure becomes greater than the blood pressure, no pulse is heard. The air in the cuff is slowly released and the height of the mercury on the manometer is noted when the pulse is first heard. This corresponds to the systolic blood pressure.

With further slow deflation of the cuff, the pulse gradually becomes softer and fades. The level of the mercury is again noted just before the pulse becomes inaudible; this represents the diastolic blood pressure. If the blood pressure is recorded as 100 mm. Hg, it simply means that the pressure of the blood on the walls of the vessel is sufficient to raise a column of mercury to a height of 100 mm. The normal systolic pressure in a healthy young adult in a sitting position is 100 to 135 mm. Hg; the normal diastolic pressure is 60 to 80 mm. Hg. Blood pressure may also be determined by a more direct method. A needle or a cannula is placed in an artery and connected to a mercury manometer on which the blood pressure is indicated. For continuous monitoring of blood pressure, the needle may be connected to a transducer for electronic recording.

FACTORS WHICH DETERMINE ARTERIAL

BLOOD PRESSURE. Arterial blood pressure is influenced by the strength of the heartbeat, volume of blood, elasticity of the vessels and the resistance offered to the flow of blood.

STRENGTH OF THE HEARTBEAT. If the myocardial strength is weakened by disease, lack of essential materials or a deficiency in stimulation, it follows that the pressure under which the blood is ejected into the arteries would be reduced, as well as the volume of blood emitted. The arterial pressure is directly proportional to the cardiac output.

BLOOD VOLUME. Any reduction in the intravascualr volume will reduce the head of pressure and the stretch and recoil of the arteries, resulting in an appreciable decrease in the pressure of the blood. Small decreases in the volume are compensated for by the contraction of vessels but, in some conditions (e.g., hemorrhage, severe dehydration, burns), the loss may be beyond compensation. In some instances, vasodilation may occur (e.g., shock, anaphylaxis), increasing the capacity of the system beyond that of the contained volume, and the blood pressure falls. A disproportion between the volume of blood and the capacity of the vascular system due to widespread vasodilatation or a diminished blood volume, as in hemorrhage, reduces the venous return to the heart. This is an important factor in determining the cardiac output, the strength of the heartbeat and the blood pressure.

Aldosterone, a hormone secreted by the adrenal cortex, produces an increase in the intravascular volume and a corresponding increase in blood pressure by its effect on kidney activity. It promotes absorption of sodium by the kidney tubules. The increased sodium concentration of the blood in turn causes more water to be absorbed by the renal tubules, increasing the total vascular volume and, as a result, the blood pressure. Conversely, a reduction in aldosterone secretion will reduce the intravascular volume, and the blood pressure falls. The mechanism that regulates the amount of aldosterone secreted by the adrenal cortices is not yet established.

ELASTICITY OF THE VESSELS. The elastic quality of the large arteries has an important role in determining blood pressure. It allows for an increase in the capacity of the arteries when the blood is ejected by each heartbeat. The stretch factor reduces the resistance offered to the flow of blood from the heart, thus reducing somewhat the demand on that organ. With ventricular diastole and the run-off of blood into succeeding vessels, the elastic arterial wall recoils. This provides some pressure on the contained blood to augment its forward movement, and helps to maintain a continuous flow of blood between ventricular contractions. The pressure of the blood at this time (i.e., during arterial recoil and between ventricular contractions) represents the diastolic blood pressure. If the elasticity of the arteries is reduced, as in arteriosclerosis, the blood is pumped into rigid, nondistensible tubes; the systolic pressure is increased because of the lack of vascular stretching and the diastolic pressure is reduced because of the reduced recoil force.

RESISTANCE TO BLOOD FLOW. The amount of resistance with which the blood is met as it flows through the vascular system depends mainly on the caliber of the arterioles and the viscosity of the blood.

Caliber of the Arterioles. The relatively large lumen of the arteries offers little peripheral resistance to the flow of blood, but their subsequent branching into numerous arterioles introduces more surface contact for the blood, which increases friction and resistance to the flow. This resistance determines the rate at which blood can flow from the arteries into the arterioles, which in turn influences the volume of blood confined in the arteries and, hence, the arterial blood pressure.

Normally the arterioles are in a constant state of partial contraction, referred to as the basic level of tone, but the caliber of the vessels may be modified by contraction or relaxation of the well developed, circular, smooth muscle in the walls in response to various factors. Obviously, with relaxation, the increased diameter of the arterioles will offer less resistance, more blood will pass from the arteries through the arterioles to the capillaries and the arterial blood pressure will tend to be normal or below normal. Conversely, with contraction of the arterioles, the decreased diameter increases the resistance to the blood flow, less blood escapes from the arteries and arterial blood pressure is maintained at a normal or above normal level. The caliber of the arterioles is controlled by nerve impulses delivered to the musculature of the arterioles and by certain chemical changes in the extracellular fluids. The latter may exercise their influence directly on the vessels or

indirectly through the autonomic nervous system.

Neural control of vasotone is exerted by the autonomic nervous system. The vessels are supplied by two types of nerve fibers; those whose impulses cause contraction of the muscle tissue of the vessel are the excitatory or vasoconstrictor nerves, and those which cause relaxation are the inhibitory or vasodilator nerves. All vasoconstrictor nerves derive from the sympathetic division of the autonomic nervous system and are thought to act on the alpha (α) receptor sites of smooth muscle. Sympathetic vasoconstrictors are located in the kidneys, skin, gut and spleen. Vasodilation may be initiated by a decrease in sympathetic innervation which allows a relaxation of the smooth muscle of the vessel or, in some instances, dilation results from impulses delivered by nerves to the vessel walls. The vasodilator, or inhibitory, nerves in some areas of the body belong to the parasympathetic division; in others the vasodilator as well as the vasoconstrictor nerves originate in the sympathetic nervous system. Sympathetic vasodilators are distributed to the vessels of skeletal muscles, the intestines, the coronary system and some areas of the skin. Parasympathetic vasodilators supply the vessels in the tongue, sweat and salivary glands, external genitalia and possibly the bladder and rectum.[6]

The principal source of the impulses that regulate the caliber of the blood vessels is the vasomotor center in the medulla. Some impulses may arise from spinal cord neurons in the thoracolumbar areas. These areas may be influenced by impulses received from the blood vessels themselves, the pressoreceptors and chemoreceptors of the carotid sinus and aortic arch, the cerebral cortex, the hypothalamus and various other regions of the body, such as the skin, muscles and viscera.

Chemical influence of the smooth muscle in the vessels may be direct or may be indirect

---

[6]Facts relating to the innervation of the blood vessels are not well established. Some controversy appears between several authoritative references (listed).

John R. Brobeck (Ed.): Best and Taylor's Physiological Basis of Medical Practice, 9th ed. Baltimore, Williams and Wilkins, 1973, pp. 3–164 to 3–188.

Alan C. Burton: Physiology and Biophysics of the Circulation, 2nd ed. Chicago, Year Book, 1972.

Robert F. Rushmer: Cardiovascular Dynamics, 4th ed. Philadelphia, W. B. Saunders, 1976.

through the nervous system. Certain chemical changes in the composition of the extracellular fluid may result in the initiation of nerve impulses which influence the blood vessels. Increased carbon dioxide or decreased oxygen tension results in vasoconstriction and a corresponding increase in resistance. Similarly, an increase in the hydrogen ion concentration (decreased pH) causes vasoconstriction.

A direct effect on the arterioles may be produced by metabolites and hormones. Metabolites produce the opposite effect locally to that caused indirectly through the nervous system. An increase in the concentration of hydrogen ions and carbon dioxide and a diminished oxygen tension in an area cause dilatation of the arterioles in that area. The indirect action of the nervous system produces a more general vasoconstriction and a rise in blood pressure, increasing the rate of flow through the locally dilated arterioles, when there is an increased need for more oxygen and nutrients, and for the removal of more metabolites.

When tissue cells are irritated or injured, chemical substances are released which produce relaxation in the local arterioles and capillaries, resulting in more blood in the area. One of these substances is identified as histamine, a strong vasodilator.

Still another chemical substance, renin, stimulates vasoconstriction and increases arterial blood pressure. It is produced by kidney tissue in response to a diminished blood supply (renal ischemia). Renin is a proteolytic enzyme which, when released into the blood stream, acts upon a globulin fraction, producing the vasoconstrictor angiotensin (hypertensin) that acts directly on the arterioles. It would appear that angiotensin has no significant role in the maintenance of normal blood pressure, since it is quickly destroyed in the healthy person. It remains active for a longer period in persons with a blood pressure higher than normal and is receiving some attention in relation to the disease of hypertension.

The hormones associated with vasomotor activity are epinephrine and vasopressin. Epinephrine, secreted by the adrenal medulla or administered parenterally, has a direct vasoconstricting effect on the arterioles in the skin, mucous membranes and the splanchnic area. At the same time, it inhibits the tone in the arterioles of the skeletal muscles and the coronary system. Guyton suggests that the effect of epinephrine on the coronaries may be indirect, since the hormone stimulates metabolism which causes the local metabolic regulatory system to increase blood flow.[7]

The secretion of the neurohypophysis or posterior lobe of the pituitary gland contains the hormone vasopressin. It excites the smooth muscle of most blood vessels, but its effect is slower than that of epinephrine.

It may be seen from the foregoing discussion of vasomotor regulation that peripheral resistance is a complex affair. Resistance is directly proportional to the length of vessels and inversely proportional to the diameter, and many factors may influence the diameter. A moderate degree of vasoconstriction is essential; most of the arterioles must be in a partial state of constriction at all times. If too many vessels relax at one time blood pressure falls to dangerously low levels, and circulation becomes seriously impaired.

Frequent and quick readjustments in the caliber of the arterioles are necessary to maintain a relatively constant level of blood pressure and to meet the changing needs of tissue cells. Increased activity of structures or areas demands more blood in those parts and vasodilation occurs. To compensate for the increased volume in one area, vasoconstriction must occur in other parts of the body to maintain a forward movement of the blood and a normal cardiac output and blood pressure. For example, when a person moves from the recumbent to the upright position, the blood tends to collect in the lower part of the body because of gravity. This causes a decrease in the blood pressure in the aorta and carotid arteries, and the pressoreceptors then initiate the reflex response of vasoconstriction in the arterioles. This response maintains an adequate circulation throughout the upper parts of the body.

Blood Viscosity. The second factor on which the resistance to the flow of blood depends is the viscosity of the blood. It is a much less significant factor than the caliber of the arterioles. Viscosity is the resistance to flow created within the fluid itself by the friction and cohesiveness between its molecules. Resistance of a fluid is directly proportional to its viscosity.

---

[7]Guyton, op. cit., p. 323.

Blood viscosity is mainly dependent on the concentration of the red blood cells and blood proteins. It is approximately 2.5 to 5 times the viscosity of water. An increase above the normal number of red blood cells (polycythemia) impedes the flow of blood and may cause an appreciable increase above normal in the arterial blood pressure. The caliber of the arterioles is subject to frequent fluctuations, but usually viscosity only changes when blood is diluted or when there is an increase or decrease in the number of red blood cells.

NORMAL VARIATIONS IN ARTERIAL BLOOD PRESSURE. Age, exercise, emotions and weight influence blood pressure.

Blood pressure changes with age. During infancy and childhood, blood pressure is lower than later in life. In the newborn infant systolic pressure is approximately 55 to 90 mm. Hg; the diastolic is approximately 40 to 55 mm. Hg. This gradually increases throughout childhood, reaching adult level about puberty. Usually in the fifties, the systolic pressure begins to show a slight increase which progresses with age, corresponding to the loss of elasticity and to the thickening of the walls of the arteries characteristic of the aging process.

Physical exertion is accompanied by a rise in the arterial blood pressure due to the increased venous return and the increased production of metabolites such as carbon dioxide and lactic acid. The systolic pressure may increase as much as 60 to 70 mm. Hg in strenuous exercise.

Emotions may also cause an elevation in blood pressure; the more excited, anxious, angry or fearful a person becomes, the higher the blood pressure goes. Vasoconstriction is increased due to sympathetic innervation and the release of epinephrine into the blood stream.

Blood pressure increases with increased body weight, especially after middle age. This is of significance in our present-day society in which overweight and hypertension have a high incidence.

Capillary Blood Pressure

The pressure of the blood on entry to the capillaries is approximately 20 to 35 mm. Hg. This varies with the constriction and dilation of the arterioles. It is this pressure that is responsible for the movement of fluid and dissolved particles through the semipermeable capillary walls into the interstitial spaces, making them available to cells. The volume of fluid that moves out into the interstitial spaces is dependent upon the capillary blood pressure and the opposing pressure exerted by the interstitial fluid. The capillary blood pressure is quickly reduced by this loss of fluid and to some extent by the resistance of the minute vessels. As a result, by the time the blood leaves the capillaries, the pressure is reduced to approximately 10 to 20 mm. Hg. The movement of fluid across the capillary walls is more fully discussed under Fluids and Electrolytes, p. 75.

Venous Blood Pressure

The pressure of the blood is reduced slowly but progressively from the time it leaves the capillaries until it reaches the right atrium.

Venous blood pressure is influenced by cardiac strength, blood volume, respirations and posture. Venous pressure is actually the force that remains of that created by the left ventricular contraction. The blood enters the venous system under a pressure of approximately 10 mm. Hg. The walls of the veins continue to offer some resistance and the blood, particularly in the lower parts of the body, must travel a considerable distance before reaching the heart.[8] As a result, the pressure is dissipated progressively, and by the time it reaches the right atrium is very low — 0 to 1 mm. Hg. Obviously, if the left ventricular systole is weak and the blood starts out at a lower than normal arterial pressure, it will tend to move more slowly in the veins toward the heart.

CARDIAC STRENGTH. Maintenance of normal pressure and flow of the venous blood are influenced by the ability of the right heart chambers to empty sufficiently to receive the volume of blood being forwarded by the large veins. If the heart cannot pass on the blood it receives, the normal volume cannot enter and there is a damming back in the veins. The resulting increased volume causes an increase in the blood pressure. Normal emptying of the right atrium actually promotes venous flow; in diastole, the empty right atrium tends to produce an aspirating effect on the large veins.

BLOOD VOLUME. The greater the volume

---

[8]Pressure is inversely proportional to frictional resistance and the length of the tube.

of blood flowing into the veins from the arterioles and capillaries, the greater will be the venous pressure. If the arterioles are constricted, the pressure in the veins will be lower. If the arterioles are dilated, as in muscular exercise, the greater volume escaping into the veins will increase the venous pressure. Normally, marked changes do not occur since the veins have the ability to adjust by either vasoconstriction or dilation to the volume of blood being received. This is accomplished mainly in the smaller veins.

RESPIRATION. On inspiration there is a decrease in intrathoracic pressure and an increase in intra-abdominal pressure. Abdominal venous pressure increases while that in the thoracic veins is lowered, causing a larger volume of blood to move into the thoracic veins. On expiration, intrathoracic pressure increases, compressing the veins and raising the pressure within them, thus helping to move the blood into the atria.

POSTURE. Due to gravity, the upright position favors an increase in venous pressure in the lower parts of the body, but continuous venous return is preserved by compensatory mechanisms. The pressoreceptors initiate reflex vascular constriction which usually preserves an adequate blood pressure. In spite of the compensatory vasoconstriction, a greater volume of blood is likely to accumulate in the lower veins during long periods of standing. This may be seen in persons who faint when required to stand for a relatively long period.

For measurement of venous blood pressure see p. 297.

Pulse

Each ventricular contraction ejects a volume of blood into the aorta, producing an increase in the blood pressure which causes an expansion of the artery. During ventricular diastole, the elastic recoil of the aorta moves the blood into the next portion of the artery, which stretches and then recoils. This alternating expansion and recoil spreads along the whole arterial system, producing a pulse wave. Each pulsation corresponds to a heartbeat and is the result of the impact of the ejected volume of blood on the arterial wall. The pulsations occur in the arteries of the pulmonary circulatory system as well as in the systemic circulation.

A pulse may be felt in arteries near the surface of the body, and is a valuable source of information about the heart and vessels. The radial artery at the wrist is the most convenient site for feeling the pulse, but it may also be felt in the temporal, carotid, brachial, external submaxillary, abdominal aorta, femoral, popliteal and dorsalis pedis arteries. When palpating a pulse, the observer notes the following:

1. The frequency per minute, which represents the number of left ventricular contractions that are strong enough to produce pulse waves that will reach the peripheral artery being used.
2. The volume, which indicates the strength of the heart contraction.
3. The rhythm, or regularity, of the intervals between pulsations.
4. The tension and thickness of the arterial wall, which gives some indication of the resistance.

The loss of pressure of the blood in arterioles and capillaries effaces pulse in the veins. There is one exception — a feeble venous pulse may be palpated in the internal jugular veins while the subject is in a recumbent position. It is caused by the atrial systole. Since no valves guard the openings of the vena caval veins into the right atrium, a small amount of blood is regurgitated into the large veins with atrial contraction, producing a weak pulse.

FETAL CIRCULATION

The circulatory pathway in the fetus differs from that established at birth (Fig. 13–7). This is a necessity, since the developing organism is dependent upon the maternal blood for its oxygen and nutrients, as well as for the elimination of its metabolic wastes.

Special Circulatory Structures

Several special structures are developed in the fetal circulatory system, and they function to support the developing organism during intrauterine life. Two umbilical arteries arise from the fetal hypogastric or internal iliac arteries and deliver fetal blood from the aorta to the placenta. One umbilical vein originates in the placenta. The blood which is transported has taken on oxygen and nu-

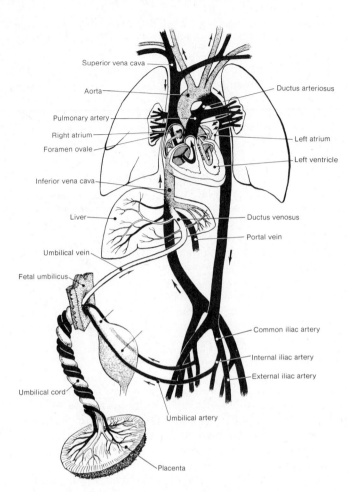

Superior vena cava

Aorta

Pulmonary artery

Right atrium

Foramen ovale

Inferior vena cava

Liver

Umbilical vein

Fetal umbilicus

Umbilical cord

Ductus arteriosus

Left atrium

Left ventricle

Ductus venosus

Portal vein

Common iliac artery

Internal iliac artery

External iliac artery

Umbilical artery

Placenta

FIGURE 13–7 Fetal circulation.

trients in the placenta in exchange for carbon dioxide and other metabolic wastes. The placenta is a mass of finger-like projections (chorionic villi) which penetrate deeply into the thick endometrium early in pregnancy. The villi become highly vascularized and lie in close contact with the maternal blood in the wall of the uterus to allow for an exchange of substances. The ductus venosus is a vein formed by a continuation of the umbilical vein along the undersurface of the liver. It receives blood from the portal vein and gives rise to a few small vessels which enter the liver. The ductus venosus terminates in the inferior vena cava. The ductus arteriosus is a short vessel between the pulmonary artery and the descending thoracic aorta. Blood flowing through this vessel bypasses the pulmonary system. The foramen ovale is an opening between the right and left atria. A valve permits blood to flow from the right atrium into

the left atrium, thus bypassing the pulmonary system.

The Circulatory Pathway in the Fetus

With these special structures in mind, the course which fetal blood takes may be outlined (Table 13–1).

Starting with the left ventricle of the fetal heart, the blood is received into the aorta and continues on the usual route. A supply is distributed through aortic branches to structures in the thoracic and abdominal regions. Some of the blood continues on to the lower limbs via the external iliac arteries, but the greater volume of it is delivered to the placenta by the two umbilical arteries which derive from the hypogastric arteries (internal iliac arteries). The umbilical arteries leave the fetus in the umbilical cord and pass to the placenta, where they divide and subdivide into thin-walled capillaries contained in the villi of the placenta. The semipermeable walls of the capillaries permit the movement of oxygen, nutrients and other substances into fetal blood from maternal blood and movement of wastes from fetal blood to maternal blood. Since this exchange is through capillary walls, there is no direct mixing of the fetal and maternal bloods.

The fetal blood is collected in the placenta into the umbilical vein and passes via the umbilical cord to the fetus. Within the fetal body, the umbilical vein proceeds toward the liver where it becomes the ductus venosus. Most of the blood bypasses the liver, continuing on into the right inferior vena cava by which it enters the right atrium.

A volume of the blood in the right atrium passes through the foramen ovale into the left atrium because the pressure of the blood in the right atrium is greater than that in the left atrium. The remainder of the blood flows into the right ventricle and out into the pulmonary artery. Only a small portion of this blood continues on through the lungs, and is eventually delivered to the left atrium by the four pulmonary veins. The larger portion is shunted through the ductus arteriosus into the arota, thus bypassing the lungs.

The shunting of the blood through the foramen ovale and the ductus arteriosus into the aorta greatly reduces the volume of blood in the pulmonary circulation. This particular pathway would seem to be so designed because the lungs of the fetus are not functioning, and no purpose would be served by having all the blood pass through the pulmonary system.

The blood in the left atrium passes into the left ventricle and out into the aorta to join that received from the ductus arteriosus. The circuit is now complete.

Changes in Fetal Circulation at Birth

After birth, the new organism must function independently, so the special structures are no longer useful. With the cutting of the umbilical cord, no blood enters either the umbilical vein or arteries. The portion of these vessels within the body contract, thrombose and eventually become fibrous cords. The ductus venosus, now nonfunctional, also becomes fibrous. All the blood in the portal vein is now directed into the liver.

When the lungs expand and become functional, a greater volume of blood enters the pulmonary circulation and flows into the left atrium. The pressure of the blood in the left atrium is now higher than that in the right atrium and the foramen ovale in the atrial septum is closed. A gradual constriction and atrophy of the ductus arteriosus takes place, and its closure is usually complete within a few weeks of birth.

TABLE 13–1 SCHEMATIC OUTLINE OF FETAL CIRCULATION

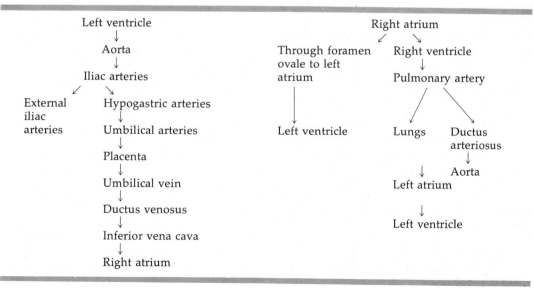

NURSING IN IMPAIRED CARDIAC FUNCTION

Heart disease is a national health problem of considerable proportions. It is the leading cause of death in Canada and the United States. Many nursing hours in hospitals, homes and clinics are devoted to patients with heart disease.

NURSE'S ROLE IN PREVENTION OF HEART DISEASE

The nurse has many opportunities to contribute to the prevention of cardiac insufficiency. Whether the work is in the hospital, clinic, home, industry or school, the role may be participation in case-finding, education or provision of care. In order to recognize and fulfill the responsibilities in the preventive program, the nurse must be informed and must make a personal effort to keep abreast of new knowledge. In addition to an understanding of the role of the heart in supplying all the cells throughout the body with materials essential to their survival and activities, a knowledge of how this function may be impaired by various pathologic processes is necessary. This information serves as the basis for the recognition of excessive demands on the heart, significant signs and symptoms and the need for medical attention. It also provides the basis for explanations and appropriate health education as well as for the planning and giving of safe and effective care.

People are urged to secure an early diagnosis and treatment of illnesses which may damage the heart. Examples of such conditions are rheumatic fever, hypertension, syphilis and hyperthyroidism. The promotion of immunization for diphtheria contributes to the prevention of heart disease because the toxin produced by the causative organisms may have a serious effect on the heart muscle.

Opportunities often arise for the nurse to discuss the hazards of obesity and its possible effects on the heart. Similarly, the advantages of such factors as moderate exercise, annual physical examinations and the reduction of animal fat in the diet are stressed. Avoidance of unaccustomed strenuous physical activities and overexcitement, particularly by persons past middle age, are stressed in health education in relation to the prevention of heart disease. All too often one reads of sudden deaths due to a heart attack suffered while shovelling snow or while participating in competitive sports. The nurse has an important role in helping both adults and children to develop good health habits and to live a balanced life of physical activity, rest, work and recreation.

Recent studies have indicated a higher incidence of coronary heart disease among cigarette smokers. Established smokers are encouraged to stop or at least reduce the number of cigarettes smoked per day. Every effort should be made to discourage young persons from starting the smoking habit.

The nurse is ever alert to the possible significance of shortness of breath, cyanosis, edema and chest pain on exertion. Recognition leading to an early diagnosis and treatment may prevent irreparable damage and eventual incapacitation of the person.

It must be understood that much heart disease can be and is cured. Many persons with a heart condition or reduced cardiac efficiency live useful, satisfactory lives by readjusting their activities. The nurse must appreciate these facts to develop an optimistic, encouraging attitude with cardiac patients. Any pessimism on her part may readily be conveyed to a patient or family who, generally, tends to be overpessimistic about heart disease. Motivation, instruction and planning to have the heart patient live within the functional ability of his heart may prevent progression of the heart disease and possible heart failure. Follow-up of patients to provide guidance in following the doctor's suggestions may prevent problems and relapses. For example, visits to the child who has had rheumatic fever may ensure the continuation of prescribed prophylactic doses of penicillin or sulfonamide.

ASSESSMENT OF IMPAIRED HEART FUNCTION

At the present time the nurse often assumes more responsibility than formerly for assessing the clinical status of patients. Assessment includes taking a clinical history, monitoring and recording physical signs and symptoms, and observing emotional and psychological reactions and administering invasive and noninvasive diagnostic tests.

The responsibility of the nurse in patient assessment varies with the practice setting. In all instances the nurse is responsible for observing, recording and reporting specific physical signs and symptoms, understanding their implications and preparing and supporting the patient for various diagnostic procedures. In some situations certain physical assessments or diagnostic measures may be delegated to the nurse by the physician — for example, electrocardiographic monitoring and/or assessing heart sounds.

Manifestations of Impaired Heart Function

Any impairment in circulation due to an abnormal heart condition is reflected in signs and symptoms which are produced by two main factors: (1) a reduced blood supply to the heart and tissues throughout the body, causing a reduced nutrient and oxygen supply and an accumulation of metabolic wastes; (2) malfunctioning of the conduction system; and (3) the inability of the heart to forward the blood it receives. The latter results in an excessive volume in the venous system, creating congestion and increased pressure that interfere with the function of tissues and organs.

The signs and symptoms of cardiac conditions vary with the degree to which circulation is impaired and with the form and location of the heart condition. All those which are discussed here do not necessarily occur in every patient, nor are they all inclusive but are the more common problems presented by cardiac patients.

ABNORMAL PULSE. The pulse rate may be abnormally fast or slow and the intervals between the heartbeats may be unequal. The volume may vary.

BLOOD PRESSURE. Arterial blood pressure is an important indicator of the patient's circulatory status. The systolic pressure depends on the cardiac output and, obviously, will fall with a reduced output by the left side of the heart. Venous pressure is frequently used to assess the ability of the heart to accept the inflow into the right side of the heart. A venous pressure in excess of the normal may indicate cardiac insufficiency or failure or an excessive intravascular volume.

DYSPNEA. The patient may experience shortness of breath or labored breathing only on exertion, or it may be present even at rest.

This is due to pulmonary congestion. The left side of the heart may not be forwarding all the blood it receives, and the blood is dammed back in the pulmonary veins. The pulmonary congestion and hypertension resist alveolar expansion, increasing the work of breathing and decreasing the vital capacity. If the congestion is of long standing, alveolar tissue changes occur; the elastic tissue is replaced with fibrous tissue, and normal gas exchange is disturbed.

Dyspnea that occurs when the patient is recumbent is referred to as orthopnea. It may be relieved when the patient sits upright.

COUGH. Fluid escapes into the alveoli from the capillaries in the congested pulmonary system and acts as a cough stimulus. This collection of transudate in the alveoli may be referred to as pulmonary edema. The fluid may be raised as a frothy sputum and in severe heart failure may contain blood.

HYPOXIA. Any impairment in circulation will create an oxygen deficiency in tissues. The cardiac output may be reduced, or a disturbance in pulmonary circulation may reduce the exchange of gases in the lung. Symptoms of an oxygen deficiency are many and varied, since the function of all structures is affected. The brain quickly reflects oxygen deprivation and reduced mental efficiency, apathy and disorientation are manifested. If the deficiency is severe, consciousness is lost and, unless the supply to the brain is promptly reestablished, there is likely to be permanent tissue damage.

Severe pain occurs when muscle tissue, such as the myocardium, is deprived of adequate oxygen. Hypoxia may also cause cyanosis, a bluish color, which is usually seen first in the lips and nail beds.

EDEMA (see p. 84). Excess fluid accumulates in the interstitial spaces of the tissues in cardiac disease when the heart cannot forward the blood it receives. The blood backs up in the veins and venules, raising the venous blood pressure. Normally, at the venous end of the capillaries, the colloidal osmotic pressure exceeds the hydrostatic pressure of the blood, and interstitial fluid moves into the capillary. However, if the hydrostatic pressure of the blood in the distal portion of the capillaries exceeds the blood protein osmotic pressure, interstitial fluid will not be moved into the capillaries.

The retention of sodium ions also contributes to the formation of edema in the cardiac

TABLE 13–2   DIFFERENTIATING CHARACTERISTICS OF CHEST PAIN

Medical Condition	Characteristics of Pain	Location
Angina	Pressing; squeezing. Precipitated by cold, physical activity, large meals, emotional upsets. Usually relieved within a few minutes by rest and/or nitroglycerin.	Retrosternal. May start in midchest and may radiate to jaw, shoulders, arms or fingers (often the left arm). May only be present in the neck, jaw, shoulders or arm(s).
Myocardial infarction	Similar pain to angina but longer-lasting and usually more severe. Not relieved by rest or nitroglycerin.	Same locations as angina.
Pericarditis	More stabbing or burning than pain of myocardial infarction. Usually aggravated by deep inspiration or turning the trunk. May be relieved by high Fowler's position or bending forward.	Substernal. May radiate to the precordium, trapezius muscle area or upper part of abdomen.
Pulmonary embolus	Small pulmonary emboli may produce no pain, but with larger emboli pain is sharp and often sudden. May be aggravated by deep breathing. Accompanied by cyanosis, dyspnea, cough, hemoptysis.	Often located laterally but may be central.
Dissecting aneurysm	Often sudden and excruciating. Described as burning or tearing.	May originate in anterior chest but often shifts to intrascapular region.

patient. The decreased sodium excretion is favored by the reduced blood flow through the kidneys which results from the impaired circulation. It is also suggested that some mechanism may exist which causes an increased secretion of aldosterone by the adrenal cortices. This hormone promotes reabsorption of sodium in the kidney tubules.

Edema is a very characteristic sign of some weakening in heart function. Considerable fluid accumulates before the edema becomes apparent; a person may retain 10 to 15 pounds of excess fluid before the edema becomes evident. It appears first in the dependent parts of the body where the venous and capillary blood pressures always tend to be greater. If the patient is ambulant, it becomes evident first in the ankles and feet but, if he is in bed, it appears initially in the sacral region.

PAIN.   The chest pain which cardiac patients experience is usually due to the deficiency of oxygen in the myocardium. It is important to determine the location, nature and precipitating or contributing factors of chest pain in order to distinguish the specific cause. The pain may be described as sharp, aching, squeezing, a feeling of heaviness or weight on the chest or a sensation of pressure within the chest. It may be mild or excruciating. It may be localized to one area or may spread across the chest, and into the back, neck, jaw, shoulders and/or arms. It may be precipitated or aggravated by activity, cold respirations or certain bodily positions, and may be relieved by resting or a change of position. Table 13–2 describes some cardiac problems and the pain often associated with them.

PALPITATION.   Change in heart function may cause the person to be conscious of his heartbeats. Palpitation may be due to the apex of the enlarged heart striking the chest wall with each contraction, or it may occur with an increased stroke volume in extrasystole, or ectopic beats (see Arrhythmias, p. 316.)

GENERAL DEBILITATION, LOSS OF STRENGTH AND DECREASED MENTAL AND PHYSICAL EFFICIENCY. Weakness, loss of appetite and weight, general apathy and reduced efficiency occur as the results of the reduced nutrient and oxygen supply, venous congestion and the accumulation of metabolic wastes. In a child, growth and development may be retarded.

ABNORMAL HEART SOUNDS. Cardiac murmurs are abnormal sounds caused by small jets of blood which create eddies in the blood stream. Movements of these currents produce audible vibrations which are referred to as murmurs. The most frequent causes of heart murmurs are stenosed and insufficient valves and openings between the right and left sides of the heart. Murmurs may also occur in an aneurysm, a localized saccular dilation of an artery.

The physician, in determining the significance of a murmur, considers when it occurs in the cardiac cycle, its intensity, quality of sound, duration, factors which alter the sound (such as respiration and change of position) and the patient's history. Murmurs in some persons may have no great significance.

Occasionally, in tachycardia, a third heart sound becomes audible, producing then a quick sequence of three sounds during each cardiac cycle. This phenomenon is referred to as gallop rhythm and is an unfavorable sign since it indicates a weakening and dilatation of the heart and often precedes heart failure.

Friction rub is a sound produced by the contact between the two pericardial surfaces with each heartbeat. Because of disease the surfaces are rough, causing audible vibrations.

Diagnostic Procedures

Although the diagnostic procedures are mainly the concern of the attending physician, the nurse requires some understanding of them in order to meet the associated nursing needs.

BLOOD TESTS. Various blood tests are used in investigating heart disease. Those used depend on the presenting signs and symptoms.

LEUKOCYTE COUNT. The number of white blood cells may be of significance, since these will be increased if there is an inflammatory process as occurs in bacterial endocarditis and rheumatic fever. Leukocytosis also occurs following a myocardial infarction as a result of the necrotic tissue.

Normal: 5,000 to 10,000 per cu. mm.

ERYTHROCYTE COUNT AND HEMOGLOBIN CONCENTRATION. These are observed to determine the oxygen-carrying capacity of the patient's blood. In congenital cardiac defects which establish an abnormal blood pathway, the red blood cells and hemoglobin may be increased as a compensatory mechanism, since areas of the body are deficient in oxygen.

An increase in erythrocytes increases the viscosity of the blood, adding to the work of the heart and predisposing to thrombus formation.

In those with rheumatic fever or bacterial endocarditis, there may be fewer erythrocytes and less hemoglobin than normal.

Normal:

Erythrocytes, 1½ to 5 million per cu. mm.

Hemoglobin, 12 to 16 Gm. per 100 ml. (varies with age and sex).

Hematocrit, males 45 to 50 volumes per cent; females 40 to 45 volumes per cent.

ERYTHROCYTE SEDIMENTATION RATE. The rate at which erythrocytes settle in a blood sample is increased in inflammatory conditions and in myocardial infarction. Periodic checking of the sedimentation rate gives information as to the progress of the disease; as the inflammatory process subsides or as the infarcted area heals, the rate decreases.

Normal:

Westergren, male, 0 to 15 mm. in 1 hour; female, 0 to 20 mm. in 1 hour.

Wintrobe, male, 0 to 9 mm. in 1 hour; female, 0 to 15 mm. in 1 hour.

BLOOD CULTURE. Studies may be made to determine the causative organism in bacterial endocarditis.

PROTHROMBIN TIME. This test indicates the amount of prothrombin in the blood. Some heart patients receive anticoagulant therapy and a frequent check must be made of the concentration of prothrombin, which serves as a guide to the dosage of the drugs. From 1½ to 2½ times the normal level is considered a therapeutic range.

Normal: 11 to 12 seconds.

TABLE 13–3   SERUM ENZYMES FOLLOWING MYOCARDIAL
INFARCTION*

Enzymes	Normal Values (units)†	Begins to Rise (hours)	Peaks (hours)	Returns to Normal
SGOT	8 to 40	6 to 8	24 to 48	4 to 8 days
LDH	150 to 300	24 to 48	48 to 72	5 to 10 days
SHBD	50 to 250	12	48 to 72	1 to 3 weeks
SCPK	0 to 4	2 to 5	12 to 24	2 to 3 days
MBCPK	0 to 2	6	8 to 16	36 hours

*SGOT: serum glutamic oxaloacetic transaminase
 LDH: serum lactic dehydrogenase
 SHBD: serum alpha-hydroxybutyrate dehydrogenase
 SCPK: serum creatinine phosphokinase
 MBCPK: cardiospecific creatine phosphokinase
†J. Willis Hurst, et al. (Eds.): The Heart, 3rd ed. New York, McGraw-Hill, 1974, pp. 1044–49.

PARTIAL THROMBOPLASTIN TIME (PTT). This test assesses the intrinsic clotting system. It defines abnormalities of certain factors usually present in the coagulation pathway. It is also used as a guide for the administration of heparin which is given parenterally, either subcutaneously or intravenously. A therapeutic level is 1½ to 2 times the normal range.

Normal range: 50 to 80 seconds.

CLOTTING TIME. This test measures the total time for fibrin formation. In some institutions it is used to monitor the administration of heparin, but it is less reliable than partial thromboplastin time.

Normal range: 5 to 10 minutes.

SERUM ENZYMES. Certain intracellular enzymes known to be present in myocardial cells are released into the blood when the cells are damaged or destroyed. Determination of the serum concentration of these enzymes provides information that assists in confirming myocardial infarction and the extent of the damage. Changes may also occur with shock and cardiac surgery. In addition, these enzymes are present in other tissues and may therefore be elevated in other than myocardial conditions (e.g., pulmonary embolus).

The enzyme tests include serum glutamic oxaloacetic acid (SGOT), serum lactic dehydrogenase (SLDH), serum creatine phosphokinase (SCPK), and serum alpha-hydroxybutyrate dehydrogenase (SHBD) (see Table 13–3).

The concentration of SGOT rises within 6 to 8 hours after a myocardial infarction, reaching a peak in 24 to 48 hours and usually returning to normal within 4 to 8 days. SGOT may also be elevated in liver cell necrosis, in acute pancreatitis and with severe skeletal muscle damage.

Normal range: 8 to 40 units.

Following an infarction, the SLDH level becomes elevated in 24 to 48 hours, reaching a peak in 48 to 72 hours. The increase persists for 5 to 10 days and then gradually returns to normal. The LDH level may also increase in patients with megaloblastic and hemolytic anemias, pulmonary infarctions and hemolysis of red blood cells. LDH may be separated into five main fractions (isoenzymes) for greater specificity. Cardiac necrosis would show an elevation of LDH-1 and LDH-2 (using standard international nomenclature). LDH-1 and 2 may rise in patients with myocardial infarction even though there is no change in total LDH.

Normal range: 150 to 300 units.

SHBD is associated with the cardiospecific isoenzymes of LDH. It is elevated within 12 hours after a myocardial infarction, peaks in 48 to 72 hours and remains elevated for up to 3 weeks. Slight elevations may also appear in liver disease, muscular dystrophy and megaloblastic anemia.

Normal range: 50 to 250 units.

CPK has a more limited distribution than the other enzymes; it is found only in skeletal muscle, brain tissue and cardiac muscle. Therefore it is considered by some to be more cardiospecific than the other enzymes. CPK begins to show a postinfarction increase in approximately 2 to 5 hours, reaching its peak within 12 to 24 hours. It usually returns to normal within 2 to 3 days. CPK is often elevated following intramuscular injections.

It may also be fractionated to isoenzymes, with MBCPK being the isoenzyme found only in the myocardium. Studies have shown that CK-MB (or MBCPK) was 100 per cent sensitive and specific for the diagnosis of acute myocardial infarction provided that it was determined between 6 and 36 hours after the onset.[9] Although total CPK may be influenced by intramuscular injections, MBCPK seems to be unaffected.[10]

Normal range: 0 to 4 units.

Normal values of serum enzymes may vary slightly from one laboratory to another depending upon the techniques and sampling methods used.

BLOOD GASES. The circulatory status of a patient is reflected in the blood concentrations of oxygen and carbon dioxide. The volumes differ in arterial and venous blood for obvious reasons. The amount of oxygen is usually expressed as tension or pressure in mm. Hg. Rarely, the volumes per cent are recorded.

Normal:

pO_2, arterial, 95 to 100 mm. Hg

O_2, arterial, 15 to 23 volumes per cent

pO_2, venous, 35 to 40 mm. Hg

O_2, venous, 10 to 16 vol. per cent

The partial pressure of carbon dioxide in the blood provides information about the pH of the body fluids and is usually given in mm. Hg. The carbon dioxide combining power indicates the available alkali and reflects the amount of carbon dioxide in the blood available to form carbonic acid.

Normal:

pCO_2, arterial, 35 to 40 mm. Hg

pCO_2, venous, 40 to 45 mm. Hg

CO_2 combining power, 50 to 58 vol. per cent

bicarbonate (alkali), 22 to 28 mEq./L.

pH is an indicator of the hydrogen ion concentration of the blood. When within the normal range, the body is said to be in a state of acid-base balance.

Normal range: 7.35 to 7.45 (pH arterial)

A pH below 7.35 signifies an increased hydrogen ion concentration, or acidosis, while a pH above 7.45 indicates a decreased hydrogen ion concentration, or alkalosis.

CIRCULATION TIME. This test measures the time it takes the blood to flow from one part of the body to another. A substance with a characteristic taste may be injected into the antecubital vein, and the time interval between the injection and when the patient first tastes the substance is noted. This interval represents the time the blood took to pass from the arm through the right side of the heart, pulmonary system and left side of the heart, into the aorta and out to the taste buds via the lingual artery. There are several different substances which may be used. A saccharin preparation may be injected to produce a sweet taste, or a bitter-tasting preparation of bile salts (Decholin) may be used. Accuracy of the test depends largely on the patient's alertness and senses.

Another method of determining circulation time is by the injection of a radioactive material into the vein of one arm. A Geiger counter is placed over the other arm and the time noted when the radioactive material is registered.

The normal time for these circuits varies from 10 to 20 seconds.

Nursing responsibilities involve an explanation of the test and what will be expected of the patient, preparing for and assisting with the injection of the test substance, and establishing the circulation time.

ELECTROCARDIOGRAPHY. Electrocardiography is the study of the electrical activity associated with heart contractions. The electrocardiogram (ECG), which produces a visible record of heart activity, provides one of the most dependable aids in assessing heart function and in diagnosing heart disease.

Each heart contraction results from electrical currents which spread from the heart through the body to its surface. These currents, which reflect the electrical activity of the heart, are detected when electrodes are placed on the external surface of the body. An application of contact jelly is made to the skin beneath the electrodes in order to facilitate conduction. The ebb and flow of the electrical forces result in a specific pattern, called a

[9]David J. Blomberg, et al.: "Creatinine Kinase Isoenzymes: Predictive Value in the Early Diagnosis of Acute Myocardial Infarction." Am. J. Med., Vol. 59, No. 4 (Oct. 1975), pp. 464–469.

[10]Robert Roberts, et al.: "An Improved Basis for Enzymatic Estimation of Infarct Size." Circulation, Vol. 52 (Nov. 1975), pp. 743–754.

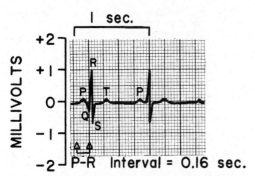

FIGURE 13–8 A normal electrocardiogram. (From Guyton, A. C.: Textbook of Medical Physiology, 5th ed. Philadelphia, W. B. Saunders Co., 1976, p. 190.)

complex or cardiac cycle. Each part of the complex represents the electrical pathway of a specific part of the heart and normally occurs over a specific period of time.

The waves for each cycle are identified as P, Q, R, S, and T, as shown in Figure 13–8, and are recorded on special graph paper. The base line of the graph represents zero electrical potential. Three of the waves (P, R and T) appear above the base line and two (Q and S) appear below.

The P wave, or first rounded contour, represents atrial depolarization. Although depolarization of the S-A node precedes depolarization of the atria, it cannot be picked up by body surface leads.

The P-R interval indicates the time from the beginning of the P wave to the beginning of the QRS complex. The QRS complex represents conduction through the ventricles. The Q wave is the initial downward (negative) deflection following the P wave, the R wave is the initial upward (positive) deflection following the Q wave, and the S wave is the downward deflection following the R wave. The S T segment is an interval of zero potential, the period between completion of depolarization and the beginning of repolarization (recovery) of the ventricles. The T wave represents the recovery phase after contraction or return of the ventricular muscular fibers to their resting state.

The horizontal axis of the graph paper represents time. Each small square indicates 0.04 second. Each large square is composed of five small squares and is therefore equal to 0.20 second.

The vertical axis of the graph indicates voltage. Each small vertical square represents 0.1 millivolt, while a large square composed of five small squares equals 0.5 millivolt.

The P wave should not be longer than 0.10 second duration, or 2 or 3 mm. in height. Normally the P-R interval is between 0.12 and 0.20 second. The QRS complex should not exceed 0.10 second in duration, or 5 to 20 or 25 mm. in height. The T wave is of 0.20 second duration and normally not above 5 to 10 mm. in height, depending upon the lead.[11]

The tracing is studied for deviations by comparing it to a tracing made by a normal heart; the direction, contour and timing of the waves and segments are noted. Information is obtained that is related to impulse formation and conduction and to the condition and response of the myocardium.

A nursing responsibility associated with this diagnostic procedure is to give the patient a brief explanation of the test. Some patients are fearful that they will receive a shock from the electrodes. The patient is advised that he should relax and that he will not feel anything as the instrument records his heart's action. If digitalis or quinidine has been prescribed for the patient, it must be noted on the requisition as well as on a conspicuous place on the patient's chart, as either drug may influence the interpretation of the tracing.

If the patient is very ill the nurse remains with him during the test. In some instances the nurse is responsible for obtaining the electrocardiogram.

EXERCISE ELECTROCARDIOGRAMS. This test is done to assist in the diagnosis of myocardial ischemia in a patient with atypical symptoms. Many patients with angina pectoris have normal electrocardiograms at rest but changes may occur during exercise. The exercise ECG is also used to assess the effect of specific treatments for angina and in rehabilitation following a myocardial infarction.

Electrodes are attached to the body and recordings taken while the patient exercises. One of the earliest stress tests was the "Master's two-step stress test," in which a person climbed two 9-inch steps a selected number of times at a specific speed. The test was considered positive if the recordings showed an S T depression of at least 0.5 mm.

Graded exercise testing has been developed in which the patient exercises on a tread-

[11] Henry J. L. Marriott: Practical Electrocardiography. 6th ed. Baltimore. Williams and Wilkins, 1976.

mill or rides a bicycle at gradually increasing speeds against a regulated amount of resistance. The exercise continues until the patient reaches a predetermined maximal heart rate (according to age and sex). The test is discontinued earlier if the patient develops chest pain, hypotension or signs of cerebral insufficiency. The test is considered positive if the electrocardiogram shows an S T segment displacement of 1 mm. or more.

ROENTGENOGRAMS. An x-ray of the chest may be made to note the size and shape of the heart. Visualization of the lungs may show a density that may indicate an increased volume of blood in the pulmonary circulation and fluid in the alveoli. The size and shape of the pulmonary artery and aorta may also be noted.

Fluoroscopic examination allows the physician to observe the heart in action. The functioning of different chambers and large vessels may be noted.

A brief explanation of the patient's role may be necessary if he is apprehensive and completely unfamiliar with the x-ray procedure.

ANGIOCARDIOGRAM. In this test, also known as a cardiopulmonary angiogram, visualization of the heart and vessels is made possible by the injection of a radiopaque dye into a vein or artery or directly into a heart chamber. The site depends on the type of abnormality suspected. A series of x-ray pictures is taken, or a fluoroscopic study is made, as the blood flows through the heart and pulmonary system. The pathway of the blood is followed, and the size, shape, and the filling and emptying of the various structures are noted. This examination is of particular importance in identifying congenital defects of the heart and large vessels.

Preparation of the patient includes an explanation of the test so that he will have some idea of what to expect. This may be given by the doctor but, if it is not, the nurse must have sufficient understanding of the procedure to be able to prepare the patient and reduce his fear.

It may be necessary to obtain a written consent for an angiocardiogram, depending on the policy of the particular hospital. Food and fluids are withheld for 6 to 8 hours previous to the hour of the test, and a sedative may be ordered 30 minutes to 1 hour before the patient is taken to the x-ray or cardiology department.

The physician usually administers a test dose of the radiopaque dye before proceeding with the angiocardiogram in case of a hypersensitivity to such substances. This examination is not done on a person with a history of asthma or allergic reaction. A reaction to the dye might be manifested by respiratory distress, fall in blood pressure, shock, urticaria, and nausea and vomiting. Antihistamines, adrenalin and oxygen should be quickly available in the event of a reaction. Postexamination care involves close observation for signs of delayed reaction. The site of injection should be examined for a few days for signs of irritation or thrombosis.

CARDIAC CATHETERIZATION. Cardiac catheterization is a useful diagnostic procedure for certain patients. It is undertaken to evaluate the severity of known cardiac lesions, such as acquired valvular heart disease, congenital defects and coronary artery disease, when these conditions might be amenable to surgical treatment. It is also used for diagnosing heart disease and for the evaluation of the long-term effects of cardiac surgery.

Under local anesthesia a long radiopaque catheter is passed into the right and left side of the heart. Pressures within the chambers of the heart and oxygen concentrations in certain chambers are determined. An example of an abnormal finding is an atrial septal defect which results in an oxygen tension higher than normal in the right side of the heart.

A contrast material or radiopaque dye is usually introduced into the heart through the catheter. The pathway of this dye is filmed, and obstructions in the coronary arteries may be evaluated. The cardiac output is also measured.

Right heart catheterization provides information about the right side of the heart and the pulmonary circulation. The catheter is introduced through a cutdown in the femoral vein of the right leg or the basilic vein of the right arm and, under a fluoroscope, is passed through the inferior or superior vena cava into the right atrium. It may then be guided through the tricuspid valve into the right ventricle and on into the pulmonary artery. An x-ray may be taken with the catheter in various positions for future studies.

In *left heart catheterization,* one of two approaches may be used. One method is the retrograde passage of the catheter into a femoral artery up through the aorta and aortic valve to the left ventricle; it may then be advanced through the mitral valve into the left atrium. It may also be directed from the aorta into the right and left coronary arteries. The other approach is transeptal. The catheter is passed through a peripheral vein into the right atrium and from there through the interatrial septum into the left atrium. The catheter may then be guided under the fluoroscope into the left ventricle.

Preparation of the patient for a cardiac catheterization includes an explanation of the procedure and obtaining a written consent. Although the doctor usually talks with the patient and family, the nurse should be conversant with the procedure. It is understandable that the patient and relatives are apprehensive. The nurse encourages them to verbalize their fears and is prepared to answer questions. The patient is informed of the equipment he may see during the procedure, the sterile precautions that will be taken, and some of the physical sensations that he will experience, such as a feeling of pressure when the catheter is introduced and the warm flush which immediately follows the injection of the dye. Although each step is usually explained during the procedure, the patient's anxiety is often decreased when given this information beforehand. Some institutions provide booklets describing the experience.

Food and fluid are withheld for a stated number of hours preceding the catheterization. A sedative may be ordered.

The patient's reaction must be observed closely during the procedure. Heart action is constantly observed on the oscilloscope, an instrument which visibly registers and traces the electrical activity of the heart. Irritation of the myocardium by the catheter may precipitate fibrillation, so a defibrillator is close at hand. The patient experiences little discomfort but may complain of a fluttering or irritation in the chest, especially during movement of the catheter. He is advised that this is a temporary sensation.

Following the catheterization, which may have taken 2 or 3 hours, the patient is given fluids and nourishment and is allowed to rest. The pulse is checked at frequent intervals — every 15 minutes for the first hour and then at gradually increased intervals if it remains normal. An irregular, rapid or weak pulse is promptly reported to the physician. If the catheter was passed through a femoral artery the patient remains flat for 12 to 24 hours, and the site where the catheter was inserted is examined frequently for possible bleeding. A sandbag is placed over the site to apply pressure.

The site at which the catheter was introduced is observed for several days for possible irritation or phlebitis, evidenced by redness and tenderness.

Patients frequently wish to discuss their feelings following the procedure. Although one probable reaction is relief that the procedure is completed, anxiety about the findings and their implications is often evident.

VITAL CAPACITY. Vital capacity represents the maximum volume of air that a person can exhale after inhaling to the maximum. The normal is approximateqy 2500 to 5000 ml. Usually it is higher in males than females, and will be greater in those accustomed to regular and fairly strenuous activity.

In the procedure, the patient is required to take a maximum breath and then exhale into the mouthpiece of a spirometer which makes a graphic record of the volume of air exhaled. The nurse advises the patient as to the value of the test and what will be required of him.

Lung capacity may be reduced in heart conditions by an excessive volume and pressure of blood in the pulmonary circulatory system. Expansion of the lungs meets with resistance and fluid escapes into the alveoli, reducing respiratory efficiency.

PHONOCARDIOGRAPHY. Heart sounds may be picked up, amplified and recorded by a microphone placed on the chest. A study of the phonocardiogram is helpful in cases in which the physician has difficulty in distinguishing heart sounds and murmurs by the usual auscultation.

ECHOCARDIOGRAPHY. This is a noninvasive test used to detect mitral and aortic valve abnormalities, pericardial effusion and some congenital defects. Through a transducer placed against the chest wall, ultrasound waves are aimed at the heart and a recording is made of the echo. As the sound waves hit various structures while passing through the heart some of them are bounced back, producing patterns characteristic of each structure. An electrocardiogram is taken simultaneously.

Although the test is painless it does require the patient to remain motionless for 10 to 30 minutes. An explanation of the purpose, procedure and equipment is given to the patient prior to the test.

MEASUREMENT OF VENOUS BLOOD PRESSURE. Venous blood pressure is an important parameter in the care of seriously ill patients. It reflects the intravascular volume and the ability of the heart to forward the blood it receives. Measurement of the venous pressure may be made in a peripheral vein, such as the medial basilic, or in a large central vein, such as the superior vena cava.

PERIPHERAL VENOUS PRESSURE. To record peripheral venous pressure a needle is inserted into a superficial vein (usually the medial basilic in the antecubital region) and is attached to a water manometer. The patient is placed in the supine position, if possible, with the arm level with the right atrium. The level to which the water rises in the manometer is noted. The pressure may be recorded in mm. of Hg but is so small that it is usually expressed in mm. or cm. of water.[12]

The normal venous pressure in an arm or leg vein in a supine adult is approximately 8 to 10 cm. of water. It is slightly lower in females and in children.

CENTRAL VENOUS PRESSURE. Central venous pressure (CVP) is more reliable than the peripheral, and is being used clinically more often in assessing the patient's condition. It may be used as a guide for fluid replacement for the dehydrated or postoperative patient, or for a critically ill patient.

An intravenous catheter is passed into the superior vena cava via a basilic or jugular vein, or into the inferior vena cava via a femoral vein. The catheter is attached to a three-way stopcock which is also connected to a water manometer and intravenous flask and tubing. In setting up the CVP line the zero level of the manometer is positioned at the level of the right atrium, which is approximately in line with the mid-axillary and suprasternal notch. The most important factor is that the equipment be at the same level for each determination, so the initial level is usually marked on the patient's skin. In most instances the changes in the venous pressure are more significant than the actual level. The patient must be in the same position for each reading. The pressure is generally recorded

hourly. When the catheter is introduced, the stopcock is adjusted to allow fluid to flow to the patient. Then, to determine the venous pressure, the stopcock is turned to direct the fluid up into the manometer to a level of 30 to 35 cm. The valve is then adjusted to close off the flow from the intravenous bottle and to establish a flow line between the manometer and the catheter. When the fluid reaches the level of the venous pressure it remains at a relatively stationary level, rhythmically rising and falling 1 to 2 cm. with respirations. Following the recording the stopcock is readjusted to allow the intravenous solution to flow to the patient.

The normal central venous presure is approximately 5 to 10 cm. of water. This varies with the patient's size, position and state of hydration. The significance of the pressure is determined in conjunction with the arterial blood pressure, the hourly output of urine, pulse rate and volume, and electrocardiograph. The nurse requires a directive regarding the levels at which the physician is to be notified, and the rate and volume of intravenous infusion.

Other nursing responsibilities include observation for complications such as inflammation at the insertion site. This may be prevented by the use of aseptic technique during catheter insertion and during the application of dressings. Interference with flow may be minimized by periodic flushing with a solution of heparin or normal saline to prevent clotting and loosely coiling the tubing to prevent it from kinking.

MEASUREMENT OF PULMONARY ARTERY PRESSURE (WEDGE PRESSURE). To obtain more specific information about the functioning of the left side of the heart, pulmonary artery and pulmonary capillary pressures are measured. This procedure is used for critically ill patients in whom early detection of left ventricular dysfunction is important.

A flow-directed (Swan-Ganz) catheter is inserted into a peripheral vein. A balloon at the tip of the catheter is partially inflated and the catheter floats into the right atrium, right ventricle and pulmonary artery at which time the pulmonary artery pressure may be measured. The catheter is then forwarded into a branch of the pulmonary artery until it becomes wedged in a pulmonary capillary. Pressure measurements are obtained which reflect pressures in the left atrium. The

---

[12]Mercury is approximately 13 times as heavy as water.

balloon is then deflated until the next pressure reading.

The nurse is responsible for monitoring pressures, reporting abnormalities and preventing complications. The normal pulmonary artery pressure is 25/10 mm. Hg, and the normal pulmonary capillary wedge pressure is 4 to 12 mm. Hg.

CLASSIFICATION OF CARDIAC PATIENTS

The required care is not the same for all cardiac patients since there are varying degrees of heart impairment and reduced efficiency, in addition to different pathologic conditions.

There are those individuals who have a slight abnormality or who have had a condition which has been cured. The heart may carry some structural change or scar, but the cardiac efficiency and reserve are such that no restrictions on activities are necessary. Some of these persons have unwarranted fears and restrict their activities unnecessarily, even though they have been advised by their physicians to live a normal, active life. The role of the nurse with these patients is to try to dispel their unsound fears and encourage them to be active. In some instances, overprotection by the family may be a problem.

A second group of persons whom the nurse may help are those who are not ill but who have a reduced cardiac reserve. The heart condition has resulted in adaptive changes (dilatation, hypertrophy and/or acceleration) to compensate for the defect in order to maintain circulation. Energy expenditure must be

THE CLASSIFICATION OF PATIENTS WITH DISEASES OF THE HEART[13]

Functional Capacity

Class I.   Patients with cardiac disease but without resulting limitations of physical activity. Ordinarily physical activity does not cause undue fatigue, palpitation, dyspnea or anginal pain.

Class II.   Patients with cardiac disease resulting in slight limitation of physical activity. They are comfortable at rest. Ordinary physical activity results in fatigue, palpitation, dyspnea or anginal pain.

Class III.   Patients with cardiac disease resulting in marked limitation of physical activity. They are comfortable at rest. Less than ordinary activity causes fatigue, palpitation, dyspnea or anginal pain.

Class IV.   Patients with cardiac disease resulting in inability to carry on any physical activity without discomfort. Symptoms of cardiac insufficiency or of the anginal syndrome are present even at rest. If any physical activity is undertaken discomfort is increased.

Therapeutic Classification

Class A.   Patients with cardiac disease whose ordinary physical activity need not be restricted.

Class B.   Patients with cardiac disease whose ordinary physical activity need not be restricted, but who should be advised against severe or competitive physical efforts.

Class C.   Patients with cardiac disease whose ordinary physical activity should be moderately restricted and whose more strenuous efforts should be discontinued.

Class D.   Patients with cardiac disease whose ordinary physical activity should be markedly restricted.

Class E.   Patients with cardiac disease who should be at complete rest, confined to bed or chair.

[13]New York Heart Association: The Classification of Patients with Disease of the Heart. New York, American Heart Association. (Available in Canada through the Canadian Heart Foundation.)

restricted to correspond to the functional capacity of the heart in order to avoid failure. Obviously, the limitations vary with the extent of pathology and physiological changes in the heart and its resulting capacity. For some it may mean only giving up strenuous competitive sports; for others, greater restrictions are necessary. The aim of the care of these persons is to have each one live within his compensatory limits and, at the same time, live as useful and satisfying a life as possible. Continuous treatment may be necessary for some to remain asymptomatic. The physician assesses each patient's capacity, and the nurse helps the patient and family accept and adjust to the necessary restrictions. Positive emphasis is placed upon certain activities, suggestions are made as to what the patient can do, remembering that appropriate amounts of work, recreation and rest are more satisfying and beneficial.

The functional capacity of some cardiac patients may be so limited that they cannot participate in any physical activity without experiencing symptoms of cardiac insufficiency. They may be restricted to self-care activities or may be confined to a chair or bed, completely dependent upon others. The nurse's role with these patients is to provide the prescribed treatment and necessary care.

The physician may use the functional and therapeutic classifications developed by the New York Heart Association and published by the American Heart Association. This serves as a general guide to the type of care required and is useful in finding suitable employment for the patient (see p. 298).

CAUSES AND TYPES OF HEART DISORDERS

Heart disorders may be classified as congenital or acquired. Various subclassifications may be used in acquired heart disease. Some authors concentrate on structure, such as pericardium, myocardium and endocardium. Others highlight the causes of heart disease, such as trauma, infections, degenerative processes, and hyper- and hypometabolic processes. This text classifies heart disorders as:

1. Congenital cardiovascular defects
2. Inflammatory diseases which may result in structural changes within the heart

3. Deficiency in the blood supply to the myocardium
4. Disturbances in conduction
5. Decompensation, or heart failure

Congenital Cardiovascular Defects

Congenital cardiovascular defect implies a structural abnormality that was present at birth in the heart or the large proximal blood vessels. It has only been within the last two to three decades that many of the congenital cardiovascular defects have been identified and successfully treated by surgery. Many are recognized shortly after birth if the infant survives. Others may go undiscovered for months or years because the heart maintains an adequate circulation by compensation. As in so many congenital deformities, the cause remains obscure. In some instances it is thought that a viral infection, such as German measles, occurring in the mother in the first trimester of pregnancy, may cause the defect. Frequently, cardiovascular malformations accompany other congenital defects such as cataract, mental retardation and deafmutism.

Many types of heart malformations occur. They may be classified into three main groups: (1) those which produce a left-to-right shunt of blood; (2) those which offer resistance to the blood flow; and (3) those which cause a right-to-left shunt (Fig. 13–9).

Anomalies Which Cause a Left-to Right Shunt

Several malformations occur which produce an abnormal pathway that permits a direct flow of blood from the left side of the heart or aorta to the right heart or pulmonary artery, creating a bypass of the systemic circulation and an overloading of the pulmonary circulation. These anomalies include patent ductus arteriosus and septal defects.

ATRIAL SEPTAL DEFECT. An opening between the two atria may be due to failure of the foramen ovale to close after birth or to a gap in the septum, either above or below the foramen ovale. Blood in the left atrium will flow through the opening into the right atrium, increasing the volume of blood in the pulmonary system. The right atrium, right ventricle and pulmonary artery enlarge. Pulmonary hypertension develops and causes dyspnea, par-

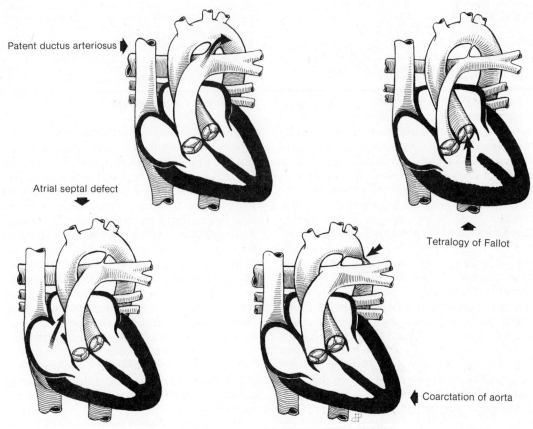

Patent ductus arteriosus

Atrial septal defect

Tetralogy of Fallot

Coarctation of aorta

FIGURE 13–9 Congenital cardiac defects.

ticularly on exertion. The reduced systemic circulatory volume retards physical and mental development and efficiency. The size of the opening may be so small that it goes undiscovered, and the patient may not experience any respiratory or circulatory difficulty.

Surgical repair of an atrial septal defect is usually accomplished by open heart surgery. Some defects may be closed simply by suturing while others may require a patch of Teflon, an inert material to which tissues do not react.

VENTRICULAR SEPTAL DEFECT. An opening in the ventricular septum results in a left-to-right shunt and produces problems similar to those cited in atrial septal defect — pulmonary hypertension, enlargement of the right ventricle and pulmonary arteries, and a deficient systemic circulation. If the defect is small and the patient is asymptomatic, surgery is not indicated. Moderate to severe defects may be closed by patching with either pericardial tissue or Teflon. Occasionally the

defect closes spontaneously in the young child.

PATENT DUCTUS ARTERIOSUS. Normally, after birth, a gradual spontaneous constriction and atrophy of the ductus takes place. If it remains open the blood in the aorta, under a pressure approximately five to six times that in the pulmonary artery, is shunted into the pulmonary artery. This increases the volume of blood entering the lungs, resulting in a high pulmonary blood pressure and dilatation of the pulmonary vessels. The patient experiences dyspnea, particularly on exertion. There is a corresponding increase in the venous flow into the left atrium and left ventricle, causing dilatation and hypertrophy of the left side of the heart. The volume of blood in the systemic circulatory system is less than normal, and the resulting oxygen and nutritional deficiencies retard normal mental and physical development.

The patent ductus arteriosus is corrected by surgical division and suturing of the two ends of the vessel.

Anomalies Which Cause Resistance to Blood Flow Within the Circuit

The seriousness of the resistance is determined by the degree of constriction or stenosis which may be found in the pulmonary artery or the aorta.

PULMONARY STENOSIS. A stenosis of the pulmonary valve or artery offers resistance to the outflow of blood from the right side of the heart. The right ventricle enlarges and the pressure in both the right ventricle and atrium is above normal. Blood may be backed up in the venous system, while the blood volume entering the pulmonary system is below normal. The latter creates an oxygen deficiency throughout the body which is manifested by fatigue, shortness of breath and, less frequently, cyanosis. Symptoms may not be present for several years.

This malformation may be treated surgically by incision of the constricted ring.

AORTIC STENOSIS. A defect comparable to pulmonary stenosis may occur in the aorta and offer resistance to left ventricular outflow. The left side of the heart enlarges and the pressure in both left chambers is above normal; this may be reflected in an increased pulmonary pressure if the restriction is severe. The cardiac output is lower and reduces arterial blood pressure and the systemic circulation as well as the blood supply into the coronary arteries. The defect may be treated by surgery, using an extracorporeal pump-oxygenator during the procedure.

COARCTATION OF THE THORACIC AORTA. Coarctation is a stricture in a segment of the aorta. Postductal coarctation occurs just beyond the obliterated ductus arteriosus and distal to the origin of the left subclavian artery. The second type, preductal coarctation, develops in the segment of aorta before the entrance of the ductus arteriosus. With this latter type the ductus usually remains patent.

Blood volume and pressure are increased behind the stricture, and the work of the left side of the heart is increased greatly. The blood volume and pressure are high in the upper extremities and head, but are abnormally low in the body parts which derive their blood supply from below the stricture. A difference in growth and development may be seen between the areas supplied from behind the stricture and those supplied from the aortic flow distal to the stricture. The patient may experience headaches, epistaxis, dyspnea on exertion, leg cramps and fatigue.

Surgical treatment of the condition involves resection of the constricted area and an end-to-end anastomosis or, in some instances, the area is excised and a graft of inert material introduced.

Anomalies Which Cause a Right-to-Left Shunt

A shunting of blood from the right side of the heart to the left involves a combination of two or more anomalies. Normally, the pressure is much higher in the left side of the heart than in the right side. A stenosis which offers resistance to flow from the right ventricle may increase the pressure in the right side to a level exceeding that in the left side. If a septal defect coexists with this increased pressure, blood is shunted from the right to the left side of the heart.

One of the most frequently seen combinations of anomalies which produces a right-to-left shunt is the tetralogy of Fallot. Tetralogy denotes a set of four conditions: pulmonary stenosis, ventricular septal defect, dextraposition of the aorta which causes it to override the septal defect, and right ventricular hypertrophy. The pulmonic stenosis produces an increased pressure in the right ventricle, causing a right-to-left shunt. The volume of blood flowing through the pulmonary system for oxygenation is reduced. Unoxygenated blood escapes into the aorta and a general systemic hypoxia occurs, manifested by cyanosis and dyspnea, especially on physical exertion, and by clubbing of the fingers. Compensatory responses to the oxygen deficiency develop in the form of polycythemia, high hemoglobin level and increased pulse and respiratory rates.

Correction of these defects is possible by means of open heart surgery and the use of the pump-oxygenator. The septal opening is patched, and the pulmonary stenosis is relieved. Occasionally the surgeon may decide not to perform corrective surgery but will proceed with a palliative surgical procedure. This consists of an anastomosis between the subclavian and pulmonary arteries (Blalock operation) or between the aorta and pulmonary artery (Potts operation). The purpose of the anastomosis is to divert a larger volume of blood through the lungs for oxygenation.

Miscellaneous Congenital Cardiac Anomalies

Only the more common anomalies that are recognized and treated have been presented here. A wide variety of anomalies can occur, many are not yet amenable to treatment, and others may be so severe that the infant cannot survive. Transposition of the great vessels is relatively common and may be treated surgically. In this anomaly, the pulmonary artery originates from the left side of the heart and conducts the oxygenated blood back to the lungs, and the aorta rises from the right ventricle, carrying unoxygenated blood into the systemic circulation.

Rarely, transposition of the pulmonary veins to the right of the heart is seen, and transplantation of the veins to the left atrium may be attempted.

Valvular atresia (absence of an opening) is another form of anomaly which occurs most frequently with the tricuspid valve but may also develop with the aortic valve. Tricuspid atresia raises the pressure within the right atrium to a level exceeding that in the left atrium, and blood flows through the foramen ovale. This anomaly frequently is accompanied by a ventricular septal defect which permits some blood to enter the right ventricle and pass into the pulmonary artery. Either the Blalock or Potts operation (see above), or an anastomosis between the superior vena cava and the pulmonary artery may be done to increase the volume of blood through the lungs.

Inflammatory Disease Involving Heart Structures

In any tissue, the inflammatory process may result in destruction of normal functional tissue followed by its replacement with scar tissue, which is fibrous in nature and less specialized.

Diseases which produce inflammatory heart lesions and impaired function include rheumatic fever, bacterial endocarditis, syphilis and pericarditis.

Rheumatic Fever

This is the most common cause of inflammation in the heart structures. Although any or all parts may be affected by rheumatic fever, the valves and the myocardium are the most frequent sites and tend to sustain greater permanent damage. The disease is a complication of a group A streptococcal infection which is usually respiratory. A period of 1 to 5 weeks may lapse between the infection and the onset of the rheumatic fever, during which time the patient may have recovered completely from the infection.

The inflammatory response, which may occur in the joints as well as in the heart, is thought to be due to a sensitivity of the affected individuals to the antibodies that were formed in response to the invading bacteria. The antistreptococcal lysin titer is found to be high in these persons at the onset of rheumatic fever. This sensitivity is only present in certain individuals, since not all those with streptococcal infection develop rheumatic fever. The symptoms of the acute stage vary in intensity and may be so mild that they go unrecognized. In some, joint involvement and fever may be predominant with no evident symptoms referable to the heart, and it is not until much later that it becomes known that cardiac tissue was involved and received permanent damage.

Rheumatic fever may cause acute myocarditis with subsequent scarred areas that reduce myocardial efficiency and impairment of the conduction system.

The valves are the most common area of the heart to be affected, and the mitral and aortic valves are the most susceptible. They frequently become scarred, distorted and functionally impaired. Both the valve ring at the opening and the valve cusps may be affected. Following the acute inflammation scarring occurs, the orifice is diminished and the edges of the cusps may fuse. These changes result in resistance to the forward movement of the blood, thus increasing the work of the heart chamber behind the obstruction. Damage of this type is referred to as a stenosis. Normally, the mitral opening in an adult is large enough to admit three fingers; in severe stenosis it can become so restricted that only one finger may be introduced.

In some instances, the scarring of the valvular cusps produces a thickening and loss of tissue that prevents them from coming together to close off the opening completely. This incomplete closure allows a regurgitation or backflow of blood through the valve, and is called valvular insufficiency. An added strain is placed on the heart chamber behind the insufficiency. Many patients with rheumatic heart disease have a combined stenosis and insufficiency in the affected valve. If the mitral valve is involved, the left atrium develops dilatation and hypertrophy to compensate for the resistance of stenosis and the backflow of insufficiency. In the case of aortic valvular damage, the left ventricle dilates and hypertrophies. Prolonged strain created by a damaged valve, increased demands on the already weakened heart, or further progress of the initial rheumatic disease process may result in decompensation or heart failure.

Treatment of rheumatic fever includes drug therapy (antimicrobial preparations, salicylates, corticosteroids), rest and possible surgery.

In the acute stage of rheumatic heart disease the patient may receive large doses of *penicillin* to destroy any hemolytic streptococci which may still be active in the body. Reactivation of the disease occurs very readily with any subsequent streptococcal infection. Rheumatic fever patients, particularly children, continue on prophylactic doses of oral penicillin or on a monthly intramuscular injection of a large dose which is slowly absorbed. For better absorption, the oral penicillin is given before food is taken in the morning and again at bedtime when the stomach is empty. Sulfadiazine may be used for prophylactic therapy instead of penicillin, and the patient is advised to drink a minimum of six to eight glasses of fluid each day to prevent precipitation of the drug in the renal tubules.

With the initial administration of penicillin the nurse is alert for symptoms of allergic reactions. If the patient has not had the drug previously, a test dose may be given intracutaneously. Any information of previous reactions or of asthma or hay fever should be passed on to the physician before the drug is given.

Sodium salicylate and acetylsalicylic acid (aspirin) are preparations commonly used in rheumatic fever. These relieve symptoms by suppressing tissue reaction. They are given orally and may produce gastric distress, so they should be given with meals or with a snack or a large volume of fluid. If the patient complains of dizziness, headache, tinnitus or dullness of hearing, the physician is informed. Frequently, enteric-coated acetyl-salicylic acid tablets are used to prevent gastric irritation.

Various preparations of *cortisone* are also used in the treatment of rheumatic heart disease. Their action is similar to that of salicylates in that they are anti-inflammatory and reduce tissue responses. While a patient is receiving a corticoid preparation his sodium intake may be restricted, since there tends to be an excessive reabsorption of sodium by the kidney tubules, leading to edema. The patient is weighed daily if possible and is observed for other indications of edema.

Activity restrictions may vary from bed rest in the acute stage to gradually increasing periods out of bed as symptoms abate.

Therapy for valvular damage includes restriction of activity to within tolerated limits, treatment of complications such as heart failure and, in some instances, surgical replacement of valves.

Bacterial Endocarditis

Inflammation of the endocardium, including the valves, may be caused by many different pathogenic organisms, but the viridans streptococcus causes the greatest number of cases.[14] Bacterial endocarditis has a higher incidence in those who have some valvular abnormality, either acquired or congenital in origin, or who have a history of rheumatic fever. Special precautions should be taken with such persons when they experience minor infections, tooth extraction, and surgery, all of which predispose to the entrance of organisms into the blood.

Bacterial endocarditis may be further defined as acute or subacute. The differentiation is based upon the causative organism and the rapidity of onset. Subacute bacterial endocarditis is most commonly caused by the viridans streptococcus and the onset of symptoms may be insidious. The acute form is caused by more virulent organisms such as *Staphylococcus aureus*, pneumococcus, group A streptococcus and gonococcus. This form of the disease progresses more rapidly and more often attacks the normal heart.

Symptoms include fever, weakness, fatigue, anorexia, chills and petechial lesions

---

[14]Paul B. Beeson: "Endocarditis." *In* Paul B. Beeson and Walsh McDermott (Eds.): Textbook of Medicine, 15th ed. Philadelphia, W. B. Saunders, 1979.

in the mucous membranes of the mouth, pharynx or conjunctiva. Cardiac auscultation usually reveals the presence of a heart murmur. In bacterial endocarditis the organisms, transient in the blood, implant on areas of the endocardium and clusters of vegetative structures form which consist of inflammatory exudate, fibrin, platelets and bacteria. These are quite friable and may break off to form an embolus which may then lodge in an artery, interrupting the blood supply to an area of tissue. Should the embolus derive from the right side of the heart, it is likely to obstruct a pulmonary artery, causing a pulmonary infarct.[15] If the embolus originates in the left side of the heart, it may enter any systemic artery, resulting in an infarction. For example, it may lodge in a cerebral artery, leading to a stroke, or in a femoral artery, interrupting the blood supply to the limb.

Treatment for bacterial endocarditis includes antibiotic therapy, the choice of drug being determined by the organism isolated in blood cultures. Antibiotics are administered in large doses, usually parenterally for at least 2 weeks, and treatment is continued for at least 4 weeks. Nursing care includes the usual nursing measures for a patient with an inflammatory condition.

As the infection subsides in endocarditis, the affected areas become scarred; if a valve was involved insufficiency is likely to develop, and the patient then has the same problems as mentioned in relation to the patient with rheumatic fever.

Syphilis

Another type of infection that may produce a valvular lesion is syphilis. Most frequently it is the aortic valve that is affected, and an insufficiency develops.

Pericarditis

Pericarditis may occur as the result of an infectious or noninfectious process, or may be due to an auto-immune reaction (see p. 315 for a discussion of hypersensitivity reaction following a myocardial infarction). Fluid accumulates in the pericardium as part of the inflammatory response. The pressure exerted on the heart by this fluid may prevent its

normal filling, creating a condition referred to as cardiac tamponade. In some instances extensive scarring of the visceral pericardium may prevent normal stretching and filling of the heart chambers.

Pericarditis is characterized by chest pain, often pleuritic in nature, electrocardiographic changes (elevation of S T segments followed several days later by T wave inversions) and a pericardial friction rub on auscultation. A paradoxical pulse may be present if cardiac tamponade has occurred.

Treatment includes salicylates and occasionally corticosteroids to combat the inflammatory response. The patient must be observed carefully for complications such as cardiac tamponade.

In the inflammatory conditions discussed in the preceding paragraphs, it can be seen that permanent heart damage can occur from the formation of scar tissue. The patient may remain active as long as his heart compensates, but may have limitations due to reduced cardiac efficiency.

Deficiency in the Blood Supply to the Myocardium (Ischemic Heart Disease)

Coronary Atherosclerosis

A narrowing or obstruction in the coronary arteries reduces the blood supply to the myocardium, and causes what is called ischemic heart disease. It results in a deficiency of oxygen and nutrients to the muscle. The reduced oxygen supply is most significant and is quickly reflected in reduced myocardial efficiency. The heart muscle can withstand only a very small oxygen debt, as it is much more susceptible to a reduced oxygen supply than skeletal muscle. In most instances the decreased blood supply to the myocardium is due to degenerative changes in the arteries that produce a narrowing of the lumen of the vessels. Fatty substances, which include cholesterol, are deposited within the intima of the arteries to cause *atherosclerosis*. These fatty plaques interfere with the nutrition of the cells in the intima, leading to necrosis, scarring and calcification, which leave the surface rough and the lumen reduced. These roughened constricted areas allow less blood through and predispose to thrombus formation and occlusion of the vessel.

---

[15] An infarct is an area of tissue which undergoes necrosis because it is deprived of its blood supply.

Atherosclerosis usually develops gradually. While the blood supply through the artery is being reduced, a collateral circulation develops in an effort to increase the supply to the myocardium, but this supplementary circulation is rarely sufficient to provide enough oxygen to the heart muscle during strenuous physical exertion.

Coronary atherosclerosis is a disease having many causes. It seems to develop as a result of a host-environment interaction; the incidence increases with age and shows a strong familial tendency. It is less common in women of childbearing age than men of the same age but after this period gradually becomes as frequent in women. A number of surveys have shown a greater incidence of coronary atherosclerosis among populations whose diet regularly contains high amounts of calories, total fats, saturated fats, cholesterol and refined sugars.

The major risk factors associated with the development of coronary atherosclerosis are hyperlipoproteinemia (especially hypercholesteremia), hypertension, cigarette smoking and diabetes mellitus. These factors may usually be controlled — hyperlipoproteinemia by diet and/or medications, and hypertension by medications. Cigarette smoking should be discontinued, although for some individuals this represents considerable difficulty. Other suggested risk factors include lack of exercise and psychosocial tensions. Obesity, although not directly associated with atherosclerosis, is associated with hypertension and diabetes.[16]

Although control of risk factors does not guarantee elimination of atherosclerotic heart disease, evidence suggests that modifying dietary, smoking and exercise habits and reducing emotional stress may decrease its incidence.

HYPERLIPOPROTEINEMIA. Blood lipids include cholesterol, triglycerides, phospholipids and free fatty acids. Cholesterol and triglycerides are of clinical significance and are transported in plasma as lipoproteins. There are four major classes of lipoproteins and each contains varying proportions of protein and the three blood lipids. As illustrated in Figure 13–10, they are chylomicrons and prebeta, beta and alpha lipoproteins,

---

[16]Mario DiGirolamo and Robert C. Schlant: "Etiology of Coronary Atherosclerosis." In J. Willis Hurst, et al.: The Heart, 3rd ed., New York, McGraw-Hill, 1974.

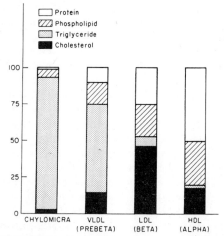

FIGURE 13–10 Approximate per cent composition of lipoproteins. (From Stone, Neil J., and Levy, Robert I.: "Hyperlipoproteinemia and Coronary Heart Disease." Progr. Cardiovasc. Dis., Vol. XIV, No. 4, Jan. 1972, p. 344.)

and they may be separated by the process of electrophoresis.

Chylomicrons are mainly of dietary origin. Prebeta lipoproteins contain a large amount of triglycerides, primarily of hepatic origin, synthesized from fatty acids and carbohydrate. Beta lipoproteins carry one-half to two-thirds of the total plasma cholesterol. Alpha lipoproteins carry little triglycerides but larger amounts of protein and an appreciable amount of cholesterol.

Hyperlipoproteinemia may be classified as Type I, II, III, IV or V. Types I and V hyperlipidemia are rare. Types II, III and IV are associated with an increased incidence of coronary heart disease. Hyperlipoproteinemia may be secondary to another disease such as obstructive liver disease, due to an excessive intake of saturated fats and cholesterol in the diet, or may result from a primary or familial disorder. Determination of serum cholesterol and triglyceride levels will detect hyperlipoproteinemia in most cases and is less costly than other laboratory procedures. However, in some instances, further studies may be warranted. Control of hypercholesteremia is directed toward lowering the serum cholesterol levels by diet and in some instances by medications.

Studies suggest that by modifying the dietary intake of fats, carbohydrate and calories, the blood lipid levels of most patients with primary hyperlipidemia can be lowered. The contribution of diet to the prevention of coronary atherosclerosis is not clear but evidence suggests that this approach might be worthwhile.

The purpose of the diet is to reduce body weight when required and to lower the intake of total fat, saturated fatty acids and cholesterol, while increasing the intake of unsaturated fatty acids. Saturated fat and cholesterol are found in high-fat meats and dairy products and in some commercially baked goods. Polyunsaturated fats are contained in vegetable and fish oils.

The modified diet emphasizes substitution of lean meat (veal, lean beef), poultry and fish for fattier meats (pork, organ meats, visible meat fat). It also includes nonfat products such as corn oil, margarine, skim milk cheese, whole grain or enriched flour products, fruits, vegetables and polyunsaturated vegetable oils.

The degree of dietary restriction depends upon the type of hyperlipidemia and the age and condition of the patient. Dietary teaching is a combined function of the physician, nurse and dietition. The dietition is the primary person involved if the diet is complex, but the nurse also needs to be informed so that she can reinforce the teaching. Some patients may require much support and understanding to continue on their diets, especially if drastic changes in eating habits are needed. Compliance will probably be greater if the diet is adjusted as much as possible to individual tastes.

Lipid-lowering drugs may be ordered for selected patients who do not respond to diet therapy alone. These include:

CLOFIBRATE (ATROMID-S). This drug interferes with cholesterol synthesis. It reduces cholesterol and triglyceride levels in patients with Types III, IV and V hyperlipidemia and, to a small degree, may alter the cholesterol levels of patients with Type II. Its side effects include weight gain, gastrointestinal upsets, gallstones and increased levels of the enzymes SGOT and SGPT. It also prolongs the prothrombin time of patients on warfarin (Coumadin) so that anticoagulant dosage of the drug may need to be adjusted.

NICOTINIC ACID. This drug inhibits cholesterol synthesis and the release of free fatty acids from adipose tissue. Almost all types of hyperlipidemia, including Type II, respond to it. Marked flushing, pruritus, nausea and vomiting are among its side effects. Liver function may be abnormally altered but this situation is reversible if the drug is discontinued. Gradual increases in dosage may prevent the side effects.

CHOLESTYRAMINE. This drug acts by binding bile acids and preventing their reabsorption in the intestine. Increased breakdown of cholesterol results. It is used for patients with familial Type II hyperlipidemia. Cholestyramine is administered with meals. Side effects include gastrointestinal disturbances.

The development of coronary atherosclerosis produces the ischemic heart diseases known as angina pectoris and myocardial infarction.

Angina Pectoris

The term angina pectoris describes a clinical syndrome characterized by chest pain. "Pectoris" indicates the general location (chest) and "angina" refers to the choking, suffocating nature of the pain. This condition arises because of a discrepancy between the oxygen being supplied to the myocardium and the energy expenditure. The pain, arising from heart muscle fibers which are deficient in oxygen, is usually precipitated by physical exertion or emotional stress which increases the workload of the heart. There is a need for a greater blood supply than is being delivered by the coronary circulation.

The patient suddenly develops chest pain substernally which may radiate to the left or both shoulders and arms and occasionally up the neck to the jaws. The pain may, however, be atypical and arise only in the arms, jaw or neck and not in the chest. It is usually relieved within a few minutes by resting and/or by nitroglycerin but may last as long as 30 minutes. The patient may become short of breath.

Angina may remain a stable condition brought about by predictable precipitating factors with no change in the severity or frequency of the attacks. It is then controlled by limiting those activities or situations known to cause pain, and by medication. The pain may progress in frequency and intensity if the atherosclerosis process in the coronary arteries proceeds more rapidly than the development of collateral circulation. Activities may then need to be curtailed greatly and the patient may even experience pain at rest.

Angina decubitus is a term applied to severe angina occurring frequently and at rest. It is sometimes difficult to alleviate with medications and often leads to myocardial infarction.

MANAGEMENT OF ANGINA PECTORIS. Immediate care during an anginal episode includes having the patient stop any activity he is engaged in, and rest, and administering medications as ordered, such as nitroglycerin. Pulse, respirations and blood pressure are checked during the episode. Occasionally the physician will want an electrocardiogram taken while the patient is having pain.

The patient is advised that strenuous physical exertion and emotional conflicts should be avoided. In many instances normal functioning can be maintained by modifying aspects of his occupation, recreation and social life. Risk factors such as smoking and obesity are eliminated in an effort to prevent progression of the disease. Smoking favors vasoconstriction and overweight increases the demand on the heart.

Moderate exercise below the point of producing pain is encouraged. Walking is excellent exercise and should be done on a regular basis. The individual should begin with short walks on level ground, gradually increasing the distance over a period of weeks. Regular, medically supervised exercise programs are recommended for some patients. Regular exercise improves muscle tone and general well-being and stimulates the development of collateral circulation in the myocardium. Normal weight is more easily maintained. The psychological benefit of exercise to the patient cannot be underestimated.

Drugs used in angina pectoris include the following (Table 13–4):

NITRATES. Nitrates act by relaxing vascular smooth muscle. This results in decreased peripheral vascular resistance and venous return, with a subsequent decrease in heart size, stroke volume and cardiac output. The net effect is a decrease in the oxygen consumption of the heart.

Glyceryl trinitrate (nitroglycerin) is a short-acting vasodilator administered in tablet form. The tablet is placed under the tongue where it is absorbed very quickly. The patient will experience a tingling feeling

TABLE 13–4   DRUGS USED IN PATIENTS WITH ANGINA PECTORIS

Drug	Action	Side Effects

Nitrates
Short-acting:
  Glyceryl trinitrate
  (nitroglycerin)
	Relaxes vascular smooth muscle, thus decreasing peripheral vascular resistance	Headache or sense of fullness in the head

Long-acting:
  Isosorbide dinitrate
  (Isordil)
		Headache
		Orthostatic hypotension

Pentaerythritol
  tetranitrate
  (Peritrate)
	Same as above	

Erythrityl
  tetranitrate
  (Cardilate)		

Beta Blocker
  Propranolol
  (Inderal)
	Decreases myocardial oxygen requirements by decreasing heart rate, depressing myocardial contractility and decreasing left ventricular tension development	Excessive bradycardia
		Congestive heart failure
		Bronchospasm

on the tongue when first taken and should obtain relief in 1 to 2 minutes. Patients should not take multiple doses to get quick relief of pain. If relief is not apparent after 3 tablets taken at 5 minute intervals, a physician should be called. Initial dosage should be 0.3 mg. This reduces the likelihood of severe headaches, which often occur in the initial stage of treatment. Persons who suffer attacks of angina are advised to carry the drug at all times. It should be replaced periodically so that a fresh supply is available when required. Pills should be kept in a dark container and those not being carried should be stored in a cool, dark place, since nitroglycerin is affected by both light and heat. The patient is advised that he may experience mild fullness, warmth or throbbing in the head, but fortunately with continued use side effects usually diminish. Nitroglycerin may also be used prophylactically 2 to 3 minutes prior to activities which are known to precipitate anginal attacks.

Isosorbide dinitrate (Isordil) is a slower- and longer-acting nitrate given sublingually in small doses or orally in larger doses. It is ordered for patients experiencing regular attacks of angina. Since it reduces vascular tone, some patients may experience hypotension on standing, especially when taking larger doses. The patient is usually started on small doses, which are gradually increased as the drug becomes tolerated. Isordil is frequently prescribed in combination with propranolol. The effects of both drugs may be complimentary; the increase in heart rate and contractility induced by nitrates is offset by propranolol.

Pentaerythritol tetranitrate (Peritrate) is also a slower-acting vasodilator and is effective for a longer period. It is given orally in doses of 80 to 320 mg. daily. Some patients may require doses of oral Peritrate and Isordil much greater than those generally recommended.

BETA-ADRENERGIC BLOCKERS. These drugs block sympathetic stimulation of the beta receptors.

Propranolol (Inderal) relieves anginal symptoms by decreasing myocardial oxygen requirements. It does this by depressing myocardial contractility and decreasing heart rate and left ventricular tension development. It significantly reduces pulse rate, sometimes to as low as 40 beats per minute.

The patient is usually started on a low dose (e.g., 10 to 20 mg.) every 6 hours which is gradually increased until relief is obtained. However, in some patients, this goal may not be achieved because of significant bradycardia or the occurrence of side effects. Because of variability in metabolism, the individual therapeutic dose of propranolol may vary from 80 to 1000 mg. per day. Patients with congestive heart failure or a history of bronchial asthma are not given the drug because it will increase the failure and its beta blocking properties will prevent dilatation of the bronchioles. Mild cardiac failure is not an absolute contraindication to the use of propranolol. The benefit-risk ratio is considered by the physician in deciding whether or not to start propranolol in these patients.

For those patients who do not obtain adequate relief with medications surgery may be indicated (see p. 343).

Acute Myocardial Infarction

Acute myocardial infarction (also known as coronary occlusion or thrombosis) is the most serious and acute form of ischemic heart disease. A coronary artery becomes blocked and the myocardial area which it supplies suffers oxygen deficiency and necrosis. It occurs suddenly, and compensation through collateral channels is inadequate to maintain the myocardial cells. The resulting area of necrotic tissue is referred to as an infarction.

The extent of the infarction varies from patches of 1 or 2 centimeters in diameter to widespread areas of necrosis. One or more layers of the heart may be involved. The area of infarction becomes soft and then eventually fills in with firm, fibrous scar tissue. Survival and the extent of subsequent restrictions depend upon the amount of myocardial damage and the area of the heart affected. Death may occur immediately or within a few hours. Obviously, the remaining viable heart tissue must compensate for the loss of functional tissue.

Occlusion may be preceded by some manifestations of coronary insufficiency such as angina, or it may occur suddenly without any previous warning.

TYPES OF MYOCARDIAL INFARCTION. It is difficult to delineate the precise area of the myocardium which is affected, but general areas can be identified. Although other areas of the heart may be involved, most infarctions occur in the left ventricle.

ANTERIOR WALL INFARCTION. The anterior wall of the left ventricle is infarcted due to an occlusion of the left anterior descending artery. The papillary muscles of the left ventricle and the intraventricular septum may also be involved. In the latter instances, the infarction would be referred to as anteroseptal.

LATERAL WALL INFARCTION. An infarction in the lateral wall of the left ventricle is associated with an occlusion of the lateral branch of the left circumflex artery. Occasionally both the anterior descending and the left circumflex branches are obstructed, and the infarction is designated anterolateral.

INFERIOR WALL INFARCTION. This term implies an infarction of the part of the left ventricle which rests on the diaphragm. It is usually due to occlusion of the right coronary artery. Occasionally it is called a diaphragmatic infarction.

POSTERIOR WALL INFARCTION. This type is usually due to occlusion of the posterior branch of either the right coronary or left circumflex artery. It is sometimes called a true posterior infarction to distinguish it from an inferior infarction.

MANAGEMENT OF PATIENTS WITH MYOCARDIAL INFARCTION. In most instances the patient suddenly becomes seriously ill, and prompt action is necessary. The physician is called immediately. The patient is kept at rest in a position that is most comfortable and facilitates breathing — usually semirecumbent. Tight clothing (collars, belts, etc.) is loosened and the patient covered sufficiently to prevent chilling. Food and fluids are withheld.

The patient is transported to a hospital and admitted to a coronary care unit where he remains for approximately 3 to 5 days. When his condition has stabilized, he is transferred to a general care ward. Hospitalization for patients without complications varies from 10 days to 3 weeks. Total convalescence ranges from 8 to 12 weeks.

The objective of care of the patient with myocardial infarction is to restore the ability of the heart to maintain adequate circulation.

A. ASSESSMENT. Constant observations of the patient are necessary in the acute stage. The nurse must be alert to significant changes and must make decisions about the need for prompt reporting, the seeking of assistance and the use of emergency measures.

Pulse. The pulse becomes rapid and weak and may be imperceptible at the time of the attack. Initially, a few patients may exhibit bradycardia, followed by tachycardia. The monitor gives more specific information about the type of disorder in rate and rhythm during the acute stage. The patient's pulse is checked every 2 to 4 hours during the acute stage and more frequently if it is showing great variability. Once the heart rate and rhythm have stabilized, the pulse is taken four times daily. Changes in rate or rhythm are reported. Pulse rate is noted in response to activity.

Blood Pressure. Due to the decreased pumping efficiency of the heart, the blood pressure falls but may be elevated in the first few hours following an attack due to an augmented sympathetic response. It is taken every 2 to 4 hours during the acute stage, and more often if there is variation or abnormality. It is also checked following the administration of medications such as morphine or meperidine (Demerol), and if the patient is experiencing signs or symptoms such as pain, faintness or cyanosis. When the acute episode is over and the patient's condition has stabilized, the blood pressure is taken four times daily. Blood pressure is checked when the patient is lying down and after assuming the upright position to detect orthostatic hypotension. Either a fall in blood pressure or continuous hypertension is reported immediately.

Pain. The most common presenting complaint of patients with myocardial infarction is severe chest pain. The nurse must ascertain the exact location and character of the chest discomfort (see p. 290 for a description of various types of chest pain), whether it is aggravated by any particular motion or change of position, and how it is relieved. The pain may last for several hours or until relieved by analgesics. It should not persist for days; prolonged pain may be an indication of pericarditis or an extending infarction.

Dyspnea. Dyspnea may be due to pulmonary congestion or pain. It may also occur as activity is increased. Relief of pain and congestion may relieve the dyspnea. It is important to note whether shortness of breath is present at all times or if intermittent, how it is precipitated and what measures relieve it. In the acute stage respirations are checked at least every 2 to 4 hours, or more often as changes occur. During the convalescent stage, they are observed and recorded four times daily and in relationship to various activities.

Skin. The skin may be cool, moist and a greyish color in response to the decreased cardiac output. The color, temperature and moistness of the skin are continually observed and any changes noted.

Nausea and Vomiting. Nausea and vomiting may be experienced at the time of the attack, lasting from several hours to 2 or 3 days. Occasionally, nausea and vomiting occur in response to the opiates being administered. The nurse notes the presence of nausea and vomiting and any possible precipitating factors.

Temperature. Myocardial necrosis causes an elevation of body temperature ranging from 37.7° to 39° C. (100° to 102° F.) The temperature usually rises within 24 to 48 hours and returns to normal by the sixth or seventh day. If the temperature persists longer, it may be due to complications. The patient's temperature is taken four times daily until it has been normal for several days. It may then be taken once or twice daily. Rectal temperatures are avoided to prevent rectal stimulation which may lead to straining at stool.

Weakness and Tiredness. Extreme weakness may be experienced and may persist for many days. Many patients complain of tiredness for weeks after their infarction. The exact cause of this is not clearly defined. Some suggest it results from decreased oxygen perfusion of the tissues due to a lowered cardiac output. It has also been attributed to weakened skeletal muscles as a result of even a brief period of immobilization. The patient may have been in a state of physical exhaustion prior to his attack or he may be emotionally exhausted from the experience.

The nurse observes the extent to which the patient tolerates any activity (such as walking). She also notes how much he sleeps during the day and how quickly he falls asleep following activities.

Psychological Reactions. A heart attack carries the threat of death or invalidism for the patient. The sudden change in his wellbeing leaves feelings of vulnerability and helplessness. The patient is required to make very rapid adjustments to both his illness and change in environment.

Anxiety is the most common psychological response. It is manifested by various overt and covert behaviors, such as tenseness, restlessness, short attention span, inability to concentrate, crying, constant talking and verbalization of feelings of anxiety. The patient may appear generally relaxed but may exhibit more subtle manifestations of anxiety such as darting eye movements. Patients may also show denial, and may be angry and/or depressed. These emotional responses may appear in varying degrees and at any time during hospitalization or may not become evident until after discharge from the hospital. The individual's interpretation of his experience and his personal coping pattern influence his responses. Continuing restlessness and apprehension are noted and reported.

Electrocardiographic Monitoring. In the coronary care unit a constant monitoring of heart action is established for continuous assessment of cardiac activity. Electrodes are applied to the chest wall and are connected to an electrocardiograph with an oscilloscope. The purpose of the monitor is explained to the patient and his family. The patient is advised that he need not lie immobile because of the electrodes. The nurse responsible for the patient must become sufficiently familiar with the monitoring system and oscilloscope graphs so that she is able to recognize changes and arrhythmias that demand prompt action. The basic rhythm of the patient's heart is observed and recorded in the nurse's notes for each shift. Any changes in the rhythm are immediately observed and decisions made as to further action required.

Diagnostic Tests. The nurse must be aware of the results of diagnostic tests and their significance following a myocardial infarction. Assessment includes noting ongoing changes in the ECG, serum enzyme and leukocyte count and erythrocyte sedimentation rate.

1. Changes in the electrocardiogram. Theoretically, three types of changes are present in the myocardium when an infarction develops. These define three areas, referred to clinically as the area of infarction, the area of injury and the zone of ischemia, resulting in a distinctive elec-

trocardiographic pattern. In the infarcted area, irreversible structural changes occur with resulting necrosis of the tissue. Since electrical impulses cannot be conducted through this tissue, electrical energy is lost, causing a relative gain of electromotive forces directed away from the necrotic area. These developments produce a negative deflection (Q wave) in electrodes facing the infarcted area, indicating that electrical forces are not being directed toward it but away from it. An increased positive deflection (R wave) will be seen in leads facing the opposite surface of the heart, indicating forces moving toward the leads and away from the infarcted area.

Surrounding the zone of infarction is an area of injury which suffers a decreased blood supply, but the damage is not permanent. Although specific abnormal electrocardiographic changes are produced, these may revert to normal if the blood supply is restored. Electrodes placed over the injured area will record an S T segment elevation.

The zone of ischemia surrounds the area of injury and may also return to normal once the blood supply is restored. Inverted T waves indicate ischemia.

S T elevations appear within several hours following an infarction and disappear in a few days. In the early stages T waves become taller and appear as an extension of the elvated S T segment. They later become inverted. Q waves appear within 1 to 2 days and persist for months

(see Fig. 13–11). The area of infarction will be reflected in leads which view that portion of the heart. Thus, inferior infarctions can be identified in leads II, III and AVF, anterior infarctions can be identified in the anterior leads V_1 to V_4, and lateral wall infarction in leads I, AVL, V_5 and V_6. Since under normal conditions, no leads face the posterior wall of the heart, diagnosis is based upon reciprocal changes in leads facing the opposite wall — that is, increased R waves in leads V_1 and V_2.

2. Serum enzymes. Diagnosis of a myocardial infarction is confirmed by the elevation of specific intracellular serum enzymes and by a characteristic electrocardiographic pattern (see p. 292 for a description of enzymes). Table 13–5 demonstrates enzyme elevations in one patient with an acute myocardial infarction. CPK and SGOT levels increased early and peaked within 48 hours. The LDH level increased more gradually and remained elevated after 7 days.

3. Leukocyte count and erythrocyte sedimentation rate. Leukocytosis and an increased erythrocyte sedimentation rate occur in response to necrosis but are nonspecific diagnostic measures. The white blood count rises a few hours after the infarction and returns to normal within 7 days. The sedimentation rate becomes elevated by the third or fourth day and may remain so for weeks.

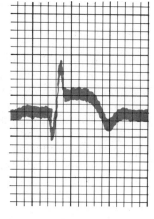

FIGURE 13–11 Electrocardiographic changes indicating acute myocardial infarction: Q wave, S-T elevation, and T wave inversion.

TABLE 13–5 SERUM ENZYME ELEVATIONS IN ONE PATIENT
FOLLOWING A MYOCARDIAL INFARCTION

Enzyme	Day of Admission	Day 2	Day 3	Day 7
CPK	6	162	5	5
SGOT	14	177	201	23
LDH	151	513	789	419

B. RELIEF OF DISCOMFORT (PHYSICAL AND
PSYCHOLOGICAL)

Pain. An analgesic such as morphine sulfate or meperidine (Demerol) is usually given to relieve the severe pain associated with myocardial infarction. The drug is administered intravenously in small doses in the emergency room and in the coronary care unit. Intramuscular injections elevate CPK readings, as this enzyme is also present in skeletal muscle and diagnosis of a myocardial infarction may be obscured. The effect of the drug on the respirations should be noted, since depression of the respiratory center may occur.

Hypoxia and Dyspnea. Oxygen is usually administered by mask or nasal catheter in order to increase arterial oxygen tension, which may help to relieve the myocardial pain caused by hypoxia and prevent extension of the infarction. Mechanical respiratory assistance may be necessary in cases of severe insufficiency.

The nurse briefly explains the procedure to the patient and remains with him until he is accustomed to the mask or nasal prongs. Observations are made of the patient's response to the oxygen. Its effectiveness will be indicated by reduced pulse rate, less dyspnea, improvement in color and less restlessness. (For details of administration of oxygen, see p. 408.)

Some degree of dyspnea may be prevented by having the patient avoid exertion. Explanations are given concerning the easiest way to move in bed, the importance of avoiding straining and the Valsalva maneuver. The patient is positioned in a low semi-Fowler's position. This allows for greater expansion of the lungs and reduces the venous return to the heart, thus reducing the stress on it.

Nausea and Vomiting. Dimenhydrinate (Gravol) may be given intravenously until the patient can tolerate it orally. Nursing measures cited on p. 491 are observed.

Anxiety. Mental rest is a considerable part of therapy for the heart patient. Anxiety may be somewhat reduced by the relief of physical symptoms. In the coronary care unit, brief and precise explanations of all equipment, routines, tests and procedures prove very helpful. Patients are also reassured by prompt attention to their needs and constant monitoring. Competent, quiet performance without apparent concern and hurry provides some reassurance for the patient. Anticipation of needs and preparedness for treatments contribute to more effective care. Articles likely to be wanted are left within reach so that the patient is neither tempted to get up nor reach for something, rather than ask.

Patients may pose direct questions about their condition, such as "Is it serious?" or "Will I recover?" Anwers should be honest and supportive. Klein and Garrity suggest a relationship between long-term survival and emotional responses as well as severity of infarction, and state that each patient must be helped to find a coping strategy appropriate to his personal situation and his own strengths and weaknesses.[17] This is done through effective communication with the patient; it is the only means by which he may influence his environment and be assisted in working out appropriate coping strategies.[18] Effective communication includes listening to the patient and responding to his cues, introducing statements to which the patient might respond and allowing the patient to discuss his feelings. Considerable help and peace of mind may be derived from the patient's spiritual adviser.

---

[17]Thomas F. Garrity and Robert F. Klein: "Emotional Responses and Clinical Severity as Early Determinants of Six-Month Mortality after Myocardial Infarction." Heart Lung, Vol. 4, No. 5 (Sept.-Oct. 1975), pp. 730–737.

[18]Ibid., p. 734.

If the patient is very upset the nurse remains with the patient until he becomes less apprehensive, and then assures him that someone is close by and will be in and out frequently. The presence of a close family member who will not disturb the patient may provide additional comfort. Occasionally, diazepam (Valium) or another antianxiety drug may be prescribed.

Family. Members of the patient's family also experience shock and anxiety in response to the patient's illness. Seeing someone close to us in pain and seriously ill is a very frightening experience. Relatives of patients have described their initial reaction as "feeling numbed and dazed." As reality sets in, anxiety about the patient's survival and future increases.

The physician and nurse speak to a family member shortly after the patient's admission to the hospital, explaining the suspected diagnosis and the treatment to be given during the next few hours. The nurse then attempts to speak to close family members whenever they visit to answer any questions and to show some understanding of the anxiety they are experiencing. Family members as well as patients are reassured by simple explanations of equipment, procedures and routines. In talking to the family, the nurse may elicit information about the patient's habits, likes and dislikes and emotional reactions which may be helpful in planning care.

Alleviating the anxieties of relatives and/or close family friends allows them to be more supportive of the patient. As with the patient, concern may prevent the family member from absorbing all that he or she is told. Explanations and instructions may have to be repeated. Family members are included in teaching programs provided for the patient or in programs specifically designed for them.

C. Reduction of Energy Demands

Rest and Restriction of Activity. This is of the utmost importance in the treatment and care of the patient with an acute myocardial infarction. The patient is placed on complete bed rest until symptoms such as pain and shortness of breath have abated, meaning that he remains in bed and all care is provided for him. This necessary dependence should be discussed with the patient as to its purpose and importance, its tem-

porary nature and what it involves. Previously, the patient remained at this level of activity for several days to several weeks. In recent years the trend has been to mobilize the patients early once pain and severe shortness of breath are no longer present. Research has shown that fewer complications occur. Also, the psychological effect of early ambulation is worth a great deal.

By the second day, strict inactivity is modified. The patient is allowed mild activities such as cleaning his teeth, washing his face and hands and feeding himself, as long as reaching is avoided. Exercising of the lower limbs to prevent venous stasis is commenced. By the second day, some patients are permitted to use a bedside commode, since this demands less energy than using a bedpan. Undisturbed rest periods are provided following short periods of activity — for instance, after eating and after bathing.

Activities and ambulation are gradually increased. In many instances, by the second or third day, the patient is allowed to dangle his legs over the side of the bed for 5 to 10 minutes. He is advised to sit up gradually to prevent feelings of dizziness or faintness. If pain-free by the third day, he may be allowed to sit in a chair for brief periods, starting with 10 to 15 minutes and increasing each day. Continual cardiac monitoring immediately identifies any arrhythmias accompanying changes in activity. Blood pressure is recorded in the lying and sitting positions and the patient is observed closely for reactions such as weakness, fatigue, shortness of breath and chest pain.

The degree to which activities and exertion are restricted varies with the patient's response, the size and location of the infarction, the presence of complications and the physician's philosophy. The body temperature, enzyme concentrations, leukocyte count, sedimentation rate and electrocardiographic changes are used as guides. An important determining principle is that activities be increased gradually, that rest periods be alternated with activities and that certain activities such as pushing, pulling, lifting or straining be avoided. By the time the patient leaves the coronary care unit (4 to 5 days postinfarction), he may be sitting in a chair three times a day for 30 to 45 minutes, using a bedside commode, feeding and bathing himself and taking short walks around his bed.

The progression in activities continues after the patient is transferred from the coronary care unit and in the weeks after he leaves the hospital. He will begin walking short distances on the ward, progressing in most cases to the length of the ward hallway by discharge. Limitations are applied to those activities which precipitate dyspnea and pain.

Once the patient is free of pain and other early symptoms, he feels quite well but must still be restricted. Time hangs heavy on his hands, so some effort is made to provide suitable diversions in which the patient is interested. Reading and radio and television programs may occupy the patient but these are selected to avoid overexcitement and fatigue. He may have some hobby he can pursue without overtaxing his heart. Visitors are restricted at first, but later they help relieve the patient's boredom. Visitor selection should be made by the family to avoid those who might excite or distress the patient. Visitors should be made aware of time limitations as it may be difficult for the patient to ask them to leave if be becomes tired.

Nutrition. Liquids are given in small amounts at first following a myocardial infarction. The diet is increased gradually to easily digested, nongas-forming solids as tolerated. Large meals are avoided. If necessary, the caloric intake is decreased. Salt is usually restricted. Fluids may be restricted if the patient is in heart failure (see p. 337).

Elimination. Constipation should be prevented and the patient cautioned against straining at stool because of the stress it places on the heart. A mild laxative or stool softener may be given as necessary.

D. Assisting the patient to understand his illness and to adjust to the imposed limitations

Patient Teaching. In order to make the best possible adjustment to his illness and recovery, the patient must have some understanding of the illness and how he can assist in recovery. Providing this information helps give the patient some control over his situation. Teaching programs are adjusted to specific patient needs and capabilities, since learning capacity varies among individuals. Patients experiencing myocardial infarctions often have many misconceptions of their condition and how it will affect their future. It is useful for the nurse to find out what the patient already knows and to obtain information about his life style. The nurse has many opportunities to reinforce and elaborate on explanations given by the physician and to respond to further questions.

During the acute stage, the patient is often too anxious to absorb much information. *Simple* explanations of equipment being used and procedures common to coronary care units are usually adequate. Following transfer to the general ward, the patient is usually better able to participate in a planned program. Written as well as verbal instruction is provided. Visual aids such as heart models or diagrams help to enhance learning. Suggested topics include basic information on how the heart functions, what happens to the heart with a myocardial infarction, how the heart heals and the purpose of treatment. For 6 to 10 weeks the patient is advised to avoid heavy lifting, pushing, mental and physical fatigue, sexual activity, driving and travel by car, bus, airplane and train. Activity and ambulation is increased gradually, interspersed regularly with rest periods. Some explanation is given of risk factors, how these factors relate to the patients, and how they may be reduced. Any prescribed special diet or medication is reviewed. In some instances the dietitian or clinical pharmacologist as well as the physician and nurse may be involved in teaching the patient.

Short sessions are necessary, as many patients with myocardial infarction tire easily. It is helpful if a family member can be present in the teaching session. Acknowledgment is made of the feelings that the patient has in response to his illness. He may wish to express verbally the feelings that he is experiencing such as discouragement, fear, anger and/or depression; the nurse provides opportunities for free expression and is a willing listener.

E. Recognition of complications. Complications following myocardial infarction include arrhythmias, congestive heart failure, pericarditis, mitral regurgitation, myocardial rupture, aneurysm and systemic or pulmonary emboli.

Arrhythmias. Arrhythmias usually occur early following a myocardial infarction (see p. 316 for a discussion of arrhythmias). The most serious arrhythmia that may be seen is ventricular fibrillation; this is treated by cardiac defibrillation. Bradyarrhythmias, such as sinus bradycardia, first degree A-V block and Wenckebach heart block are most often associated with inferior wall infarctions. Since the S-A node and the A-V junctional tissue are most often supplied by the right coronary artery, occlusion of this vessel will lead to their decreased functioning. Anterior myocardial infarctions are more prone to heart failure and arrhythmias that accompany it, such as sinus tachycardia and rapid atrial arrhythmias, and to intraventricular conduction disturbances, such as Mobitz Type II block.[19]

Heart Failure. Mild congestive heart failure occurs in many patients due to the decreased efficiency with which the heart contracts. Gross left ventricular failure is more common following an anterior infarction. Heart failure is diagnosed by the presence of rales on chest auscultation, complaints of shortness of breath and a chest x-ray. (See p. 333 for management.)

Pericarditis. Pericarditis following a myocardial infarction is thought to be due to an autoimmune reaction in which antigens originate from the injured myocardial tissue, initiating inflammation of the pericardium. It may occur as early as 24 hours after the infarction. The pain which accompanies pericarditis is similar to that of a myocardial infarction but is sometimes more excruciating. It is alarming to the patient, who may think that he is having another heart attack. A distinction may be made if the pain is increased by deep breathing or twisting the trunk, or if it is relieved by leaning forward, lying on the right side or sitting in an upright position with the trunk straight. A friction rub may be heard on auscultation but is not always present in the early stages. The patient's temperature may remain elevated beyond 1 week. Treatment is usually enteric-coated acetylsalicylic acid (aspirin) given in divided doses, and a corticosteroid preparation may be employed.

Mitral Regurgitation. This complication may occur when a papillary muscle dysfunctions or ruptures, causing the valve to become incompetent. This is a grave complication which may be corrected by surgery. Less severe mitral insufficiency may be due to infarction of the papillary muscle.

Myocardial Rupture. Myocardial rupture, when present, usually occurs within 7 days. It is more often seen in patients with transmural infarctions. Rupture of the interventricular septum usually occurs within the first 2 weeks and is a very grave prognostic sign. Instead of flowing normally from the left ventricle into the aorta, blood is rerouted to the right ventricle, increasing the demands on it and flooding the lungs. Immediate surgery is the only effective treatment.

Aneurysm. An aneurysm is a ballooning out of the infarcted myocardial tissue, causing the heart to contract in a disruptive fashion. If large, it seriously impedes the maintenance of normal cardiac output. The extent of the aneurysm may be determined by a myocardial scan and in some instances may be corrected by surgery.

Emboli. Emboli occur because clots formed in the healing area of the myocardium break loose and escape into the circulation. Pulmonary emboli may arise in the leg veins due to circulatory stasis, and may be prevented by exercising the limbs. The treatment for emboli includes anticoagulant drugs.

Shoulder-Hand Syndrome. In the weeks following a myocardial infarction a few patients may develop a stiffness or tenderness in the left arm and shoulder. Immobility during the early period of recovery has been suggested as a cause.

F. TRANSFER FROM THE CORONARY CARE UNIT. Transfer out of the coronary care unit is often a difficult period of adjustment for patients. Klein et al. documented increased urinary catecholamine levels in myocardial infarction patients at the time of transfer to a general ward and again just before discharge home.[20] These are obviously periods of great anxiety for patients.

Although interpreting transfer as a sign of progress, patients often miss the security of constant observation by the staff as well as their continual contact. Concern may also be related to the increased independence expected, particularly in relation to physical care and decision making. This transition is much less difficult if the patient is prepared for it and if the change to independence is not abrupt. When explanations are given as to why the patient no longer needs to be monitored and

[19]Louis Lemberg and Susan Hamer: "Arrhythmias Complicating an Acute Myocardial Infarction: A Self-teaching Program." Heart Lung, Vol. 5, No. 4 (July-Aug. 1976), pp. 576–584.

[20]Robert F. Klein, et al.: "Transfer From a Coronary Care Unit." Arch. Int. Med., Vol. 122, No. 2 (Aug. 1968), pp. 102–106.

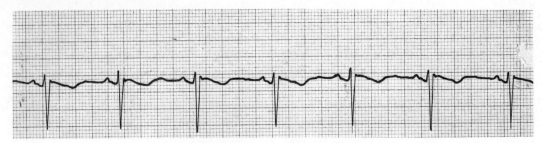

FIGURE 13–12   *A*, Normal sinus rhythm.

what schedules and routines he might expect on the ward, adjustment is much easier. A gradual reduction in the amount of physical care provided and a gradual increase in the amount of responsibility assumed by the patient helps him to feel more secure. Specific information about the patient's regimen, likes and dislikes and problems should be communicated by the coronary care staff to the nurses assuming responsibility for the patient. This helps to facilitate continuity of care.

Arrhythmias and Conduction Disturbances

Normally, the rate and rhythm of the heart contractions are established by impulses generated in the S-A node at a rate between 60 and 100 beats per minute (Fig. 13–12*A*) A disorder of rate or rhythm is referred to as a cardiac arrhythmia, and is due to some disturbance in the formation or conduction of impulses. The arrhythmia may be of short duration or persistent and may be functional in origin, result from organic heart disease or be associated with an electrolyte imbalance, such as hypokalemia.

An arrhythmia may have significant hemodynamic consequences. For example, an excessively slow or fast heart rate may decrease the cardiac output and blood pressure, thus compromising the perfusion of vital organs such as the brain, kidneys, liver and heart itself. Arrhythmias may also predispose the patient to thrombus formation.

Common irregularities include tachycardia, bradycardia, ectopic beats (extrasystoles), flutter, fibrillation and heart block. The arrhythmia is further defined by the site of its origin; sinus arrhythmia originates in the S-A node, atrial originates in an atrium, nodal or junctional originates in the A-V node, and ventricular originates in the ventricle.

Tachycardias

SINUS TACHYCARDIA.   In this rhythm the heart rate is greater than 100 beats per minute, and the impulse originates in the sinoatrial node. It is not always an abnormal rhythm, since it occurs during and after exercise and in response to emotional stress. It may be due to an abnormal state such as fever, anemia, infection, hyperthyroidism, myocardial infarction and heart failure. It also may result from medications — for example, atropine, epinephrine, isoproterenol hydrochloride and thyroid extract, or other drugs such as alcohol and nicotine (see Fig. 13–12*B*).

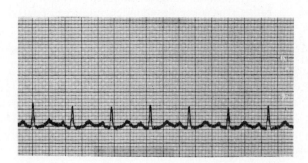

FIGURE 13–12   *B*, Sinus tachycardia: rate over 100/min.; P wave and QRS are normal and in 1:1 relationship.

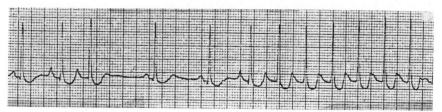

FIGURE 13–12 *C,* Paroxysmal atrial tachycardia.

Tachycardia is significant for two reasons. Coronary blood flow occurs predominantly during diastole. With tachycardia the diastolic time is shortened, reducing the time for perfusion of the myocardium. Also, an increased heart rate increases the need of the myocardium for oxygen. In someone with narrowed coronary arteries, tachycardia may precipitate myocardial ischemia.

Treatment may be directed at correcting the underlying cause or it may be necessary to reduce the rate by giving a drug such as a digitalis preparation or propranolol (Inderal).

PAROXYSMAL ATRIAL TACHYCARDIA (P.A.T.). This is an abrupt onset of a very rapid heart rate, usually 150 to 250 beats per minute, initiated in the atria. It may last a few seconds or longer. Such attacks cannot be explained in some persons; in others they may be related to organic heart disease (Fig. 13–12*C*).

A rapid heart rate of this type is serious if imposed on a diseased heart. When this arrhythmia occurs, the patient is advised to rest and the physician is notified. If the patient is subject to recurring attacks, he is encouraged to recognize and avoid possible precipitating factors such as fatigue, emotional stress, reaching, or excessive smoking or coffee drinking. In some instances an attack may be relieved by measures that increase parasympathetic (vagal) innervation to the heart. Among those suggested is pressure on the carotid sinus or eyeballs. *Caution must be used in relation to both these maneuvers.* Carotid sinus massage applied injudiciously may result in asystole; too frequent and too heavy pressure on the eyeballs may predispose to retinal detachment in the eye.

Some who experience paroxysmal tachycardia find that it may be checked by assuming a certain position, such as flexion of the trunk or holding the arms over the head. The Valsalva maneuver, which involves an inspiration followed by voluntary closure of the glottis and an effort to exhale, may prove helpful. This reduces the venous return from the extremities and head, thus reducing the volume of blood entering the heart which in turn, decreases the cardiac output and the arterial blood pressure. An antiarrhythmic drug such as quinidine, procainamide hydrochloride (Pronestyl), digoxin or propranolol (Inderal) may be prescribed. These drugs reduce the myocardial excitability and slow the rate.

VENTRICULAR TACHYCARDIA. Usually the term ventricular tachycardia refers to a run of rapidly repeated ventricular beats, essentially regular in rhythm, at a rate of 150 to 210 per minute. Any rate above 60 per minute which is initiated in the ventricles might be considered tachycardia, because the ventricles normally do not initiate impulses at more than 25 to 40 beats per minute. However, rates between 60 and 100 per minute are usually distinguished from the faster rates. Marriott refers to them as "accelerated idioventricular rhythms"[21] but they are also called "slow ventricular tachycardia" or "nonparoxysmal ventricular tachycardia." (See Fig. 13–12*D*.)

Ventricular tachycardia is a more serious arrhythmia than atrial tachycardia, as there is always the danger it will lead to ventricular fibrillation. It is usually due to ischemic heart disease and is frequently present following a myocardial infarction.

Treatment includes electrical countershock and/or antiarrhythmic drugs such as intravenous lidocaine and parenteral or oral procainamide hydrochloride (Pronestyl), quinidine and diphenylhydantoin (Dilantin).

---

[21]Marriott, op. cit., p. 116.

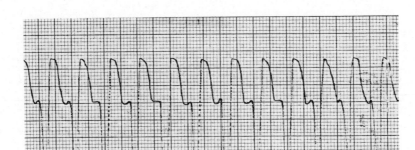

FIGURE 13–12 *D*, Ventricular tachycardia: series of broad, ventricular beats at rate of 175/min.

Bradycardias

SINUS BRADYCARDIA. This is the term used for an abnormally slow pulse rate. It is applied when the pulse rate is below 59 per minute in an adult, less than 80 per minute in a child and less than 100 per minute in an infant. (Fig. 13–12*E*).

Circulation may be adequately maintained by an increased stroke volume in a person with bradycardia. With fewer contractions more blood collects in the heart chambers to produce greater stretching of the myocardial fibers, resulting in a stronger contraction and increased output. Obviously this can only occur if the myocardium is in good condition. If the heart rate is less than 30 to 40 per minute circulatory insufficiency is likely to occur, especially with physical activity.

The most common causes of bradycardia are a decreased blood supply to the S-A node, increased vagal tone, old age, head injury, amyloidosis and obstructive jaundice. Circulatory reflexes may initiate a compensatory increase in the heart rate but, if the cause persists and becomes progressively severe, the heart muscle will gradually become weaker and less responsive, producing fewer contractions. Any disturbance which initiates an increase in vagal nerve impulses to the heart will produce a decrease in the heart rate. An example of this would he bradycardia produced by carotid sinus massage or in some persons by vomiting. Other examples of conditions in which slowing of the heart rate may be secondary are increased intracranial pressure and myxedema (a deficiency of thyroid secretion).

The pulse rate may normally be slower in those with well developed cardiac reserve, such as well trained athletes. In such persons, the venous return is of greater strength, producing an increased stroke volume with each contraction.

Ectopic Beats

When impulses which influence the heart rate and rhythm are generated elsewhere than in the S-A node, the contractions are called *ectopic or premature beats or extrasystoles*. The ectopic or premature beat occurs when the myocardial fibers are in the relative re-

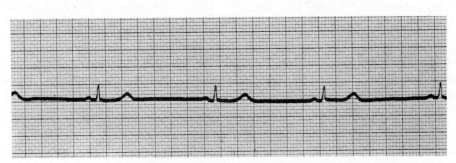

FIGURE 13–12 *E*, Sinus bradycardia.

fractory period following a normal contraction. The impulse from the S-A node for the succeeding normal contraction is ineffective, since it arrives when the muscle fibers are in the absolute refractory period following the premature beat, and no contraction takes place. This causes a longer than normal pause before the next normal contraction and the heart "misses" a beat. The next normal contraction may be stronger because of the prolonged filling period. The time between the normal heart contraction which precedes the extrasystole and the one that follows is equal to two normal cardiac cycles. The subject usually describes the experience as his heart "missing a beat and then a thud."

Extrasystoles, or premature beats, may be due to ischemic areas or to inflammation in the heart muscle. The fibers may also become irritated and hypersensitive as a result of certain toxic conditions, such as may occur with the excessive use of tobacco, coffee, tea or alcohol. The extrasystoles may occur irregularly, with varying lengths of time between them. The incidence may be so rare as to have no clinical significance but they should be investigated if persistent, even though they occur irregularly and at relatively long intervals. Premature beats may arise regularly and at a rate in excess of that of the normal S-A pacemaker, resulting in paroxysmal tachycardia.

ATRIAL PREMATURE BEATS.   The ectopic focus is in the atria and the complex occurs earlier than expected. Atrial premature beats are significant because, if they occur during the vulnerable period of the atria, they may precipitate more serious atrial arrhythmias, such as atrial flutter or atrial fibrillation. They may or may not be conducted to the ventricles, depending upon the state of conduction through the A-V node and the refractory period at which they occur. Treatment is usually not required unless they occur with great frequency or unless progression to more serious arrhythmias is feared, as may occur following a myocardial infarction. Digitalis or quinidine may be prescribed. If a precipitating cause is recognized, it should be eliminated. (See Fig. 13–12F.)

VENTRICULAR   PREMATURE   BEATS (VPBs).   The ectopic focus is in the ventricle, and therefore there will be no related P wave on the electrocardiogram. Occasional ventricular premature beats may be innocuous but they may also precipitate ventricular tachycardia and/or fibrillation. If they occur in a diseased heart, in groups of two, three or more, more frequently than five per minute, arise from more than one focus (multifocal) or are on the T wave of the preceding complex, they are considered serious and require treatment. The usual immediate treatment is lidocaine (Xylocaine) by intravenous injection and/or continuous intravenous drip. Quinidine sulfate may be substituted and the patient gradually tapered off lidocaine. (See Fig. 13–12G.)

Flutter

ATRIAL FLUTTER.   As with atrial tachycardia, atrial flutter is due to a rapidly firing ectopic focus in the atria. There is some dispute as to whether atrial flutter should be differentiated from atrial tachycardia; some cardiologists describe both as supraventricular tachycardia, while others differentiate on the basis of rate and pattern. The rate

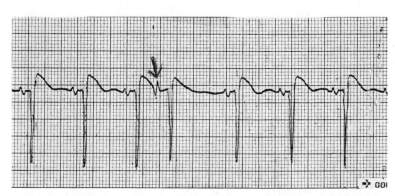

FIGURE 13–12   *F*, A trial premature beat: the fourth beat occurs earlier than expected, followed by a compensatory pause before the next beat.

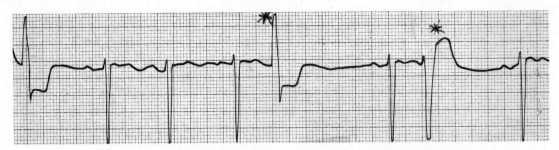

FIGURE 13-12 *G,* Ventricular premature beat: no related P wave with widened QRS complexes.

usually falls between 250 and 350 beats per minute and a characteristic sawtooth pattern is seen on the electrocardiogram. A-V block is usually present, so that the ventricular response may vary from 150 to 175 beats per minute. (See Fig. 13–12*H*.) Atrial flutter may occur with mitral stenosis, ischemic heart disease and chronic obstructive pulmonary disease. The usual treatment is countershock in emergency situations or the administration of digitalis, which blocks impulses at the A-V node.

Fibrillation

This is an arrhythmia in which the normal rhythmic contractions of the myocardium of either the atria or ventricles are replaced by extremely rapid (250 to 500 per minute), ineffective contractions, irregular in force and rhythm. Some area of the heart gives rise to very rapid and irregular impulses, and the myocardial contractile fibers do not achieve the contraction and relaxation that permit normal emptying and filling of the chambers.

ATRIAL FIBRILLATION. Atrial fibrillation is a fairly common arrhythmia in which electrical activity in the atria is totally disorganized. It is due to some myocardial weakness or disease which may be the result of coronary insufficiency, rheumatic heart disease, thyrotoxicosis or acute infection. The atria are never completely empty, and normal filling cannot occur. Since little pressure is created by the atrial contractions, the flow of blood into the ventricles is due mainly to the pressure created by the volume of blood. Circulation may become seriously impaired. Only a proportion of the impulses arising in the atria are conducted through the A-V node to the ventricles, but those that do pass through may far exceed the normal in frequency, and are irregular. (See Fig. 13–12*I*.) Normal filling and emptying of the ventricles do not take place, cardiac output is reduced, arterial blood pressure falls and the blood is backed up in the large veins.

The pulse is very rapid, weak and irregular. With some ventricular contractions, the stroke volume may be so reduced that radial pulsation does not occur. This sets up a *pulse deficit,* defined as the difference between the apical and radial pulses. To determine a pulse deficit accurately, the ventricular rate is counted for a full minute, using a stethoscope placed over the apical region of the heart. At the same time, a second person counts the radial pulse for a full minute. If two people are not available, one may count one pulse and then the other, each for a full minute.

Atrial fibrillation may be treated with a digitalis preparation or quinidine sulfate. Digitalis slows the heart rate by depressing the impulse conduction through the A-V node and by increasing vagal nerve stimulation. The myocardial contractions are strengthened, resulting in more efficient emptying of the heart chambers. Quinidine prolongs the

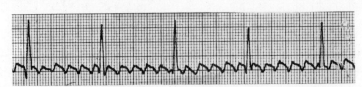

FIGURE 13-12 *H,* Atrial flutter: high degree of A–V block with a ventricular rate of 58/min.

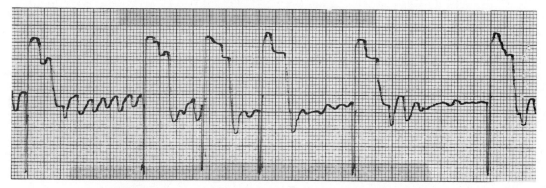

FIGURE 13–12 *I*, Atrial fibrillation with varying ventricular response.

refractory period of the myocardial fibers and is used to restore normal sinus rhythm. The latter drug is less predictable as to the patient's reaction, close observation of the patient and frequent checking of the heart action are necessary. Direct current (DC) countershock may be employed when an immediate reversion is required and if drug therapy has not been effective.

A complication that may follow atrial fibrillation is embolism. The blood that was not forwarded into the ventricles during fibrillation may have formed a thrombus in an atrial chamber and then, when normal heart action is reestablished, the thrombus may be moved out into the circulation.

VENTRICULAR FIBRILLATION. In ventricular fibrillation very rapid, asynchronous contractions arise in the ventricular myocardium because the electrical activity occurs in a totally disorganized sequence. (See Fig. 13–12*J*.) The contractions are so ineffective in pumping that the condition may very quickly prove fatal. The pulse and blood pressure become unobtainable in a few sec-onds, the patient quickly loses consciousness, his pupils dilate and his reflexes are lost. Prompt emergency treatment may reestablish circulation. If the patient is being monitored in a coronary care unit, the arrhythmia may be identified immediately at onset and treatment would consist of immediate countershock (defibrillation). In many coronary care units nurses who are taught this procedure implement it. *Hospital policy will dictate who may defibrillate a patient.* An important guideline is that it must be initiated within minutes.

Although an electrical shock may cause fibrillation, it may also be used to stop it. In defibrillation two electrodes ("paddles") are placed on the chest wall, one on each side of the heart or one on the ventral wall with a second on the dorsal wall. A strong current (approximately 400 volts) is passed through the electrodes for a brief period. All the muscle fibers of the myocardium are thrown into contraction together and then enter a refractory period simultaneously. This quiescent period may give the normal pacemaker, the

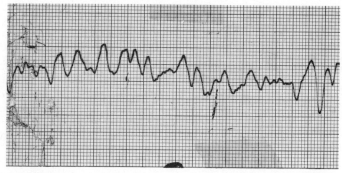

FIGURE 13–12 *J*, Ventricular fibrillation: chaotic ventricular activity.

S-A node, an opportunity to take over. It is important to make sure that no one is touching the bed or the patient during the electrical discharge to prevent their receiving a severe shock. When a defibrillator is not available, cardiac massage accompanied by artificial respiration may sustain life and restore circulation (see "Cardiac Arrest," p. 331).

Ventricular fibrillation may occur with irritation of the heart during heart catheterization because of coronary occlusion by the catheter, myocardial infarction, hypothermia, hypoxia, hypokalemia and electrical shock. Very frequently ventricular fibrillation is preceded by ventricular premature beats. Prompt administration of an antiarrhythmic drug such as lidocaine (Xylocaine) or procainamide hydrochloride (Pronestyl) may prevent serious ventricular tachycardia and fibrillation.

Heart Block

This is a condition in which impulse formation is depressed or impulse conduction is blocked. Although conduction may be interrupted between the S-A node and the atria, the term "heart block" usually refers to a disorder of conduction at the junctional tissues, which are the atrioventricular node and the common bundle (bundle of His) and its branches. The S-A node or the conduction pathway may be damaged by inflammatory disease such as rheumatic fever, coronary insufficiency, pressure from scarred or calcified tissue, or surgical trauma.

SINOATRIAL BLOCK. In sinoatrial block impulses either are not formed in the S-A node, fail to be conducted from it or emerge very slowly. If sinoatrial impulses are not received by the atria, occasional beats may be dropped, cardiac standstill may occur or the ventricles may respond to impulses arising from a lower pacemaker, such as the junctional tissue. In the latter instance a junctional rhythm will result. (See Fig. 13–12K.)

The seriousness of an S-A block depends on the extent to which the heart rate is slowed and cardiac output is decreased. A slow rate may precipitate other arrhythmias. Specific precipitating causes include the drugs digitalis, quinidine and salicylates, coronary artery disease, myocardial infarction and increased vagal tone.

Treatment is directed at removing the cause, when possible, and improving conduction between the S-A node and the atria by drugs such as atropine and isoproteronol (Isuprel). If drug therapy is not effective, artificial pacing may be required.

Heart block at junctional tissues occurs in varying degrees of severity and may be categorized as first degree, second degree — Type I and Type II — and third degree, or complete heart block. Conduction may be impaired in the bundle branches, referred to as right or left bundle branch block.

FIRST DEGREE HEART BLOCK. First degree heart block is usually due to delayed conduction through the A-V node, and the interval between atrial and ventricular contractions is lengthened. This is exhibited on the electrocardiogram by a prolonged P-R interval (greater than 0.20 second) (Fig. 13–12L). It may be caused by increased vagal tone in the normal person, fatigue in the conduction system because of prolonged tachycardia, digitalis intoxication, inflammatory heart disease, or coronary artery disease. Although the patient often has no characteristic physical symptoms, auscultation may reveal a decline in the intensity of

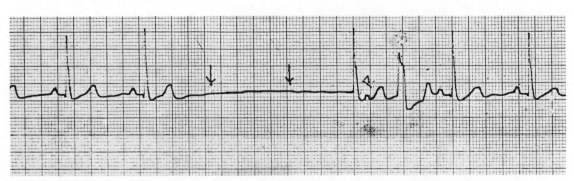

FIGURE 13–12   K, Sinoatrial block: two P waves do not emerge (arrows). A junctional beat follows.

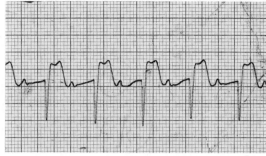

FIGURE 13–12 *L,* First degree heart block: The P–R interval is prolonged to 0.28 sec.

the first heart sound. First degree heart block may progress to second and third degree heart block but in the absence of evidence of disease requires no treatment. Digitalis may be discontinued or the dosage reduced.

SECOND DEGREE HEART BLOCK. Second degree or partial heart block refers to a more advanced disturbance in which some of the sinus impulses fail to get through and activate the ventricles. It may be divided into Mobitz Type I or Wenckebach and Mobitz Type II.

In Wenckebach block the period of time between atrial and ventricular conduction becomes progressively longer, until finally an atrial impulse is completely blocked. The electrocardiogram shows progressively longer P-R intervals, until finally a P wave is not followed by a QRS complex. The P-R interval following this dropped ventricular beat is close to the normal range, but with each successive beat it lengthens and the cycle repeats itself. The patient may be conscious of a decreased ventricular rate if the change occurs suddenly but may exhibit no physical symptoms. On examination, the intensity of the first heart sound may be weak or

may decrease over several beats. (See Fig. 13–12*M.*)

Type II, second degree block, is usually more serious than Type I. At definite intervals impulses are blocked at the A-V node and an atrial beat fails to be followed by a ventricular beat. The ratio of atrial to ventricular beats may vary — for example 2:1, 3:1, 4:3, 3:2. The P-R interval is fixed and unvarying. The patient may experience syncopal (fainting) attacks. (See Fig. 13–12*N.*)

Both second degree blocks may be due to inflammatory or fibrotic processes, coronary artery disease, infarction, or drugs such as digitalis.

THIRD DEGREE HEART BLOCK. In this block conduction is so disturbed that no impulses reach the ventricles and the atria and ventricles beat independently at their own inherent rhythms. The block may occur at the A-V node, main bundle or one of the bundle branches. It is a more advanced block and may be caused by any of the disorders responsible for Type II partial blocks. Since atrial impulses are unable to penetrate the A-V node, a lower pacemaker takes over and controls the ventricles. If this "rescuing" pace-

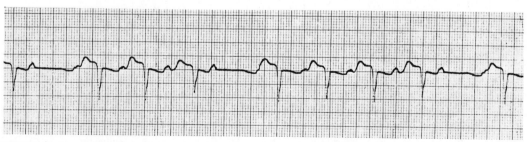

FIGURE 13–12 *M,* Wenckebach block: P–R interval becomes progressively longer until the fourth P wave is not followed by a QRS complex.

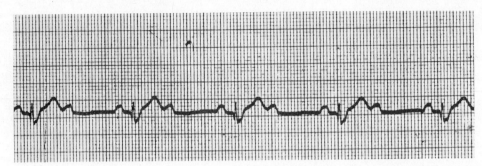

FIGURE 13–12   N, Type II second degree block in a 2:1 pattern.

maker is initiated in the junctional tissue, the electrocardiogram will show a QRS complex which is normal in appearance and not wide unless there is an associated bundle branch block. If the pacemaker is in the ventricles, the QRS complexes will be wide and abnormal in shape. (See Figs. 13–12*O*.)

Palpation of the pulse will usually reveal a rate of 45 or less because the rhythm is ventricular. On physical examination, the first heart sound varies markedly from beat to beat and may occasionally be quite loud (bruit de canon) when the ventricular contractions happen to follow very quickly after the atrial. The prognosis for complete heart block is uncertain but, in the event that Stokes-Adams syndrome occurs, it is poor without immediate treatment.

Heart block may be a temporary or permanent condition. If it is permanent, the independent ventricular rhythm may become firmly established and, with some restrictions of activities, the patient may live a fairly normal life. In some instances the ventricular rhythm may be irregular and episodes of cardiac arrest may threaten the patient. Cardiac asystole lasting 10 seconds or longer may occur, reducing the cardiac output to a level that causes cerebral ischemia. The patient becomes dizzy and may faint or convulse, or sudden death may occur. This type of episode is referred to as a Stokes-Adams attack or syndrome.

Treatment

Treatment of heart arrhythmias includes the use of a pacemaker and/or drugs.

ARTIFICIAL CARDIAC PACEMAKERS. In serious conduction defects, electrical stimulation may be provided by an electronic battery-operated pacer to stimulate or control cardiac contractions. The pacemaker consists of a power unit which generates electrical impulses and two fine insulated wires, each terminating in an electrode (one positive and the other negative, to complete the electrical circuit). The pulse-generating system of most pacemakers consists of small mercury or transistor batteries which last approximately 18 to 30 months. Exhaustion of the batteries necessitates surgical replacement.

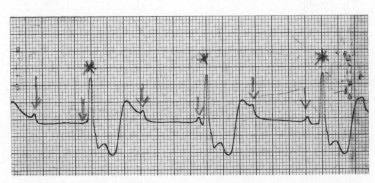

FIGURE 13–12   O, Third degree heart block: Atria *(arrows)* beating at a rate of 90/min. Ventricles *(asterisks)* beating independently at 40/min.

Lithium and nuclear power batteries are other generating sources available. These last a great deal longer than the mercury batteries but are very expensive; the greater cost limits their availability and use. The strength (milliamperes) of the power impulses and the rate at which they are discharged by the artificial pacemaker are adjustable and are preset on an individual basis. The electrodes of the early pacemakers were applied externally to the chest wall over the heart. More recent models deliver the charges by an electrode placed in direct contact with the heart (see Fig. 13–13).

If the conduction defect is transient, a *temporary pacemaker* is used. A pacing electrode is introduced through the external jugular, subclavian, antecubital or femoral vein and advanced into the right ventricle under fluoroscopy. The electrode wire is connected to an external battery pacer control unit that is strapped securely to the patient (Fig. 13–13*A*).

When the conduction defect is irreversible, a *permanent pacemaker* is implanted within the body. The electrode is introduced transvenously, usually through the right cephalic or the right external jugular vein, and the battery unit is implanted subcutaneously in the patient's chest. This requires a small incision (Fig. 13–13*B*).

There are three types of pacemakers, according to their pattern of activity. The pacemaker may be preset to discharge at a fixed rate, by demand, or at a rate that corresponds to atrial contractions.

In *fixed-rate pacing*, which may also be referred to as asynchronous pacing, the pacemaker delivers a predetermined fixed number of electrical impulses per minute regardless of the number of impulses generated by the heart itself. In other words, fixed-rate pacing is not synchronized with generic cardiac activity. There is a risk of causing tachycardia or ventricular fibrillation due to additional spontaneous impulse formation as the condition of the heart improves. A second disadvantage of fixed-rate pacing is that it will not increase or decrease heart activity to correspond with body activity and demands.

The *demand or standby pacemaker* is preset to discharge impulses only when the patient's heart rhythm falls below a preset rate. A device in the power unit of the demand pacemaker is sensitive to the electrical currents generated by spontaneous heart impulses. These electrical stimuli are conveyed via the electrode wire to the sensor and inhibit the release of impulses by the power unit. If no stimulation of the sensory device is generated by spontaneous heart impulses, the pacemaker is activated to discharge at a constant preset rate. The advantage of demand (standby) pacing is the elimination of the risk of intrinsic impulses in addition to pacemaker impulses, resulting in an arrhythmia .

A pacemaker capable of varying the rate of impulses discharged, producing *synchronous* pacing, is also available. A device sensitive to the atrial contraction is placed in the right atrium. The stimulus is conveyed to the power unit of the pacemaker and an impulse is initiated and conveyed to an electrode in the right ventricle, resulting in a ventricular contraction (see Fig. 13–13*C*). This arrangement produces a delay in the delivery of the impulse to the ventricle similar to that normally occurring in the A-V conduction system. It also provides a means by which ventricular contractions correspond with the impulses initiated by the S-A node and atrial contractions. Normally the S-A node responds to increased physiological needs, as in exercise and fever, by discharging more impulses; this is evidenced by an increase in the pulse rate. Conversely, the rate of discharge by the S-A node becomes slower with a decrease in physiological demands (e.g., during rest). Thus, the synchronous type of pacemaker has the distinct advantage of varying the rate according to the patient's physiological needs, and synchronizes ventricular contractions with the intrinsic atrial impulses and contractions.

NURSING CARE OF THE PATIENT WITH A PACEMAKER. Nursing care involves assisting in the preparation of the patient for implantation. He may be apprehensive because of the symptoms he is experiencing, such as dizziness and fainting, and may also be fearful of the procedure and his dependence on a mechanical device. When explaining the need for a pacemaker the physician reviews the procedure with the patient. The nurse reinforces this explanation and answers any further questions before having him sign the consent. Explanations are also given to the family.

The patient receives a sedative before the implantation. Temporary pacemakers are usually implanted under local anesthetic in a

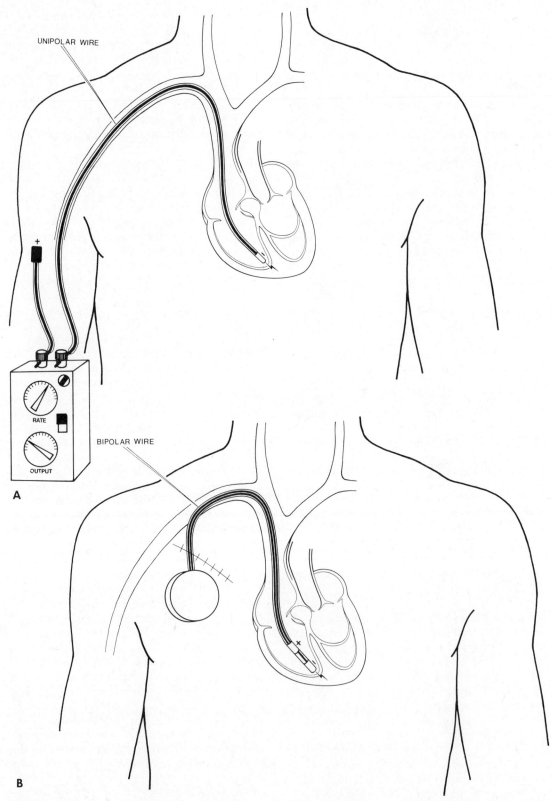

FIGURE 13–13 *A,* Temporary electronic pacemaker. *B,* Permanent electronic pacemaker. *C,* Pacemaker for synchronous pacing.

Illustration continued on the opposite page

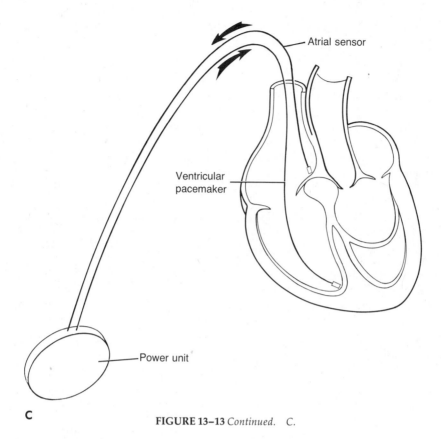

Atrial sensor

Ventricular
pacemaker

Power unit

C

FIGURE 13–13 *Continued.   C.*

heart catheterization laboratory, in the radiology department or occasionally, in an emergency, at the bedside. Permanent pacemakers are inserted in the operating room.

Following the implantation of a permanent pacemaker, the patient is monitored continuously until it has been established that the pacemaker is functioning properly. Bed rest is indicated for the remainder of the day. If a temporary pacemaker has been inserted ambulation is delayed, depending upon the site of insertion as well as the patient's general condition. Cardiac monitoring is continued as long as the temporary pacemaker is being used.

The nurse is responsible for monitoring and reporting the patient's rhythm, for checking the operative site and cleansing the wound as necessary, for assessing and reporting any complications and for supporting the patient and providing him with information as needed.

Complications include mechanical malfunction of the pacemaker, perforation of the myocardial wall by an electrode, breakage or dislodgement of the electrodes, thrombus formation, and infection, such as phlebitis, endocarditis or septicemia. Mechanical malfunctions may occur because the pacemaker fails to fire, fires too rapidly or fires erratically. Malfunctioning may be detected by cardiac monitoring or by an electrocardiogram, as well as by the presence of certain physical signs and symptoms, such as decreased pulse rate, dizziness and/or fainting.

Following perforation of the myocardium blood seeps into the pericardium, causing cardiac tamponade. The resulting compression of the heart causes low blood pressure, tachycardia, increased central venous pressure and distended neck veins. The electrode may also stimulate innervation to the upper abdominal or lower chest muscles, resulting in spasm. Breakage or dislodgement of the electrode will result in a change in the shape of the QRS complex and in the heart rate.

The nurse is also alert to electrical hazards in the environment. Electrical equipment in the patient's environment must be properly grounded and the external pulse generator of temporary pacemakers must be kept dry.

Caution regarding electrical hazards includes avoiding close contact with large electrical motors; for example, in a machine shop the patient may develop arrhythmias as a result of the electrical interference. Microwave ovens may cause similar interference with some pacemakers. Small home appliances, if properly grounded, produce no untoward effects. Contact sports are avoided, although other sports might be allowed on the physician's advice. The patient's dentist should be advised that he is wearing a pacemaker before any electrical equipment is used.

The amount of information given to the patient depends upon his interest and capacity for learning. Certain points are reviewed with him and a member of his family. Basic information is given on the functioning of the heart, the way in which the pacemaker works, activities allowed, battery changes, and precautions regarding electrical hazards. A follow-up appointment is made for the patient to visit the pacemaker clinic or the physician's office, and it is stressed to the patient that regular checkups are necessary.

The patient should carry an identification card indicating the type of pacemaker he is wearing and the physician to be notified in case of difficulty. Before travelling he should obtain the name of a local physician or clinic in case of an emergency.

DRUGS USED IN CARDIAC ARRHYTHMIAS. Drugs commonly used (Table 13–6) include:

DIGITALIS. This drug is used to strengthen and slow the myocardial contraction without increasing oxygen utilization by the myocardium, thereby increasing cardiac output.

TABLE 13–6 DRUGS USED IN CARDIAC ARRHYTHMIAS AND FAILURE

Drug	Action	Clinical Uses	Toxic Effects
Cardiac Glycosides			
Digoxin	Increases force of contraction without significantly increasing oxygen utilization; decreases conduction through the A-V node; increases vagal stimulation	Congestive heart failure; atrial arrhythmias (e.g., fibrillation)	Anorexia; nausea and/or vomiting; diarrhea; blurred or colored vision; arrhythmias (e.g., junctional rhythms and blocks)
Digitoxin	As above		
Ouabain	As above		
Antiarrhythmic Drugs			
Quinidine sulfate	Decreases automaticity; slows conduction; acts as a vasodilator; decreases contractility	Paroxysmal atrial tachycardia; atrial flutter and fibrillation; premature ventricular contractions	Nausea and/or vomiting; Diarrhea; Visual disturbances; Arrhythmias, e.g., ventricular tachy-arrhythmias and A-V block
Quinidine polygalacturonate (Cardioquin)	As above		
Procainamide (Pronestyl)	Similar to quinidine	More useful in ventricular than atrial arrhythmias	Gastrointestinal symptoms; lupus erythematosus syndrome
Lidocaine (Xylocaine)	Depresses ventricular ectopic foci	Premature ventricular contractions	Central nervous system disturbances (e.g., convulsions).
Dysopyramide (Norpace)	Similar to quinidine	Ventricular arrhythmias	Dry mouth, urinary hesitancy, constipation, blurred vision

It slows the pulse rate by depressing the A-V conduction and by increasing vagal nerve stimulation. The resulting fewer contractions give the heart muscle time to rest and recover.

A secondary action is diuresis. As it improves circulation, the urinary output increases and helps to reduce edema, if present.

There are many preparations of digitalis; digitalis, digitalin, digitoxin, digoxin and digifolin are a few. There are preparations for intravenous and oral administration. A large dose may be prescribed for the first 2 to 3 days in order to achieve a therapeutic concentration of the drug in the blood; this is referred to as digitalization. The dosage is then reduced to a smaller maintenance dose.

Nursing responsibilities in administering digitalis preparations include assessing and reporting changes in physical signs and symptoms, such as less dyspnea and decreased fatigue. Observations are also made for signs of toxicity such as anorexia, nausea and vomiting, diarrhea, abdominal discomfort and visual disturbances. The cardiovascular signs of toxicity are extreme slowing of the pulse and/or a sudden change in rhythm. Patients with hypokalemia are predisposed to cardiac arrhythmias when receiving digitalis.

The radial pulse is taken before each dose. If it has slowed considerably the apical pulse is checked. If the apical pulse is also very slow the physician is consulted before giving the drug. A rate below 60 is usually given as the point at which to notify the physician, but some patients may have a rate as low as 50 without toxicity. Specific arrhythmias cannot be determined without an electrocardiogram and one should be obtained if there is concern.

Digitalis should be given at the same time every day. Occasionally, serum digitalis levels are determined for patients who become toxic or who do not show a therapeutic response with normal dosage. In these situations the serum levels help the physician to decide whether to increase or decrease the dosage.

Digitalis should not be given intramuscularly because it causes intense local pain and because of unpredictable and erratic absorption from this site. Parenteral preparations should not be added to intravenous fluids since precipitation of the drug may occur. Patients are instructed to take their drug every day at the same time and not to miss doses.

QUINIDINE SULFATE. This drug is most frequently prescribed in the treatment of atrial flutter or fibrillation, recurrent paroxysmal atrial tachycardia and ventricular ectopic beats. It slows the rate by decreasing automaticity and conduction at the S-A node and ectopic pacemakers. It also depresses the excitability of both atrial and ventricular myocardium and has vasodilator effects, which may result in hypotension.

The drug is administered by mouth and radial and apical pulses are taken before each dose. The blood pressure should also be checked. Reactions to the drug may include nausea, vomiting, diarrhea, tinnitus, headache, visual disturbances and fever. Cardiovascular abnormalities include heart block and ventricular rhythm disorders (e.g., ventricular fibrillation). A patient may have an idiosyncrasy to the drug and the nurse is required to observe him closely for any toxic effects. Oral membranes are inspected frequently for signs of petechial hemorrhages which may indicate thrombocytopenic purpura.

DISOPYRAMIDE (NORPACE, RHYTHMODAN). This agent has no chemical similarities to other existing antiarrhythmic agents but it resembles quinidine in its activity. It is as effective as quinidine and procainamide in controlling certain arrhythmias and is generally better tolerated. The most common side effects of disopyramide are primarily related to its anticholinergic action. These include dry mouth, urinary hesitancy, constipation, and blurred vision. The usual dose is 100 to 200 mg. every 6 hours.

PROCAINAMIDE HYDROCHLORIDE (PRONESTYL). This drug has a similar action to quinidine. It was originally used for both atrial and ventricular arrhythmias but is more useful for ventricular disorders. It may be given intravenously, intramuscularly or orally. Because of the short half-life of the drug, it is usually given at frequent intervals — for example, every 3 to 4 hours. The blood pressure is checked during intravenous administration and the patient is observed closely for any indication of hypersensitivity. This may be manifested by a chill, joint pain, itching, weakness, dizziness or gastrointestinal disturbances. Norepinephrine and epinephrine are readily available in the event of a reaction.

Patients on moderate to large doses of procainamide over a long term frequently develop a lupus-like syndrome, with muscle pain and arthralgic-type symptoms. This usually disappears after a period of time when the drug is discontinued.

LIDOCAINE HYDROCHLORIDE (XYLOCAINE). This preparation is commonly used to decrease premature ventricular contractions which frequently precede ventricular fibrillation. It depresses the rate of impulse discharge and conduction. Lidocaine is ad-

ministered intravenously. An initial dose of 50 to 100 mg. by direct intravenous injection may be given followed by an intravenous infusion at the rate of 1 to 4 mg. per minute.

The drug acts rapidly within a matter of 2 to 4 minutes. The patient is observed closely for possible hypotension and the heart action is checked by monitor. It is kept readily available for use following a myocardial infarction, during a cardiac catheterization and following cardiac surgery.

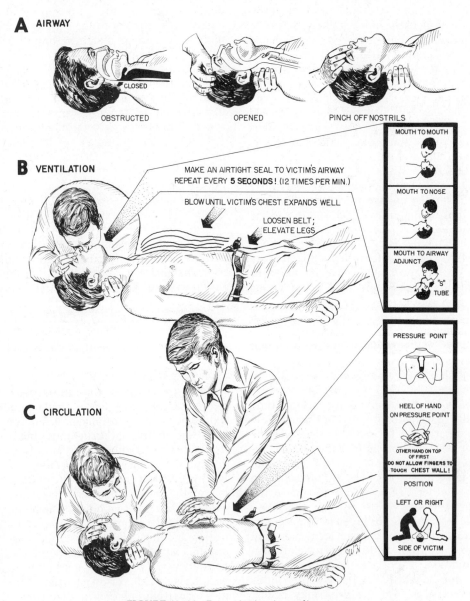

FIGURE 13–14 Resuscitation in cardiac arrest.

Cardiac Arrest

Cardiac standstill or arrest means the sudden cessation of effective ventricular contraction. It includes ventricular fibrillation and ventricular asystole. Possible causes are myocardial ischemia, respiratory insufficiency, heart block, electric shock, metabolic acidosis and adverse reactions to an anesthetic or a drug.

The condition must be recognized as an emergency. It is urgent that circulation be sufficiently reestablished to deliver oxygen to the brain within 4 minutes to prevent permanent cerebral damage. Cardiac arrest may be manifested by sudden collapse and loss of consciousness, an absence of pulse in the radial, carotid and femoral arteries, apnea and dilatation of the pupils.

Cardiopulmonary resuscitation (CPR) must be commenced at once. This comprises external cardiac massage and artificial respiration (Fig. 13–14).

External Cardiac Massage

External cardiac massage consists of the intermittent application of vertical pressure over the lower third of the sternum. The pressure stroke compresses the heart between the sternum and the spine and empties the ventricles. To be effective, the compression must force a volume of blood into the arteries sufficient to produce pulsation in the carotid and femoral arteries. The pressure should depress the sternum 1 to 2 inches and is exerted about once a second. The thoracic cage is quite flexible in an unconscious person, and thus the possibility of injury to the ribs is reduced. Relief of the pressure allows the heart to refill. This technique of resuscitation is simple, requires no special equipment and may be done anywhere.

Artificial Respirations (Mouth-to-Mouth)

Since cardiac arrest causes respiratory failure, artificial respirations must accompany cardiac massage; otherwise, the persisting oxygen deficiency to the cardiac muscle will prevent its response and increase the possibility of cerebral damage.

The most important factor for successful resuscitation is immediate opening of the air-way. This can be accomplished easily and quickly by tilting the victim's head backward as far as possible. The mouth-to-mouth method of artificial respiration is the one of choice unless the victim is in a situation where a self-inflating (Ambu) bag is available. If a second person is not available to perform the respiratory resuscitation efforts, cardiac massage is interrupted every 15 pressure strokes to ventilate the victim's lungs twice. In a hospital, mouth-to-mouth respirations may be replaced by an intermittent positive pressure respirator which will deliver a higher concentration of oxygen.

Once cardiopulmonary resuscitation has begun, diagnosis and definitive therapy are attempted. One member of the team attaches electrodes to the patient and continuous cardiac monitoring is begun to determine the underlying cardiac rhythm. Another member of the team inserts an intravenous line for the infusion of medications. If ventricular fibrillation has caused the arrest, an electric defibrillator is used whereby an electric current is delivered through electrodes into the chest wall.

Since metabolic acidosis rapidly develops, Hurst advises that "an immediate injection of 44 mEq./L. of sodium bicarbonate (HCO_3^-) is given and repeated at 10-minute intervals as long as resuscitation efforts are continued."[23] Arterial blood is withdrawn for blood gas analysis; the carbon dioxide level serves as a guide for the sodium bicarbonate administration. Other emergency drugs are given as required.

Every institution has written policies governing the responsibilities of medical and nursing personnel and members of the Cardiac Arrest team. The nurse should review and be aware of which responsibilities and procedures she is expected to assume, and those for which she is not legally responsible.

Care Following Resuscitation

The patient who has been resuscitated requires constant observation of the vital signs. If possible, he is transferred to an Intensive Care Unit and continuous monitoring of heart action is established. A pacemaker may be applied which will deliver a stimulus

[23]Marvin M. McCall, III: "Cardiopulmonary Resuscitation." In J. Willis Hurst, et al.: The Heart, 3rd ed. New York, McGraw-Hill, 1978.

CARDIOPULMONARY RESUSCITATION[22]

Cardiopulmonary resuscitation is an emergency first aid measure, and must proceed in an organized manner. It includes assessing the need for both artificial ventilation and artificial circulation. The steps which should be started and the order in which they should be performed are:
1. Establishing an open airway
2. Initiating artificial ventilation
3. Initiating external cardiac massage

Steps in Artificial Ventilation

1. The mouth is cleared of any foreign matter.
2. The head is hyperextended, the lower jaw held forward and the nostrils pinched.
3. The operator takes a large breath, places his mouth tightly over the patient's mouth and blows out his breath to inflate the patient's lungs. In the case of a small child, the operator's mouth is placed over the mouth and nose. If effective, the chest will rise with each blowing.
4. The operator removes his mouth. Air should be heard escaping from the patient's lungs, and the chest should fall.
5. The procedure is repeated approximately 12 times per minute.
6. If the patient's chest does not rise with the first respiration, the position of the head, neck, and lower jaw are checked again to ensure an open airway. If air still does not enter the patient's lungs, check the mouth for mucus and turn him to one side. Several sharp blows with the heel of the hand are then struck between the shoulder blades to dislodge a mucus plug or foreign substance which may be blocking the airway.
7. The artificial respirations and the pressure strokes of the cardiac massage must be coordinated. About one respiration to five pressure strokes is given, and the blowing in of air must occur during the release of sternal pressure. When there is only one rescuer, two respirations are given after every 15 pressure strokes.

Steps in External Cardiac Massage

1. Someone is dispatched for the necessary medical assistance and equipment.
2. The victim is placed on his back on a firm surface, such as the floor or ground. In the case of a bed patient, a board is placed under the patient. Each hospital ward is usually equipped with an "emergency board" that is easily handled and may be quickly placed under the upper half of the patient's trunk.
3. The operator places the heel of one hand over the lower one-half of the sternum and the heel of the other hand over the first hand. The hands should not be placed over the lower tip of the sternum (the xiphoid process). Pressure is applied vertically downward, depressing the sternum 1 to 2 inches about once each second. The pressure should be sufficient to produce a carotid and femoral pulse, which may be checked by a second person. Less pressure is required in cardiac massage for children up to 10 to 12 years, since the thoracic cage is very flexible. The pressure delivered by the heel of one hand is sufficient. In infants, the pressure is exerted by the fingers of one hand.
4. At the end of each pressure stroke, the hands are completely relaxed but kept in position.
5. Mouth-to-mouth respirations are started as soon as possible if assistance is at hand. If the person doing the cardiac massage is alone he initially gives four quick ventilations and then interrupts the massage approximately every 15 pressure strokes (every 15 seconds) to give two artificial respirations.
6. The massage is continued until heart action resumes and is producing a strong peripheral pulse or until some other form of treatment is instituted. As circulation is restored, spontaneous respirations and constriction of the pupils should occur.

---

[22]Canadian Heart Foundation: Cardiopulmonary Resuscitation (CPR). Part I, Recommended Standards for Basic Life Support. Aug. 1976.

to the heart in the event of recurring asystole. Peripheral pulses are checked for volume, rhythm and rate.

Respirations and blood pressure are noted and recorded at frequent intervals (every 15 minutes); the temperature is checked hourly. The defibrillator and mechanical respirator are kept nearby and ready for immediate use.

The patient will be very apprehensive. He is advised of improvement in his condition and of the importance of rest and minimal emotional stress, and is assured that someone will either be with him or close by so that treatment may be quickly instituted should he need it.

Heart Failure or Decompensation

The ability of the heart to dilate and hypertrophy to compensate for an abnormal condition is limited. Excessive dilatation overstretches the muscle fibers to the point of injury; increasing hypertrophy creates a need for a corresponding increase in oxygen and nutrients, but there is no proportional increase in the coronary blood supply.

Prolonged strain, progressive disease and demands exceeding the individual's cardiac compensation are likely to lead to a reduced cardiac output that will not meet the needs of the body. The heart is then said to be *decompensated or in failure*. Heart failure may be designated as left-sided or right-sided heart failure, acute or chronic failure, or congestive heart failure.

Failure of the heart to forward the volume of blood it receives is usually confined to one side of the heart, although the other side may later fail as a result of the primary failure. The side affected is determined by the site of the causative lesion. If the *left side of the heart* cannot forward the blood offered to it, blood is backed up in the pulmonary circulatory system. The vessels become engorged and fluid escapes into the alveoli, producing acute pulmonary edema manifested by dyspnea and cough. In severe failure of the left side of the heart, more blood is pumped into the pulmonary system than the left side of the heart can receive and forward. The vessels become congested, and the alveoli gradually fill with serous fluid and blood. Unless this is checked the respiratory exchange is cut off and the patient literally drowns in his own secretions.

This may be referred to as acute pulmonary edema. Left cardiac failure precipitates an emergency which demands prompt action. Efforts are made to reduce the venous return to the heart and, at the same time, strengthen the heart in order to increase the output from the left side.

Right-sided failure may be secondary to that of the left side, or it may occur independently. If the right heart chambers cannot forward the blood being returned to the heart by the venae cavae, the system becomes congested and edema develops in the tissues and organs.

Acute cardiac failure occurs suddenly and is considered a more serious threat to the patient's life. Chronic heart failure develops gradually and may only appear when the patient increases his activities and energy expenditure.

The term congestive is applied to cardiac failure to describe the condition in the circulatory system behind the failure. It implies an excessive accumulation of blood in the system because the heart cannot accept and forward it.

Specific precipitating causes of heart failure include myocardial infarction, systemic hypertension, pulmonary emboli, cardiac arrhythmias, anemia, chronic obstructive pulmonary disease, thyrotoxicosis and pregnancy with underlying heart disease.

Nursing Care in Heart Failure

Nursing care in heart failure is directed towards: (1) assessment, by observing, recording and reporting significant signs, symptoms and patient reactions; (2) improving cardiac output; (3) improving the oxygenation of the tissues; (4) reducing excess fluid accumulation; (5) reducing energy demands on the body, thus minimizing the work of the heart and providing comfort; and (6) helping the patient to live within his cardiac capacity.

Assessment

RESPIRATIONS. Dyspnea is the most common symptom of heart failure. Pulmonary edema impairs gas exchange and may induce hypoxia. In mild or early failure, dyspnea may only be experienced with exertion. With severe heart failure, it is present at rest. With acute pulmonary edema, it is severe. The respirations are checked every ½ to 1 hour in acute failure and every 4 hours in moderate or mild failure. With breathlessness related to activity, the degree of exertion is noted. The lungs are auscultated for the presence of rales or rhonchi. This is done frequently by the physician and in some instances is done by the nurse.

PULSE. The pulse may be rapid, weak and irregular, as tachycardia frequently accompanies severe heart failure. The strength, rate and rhythm of the pulse are noted frequently and in relation to activities.

COUGH. Due to congestion and fluid in the alveoli and bronchial tubes, cough may be present. The frequency, characteristics and amount of sputum are noted. Frothy, colorless sputum occurs in pulmonary edema, and blood may appear from the rupture of capillaries and arterioles in severe congestion.

COLOR. The color of the lips, nail beds and skin is observed frequently, and any changes noted. There may be cyanosis of lips and nail beds. The skin may show pallor due to generalized vasoconstriction.

BLOOD PRESSURE. The blood pressure is checked frequently since it reflects the cardiac output.

BODY TEMPERATURE. Many patients with cardiac insufficiency register a subnormal temperature, since their heat production is reduced because of inadequate circulation, deficiency in oxygen and resulting decrease in metabolism.

GENERALIZED EDEMA. Failure of the right side of the heart causes fluid to accumulate in the systemic venous circulation. The reduced venous return to the heart leads to a reduction in left ventricle output and compensatory mechanisms occur in an attempt to maintain adequate perfusion of vital organs. This causes further retention of fluid. Systemic venous and capillary pressures are raised due to the inability of the heart to receive the blood. Fluid escapes from the vascular system into the interstitial tissues, resulting in edema.

One looks for edema in the dependent areas of the body. If the person is ambulatory, swelling first appears in the feet and ankles, but, if he is confined to bed, edema may first become apparent in the back and sacral region. As it becomes more severe all body tissues become affected, and even ascites and hydrothorax may develop. The latter further embarrass the patient's breathing.

The most accurate method of observing the patient for edema is by weighing him daily if his condition makes this possible. He should be weighed at the same time each day with the same weight of clothes. Before edema becomes apparent, 10 to 15 pounds of water may be retained.

FLUID BALANCE. An accurate record is kept of the patient's fluid intake and output. A positive balance is brought to the attention of the physician, particularly if the urinary output is decreased to 20 to 25 ml. per hour. The amount of diaphoresis is noted, as a large amount of fluid may be lost in this manner.

FATIGUE. The degree of fatigue is noted at rest as well as in relationship to specific activities.

ORIENTATION AND LEVEL OF CONSCIOUSNESS. When circulation and/or the oxygen content of the blood perfusing the brain is inadequate, the patient's cerebral functioning may decrease. Observations are made as to the patient's level of consciousness, his orientation to person, time and surroundings, and his response to stimuli such as questioning.

ANXIETY. It is very important to observe the patient for fear and apprehension. Anxiety may initiate the release of epinephrine which increases the demands on the heart. The patient's apprehension may indicate a need for information, explanations or sedation.

ANOREXIA. The patient may not eat because of lack of strength to feed himself or because of dietary restrictions which make meals unpalatable. Congestion of internal organs due to edema may contribute to loss of appetite. Anorexia may also result from drug toxicity (e.g., digitalis). The amount and type of food the patient eats is observed at every meal.

CHEST OR ABDOMINAL PAIN. Chest pain and any apparent precipitating causes are observed and reported immediately. Abdominal pain may be due to the congestion and poor perfusion of internal organs. Abdominal distention may be associated with reduced peristalsis as a result of congestion and reduced blood supply.

IMPROVING CARDIAC OUTPUT. Heart contractility is improved by pharmacological agents ordered by the physician. The nurse is responsible for administering them and observing their effects and possible side effects. The drugs commonly used are cardiac glycosides (see p. 328).

OXYGENATION OF THE TISSUES. Oxygen may be administered by mask or catheter to increase arterial oxygen concentration. It will only be effective if delivery to the tissues is improved.

The nurse explains the procedure to the patient briefly and remains with him until he is accustomed to the nasal catheter, cannulae or mask. Observations are made of the patient's response to the oxygen. Its effectiveness will be indicated by reduced pulse rate, less dyspnea, improvement in color and less restlessness. (For details of administration of oxygen see p. 408.)

In severe pulmonary edema, the physician may administer oxygen under positive pressure to counteract the movement of fluid from the capillaries into the alveoli.

REDUCING EXCESS FLUID ACCUMULATION. Measures directed toward reducing the edema associated with cardiac failure include tourniquet, phlebotomy, drugs and therapeutic diet. The selection of measures is dictated by the severity and location of the edema. In the case of sudden left-sided cardiac failure, acute pulmonary edema develops quickly. Prompt treatment is necessary to save the patient's life. The nurse, advised that such a patient is to be admitted, quickly assembles the necessary equipment and medications for treatment so there will be no delay.

The patient with severe pulmonary edema is naturally very fearful, which further aggravates the primary condition. The physician will probably administer morphine intravenously to reduce pulmonary artery pressure and to provide sedation, digitalis to strengthen myocardial contractions, and a diuretic intravenously to decrease circulating blood volume further. Additional efforts to reduce venous return may be made by the application of tourniquets and a phlebotomy.

Generalized edema generally develops gradually and is usually associated with right-sided failure.

Measures used to reduce edema include tourniquets, phlebotomy, diuretic drugs, and special diet.

TOURNIQUETS. A reduction in venous return to the heart may be achieved by rotating application of tourniquets. Three tourniquets are necessary; one is applied to the upper part of three extremities with just enough pressure to interfere with superficial venous circulation. One tourniquet is moved to the free limb every 10 to 15 minutes and a definite pattern, either clockwise or counterclockwise, is established (see Fig. 13-15). The physician will indicate the period between moves and how long the tourniquet procedure is to be used. Too long a period of venous compression may produce the risk of phlebothrombosis and embolism.

PHLEBOTOMY. The second emergency measure that may be used to reduce venous return and total blood volume is phlebotomy. The physician withdraws 250 to 700 ml. of blood from a vein. A blood donor set is quickly made available for this procedure, and the blood may be donated to the blood bank.

DRUGS TO PRODUCE DIURESIS. There are various groups of diuretics which act directly on the kidneys and are administered orally and/or parenterally. They increase the rate of urine formation and indirectly cause the removal of fluid from the tissues. Commonly used diuretics include the following (see Table 13-7):

Thiazides. The thiazide diuretics are the most widely used because of their effectiveness and the fact that they may be administered orally and are well tolerated. This group of drugs inhibits the reabsorption of sodium and chloride ions, and therefore water, by the distal renal tubules. Potassium depletion also occurs and potassium supplements are usually given. Hypokalemia is particularly important in patients taking digoxin because a low potassium level can predispose a patient to digitalis toxicity. Other complications associated with thiazide therapy include hyperglycemia, hyperuricemia and rarely cholestatic hepatitis and hypersensitivity. Preparations currently in use include chlorothiazide (Diuril) and hydrochlorothiazide (hydro-Diuril).

Furosemide (Lasix). This sulfonamide derivative inhibits sodium reabsorption, especially in the ascending loop of Henle. It acts quickly, producing diuresis in ½ to 1 hour following oral administration. It is approximately five times more potent than hydrochlorothiazide. For patients in acute pulmonary edema it is administered intravenously. The rate of intravenous administration should not exceed 5 mg. per minute, since rapid

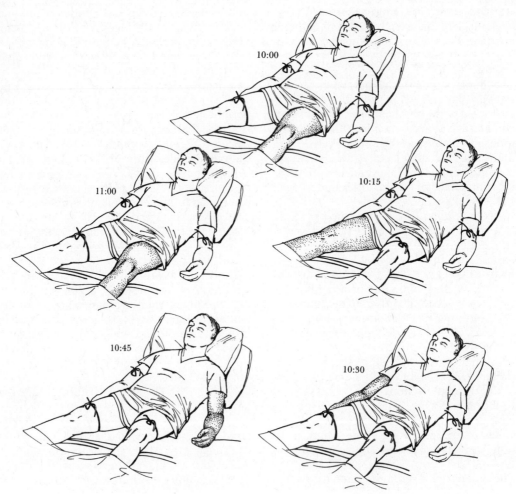

FIGURE 13–15 Rotation of tourniquets at 15-minute intervals.

intravenous administration may result in deafness. Because the low pH of dextrose solutions may cause precipitation of furosemide, every effort should be made to dilute it in normal saline. A close check is kept on serum electrolyte levels. Furosemide is often ordered for patients with severe heart failure who might be refractory to the thiazide diuretics.

Ethacrynic Acid (Edecrin). This is a very potent diuretic which inhibits sodium reabsorption at the ascending loop of Henle. It is well absorbed when administered orally and may also be given intravenously. With the intravenous route extravasation should be avoided, as it is very irritating to the superficial tissues. It should not be given intramuscularly. Serum electrolyte levels are monitored closely as chloride, potassium and

hydrogen ions are also excreted. Because of its powerful effect the patient may become hypovolemic. Ethacrynic acid and furosemide are the agents of choice for patients with severe heart failure refractory to thiazides.

Mercurial Diuretics. The potency and effectiveness of furosemide when given orally and its relatively low incidence of side effects has resulted in the virtual abandonment of the use of the mercurial preparations. They may occasionally be ordered.

Thiomerin and Mercuhydrin require parenteral administration because they are poorly tolerated and absorbed when taken orally. They act to depress sodium reabsorption beyond the proximal tubules of the kidneys. Their administration may result in metabolic alkalosis but potassium loss is less than with

TABLE 13–7   DIURETICS

Name	Action	Onset of Action	Length of Action	Possible Side Effects
Chlorothiazide (Diuril)	Inhibits sodium and chloride and therefore water reabsorption by the distal renal tubules	Within 2 hours	6 to 12 hours	Hypokalemia; hyperuricemia; hyperglycemia; skin rashes
Hydro-chlorothiazide (Hydro-diuril)	As above	As above	As above	As above
Furosemide (Lasix)	Inhibits sodium and chloride reabsorption; acts primarily at ascending loop of Henle	½ to 1 hour	6 to 8 hours	Hypokalemia; hyponatremia; hypovolemia
Ethacrynic acid (Edecrin)	As above	1 hour	6 to 8 hours	hypokalemia; hyponatremia; hypovolemia; skin rash; granulocytopenia
Mercuhydrin; Thiomerin	Reduce sodium reabsorption in distal tubule	1 to 2 hours	3 to 20 hours	Dermatitis; flushing; nausea and vomiting
Spironolactone (Aldactone A)	Aldosterone antagonist in distal renal tubule	24 to 48 hours	2 to 3 days	Hyperkalemia; gastrointestinal upsets; gynecomastia; drowsiness
Triamterene (Dyrenium)	Blocks sodium reabsorption and potassium excretion at distal exchange sites	24 hours	Several days	Hyperkalemia; gastrointestinal upset; megaloblastic anemia

other diuretics. They act quickly within 1 to 2 hours, but excretion of the drug begins in 3 hours.

Spironolactone (Aldactone A). This diuretic acts by inhibiting the action of aldosterone; this is secreted by the cortex of the adrenal glands and promotes the absorption of sodium ions and water by the kidney tubules and the excretion of potassium. By inhibiting the action of aldosterone, spironolactone promotes the excretion of sodium and water and the retention of potassium. Hyperkalemia may result if spironolactone is administered concomitantly with potassium supplements, or it may occur in patients with uremia. Occasionally gynecomastia (enlargement of the mammary glands in the male) may develop. Spironolactone is most effective when administered with thiazide diuretics. It is contraindicated (unless administered with other diuretics) for patients with hyperkalemia. It has a slow onset of action and does not reach peak effectiveness for 2 to 3 days.

Triamterene (Dyremium). This drug acts directly on the kidney tubule to cause sodium excretion and potassium retention but, unlike spironolactone, its effect is independent of that of aldosterone. Diuresis may occur within 24 hours but maximum effect may not be seen for several days. Side effects include gastrointestinal upsets, headache, hyperkalemia and megaloblastic anemia.

NUTRITION AND FLUIDS. Modifications in the diet for patients with heart failure are based first on their retention of an excess of sodium which causes the formation of edema, and secondly on the knowledge that overeating and overweight increase the work load of the heart.

Low-sodium diets are prescribed to reduce

edema and to prevent further accumulation of fluid in the tissues. The sodium restriction varies with patients, depending upon their heart efficiency and amount of edema. Normally the average daily salt intake is 10 to 12 Gm. If no salt is added to food either at the table or in cooking and no salted foods are used, the intake may be reduced to approximately 3 Gm. In congestive heart failure more stringent restrictions are sometimes necessary, and foods are selected that will provide still less sodium. Diets that contain as low as 0.25 Gm. can be prepared.

Low-sodium diets are unpalatable, and the patient finds it difficult to adhere to the prescribed restriction. Frequently the result is that he does not take sufficient food to meet his nutritional needs. The nurse explains the purpose of the diet and relates it to symptoms the patient is experiencing. There are many spices and foods allowable that help to make a low-sodium diet more palatable. In prolonged, severe restriction of sodium, the patient may develop a sodium deficiency. The physician is informed of any complaints of muscular cramps and weakness.

Hurst and Logue suggest that with the advent of the newer and more potent diuretic drugs, severe dietary sodium restriction is not as mandatory as previously for the average patient with heart failure.[24] Obviously salty foods, however, should be avoided, as well as extra salt at the table.

Braunwald suggests that the normal daily salt intake may be reduced by half by eliminating salt-rich foods and salt added at the table.[25] This reduction would be required for the patient with mild or moderate heart failure. Omitting all salt from cooking reduces salt intake to one-fourth of the normal. Even further reductions to between 500 and 1000 mg. may be obtained for the patient in severe heart failure by eliminating milk, cheese, bread, cereals, canned vegetables and soups, some salted cuts of meat and fresh vegetables such as spinach, celery and beets that have a high sodium content.

If the patient with heart failure is overweight, the caloric intake is reduced in an effort to reduce the weight to normal. A maintenance diet is then prescribed. The lower-calorie diet should contain less fat but enough of the other food principles to meet nutritional requirements.

REDUCING ENERGY DEMANDS ON THE HEART

REST. Rest is important in the treatment of the patient with heart failure since it reduces the demand on the heart by reducing body requirements for oxygen. For the patient in failure, rest in bed is necessary until the edema is decreased. The physician's order may read "complete (or absolute) bed rest" or simply "bed rest." These usually mean something different, and the nurse determines exactly what is meant by each in the particular situation. Generally, "complete bed rest" is interpreted as absolute minimal activity on the patient's part, with the nurse doing everything possible for him. He is fed, bathed, turned, and assisted on and off the bedpan; his teeth are cleaned and his hair combed. "Bed rest" usually means that the patient may participate to some degree in his personal care, and the nurse observes the effects of such activities on the patient. If they produce shortness of breath, an increase in pulse rate and excessive fatigue, his activities are reduced.

Once the acute episode has passed the patient is allowed out of bed for gradually increasing intervals. Intermittent rest periods during the day and following activities are arranged, and the patient rests before and after meals and between procedures.

PSYCHOLOGICAL SUPPORT. Mental rest is as important as physical rest, but is often difficult to promote. The common knowledge that the heart is a most vital organ and that heart disease is a frequent cause of death produces a greater emotional reaction in the person advised of a diagnosis of a heart failure. He becomes fearful and apprehensive: his life, his job, his family's security and his whole future are threatened. Rarely does any other condition, even though it may be an equally severe threat, engender as much fear and concern. Frequently the anxiety reaction may be completely out of proportion to the actual threat. Emotional reactions increase respirations and the work load of the heart. A patient may appear to be at rest but is actually in mental turmoil. The sensitive, observant

[24]J. Willis Hurst and R. Bruce Logue (Eds.): The Heart, Arteries and Veins, 3rd ed. New York, McGraw-Hill, 1974.

[25]Eugene Braunwald: "Heart Failure." in George W. Thorn, et al.: Harrison's Principles of Internal Medicine, 8th ed. New York, McGraw-Hill, 1977.

nurse who understands the possible implications that illness has for this patient is likely to detect his mental unrest and endeavors to promote the peace of mind essential to optimum rest.

The nurse who understands the patient's condition, knows what to look for, and knows what to do usually displays calm and composure which contribute to the patient's confidence and security. A quiet, controlled atmosphere does more toward allaying fear than verbal reassurance.

It is helpful to have someone remain with the anxious patient; alone, he may panic, thinking he is cut off from help. If a nurse is not available, the presence of an auxiliary worker or a member of the family will provide some reassurance. Emotionally disturbed relatives should not be permitted to visit or remain with the patient unless they can conceal their feelings and control their reactions.

There may be a problem at home that contributes to the patient's unrest. Some solution may be suggested or arrangements made for assistance from a social service agency. The nurse encourages the patient to express his anxieties and tries to identify his feelings and his problems as he sees them. Frequently, verbal expression of concerns may reduce their proportions; having shared them, he now has the support of someone who knows his problems. It may be necessary with some patients to seek the assistance of the physician or the patient's religious adviser to deal with questions or expressions of fear.

In the interest of providing optimum rest for the patient, consideration is given to placement on the ward. He is not located next to disturbing persons and will most likely feel more secure if he is close to the nursing station. A light left burning at night may contribute to a feeling of security, as well as make it easier for the nurse to make frequent, reassuring visits and the necessary observations. If his degree of activity permits, reading or listening to the radio may provide diversion and relaxation.

There is no specific formula for dealing with the cardiac patient's anxiety in order to provide the much needed rest. The nurse must be alert to the problem and work at it; that which proves successful with one patient will not be the answer for all.

Physical comfort will contribute to the patient's rest and may be promoted by change of position, back rub, bathing, warmth, etc. Anticipation of need and the planning and provision of undisturbed rest periods are important. Cooperation is sought from the laboratory, dietary and housekeeping staffs to control the interruptions. A sedative may be prescribed to reduce anxiety and restlessness, and the nurse provides the necessary attention to ensure maximum benefits from the drug.

ACTIVITY. Rest has been emphasized as an important phase of the treatment of cardiac patients, but it is well known that there are certain disadvantages inherent in bed rest. The limbs should be put through passive movements to promote venous drainage and prevent phlebothrombosis. Gentle massage will also be helpful. If the patient's condition permits, the physician will have him gradually commence foot, leg and arm exercises. The patient is also encouraged to take five to ten deep breaths every 1 to 2 hours. As soon as possible he is allowed to get out of bed to use a commode, since the use of a bedpan for defecation places considerable strain on the patient.

Observations are made of reactions to any activity so that undue stress on the heart may be avoided. These will also assist the physician in defining the patient's future activities and the amount of rest and restriction that will be necessary.

POSITIONING. The position the patient with heart failure finds most comfortable in bed is determined by his breathing. The patient who is experiencing dyspnea will be more comfortable with the head of the bed elevated, but the height of elevation should only be that at which the dyspnea is minimal.

Patients with congestive failure manifest orthopnea — that is, less difficulty in breathing with the trunk in the upright position. Semi- or high Fowler's position increases the vital capacity and tends to reduce the volume of blood returned to the heart and to the pulmonary system. Pressure of abdominal viscera on the diaphragm is reduced. Some patients may be still more comfortable in a true sitting position — that is, with the lower limbs down. A special cardiac bed on which the foot of the bed can be lowered to provide a chair-like support is available. The sitting position promotes the formation of peripheral edema in the dependent parts but relieves the pulmonary congestion to some extent; peripheral edema is much less serious than pulmonary edema.

In the sitting position a pillow placed longitudinally at the patient's back may help provide some comfort. Pillows should be used at the sides to support the arms and relieve the fatiguing pull on the shoulders. A change may be effected by arranging a table and pillow over the bed in front of him, upon which he may rest his head and arms. Side rails are kept up on the bed to safeguard the patient when he is in the upright position, since he may become drowsy and fall to the side, or may experience cerebral hypoxia which causes disorientation. The sides are also useful when a change of position is made since they may be grasped by the patient and used for added support. Patients in the upright position are encouraged to assume the recumbent position for brief periods to help reduce circulatory stasis and edema in the lower parts of the body. This should not be forced in severe dyspnea.

In heart patients, as with all patients, the general principles of positioning apply. Good body alignment is respected to prevent contractures, hyperextension and circulatory stasis. *Even a slight change in position* every 1 to 2 hours is helpful. A footboard is used to prevent foot drop.

ELIMINATION. Constipation and straining at defecation are to be avoided because of the undue strain placed on the heart. A mild laxative may have to be given to keep the stool soft. If constipation does occur, an oil enema may be given. Abdominal distention is also to be avoided, since it raises the diaphragm and further embarrasses the patient's breathing. It has been shown that the use of the bedpan requires more energy than getting out of bed and using a commode. Therefore the physician may prefer to have the patient use a bedside commode for defecation.

When a patient receives a diuretic it will mean frequent use of the bedpan or commode, which can be very exhausting. The nurse provides the necessary assistance, and the patient is allowed to rest undisturbed between voidings.

CARE OF THE MOUTH AND SKIN. The dyspnea and retention of sodium experienced by the cardiac patient cause a decrease in normal salivary secretions. The tongue is rough and dry, and a thick mucus accumulates and adheres to the teeth and mucous membrane, providing a medium for organisms. Under such conditions, older patients are especially predisposed to parotitis. The mouth is cleansed every 2 to 3 hours and is kept moist.

The poor circulation, edema, bed rest and restricted activity necessitate special skin care to prevent pressure sores. Bony prominences and pressure areas are kept clean and dry and are massaged gently but with sufficient pressure to promote circulation. The alternating air pressure mattress is useful in protecting pressure areas but, if not available, a sponge rubber mattress may be used, or a piece of sponge rubber or sheepskin may be placed under pressure areas such as the sacrum, buttocks and heels.

REHABILITATION OF THE PATIENT WITH CARDIAC DYSFUNCTION. The philosophy and principles of rehabilitation are applicable to heart patients just as they are to patients with other conditions in which there is some residual damage or progressive disease. These persons may require help to learn to live within the limits of their cardiac capacity and, at the same time, achieve personal satisfaction and be able to function as productive members of society.

When a patient learns that he has a heart condition or recovers from an acute heart illness, he is advised as to whether he may resume his former activities or if it will be necessary for him to curtail some activities. The amount of activity and necessary restrictions are defined by the physician on the basis of the functional capacity of the heart (see p. 298. Many of these persons consider themselves doomed to complete invalidism and an early death. They may have an unjustified fear of another attack or of participating in any activity and may become helpless and dependent, creating unnecessary problems and hardships for themselves and their families.

Heart disease does not differ from many other diseases in that the patient may recover and take up his life where he left off. Some may find that a few simple adjustments in their pattern of living are necessary, while others are more restricted.

The physician has several ways of assessing the patient's capacity for activity and his limitations. He may observe the patient's responses to a gradual increase in energy expenditure. This will probably begin with self-care activities which are progressively extended to include more strenuous efforts. The assessment program may go on over several weeks or months, and the patient may require considerable encouragement to persevere.

An evaluation by standardized tests may be made in a heart clinic. In some situations, work evaluation clinics are established and serve to determine how much activity the patient's heart will permit. Following an assessment, a functional and therapeutic classification may be made (see p. 298). This is particularly useful in placing the patient in employment.

The nurse may assist in the assessment of the patient by observing and recording his responses to various activities. Any complaint or shortness of breath, palpitation, fatigue or an undue increase in the pulse rate are reported, and the effort is discontinued until the patient is checked by the doctor.

It is sometimes helpful to have the patient list his accustomed pattern of activities. The doctor may then indicate what changes, if any, are necessary. This is useful in getting the patient to think and talk about how much he will be able to do. It encourages him to plan independently and to reach a compromise between activity and restrictions.

The patient should realize that he has some responsibility for his future. The length of time he will live, and with what degree of satisfaction, depends largely on his own efforts. Each person reacts differently to illness and to restrictions. One may refuse to take advice or accept limitations and decide to "live it up." Another may become depressed or may display hostility, and still othere become overdependent. It is usually more difficult for the adult patient to accept and adjust to restrictions. Heart disease so often occurs just when the patient has reached a high position in his job and when life has become easier. The adult required to change to a less strenuous occupation finds it difficult to face a retraining program. Often his age makes it difficult for him to get another job.

With emphasis on the positive aspects, the nurse helps the patient and family understand and accept the decision of the doctor and to plan for the necessary adjustments. In the following paragraphs, consideration is given to the planning for assistance and guidance for these patients, remembering that every program must be planned in relation to each individual.

The nurse should have a copy of the many useful pamphlets and booklets available from the Heart Foundation. Many of these deal with rehabilitation, and appropriate copies may be given the patient to read with the doctor's approval.

Progressively increased activity is encouraged and directed by the nurse to condition the patient to the level of activity that corresponds to his heart's ability.

Changes may be necessary in the patient's home if he is not allowed to use stairs. It may be helpful to have a visiting nurse or social worker assess the home situation before the patient returns to it. Suggestions may be made in the interest of the patient and those who will be caring for him. For example, a bedroom and bathroom may have to be provided on the ground floor. Distance from public transportation and work may be factors that require consideration for some patients.

It should be pointed out to the patient and his family that moderation in everything is a good rule for persons who have had a heart illness. Some work, exercise, rest and recreation are important for everyone. Situations that are likely to add undue strain should be anticipated and avoided. Enough time should be allowed to prevent rushing. For example, rather than run the risk of running for a bus, the patient should plan to leave earlier. Climbing, walking against a strong wind, lifting, pushing and fatigue are to be avoided. Constipation, infections and emotional upsets also tend to increase the demands on the heart. The patient should strive for equanimity and develop the philosophy that what cannot be changed must be accepted. Suitable recreational activities, which meet both his interests and his cardiac funcitonal capacity, may be suggested. Some exercise is beneficial and appropriate forms are discussed. Walking is considered a good exercise. Regular hours of rest at night and, if necessary, a rest period during the day are recommended.

The physician, a social worker or the nurse may discuss necessary adjustments in the person's work situation with his employer or the industrial nurse. Assistance might be given to find suitable employment or to obtain retraining if a change in occupation is indicated.

Since smoking, particularly cigarettes, is found to be vasoconstricting, the heart patient is well advised to discontinue smoking.

Shortness of breath, palpitation, faintness, persisting fatigue, pain and edema are indications for the person to slow up and report to the the clinic or his physician.

Clarification of the prescribed diet is made. Many heart patients are advised to continue with a low sodium intake and a limited number of calories. Foods allowed, those restricted and meal planning are discussed. The importance of keeping the weight normal and avoiding large meals is explained. Preferably, the discussion of the diet should be with the homemaker as well as the patient. Directions and suggestions are given to the patient in writing, and an appropriate diet booklet is obtained from the Heart Foundation.

The medications that are to be continued are discussed, and written instructions are provided. Early signs of untoward reactions are cited, and included with these are directions about what to do if they develop. For example, if an anticoagulant such as dicoumarol is to be continued, the patient and a family member are advised of the action of the drug and the necessary observations to recognize bleeding. They are told that bleeding from body orifices, discolored areas of the skin (bruises and petechiae), bleeding gums, and persistent bleeding from minor cuts or injuries are to be reported immediately to the doctor or clinic. If he is to have dental work done, the patient should advise his dentist that he is receiving dicoumarol. He is given an identification card to carry which states that he is receiving dicoumarol. A weekly visit to clinic for prothrombin time evaluation is usually requested by the physician.

Many heart patients are required to take digitalis continuously and should understand that loss of appetite, nausea or diarrhea may indicate the need for some adjustment in the dosage of the drug. If the patient is an elderly person who lives alone, he is advised to keep a calendar available with the days that he is to take a medication clearly marked. It is stressed that he adopt the habit of marking off the medication as soon as he takes it.

Some follow-up service is important. The patient and family are advised of the resources outside the hospital, and a referral may be made to the visiting nurse or public health agency. Home visits by a nurse can be very helpful; they provide an opportunity for the patient and family to ask questions and receive counseling on the various aspects of care. At the same time the patient's condition and progress are noted.

If the patient's heart condition demands fairly stringent restrictions on his activities, it may be necessary to assist the family in planning how they will provide the required care. Some patients need provision made for their ordinary personal care. The family is advised about the amount of care needed, how to provide it and how to protect their own health. They are encouraged not to overprotect the patient or foster an overdependent role. The family should plan together and all share in the necessary care. The nurse may recognize that the care of the patient will impose too heavy a burden on the family and help them to seek some other solution. A referral may be made for home care service or the patient may be transferred to a nursing home. Circumstances might necessitate the family receiving social welfare assistance. The nurse may have to help the patient accept this situation.

The importance of regular medical supervision is stressed. The severely handicapped person may have difficulty getting to the clinic or doctor's office; transportation may be requested of a voluntary organization such as the Red Cross Society or a service club.

The homemaker with a cardiac condition is given assistance in learning to continue her home functions within her heart capacity. Again, the reader is referred to the appropriate publications available through the American Heart Association or Canadian Heart Foundation.[26] Much work has been done on work simplification in the home, and there are many simple and inexpensive ways of making it possible to achieve more with less effort. In some communities, a consultant is available through the Heart Association or a rehabilitation unit who will visit the home and make suggestions as to how the housekeeper's work can be made easier. Some physical changes, a reorganization in the placement of equipment, elimina-

---

[26]Example: "The Heart of the Home." Published by the American Heart Association, New York. Available in Canada through the Canadian Heart Foundation.

tion of unnecessary chores, and the management of many tasks to economize on time and motion may be suggested and demonstrated. The success of rehabilitating the homemaker is largely dependent on how willing she is to change her way of doing things. The nurse and rehabilitation worker may find that much time will have to be devoted to persuasion.

The patient's health and degree of satisfaction in living will depend to a large extent on his recognition and acceptance of the limitations imposed.

NURSING THE CARDIAC SURGICAL PATIENT

Significant advances have been made in the field of cardiac surgery, in correcting both congenital and acquired heart defects. Correction of acquired heart disease includes surgery for coronary artery disease and for stenosed or incompetent cardiac valves. The fact that the heart must function immediately after the surgery presents a problem different from that in many areas of the body. It must heal while continuing to maintain adequate circulation. This creates the need for greater support and for minimizing physiological demands.

Progress in this area of surgery was delayed until the introduction of the pump-oxygenator. This machine permits extracorporeal oxygenation of the blood and maintenance of circulation while the heart is arrested and opened to provide a direct approach to defects within the heart. Circulation bypasses the heart and lungs. The venae cavae are cannulated, and the blood passes from them into tubes leading to the mechanical oxygenator, which takes the place of the lungs. It is then pumped through a heat exchanger and filtered into a femoral or subclavian artery. The blood flows in a reverse direction in the aorta, keeping the aortic valve closed. Sufficient blood enters the coronary system to sustain the myocardial cells. The blood is heparinized in order to prevent coagulation and thrombus formation. On completion of the cardiopulmonary bypass, the heparin is neutralized by the administration of protamine sulfate.

Hypothermia may be used to reduce the metabolic activity of the heart so the cells can survive interruption of the coronary circula-tion. Reducing the body temperature to within a range of 20 to 30° C. (hypothermia) may be used in heart surgery either alone or as an adjunct to the extracorporeal circulation. It reduces the metabolic activity of cells throughout the body and therefore their oxygen and nutritional needs. Hypothermia prevents damage to the brain and other vital organs when an interruption of circulation or a reduction in oxygenated blood to a dangerously low level is anticipated (see section on hypothermia, p. 110).

Surgery for Coronary Artery Disease

Both direct and indirect methods are used to revascularize the myocardium. The indirect method, or Vineberg procedure, involves implanting the internal mammary artery into the myocardium. Collateral circulation develops over a period of months; revascularization is not immediate. Consequently, infarction and mortality rates are higher during this period than with direct revascularization procedures.

The most popular procedure is the aortocoronary bypass surgery, in which one end of a resected saphenous vein is anastomosed to the aorta and the other to the coronary artery beyond the point of obstruction. The blood supply to the myocardium is immediately improved.

Surgery for Diseased Valves

The surgeon can significantly enlarge the size of the orifice of stenosed valves in some individuals by dilating the valve, either manually or instrumentally. Others, however, may require valve replacement.

Certain patients with regurgitation of the aortic, mitral and/or tricuspid valves, who no longer respond to medical treatment, require total replacement. This is accomplished with an artificial valve prosthesis or the use of tissue homografts.

Preoperative Nursing Care

The preoperative preparation for cardiac surgery may extend through days to weeks, while the patient is thoroughly investigated and his physical and mental conditions are improved.

PSYCHOLOGICAL   PREPARATION.   In

most instances, heart surgery carries more than the ordinary risk. The incision may be midsternal, which avoids entrance into the left pleural cavity and collapse of the left lung, or it may be through the left chest and may result in collapse of the left lung. Because of the tremendous emphasis placed on the heart by the average person, it is understandable that the patient and his family will be very apprehensive. The surgeon describes the patient's condition to the patient and his family, and the likely prognosis if he continues untreated. An explanation is then made of what can be done surgically and the inherent risk.

It takes courage to face heart surgery; the patient or (in the case of a child) the parents may find it difficult to arrive at a decision. They require a great deal of emotional support. The nurse assesses the patient's anxiety and fears, and efforts are directed towards minimizing them, since they will affect the patient's reaction to surgery and his postoperative progress. He is encouraged to talk about his concerns and to ask quesitons. Worries may become less significant through verbalizing them and being able to share them. Socioeconomic problems may come to light which necessitate voluntary or welfare assistance for the patient and family. The patient may fear death and may wish to talk about this. A visit from the patient's spiritual adviser may provide considerable support.

Acquainting the patient with what to expect when he goes to the operating room and after the surgery will reduce some of his fear of the future. As the patient talks more and more about the whole major event, he will begin to accept it with less stress. In all discussions with the patient and family, what is said should be informative, in understandable terms, and judiciously selected to prevent inducing unnecessary anxiety. Sincere interest and understanding of their problems are frequently better expressed by feeling tones than by words.

To prevent unnecessary concern, the patient is advised of the multiple and complex equipment that will surround him after his operation. It may be helpful with some patients to actually let them see some of the equipment in this preoperative period. The patient is told that he will have a tube in his throat (endotracheal) so that he may receive oxygen by a respirator which will reduce the work of breathing, that his blood pressure and pulse will be taken at very frequent intervals to reveal information about his condition, and that there will be a tube in the chest as well as an intravenous tube and an indwelling catheter. The nurses will be making frequent checks of these tubes and the drainage. He is advised that he will likely experience a sensation of heaviness and tightness as well as some pain in the chest, and is reassured that the staff will do everything possible to provide relief. In many hospitals, the patient is visited the day before surgery by the nurse who will be caring for him in the intensive care unit. This preoperative visit establishes a contact for the patient as well as helping the nurse to know him better.

OBSERVATIONS. During the preoperative period vital signs, fluid intake and output, daily weight and reactions to any exertion are noted. The patient is also observed closely for indications of any condition, such as a cold or skin infection, which could cause serious postoperative complications. A detailed knowledge of the patient and his vital signs serves as a basis for comparison postoperatively.

OPERATIVE CONSENT. The patient, if responsible and of age, will sign his consent for operation. In some situations, the hospital and/or the surgeon may also require the signature of a close relative on the consent. The patient and family should have had a description of the operation and its expected outcome before being asked to sign the operation permit. In the case of a minor, both parents may be required to give permission.

FUNCTIONAL TESTS (see p. 291). Cardiac and respiratory functional tests, as well as complete blood studies, are done to further assess the patient's condition. The blood work will include typing and crossmatching so that compatible blood will be available at the time of operation. Serum electrolytes, cardiac enzymes, serum creatinine and blood urea nitrogen determinations are also performed, and blood clotting tests such as prothrombin time and partial thromboplastin time are done. A preoperative urinalysis is carried out.

The nurse explains the tests to the patient and provides the required preparation and aftercare applicable to each one. For 2 to 3 days following the more complex cardiac tests, such as heart catheterization, close observation is necessary for manifestations of reactions or complications. Bleeding or irritation at the site of entrance into the blood vessel, reaction to the radiopaque substance, fibrillation and cardiac arrest occur rarely.

For some patients, tests such as cardiac catheterization may be done several weeks preoperatively, and the patient may reenter the hospital 1 to 3 days prior to surgery.

PHYSICAL PREPARATION. Optimum nutritional status is important; attention is directed to having the patient take adequate meals. Protein and vitamin C are particularly important, for they contribute to tissue repair. If the patient has been on a low-sodium diet previously, this will be continued. Optimum hydration is desirable; a daily intake of 2000 to 2500 ml. is encouraged as long as his output is adequate.

The patient is advised that he will be required to cough, take five to ten deep respirations, change position and do some simple leg and foot exercises frequently, for several days after the operation. Arm and shoulder exercises will also be necessary later. The purposes of these activities are explained. Instructions are given on how to cough and do the exercises, and the patient is encouraged to practice. To cough, he is instructed to take a deep breath, contract the abdominal muscles and then cough with the mouth and throat open. Postoperative coughing and deep breathing promote expansion of the lungs, the removal of secretions from the respiratory tract and the removal of air and fluid from the thoracic cavity. The foot and leg exercises are to prevent phlebothrombosis. The arm exercises promote a return to the full range of motion of the arms, since the patient will tend to favor them following the operation.

Particular attention is paid to skin and oral hygiene during this period. Daily bathing with a mild antiseptic solution or soap minimizes the possibility of staphylococcal wound infection. This will be done 1 to 2 days prior to surgery. Antiseptic mouthwash will help to prevent mouth and respiratory infection.

IMMEDIATE PREOPERATIVE CARE. Extra precautions are taken with these patients in preparing the skin. Infection superimposed on their surgery could prove fatal. The day before operation almost the whole trunk is shaved and cleansed, including the axillae. Since a femoral artery is cannulated, the perineum and upper thighs are also prepared. The surgeon will indicate what antiseptic, if any, is to be applied; following the shave, the patient may be given an antiseptic bath and placed in fresh bed linen. Care is taken during the shave to keep the skin intact. It is important that the fingernails are free of nail polish so that their true color may be detected.

Solid food is withheld for 10 to 12 hours previous to operation and the meal preceding this period should be light. Water may be given up to 4 to 6 hours prior to operation.

The doctor may or may not want the patient to have a small cleansing enema the afternoon before operation. A sedative is prescribed to ensure the patient a good sleep the night before operation. The nurse makes a final check to see that the required blood is available, the urinalysis report and vital signs are satisfactory, and that the operative consent has been signed.

The morning of operation the patient may be required to take an antiseptic bath, and he empties his bladder just before the sedative is given. All procedures are completed before the patient receives his preoperative medication so that he may be left undisturbed to derive the maximum benefit from the drug. A nurse accompanies the patient to the operating room and remains with him until the anesthetist or operating room staff takes over.

In the operating room, a Foley catheter is inserted into the patient's bladder and attached to a drainage tube and bag, a venous catheter is forwarded into the right heart for measurement of central venous pressure, and an arterial catheter is inserted to be used postoperatively to obtain samples of arterial blood for measurement of blood gases and to monitor blood pressure. Some patients may require a Swan-Ganz catheter for assessment of pulmonary artery and pulmonary capillary pressures.

FAMILY. Consideration is given to the relatives during this stressful situation. A spouse, parent or someone close whom the patient wishes to have may be allowed to visit before the preoperative medication is administered. The family may wish to remain at the hospital during the operation, or may decide to return home to await word by telephone. If they remain, they are shown to a sitting room where an understanding hostess may be provided to help them through the difficult hours. If there is no hostess, the nurse should take a few moments at intervals to go and speak with them and to see that they have refreshments. Recognition on the part of the nurse or others that this is a difficult time will help. Many surgeons, knowing the family's stress, may forward a message from time to time to reassure them.

Postoperative Nursing Care

The patient who has had cardiac surgery is cared for in an intensive care unit where the necessary special equipment is assembled. Continuous observation and constant, expert nursing care are required. The patient becomes very anxious and fearful if left alone for even a very brief period the first day or two.

The care must be adapted to the patient's particular needs and the surgeon's directives. The following points of care may not be applicable nor complete in all situations, but may serve as a guide to the nurse who is planning and providing care for the surgical cardiac patient.

PREPARATION TO RECEIVE THE PATIENT. During the operation the necessary equipment is assembled at the patient's bedside. In many intensive care units, much of the monitoring equipment is attached to the wall beside the patient's bed.

RECEPTION OF THE PATIENT. The closed chest drainage, urinary drainage, intravenous infusion, arterial line, and central venous and pulmonary arterial pressure lines are checked for function. The endotracheal tube is attached to the mechanical respirator and respiratory support and the administration of oxygen are continued as ordered. Limbs with infusions are secured and continuous cardiac monitoring is started.

POSITIONING. The patient is kept flat until the systolic blood pressure is 100 mm. Hg or more. He is raised gradually and his responses noted. Unless otherwise directed, his position is changed every 2 hours from back to left side to back and to right side, etc. Precautions are necessary to avoid dislodging any tubes when turning the patient.

OBSERVATIONS. A constant monitoring of the heart action is used so that cardiac arrhythmias and change of rate may be quickly detected. Blood pressure, radial and apical pulses, respirations and color are checked and recorded every 15 minutes at first and every hour once the vital signs become stabilized.

Venous pressure readings are taken hourly as an indication of intravascular volume and right heart function. Pulmonary artery and pulmonary capillary wedge pressures, when ordered, are measured hourly as an indication of left heart functioning. These measurements are continued for at least 48 hours following surgery.

Initially the patient is supported by mechanical ventilation, either pressure- or volume-controlled. The adequacy of this ventilation is assessed by measurement of arterial blood gases as well as by observation of the patient's responses which include color, blood pressure, restlessness and pulse rate. The nurse collects arterial blood specimens from the interarterial line when the patient is first admitted to the intensive care unit and periodically thereafter as indicated. Observations related to the respirator are discussed on p. 426. The arterial line is flushed with normal saline hourly.

Movement of both sides of the chest is noted; unequal expansion of the two sides, audible moist sounds and dyspnea should be reported.

Continuous recording of the body temperature by an electric thermometer may be used for the first day or two; if not, the rectal temperature is taken every 2 hours. The wounds are observed at frequent intervals for possible bleeding.

Orientation, level of consciousness, restlessness and anxiety are significant and should be noted. Stasis of circulation during surgery may have resulted in the formation of a thrombus which later may move out as an embolus. Also, a small amount of air left in the heart on closing may cause an air embolism. For these reasons the patient's ability to move his limbs and his speech are tested every 1 to 2 hours. Any weakness or loss of function is promptly reported. Peripheral pulses in the limbs, as well as the radial pulse, are checked (dorsalis pedis, femoral and posterior tibial). The absence of one of these may point to a thrombosis or embolism.

Fluid intake and output are recorded. When his condition permits, the patient is weighed daily to detect possible retention of fluid.

Respiratory tests may be required at frequent intervals; the expiratory volume per minute may be estimated by the use of a respirometer. Blood specimens are collected for determination of blood gases, electrolyte concentrations, hemoglobin, and hematocrit.

ASSISTING RESPIRATORY FUNCTION. As mentioned, the patient's endotracheal tube is attached to a mechanical respirator. While the endotracheal tube is in place the patient is suctioned every 2 hours, or more often if necessary. The secretions are assessed for amount, color and consistency. Suctioning can be a very frightening experience for the patient, so the procedure is explained before it is carried out. Careful aseptic technique is observed and each suctioning should not exceed 10 seconds.

After 24 hours the patient is assessed to see if he can breathe spontaneously and adequately. If lung expansion is adequate and arterial blood gases are within acceptable limits, the endotracheal tube is removed. The patient then receives warm, moisturized oxygen. If the patient is unable to be weaned from the respirator after 48 hours, a tracheostomy is performed and mechanical respiratory support is continued.

Coughing every 1 to 2 hours is started as soon as the blood pressure is stabilized. The nurse assists the patient by elevating him to a sitting position and supporting the chest, back and front. If the coughing is not productive, and it is evident that secretions are present, suctioning is used.

Intermittent positive pressure breathing may be used prior to chest physiotherapy to help loosen and moisten secretions and to help in lung expansion. When the patient is not on a respirator, he is encouraged to take five to ten deep breaths every 1 to 2 hours.

Deep breathing, coughing, turning and skin care are done at one time in order to provide a longer, undisturbed period for the patient.

CARE OF DRAINAGE TUBES. Drainage tubes are inserted into the thoracic cavity at the end of surgery to promote the drainage of blood and secretions. These tubes are connected to a tube which extends into the fluid in a drainage bottle or bag. Disposable pleurovac drainage systems are frequently used. Keeping the end of the tube submerged in the water allows fluid and air to escape from the chest cavity but prevents air from entering the chest. (For details of closed, water-sealed drainage in chest surgery, see p. 463.) The system is observed at frequent intervals for functioning; the level of the fluid should fluctuate in the tube in the bottle, with respirations and with coughing. To prevent blockage by a clot the tubes are "milked" or stripped every hour for the first 24 hours. If the tubes are not draining it is reported promptly, since an accumulation of fluid in the thoracic cavity could cause serious cardiac embarrassment. The drainage is examined for possible bleeding, and the volume is measured. The tube must be clamped with two hemostats close to the chest wall in the event of any disruption of the system.

The urine drainage is checked hourly for the first 24 to 36 hours, particularly if the blood pressure is low. An hourly output of 25 ml. or less is brought to the doctor's attention since it may indicate the onset of a renal shutdown. The physician may require the bladder to be irrigated once or twice daily as long as the patient has an indwelling catheter.

The total 12-hour or 24-hour output is recorded and the fluid balance determined.

NUTRITION AND FLUIDS. For the first 24 to 48 hours the patient is maintained on intravenous infusion. The maximum amount to be given in an hour is specified and the rate of flow carefully controlled to prevent overloading the circulatory system and increasing the demand on the heart. The intravenous fluid is usually glucose in distilled water rather than saline.

Sips of water may be permitted to relieve the thirst sensation once the endotracheal tube is removed and the patient is able to swallow. Frequent mouth care also helps and is necessary to prevent infection. All fluid intake is measured and recorded. A positive balance may necessitate restricting the fluid intake to a prescribed volume.

The diet progresses from fluids to soft foods and then to light solid foods as tolerated. Frequent small amounts are more acceptable than larger amounts less often. Gas-forming foods are to be avoided, and sodium restriction may be indicated.

REST. Uninterrupted periods of rest are important to reduce the demands on the heart. The various observations that must be made and the treatments, tests and doctors' visits sometimes make it difficult for the patient to get sufficient rest. The nurse should be alert to the problem and, if necessary, consult the physician.

PSYCHOLOGICAL CARE. The patient who has had considerable preparation for what will follow the operation tends to accept the postoperative situation with less anxiety than patients who have not had a similar preparation. It is important that his questions are answered and that he receive some information as to his progress. Brief explanations of what is going to be done are appreciated by the patient and a visit from a family member is also reassuring.

It is not uncommon for the patient's spirits to fluctuate; he may have brief periods of depression and may become very irritable. Patience and understanding on the part of the nurse are important. An expression that indicates to the patient that she knows how he feels may provide some support.

MEDICATIONS. Analgesics and sedatives are used sparingly with the cardiac surgical patient since they tend to depress respirations and the cough reflex.

A small dose of morphine or meperidine hydrochloride (Demerol) may be ordered for the relief of pain. Close observation of the patient's response to the drug is necessary; respirations are checked before the administration and during the period following. Very judicious use of these drugs is necessary; to withhold the drug unnecessarily may be harmful, since pain and the patient's response to it may increase the demands on the respiratory system and the heart. The narcotic ordered by the doctor should be used only for pain — not for restlessness. The latter condition indicates the need for increased observation to determine its cause; it may be due to hypoxia or hemorrhage and should be reported.

A prophylactic antibiotic may be administered for a period of 5 to 10 days. The number of days will depend on the patient's history; if he has had rheumatic fever and rheumatic heart disease he will probably receive the antibiotic for a longer period to prevent reactivation of the rheumatic disease.

Digitalis may be prescribed to strengthen the heart. Quinidine sulfate or another antiarrhythmic drug may be necessary to treat fibrillation.

EXERCISES AND MOBILITY. To prevent circulatory stasis and thrombus formation some activity is desirable. Passive movements of the limbs are initiated first and are followed by active foot and leg exercises when indicated by the doctor. Later, active exercises are extended to include the arms and shoulders. A pull cord by which the patient may pull himself up may be attached to the foot of the bed. His next move will be to the side of the bed, then to a chair, and finally to self-care activities and walking.

The patient tends to immobilize the shoulders and arms and may develop "frozen shoulders." Gentle passive movement is all he may tolerate at first, but as soon as possible he is encouraged to use his arms and put them through a full range of motion as he was instructed preoperatively.

The starting of exercises and the rate of progression and degree of mobility will be decided by the doctor for each patient. For example, the patient who has had surgical correction of a coarctation of the aorta must remain inactive for a much longer period than many other patients. The patient's responses will also be a factor in determining the amount of activity and when it should be started.

THE FAMILY. When the operation is completed, the surgeon sees the family, informs them as to what was done and advises them of the patient's condition. It is then helpful if they may see the patient without disturbing him. Before taking them to the patient's room, a brief description of some of the equipment in use may reduce their concern when they enter the room. A close family member may wish to remain in the hospital for most of the day and may be allowed to look in on the patient briefly at intervals. The nurse who stops to speak briefly with the family and inform them of the patient's condition conveys to them an understanding of their anxiety.

TRANSFER FROM THE INTENSIVE CARE UNIT. When patients are moved through various wards as their condition changes, the problem arises of the patient's adjustment to different environments and variations in the nursing care provided. In studying the effect of changes in location on cardiac surgical patients, Kimball was impressed by the frequency with which patients experienced discomfort and anxiety upon leaving the intensive care unit. He noted that it was important "to emphasize that return to the general nursing unit from the I.C.U. can be a time of stress and anxiety.''[27] In a study by Jarvis, most patients related difficulties after transfer to the decreased observations and attention of staff.[28] The adjustment required may seem abrupt to the patient. Although requiring less monitoring and technical support, patients still need measures for relief of pain and fatigue, assistance with hygienic care, teaching and guidance regarding activity, medications and diet, and opportunities to express emotional reactions to the experience of heart surgery. To make the transition as smooth as possible, communication is required between the staff of the units involved as to the patient's progress, individual reactions and needs.

CONVALESCENCE AND REHABILITATION. While the patient's physical activity is increased, his tolerance is noted. Any shortness of breath, cardiac pain, or edema is promptly reported and activity is stopped until the doctor has seen the patient.

Prescribed exercises are continued throughout convalescence and rehabilitation. A member of the family and the patient are given instructions about his care after discharge. How long he must curtail his activities and to what extent will depend on the patient's condition before and after the operation and on his responses to activity.

Planning for his return home and his rehabilitation should include consideration of the factors suggested on page 340 under Rehabilitation, recognizing of course that every program must be determined on an individual basis.

SYSTEMIC DISEASE

Cardiac disease may be a secondary development in a disease in an area other than the heart. The primary disease may have placed an added strain on the circulation, or may have produced toxins or deficiencies in essential materials. Examples of these are diphtheria, hyperthyroidism, anemia, septicemia and pneumonia. Diphtheria produces a toxin that may cause myocarditis or may damage the conduction system. Diseases in which there is a prolonged and marked increase in the metabolic rate, as in hyperthyroidism, place an increased demand on the circulatory system to keep the overactive body cells supplied. Pulmonary conditions, such as pneumonia and emphysema, may produce a respiratory insufficiency that results in an inadequate oxygen supply to the heart muscle and a consequent cardiac inefficiency. They may also increase pulmonary pressures, putting an added strain on the heart.

HEART DISEASE IN PREGNANCY

The woman with a heart disease who contemplates having a child should consult a cardiologist. Many such women are quite able to bear a child and come through safely if they are closely supervised throughout pregnancy and follow the doctor's instructions. For others, pregnancy may carry considerable risk, since it creates increased demands on the heart.

During pregnancy, the total blood volume is increased as much as 25 per cent by the seventh or eighth month. This increases the work load of the heart and persists 24 hours of the day, not just with physical activity. Some enlargement of the heart usually occurs in the normal pregnant woman. The changes in the concentration of certain hormones in pregnancy cause some retention of sodium. This varies in different women but does produce a hazard for the heart patient who, because of some cardiac insufficiency, may already be retaining an excess of sodium. The pregnant woman also experiences some shortness of breath as the enlarging uterus rises in the abdominal cavity, causing pressure on the diaphragm.

The nurse may be asked by the woman with a heart condition whether it is safe for her to become pregnant. She is advised to go to a heart clinic or to consult her doctor. If the woman confides in the nurse that she thinks she is already pregnant, she is urged to see her doctor or go to the clinic at once. A thorough history is taken, and her heart's

[27]Chase Patterson Kimball: ''Psychological Responses to Open-Heart Srugery.'' A.O.R.N.J., Vol. II, No. 2 (Feb. 1970), pp. 75–84.

[28]Dorothy Jarvis: ''Open-Heart Surgery: Patients' Perceptions of Care.'' Am. J. Nurs., Vol. 70, No. 12 (Dec. 1970), pp. 2591–2593.

functional capacity is assessed. The doctor may tell her he believes it would be safe for her to have a child, but that it will be necessary for her to follow his instructions closely. The fact that pregnancy imposes an increased work load on the heart and that she has a reduced cardiac reserve should be explained to her and to her husband. Pregnancy for her will necessitate reduced activity, longer and more frequent rest periods, avoidance of infection and emotional stresses, weight control and restricted salt intake.

The patient and her husband will be instructed to get in touch promptly with the doctor if she experiences shortness of breath, palpitation, vomiting, any infection or gain in weight in excess of that suggested by the doctor. Frequent visits to the obstetrician and cardiologist are necessary. Weekly visits alternating between these two physicians may be requested.

If the woman develops any signs of cardiac failure, she is put to bed, and digitalis and a diuretic are prescribed. More stringent restrictions of sodium will be used. The visiting nurse can give this patient a great deal of help and support and should know that the strain on the heart reaches a peak in the seventh and eighth months. During these later months of pregnancy, closer observation of the patient and a strict regimen are very important.

The patient may be allowed to go to full term, or the doctor may think it advisable to induce labor a few weeks before term. In caring for the patient during labor, the nurse is alert for early signs of cardiac failure. The pulse, blood pressure and respirations are noted at frequent intervals. Every effort is made to prevent unnecessary exertion and to provide the patient with as much rest as possible. Fluid intake and output are measured and recorded. The equipment and supplies used in the treatment of any heart patient are kept at hand.

Following delivery, close observation for manifestations of cardiac insufficiency and precautions to reduce the work load of the heart are continued.

THE SURGICAL PATIENT WITH IMPAIRED CARDIAC FUNCTION

The person with some cardiac insufficiency may require an operation. Unless it is an emergency, time is taken to assess carefully the functional capacity of the heart. Several tests are likely to be done which bear nursing responsibilities as discussed on page 291. The patient is closely observed during the period of preparation for any signs of failure; the recognition of such signs may influence his treatment and the risk which the surgery may carry.

This patient, knowing he has a heart condition, is likely to be more fearful than other surgical patients. The nurse encourages him to verbalize his concerns and takes time to help him work through them. He should be advised that there will be a nurse with him constantly until he is conscious, that when he regains consciousness one will remain close by and visit him at frequent intervals, and that a doctor will be notified promptly of any change in his condition.

Surgery carries less risk for these patients than it did formerly; recent knowledge and new and improved techniques, equipment and anesthetics have made surgery safer and provide more physiological support.

Postoperatively, the nurse provides even closer attention for this patient, since his condition could change suddenly. Frequent checking of vital signs, color, level of consciousness and accurate recording of the fluid intake and output are necessary for several days longer than for most surgical patients. Any dyspnea, cyanosis, abnormal pulse rate, rhythm or volume, positive fluid balance, apathy and loss of consciousness are reported to the physician promptly since they may indicate reduced cardiac function. If the patient is to receive intravenous fluids, the rate of flow and volume must be carefully controlled to avoid a sudden increase in the intravascular volume and an overloading of the impaired heart. Any surgical complications, such as infection and phlebitis, are extremely hazardous because they may precipitate failure.

NURSING IN VASCULAR DISEASES

Disturbance of circulation within the vascular system may originate in the arterial system (arteries and arterioles) or in the veins. In the case of the former, a partial or complete occlusion reduces the volume of blood into the part which the vessel supplies, and the tissues suffer oxygen and nutritional deficiency. If the site of the vascular problem is the veins, there is interference with the normal outflow of venous blood, causing congestion and edema within the tissues. Vascular conditions may be chronic, developing slowly over a considerable period of time, or they may be sudden and acute.

ARTERIAL DISORDERS

Aortic Aneurysm

An aneurysm is a saccular dilatation of the wall of an artery and develops as a result of weakness in the wall of the vessel in that area. The weakness in the majority of cases is due to arteriosclerosis, but may also be caused by an infectious disease (e.g., syphilis), congenital defect or trauma. The aorta and cerebral arteries are the most common sites of aneurysms.

The aneurysm that does not extend completely around the artery is referred to as a *saccular aneurysm.* If it involves the complete circumference, it is classified as a *fusiform aneurysm.*

Separation of the layers of the aorta is referred to as a *dissecting aortic aneurysm,* even though no dilatation may be present. The tear is often in the intima and may be due to bleeding in the medial layer from the vasa vasorum. The dissection may extend lengthwise for a considerable distance and may involve branches of the aorta. The aortic aneurysm may also be classified according to the section of the artery in which the defect is located; for example, it may be designated as a thoracic or abdominal aortic aneurysm. The former may be further categorized as an ascending thoracic aortic aneurysm, a transverse thoracic aneurysm or a descending thoracic aortic aneurysm.

A serious threat to any patient with an aneurysm is rupture of the weakened vascular area; the rapid loss of blood almost always proves fatal.

MANIFESTATIONS. Signs and symptoms may be absent until the aneurysm is large enough to compress adjacent structures. The patient with a thoracic aneurysm may experience chest pain, dyspnea, hoarseness due to vocal cord paralysis and/or congestion of the veins in the neck because of pressure on the superior vena cava. With an abdominal aneurysm, the patient may complain of midabdominal, lumbar or pelvic pain, often severe. Physical examination may reveal an expansile, abdominal mass. Femoral pulses may be reduced. Careful physical examination, x-rays, echocardiograms and/or aortography are means of confirming the diagnosis.

Symptoms of a dissecting aortic aneurysm include pain, often described as ripping or tearing in nature, and may involve the chest, back and/or abdomen. Blood pressure drops and there may be a discrepancy in pulses in various locations in the body.

TREATMENT. In recent years, encouraging advances have been made in the surgical treatment of aneurysms. If a small blood vessel is affected, it may be tied off and the flow of blood is diverted to another artery. In treating an aortic aneurysm, the area is resected and replaced with a graft of inert synthetic material such as Teflon or Dacron which does not cause tissue reaction. In most instances the surgery involves a cardiopulmonary bypass to maintain adequate oxygenation of the body tissues during the period the aorta is clamped. The patient is placed on an extracorporeal system (see p. 343).

Nursing management of the patient is similar to that for the patient having heart surgery (see p. 343).

Acute Arterial Occlusion

Acute occlusion occurs suddenly as a result of external compression, thrombosis or embolism. It is serious because there is a lack of collateral circulation to the tissues supplied by this artery.

Arterial thrombosis occurs with the formation of an abnormal blood clot (thrombus) within an artery, usually as the result of narrowing of the lumen of the artery by atherosclerotic changes. The stasis in the blood flow predisposes to the formation of the clot, partially or completely blocking the vessel. If the vessel is not completely blocked, treatment is directed toward preventing the clot from enlarging to occlude the vessel and toward keeping it at the site of formation to prevent an embolism.

Arterial embolism is the blocking of an artery by a foreign mass that has been carried by the blood stream until it reaches an artery too small for it to pass through. The foreign mass is referred to as an embolus.

Most frequently it is a thrombus that breaks loose from its site of origin, but it may consist of air, fragments of vegetations from diseased cardiac valves, fat, atherosclerotic plaques or small masses of tissue or cancerous cells. The effects of an embolism are determined by the localization of the embolus. The vessel which the embolus obstructs depends upon the size of the embolus, its origin, and whether the artery blocked is an end-artery or one that anastomoses above the block with smaller vessels in the part supplied. Obviously, if it is an end-artery, the tissue entirely dependent upon it becomes necrotic. An embolus originating in a vein or the right side of the heart is likely to cause a pulmonary embolism (see p. 467). One arising from the left side of the heart or a large systemic artery may produce a cerebral embolism or may plug a smaller arterial artery. The site of arterial occlusion by an embolus may also be a lower extremity.

Chronic Arterial Occlusion

This most frequently develops as a result of gradual changes in the walls of the vessels, causing narrowing of the lumen. It may also be of functional origin due to a hyperactivity of the sympathetic nervous system, causing an excessive vasoconstriction. Gradual occlusion of the vessels allows for collateral circulation to be established, lessening the problem of deprivation in the tissues distal to the occlusion.

The most common causes of chronic occlusion are atherosclerosis and arteriosclerosis. The arteries in any area of the body may be affected, but the coronary, cerebral and renal arteries are frequent sites. The problems caused by their insufficiency are discussed under disorders of the relative structures. When the abdominal aorta and/or medium- and large-sized arteries are involved, the condition may be referred to as *arteriosclerosis obliterans*. The arteries of the extremities are also a relatively frequent site of chronic occlusion that may be referred to as *peripheral vascular disease*. Two common forms of peripheral vascular disease are Raynaud's disease and thromboangiitis obliterans.

Raynaud's disease is a condition in which episodes of excessive vasoconstriction occur in the digits of the hands and/or feet. The cause is obscure, but the episodes are most frequently precipitated by cold or emotional stress. The disease is more common in females, usually develops before the age of 40 to 45 years and is bilateral.

Thromboangiitis obliterans (Buerger's disease) is a chronic occlusive disease in which there is an inflammation and thickening of the walls of limb arteries, predisposing to thrombosis. It has á higher incidence in young males and in Jewish persons. The parts are very tender and painful, and necrotic areas develop in the distal portions of the digits. The condition is seriously aggravated if the person smokes. The cause of this disease is unknown.

MANIFESTATIONS OF ARTERIAL INSUFFICIENCY IN THE EXTREMITIES. These manifestations are due to the deficiencies in oxygen and nutrients to the tissues resulting from the decreased blood supply into the limb. If there is a complete deprivation, the tissue cells die, and necrosis occurs in the form of ulceration or gangrene.

PAIN. The patient may experience intermittent claudication. This is pain that occurs on exercise and is relieved by rest. The blood supply is sufficient to meet the tissue needs only when the part is at rest; on exercise, oxygen demands cannot be met. The pain may be constant even with the part at rest, indicating a decreased blood flow into the tissues or a complete obstruction. The pain may be described as aching or cramp-like and is often severe. The patient may complain of a numbness or tingling in the extremity.

PULSE. A weakness or absence of peripheral pulses may be evident. In the arm, the radial, ulnar, brachial or axillary artery may be palpated with the fingertips, and in the leg the dorsalis pedis, popliteal or femoral artery may be felt. An oscillometer may be used to palpate the pulsation of arteries in an area where the vessels are deeper and cannot be palpated by the fingers. A comparison is made of the pulse in the different arteries and would reveal a partial block if one were present. Complete occlusion would be indicated by an absence of the pulse.

COLOR. A difference in the color of the two extremities or an abnormal change in both extremities, if both are involved, will most likely be present. The skin may become white and blanched, or it may become a dusky red or cyanosed, depending on the amount of blood in the capillaries and the amount of unsaturated hemoglobin in the blood. On being raised, the limb becomes even paler as the venous drainage increases but, on being lowered, it fails to increase its color as the normal limb would do quickly with the rush of arterial blood into it. The superficial veins are slow in filling when the limb is lowered; normally, they fill in approximately 5 seconds.

SKIN TEMPERATURE. The skin temperature and moisture may be different in the two limbs. The affected one exhibits a coldness to the touch and may be unusually moist. The warmth of the skin is dependent on the heat brought to the part by the blood. The moisture may point to excessive sympathetic stimulation, causing vasospasm.

ATROPHY OF TISSUES. Limb tissues may atrophy, causing the affected limb to become smaller than the other. The skin becomes dry and shiny and loses its hair. Nails thicken and become brittle and ridged.

NECROSIS. Ulcerated or gangrenous areas may develop, denoting areas of tissue completely deprived of a blood supply. Ulceration is a superficial area of devitalized tissue; gangrene is a more massive area of dead tissue.

DIAGNOSTIC PROCEDURES. Hurst states that "... the diagnosis of chronic occlusive arterial disease can be established with certainty in well over 95 per cent of cases without the aid of special laboratory procedures" by correlating the findings of "...characteristic ischemic pain with other physical findings of occlusive arterial disease such as absence of pulses, postural color changes and nutritional changes in the extremity."[29]

Various tests may be used by the physician in diagnosing and assessing vascular disease.

EXCERCISE TOLERANCE. The patient is required to walk or perform some form of exercise until intermittent claudication occurs. The length of time from the start of activity until the occurence of pain is noted.

ANGIOGRAPHY. The method frequently used to locate the site of occlusion precisely is angiography, either aortography or selective arteriography. A radiopaque dye is introduced into the arteries, and roentgenograms are made of the vessels. The site of narrowing or obstruction may be located in this way, and some information as to the amount of collateral circulation present may also be obtained.

ULTRASONIC ARTERIOGRAPHY.[30] By ultrasonic technique images of arteries are produced which are comparable to x-ray angiography. By this noninvasive method, the dimensions and configurations of arteries are mapped.

REACTIVE HYPEREMIA. In this test, the flow of blood into the limb is reduced by the application of a tourniquet or blood pressure cuff for 2 to 3 minutes. On release, vasodilation normally follows, and blood flows in very quickly to produce warmth and flushing of the skin. In arterial insufficiency the flow of blood into the part is delayed.

RADIOGRAPHY. If the problem is arteriosclerosis, calcified deposits may show up in x-ray pictures but this does not necessarily indicate an obstruction to blood flow.

TREATMENT AND NURSING CARE OF THE PATIENT WITH ARTERIAL OCCLUSIVE DISEASE

The aims in the care of the patient are:
1. To prevent further progress of the condition causing the ischemia in the limbs.

2. To prevent complications, such as dryness and cracking of the skin, infection and ulceration, since the resistance of the tissues is lower.

3. To increase the blood supply to the extremities.

4. To keep the demands of the tissues within the limits of the existing blood supply into the limb.

Arterial occlusive disease (peripheral vascular disease) is a chronic condition, and the patient will most likely have to continue with the prescribed care and precautions indefinitely. It may create considerable hardship for the patient and his family, depending on the

---

[29]J. Willis Hurst, et al.: The Heart, 4th ed. New York, McGraw-Hill, 1978, p. 1604.

[30]D. J. Mozersky, et al.: "Ultrasonic Arteriography," Arch. Surg., Vol. 103, No. 6 (1971), pp. 663–667.

severity of the disease and the limitations it imposes. Adjustments may have to be made in his occupational and social life; he may become partially or completely dependent financially and for his personal care. The patient will certainly find it difficult to accept the situation and will react accordingly. The nurse will be alert to the possible implications for the patient and family and will provide the necessary assistance and guidance.

The patient and a family member are instructed in the necessary care. They should understand that adherence to the physician's suggestions and regular supervision are all important in preventing serious complications.

DIET. Obesity should be avoided, since excess tissue always increases the demands on the circulatory system. Overweight persons tend to be less active, which does not favor circulation. Protein and vitamin C are usually increased for maximum maintenance and support of the tissues suffering a degree of ischemia. An increase in B vitamins may be recommended, especially if there is peripheral nerve involvement and the patient is experiencing peripheral neuritis. The saturated fat and cholesterol content of the diet will probably be reduced and vegetable fat substituted for most of the animal fat if the arterial insufficiency is due to atherosclerosis.

An optimum fluid intake is important in maintaining a normal vascular volume and in preventing possible hemoconcentration predisposing to thrombus formation.

SMOKING. The use of tobacco is discontinued, since it promotes vasoconstriction and aggravates the disease. The close relationship between thromboangiitis obliterans and cigarette smoking implicates tobacco as an etiologic agent in this condition.

PROTECTION FROM COLD. Exposure to cold with lowering of normal body temperature incites undesirable responses —namely, peripheral vasoconstriction and increased metabolism. Special precautions are necessary in cold weather. Extra, warm clothing should be worn, and a change of residence to a warmer climate may be helpful. If exposure to cold precipitates an episode, the patient is advised to take a warm drink and seek a warm environment. A warm bath or a heating pad to the abdomen may be used to pro-

duce reflex vasodilation in the limbs. Local heat applications to the affected parts are discouraged because the tissue resistance is lowered and, frequently, there is a reduced nerve sensitivity. The patient is advised to wear warm socks or to wrap his feet in a warm blanket rather than applying a hot water bottle.

PROTECTION OF THE AFFECTED LIMBS. Extra precautions are necessary to protect the affected limbs from trauma and infection. Daily bathing in comfortably warm (not hot) water using a mild soap is recommended. Gentle and thorough drying is important, and special attention is given to the areas between the digits. If the skin is dry, the limbs may be gently massaged with lanolin or some light emollient. Nails are cut straight across but not right down to the soft tissue. A pumice stone may be used on calluses, but corns should be removed by a physician or podiatrist; the patient should not undertake to "pare" them with sharp instruments. The extremities, especially the terminal portions, are examined daily for changes; any discoloration, blister, broken area of skin, tenderness and swelling are to be promptly seen by the doctor.

The patient is advised of the importance of well-fitting shoes and socks or stockings. Socks should be loose and are changed daily. The patient is instructed to avoid walking about in bare feet; a cut, abrasion, sliver or infection could be quite serious, since the tissue resistance is lowered and healing is poor. If injury does occur, even of a minor nature, it should receive prompt medical attention. Anything tight or restricting, such as round garters, must not be worn. The pressure of bedclothes can be prevented by using a footboard at the foot of the bed.

POSITIONING. The horizontal position is used when the patient rests unless the doctor suggests otherwise. Occasionally, raising the head of the bed may be used to encourage the flow of blood into the lower limbs by gravity. Position should be changed at frequent intervals throughout the day, and long periods of standing must be avoided. The patient is advised not to cross his legs and, when sitting, pressure on the popliteal region is avoided. If ambulatory, he sits or lies down every 2 to 3 hours and elevates his feet for 10 to 15 minutes.

MEASURES TO INCREASE THE BLOOD SUPPLY TO THE EXTREMITIES

ACTIVITY. Many authorities indicate the most effective treatment for intermittent claudication is physical exercise, especially walking. It is suggested that the patient should exercise 20 to 30 minutes daily. He may do this by walking to the point of distress, stopping until the discomfort disappears and then continuing to walk until the distress develops again. The patient repeats this exercise for the prescribed period. The underlying theory is that exercise increases collateral circulation.

EXERCISES. Buerger-Allen exercises may be used for arterial insufficiency in the lower limbs. The leg is raised to approximately 45° above the horizontal and held until it blanches (1 to 2 minutes). It is then lowered to below the horizontal (over the side of the bed) until it becomes pink and then returned to the horizontal level for 1 to 2 minutes. This is repeated five to ten times every 6 or 8 hours. A padded support at the required height is provided for the elevation part of the cycle. The timing is determined by how long it takes for venous drainage and for refilling of the vessels, so the color must be observed closely and timed at first.

Passive and active exercises may also be prescribed; flexion and extension of the legs, feet and toes may be used for lower limbs, and similar exercises may be employed for the arms and fingers if these are the sites of the arterial insufficiency. Exercises promote emptying and filling of the vessels and stimulate the development of collateral circulation.

REFLEX DILATATION. Warm baths or increasing general body warmth by a higher environmental temperature may produce a reflux vasodilataion.

OSCILLATING BED. Alternate raising and lowering of the limbs to promote more efficient emptying and filling of the blood vessels may be achieved passively by placing the patient on an electric oscillating bed. A rocking motion is produced by a motor that can be set to tilt the bed longitudinally at a definite rate. The length of the period for operation may gradually be increased as the patient adjusts to the repeated tilting. It may be operated day and night and is helpful in relieving and preventing the pain which is associated with immobility. The patient is taught how to operate the motor, since the switch is readily available to him.

DRUGS. Vasodilating and anticoagulant drugs have been used to treat patients with arterial occlusive disease.

Vasodilators. Examples of vasodilators used are isoxuprine (Vasodilan), cyclandelate (Cyclospasmol) and papaverine. Coffman and others have indicated that none of these drugs is capable of selectively dilating the vessels supplying an ischemic limb.[31] The vasodilatation is general, often causing side effects of hypotension, tachycardia and syncope. Whiskey 30 to 60 ml. 3 or 4 times daily has been suggested as a sedative and analgesic.

Anticoagulant Drugs. Anticoagulants may be prescribed to prevent and treat thrombosis. The most widely used anticoagulants are heparin, warfarin (Coumadin), aspirin and sulfinpyrazone (Anturan). Heparin is given parenterally since it has no effect orally. It is thought to block the effect of thrombin on fibrinogen, thereby preventing clot formation. Heparin begins to be effective within minutes after administration and is prolonged for 3 to 4 hours. It may be given in a continuous intravenous drip or at regularly spaced intervals. Heparin therapy is usually extended over several days and then gradually replaced by a warfarin preparation given orally. Warfarin takes effect in approximately 48 hours, so it is started before the heparin is withdrawn.

The dosage and frequency of warfarin administration is dependent each day upon the prothrombin time of that day. The dosage of heparin is decided by the partial thromboplastin time (PTT). A therapeutic level is generally considered to be one and one-half times to twice the normal values for the PTT. A clotting time is done when partial thromboplastin time cannot be measured.

These drugs produce the risk of bleeding but their therapeutic value may be considered to outweigh this risk.

The nurse's responsibilities include close observation for signs of hemorrhage. Profuse bleeding from minor cuts, bleeding gums, hematuria, hematemesis, blood in the stool, pe-

---

[31] J. O. Coffman and J. A. Mannick: "Failure of Vasodilator Drugs in Arteriosclerosis Obliterans." Ann. Int. Med., Vol. 76, No. 1 (Jan. 1972), p. 35.

techiae and abnormal vaginal bleeding are reported promptly. In the event of bleeding the drug is discontinued, and vitamin K and a blood transfusion may be given to counteract the reduced coagulation. Protamine sulfate, a heparin antagonist, is given if severe bleeding occurs as a result of heparin administration.

Each day the nurse makes sure that the prothrombin or partial thromboplastin time is determined before the anticoagulant drug is administered, and that the physician is notified promptly if these tests are not within the desired range previously indicated by him. Patients outside the hospital on an anticoagulant are usually required to report to the clinic weekly for a prothrombin time check. More recently, drugs which prevent platelet aggregation, such as aspirin and sulfinpyrazone (Anturan), are being used to prevent arterial thrombosis.

SURGICAL TREATMENT AND CARE. If there is evidence of a decrease in vasomotor tone and improved circulation in the limbs in a diagnostic sympathetic block, a lumbar sympathectomy (removal of the second, third and fourth ganglia) may be performed.

A direct surgical approach may be employed in which the surgeon chooses to do an endarterectomy, a bypass or a graft. An endarterectomy is the removal of the thickened intima and atheromatous plaques from the artery and is used when the disease is localized to a relatively small area. The establishment of a bypass channel in order to reduce the arterial insufficiency may be achieved by transplanting one end of another artery into the occluded artery below the site of obstruction or by an autogenous venous graft. The latter consists of the removal of a section of a vein (usually the saphenous), reversing it (because of the valves) to ensure flow in the right direction and attaching it to the affected artery above and below the occlusion. The surgeon may elect to resect the affected segment of the artery and replace it with an inert synthetic (Teflon or Dacron) graft. This type of graft is relatively porous and is eventually incorporated into host tissues. An intima develops within it fairly quickly as cells proliferate through the interstices and from the host intima of the artery at each end of the graft. A layer of fibrous tissue also develops on the exterior surface, reinforcing the tube.

The most frequent site of major vascular surgery for occlusive disease is the aorta and the iliac and femoral arteries.

Nursing responsibilities in the care of a patient having major vascular surgery include those applicable to most surgical patients, as cited in Chapter 10, as well as the following considerations.

Preoperative Preparation. Local preparation involves the shaving and cleansing of the skin from the nipple line to the knees. The patient's blood is typed and crossmatched in readiness for transfusions during and after the operation.

The patient and family are advised that he will be taken to the intensive care unit following surgery. To avoid unnecessary concern later, they are given some information about the nasogastric tube and the suction-siphonage decompression, intravenous infusion, urinary catheter drainage, cardiac monitoring and frequent checking of pulse and blood pressure that will follow surgery.

Postoperative Care. It is very important that the nurse understand the patient's disease process and the corrective surgical procedure used.

Observations. The nurse is alerted to the possible complications of thrombosis in the graft, hemorrhage and embolism. Heart action is constantly monitored so that any adverse change is quickly detected. Arterial pressures are recorded at frequent intervals.

Peripheral pulses in the lower limbs are checked frequently. Those in the feet are not usually detectable for 6 to 8 hours after surgery but, if they cannot be felt after this period, it is brought to the surgeon's attention. The pulses used are the femoral, popliteal, dorsalis pedis and posterior tibial. The femoral pulse may be felt in the middle of the groin, and the popliteal is located behind the knee. The dorsalis pedis pulse is found in the central region of the dorsum of the foot, and the posterior tibial behind the medial malleolus. With the latter two, it is helpful to mark the location on the skin so they can be readily checked. When only one limb has been affected, a comparison of the distal pulse is made with that of the unaffected limb.

Skin temperature and color are assessed and, where applicable, a comparison is made between the affected and unaffected limbs. Blanching or cyanosis and a lowering of the temperature in areas distal to the operative site must be reported quickly.

Restlessness, general pallor, a rapid pulse of decreased volume, increased respirations and a fall in arterial blood pressures associated with bleeding necessitate prompt medical attention.

The patient's level of consciousness, speech, strength of hand grip and ability to move his limbs are checked frequently. A disturbance in any one area may indicate a cerebral embolism.

Positioning. The revascularized area is usually elevated to a level above that of the heart to promote venous and lymphatic drainage and to prevent edema. The sudden increase in the blood supply may exceed the drainage capacity unless it is assisted by gravity.

When vascular grafts cross flexion lines, such as the groin and knee, precautions are taken to prevent flexion for 7 to 10 days. The patient is rolled to either side as though he were one straight rigid piece. It may be necessary to get him out of bed in a stiff legged fashion to stand and walk. An explanation to the patient of the need to avoid flexion is necessary. Padded splints or restraints may be necessary to ensure nonflexion for the required length of time. When flexion is permitted, it is for very limited periods.

Care of Affected Limb. The skin breaks down very easily, necessitating special protective measures against pressure and trauma. A padded bed cradle is used to relieve the limb of the weight of bedclothes, and the foot rests on sheepskin. The toes are separated by loose absorbent cotton to prevent maceration. The skin is bathed and handled gently. A light application of lanolin may be used to relieve dryness and scaling.

Coughing and Exercises. The patient is required to breathe deeply and cough hourly to improve pulmonary ventilation. The ankles and toes are flexed 10 times hourly to prevent venous stasis. These flexion exercises may have to be passive until the patient is sufficiently responsive to carry them out himself.

Fluids and Nutrition. The patient is sustained by intravenous infusions of 5 to 8 per cent glucose in water. Saline solutions are avoided with most patients with circulatory problems because of their tendency to retain the sodium.

The suction-siphonage decompression is discontinued and the nasogastric tube removed 2 or 3 days after surgery if there is no nausea or abdominal distention. The patient receives clear fluids at first and, if these are tolerated, the diet is gradually increased. High protein and vitamin C content contribute to the healing and resistance of affected tissues.

Instruction. In preparation for the patient's discharge from hospital, he is advised of his need to avoid sitting with his hips and knees flexed for long periods. If necessary, continued abstinence from smoking is stressed. He is made aware of ominous changes (pain, discoloration, cold, abrasions, edema) in his limbs that would necessitate prompt medical attention. The physician gives him some idea of when he may expect to resume former activities and makes an appointment for a follow-up visit to him or the clinic.

VENOUS DISORDERS

As stated earlier, interference with the flow of blood through the veins reduces venous return from the part, inducing congestion and edema, which interfere with normal cell function and eventually prevent a normal arterial volume from reaching the tissue cells. Common venous conditions are varicose veins, thrombophlebitis and phlebothrombosis.

Varicose Veins

When venous blood meets with increased resistance to its forward flow, the walls of the veins become dilated and tortuous, the valves become damaged and incompetent and the blood tends to pool and stagnate. The condition may be referred to as varicosities, or as varicose veins. The superficial veins of the lower extremities are most susceptible. Because of our upright position, the venous pressure in the lower limbs is increased by gravity. Other common sites of varicosities are the veins of the anal canal (hemorrhoids), spermatic veins (varicocele), esophageal veins, and the vulvar veins in pregnant women due to pressure from the enlarging uterus. Although resistance to the flow of blood is the main cause of varicosities, an inherited weakness of the valves of the veins is said to be a factor. Long periods of standing also predispose to the development of varicose veins in the lower extremities.

The overfull veins result in local edema of the tissues, crampy pains or aching, and a full, heavy feeling in the affected area. The congestion and edema in the tissues interfere with the normal supply of oxygen and nutrients reaching the cells, leading to fibrosing of subcutaneous tissues and, in some instances, necrosis of superficial tissue, producing what is referred to as a varicose ulcer. The affected area appears swollen and discolored, and the veins are seen as tortuous, bulbous protusions. These veins readily develop phlebitis, and occasionally the vessel wall ruptures, causing hemorrhage.

The test most frequently done for varicosities in the lower limbs is the Trendelenburg test. While the patient is in the horizontal position, the leg is elevated above the level of the pelvis until the superficial veins appear to be empty. The patient then stands, and the veins are observed as they fill. Normally they fill relatively slowly from below; in varicosities, the incompetent valves allow them to fill from above as well.

TREATMENT AND NURSING CARE OF A PATIENT WITH VARICOSE VEINS. Treatment may be conservative. The patient is instructed to avoid situations and factors that tend to increase the resistance to venous flow, to provide support to the veins and tissues by bandages or special hose, and to assist drainage by elevation of the limb at intervals.

If the varicosity is not extensive, the physician may inject a sclerosing agent (e.g., sodium morrhuate, sodium tetradecyl sulfate) into the veins. The varicosed segment becomes inflamed, scarred and thrombosed by the sclerosing agent. Antihistamines and the emergency drug tray are kept readily available in the event of a reaction.

With more severe varicosities in the lower limbs, surgical treatment in the form of ligation and stripping of the veins may be employed under local anesthesia. The affected vein is ligated above the varicosity, its connecting branches are severed and tied, and the vein removed. The venous blood then returns via the deep veins. The great saphenous vein is the one most frequently ligated and removed from the groin to the ankle. This necessitates several small horizontal incisions along the course of the vein. Elastic bandages are applied from the foot to the groin after the operation, and the foot of the bed is elevated. Beginning soon after operation, usually the day following surgery, the patient will be required to get up at regular intervals and walk about to prevent thrombosis. He may experience stiffness and some pain on movement and is given the necessary assistance and support. Early regular activity is very important and is explained to the patient in order to gain his cooperation.

In the postoperative period, the nurse observes the limb at regular, frequent intervals. The wound areas are checked for bleeding, and the distal parts and digits are examined for color, warmth and sensation, so that any disturbance in the circulation will receive early recognition. If there is bleeding, if the distal parts are cold or cyanosed, or the patient experiences numbness, pain or "pins and needles," the surgeon is informed promptly.

The patient is usually only hospitalized for a brief period of 2 to 3 days. He is advised as to how long to continue the alternating periods of rest and walking and the bandaging and elevation of the limbs. He is taught how to apply and care for the elastic bandages or stockings and is told when to return to the doctor or clinic. Since the superficial tissue continues to be tender and has less resistance, he is instructed to use precautions against injuries and abrasions. Long periods of standing are still to be avoided.

All patients with leg varicosities should avoid constricting clothing, such as round garters and tight girdles. They are also advised not to sit with their legs crossed. As with all circulatory conditions, obesity is to be avoided.

Varicose ulcers develop very easily with the circulatory stasis but are very slow to heal. The patient may have to rest in bed with the affected leg elevated or, if he remains active, an elastic bandage or stocking is applied in an effort to reduce the edema and congestion.

Moist antiseptic dressings may be applied to the ulcer, and when it is free of infection and necrotic tissue, the physician may enclose the foot and leg in a "boot" of Unna's paste. A mixture of gelatin, zinc oxide, glycerine and water is prepared and applied, along with bandages, to the foot and leg. The ulcer is protected by a thin sterile dressing and a layer of paste is then applied with a brush directly to the skin. This is followed with a layer of bandage and the two are alternated until three or four layers of each are applied. The "boot" provides even pressure to the veins and protects the ulcer. It dries to a firm support in approximately ½ hour, but the patient remains where the nurse may check the exposed distal portions of the limb for circulation and sensitivity. The toes should be warm, a normal color, sensitive to touch and comfortable. The boot is usually changed every 12 to 14 days until the ulcer heals. Large ulcers that are difficult to keep uninfected and are resistant to healing may be treated by skin grafts.

Thrombophlebitis and Phlebothrombosis

Phlebitis is an inflammation of the walls of a vein and may be caused by injury, prolonged pressure or infection. The endothelial lining is damaged and a thrombus develops at the site of inflammation, producing a secondary condition known as thrombophlebitis.

Phlebothrombosis is the formation of a blood clot within a vein with no associated inflammation and for this reason may be referred to as a bland or silent thrombosis. It is nearly always due to slowness or stasis of the circulation, such as occurs with prolonged bed rest, inactivity or pressure causing resistance to the venous blood flow. The serious factor in both phlebothrombosis and thrombophlebitis is the blood clot, which becomes a potential embolus. The silent thrombus or that associated with inflammation may be carried along in the blood stream and may eventually lodge in an artery to cause an embolism. Phlebitis and venous thrombosis may occur in any vein, but the most frequent site is the saphenous veins of the legs.

MANIFESTATIONS. Thrombophlebitis in superficial veins produces local pain, tenderness and swelling. The pain may vary from moderate discomfort on touching the limb to severe cramping. If the leg is involved, there may be calf pain during dorsiflexion of the foot (Homans' sign). Systemic symptoms such as fever, headache, and general malaise develop. If the vein is superficial, the overlying skin becomes red and hot. It may be taut and shiny.

With deep vein thrombosis, the process may be silent. No symptoms may be present until the thrombus is swept along and causes an embolism. In either phlebothrombosis or thrombophlebitis, the thrombus may become large enough to block the vein, causing severe congestion, edema and pain.

PREVENTION. Circulatory stasis in the lower limbs is the principal cause of phlebothrombosis, so efforts are directed toward avoiding prolonged inactivity and positions which favor its development. Passive movement and active exercises, especially of the lower limbs, and frequent change of position are used for patients who are inactive or confined to bed. Early ambulation is always to be encouraged when the condition permits. A dorsal recumbent position with the knees flexed and supported by a pillow or elevated Gatch frame is always contraindicated, since it promotes a venous stasis in the legs. Sitting for hours is discouraged because the legs are dependent and there is a risk of pressure on the veins in the popliteal region. Sitting should be altered with periods of walking around or lying down. The patient is instructed not to sit with his legs crossed, but to extend his legs, rotate his feet at the ankles, and flex and extend his toes five to ten times hourly when sitting for an extended period. Persons with leg varicosities are predisposed to phlebothrombosis and thrombophlebitis. Bandaging their lower limbs up to the groin with elastic bandages or stockings provides support to the veins and promotes venous return when they are nonambulatory.

TREATMENT AND NURSING CARE OF A PATIENT WITH THROMBOPHLEBITIS. When thrombophlebitis develops, care is directed toward preventing an embolism and relieving the congestion and edema of the tissues. The patient is confined to bed, and the affected limb immobilized in an elevated position to promote venous and lymphatic drainage. Active exercise and massage of the limb are contraindicated to avoid possible dislodging of the thrombus and ensuing embolism, but are applied to unaffected extremities. All strenuous activity, straining at stool, coughing and deep breathing are discouraged. The circulation of the affected extremity is checked frequently.

Local heat applications, moist or dry, may be prescribed. Precautions are taken to avoid burns since the skin is very susceptible to injury. A footboard or cradle is used to keep the weight of the bedclothes off the limbs.

Anticoagulant therapy is started as soon as the thrombosis is recognized (see p. 355). Rarely, if the patient is experiencing severe pain from vascular spasm, a sympathetic ganglionic block may be done to relax the veins. Analgesics are ordered for the relief of pain.

If the clot is dislodged, it will be carried along by the venous blood through the right side of the heart into the pulmonary circulation, where it is likely to cause a pulmonary embolism. Pain in the chest, dyspnea, coughing, hemoptysis, rapid weak pulse and pallor are reported promptly. A lung scan (see p. 405) may be done to confirm the diagnosis.

After 7 to 10 days, if the symptoms have subsided, ambulation is permitted. An elastic bandage or antiembolic stocking is applied before the patient gets out of bed. Activity is alternated with periods of rest. During the rest period the limb is elevated to the horizontal position or higher. The leg is examined for swelling and discoloration following ambulation and following a period of sitting. The patient may have to wear an elastic support indefinitely and must plan to avoid prolonged periods in which the limb is in the dependent position. The doctor may suggest that it is important that the limb be elevated above heart level for several brief periods through the day. This is more often necessary following a thrombosis of the larger deep veins. Before going home, the nurse teaches the patient the application and care of the bandages or elastic stockings. He is helped to understand the importance of the prescribed periods of elevation of the limbs and that he must be in the dorsal recumbent position to do this. The patient is also advised not to stand for long periods of time, to alternately flex and extend the legs frequently when sitting, to avoid constricting clothing, not to smoke and to report any further symptoms to his physician immediately. If discharged on anticoagulant medication, the purpose, dosage, times of administration and side effects are reviewed with the patient and, if possible, a member of his family or other significant person. The patient is followed closely in the clinic or the doctor's office for some time following the phlebothrombosis.

NURSING IN HYPERTENSION

Hypertension is a condition in which there is a sustained elevation of the arterial blood pressure. The level at which the normal blood pressure becomes abnormally high is not firmly established, but Jagger and Braunwald state that hypertension is present when an adult resting in the supine position has an arterial pressure of 160/95 mm. Hg or higher.[32] Julius classifies hypertension as an arterial pressure greater than 160/100 mm. Hg and borderline hypertension as pressures between 140/90 and 160/100 mm. Hg, allowing for the age of the individual.[33] The diastolic pressure is the more significant since it reflects the degree of peripheral resistance.

Hypertension is a serious condition; it is a common cause of heart failure and cerebral vascular hemorrhage. The sustained elevation in the arterial blood pressure seriously increases the work load of the heart and causes organic changes in the arteries. The myocardium hypertrophies in response to the increased demands, but there is not an adequate increase in the coronary blood supply and eventually some failure develops. The changes in the arterial walls involve thickening and sclerosis which alter the blood supply to tissues and ultimately may reduce their functional ability. The arteries may develop necrotic areas that weaken and tend to rupture under the high pressure of the blood, or they may thicken and narrow the lumen, predisposing to thrombosis. The areas of most serious damage are the heart, kidneys, brain and eyes, and these most often account for the symptoms seen in hypertensive patients. Cerebral hemorrhage (stroke) is a common sequela. Kidney function becomes impaired as the result of sclerosing hemorrhage or thrombosis of the renal arteries which destroys functional tissue. Retinal hemorrhages and edema of the optic disc occur frequently, resulting in degenerative changes in the eyes. Thickening and sclerosis of the coronary arteries may cause ischemic heart disease; the patient may experience angina pectoris or suffer a coronary occlusion in addition to developing the myocardial hypertrophy previously mentioned.

[32]Paul I. Jagger and Eugene Braunwald: "Hypertensive Vascular Disease." In Maxwell M. Wintrobe, et al. (Eds.): Harrison's Principles of Internal Medicine, 8th ed. New York, McGraw-Hill, 1978.

[33]Steve Julius: "Borderline Hypertension: An Overview." Med. Clin. North Am., Vol. 61, No. 3 (May 1977), pp. 495–509.

TYPES OF HYPERTENSION

Hypertension may be classified as primary (essential) or secondary. Approximately 90 per cent of the persons with hypertensive disease are said to have essential hypertension; the remaining 10 per cent have secondary hypertension.[34]

Primary or Idiopathic Hypertension

Primary hypertension is most frequently referred to as essential or idiopathic hypertension. The cause of this type of hypertensive disease is not known; no initial disturbance in the areas commonly associated with secondary hypertension has been established. It may cause cardiac or kidney disease but is not preceded by either. Heredity is though to be a factor, since most persons with the condition have a history of a parent or grandparent having had it. There is a higher incidence in females, and the majority of hypertensive women are overweight.

Essential hypertension may be referred to as benign or malignant. The term benign, rarely used, is applied to essential hypertension that persists over 10 to 20 years without causing serious problems. Malignant indicates a rapidly progressive and serious condition. The patient develops kidney and heart complications and other sequelae very quickly and survives only a few months to 1 or 2 years at the most.

Essential hypertension may be classified according to the degree of severity of the disease. The numerical grading is based on changes in the ocular fundi, the response to treatment, the amount of cardiac hypertrophy and the effect on kidney function. Grades 3 and 4 are considered serious, and the patient with a Grade 4 hypertension as well as papilledema may be said to have a malignant hypertension.

Secondary Hypertension

Causes of secondary hypertension include the following:

COARCTATION OF THE AORTA. Obviously, a congenital stricture of an area of the aorta increases the resistance to the flow of blood through the vessel, causing an increase in the arterial pressure behind the coarctation. This may be corrected by surgery.

DISTURBANCES WITHIN THE CENTRAL NERVOUS SYSTEM. Interference with the vasomotor center or with pathways from the center may result in an increased vasoconstriction and peripheral resistance. Space-occupying lesions, such as a brain tumor, increased intracranial pressure, a cerebral thrombosis or poliomyelitis are examples of conditions which may lead to the malfunctioning of the vasomotor center or pathway.

ENDOCRINE DISTURBANCE. A pheochromocytoma is a tumor of the adrenal medulla. Tumors may be single or multiple. The tumor cells secrete epinephrine in the same way as normal medullary cells, which produces vasoconstriction and an increased cardiac output with a corresponding elevation in arterial blood pressure. Removal of the tumor restores a normal blood pressure.

An increased output of aldosterone by the cortex of the adrenal glands may also be responsible for hypertension. The increased secretion may be idiopathic or may be due to a tumor. Aldosterone increases the reabsorption of sodium by the kidney, leading to water retention and an expansion of the intravascular volume, increasing the arterial blood pressure. It is suggested that aldosterone may also have a direct vasoconstricting effect. A general increase in the secretion of all of the adrenocorticoids causes Cushing's disease, which is also accompanied by hypertension.

ORAL CONTRACEPTIVES. Some women taking oral contraceptives may develop hypertension. It is thought that the estrogen component of the pills may be responsible by stimulating hepatic synthesis of angiotensinogen which leads to increased amounts of angiotensin.[35] The contraceptive agents are discontinued for 6 months and the blood pressure usually returns to normal.

KIDNEY DISTURBANCE Any condition which reduces the blood flow through the kidneys or destroys renal functional tissue causes hypertension. Examples of such conditions are sclerotic changes or stenosis of a renal artery, nephritis and polycystic disease. The ischemic kidney reacts by secreting a proteolytic enzyme called renin (Table 13–8).

---

[34]Guyton, op cit., p. 289.

[35]Hurst, op. cit., p. 1504.

TABLE 13-8 SCHEMATIC OUTLINE OF THE RENIN-HYPERTENSION MECHANISM*

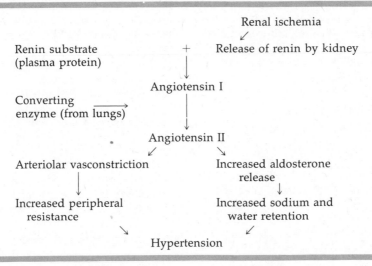

*Arthur C. Guyton: Textbook of Medical Physiology, 5th ed. Philadelphia, W. B. Saunders, 1976, p. 276.

In the blood stream, renin acts upon a plasma protein to produce angiotensin I which is then converted to angiotensin II by another enzyme. This angiotensin II causes widespread vasoconstriction of the arterioles and increased peripheral resistance, leading to an elevation in arterial blood pressure. Angiotensin II is also alleged to increase the secretion of aldosterone by the adrenal glands[36] which, as previously cited, increases the blood pressure through its influence on sodium and water retention.

TOXEMIA OF PREGNANCY. Hypertension is a feature of toxemia in pregnancy in which there is renal involvement.

MANIFESTATIONS OF HYPERTENSION

A person may have an abnormally high arterial blood pressure for a long period without symptoms. The condition is often discovered on a routine physical examination. Some persons may exhibit a higher than average normal blood pressure and, on investigation, may produce a higher than average response to stimuli that normally elicit an increase in blood pressure. The stimuli under which persons are observed are generally cold and exertion. Those who manifest an excessively

high response are said to have vascular hyperactivity and are most likely headed for hypertension.

Those who do experience symptoms may complain of a throbbing occipital headache, especially on wakening in the morning, dizziness, visual disturbance, fatigue, irritability and restlessness, vomiting, emotional instability or epistaxis. Patients with pheochromocytoma often have pounding headaches, excessive sweating and flushing of the face, and are often under the age of 30. Later, more serious manifestations appear as the heart, kidneys, brain or eyes become damaged by the persisting hypertension. The person who manifests even a slight elevation above the normal in both systolic and diastolic blood pressures undergoes careful investigation to determine a possible primary cause.

DIAGNOSTIC PROCEDURES

Several systems may be investigated in an attempt to identify the cause of the hypertension. The renal and endocrine systems are the more important of these.

Renal System

Blood levels of creatinine and urea nitrogen (BUN) are determined. Twenty-four-hour urine collections may be ordered and exam-

---

[36]Guyton, op. cit., pp. 469–470.

ined for proteins, creatinine and electrolytes. When the renal system is damaged proteins not normally present may leak into the urine. An intravenous pyelogram may be ordered in which serial 1-minute films are taken. The differential secretion rates of the two kidneys are studied. Minor differences may be apparent in rapid films that might go unrecognized in the standard 5-, 10- and 20-minute films. A renal scan and renal arteriograms are occasionally ordered.

Endocrine System

ADRENAL SECRETIONS. A 24-hour urine collection is tested for levels of 17-ketosteroids and 17-hydroxycorticosteroids. The former is the excreted form of the androgen hormone and the latter is the product of the breakdown of the hormones cortisone and hydrocortisone. A more precise screening test for Cushing's syndrome is the dexamethasone suppression test. When dexamethasone 0.5 mg. is given every 6 hours for 48 hours to persons with normally functioning adrenal glands, adrenal corticoid production is suppressed, as evidenced by decreased amounts of cortisol in the urine. This does not occur in persons with bilateral adrenal hyperplasia.

The 24-hour urine collection is also tested for electrolytes. With increased mineralocorticoid production, sodium excretion is decreased while potassium excretion is increased. Tests for sugar, serum cortisol and serum electrolytes are also done. With Cushing's disease, the blood sugar and cortisol levels are elevated. Serum potassium will be below normal.

TEST FOR PHEOCHROMOCYTOMA. The urine is collected over 24 hours and examined for the presence of vanillylmandelic acid (VMA). The latter is a metabolite of catecholamines which is secreted in the urine. In some institutions, the patient is put on a special diet for 3 days before the test and foods such as bananas, coffee, tea, chocolate and vanilla are excluded. The urine is collected in a bottle containing hydrochloric acid as a preservative and is refrigerated during the collection period. When a tumor of an adrenal gland is present the level of vanillylmandelic acid in the urine is elevated above normal.

Occasionally, a Regitine test is ordered. The arterial blood pressure is recorded before the test. Phentolamine (Regitine) 5 mg., an adrenergic blocking drug, is given intravenously. The blood pressure is then checked every 30 seconds for 5 to 10 minutes. The test is considered positive for pheochromocytoma if the fall in systolic pressure is greater than 35 mm. Hg and the diastolic pressure falls more than 25 mm. Hg, and if they remain decreased for more than 3 to 4 minutes.

TREATMENT AND NURSING CARE OF HYPERTENSION

If the hypertension is secondary, treatment is directed toward correcting the primary condition. In essential hypertension, treatment is directed at: (1) lowering the blood pressure in an effort to prevent serious complications; and (2) having the patient adjust his life to reduce the demands on the cardiovascular system and kidneys. The treatment depends on the height and constancy of the blood pressure and the signs and symptoms of impaired function in vulnerable organs. The patient with mild hypertension may simply be advised to reduce his weight to normal, avoid overwork and overexcitement, and decrease his salt intake to a prescribed level in order to prevent the development of hypertension.

Persons with more severe hypertension may receive a drug to lower the blood pressure and are likely to be more restricted in activities and diet. The patients seen in the hospital are usually those with Grade 3 or Grade 4 hypertension and those with cardiac, cerebral or renal complications.

OBSERVATIONS. The blood pressure is determined at regular intervals with the patient in the same position each time. The doctor may request several casual readings at times when the patient is not anticipating the recording. A record of the pressure each morning before the patient moves about may also be necessary and, in some instances, there may be a request to obtain a reading while the patient is asleep. The nurse should know the patient's activities or experiences for the period preceding any reading. If frequent recordings cause anxiety, this is brought to the physician's attention. Fluid balance is noted, as a positive balance may point to either renal or cardiac failure. The patient's weight is recorded daily, either to indicate progress to his normal weight level or to indicate possible sodium and water retention. The pulse rate and volume are recorded at least twice daily, and the respirations are observed for any signs of dyspnea, particularly on exertion. Any complaint of headache or pain is reported.

REST AND ACTIVITY. The amount of rest needed, and whether it must be bed rest or not, will depend on the severity of the hypertension. Moderately severe hypertensive patients may require a period of bed rest. A sedative such as amobarbital (Amytal) or phenobarbital may be prescribed to encourage relaxation and rest. When activity is permitted, it is graduated and the patient's blood pressure response noted. Moderate exercise, such as walking and golfing, is encouraged once the blood pressure has been somewhat lowered, and as long as there is no dyspnea nor undue fatigue.

DIET. The caloric intake is reduced to 1000 to 1200 calories daily until the weight is normal; then a maintenance diet is established. The sodium intake is usually reduced, and the degree of restriction depends upon the severity of the patient's disease. If the salt restriction is prolonged, one should be alert for sodium deficiency, which is manifested by muscular cramps, weakness, nausea and vomiting. The amount of coffee, tea and alcohol is usually limited with most hypertensive persons.

ELIMINATION. Constipation is to be avoided since straining raises the blood pressure and could cause the rupture of a damaged sclerosed artery.

MEDICATIONS. Drugs comprise the main treatment of essential hypertension at present. Drug therapy is directed toward decreasing peripheral vascular resistance by vasodilation or by adrenergic blockade, decreasing the blood volume, or decreasing cardiac output. Drugs commonly used are diuretics, vasodilators, postganglionic blocking agents and beta-adrenergic blocking agents.

DIURETICS. A thiazide diuretic or furosemide is frequently given to hypertensive patients to produce a negative sodium and water balance. It may be given in conjunction with a sodium restricted diet and a hypotensive drug. If adminstration is prolonged, the patient is observed for possible potassium deficiency and skin rash. As with the administration of any diuretic, the urinary output is measured and the patient is weighed daily during hospitalization (see p. 335).

VASODILATORS

Hydralazine (Apresoline). This drug acts primarily on the arterioles, rather than on the nervous system, causing smooth muscle relaxation. Peripheral vascular resistance is lowered and arterial pressure falls. It may cause sodium and water retention and is much more effective when combined with a diuretic. In addition, it can cause reflex tachycardia and therefore is used cautiously for patients with angina. This reflex increase in sympathetic discharge may be offset by combining it with a drug which blocks the sympathetic nervous system, such as propranolol. Toxic reactions are manifested by headache, dizziness, rapid pulse, palpitation, precordial pain and shortness of breath. Large doses, in excess of 200 mg. daily, have been associated with a lupus erythematosus-like syndrome.

Diazoxide (Hyperstat). This is a fast-acting vasodilator used for the emergency treatment of hypertensive crisis. It is usually given as a 300 mg. bolus within 15 to 30 seconds and the effect lasts approximately 5 to 8 hours. The typical response is an immediate and precipitous fall in blood pressure, which comes back up a little in the next few minutes. To prevent this rapid drop in pressure, which may compromise the blood flow to the heart and brain in patients with atherosclerotic coronary and cerebral disease, diazoxide may be given by slow infusion over 10 to 30 minutes or smaller boluses (75 to 100 mg., I.V.) may be given every 5 to 10 minutes. Diazoxide also causes sodium and water retention and is usually given with furosemide (intravenously) to counteract these effects. Reflex tachycardia similar to that observed with hydralazine can be controlled with the use of parenteral propranolol (Inderal). It is used with caution for patients with angina. Extravasation must be avoided.

Sodium Nitroprusside. This drug is also used to treat hypertensive crisis. The hypotensive response to this potent vasodilator occurs within seconds, so blood pressure must be monitored very frequently. Fifty to 100 mg. is added to 1000 ml. of 5 per cent glucose in water. The drug is started as a continuous drip at the rate of 10 drops per minute. The concentration and rate of administration is then adjusted to maintain the desired level of blood pressure. Adverse effects include nausea, vomiting, muscle twitching, apprehension and sweating. Since sodium nitroprusside is air- and light-sensitive, the infusion bottle should be protected from light during administration. A fresh solution should be prepared after 4 hours.

PERIPHERAL SYMPATHETIC BLOCKERS

Reserpine (Serpasil). These preparations deplete the stores of norepinephrine at nerve endings. They are given orally in the treatment of patients with mild to moderate hypertension. When given parenterally they also directly affect vascular smooth muscle, causing vasodilation. For this reason they are sometimes given intravenously in hypertensive emergencies. Undesirable side effects include nasal stuffiness, flushing of the skin, increased gastrointestinal motility, impairment of sexual function, dizziness, drowsiness and mental depression. These drugs should not be given to patients with a history of depression or mental illness. Some preparations are combined with diuretics (Serpasil-Esidrix and Hydropres).

Guanethidine (Ismelin). This agent has generally been reserved for severe or resistant hypertension, although it may be useful in selected patients with less severe disease. It acts by inhibiting the release of norepinephrine at sympathetic neuroeffector junctions and by depleting tissue stores of catecholamines. The patient should be warned against activities that cause vasodilation, such as taking hot showers, drinking liquor and long exposure to the sun, as they may result in severe orthostatic hypotension. Patients are advised to avoid sudden changes in posture. Ismelin has a long period of onset of action (1 week) and a long duration of action. When the patient is being changed from this to another antihypertensive drug, a few days without Ismelin are advisable before he is started on the new drug.

Side effects are dose-related and include diarrhea (often severe) and sexual problems in men, such as inhibition of ejaculation or retrograde ejaculation, as well as orthostatic hypotension. Like other antihypertensive agents, it is more effective when combined with a diuretic.

Bethanidine (Esbaloid). This drug acts similarly to guanethidine and has comparable potency and produces similar side effects, except that it causes less diarrhea. The main difference is its shorter duration of action, 8 to 12 hours, so that alteration of dosage is easier.

Debrisoquine (Declinax). This drug is another adrenergic neuronal blocker with a shorter duration of action than guanethidine.

Prazosin (Minipress). Although originally considered to be a vasodilator, prazosin acts as an alpha-adrenergic blocker. It is moderately effective in lowering blood pressure in hypertensive patients. The drug seems equivalent to alpha-methyldopa in antihypertensive potency and side effects. Prazosin is frequently combined with beta-blockers and diuretics. To prevent profound hypotension and collapse, the initial dose should not exceed 0.5 mg., preferably taken at bedtime. Other side effects include lassitude, edema, anticholinergic effects and CNS symptoms (headache, drowsiness and nervousness).

CENTRALLY ACTING VASODILATORS

Alpha-methyldopa. It is currently believed that this drug lowers blood pressure primarily by acting on vasomotor centers in the brain, resulting in decreased sympathetic outflow. Peripheral sympathetic inhibition may add to the cardiovascular effect of the drug. It is used in the treatment of patients with mild to moderate hypertension. The most common side effects are drowsiness and fatigue. In approximately 20 per cent of patients it causes a positive reaction to the direct Coombs' test.[37] Occasionally patients develop hemolytic anemia and hepatitis. The hepatic damage seen with alpha-methyldopa is generally preceded by a flu-like syndrome characterized by chills, fever and muscle aches. If these occur, the drug should be discontinued immediately. Some patients may experience an inability to concentrate and a marked slowing of mental performance.

---

[37]Thorn, G. W., et al. (Eds.): Harrison's Principles of Internal Medicine, 8th ed. New York, McGraw-Hill, 1977, p. 1242.

Clonidine (Catapres). Clonidine is a centrally acting antihypertensive agent. It reduces blood pressure by inhibiting the outflow of adrenergic impulses, resulting in decreased sympathetic stimulation of the heart, kidney and peripheral vasculature. It is effective in moderate to severe hypertension. The onset of action is usually within 30 minutes and maximum effect occurs within 2 to 4 hours. The most frequent side effects associated with clonidine are sedation and dry mouth. These usually disappear as the patient develops a tolerance for the drug. An unusual reaction attributed to clonidine is rebound hypertension following abrupt discontinance of the drug. Patients should be warned against sudden withdrawal of the drug. Dosage reduction is gradual over a period of a week.

BETA-ADRENERGIC BLOCKING AGENT

Propranolol(Inderal). Propranolol works directly on the heart to slow the rate and force of contraction. It is also thought to interfere with renin release from the kidney and to have a central mechanism of action. It may be combined with other agents in the treatment of hypertensive patients (see p. 308).

SEDATIVES. Frequent small doses of a tranquilizing drug may be ordered for the hypertensive patient to promote relaxation and rest.

PRECAUTIONS. When a patient is receiving a hypotensive drug, he must be observed for the particular side effects that are associated with the drug he is receiving. If they occur, the physician is informed promptly. Most of these drugs can cause orthostatic hypotension — a sudden fall of blood pressure to below the normal when a patient assumes the upright position. The nurse instructs the patient to move slowly and to assume the recumbent position on the first feeling of faintness. When getting up, he should sit on the side of the bed for a few minutes before standing.

The blood pressure is recorded at frequent intervals as indicated by the physician. The nurse may be requested to take the blood pressure with the patient standing, especially if the patient is on ganglionic blocking drugs. It may be necessary to take the blood pressure before each dose of the drug. The level frequently determines whether the drug should be given and in what dosage. The antihypertensive drug and the dosage are prescribed individually; one drug may be more effective than another with one patient, and the effective dosage will often vary from one patient to another.

If the patient develops a fever or a spell of hot weather occurs, the dosage of the antihypertensive drug may have to be reduced, since a higher temperature seems to intensify the effect of the drug.

HYPERTENSIVE CRISIS

Hypertensive crisis is a syndrome characterized by a sudden elevation of the blood pressure accompanied by severe headache, nausea, vomiting, visual disturbances, transient neurological disturbances, disorientation and drowsiness which may progress to coma. The retinopathy seen in malignant hypertension is often present. The blood pressure is extremely high, often as great as 250/150 mm. Hg. Rarely, hypertensive encephalopathy occurs. This is associated with cerebrovascular spasm and ensuing ischemia, edema and possibly thrombosis. It constitutes a medical emergency requiring prompt treatment.

Immediate treatment for the patient in a hypertensive crisis includes the intravenous administration of diazoxide or sodium nitroprusside and furosemide. Because of the potency of the medications being used, the patient is observed for sudden hypotension. The blood pressure is monitored every 5 to 10 minutes or more often. Anticonvulsant medications or sedatives may be required. The patient is maintained on bed rest. The pulse, respirations and neurological signs are checked every 5 to 10 minutes and the intake and output of fluids measured. It is important to maintain a calm, quiet environment.

References

Books

Andreoli, K. G., et al.: Comprehensive Cardiac Care. St. Louis, C. V. Mosby, 1975.

Beeson, Paul B., and McDermott, Walsh (Eds.): Textbook of Medicine, 15th ed. Philadelphia, W. B. Saunders, 1979.

Beland, I. L., and Passos, J. Y.: Clinical Nursing: Pathophysiological and Psychosocial Approaches, 3rd ed. New York, MacMillan, 1975, pp. 533–686.

Brobeck, J. R. (Ed.): Best and Taylor's Physiological Basis of Medical Practice, 9th ed. Baltimore, Williams and Wilkins, 1973. Section 3, Chapters 1–11.

Burton, A. C.: Physiology and Biophysics of the Circulation, 2nd ed. Chicago, Year Book Medical Publishers, 1972.

Ganong, William F.: Review of Medical Physiology, 7th ed. Los Altos, Cal., Lange, 1975. Chapters 28–33.

Goodman, Louis S., and Gilman, Arthur (Eds.): The Pharmacological Basis of Therapeutics, 5th ed. New York, MacMillan, 1975.

Guyton, Arthur C.: Textbook of Medical Physiology, 5th ed. Philadelphia, W. B. Saunders, 1976. Chapters 13–29.

Hurst, J. Willis, et al. (Eds.): The Heart, Arteries and Veins, 3rd ed. New York, Blakiston Division, McGraw-Hill, 1974.

Lancour, J., and Dressler, D.: Nursing Care of the Cardiovascular Surgical Patient. Milwaukee, St. Luke's Hospital, 1975.

Levine, Donald, et al.: Chest Pain: An Integrated Diagnostic Approach. Philadelphia, Lea and Febiger, 1977.

Marriott, Henry J. L.: Practical Electrocardiography, 6th ed. Baltimore, Williams and Wilkins, 1977.

Melmon, K., and Morelli, H. (Eds.): Clinical Pharmacology. New York, MacMillan, 1972, pp. 142–261.

Phillips, Raymond E., and Feeney, Mary K.: The Cardiac Rhythms: A Systematic Approach to Interpretation. Philadelphia, W. B. Saunders, 1973.

Ravel, R.: Clinical Laboratory Medicine: Application of Laboratory Data, 2nd ed. Chicago, Year Book Medical Publishers, 1973.

Redmond, Barbara K.: The Process of Patient Teaching in Nursing. St. Louis, C. V. Mosby, 1976.

Rushmer, Robert F.: Cardiovascular Dynamics, 4th ed. Philadelphia, W. B. Saunders, 1976.

Sanderson, Richard G. (Ed.): The Cardiac Patient. Philadelphia, W. B. Saunders, 1972.

Tana, J., and Judge, R. D.: Physical Appraisal Methods in Nursing Practice. Boston, Little, Brown, 1975.

Thorn, G. W., et al. (Eds.): Harrison's Principles of Internal Medicine, 8th ed. New York, McGraw-Hill, 1977.

Periodicals

Cardiac

Adler, J., and Brown, G. E.: "Patient Assessment: Abnormalities of the Heartbeat — Programmed Instruction." Am. J. Nurs., Vol. 77, No. 4 (April 1977), pp. P.I. 1–26.

American Heart Association: Cardiopulmonary Resuscitation — Emergency Cardiac Care. Critical Performance Rationale. Pamphlet, New York, 1975.

Aranda, Juan M., et al.: "His Bundle Recordings: Their Contribution to the Understanding of Human Electrophysiology." Heart Lung, Vol. 5, No. 6 (Nov.-Dec. 1976), pp. 907–918.

Barold, S. Serge: "Modern Concepts of Cardiac Pacing." Heart Lung, Vol. 2, No. 2 (March-April 1973), pp. 238–252.

Barstow, Ruth E.: "Nursing Care of Patients with Pacemakers." Cardiovasc. Nurs., Vol. 8, No. 2 (March-April 1972), pp. 7–10.

Biddle, Theodore L., and Yu, Paul N.: "Understand and Treating Arrhythmias Accompanying Myocardial Infarction." Nurs. Clin. North Am., Vol. 7, No. 3 (Sept. 1972), pp. 481–490.

Blomberg, David J., et al.: "Creatinine Kinase Isoenzymes: Predictive Value in the Early Diagnosis of Myocardial Infarction." Am. J. Med., Vol. 59, No. 4 (Oct. 1975), pp. 464–469.

Bolognini, V.: "The Swan-Ganz Pulmonary Artery Catheter: Implications for Nursing." Heart Lung, Vol. 3, No. 6 (Nov.-Dec. 1974), pp. 976–981.

Brammel, H. L., and Niccoli, Arlene: "A Physiologic Approach to Cardiac Rehabilitation." Nurs. Clin. North Am., Vol. 11, No. 2 (June 1976), pp. 223–236.

———.: A Physiologic Approach to Cardiac Rehabilitation." Nurs. Clin. North Amer., Vol. 11, No. 2 (June 1976), pp. 237–250.

Brogan, Mary R.: "Nursing Care of the Patient Experiencing Cardiac Surgery for Coronary Artery Disease." Nurs. Clin. North Am., Vol. 7, No. 3 (Sept. 1972), pp. 517–527.

Bunke, Betty: "Respiratory Function after Acute Myocardial Infarction: Implications for Nursing." Cardiovasc. Nurs., Vol. 9, No. 3 (May-June 1973), pp. 13–18.

Canadian Heart Foundation: Cardiopulmonary Resuscitation (CPR). Part I, Recommended Standards for Basic Life Support.

Castellanos, Agustin, et al.: "Didactic Vectorcardiography: General Concepts." Heart Lung, Vol. 4, No. 5 (Sept.-Oct. 1975), pp. 697–723.

Clark, M. C.: "Chest Pain." Heart Lung, Vol. 4, No. 6 (Nov.-Dec. 1975), pp. 956–962.

Clark, N. F.: "Pump Failure." Nurs. Clin. North Am., Vol. 7, No. 3 (Sept. 1972), pp. 529–539.

Coats, K.: "Non-Invasive Cardiac Diagnostic Procedures." Am. J. Nurs., Vol. 75, No. 11 (Nov. 1975), pp. 1980–1985.

———.: "Techniques in Cardiac Diagnosis." Nurs. Clin. North Am., Vol. 11, No. 2 (June 1976), pp. 259–269.

Cortes, Tara Siegal: "Pacemakers Today: All About Various Kinds, Nursing Implications and Counselling Problems." Nurs. '74, Vol. 4, No. 2 (Feb. 1974), pp. 22–29.

Cullard, George M., and Jude, James R.: "Cardiopulmonary Resuscitation in the Cardiac Care Unit." Nurs. Clin. North Am., Vol. 7, No. 3 (Sept. 1972), pp. 573–585.

Delaney, M. T.: "Examining the Chest." Nurs. '75, Vol. 5, No. 9 (Sept. 1975), pp. 41–46.

Diethrieh, Edward B.: "Aortocoronary Bypass — Classification and Results." Heart Lung, Vol. 4, No. 3 (May-June 1975), pp. 381–389.

Edwards, M., and Payton, V.: "Cardiac Catheterization: Technique and Teaching." Nurs. Clin. North Am., Vol. 11, No. 2 (June 1976), pp. 271–281.

Ehrlich, Ira B.: "Patient Selection and Pre-Operative Evaluation." Heart Lung, Vol. 4, No. 3 (May-June 1975), pp. 373–380.

Finnigan, M., and Warm, J.: "Ventilatory Considerations in Cardiac Patients." Nurs. Clin. North Am., Vol. 7, No. 3 (Sept. 1972), pp. 541–548.

Foster, S., and Andreoli, K. G.: "Behaviour Following Acute Myocardial Infarction." Am. J. Nurs., Vol. 70, No. 11 (Nov. 1970), pp. 2344–2348.

Garrity, Thomas F., and Klein, Robert F.: "Emotional Responses and Clinical Severity as Early Determinants of Six-Month Mortality After Myocardial Infarction." Heart Lung, Vol. 4, No. 5 (Sept.-Oct. 1975), pp. 730–737.

Gentry, W. D., and Haney, T.: "Emotional and Behavioral Reaction to Acute Myocardial Infarction." Heart Lung, Vol. 4, No. 5 (Sept.-Oct. 1975), pp. 738–745.

Gernert, C. F., and Schwartz, S.: "Pulmonary Artery Catheterization." Am. J. Nurs., Vol. 73, No. 7 (July 1973), pp. 1182–1185.

Gordon, M.: "Assessing Activity Tolerance." Am. J. Nurs., Vol. 76, No. 1 (Jan. 1976), pp. 72–75.

Green, Andrew W.: "Sexual Activity and the Post-Myocardial Infarction Patient." Am. Heart J., Vol. 89, No. 2 (Feb. 1975), pp. 246–252.

Harding, A. Laurie, and Morefield, Mary-Ann: "Group Intervention for Wives of Myocardial Infarction Patients." Nurs. Clin. North Am., Vol. 11, No. 2 (June 1976), pp. 339–347.

Jarvis, Dorothy: "Open-Heart Surgery: Patients' Perceptions of Care." Am. J. Nurs., Vol. 70, No. 12 (Dec. 1970), pp. 2591–2593.

Johnston, Barbara L., et al.: "Eight Steps to Inpatient Cardiac Rehabilitation. The Team Effort — Methodology and Preliminary Results." Heart Lung, Vol. 5, No. 1 (Jan.-Feb. 1976), pp. 97–111.

Kay, Gloria, and Kearns, Patricia: "Monitoring Central Venous Pressure: Principles, Procedures and Problems." Can. Nurs., Vol. 72, No. 7 (July 1976), pp. 15–17.

Kimball, Chase Patterson: "Psychological Responses to Open-Heart Surgery." A.O.R.N.J., Vol. II, No. 2 (Feb. 1970), pp. 75–84.

Kise, Monica Swartz: "Drug Therapy in the Treatment of Angina Pectoris." Nurs. Clin. North Am., Vol. 11, No. 2 (June 1976), pp. 309–317.

Klein, Robert F., et al.: "Transfer from a Coronary Care Unit." Arch. Int. Med., Vol. 122, No. 2 (Aug. 1968), pp. 102–106.

Lawson, B. N.: "Clinical Assessment of Cardiac Patients in Acute Care Facilities." Nurs. Clin. North Am., Vol. 7, No. 3 (Sept. 1972), pp. 431–444.

Lehman, Sister J.: "Auscultation of Heart Sounds." Am. J. Nurs., Vol. 72, No. 7 (July 1972), pp. 1242–1246.

Lemberg, Louis, and Hamer, Susan: "Arrhythmias Complicating an Acute Myocardial Infarction: A Self-Teaching Program." Heart Lung, Vol. 5, No. 4 (July-Aug. 1976), pp. 576–584.

Levitt, Barrie, et al.: "The Clinical Pharmacology of Antiarrhythmic Drugs, Part I. Lidocaine and Procainamide." Cardiovasc. Nurs., Vol. 10, No. 5 (Sept.-Oct. 1974), pp. 23–26.

———.: "The Clinical Pharmacology of Antiarrhythmic Drugs, Part II. Quinidine, Propanolol, Diphenylhydantoin and Bretylium." Cardiovasc. Nurs., Vol. 10, No. 6 (Nov.-Dec. 1974), pp. 27–31.

Long, Madeline, et al.: "Cardiopulmonary Bypass." Am. J. Nurs., Vol. 74, No. 5 (May 1974), pp. 860–867.

Mannaring, Mary: "What Patients Need to Know About Pacemakers." Am. J. Nurs., Vol. 77, No. 5 (May 1977), pp. 825–830.

Mechner, F., and Brown, G. E.: "Patient Assessment: Examination of the Heart and Great Vessels." Am. J. Nurs., Vol. 76, No. 11 (Nov. 1976), pp. 1–24.

————.: "Patient Assessment: Auscultation of the Heart — Programmed Instruction." Am. J. Nurs., Vol. 77, No. 2 (Feb. 1977), pp. 1–24.

Miller, Richard, et al.: "Procainamide: Reappraisal of an Old Antiarrhythmia Drug." Heart Lung, Vol. 2, No. 2 (March-Apr. 1973), pp. 277–283.

Mozersky, D. J., et al.: "Ultrasonic Arteriography." Arch. Surg., Vol. 103, No. 6 (Dec. 1971), pp. 663–667.

Naagar, C. L.: "Ultrasound in Medical Diagnosis. Part I, Applications in Cardiology." Heart Lung, Vol. 5, No. 6 (Nov.-Dec. 1976), pp. 895–906.

Powell, A. H.: "Physical Assessment of the Patient with Cardiac Disease." Nurs. Clin. North Am., Vol. 11, No. 2 (June 1976), pp. 251–257.

Rasmussen, Susan, et al.: "The Pharmacology and Clinical Use of Digitalis." Cardiovasc. Nurs., Vol. 11, No. 2 (Jan.-Feb. 1975), pp. 23–28.

Roberts, Robert, et al.: "An Improved Basis for Enzymatic Estimation of Infarct Size." Circulation, Vol. 52, (Nov. 1975), pp. 743–754.

Romhilt, D. W., and Fowler, N. O.: "Physical Signs in Acute Myocardial Infarction." Heart Lung, Vol. 2, No. 1 (Jan.-Feb. 1973), pp. 74–80.

Shapiro, Ruth Mayer: "Anticoagulant Therapy." Am. J. Nurs., Vol. 74, No. 3 (March 1974), pp. 439–443.

Smith, A. M., et al.: "Serum Enzymes in Myocardial Infarction." Am. J. Nurs., Vol. 73, No. 2 (Feb. 1973), pp. 277–279.

Stone, N. J., and Levy, R. I.: "Hyperlipoproteinemia and Coronary Heart Disease." Prog. Cardiovasc. Dis., Vol. 14, No. 4 (Jan. 1972), pp. 341–356.

Sweetwood, Hannelore: "Patients with Pacemakers." Nurs. '77, Vol. 7, No. 3 (March 1977), pp. 44–51. 51.

Tanner, G.: "Heart Failure in the Myocardial Infarction Patient." Am. J. Nurs., Vol. 77, No. 2 (Feb. 1977), pp. 230–234.

Vlodaver, Z., and Edwards, J.: "Pathology of Coronary Atherosclerosis." Prog. Cardiovasc. Dis., Vol. 14, No. 3 (Nov. 1971), pp. 256–272.

Walton, Christine, and Hammond, Betsy: "Angina — Teaching Your Patient How to Prevent Recurrent Attacks." Nurs. '78, Vol. 8, No. 2 (Feb. 1978), pp. 32–38.

Warkentin, Eleanor: "Programmed Learning: Cardiac Depressants." Can. Nurs., Vol. 73, No. 5 (May 1977), pp. 30–37.

Watts, Rosalyn Jones: "Sexuality and the Middle-Aged Cardiac Patient." Nurs. Clin. North Am., Vol. 11, No. 2 (June 1976), pp. 349–359.

Waxler, R.: "The Patient with Congestive Heart Failure." Nurs. Clin. North Am., Vol. 11, No. 2 (June 1976), pp. 297–308.

Westfall, Una Elizabeth: "Electrical and Mechanical Events in the Cardiac Cycle." Am. J. Nurs., Vol. 76, No. 2 (Feb. 1976), pp. 231–235.

Winslow, Elizabeth H.: "The Role of the Nurse in Patient Education, Focus: The Cardiac Patient." Nurs. Clin. North Am., Vol. 11, No. 2 (June 1976), pp. 213–222.

————, and MacVaugh, Horace: "Coronary Artery Surgery: Operative Technique and Patient Education." Nurs. Clin. North Am., Vol. 11, No. 2 (June 1976), pp. 371–383.

————, and Marino, Lynn B.: "Temporary Cardiac Pacemakers." Am. J. Nurs., Vol. 75, No. 4 (April 1975), pp. 586–591.

Wishnie, H. A., et al.: "Psychological Hazards of Convalescence Following Myocardial Infarction." J.A.M.A., Vol. 215, No. 8 (Feb. 22, 1971), pp. 1292–1296.

Zoll, Paul M.: "Historical Development of Cardiac Pacemakers." Prog. Cardiovasc. Dis., Vol. 14, No. 5 (March 1972), pp. 421–428.

Vascular

Aagaard, George N.: "Treatment of Hypertension." Am. J. Nurs., Vol. 73, No. 4 (April 1973), pp. 621–623.

Coffman, J. O., and Mannick, J. A.: "Failure of Vasodilator Drugs in Arteriosclerosis Obliterans." Ann. Int. Med., Vol. 76, No. 1 (Jan. 1972), pp. 35–39.

Dhir, Sisir K., and Friedman, Philip: "Clinical Management of Hypertensive Emergencies." Heart Lung, Vol. 5, No. 4 (July-Aug. 1976), pp. 571–575.

Eddy, Mary Elizabeth: "Teaching Patients with Peripheral Vascular Disease." Nurs. Clin. North Am., Vol. 12, No. 1 (March 1977), pp. 151–159.

Fagan-Dubin, L.: "Atherosclerosis — A Major Cause of Peripheral Vascular Disease." Nurs. Clin. North Am., Vol. 12, No. 1 (March 1977), pp. 101–108.

Federspiel, Billie: "Renin and Blood Pressure." Am. J. Nurs., Vol. 75, No. 9 (Sept. 1975), pp. 1462–1464.

Fenn, John E.: "Reconstructive Arterial Surgery: For Ischemic Lower Extremities." Nurs. Clin. North Am., Vol. 12, No. 1 (March 1977), pp. 129–142.

Fuhs, Margaret F.: "Smoking and the Heart Patient." Nurs. Clin. North Am., Vol. 11, No. 2 (June 1976), pp. 361–369.

Gluck, Joan: "Hypertension — Caring for the Patient who Feels Well." Nurs. '74, Vol. 4, No. 9 (Sept. 1974), pp. 74–76.

Jones, Linda Newell: "Hypertension: Medical and Nursing Implications." Nurs. Clin. North Am., Vol. 11, No. 2 (June 1976), pp. 283–295.

Julius, Steve: "Borderline Hypertension: An Overview." Med. Clin. North Am., Vol. 61, No. 3 (May 1977), pp. 495–509.

Kessro, Bonnie: "Peripheral Arterial Insufficiency: Post-Operative Nursing Care." Nurs. Clin. North Am., Vol. 12, No. 1 (March 1977), pp. 143–149.

Lancour, Jane: "How to Avoid Pitfalls in Measuring Blood Pressure." Am. J. Nurs., Vol. 76, No. 5 (May 1976), pp. 773–775.

Long, Madeline, et al.: "Hypertension: What Patients Need to Know." Am. J. Nurs., Vol. 76, No. 5 (May 1976), pp. 765–780.

Mitchell, Ellen Sullivan: "Protocol for Teaching Hypertensive Patients." Am. J. Nurs., Vol. 77, No. 5 (May 1977), pp. 808–809.

Page, L., et al.: "Drugs in the Management of Hypertension, Part II." Am. Heart J., Vol. 92, No. 1 (July 1976), pp. 114–118.

Robinson, Alice M.: "Detection and Control of Hypertension: Challenge to All Nurses." Am. J. Nurs., Vol. 76, No. 5 (May 1976), pp. 778–780.

Skinner, J. S., and Strandness, D. E.: "Exercise and Intermittent Claudication. I. Effect of Repetition and Intensity of Exercise." Circulation, Vol. 36, No. 1 (July 1967), pp. 15–22.

————.: "Exercise and Intermittent Claudication. II. Effect of Physical Training." Circulation, Vol. 36, No. 1 (July 1967), pp. 23–25.

Taggart, Eleanor: "The Physical Assessment of the Patient with Arterial Disease." Nurs. Clin. North Am., Vol. 12, No. 1 (March1977), pp. 108–117.

Zell, Paul M.: "Rational Use of Drugs for Cardiac Arrest and After Cardiac Resuscitation." Am. J. Cardiol., Vol. 27 (June 1971), pp. 645–649.

14

Nursing in Shock

INTRODUCTION

Shock is a pathophysiological condition, characterized by inadequate tissue and organ perfusion, which seriously reduces the delivery of oxygen and other essential substances to a level below that required for normal cellular activities. Cellular injury or destruction may occur, and tissue and organ functions deteriorate.

Causes of Shock

The basic pathophysiological mechanisms involved in the production of shock are:

1. Widespread vasoconstriction or vasodilation which alters the peripheral vascular tone and resistance.
2. Reduction in the intravascular volume (hypovolemia).
3. Inadequate cardiac output.

The disturbance or initiating event may occur in any portion of the cardiovascular system but will inevitably be reflected in a reduction in the microcirculatory or capillary flow throughout the body.

Shock may be associated with any trauma or stress, regardless of its clinical orientation. The causative factor in alteration of the peripheral vascular tone and resistance may be anaphylaxis, neurogenic trauma, or sepsis. In the case of hypovolemia the cause may be hemorrhage, plasma loss as in burns and peritonitis, or dehydration. Inadequate cardiac output may be the result of myocardial infarction, congestive heart failure, cardiac arrhythmia, obstruction of a major arterial pathway as in pul-

monary embolism, cardiac tamponade or tension pneumothorax.[1]

Types of Shock

Hypovolemic shock implies a deficiency in the intravascular volume which may be due to hemorrhage, dehydration as a result of vomiting, diarrhea, loss of plasma in burns or into the peritoneal cavity in peritonitis, inadequate fluid intake, or excessive urinary output caused by adrenal crisis or overdosage of a diuretic.

Cardiogenic shock indicates an inadequate cardiac output and may be associated with congestive heart failure, cardiac arrhythmia, myocardial infarction, pulmonary embolism, pericardial tamponade or pneumothorax.

Neurogenic shock is produced by autonomic nervous system activity in response to the primary trauma or stress, resulting in reflex vasodilation and loss of arteriolar tone with consequent pooling of blood and a reduction in the venous return to the heart. This type of shock may be caused by spinal cord injury, spinal anesthesia, severe pain (e.g., renal colic), accidental injury, or extreme fright.

Septic or bacteremic shock is caused by an overwhelming infection. The offending organisms are most often gram-negative (e.g., intestinal bacilli) and release an endo-

---

[1] *Tension pneumothorax* is caused by the escape of air from the lung into the pleural cavity where it progressively accumulates, increasing the intrapleural pressure and compressing the heart as well as the lung.

371

toxin that causes an initial brief vasoconstriction followed by vasodilation and pooling of blood. The toxemia also has a direct depressant effect on the heart.

Anaphylactic shock is the result of an antigen-antibody reaction that causes the release of toxic substances (e.g., histamine) that produce vasodilation and pooling of blood (see p. 51).

The terms *reversible* and *irreversible* may also be used to classify shock according to the patient's progress. Shock is said to be reversible when the patient's condition stabilizes and he recovers independently or in response to treatment. It is labeled irreversible when the condition is not amenable to treatment and death ensues.

Concept of Pathophysiological Responses in Shock

Whatever the primary cause or type of shock, the body responses follow a similar pattern. The pathophysiological process is not clearly understood but, at the present time, medicine and pathology indicate that the following responses occur.

Initially, the response to the initiating disturbance in the circulation is stimulation of the sympathetic nervous system and the release of catecholamines (epinephrine and norepinephrine) which cause widespread vasoconstriction of arterioles and venules. The vasoconstriction is selective, occurring in the skin, lungs, gastrointestinal tract, liver and kidneys to ensure a greater volume in the coronary and cerebral circulation. In the areas of abnormal vasodynamics tissue perfusion is reduced, leading to ischemic hypoxia. Lack of available oxygen incurs anaerobic metabolism and the accumulation of abnormal, harmful metabolites, such as pyruvate, lactic acid, CO_2, and hydrogen ions. The pH of the blood decreases and metabolic acidosis develops. The presence of abnormal metabolites and the lowered pH are thought to cause vasodilation of the arterioles while the venule constriction continues. Pooling of the blood ensues, and stagnant hypoxia becomes a problem. Cellular metabolic disturbances result in failure of the active (energy-requiring) transport system of cell membranes. Enzymes, potassium and other cellular components move out. In severe shock, tissue and

organ perfusion may be further compromised by disseminated intravascular coagulation (see p. 262).

Unless the process is reversed, the hypoxia and acidosis worsen, myocardial activity becomes weaker, blood pressure continues to fall, organ functioning is seriously impaired by infarctions and death occurs.

Manifestations of Shock

The degree of shock is not always the same for all persons following stress and injuries of equal intensity. There is considerable variation in the response and also in the rapidity with which some progress to the irreversible stage. Those who are elderly or very young, have chronic disease or infection or are of lesser emotional stability are more susceptible to shock. Signs of shock reflect failure in the perfusion of vital organs and the responsive mechanisms set in operation.

It is important that the nurse be constantly alert for early changes in patients' conditions that may indicate shock, especially in those with conditions in which it is more likely to develop (e.g., burns, trauma, hemorrhage, dehydration and severe infection). Early recognition and treatment substantially increase the patient's chance for survival.

BEHAVIORAL AND RESPONSE CHANGES. Unless the shock is very severe and develops very quickly, premonitory signs are restlessness, apprehension and anxiety. Later, the restlessness and apprehension may be replaced by listlessness, apathy and decreased mental alertness or confusion, which may progress to loss of consciousness due to increasing cerebral hypoxia as a result of the reduction in cardiac output. A depression of reflex responses also occurs.

SKIN. Initially, the skin is ashen pale and cold due to increased peripheral vascular resistance and decreased perfusion of the superficial tissues. Cyanosis develops, reflecting a reduction in the cardiac output (as in cardiogenic and progressive shock) and decreased oxygen saturation. The latter occurs because of the pooling of blood and the diminished flow of blood through the lungs for oxygenation. If the skin vessels are blanched by pressure, they refill slowly.

The skin may be moist (clammy) due to

the sympathetic innervation of the sweat glands. In the case of septic shock, the skin is warm, dry and less pale.

VITAL SIGNS. The pulse is rapid and thready. The tachycardia is a compensatory response to the decreased volume in cardiac output. If the shock is cardiogenic or is not reversed, the pulse progressively weakens, becoming slower and irregular and eventually imperceptible.

The systolic blood pressure falls, followed later by a decrease in the diastolic pressure. A systolic pressure of less than 90 mm. Hg or a fall of more than 30 mm. Hg in the systolic pressure indicates shock. If one is not familiar with the patient's previous blood pressure and he has been hypertensive, the blood pressure may appear to be normal; other factors (patient's responses, color, etc.) must always be taken into consideration. A decrease in pulse pressure to below 30 mm. Hg is an early sign.

Respirations increase in response to the hypoxia. If the initial cause is a loss of intravascular volume (e.g., hemorrhage) the patient may manifest air hunger. In severe and progressive shock, depression of the respiratory center causes slower, shallow and possibly irregular respirations.

The body temperature is usually subnormal; cellular metabolism and heat production are reduced by hypoxia. The exception to this occurs with a patient in whom the primary cause of the shock is infection. This type of shock may be referred to as hyperdynamic or warm septic shock.

URINARY OUTPUT. Renal output is diminished as a result of decreased renal perfusion. The output may become less than 30 ml. per hour; urea nitrogen and creatinine are retained, as indicated by increasing blood levels.

THIRST. This is very distressing, especially in hypovolemic shock. The mouth becomes parched as a result of the increased withdrawal of fluid from the interstitial spaces into the intravascular compartment.

DIFFUSE INTRAVASCULAR CLOTTING. Prolonged and severe shock, especially that of septic origin, is frequently complicated by diffuse intravascular clotting. The coagulation and formation of thromboses block small vessels and may cause serious tissue necrosis. Clotting elements may become depleted and then diffuse bleeding occurs. The condition is suspected with the appearance of petechiae and ecchymoses or bleeding from the nasal or oral mucous membrane. It may go unrecognized until there is evident hemorrhage (e.g., epistaxis, gastric, rectal, bladder). Blood studies reveal a prolonged prothrombin time, reduced number of platelets, and deficiency of fibrinogen. Multiple coagulation factors may be involved.

ACIDOSIS. Changes that occur in the patient's responses and vital functions are worsened by the rapid development of acidosis associated with shock. As mentioned previously, the impairment of tissue perfusion and the resulting hypoxia incur anaerobic metabolism; metabolic acids accumulate and interfere with normal cell functioning. Cardiac arrhythmia and myocardial failure are likely to develop if acidosis persists.

NURSING THE SHOCK PATIENT

The treatment of shock is urgent and should be instituted as soon as possible to prevent the condition from progressing to an irreversible phase. The nurse, who is with the patient for longer periods than the doctor, may recognize early changes and may be instrumental in the patient receiving early treatment.

The patient in shock is usually cared for in an intensive or critical care unit; constant nurse attendance is necessary. Planning and implementing the care involves: (1) ongoing assessment of the patient's condition; and (2) carrying out the prescribed therapy and meeting the individual's basic needs.

ASSESSMENT OF THE PATIENT'S CONDITION

Shock is an unstable, dynamic state in which the patient's condition either improves or worsens. Continuous monitoring is essential to identify changes which dictate necessary therapeutic and care measures.

The blood pressure, pulse, respiratory status, color and hourly urinary output are noted immediately when taking over a patient. It is important to have a baseline in order to determine whether changes indicate improvement or further deterioration. Changes are frequently of greater significance than absolute values.

The nurse requires an understanding of the importance of the data obtained in assessment procedures and monitoring in order to take appropriate action. Various parameters and observations are used to assess the cardiovascular status, respiratory functions and certain biochemical levels.

Cardiovascular Assessment

Assessment of the patient's cardiovascular status includes the following procedures.

BLOOD PRESSURE AND PULSE. These are recorded at 15-minute intervals, and the intervals are lengthened only as the patient's condition improves. They reflect cardiac functioning and cardiac output.

The arterial blood pressure may be monitored by the syphygmomanometer but is likely to be lower than that obtained by intra-arterial measurement because of the peripheral vasoconstriction. Direct measurement by means of an intra-arterial catheter is more reliable. A catheter is passed via the radial or brachial artery into the subclavian artery. It is attached to a transducer which converts the mechanical pressure exerted by the blood to electrical impulses that appear on the monitor.

The pulse is counted and evaluated for a full minute. The radial artery may be used but, if it is inaccessible, the carotid, femoral or pedal pulses may be used. A stethoscope may be used to determine cardiac rhythm and apical rate.

ELECTROCARDIOGRAPH. Continuous electrocardiographic monitoring is employed for early detection of arrhythmias and arrest.

PULSE PRESSURE. The pulse pressure, which is the difference between the systolic and diastolic blood pressures, is noted. It decreases with a decrease in cardiac output. There is concern when it becomes less than 30.

JUGULAR VEINS. The jugular veins are observed for distention, pulsation or reflux, which would indicate cardiac insufficiency in receiving and forwarding the venous return.

CENTRAL VENOUS PRESSURE. A line may be established by which central venous pressure (CVP) is determined hourly. A catheter is passed into the superior vena cava and attached to an intravenous infusion setup and a manometer using a three-way stopcock (see p. 297 for details). The pressure indicated on the manometer reflects the intravascular volume and the venous return to the right side of the heart. The normal value is 10 to 12 cm. of water; an increase above normal may indicate weakening or failure of the right side of the heart, or may be due to an excessive intravascular volume that may be the result of too rapid fluid infusion. A pressure below 5 to 6 cm. of water usually reflects an intravascular volume deficit.

PULMONARY ARTERY PRESSURE (PAP). This determination provides information about the pressure within the pulmonary vascular system and the functional ability of the heart. A floating balloon-tipped (Swan-Ganz) catheter with two or more lumens is passed into the superior vena cava. The balloon is then inflated, and the catheter is carried by the blood stream through the right side of the heart into the pulmonary artery. The nonballoon lumen of the catheter is filled with water or saline which recedes in a monitoring tube until the pressure of the blood that it meets is equal to its pressure. The normal range of the PAP is 15 to 30 mm. Hg during systole and 5 to 15 mm. Hg during diastole, with a mean value of 10 to 20 mm. Hg, and in shock it is recorded every 1 to 2 hours.

PULMONARY ARTERY WEDGE PRESSURE (PAWP; PULMONARY CAPILLARY PRESSURE). This is obtained to provide information about the functional ability of the left side of the heart. A catheter similar to that used in measuring the PAP is introduced into the pulmonary artery and advanced until the inflated balloon wedges in a branch of the artery. The tip of the open lumen is closed off from the pressure in the proximal pulmonary artery which is that created by the right side of the heart. When correctly positioned the balloon is *promptly deflated*, since it obstructs blood flow beyond that point. The pressure is measured every 1 to 2 hours by the same procedure as that used in PAP determination.

The procedure must be carried out quickly, the balloon is inflated, the pressure recorded and the *balloon deflated immediately.* During inflation of the balloon, the lung tissue supplied by that branch of the pulmonary artery is deprived of its blood supply.

The PAWP is the back pressure of the blood being delivered to the left side of the heart and reflects the ability of the left atrium and left ventricle to receive and forward the blood. The normal is approximately 5 to 12 mm. Hg.

URINE OUTPUT. The hourly urinary output serves as a useful parameter in assessing a patient's cardiovascular status. An indwelling catheter is passed, and the urine excreted per hour is measured. The output reflects renal perfusion.

Normal ranges are:

Age	*ml./hour*
Infant	8 to 20
1 to 4 years	20 to 25
4 to 7 years	25 to 30
7 to 10 years	25 to 30
Adult	30 to 60

SKIN. The color and temperature of the skin are noted frequently. Lessening of the pallor, warming, and quick refilling of the capillaries and veins following compression are favorable signs. In severe shock and that associated with sepsis, the nurse is alert for petechiae or other signs of subcutaneous bleeding that may indicate disseminated intravascular coagulation (DIC).

PATIENT'S RESPONSES. The patient's responses, orientation, level of consciousness and strength of movement are observed at intervals, since they reflect cerebral perfusion and the oxygen supply.

Respiratory Assessment

This is necessary at frequent intervals.

RATE AND VOLUME OF RESPIRATIONS. These are recorded every 15 to 30 minutes. Hyperventilation may develop in the early stages of shock in response to the metabolic acidosis, and this greatly increases the work of breathing. As cited previously, respirations may become slow, irregular and shallow as a result of ischemia of the respiratory center and weakness of the respiratory muscles.

ARTERIAL BLOOD TESTS. Arterial blood specimens are collected every 2 to 3 hours for blood gas and pH determinations (see p. 405). The reports are followed closely by the nurse; unfavorable changes may occur quickly and should be brought to the physician's attention promptly so that appropriate therapeutic measures may be instituted. A paO_2 of 80 mm. Hg or less necessitates the administration of oxygen and, if it falls to 60 mm. Hg or less, mechanical ventilatory assistance may be indicated (see p. 424). The pH is likely to be below normal but the $paCO_2$ may remain within the normal range, indicating compensated acidosis. The serum bicarbonate level will likely be below normal, since it is being used for buffering the increased carbonic acid. If the $paCO_2$ rises and the serum bicarbonate and pH remain low, respiratory compensation is inadequate and the physician is notified. Ventilatory assistance may be necessary to remove the excess carbon dioxide.

PULMONARY DYSFUNCTION. Many patients in shock develop serious pulmonary dysfunction characterized by pathophysiological changes in the lungs. These changes are usually not manifested until 3 to 6 days after the shock-initiating event, and include a decrease in the secretion of surfactant with a concomitant increase in surface tension that results in areas of atelectasis, interstitial edema, congestion, diffuse intravascular coagulation, thromboses and pulmonary emboli. Pulmonary capillary perfusion is greatly reduced and oxygen and carbon dioxide transport across the alveolar membrane progressively decreases; severe hypoxemia and hypercarbia develop. The complication may be referred to as "low-flow lung syndrome," "shock lung" and, rarely, as "wet lung" (see p. 430).

When assessing the patient the nurse is aware of the serious changes that may develop in the lung in shock. Alternate intercostal ballooning and retraction, asymmetry in chest movement and dyspnea are reported. Auscultation of the anterior and posterior chests is used to assess air entry and to listen for sounds of moisture in the airways. The presence of secretions and/or nonventilated areas requires prompt attention.

If ventilatory dysfunction occurs, the tidal volume is measured by means of a

Wright respirometer and mask every 1 to 2 hours.

Biochemical Levels

The levels of certain *biochemical factors* provide necessary information about the patient's progress, as well as serving as a basis for some therapeutic measures. Considerable laboratory blood work is performed. Blood specimens are collected for determination of lactic acid, bicarbonate, potassium, chloride, sodium and calcium levels. These indicate the degree of anaerobic metabolism, acidosis and the disturbance or breakdown in cells. Determinations of blood urea and creatinine are also made for evaluation of tissue damage, kidney function and waste retention. Serum enzyme levels may be requested, since they reflect the amount of tissue damage and are especially significant in cardiogenic shock (see p. 311).

TREATMENT AND NURSING MEASURES

Therapy is directed toward improving tissue perfusion and oxygenation and correcting the specific cause. The treatment and care presented here relate to shock and do not deal in detail with the spcific initiating factor, although one is conditioned by the other.

Objectives of Treatment

In cardiogenic shock, the treatment focusses on strengthening the heart to increase the cardiac output and preventing arrhythmias by the use of certain drugs. Immediate attention is also given to the correction of acidosis.

In hypovolemic shock, the objective is expansion of the intravascular volume. For example, if the cause of the shock is hemorrhage, the treatment is directed toward arresting the bleeding and replacing the blood lost to increase blood pressure and restore tissue perfusion. The intravenous infusion solution of choice is compatible whole blood.

Septic shock is treated by an appropriate antibiotic to combat infection and a cortico-steroid drug in conjunction with attempts to improve tissue perfusion and oxygenation.

Neurogenic shock is usually associated with a spinal cord injury or may be incurred by spinal anesthesia. Since there is a widespread loss of vasomotor tone and a disproportion between intravascular capacity and intravascular volume, intravenous infusion is given to increase intravascular volume and a vasoconstrictor drug such as methoxamine (Vasoxyl) is administered.

Treatment and Care

Treatment and care of the patient in shock include the following considerations.

INTRAVENOUS INFUSION. An intravenous line is established immediately so that fluids may be administered to expand the intravascular volume, blood loss may be replaced, and a readily accessible channel is provided for the administration of medications. Initially, glucose 5 per cent in distilled water is used while the patient is being assessed. The physician then prescribes the appropriate solution, volume, and rate of administration according to the cause of shock, clinical manifestations and laboratory reports of the hematocrit, electrolyte, blood gas and pH levels. Solutions that may be used include whole blood, dextran, plasma, and electrolyte preparations. The volume and rate of administration of fluids are based on the blood pressure, central venous pressure, pulmonary artery pressure and pulmonary artery wedge pressure.

RESPIRATORY ASSISTANCE. Immediate attention is given to establishing and maintaining a patent airway. Oxygen is given by nasal prongs or mask, unless the blood gas determinations indicate the need for delivery of a higher and more controlled concentration of oxygen by means of an endotracheal tube and mechanical respirator. The aim is to restore and maintain a paO_2 level of at least 90 mm. Hg. If intubation and ventilatory assistance are still necessary after 48 to 72 hours, a tracheostomy may be done to replace the endotracheal tube. Intubation by either means and the use of mechanical ventilation have several distinct advantages. They: (1) provide better control of ventilatory volume and oxygen concentration; (2) decrease the work of breathing; (3) provide a means by which the elimination of carbon dioxide may be regulated; and (4) permit more effective deep suctioning and clearance of the airway (see p. 413).

MEDICATIONS USED IN SHOCK. The choice of drugs used in the treatment of shock depends upon the cause and severity of the hypotension. They are given intravenously and the patient's cardiac function and central venous pressure (CVP) are monitored closely.

VASOACTIVE DRUGS. Those that may be prescribed include:

Vasopressors. Examples of these are norepinephrine (Levophed), epinephrine (Adrenalin), methoxamine (Vasoxyl), metaraminol (Aramine), and mephentermine (Wyamine). These drugs produce peripheral vasoconstriction and increase the blood pressure. When a vasopressor drug is used it is discontinued gradually and the patient kept under close observation, since sudden severe hypotension may occur when the drug is withdrawn.

Vasodilators. Examples are phentolamine (Regitine) and phenoxybenzamine (Dibenzyline). These drugs are administered to improve tissue perfusion by relaxing the vasospasm that may develop in shock. It is important that the patient be observed closely; the CVP is monitored and the intravenous infusion rate regulated to maintain an adequate CVP to prevent sudden severe hypotension.

DRUGS FOR IMPROVING CARDIAC FUNCTION AND OUTPUT. These include isoproterenol, dopamine, and digitalis.

Isoproterenol (Isuprel) causes widespread vasodilation and an increased cardiac rate (chronotropic effect) and output (inotropic effect). A close check is kept on the pulse or cardiac monitor; if tachycardia or arrhythmia develops, the infusion of the drug is discontinued and the response reported. It is suggested that a defibrillator should be readily available in the event of fibrillation.

Dopamine may be used to improve myocardial contractility and rate of contractions. In small doses it selectively dilates the coronary, cerebral and renal vessels.

A *digitalis glycoside* (e.g., digoxin) may be administered to increase the strength of the heartbeat while decreasing the frequency of contractions. Cardiac function is monitored constantly.

ANTICOAGULANT. Heparin is given if the patient's shock is complicated by disseminated intravascular coagulation (DIC). The prothrombin and coagulation times are monitored.

DIURETICS. These may be prescribed if pulmonary edema develops or if there is evidence of renal insufficiency. The preparation used may be furosemide (Lasix) or mannitol. The fluid intake and output are recorded to determine the effectiveness of the drug. Serum electrolyte levels are monitored, especially that of potassium.

ANALGESICS. These may be necessary if the patient is experiencing severe pain which is contributing to the state of shock. A small dose of meperidine (Demerol), Pantopon or morphine may be prescribed. The patient's respirations are monitored frequently, especially if morphine is used, since it is a strong respiratory depressant.

CORTICOSTEROIDS. These may be prescribed in septic shock. Methylprednisolone (Solu-Medrol) or dexamethasone (Decadron) may be used.

POSITION. Until recently the practice was to elevate the lower limbs or place the patient in the Trendelenberg position. The consensus now favors the supine position which prevents possible interference with the descent of the diaphragm during inspiration. This position also reduces possible aortic and carotid sinus baroreceptor reflexes that result in vasoconstriction of cerebral vessels. If an order is received to elevate the lower limbs, the position is not recommended for longer than 24 hours.

Although minimal energy demands on the patient are important and therapy may necessitate lying on the back, it should be remembered that immobility predisposes the patient to serious complications, such as stasis of circulation, thrombosis, retention of urine and accumulation of pulmonary secretions, atelectasis and decubitus ulcer. If possible the patient is turned, if only for a brief period, every 2 hours and passive movements of the limbs (especially of the lower limbs) are carried out. Active limb exercises are encouraged when the condition permits.

MINIMAL ENERGY DEMANDS. Monitoring, treatments and care are organized to permit uninterrupted rest periods. The patient's energy expenditure is kept to a minimum by anticipating his needs, reducing discomfort and apprehension and providing adequate assistance when turning or lifting. Environmental stimuli (e.g., conversation, visitors, noise) are controlled to reduce disturbances.

BODY TEMPERATURE. The patient is kept comfortably warm by the use of light covers and control of room temperature. Heat applications are not used because they increase peripheral vasodilation and body fluid loss. It is important to avoid overheating and chilling; extremes of temperature involve increased metabolism and, as a result, a greater demand for oxygen and increased carbon dioxide production. If hyperpyrexia develops the patient receives temperature sponges and is exposed to cool air, or a hypothermia blanket may be used.

NUTRITION AND HYDRATION. The patient is sustained by intravenous infusions. If the shock state is prolonged, intravenous alimentation may be used to provide adequate nutrition (see p. 504). An accurate record of the fluid intake and output is necessary to determine the fluid balance. The patient may experience thirst but, because of intubation or his condition, oral fluids are not permitted. Moist swabbing of the tongue and oral cavity and moist compresses over the lips may be helpful.

ELIMINATION. As cited earlier, an indwelling urinary catheter is introduced in order to determine the hourly urinary output, since renal failure or shutdown is a possible complication in shock. If renal insufficiency develops, peritoneal dialysis or hemodialysis may be necessary to remove water, urea, creatinine and other wastes.

Bowel elimination is of less concern but distention may develop as a result of depressed peristalsis. The abdomen is examined for distension since it can embarass respiratory function.

PSYCHOLOGICAL SUPPORT. The responsibilities associated with the complex monitoring and technical therapeutic measures in the care of the patient in shock tend to completely occupy the nurse, and the patient's anxiety and apprehension may go unrecognized. This is a critical and life-threatening situation to the patient; what it means to him and the effect of his fear and concerns on his condition may be underestimated. Anxiety aggravates respiratory distress and increases catecholamine secretion. There is a need for compassionate understanding in addition to scientific and technical ability.

The patient in shock is usually cared for in a critical care unit and experiences loss of privacy and independence, strange sights and sounds, the absence of familiar persons and meaningful stimuli and a sense of aloneness.

Planning and implementing care gives consideration to identifying the individual's emotional responses and to reducing his apprehensions and fears.

Simple, direct communication is important in developing or reinforcing a positive relationship between the patient and nurse. The patient who is advised of his progress and what is going to be done and why is generally less fearful and more cooperative.

If the nurse is required to leave the patient alone, he is advised that it will be brief and that there are resources of assistance available during that period if they become necessary. A reliable, composed relative or friend may remain quietly in the unit. This familiar person's presence may provide reassurance and alleviate aloneness. An effort is made to learn what is troubling the patient and to solve the problem(s). Inability to speak because of intubation or a tracheostomy does not prevent the nurse from speaking to him. If his condition permits, a means of communication using writing may be provided for him.

Conversation with other workers within the patient's hearing should be guarded. Unnecessary concern may arise because the patient hears something and misinterprets it, or applies it to himself even though it is irrelevant to him and his situation. The usual 24-hour cycles of day and night should be respected; a minimum of noise and as little disturbance as possible at night (consistent with essential monitoring and treatment) contribute to rest and minimal energy expenditure.

PERSONAL HYGIENIC CARE. Bathing promotes relaxation and rest. Frequent special attention is given to skin, especially over pressure areas, to prevent pressure sores.

Frequent mouth care is important in contributing to patient comfort and in preventing sores and infection.

FAMILY. The family members also need

consideration and support. Illness of a member is a stressful, threatening event which creates a crisis situation for the family. Fear and concern for their loved one, the disruption of their accustomed pattern of living and additional burdens may disorganize their resources. They may suddenly be unable to cope and may need help.

The nurse conveys understanding and acceptance of their concern and reactions. They are kept informed about the patient's treatment and progress. Time is taken to listen to and answer their questions.

The family is advised where they may wait, of the location of a telephone they may use and where they may get a meal if they plan to remain in the hospital. They should not be left for long periods without contact with someone who can talk to them about the patient. Brief visits to the patient will mean much to them as well as indicate the nurse's appreciation of their feelings. They should receive assistance to mobilize their own resources. Guidance is provided, but they should be involved in solving their own problems if possible.

Recovery Period

When treatment has been instituted the nurse observes the patient closely for signs of its effectiveness. Criteria for effectiveness are an increase in the blood pressure and pulse volume, a decrease in pulse rate, an increased urinary output, improved color and the recovery of normal responses. When the patient's condition has improved and he is permitted to move or be moved, any change in position should be assumed slowly. It may take some time for the circulatory system to recover its ability to adjust to postural changes.

Renal ischemia incurred during the period of hypotension may result in residual damage to the tubular cells, reducing kidney efficiency. The urinary output should still be measured, and tests may be ordered to check the ability of the kidneys to concentrate solid wastes.

The skin may have suffered as a result of the period of immobility, impaired circulation and hypoxia. It is carefully examined, and the necessary care taken to improve its general condition.

Transfer and Rehabilitation

With reversal of the shock state, the patient is transferred from the critical care unit to a general care ward. This usually engenders considerable apprehension and concern even though it indicates favorable progress. The patient has been under constant observation and care. In this new situation he will likely be left to himself for lengthy periods.

The move is discussed with him in the critical care unit. The staff in general care should have some knowledge and appreciation of what the patient and family have experienced during the acute shock state, and should be aware of any residual problems.

Preparation for discharge includes a discussion of the resumption of activities and the necessary care. There may be a tendency following such a severe illness for the patient to be fearful of doing some things and for the family to be overprotective.

References

Books

Beeson, Paul B., and McDermott, Walsh (Eds.): Textbook of Medicine, 15th ed. Philadelphia, W. B. Saunders, 1979.

Boedeker, Edgar C., and Dauber, James H.: Manual of Medical Therapeutics, 21st ed. Boston, Little, Brown, 1974, pp. 409–417.

Chaney, Patricia S. (Ed.): Assessing Vital Functions Accurately. (Nursing Skillbook Series.) Pennsylvania, Intermed Communications, 1977, pp. 153–164.

Krupp, Marcus A., and Chatton, Milton J.: Current Medical Diagnosis and Treatment. Los Altos, Cal., Lange, 1975, pp. 2–7.

Sabiston, David C., Jr. (Ed.): Davis-Christopher: Textbook of Surgery, 11th ed. Philadelphia, W. B. Saunders, 1977.

Periodicals

Adams, Crawford W.: "Recognition and Evaluation of Cardiogenic Shock." Heart Lung, Vol. 2, No. 6 (Nov.-Dec. 1973), pp. 893–895.

Beaumont, Estelle (Ed.): "Septic Shock in a Burn Patient," Nurs. '76, Vol. 6, No. 1 (Jan. 1976), pp. 39–43.

Boericke, Peter H.: "Emergency (Part 2)." Nurs. '75, Vol. 5, No. 3 (Mar. 1975), p. 44.

Cook, William A.: "Shock Lung: Etiology, Prevention and Treatment." Heart Lung, Vol. 3, No. 6 (Nov.-Dec. 1974), pp. 933–938.

Craven, Ruth Falk: "Anaphylactic Shock." Am. J. Nurs., Vol. 72, No. 4 (April 1972), pp. 718–721.

Dorr, Kathleen Scesa: "The Intra-aortic Balloon Pump." Am. J. Nurs., Vol. 75, No. 1 (Jan. 1975), pp. 52–55.

Egdahl, Richard H., et al.: "The Importance of the Endocrine and Metabolic Responses to Shock and Trauma." Crit. Care Med., Vol. 5, No. 6 (Nov.-Dec. 1977), pp. 257–261.

Jahre, Jeffrey, et al.: "Medical Approach to the Hypotensive Patient and the Patient in Shock." Heart Lung, Vol. 4, No. 4 (July-Aug. 1975), pp. 577–587.

Lucas, Charles E.: "Resuscitation of the Injured Patient: The Three Phases of Treatment." Surg. Clin. North Am., Vol. 57, No. 1 (Feb. 1977), pp. 3–15.

Moyer, John H., and Mills, Lewis C.: "Vasopressor Agents in Shock." Am. J. Nurs., Vol. 75, No. 4 (April 1975), pp. 620–625.

O'Rourke, M. F.: "Cardiogenic Shock following Myocardial Infarction." Heart Lung, Vol. 3, No. 2 (March-April 1974), pp. 252–257.

Royce, Judith A.: "Shock." Nurs. Clin. North Am., Vol. 8, No. 3 (Sept. 1973), pp. 377–387.

Stude, Carol: "Cardiogenic Shock." Am. J. Nurs., Vol. 74, No. 9 (Sept. 1974), pp. 1636–1640.

Sun, Rhoda Lee: "Trendelenburg's Position in Hypovolemic Shock." Am. J. Nurs., Vol. 71, No. 9 (Sept. 1971), pp. 1758–1759.

Tharp, Gerald D.: "Shock: The Overall Mechanisms." Am. J. Nurs., Vol. 74, No. 12 (Dec. 1974), pp. 2208–2211.

Wiley, Loy (Ed.): "Staying Ahead of Shock." Nurs. '74, Vol. 4, No. 4 (April 1974), pp. 19–31.

————.: "Shock — Different Kinds . . . Different Problems." Nurs. '74, Vol. 4, No. 5 (May 1974), pp. 43–52.

15

Nursing in Respiratory Disorders

RESPIRATION

A constant exchange of oxygen and carbon dioxide between the living organism and its environment is essential for survival. Respiration is the process which performs this function. The exchange takes place between the total organism and the external environment and between the tissue cells and the blood. The former involves pulmonary ventilation and diffusion of the gases through the alveolar membrane of the lungs. The exchange between the cells and the blood (sometimes call internal or tissue respiration) requires transportation of the gases by the blood and an exchange of oxygen and carbon dioxide between the capillaries and tissue cells.

Pulmonary ventilation or breathing consists of the movement of air into and out of the lungs (inspiration and expiration). Diffusion involves the movement of gases between the air in the pulmonary air sacs (alveoli) and the blood in the pulmonary capillaries in the direction of the lower pressure or concentration.

In addition to providing oxygen for cellular metabolism and removing the cellular metabolite carbon dioxide, the respiratory system also plays an important role in voice production, regulation of the pH of body fluids and the elimination of heat and water. Ventilation enhances venous return to the right side of the heart by alternating positive and negative intrathoracic pressure, and also contributes to compression of the abdominal viscera to aid in parturition and defecation.

RESPIRATORY STRUCTURES

The structures concerned with ventilation are the upper and lower respiratory tracts, respiratory muscles and thorax (Fig. 15–1).

Upper Respiratory Tract

The upper airway is formed by the nose, mouth, pharynx and larynx. It serves as a passageway for air being inspired and expired, filters, warms and moistens the inhaled air, and provides the protective reflexes of sneezing and the closing off of the larynx to prevent aspiration of fluid and solids. Irritation of the pharynx and larynx may also initiate the cough reflex.

NOSE. The nose has a highly vascularized and ciliated mucous membrane lining which serves to moisten, warm and filter inhaled air. The nasal cavities and their connecting sinuses act as resonating chambers in sound production. The posterior portion of the cavities contains olfactory receptors concerned with the sense of smell (olfactory sense). The external orifices are called the nostrils, or anterior nares.

PHARYNX. The pharynx, a muscular

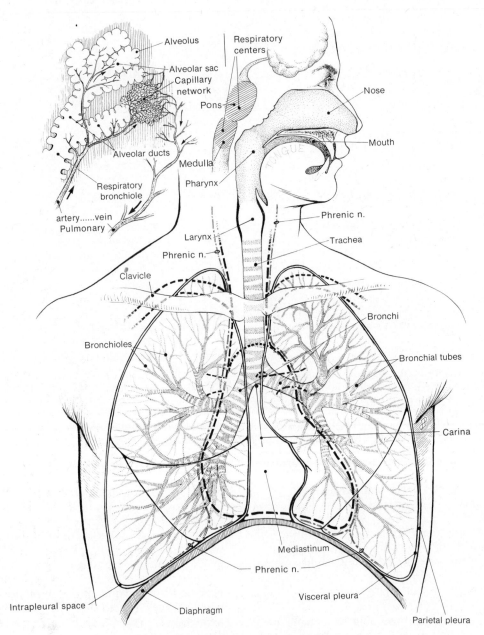

FIGURE 15–1 The respiratory system.

tube lined with mucous membrane, provides a common passageway for air entering the larynx and food entering the esophagus. Air reaching the pharynx passes readily into the larynx, but the presence of food or fluid stimulates a reflex contraction of the pharyngeal tube. The posterior nares (openings into the nasal cavities) are then blocked off and the larynx is closed off by a lowering of the leaf-shaped structure, the *epiglottis*. These closures prevent the entrance of food or fluid into the nose and lower respiratory tract. As a result of the contraction, the pharyngeal content is directed into the esophagus.

LARYNX. The larynx is composed of muscle tissue and cartilage and is lined with mucous membrane. It functions as an air passage and contains the *vocal cords*, which are responsible for sound production. The laryngeal passageway is narrowed in one area by membranous folds reflected over the vocal cords. The slit-like space between these two folds is referred to as the *glottis* and is varied in size to produce the different levels of pitch in voice production. In normal quiet inspiration and expiration the vocal cords are relaxed and the glottis is open.

Lower Respiratory Tract

The lower tract consists of the trachea, bronchi and two lungs.

TRACHEA. The trachea is a continuation of the inferior end of the larynx and divides into two tubes — the right and left bronchi. The right bronchus is shorter and more vertical than the left; this accounts for aspirated foreign particles entering the right bronchus more often than the left. The tracheal walls are composed of fibroelastic tissue in which incomplete cartilaginous rings are imbedded to prevent collapse of the tube. The trachea simply serves as an air passageway.

BRONCHI, BRONCHIAL TUBES AND BRONCHIOLES. Each bronchus enters a lung where it branches like a tree to form the bronchial tubes and, eventually, the very small tubes, the bronchioles. As the branches become more distal, the lumen of the tubes narrows and the walls change structure. The bronchi and bronchial tubes are similar in structure to the trachea except for the addition of plain muscle tissue

in their walls. In the bronchioles, the cartilaginous tissue disappears and the smooth muscle tissue becomes more abundant.

The trachea and bronchial air passages are lined by a ciliated mucous membrane continuous with that of the upper air passages. The cilia are hair-like projections of protoplasm which alternately bend in one direction and straighten, providing a sweeping motion to remove the mucus secreted and any foreign particles that may have been inhaled. Excessive secretions may initiate the cough reflex, which is a defense mechanism to rid the tract of such substances (see p. 396).

ALVEOLI. The bronchioles divide and subdivide, progressively becoming smaller. Each bronchiole eventually gives rise to a spray of microscopic tubes known as *alveolar ducts*. Each duct terminates in clusters of microscopic sacs called *alveoli* (singular, alveolus). The walls of the alveoli consist of thin epithelial and elastic connective tissue and a network of capillaries. The air in the alveoli is separated from the blood in the capillaries by very thin semipermeable tissue which permits diffusion of the respiratory gases oxygen and carbon dioxide through it. The expanse of the alveolar surface is very great and is estimated to be approximately 30 to 40 times that of skin surface.

LUNGS. Each lung is made up mainly of bronchial tubes with their successive branches, alveoli and many blood vessels of the pulmonary circulatory system. The right lung is divided into three lobes, and the left is divided into two lobes only. The portion of lung derived from each main bronchial tube is referred to as a *bronchopulmonary segment* (Fig. 15–2). Each lung is enclosed in an adherent serous membrane called the *visceral pleura,* which is continuous from the hilum of the lung with a similar layer that lines the thoracic wall and is known as the *parietal pleura.*

BLOOD SUPPLY TO THE LUNGS. Blood from two sources enters the lungs. The bronchial arteries convey blood from the aorta to nourish the respiratory structures. The pulmonary artery delivers the blood from the right side of the heart to the lungs to be oxygenated. The blood from both sources is then collected from the capillaries around the alveoli and other structures into veins and is returned to the left

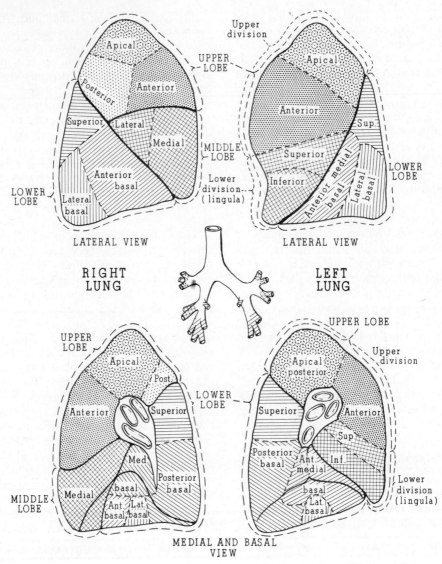

FIGURE 15-2 Bronchopulmonary segments of the lungs. (From Jacob, S. W. and Francone, C. A., and Lossow, W. J., Structure and Function in Man. 4th ed., Philadelphia, W. B. Saunders Co., 1978.)

side of the heart by the four pulmonary veins.

THORAX. The lungs are well protected by the bony thoracic cage which is formed by the sternum, ribs and thoracic vertebrae. The apices of the lungs extend about 1 inch above the clavicles. The thorax acts as an airtight box in which the lungs are suspended and in which pressure can be varied by contraction of respiratory muscles, altering the thoracic cavity dimensions.

Secretions

The respiratory tract produces two secretions, *mucus* and *surfactant*. The inner surfaces of the alveoli and alveolar ducts are covered with a film of fluid called *surfactant*, a phospholipid compound synthesized by special epithelial cells in the walls of the alveoli. The composition of this solution is such that it reduces the surface tension, facilitating inflation and preventing collapse of the alveoli on expiration. Surfactant also prevents the movement of fluid from the capillaries into the alveoli (pulmonary edema) by reducing the surface tension.

Inactivation of surfactant or a deficiency in the amount secreted increases the surface tension, resulting in resistance to the inflow of air and reduced lung expansion. The condition may be congenital, and is referred to as hyaline membrane disease or respiratory distress syndrome of the newborn. Inactivation of the secretion or a deficiency may also be associated with hypoxia, excessively high concentrations of oxygen, acidosis or inadequate perfusion (flow of blood through the capillaries).

The *mucus* which is secreted by the glandular cells of the mucous membrane lining of the respiratory tract serves to protect the organism in several ways. It provides a protective barrier against inhaled irritants and traps foreign particles, facilitating their removal by the cilia. It also waterproofs the surface, thus diminishing the loss of body water as well as setting up a barrier to inhaled organisms. Insufficient secretion of mucus or the production of a thick tenacious mucoid such as occurs in the congenital disorder mucoviscidosis (fibrocystic disease of the newborn) prevents the action of the cilia, predisposing to infection and partial or complete obstruction of bronchial tubes and bronchioles.

Chest Cavities and Their Pressures

The spaces between the visceral and parietal pleurae form the intrapleural or *pleural cavities*. (Each lung has its own closed pleural cavity.) Each pleural cavity is only a potential space since the visceral and parietal pleurae are separated normally by just a thin film of fluid that moistens the surfaces. The surfaces of the lungs are in close apposition with the chest walls. The pressure within the pleural cavities is approximately 5 mm. Hg less than atmospheric pressure, which is 760 mm. Hg at sea level. It may also be expressed as a negative pressure equal to that exerted by a column of water 10 cm. in depth.

The *intrapulmonic cavity* is the space within the lungs and, since it communicates with atmosphere, the intrapulmonary pressure varies above and below atmospheric pressure during expiration and inspiration, respectively. Between expiration and inspiration, when there is no movement of air, the intrapulmonic pressure is the same as that of the atmosphere.

The space in between the two lungs and their pleurae is known as the *mediastinum*. It contains the large blood vessels, heart, esophagus, trachea, bronchi, and lymphatic ducts and nodes.

Respiratory Muscles

The muscles used in normal breathing are principally the diaphragm and the intercostal muscles. The *diaphragm* is a dome-shaped muscular partition between the thoracic and abdominal cavities and is the most important respiratory muscle. When the diaphragm is relaxed, its thoracic surface is convex. On contraction, the convexity is reduced and the thoracic cavity is lengthened. The diaphragm also functions in coughing and sneezing and, in conjunction with the abdominal muscles, is used in defecation, vomiting and parturition.

The *external intercostal muscles* increase the lateral and anteroposterior diameters of the thoracic cavity by elevating the sternum and moving the ribs into a more horizontal position.

Accessory muscles may be used to facilitate breathing. In labored and forced inspiration, the sternocleidomastoid, scalene and pectoralis muscles contract to raise the upper ribs. At the same time the nostrils dilate and the glottis widens. Forced or difficult expiration involves the abdominal and internal intercostal muscles. The abdominal muscles contract to raise the relaxed diaphragm higher in order to compress the lungs.

RESPIRATORY FUNCTIONS

Mechanics of Pulmonary Ventilation

Each respiration involves inspiration and expiration. Inspiration is an active phase during which air moves into the lungs. Expiration, in normal breathing, is a passive phase during which air moves out of the lungs. Pulmonary ventilation is made possible by rhythmic variations in the dimensions of the thoracic and intrapulmonic spaces brought about by the alternating contraction and relaxation of the respiratory muscles.

Gases possess certain physical properties which explain the movement and exchange of respiratory gases. They differ from fluids in that their molecules spread out to fill the space available to them. The molecules of a gas are in a ceaseless movement and strike the walls of the container, creating a pressure. Within a given space, the greater the number of molecules of gas, the higher is the pressure produced. *The pressure of a gas varies inversely with the space in which it is contained if the temperature remains constant* (Boyle's law). If the space in which the volume of gas is confined is reduced, more gas molecules strike a smaller area of the container, increasing the pressure. Conversely, if the space is increased, the pressure of the gas is decreased. *Gas molecules move from an area of higher pressure to one of lower pressure.*

According to Dalton's law of partial pressure, *each gas in a mixture of gases exerts the same pressure that it would exert if it were not in a mixture, and that pressure is proportional to its concentration.* The pressure of the mixture is the sum of the pressures of the constituent gases. The pressure of each gas in the mixture is termed the partial pressure of that gas, and is indicated by a "p" preceding the gas symbol. For example, the pressure of oxygen in a mixture of gases is recorded as pO_2.

The amount of a gas absorbed by a fluid (i.e., its solubility) *is directly proportional to the partial pressure of the gas.* The fluid will absorb the gas until the pressure of the gas is the same as that at the surface. This is referred to as Henry's law of the solution of gases.

INSPIRATION. The diaphragm and external intercostal muscles contract, increasing the closed, airtight thoracic space and resulting in a pressure decrease of approximately 4 to 5 mm. Hg within the cavity. The moist visceral and parietal pleurae are apposed and resist separation in the same way that two pieces of plastic or glass whose surfaces are wet are difficult to separate but slide readily on each other. As the adherent moist parietal pleura moves out with the thoracic walls, the visceral pleura follows because of the cohesion between the two moist serous surfaces. The pressure in the intrapulmonic space is atmospheric and is greater than that of the expanded thoracic cavity. This pressure differential, combined with the cohesion of the pleurae, promotes a stretching of the elastic alveoli, resulting in the expansion of the lungs. The intrapulmonic space is now increased and the pressure of the contained air is reduced. A pressure gradient is produced between the atmospheric air and that in the lungs, so air moves into the respiratory tract, producing an inspiration.

EXPIRATION. Relaxation of the respiratory muscles reverses the above process. As the intrathoracic space decreases with the muscular relaxation, the pressure within the cavity increases. The elastic alveoli which were stretched now recoil also, diminishing the intrapulmonic space. The pressure of the air within the lungs is increased then to a level above that of the atmospheric air. This causes air to move out until the intrapulmonic pressure is equal to that of the atmosphere, thus producing an expiration. Normally, this cycle of inspiration and expiration is completed 14 to 18 times per minute in the adult.

THE WORK OF BREATHING. The inspiratory phase of breathing requires energy to overcome the elastic forces in the lungs and thorax and the flow-resistant forces within the air passages. Owing to their elastic property, the lungs and chest wall constantly tend to maintain the position they occupy at the end of a normal expiration. When the respiratory muscles contract to expand the intrathoracic and intrapulmonic spaces to provide inhalation, they must overcome this elastic resistance. *Compliance* is the term used to indicate the distensibility of the lungs and the thorax, or the ease with which they are stretched. Pulmonary disease may produce changes in the lung tissue that make it "stiffer" and less elastic, causing a reduction in compliance. Similarly, the compliance of the thorax may be decreased by disorders affecting the chest wall.

Some energy is also necessary to overcome the frictional and viscous resistance offered by the surface tissues in the air passages. Any condition which reduces the caliber of the passages, causes an excessive production of mucus, or increases the surface tension increases the flow-resistant forces. These changes create a demand for greater energy to move air in and out in ventilation.

CONTROL OF VENTILATION. The control of ventilation is complex, and knowledge of this control is incomplete and unclear. Respirations are regulated by both nervous and chemical mechanisms.

NEURAL REGULATION. Inspiration and expiration are dependent upon alternate contraction and relaxation of muscles which are subordinate to impulses initiated by groups of neurons in the medulla and pons of the brain stem. These groups of neurons make up the *respiratory centers* (see Fig. 15–1).

The *medullary center* is considered responsible for spontaneous, rhythmic respiration. Some neurons in this center discharge impulses that result in contraction of the respiratory muscles and inspiration; others discharge impulses that cause relaxation of the muscles and expiration. The rhythmic discharge of the neurons in the medulla may be modified by impulses generated by groups of neurons (centers) in the pons (*pontine center*) and by impulses transmitted to the medullary centers by afferent (sensory) nerve fibers of the vagus nerves. These nerve fibers transmit impulses from receptors in the lungs that are sensitive to stretching (pulmonary stretch receptors). Stretching of the lungs by inflation produces impulses that have an inhibitory effect on the neurons that generate inspiratory impulses. The pulmonary stretch stimulus and ensuing inhibitory response is known as the *Hering-Breuer reflex*. It is more active in infants and young children and is quite weak in adults.

Impulses from the respiratory center descend into the spinal cord. Those carried to the diaphragm are transmitted by the phrenic nerves, which originate with the third, fourth and fifth cervical spinal nerves. The impulses to the intercostal muscles are delivered by the intercostal nerves that arise from the spinal cord with the third, fourth, fifth and sixth thoracic spinal nerves. The activity of the respiratory center is influenced by the level of activity of the reticular formation. Mental alertness and wakefulness normally have a stimulating effect on breathing, but sleep, sedatives and anesthesia tend to reduce the rate and volume of ventilation.

Respiratory muscle activities may be modified by impulses originating in the cerebral cortex that are delivered to the respiratory centers. For example, breathing may be controlled voluntarily for a limited period, as in breath-holding or the taking of large deep breaths. Voluntary control and a high level of central nervous system coordination and integration are needed in speaking and singing. Changes in the rhythm, rate and depth of respirations are frequently associated with emotional states (e.g., excitement, laughing, crying, depression, fear).

Certain sensory impulses may influence respirations. Severe pain produces faster and deeper respirations. Muscle activity increases respirations; this is attributed both to an increase in carbon dioxide production and to impulses originating in the stretch and pressure receptors of muscles, tendons and joints. A sudden cold application to the body produces a brief reflex apnea (cessation of breathing) followed by increased ventilation.

CHEMICAL REGULATION. The major chemical factors that exert a control on ventilation are the pCO_2, pH and pO_2 of the blood.

The *arterial carbon dioxide* tension plays an important role in the regulation of breathing. An increase above the normal pCO_2 results in an increase in the activity of the respiratory centers and a corresponding increase in the volume and frequency of respirations. A decrease below the normal slows the respiratory rate. An increase in the *hydrogen ion concentration* (decrease in the pH) produces a similar response as that to an increase above normal in the pCO_2. The *arterial oxygen tension* influences respirations to a lesser extent than the carbon dioxide content. The cells which are sensitive to changes in these chemicals are not highly sensitive to slight variations in pO_2; the oxygen content may fall below 14 volumes per cent before there is a noticeable increase in respiratory activity.

Changes in the pH and tensions of carbon dioxide and oxygen in the blood bring about respiratory changes through *respiratory chemoreceptors*. These are groups of cells that are sensitive to certain changes in the chemistry of the blood. According to their location in relation to the nervous system the chemoreceptors are of two types, peripheral and central.

The peripheral chemoreceptors are located in the carotid and aortic bodies[1] and are sensitive to changes in the pO_2, pCO_2 and hydrogen ion concentration of the blood. Impulses are initiated in these receptors and are then transmitted to the respiratory neurons via the glossopharyngeal and vagus nerves, resulting in changes in the rate and volume of respirations. Central chemoreceptors which are located within the medulla are also sensitive to changes in the blood chemistry.

When body metabolism increases, more oxygen is used by the tissues and more carbon dioxide and acid metabolites are produced. Normally, this decreases the pO_2 and increases the pCO_2 and hydrogen ion concentration of the blood, and a corresponding increase in the rate and volume of respirations occurs.

OTHER FACTORS INFLUENCING RESPIRATION. Other factors which influence ventilatory activity include blood pressure changes, changes in body temperature, drugs, and age.

Pressoreceptors in the aortic and carotid bodies are sensitive to changes in blood pressure. When they are stimulated, impulses are delivered to the respiratory centers which produce the appropriate response. A fall in blood pressure produces increased ventilation and, conversely, an elevated blood pressure generates impulses that give rise to a slower respiratory rate.

A high fever produces a noticeable increase in respiration which may be attributed principally to the increased oxygen consumption and carbon dioxide production by the accelerated cell metabolism. A decrease in temperature well below the normal, such as is produced in hypothermia, results in shallow, slow respirations.

Some drugs are known to depress the respiratory center, and overdosage may prove fatal for this reason. Narcotics such as morphine, barbiturates, anesthetics, alcohol and some tranquilizers are examples of drugs that reduce respiratory activity.

---

[1]The *carotid bodies* lie in the bifurcations of the carotid arteries; the *aortic bodies* are located on the wall of the aortic arch.

Certain drugs have the reverse effect and in excess may cause hyperpnea (increased rate and volume of respiration). This could lead to exhaustion and respiratory alkalosis because of the excessive elimination of carbon dioxide. Salicylate preparations are perhaps the most common offenders in this area.

RATE OF RESPIRATION. Respiratory rate varies with age; it is more rapid in the young, decreasing with age. The rate at birth may be 40 to 70 respirations per minute, at 5 years of age it is approximately 25 to 30 per minute, at 10 years it is 20 to 22 per minute, and at 15 years of age and older it is 16 to 20 per minute.

Composition of Inspired, Expired and Alveolar Air

INSPIRED AIR. Dry, inspired or atmospheric air at sea level is composed of nitrogen, oxygen and carbon dioxide in the following proportions:

oxygen	20.95 volumes per cent
carbon dioxide	0.04 volume per cent
nitrogen	78 volumes per cent

Various quantities of water vapor, dust particles, and insignificant amounts of rare gases such as argon, neon and ozone may be present. Oxygen and carbon dioxide are the respiratory gases; nitrogen is not of concern since it is inert in the body. Some nitrogen does diffuse in and out of the blood, but under normal atmospheric pressures it has no physiological significance.

EXPIRED AIR. This shows a reduction in oxygen and an increase in the carbon dioxide as compared with atmospheric air. It is a mixture of alveolar air and atmospheric air from the passages above the alveoli. No exchange of gases is made in the air passages above the alveoli. This nonrespiratory area is called the *anatomical dead space* and air contained in it may be referred to as dead air. If any alveoli are not perfused by capillary blood flow, those alveolar spaces combined with the anatomical dead space compose the *physiological dead space*. If a person breathes through a tube, the dead space is increased; less of the inspired air reaches the alveoli.

ALVEOLAR AIR. Since it is at this level that an exchange of the respiratory gases takes place with the capillary blood, the

TABLE 15-1 TENSIONS OF RESPIRATORY GASES IN INSPIRED, EXPIRED AND ALVEOLAR AIR

	Volumes Per Cent		Partial Pressure (mm. Hg)	
	Oxygen	Carbon Dioxide	Oxygen	Carbon Dioxide
Inspired (atmospheric) air	20.95	0.04	159	0.3
Expired air	16.3	4.5	116	28.0
Alveolar air	14.0	5.6	100	40.0

volume of oxygen in the contained air is reduced and that of carbon dioxide increases. Air that moves into the alveoli with each inspiration is a mixture of newly inspired air and air that moved into the dead space from the air sacs on previous expirations. In other words, as inspiration begins, alveolar air which had moved into the dead space on expiration is drawn back into the alveoli mixed with a portion of newly inspired air. Thus air entering the alveoli does not have exactly the same composition as inspired atmosphere air.

A comparison of the approximate volumes of respiratory gases in inspired, expired and alveolar air may be made from Table 15-1.

Alveolar ventilation may be increased by increasing the inspiratory volume and the frequency of respirations per minute. The latter will only be effective if the inspiratory volume is increased at the same time. Rapid shallow respirations simply ventilate the dead space and expend considerable muscular energy to no avail. In exercise, when more oxygen is being used and more carbon dioxide is being produced, both the frequency of respirations and the inspired volume are automatically increased. These factors have a practical application in caring for inactive patients and emphasize the importance of having them take several deep breaths at regular intervals in order to ventilate the alveoli adequately.

Diffusion and Transportation of Respiratory Gases

DIFFUSION. The diffusion component of pulmonary respiration is the interchange of oxygen and carbon dioxide across the alveolar and capillary membranes. Gases move rapidly from areas of higher to lower pressure. A pressure differential occurs between the oxygen in the alveolar air and that in the blood in the pulmonary capillaries and, as a result, oxygen moves from the alveoli into the blood. Carbon dioxide moves in the opposite direction for the same reason.

Blood enters the vast number of pulmonary capillaries with the pO_2 at about 40 mm. Hg and the pCO_2 at approximately 46 mm. Hg. Alveolar air has a pO_2 of approximately 100 mm. Hg and a pCO_2 of about 35 to 40 mm. Hg. As a result of the diffusion exchange that quickly takes place as the blood flows through the pulmonary capillaries, blood enters the pulmonary veins with a pO_2 of 95 to 100 mm. Hg and a pCO_2 of approximately 40 mm. Hg (see Table 15-2 and Fig. 15-3).

TRANSPORTATION OF RESPIRATORY GASES BY THE BLOOD. *Oxygen* is transported by the blood in solution in plasma and as a chemical compound in the red blood cells. The amount of gas that can be carried in solution is very limited; in order to carry sufficient oxygen through the body to meet the needs of the cells, most of the gas that enters the blood in the alveoli diffuses from the plasma into the red blood cells where it combines loosely with the hemoglobin to form the compound oxyhemoglobin. If the hemoglobin has its normal complement of iron, each gram can carry 1.34 ml. of oxygen and is completely saturated. The chemical process that produces oxyhemoglobin is reversible so that as the oxygen in solution is used up by the tissues, more is made available by the dissociation of the unstable oxyhemoglobin ($Hb + O_2 \leftrightarrows HbO_2$). Of the 20 volumes per cent of oxygen in the arterial blood, only about 0.5 volume per cent remains in solution in plasma; the remaining 19.5 volumes per cent is carried as oxyhemoglobin.

TABLE 15-2 PARTIAL PRESSURES OF RESPIRATORY GASES

	pO_2 (mm. Hg)	pCO_2 (mm. Hg)
Alveolar air	100	40
Venous blood	40	46
Arterial blood	95	40

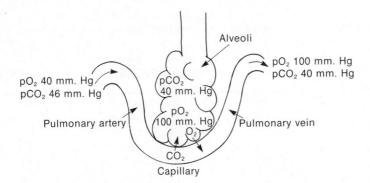

pO_2 40 mm. Hg
pCO_2 46 mm. Hg

Pulmonary artery

Alveoli

pO_2 100 mm. Hg
pCO_2 40 mm. Hg

pCO_2 40 mm. Hg

pO_2 100 mm. Hg

O_2

CO_2

Pulmonary vein

Capillary

FIGURE 15–3 Oxygen and carbon dioxide exchange through alveolar-capillary membranes.

The rate at which hemoglobin combines with oxygen and the rate of dissociation of oxyhemoglobin is influenced by the pO_2 and pCO_2 of the plasma. An increase in the pO_2 and a decrease in the pCO_2 hasten the formation of oxyhemoglobin. Conversely, a decrease in the pO_2 and an increase in the pCO_2, as occurs in the systemic capillaries, promote the release of oxygen from hemoglobin; the saturation of hemoglobin declines. The pH of the blood has a significant effect on the dissociation of oxygen and hemoglobin. A decrease in the alkalinity below the normal (i.e., a decrease in the pH) promotes release of oxygen from the hemoglobin molecule. Body temperature also influences oxygen-hemoglobin dissociation. An elevated temperature also promotes the release of oxygen from oxyhemoglobin.

Carbon dioxide is produced within the body by cellular metabolism and diffuses out of the cells through the tissue fluid into the blood, where it is carried in several forms. Only a very limited amount remains in solution in plasma; the larger proportion is carried in the form of bicarbonate (HCO_3^-) and in combination with hemoglobin and plasma proteins (carbamino compounds). About two-thirds of the total blood carbon dioxide is carried as sodium bicarbonate ($NaHCO_3$) in the plasma and serves to maintain the normal blood alkalinity (pH 7.4). A small, essential amount of potassium bicarbonate ($KHCO_3$) is found in the erythrocytes.

The chemical compounds are unstable and tend to dissociate with changes in the pressures of the gases in the blood. As the blood is circulated through the tissues, the increasing pCO_2 and decreasing pO_2 promote the formation of the compounds. A reverse of the pressure of these gases promotes dissociation of the compounds. In the pulmonary capillaries, where the pO_2 increases and pCO_2 decreases, a rapid dissociation takes place to release some of the CO_2.

TISSUE RESPIRATION. The exchange of carbon dioxide and oxygen which takes place between the cells and the blood in the systemic capillaries throughout the body comprises tissue or internal respiration. The basis of the gaseous exchange is the pressure gradient of each of the respiratory gases between the cells and the tissue fluid, and between the tissue fluid and the blood. The pO_2 of the arterial blood when it enters the systemic capillaries is approximately 95 mm. Hg (20 volumes per cent) and is much higher than that of the interstitial fluid, so oxygen diffuses from the plasma into the tissue fluid. Continuous cell activity uses oxygen, so the higher pO_2 of the tissue fluid results in a movement of the oxygen into the cells. As the oxygen tension is reduced in the plasma, the loosely combined oxyhemoglobin dissociates to free oxygen. By the time the blood again reaches the pulmonary capillaries the oxyhemoglobin has given up considerable oxygen.

The chemical activities of the cells (metabolism) produce carbon dioxide. Its concentration in the cell produces a pressure gradient that results in its movement into the tissue fluid. From here, because of the pressure difference, it moves into the capillary blood and gradually accumulates a higher concentration in the venous blood than that of alveolar air. This promotes the diffusion of carbon dioxide from the pulmonary capillary blood into alveolar air.

The amount of gas exchanged in tissue respiration varies in different tissues and organs and with a decrease or increase in activity. The brain tissue, myocardium and skeletal muscles require a constant supply of oxygen. Any deficiency is quickly reflected in impaired function of these structures.

Chemical Reactions in Respiration

Several chemical reactions are involved in the transport and exchange of oxygen and carbon dioxide and occur continuously with great speed in the blood throughout all the tissues. A brief summary of the reactions follows and, since the reactions of oxygen and carbon dioxide are interrelated, they are considered together.

IN THE TISSUES. Potassium oxyhemoglobin ($KHbO_2$) in red blood cells dissociates in the systemic capillaries to release O_2 which diffuses through the plasma into the interstitial fluid and on into the cells:

$$KHbO_2 \longrightarrow KHb + O_2$$

Carbon dioxide diffuses from the tissues into the plasma and on into red blood cells where the enzyme carbonic anhydrase promotes a reaction with water to form carbonic acid:

$$CO_2 + H_2O \xrightarrow{\text{carbonic anhydrase}} H_2CO_3$$

This is a very unstable acid and readily ionizes to hydrogen (H^+) and bicarbonate (HCO_3^-) ions. Some of the HCO_3^- ions move out into the plasma and form sodium bicarbonate ($NaHCO_3$). The H^+ ions unite with the hemoglobin (HHb):

$$H_2CO_3 \longrightarrow H^+ \cdot HCO_3^-$$
$$HCO_3^- + Na^+ \longrightarrow NaHCO_3$$
$$H^+ + Hb \longrightarrow HHb$$

Chloride (Cl^-) ions released by dissociation of NaCl move into red blood cells from the plasma to replace the HCO_3^- ions to maintain ionic equilibrium. They react with potassium hemoglobin (KHb) and form potassium chloride (KCl) and hemoglobin (Hb):

$$Cl^- + KHb \longrightarrow KCl + Hb$$

Some bicarbonate (HCO_3^-) ions which remain within the red blood cells also react

with KHb when it gives up O_2 to form potassium bicarbonate:

$$HCO_3^- + KHb \longrightarrow KHCO_3 + Hb$$

Some of the CO_2 entering the red blood cells unites with Hb, forming carbaminohemoglobin ($HbCO_2$):

$$CO_2 + Hb \longrightarrow HbCO_2$$

The above reactions at tissue level result in:

1. O_2 being released from Hb
2. The formation of $NaHCO_3$ and $KHCO_3$
3. The formation of $HbCO_2$

IN THE LUNG CAPILLARIES. The O_2 diffuses from the plasma into the red blood cells where it combines with HHb to form oxyhemoglobin ($HHbO_2$). The H^+ ion makes this compound acidic, so it reacts with $KHCO_3$, yielding potassium hemoglobin ($KHbO_2$) and carbonic acid (H_2CO_3):

$$HHb + O_2 \longrightarrow HHbO_2$$
$$HHbO_2 + KHCO_3 \longrightarrow KHbO_2 + H_2CO_3$$

Dissociation of H_2CO_3 is promoted by carbonic anhydrase, and CO_2 and H_2O are produced. The CO_2 diffuses out of the red blood cell through the plasma into the alveolar air because of the pressure gradient.

$$H_2CO_3 \xrightarrow{\text{carbonic anhydrase}} H_2O + CO_2$$

With the loss of HCO_3^- ions in these reactions the ionic equilibrium is disturbed so dissociated Cl^- ions move out of the red blood cells into the plasma where they react with $NaHCO_3$ to form NaCl and bicarbonate (HCO_3^-):

$$Cl^- + NaHCO_3 \longrightarrow NaCl + HCO_3^-$$

Much of the HCO_3^- diffuses into the red blood cells and combines with the KHb to form $KHCO_3$.

As cited above, $KHCO_3$ reacts with the acidic oxyhemoglobin ($HHbO_2$) to yield carbonic acid (H_2CO_3).

The above reactions in lung capillaries result in:

1. Formation of oxyhemoglobin (HbO_2)
2. The formation of H_2CO_3

3. The dissociation of H_2CO_3 to H_2O and CO_2
4. Diffusion of CO_2 into the alveoli.

FACTORS WHICH INFLUENCE PULMONARY DIFFUSION. The volumes of oxygen and carbon dioxide which diffuse across the pulmonary membrane depend upon the pressure gradient of each gas between the alveolar air and capillary blood. Alveolar ventilation must be adequate to maintain an effective pO_2 to drive oxygen into the blood. Sufficient elimination of carbon dioxide in expiration to reduce the pCO_2 in the alveolar air is necessary to promote the movement of carbon dioxide out of the blood into the alveoli. Increased respiratory rate alone does not necessarily provide alveolar ventilation. If the respirations are shallow, it is mainly the dead space that is being ventilated.

Diffusion is greatly influenced by the ventilation-perfusion ratio. Normally, ventilation of the alveoli and perfusion (flow of blood) are relatively uniform. Any disparity that incurs underperfusion or underventilation results in reduced diffusion, which results in decreased blood pO_2 and possibly an increased pCO_2.[2] A disturbance in the ventilation-perfusion ratio may be referred to as the mismatching or imbalance of ventilation and blood flow. Mismatching may be caused by such conditions as pulmonary embolism, which causes underperfusion, and emphysema, bronchial constriction or pneumonia, which result in a number of alveoli being underventilated.

Diffusion may be decreased by the presence of increased fluid in the alveoli, collapse of the alveoli or, rarely, by alveolar tissue changes resulting from chronic pulmonary disease (e.g., pulmonary fibrosis).

Any reduction in the alveolar surface area such as occurs with lobectomy, pneumonectomy or emphysema obviously greatly diminishes the diffusion of the respiratory gases.

Respiration and High Altitude

Atmospheric pressure decreases as the distance above sea level increases. The corresponding decreases in the partial pressure of oxygen at high altitudes reduces the pressure of oxygen in alveolar air and less oxygen diffuses into the blood, causing a deficiency throughout the body. The height at which symptoms of hypoxia (deficiency of oxygen) are first experienced varies somewhat with different individuals and according to the speed with which they ascend. A rapid ascent to 10,000 feet where atmospheric pressure is approximately 523 mm. Hg and the pO_2 in alveolar air is 67 mm. Hg produces symptoms of oxygen deficiency in the brain. The person manifests reduced mental efficiency and a decrease in visual and auditory acuity. Greater heights produce further deterioration, and at 20,000 to 25,000 feet the person lapses into coma.

In a gradual ascent to a high altitude the person's physiology makes some adjustments to acclimatize. Respirations increase in rate and volume and the heart rate and output are increased. The number of red blood cells and the amount of hemoglobin are increased when one is exposed to a higher altitude for a period of 1 or more weeks. Since more carbon dioxide is lost at these heights, owing to the lower carbon dioxide pressure in the air and the increased respirations, blood alkalinity is increased. More base ions are excreted by the kidney in an effort to maintain a normal pH of the body fluids.

In aviation, the low atmospheric pressure of high altitudes is overcome by breathing pure oxygen to increase the oxygen concentration in the alveolar air or by pressurizing the cabin of the plane.

Respiration and High Atmospheric Pressure

Atmospheric pressure increases as the distance below sea level increases. A depth of 33 feet below sea level doubles the atmospheric pressure. An abnormally high atmospheric pressure is experienced by deep-sea divers and by workers in chambers or tunnels which are filled with compressed air to prevent cave-ins that might result from the increased pressure from without. The high pressure of the air causes greater amounts of oxygen and nitrogen to diffuse into the blood.

Excessive amounts of these gases are

---

[2]Carbon dioxide is much more soluble than oxygen, so it diffuses more rapidly. Impaired diffusion is likely to cause hypoxia before hypercapnia.

carried in solution in the body fluids. The high oxygen concentration may interfere with normal cellular activity; impaired brain function may be manifested by twitching, convulsions, confusion, stupor and coma. The excessive volume of nitrogen may also affect behavior. Most frequently, it has a depressing or anesthetizing effect on the central nervous system and the person becomes very drowsy and inefficient. Nitrogen frequently causes more problems when the person ascends to normal atmospheric pressure. While exposed to the greater pressure the nitrogen remains in solution, but when the individual ascends to the surface the decreased pressure on the body causes the nitrogen to expand and form bubbles in the tissues or fluids. These may cause an embolism and tissue damage in any area of the body; severe pain, brain damage, paralysis or severe gastrointestinal distention may occur. To prevent bubble formation, the person is brought to sea level very slowly or is confined within a chamber in which the pressure is very gradually decreased while the excess nitrogen escapes.

Deep-sea divers prevent the entry of excess gases into their blood by reducing the amount of oxygen in the gas they breathe, and in some instances they add helium. Disturbances due to extremely high atmospheric pressure may be referred to as *caisson disease, decompression sickness or the bends*.

Pulmonary Volumes and Capacities

The volume of air breathed in and out varies with the activity and demands of the body, the age and size of each individual and the condition of the respiratory system. The figure given with each of the following respiratory volumes is the average for normal male adults; for the normal average adult female the volumes are approximately 20 to 25 per cent less.

TIDAL VOLUME (V_T). This represents the volume of air inspired or expired with each breath. During normal, quiet breathing the tidal volume measures about 500 ml. Approximately 150 ml. of this fills the anatomical dead space and does not exchange gases with the blood. The dead space gas is symbolized by V_D.

MINUTE RESPIRATORY VOLUME (MRV, MV, OR V MIN.). This is the total volume of air moved in or out of the lungs in 1 minute and is determined by multiplying the tidal volume by the respiratory rate per minute ($V_T \times f$).

INSPIRATORY CAPACITY (IC). This term indicates the maximum amount of air which can be inhaled in one breath. The normal is approximately 3500 ml.

INSPIRATORY RESERVE VOLUME (IRV). This is the portion of the inspiratory capacity in excess of the tidal volume and is approximately 3000 ml.

EXPIRATORY RESERVE VOLUME (ERV). The maximum quantity of air that can be forcibly exhaled after an ordinary expiration is approximately 1000 to 1100 ml.

FORCED EXPIRATORY VOLUME (FEV). This is the maximum volume of air that can be rapidly exhaled following a maximum inspiration. It is usually recorded in liters per second.

RESIDUAL VOLUME (RV). The volume of air remaining in the lungs after maximum expiration is referred to as residual air. The average normal volume is approximately 1200 ml. The lungs cannot be completely emptied of air if the chest cavity remains closed.

VITAL CAPACITY (VC). This is the maximum volume of air that can be expired after an inspiration of maximum capacity. It equals the tidal volume plus the inspiratory and expiratory reserve volumes. The normal is approximately 4000 to 5000 ml.

TOTAL LUNG CAPACITY (TLC). The residual volume plus the vital capacity volume represents the total lung capacity. The normal amounts to approximately 5200 to 6000 ml.

RESPIRATORY DISORDERS AND THEIR ASSESSMENT

There are many different disorders which may adversely affect the movement of a normal volume of air in and out of the alveoli or interfere with the diffusion of the respiratory gases across the alveolar-capillary membrane. Acute and chronic respiratory disorders have a very high incidence and account for a large part of absenteeism at work and school as well as for permanent disability and dependence. The site of the problem may be within the upper or lower respiratory tract, or it may be extrinsic in areas such as the respiratory center (brain stem), respiratory muscles, chest wall and nonrespiratory structures within the mediastinum. The dysfunction may be primary or secondary.

The system is vulnerable to a wide variety of causative factors. A large proportion of the diseases are infectious and communicable; the infected person coughs or exhales contaminated droplets and air into the atmosphere which may then be inhaled by other persons in the environment. Other causes of respiratory disorders include allergic reaction, inhalation of irritating gas or dust, aspiration of foreign material or a foreign body, neoplasms and trauma. In many instances the disorder is not of a serious nature but can be responsible for considerable discomfort for the affected person. Also, it must be remembered that the continuity and close relationship of the various respiratory structures predispose to a minor disorder spreading to another part and becoming a more serious problem.

Regardless of the etiologic factor, the primary concern, especially when the lower tract is involved, is whether ventilation is adequate and whether the diffusion is sufficient to maintain normal blood gas levels (i.e., normal paO_2 and $paCO_2$).

CHEST EXAMINATION

Physical examination of the chest involves inspection, palpation, percussion and auscultation.

Inspection

The examination usually commences with simple visual observation. Factors noted include the following:

SHAPE OF THE THORAX. Scoliosis or kyphosis may interfere with normal breathing. It is important to note any apparent abnormality in the shape or bony framework of the thorax. Chest expansion may be restricted or bony structure may be imposed on the airway. If the chest is barrel-shaped, it may indicate chronic obstructive pulmonary disease (COPD).

CHEST MOVEMENTS ASSOCIATED WITH RESPIRATIONS. The frequency, rhythm and depth of respirations are noted by observing the chest. If the individual's breathing is labored, the intercostal spaces are observed for any "ballooning out" during exhalation or retraction during inspiration. Either indicates a serious respiratory problem.

The supraclavicular and suprasternal areas are observed for retraction and the shoulders for elevation during inspiration. These movements are present with the use of accessory respiratory muscles in labored breathing.

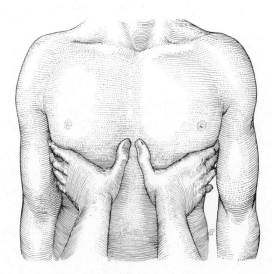

FIGURE 15–4 Assessing the chest excursion on inspiration.

The chest excursion on inspiration reflects the extent of expansion and depth of respiration. It may be assessed by placing the hands on the chest with the fingers slightly outspread and the thumbs just meeting at the midline (see Fig. 15–4). As the patient breathes in, the hands are normally separated by the chest expansion. Whether the range of the chest excursion is the same on both sides is also noted; if equal, the thumbs will be moved an equal distance from the midline on each side. Normally the movements of the two sides are symmetrical.

Palpation

This method of examining the chest assesses the presence and intensity of vibrations produced in the chest wall by voice sounds. The vibrations are conducted throughout the air passages to the chest wall and are referred to as *vocal fremitus*. They may be felt by the examiner's hand (tactile fremitus) or may be heard through a stethoscope (auditory vocal fremitus).

In the tactile method of chest palpation, the examiner places a hand on the chest and, beginning in the apical region and working down, moves from one side of the chest to the other. The patient is asked to repeat "ninety-nine" during the examination. Auditory fremitus simply requires the use of a stethoscope in place of the hand.

The vibrations are more intense in the areas of the larger bronchial tubes and are weakest in the areas of the lung bases. They are more prominent when conducted through solid matter and are not conducted as well through air and fluid. Decreased fremitus may be due to trapped air, as in emphysema or asthma, or to pleural effusion or pneumothorax. Increased fremitus occurs when underlying tissues become more dense, as in atelectasis, pneumonia or a newgrowth.

Palpation may also detect sensitive areas or a mass in the chest wall.

Percussion

This procedure involves tapping the chest with the fingertips to elicit sounds that reflect the density of underlying structures. The chest is examined anteriorly and posteriorly, going from apex to base over each side. The percussion sounds are compared with those produced on the contralateral side. Those structures that contain air result in low-pitched, resonant percussion sounds. Solid tissue and inflammatory exudate produce a higher-pitched, dull sound. Percussion helps to determine the location, size and density of underlying organs.

Percussion may be performed by placing the palmar surface of the middle finger over an intercostal space. Then, with the index or middle finger of the other hand, a sharp tap is delivered to the finger on the chest, and the sound noted. This method is called mediate percussion. A more direct method may be used by tapping the chest directly (immediate percussion).

Auscultation

Normal respirations present characteristic sounds as air enters and leaves the lower respiratory tract. Listening to the breath sounds is done through a stethoscope and the process is known as auscultation.[3]

The sounds heard in normal respirations are called *vesicular breath sounds*. They produce a soft, breezy noise and are heard over all the lung areas except over the apex of the right lung. This is because of the proximity of the large bronchial tubes to the chest wall. The inspiratory phase of a vesicular sound is longer and louder than the expiratory phase. The differences may be attributed to the movement of inspiratory air into progressively smaller air passages (and vice versa in the case of the air being exhaled).

Bronchial breath sounds are associated with a short inspiratory phase and a longer expiratory phase. The sounds are higher-pitched and equally loud in both phases. They are abnormal, and indicate some disease process such as pneumonia in the lung.

Bronchovesicular breath sounds are characterized by inspiratory and expiratory phases of equal duration. The expiratory sound is louder and higher-pitched than the vesicular breath sounds. Some alveoli may not be functioning. Bronchovesicular sounds are heard normally over the trachea and where the bronchi are close to the chest wall (e.g., between the scapulae).

---

[3]*Auscultation* is defined as the listening to sounds produced by an organ within the body. The procedure is used most frequently in the assessment of cardiac and pulmonary function but it may also be used to evaluate gastrointestinal activity.

In auscultation, the examiner first listens to the upper lobes of the lungs and progresses in a symmetrical manner to the lung bases. An assessment is made of the equality of air entry on both sides of the chest and any abnormal sounds or absence of sounds is noted. During the examination the patient is asked to breathe deeply with his mouth open. The environment should be as quiet as possible and the patient protected from chilling and unnecessary exposure. The diaphragm of the stethoscope should be warmed before being placed on the patient.

Some abnormal sounds resulting from a disease process within the tracheobronchial tree and/or lungs may be referred to as *adventitious sounds*. These include the following.

Rales are short, interrupted, bubbling sounds produced by the movement of air with mucus or exudate or by the inspiratory rush of air through bronchioles that were constricted or closed down and suddenly opened. They are heard most readily during inspiration and may be classified as coarse, medium or fine (crepitant). Coarse rales are heard at the start of inspiration and resemble a gurgling sound. They may be associated with secretions in the upper, larger air passages. Medium rales are heard about halfway through the inspiratory phase and usually occur with a disorder in the smaller, more distal tubes. Fine rales or crepitations are heard just near the end of an inspiration as fine crackling sounds similar to those produced by rubbing a few hairs together between the fingertips. They are usually produced by congestion or some disease process in terminal bronchioles and/or alveoli.

A *wheezing* or whistling sound may frequently be heard with the naked ear as well as with a stethoscope in patients with narrowing or obstruction of the lower air passages or bronchospasm. It is usually heard in the expiratory phase of a breath.

Rhonchi are coarse, wheezing sounds that tend to be more predominant during expiration. They are associated with a narrowed portion of the tracheobronchial tree.

Pleural friction rub is a characteristic sound produced when inflamed roughened pleurae rub against each other on inspiration. It becomes audible during the latter part of the inspiratory phase.

Absent or diminished breath sounds may occur over an area of a lung in which there is an obstruction that prevents air entry, atelectasis or pneumothorax.

Stridor is a crowing-like or high-pitched sound that is emitted with each inspiration as air passes through a markedly constricted larynx or trachea. It is easily recognized by the naked ear.

MANIFESTATIONS OF RESPIRATORY DISORDERS

Cough

A cough is a sudden, expulsive expiration for the purpose of removing an irritant from the air passages. It is a protective reflex that indicates the presence of some irritation in the tract.

MECHANISM. The cough mechanism involves stimulation of receptors in the mucous membrane of the bronchial tubes, trachea, larynx or pharynx or stimulation at a point along the vagus nerve. The impulses travel via afferent fibers of the vagus nerve or the glossopharyngeal nerve to the cough center, formed by a group of neurons in the medulla of the brain. Responsive impulses are initiated in the center and travel to the respiratory muscles and the larynx, producing, in succession, a quick inhalation, closure of the glottis, relaxation of the diaphragm and contraction of the abdominal and internal intercostal muscles to increase the intrathoracic and intrapulmonic pressures. The latter is exerted against the closed glottis which opens suddenly, releasing a forceful gust-like expiration. A review of the sequence of activities shows three phases — namely, the inspiratory, compressive and expulsive phases. During the compressive phase, pressure is placed on the alveoli and their secretions are moved into the small bronchial tubes. The increased velocity of the airflow in the expiratory phase results in secretions being expelled from the air passages.

The cough is generally an involuntary response, although some voluntary control may be exerted to inhibit it or produce it. If a cough is unproductive, it may be helpful to instruct the patient to make an effort to inhibit the cough in order to conserve his energy and prevent exhaustion. In other instances, the patient may be required to initiate a series of coughs at regular intervals to prevent the accumulation of secretions in the air passages. The strength or vigor of a cough is determined by the volume of the precough inspiration, the strength of the compression and the rate of expulsion of air.

CAUSES. The origin of the cough stimulus may be within the respiratory tract or may be extrinsic to it. *Intrinsic stimuli* include inflammation, secretions, fluid, scar tissue which causes traction on the nerve endings, newgrowths, inhaled or aspirated particles of dust, irritating gases and foreign bodies and very cold or very hot air. *Extrinsic stimuli* are abnormal conditions in neighboring structures which exert pressure on some area of the tracheobronchial tree. Pleurisy, newgrowths of the esophagus, enlarged lymph nodes in the mediastinum and aortic aneurysm are examples of extrinsic causes. Rarely, a cough is psychogenic. Emotional tension may result in a failure of the epiglottis to close in swallowing, allowing saliva, fluid or food to enter the respiratory tract. Occasionally, a cough is used as an attention-seeking device or as a release of nervous tension.

IMPLICATIONS FOR NURSING. A persistent cough should always be considered as an indication of something abnormal that requires investigation. It is not unusual to find persons ignoring a cough until some more distressing sign or symptom appears, at which time the cause may have progressed to a serious or advanced stage.

The treatment of a patient's cough depends upon its cause. Few coughs should be suppressed; coughing is a reflex protective mechanism designed to remove foreign and irritating matter from the respiratory tract. It has been said that more deaths occur due to failure to cough than ever result from coughing. Efforts are directed toward making the cough less difficult and more effective. The patient may be instructed to extend the interval between paroxysms of coughing by exerting voluntary control and by remaining quiet and at rest for a period of 1 to 2 hours. He will then produce more forceful expiration and will raise more secretions than he could with frequent, shallow, hacking coughs. The fluid intake may be increased and medications prescribed to increase the secretions and make them less tenacious and easier to raise. If the cough is unproductive, frequent and exhausting, a drug may be ordered to depress the cough center.

Certain observations are made and recorded by the nurse. The *frequency* of the cough is noted as well as whether it is productive or nonproductive. Any *sputum* raised is observed as to the amount, character (mucus, watery, purulent, tenacious, frothy, caseous or blood-streaked) and odor. The sound of the cough may be important; it may be hard and racking, croupy, hacking, shallow, deep and rattling or may have a whooping sound.

The cough may be worse at certain *times of the day*. Frequently, secretions accumulate during the night, and when the patient rouses and moves in the morning severe paroxysms of coughing are precipitated. If pain is experienced with coughing, its location and quality are ascertained.

Finally, it is important to assess the *effect of the cough on the patient*. If the physical exertion and disturbance of rest are exhausting or if the cough is creating anxiety in the patient, the physician is informed. Its frequency may interrupt the patient's meal to the point that he gives up and does not take sufficient nourishment.

Some patients inhibit their cough because it causes pain; support may be given by the nurse who places a hand to the anterior and posterior chest walls in the painful area. If the pain is due to pleural irritation, the doctor may reduce the chest excursion by strapping the affected side with adhesive. Each strap is applied following an expiration when the lung is deflated.

Coughing and expectoration should always be considered potentially infectious. The mouth and nose should be covered by the patient with a tissue during a cough. Paper tissues are made available to receive the expectoration, and provision is made for the prompt disposal of used tissues in a paper bag kept within the patient's reach. If the sputum is profuse or is to be measured, a covered sputum container is used. Such containers may have a disposable liner but the outer part requires daily cleansing and disinfection.

The patient is encouraged to take a daily fluid intake of 2000 to 2500 ml. unless contraindicated. Adequate fluids make the secretions less tenacious and facilitate their removal. Expectorants — drugs that increase and liquefy the secretions (e.g., ammonium chloride) — and humidification of the air also make it easier for the individual to cough up the secretions.

If the cough is nonproductive and exhausting, an antitussive drug may be prescribed to depress the cough reflex (e.g., codeine, dextramethorphan hydrobromide).

Abnormal Breathing

Normal involuntary respirations are regular, effortless and quiet. Irregularities in breathing may relate to rate, volume, rhythm or the ease with which the person breathes. The following terms are used to indicate characteristic breathing patterns.

Eupnea represents quiet normal breathing at the rate of about 16 to 20 times per minute in the adult. Respirations are more rapid and shallow in the infant and preschool child; they vary from 30 to 50 per minute in infancy, gradually decreasing to adult levels by the age of 10 to 12 years.

Apnea is a temporary cessation of breathing.

Tachypnea is rapid breathing with the volume of the respirations usually below normal.

Bradypnea is an abnormally slow rate of respirations.

Hyperpnea is an increase in the volume of air breathed per minute due to either an increase in the rate or depth of respirations or to both.

Dyspnea refers to a subjective awareness of a disturbance in breathing. The patient experiences discomfort and/or the need for increased effort or work in ventilation. The individual's perception of difficult breathing or shortness of breath may be due to physiological or psychological stress. The experience is anxiety-provoking, since the person knows that breathing is essential to life; the emotional reaction tends to aggravate and perpetuate the problem further. The individual may describe it as "a tightness in the chest," "shortness of breath," "unable to get enough air," or "suffocating." The dyspneic patient frequently has a distressed appearance, is restless and may be perspiring. It may only be present on exertion and may be episodic. The frequency of the episodes and whether their occurrence is related to a particular time of day or certain situations or factors are noted.

Orthopnea is dyspnea which is present in the recumbent position but is relieved to some extent by elevation of the trunk.

Cheyne-Stokes respirations are characterized by a few seconds of apnea followed by respirations that gradually increase in frequency and volume to a peak intensity, and then gradually subside to a period of apnea. This pattern is cyclic.

Biot's pattern of breathing is characterized by a few respirations varying in volume, followed by a prolonged period of apnea.

Kussmaul's respirations are rapid and very deep.[4]

Apneustic breathing is typified by prolonged, gasping inspirations which are held for an abnormal length of time and followed by very short inefficient expirations.

Abnormal Breath Sounds

Normal respirations present characteristic sounds as air enters and leaves the lower respiratory tract. Absence of such sounds or the accompaniment of other sounds may indicate excessive secretions or fluid in an area or constriction or blockage of a section of the system (see Chest Examination, p. 394).

Chest Pain

Pain associated with respiratory disorders originates mainly in the upper air passages or in the pleurae. Inflammation of the trachea or bronchial tubes causes a burning "raw" type of pain which is not affected by respirations but becomes worse on coughing. Pleural pain tends to be localized to one side of the chest and is due to the stretching of the affected pleura. It is sharp and stabbing on inspiration, causing the patient to take shallow breaths.

Abnormal Chest Movements

Unequal participation of the two sides of the chest in respiratory movements may be evident, or unusual retraction or ballooning of the intercostal spaces may occur. For example, in atelectasis or pneumothorax, in which a part or all of the lung is not being

---

[4]Kussmaul's respirations are usually associated with metabolic acidosis.

inflated, there is diminished movement of the chest wall on the affected side. Similarly, this may occur if a large section of alveoli is consolidated with fluid or secretions. Excessive retraction or ballooning is associated with extreme difficulty in getting air in or out of the air passages.

Secretions

Normally, the adult raises about 100 ml of mucus daily. This may be increased when there is some irritation in the air passages and may change in color and consistency. The expectoration of blood occurs in many respiratory disorders and in varying degrees of severity. There may be only a slight streaking of the mucus with blood or there may be expectoration of frank blood. The latter is referred to as *hemoptysis*. Blood in the sputum is commonly associated with inflammatory conditions and lesions which cause erosion and necrosis of the tissues and blood vessels, such as bronchitis, pneumonia, tuberculosis, carcinoma and pulmonary infarction.

Clubbing of the Fingers and Toes

Occasionally, this unusual sign develops in chronic respiratory disease and, although its cause is not definitely known, it is thought to be due to increased vascularity in response to hypoxia.

Cyanosis

A dusky bluish color of the mucous membranes, skin and nail beds may be associated with respiratory disease due to excessive deoxygenation of the hemoglobin. When more than the usual amount of dissociation occurs, the hemoglobin presents a dark blue color. The absence of cyanosis is not always a reassuring sign unless the hemoglobin level is known. In a person with 50 per cent or less of the normal complement (13 to 15 Gm. per cent), the reduced hemoglobin may not be sufficiently concentrated to be reflected through superficial tissues.

Constitutional Symptoms in Respiratory Disorders

If the respiratory disturbance is due to infection or trauma, or if there is degenera-

tion of tissue as in pulmonary infarction, the patient usually develops a fever and a corresponding increase in pulse rate. General debilitation occurs quickly in most respiratory disease; the patient complains of anorexia, weakness and fatigue and loses weight.

Abnormal Blood Gas Levels

Manifestations of disturbances in respiratory ventilation and/or gas exchange may be reflected in changes in the arterial pO_2, pCO_2 and pH. For normal values see page 389.

DIAGNOSTIC AND ASSESSMENT PROCEDURES

Investigation and assessment of the patient with a respiratory disorder includes observation of the rate, rhythm and depth of the respirations and the associated chest movements, sounds and use of accessory muscles. A knowledge of familial incidence of respiratory disturbances and information about the patient's occupation, living customs and special concerns are important and an essential part of the investigation. The nutritional status and hydration are quite significant; the former influences the individual's resistance and recuperative capacity. Dehydration may result in thick, tenacious secretions which are not readily raised and predispose to infection and obstruction of the airway. On the other hand, overhydration and edema may increase the alveolar fluid content and interfere with ventilation and diffusion.

Assessment of a patient's condition includes inspection, percussion and auscultation (see above). The investigative procedures used vary with each patient. In some instances the diagnosis is based on the physical examination and the patient's history alone. In others, blood tests and special radiologic, endoscopic, bacteriologic and cytologic studies are required. Similarly, respiratory function tests are necessary with some patients to determine to what extent, if any, they are experiencing airway resistance and ventilatory insufficiency.

Roentgenogram of the Chest

Radiologic studies of the chest may reveal a lesion in the respiratory tract or thoracic cavity, its location, the size of the area involved and something of the nature of the lesion. They also provide information about the mediastinum, the structure of the thorax, the size of the heart and aorta and the level of the diaphragm. The initial films requested are usually antero-posterior (AP) and lateral (L) views. If certain chest or lung areas are suspected of being pathologic, films may be requested that provide views from special positions. For example, right and left anterior oblique films will visualize the mediastinum and some areas of the lung that are not seen in AP and L films.

The procedure is explained to the patient if it is unfamiliar to him so he will know what to expect. His clothing is removed to the waist to prevent the possibility of objects such as buttons restricting the entrance of x-rays. If the patient is wearing an identification tag or a necklace, it is also removed. The patient is given a cotton gown or drape to prevent exposure. He is advised to take a deep breath and hold it while the x-ray is being taken, and then to breathe normally.

Radiologic investigation may include making a series of films of the lungs at different planes. This type of radiology is referred to as *tomography* or *stratigraphy*. In these films the lung tissue is visualized at different depths. They provide details that are not revealed in ordinary x-rays because of overlying structures. Tomographs are helpful in recognizing solid or calcified lesions and cavitations.

A *stereoscopic* (three-dimensional) x-ray picture may be used to delineate or confirm the presence and location of a lesion.

Fluoroscopic examination (direct viewing by x-ray) of the chest without taking a film may be done to view lung expansion and the respiratory excursion of the diaphragm.

The patient may be too ill to be moved to the x-ray department to be x-rayed. A portable x-ray machine is brought to the bedside and a film of the chest is made. Staff members leave the room while the x-ray is taken to avoid unnecessary radiation exposure.

Sputum Examination

Sputum is examined microscopically in a smear or by culture for disease organisms,

bronchial casts, eosinophils and cancer cells. Tests are also done to identify the antimicrobial drug(s) (usually antibiotics) to which the infecting organisms present in the sputum are sensitive. This denotes the drug that will be effective for the patient.

The physician may request that the sputum specimen be collected first thing in the morning, since the secretions that accumulate during the night may have a higher concentration of organisms. The mouth should be clean and free of residual food particles. The patient is given a wide-mouthed container, which is provided by the laboratory especially for a sputum specimen, and is instructed to cough deeply to raise the sputum from the lungs. A paper towel may be wrapped around the bottle to prevent contamination of the outside of the container. The specimen container is kept covered for esthetic reasons and to prevent air contamination by the sputum and vice versa. When the specimen is obtained, the container is removed from the paper covering, labeled and delivered to the laboratory.

If the patient is unable to raise a satisfactory amount of sputum, a specimen of the gastric content may be requested, since some sputum may have been swallowed while sleeping. A gastric aspiration is done in the morning before anything is taken by mouth. A sterile gastric tube is passed and a syringe is used to withdraw a specimen. The fluid is placed in a sterile container.

Pleural Fluid

Pleural fluid obtained by aspiration that is to be used for bacteriologic or cytologic examinations is placed in a sterile bottle or test tube and sealed with a sterile bottle cap or cork and labeled. The specimen is obtained by thoracentesis (see p. 429).

Endoscopic Investigation

An endoscope is a hollow instrument which is equipped with a light and is used for direct examination of an area within the body. Each one is constructed for use in specific body areas; examples are the laryngoscope, bronchoscope, gastroscope, cystoscope, and colonoscope. These instruments have been improved markedly in recent years; all except the laryngoscope are made of flexible fiberoptic material and are

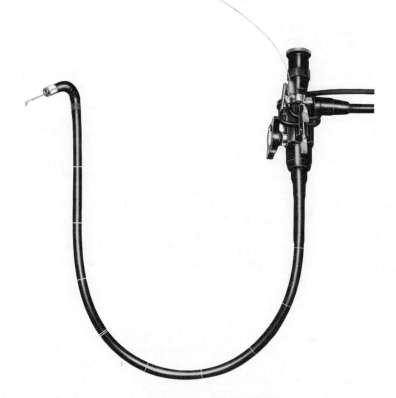

FIGURE 15–5 A fiberoptic endoscope. (From Luckmann, J., and Sorensen, K. C., Medical-Surgical Nursing. A Psychophysiologic Approach, Philadelphia, W. B. Saunders Co., 1974, p. 1058.)

smaller in diameter, which makes possible their direction into areas that could not formerly be examined with the original rigid metal endoscopes. Their flexibility and size make them less traumatizing than the previous models and the procedure less painful and uncomfortable for the patients.

The fiberoptic endoscope contains two fiberoptic bundles; one transmits light from a remote source into the field being viewed. The second bundle, which has a lens at each end, transmits the image to the proximal lens which focuses and magnifies the image, resulting in clearer viewing of the area (Fig. 15–5).

In addition to permitting direct examination of a part, endoscopy may also include an aspiration or excision biopsy; specially constructed instruments are available that may be introduced through the endoscope to obtain the specimen for biopsy.[5] Investigation of a patient with a respiratory disorder may include a laryngoscopy or a bronchoscopy.

LARYNGOSCOPY. The laryngoscope used in direct examination of the larynx is a short, hollow metal tube with a light at the distal end. It is passed through the mouth and pharynx to the area beyond the epiglottis. In some instances, an operating microscope may be used by the physician during the examination. The microscope allows binocular vision and provides magnification of the tissues.

Preparation of a patient for a laryngoscopy includes an explanation of the procedure and the signing of a consent. He is advised of the purposes, that he will be on his back with his head hyperextended and that he will remain conscious throughout the procedure since only topical anesthesia is used to introduce the instrument. The patient should know that the room will be darkened and his eyes covered.

Food and fluids are withheld for the 6 to 8 hours previous to the scheduled examination time to avoid vomiting and aspiration. Dentures are removed and atropine is generally prescribed to reduce secretions. Some sedation may also be ordered to promote relaxation and reduce the patient's anxiety.

---

[5]Frank N. Marici: "The Flexible Fiberoptic Bronchoscope." Am. J. Nurs., Vol. 73, No. 10 (Oct. 1973), pp. 1776–1778.

Following the examination the head of the bed is elevated, and the patient is encouraged to lie on either side to promote the drainage of secretions and prevent aspiration. An ice collar may be used to reduce soreness and possible laryngeal edema. The swallowing and gag reflexes are usually absent for a few hours because of the local anesthesia used; fluids and food are withheld until they return. Restoration of the reflex may be determined, after a minimum of 2 hours, by having the patient try to swallow a small amount of water from a teaspoon or by gently touching the post-pharyngeal wall with an absorbent-tipped applicator. When the normal reflex is reestablished, small amounts of fluids are given and are gradually increased if there is no vomiting. The patient is usually able to take a soft diet in 8 hours and his regular diet by the end of 24 hours. He is encouraged to rest quietly and not attempt to talk, cough or clear his throat.

Trauma of the larynx may produce hoarseness or loss of the voice; the patient needs reassurance that either is only temporary, and he is given a pencil and paper by which he can communicate.

The sputum may be streaked with blood if a biopsy was done but should clear in 24 to 48 hours. Any excessive amount of blood is reported promptly as it may manifest hemorrhage from the biopsy site.

A tracheostomy tray is kept close at hand following a laryngoscopy because, occasionally, laryngeal spasm or edema and difficulty in breathing develop. The patient is kept under close observation for several hours. Any indication of respiratory distress is brought to the physician's attention immediately.

BRONCHOSCOPY. The bronchoscope used most commonly is a flexible fiberoptic tube that permits direct visual examination of the trachea, the left and right bronchi, the lobar and segmental bronchi and the bifurcations of their smaller subdivisions.

A topical anesthetic (e.g., cocaine 5 per cent) is applied to the tongue, pharynx and epiglottis, and an endotracheal tube is passed. The bronchoscope is then introduced through the endotracheal tube.

The purpose of the bronchoscopy is to inspect accessible parts of the respiratory tract visually, aspirate secretions and exudate that are obstructing air passages, remove a foreign body or obtain a biopsy specimen.

The care of the patient before and after the bronchoscopic examination is similar to that cited above for the patient having a laryngoscopy.

Bronchography

This involves the introduction of a radiopaque liquid into the tracheobronchial tree through a catheter passed through the pharynx and larynx. The patient is then placed in various positions to distribute the fluid, and x-rays are taken in which the trachea and bronchial tubes are outlined.

The procedure may be combined with a bronchoscopy. With the fiberoptic bronchoscope, the dye may be confined to a particular lobe or segment of a lung. The bronchogram is used to confirm bronchiectasis or locate obstruction, constriction or malformation of the air passages.

The procedure is explained to the patient beforehand and usually a signed consent is required. No food or fluid is given for 6 to 8 hours preceding the bronchogram. Postural drainage (see p. 414) may be necessary before the procedure to clear the smaller distal tubes so the fluid can enter them. Dentures are removed, a mouthwash is given, and a sedative may be ordered.

Following the bronchogram, postural drainage is used to promote drainage of the fluid from the bronchial tree. Food and fluid are withheld until the swallowing reflex returns, and the same precautions are used as cited above for aftercare following a bronchoscopy.

Pulmonary Angiogram

A film of the pulmonary vessels may be made to confirm the presence of thrombi or an embolism, detect abnormalities in the pulmonary vasculature or assess perfusion in pulmonary disease. A radiopaque liquid is injected rapidly through a catheter into a large systemic vein, the right heart chambers or pulmonary artery. A film is then made to show the distribution of the opaque material throughout the pulmonary vasculature.

The site through which the catheter was

introduced into the body is observed for any local reaction and signs of inflammation.

Pulmonary Function Tests

Respiratory function tests reveal the individual's ability to move air in and out of the lungs (mechanics of respiration) and indicate the status of gas exchange across the alveolar-capillary membrane. Impaired function may be detected and information obtained concerning the nature and extent of the defect. Diffusion and exchange of the respiratory gases are reflected in the arterial oxygen and carbon dioxide tensions, hydrogen ion concentration (pH) and oxyhemoglobin saturation. These are referred to under blood studies on pages 405. Evaluation of the ventilatory functions includes the following:

MEASUREMENTS OF LUNG VOLUMES. The more common ventilatory measurements are made with a spirometer. The normal values for the different lung volumes have been established from studies made on normal subjects. They vary with height, age and sex; procedures have been developed for the calculation of the normal values according to these parameters.

Vital capacity (VC) is represented by the maximal volume of air exhaled following a maximal inspiration. To determine the VC, the individual breathes through a mouthpiece which is connected to a tube leading to a spirometer. During the process, his nasal passages are closed off by a clip placed on his nose and he is asked to keep his lips closed tightly around the mouthpiece during exhalation to prevent air leakage. The normal VC ranges from 3500 to 5000 ml.

The VC provides information about the compliance, since the person made an effort to expand his lungs fully when taking the maximal inspiration.

Vital capacity is below normal in obstructive lung disease (e.g., emphysema) because the airways reduce the volume of air exhaled. It is below normal in restrictive lung disease (e.g., fibrosis or limited chest expansion due to neuromuscular defects or weakness) because of the limited expansion of the lungs which reduces the volume of air inspired and exhaled.

Tidal volume (V_T) is the volume of air exhaled following a normal breath. It is determined by using the same method as cited above, except that the individual breathes quietly and is *not* asked to take a maximal inspiration and force out as much air as possible. The normal is usually stated as being 450 to 500 ml. with the individual at rest, but varies with individuals and their activities. *Minute ventilation* (or minute respiratory volume) is determined by multiplying the tidal volume by the number of respirations per minute.

Forced vital capacity (FVC) is the maximal volume of air that can be forcibly and rapidly exhaled following a maximal inspiration. The patient's nasal passages are closed off and he is asked to take a maximum inspiration through his mouth, and then rapidly and forcibly to exhale as much air as possible into the spirometer.

Timed forced expiratory volume (FEV_T) records the percentage of vital capacity that can be expelled in 1 second (FEV_1), 2 seconds (FEV_2) and 3 seconds (FEV_3). The individual inhales as deeply as he can and then exhales as quickly and as much as possible into the spirometer; the volume is noted for the indicated time interval. A calculation is then made to determine what percentage the volume is of the individual's vital capacity. Normally about 80 per cent of the vital capacity is expired in 1 second, 90 per cent in 2 seconds and 95 per cent within 3 seconds.

Timed forced expiratory volumes provide information about the resistance to expiratory airflow. In obstructive airway disease such as asthma the FEV and FEV_T volumes are reduced. In restrictive airway disease such as pulmonary fibrosis in which the compliance is reduced, with a resulting decrease in vital capacity, the expiratory airflow is usually normal.

Maximal voluntary ventilation (MVV) represents the maximal volume of air that can be inhaled in a given time interval. The individual is requested to breathe rapidly and deeply for 10 to 15 seconds. The volume reported is usually that for 1 minute.

Residual volume (RV) is the volume of gas remaining in the lungs at the end of a maximal expiration.

Functional residual capacity (FRC) is the air remaining in the lung after passive exhalation in normal breathing; no forceful or increased effort is used.

Measurement of the residual volumes RV and FRC involve more complex procedures, since they cannot be determined by spirometry. They may be measured by a plethysmograph. The patient sits in a closed, booth-like structure and, using a mouthpiece fitted with a valve and pressure gauge, breathes the air in the cabinet. The technician initiates the closure of the valve in the mouthpiece at a given time. The air pressure in the lungs and within the plethysmograph is recorded as the individual exhales.

The plethysmograph may also be used to measure airway resistance and blood flow in the pulmonary capillaries.

CARBON MONOXIDE (CO) TEST. This test provides information about the respiratory diffusion capacity, and is based on the particular affinity of hemoglobin in the blood for carbon monoxide. The subject inhales a very low concentration of carbon monoxide (approximately 0.1 per cent), and the rate of uptake by the blood is determined. This is estimated by the difference beweeen the concentrations of CO in the inhaled and exhaled air. The patient is asked to hold his breath for a period of 10 seconds. Calculations may be made on a minute of regular breathing. The diffusing capacity is expressed as mm. of CO diffused per minute per mm. Hg of the partial pressure of CO in the alveolar gas. The normal value for someone at rest is approximately 2.0 ml. per minute per mm. Hg.

PATIENT CARE IN PULMONARY FUNCTION TESTS. If the patient is in the hospital he is advised of the purpose of the tests and what to expect before he is taken to the pulmonary laboratory. Before each test, the technician explains what is to occur and gives the patient instructions how to carry out his role. The patient should not be rushed; the application of the nose clip to close off the nasal passages and the use of the mouthpiece produce anxiety in some patients. Fear can affect the results obtained. The patient is told that the tests may be repeated following the inhalation of a bronchodilator.

The tests can be very exhausting for the patient; the repeated maximal inspirations and rapid forceful exhalations are energy-demanding. Observations are made of the patient's condition and reactions to the various tests; he may require assistance to move from one place to another. A rest period should be provided following such a series of tests. The patient will also want information about the results.

Bronchospirometry

This is used to determine the capacity of each lung separately as well as the gas exchange between the alveoli of each lung and the blood. This is a more complex procedure than measuring the vital capacity. A double lumen tube is passed into the trachea and each bronchus is cannulated, so that one lumen connects with the right bronchus and the other with the left bronchus. One lumen is occluded in turn to measure the ventilatory capacity of the other lung; the proximal end of the tube is connected to the spirometer.

Care of the patient before and after bronchospirometry is the same as in bronchoscopy.

Blood Studies

The following blood analyses may be made in investigating the patient with respiratory disturbances.

LEUKOCYTE COUNT. A total and differential count of the white blood cells may be ordered since this information may be useful in confirming infection and distinguishing between an acute disease, such as pneumonia, and a chronic one, such as tuberculosis. A leukocytosis, with the increase being mainly in the polymorphonuclear granulocytes is generally associated with an acute infection. In chronic infection there is usually only a slight increase above the normal in the total number of leukocytes, and it is usually the lymphocytes that account for any increase. The eosinophils are increased in allergic asthma. Normal value is 5000 to 10,000 per cu. ml.

ERYTHROCYTE COUNT, AND HEMOGLOBIN AND HEMATOCRIT DETERMINATION. It is important to know if the erythrocyte count is normal since erythrocytes contain the hemoglobin which carries the oxygen (normal: 4,500,000 to 5,000,000 per cu. ml.). Similarly, an assessment of the patient includes a determination of the hemoglobin concentration (normal: 14 to 16 gm. per 100 ml.). Obviously, a deficiency of red blood cells or hemoglobin may produce an oxygen deficiency. The hematocrit represents the volume percentage of erythrocytes (normal: 40 to 50 volumes per 100 ml.).

BLOOD GAS ANALYSIS. Determinations of the partial pressures of oxygen and carbon dioxide, the hydrogen ion concentration (pH) and the oxygen-hemoglobin saturation of the arterial blood are useful in diagnosis and in on-going assessment of patients with respiratory insufficiency.

Normal values are:

paO_2	85	to 100 mm. Hg
$paCO_2$	35	to 40 mm. Hg
pH	7.35	to 7.45
Plasma CO_2	20	to 32 mEq./L.
Arterial oxyhemoglobin saturation	95	to 97 per cent

A blood specimen for gas analysis is withdrawn from an artery with a syringe that has been rinsed with heparin or is received in a heparinized vacuum tube. If frequent analyses are necessary, an indwelling arterial catheter may be introduced to avoid repeated arterial punctures. The site used for the withdrawal of blood may be a femoral, radial or brachial artery.

It is very important that the specimen does not become exposed to air in order to obtain an accurate gas measurement. This is insured with the use of the vacuum tube. If a syringe is used, all air must be excluded before withdrawal of the specimen and, when the needle is withdrawn, it must be capped *immediately* or plunged into a rubber stopper.

The tube or syringe is placed in a small basin of ice, labelled and delivered promptly to the laboratory.

Firm pressure is applied to the arterial puncture site for a least 5 minutes; it is then protected with a sterile dressing. Frequent observation is made of the site for bleeding. If the patient has been receiving an anticoagulant preparation, it is necessary to apply pressure to the site for 15 to 20 minutes, or longer if necessary. The arm or lower limb in which the arterial puncture was made is checked for adequate blood supply in the distal part in case of arterial occlusion.

If an arterial catheter or cannula is used, it is closed off following the blood withdrawal. It is kept patent by periodic flushing with a heparin solution.

As cited previously, an important function of the respiratory system is the provision of *oxygen* which is essential to all cells for normal metabolism. If the oxygen tension is inadequate, cellular metabolism becomes abnormal and anaerobic; lactic acid is produced and accumulates, decreasing the blood pH and causing metabolic acidosis. In assessing the arterial oxygen tension, the *oxyhemoglobin saturation* is also determined. Only a small amount of oxygen is in solution in plasma; the remainder is combined with hemoglobin. If the plasma concentration is lowered, oxygen is dissociated from the hemoglobin and moves out into the plasma. The hemoglobin is no longer saturated and the total amount of oxygen is less.

A second important function of respiration is the removal of *carbon dioxide* from the blood, keeping the $paCO_2$ within a very narrow range. Impaired ventilation or gas exchange that causes an increase above or a decrease below the normal $paCO_2$ produces an acid/base imbalance which is reflected in the pH. If ventilation or diffusion is decreased, less carbon dioxide is removed from the blood; the hydrogen ion concentration is increased (the pH is below normal), and respiratory acidosis develops.

Hyperventilation removes carbon dioxide in excess of the normal. The $paCO_2$ and plasma CO_2 concentration fall below normal, the pH is above normal and respiratory alkalosis develops.

LACTIC DEHYDROGENASE (LDH) LEVEL. This is a cellular enzyme which promotes the conversion of lactic acid to pyruvic acid in metabolism. Injury or destruction of cells containing LDH results in its release into the plasma. Since this enzyme is characteristic of lung tissue cells, an elevation in its plasma concentration may confirm suspected cellular destruction such as occurs in pulmonary infarction.

Normal: 165 to 300 units.

Lung Scan (Pulmonary Scintigram)

A lung scan involves the administration of a radioisotope by inhalation or intravenous injection (e.g., Xenon[133], radioiodinated albumin). A scintiscanner[6] is then used to

---

[6]A *scintiscanner* is a machine that is sensitive to gamma rays and records the concentration of the radioisotope emitting the rays.

make a graphic record of the concentration of the isotope in the lungs. The scan provides information about the equality of ventilation throughout the lung if the radioisotope is inhaled. If administered intravenously, perfusion is evaluated.

HYPOXIA

Hypoxia means that the supply of oxygen available to the tissues is insufficient to meet cellular needs for normal metabolism.

Causes of Hypoxia

The causes of hypoxia may be inadequate oxygenation of the blood, impaired delivery of oxygen to the tissues, increased oxygen demand by the body cells or inability of the cells to use the oxygen.

INADEQUATE OXYGENATION OF THE BLOOD. This may be the result of:

HYPOVENTILATION. If less than the normal volume of air enters the alveoli, then obviously the exchange of gases is decreased. This may occur as a result of weak shallow respirations which may be due to a disorder of the nervous system that depresses the respiratory centers or gives rise to paralysis of the respiratory muscles. Hypoventilation may also develop because of a reduction in functional alveoli due to atelectasis (collapse of alveoli) or a collection of exudate in the air sacs, as in pneumonia, pulmonary fibrosis which restricts lung expansion and ventilation, or obstructive lung disease such as asthma and emphysema.

LOW ATMOSPHERIC TENSION. A decline in the oxygen tension in the atmosphere, as at high altitudes, is a cause of inadequate oxygenation of the blood. Hemoglobin saturation decreases gradually after an altitude of about 5,000 feet above sea level is reached. Johnson states that the hemoglobin does not fall below 90 per cent until an altitude of 10,000 feet is reached.[7]

DEFECTIVE PERFUSION OF THE ALVEOLI. Some alveolar capillaries may not be perfused; the alveoli are ventilated but inadequate blood perfusion results in a reduction in the oxygenation of the blood. This condition may be referred to as mismatching or inequality of perfusion and ventilation.

DIFFUSION DEFECT. Fibrosing changes or edema of the alveolar walls produces a decrease in the amount of oxygen that diffuses from the alveolar air into the blood. Oxygen is less soluble than carbon dioxide, and is 20 times slower in its transfer to the blood than is carbon dioxide in its diffusion from the blood into the alveoli.

VENOARTERIAL SHUNTS. A shunt within the circulatory system that causes a mixing of arterial (oxygenated) and venous (reduced oxygen) bloods reduces the oxygen tension of the blood delivered to the tissues. The blood that is shunted bypasses the lungs so is not oxygenated. The cause is usually a congenital cardiac or large vessel defect.

IMPAIRED TRANSPORTATION OF OXYGEN TO THE TISSUES. This may be due to:

ANEMIA. Fewer than the normal number of erythrocytes or less than a normal complement of hemoglobin reduces the amount of oxygen uptake by the blood.

ABNORMAL HEMOGLOBIN. Hypoxia may be caused by a chemical alteration of the hemoglobin to a form that reduces its oxygen-carrying capacity (e.g., as seen in carbon monoxide poisoning). The offending gas unites with hemoglobin even more readily than oxygen to form a compound (carboxyhemoglobin) that is more stable than oxyhemoglobin.

Certain drugs may also alter hemoglobin and prevent its combination with oxygen. Examples of these drugs are sulfathiazole, phenacetin and acetanilide.

CARDIAC FAILURE. Failure of the heart to pump blood throughout body tissues results in stagnation. The oxygen becomes depleted and is not being replaced.

Inadequate transportation of oxygenated blood may be limited to a certain area of the body (ischemia) as a result of thrombosis or embolism, and the tissues in that area experience hypoxia.

INCREASED OXYGEN REQUIREMENT. This may develop in:

SEVERE HYPERTHYROIDISM. The utilization of oxygen is increased in severe hyperthyroidism by the rapid rate of metabolism. Similarly, hypoxia may also develop in the person with a high fever; an excessive amount of oxygen is used by the cells in accelerated metabolism and the production of increased body heat.

[7]Paul B. Beeson and Walsh McDermott (Eds.): Textbook of Medicine, 14th ed. Philadelphia, W. B. Saunders, 1975, p. 79.

TISSUE CELL IMPAIRMENT. This may result in the cells being unable to use the oxygen that is in the blood. The cellular defect is usually in the enzyme system, and is such that the normal oxidative processes are inhibited. This may occur in narcotic or cyanide poisoning.

Classification of Hypoxia

Hypoxia may be classified according to the above causes as:

Arterial hypoxia, which indicates inadequate oxygenation of the blood.

Anemic hypoxia, which is an oxygen deficiency in the blood due to a reduction in its oxygen-carrying power.

Circulatory hypoxia, which is characterized by a decline in the delivery of an adequate volume of oxygenated blood to the tissues.

Metabolic hypoxia, which is an imbalance between the oxygen demands of the tissue cells and the quantity of oxygen available.

Histotoxic hypoxia, which occurs when the cells become defective due to a toxic substance and, as a result, are unable to utilize oxygen.

Effects and Symptoms of Hypoxia

The effects and symptoms of hypoxia depend upon the severity of the hypoxia and the causative condition, and whether the oxygen deficiency is acute or chronic. If it is chronic, physiological adaptation by increasing the number of red blood cells (polycythemia) may occur, such as when a person resides at a high altitude.

General hypoxia produces some impairment of cellular activities throughout the body. The brain, heart, kidneys and liver are the most sensitive structures, and may suffer permanent damage due to the restricted oxygen supply. Metabolic processes are incomplete; the anaerobic situation results in an accumulation of lactic acid, producing tissue acidosis.

Initially an acute deficiency of oxygen in the blood (hypoxemia) induces an increased cardiac output and dilates the peripheral vessels. The pulse rate and blood pressure increase; then the pulse weakens as the myocardium suffers hypoxia. The patient may experience nausea and vomiting and complain of precordial pain.

The cerebral hypoxia and general reduction in metabolism produce a large range of symptoms. Early manifestations may be headache, restlessness, weakness, muscle incoordination, and loss of visual acuity. If the oxygen deficit continues, reduced cerebral efficiency may progress through confusion and stupor to coma. Respirations may be increased, especially if there is a concomitant increase in the carbon dioxide content of the blood. They may be interspersed with sighing and yawning, and the patient may complain of dyspnea. If the hypoxia persists, respirations gradually fail as the respiratory centers become depressed.

Cyanosis (bluish color of mucous membranes and skin) is seen due to an excessive reduction of oxyhemoglobin. Since it is dependent upon the presence of reduced hemoglobin, cyanosis is not present in individuals whose hemoglobin is reduced to 5 to 6 grams per cent or less.

Treatment of Hypoxia

Oxygen administration is used to increase the arterial oxygen tension in conjunction with treatment directed toward the cause of the hypoxia. The patient is kept at rest to reduce oxygen needs to a minimum.

Oxygen is not usually prescribed for patients unless their paO_2 is 60 to 70 mm. Hg or less, or unless they experience an acute and sudden lack of oxygenation that rapidly lowers the oxygen content of the blood. As with any medication, it should not be used indiscriminately. For instance, the administration of oxygen, except in a very low concentration, could be fatal to the patient with hypoxia associated with chronic pulmonary disease, such as chronic bronchitis and emphysema. This is because this patient usually has some retention of carbon dioxide (chronic hypercapnia). Normally, increased carbon dioxide tension stimulates the respiratory centers and elicits a ventilatory response that increases carbon dioxide elimination. The sensitivity of the chemoreceptors to hypercarbia is diminished in chronic hypercapnia and the patient becomes dependent upon hypoxia as a respiratory stimulus. If oxygen is given to correct the hypoxemia, the patient's "respiratory drive" is removed, hypoventilation develops and carbon dioxide retention is increased.

The concentration of oxygen administered

to raise the oxygen level depends upon the patient's paO_2 and general condition. Commonly, the flow rate per minute is set to deliver an oxygen concentration of about 30 to 40 per cent. A frequent policy observed is to commence therapy with a low concentration (the flow rate will depend on the method used to deliver the oxygen), and in 30 minutes have a determination made of the arterial blood gases and pH. The flow rate is then adjusted on the basis of the findings. The arterial blood gases and pH are monitored at frequent intervals throughout oxygen therapy to indicate progress and any adjustment to be made in the concentration of oxygen administered.

When using oxygen, it should be remembered that it is colorless, odorless, tasteless and heavier than air, and that it is hazardous because it supports combustion. Certain *precautions* must constantly be observed to avoid possible fire: (1) smoking is prohibited in the area, and signs indicating the restriction are posted; (2) cigarettes, pipe and matches are removed from the patient's bedside; (3) the use of woolen blankets and other equipment which may produce static electricity is restricted; and (4) inflammable solutions and electrical equipment (e.g., electric razor) may not be used in the room as long as oxygen is being given. Compressed oxygen is very dry and must be humidifed before reaching the patient.

METHODS OF ADMINISTERING OXYGEN. Oxygen may be administered by an open or closed method.

OPEN METHOD. If the open method is used, the oxygen may be delivered by face or nasal mask, face tent, nasal catheter, nasal prongs (cannula), or tent.

Face Mask. The face mask (Fig. 15–6) covers the nose and mouth and may be used to deliver low or relatively high concentrations of oxygen, depending upon the type of mask used. Some models permit fairly precise control of the oxygen concentration; some have a rebreathing or reservoir bag which has a capacity of about 1500 ml.

Those with no rebreathing bag have openings and flutter valves that permit the entry of air on inhalation, as well as allowing the escape of the exhaled gas. The air that enters mixes with the oxygen.

A popular model (Ventimask) currently in use is designed so that a fairly constant air and oxygen mixture can be maintained. This mask is available for the administration of 24, 28, 35 and 40 per cent oxygen.

The mask with a bag may permit partial or no rebreathing. The partial rebreathing bag traps the first part of the exhaled gas in the bag, where it mixes with oxygen. The re-

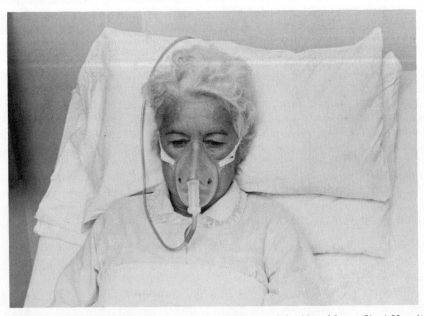

FIGURE 15–6 Oxygen administration by a face mask. (Courtesy of the New Mount Sinai Hospital, Toronto.)

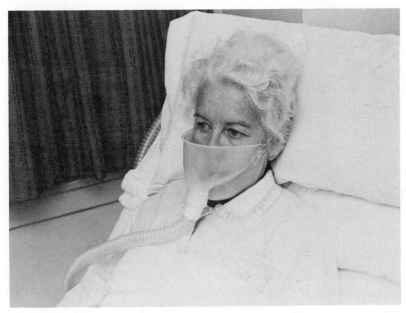

FIGURE 15–7   A face tent used for administering oxygen. (Courtesy of the New Mount Sinai Hospital, Toronto.)

mainder of the exhalation is allowed to escape through openings in the mask. The rationale for this procedure is that approximately one-third of the exhalation is composed of dead air; it is that portion of the inspired gas that did not enter the areas of the lung where gas exchange takes place. The mask must fit closely to the face and the flow rate of oxygen kept at 8 or more liters per minute. Concentrations of 40 to 70 per cent may be delivered with this type of mask.

The nonrebreathing mask has a reservoir with only one-way valves. These allow the exhaled gas to escape and prevent rebreathing. This type of mask is used for the administration of 100 per cent oxygen or premixed gases such as helium and oxygen or carbon dioxide and oxygen. The newer masks, such as the Ventimask, have the advantages of being light and disposable. The masks with a rebreathing bag or reservoir are less comfortable because they must fit more closely and are secured by straps around the head. They are removed at least every 2 hours and the skin bathed, dried, powdered and massaged to prevent irritation and pressure necrosis of the tissues.

Nasal Mask.   Occasionally a mask may be used that covers only the nose. The patient must be aware of the need to inhale through the nose with the mouth closed. The advantage of the nasal mask is that the patient can take fluids by mouth and communicate readily.

Face Tent.   The face tent is a transparent, firm plastic mask that fits under the chin and extends up over the mouth, nose and sides of the face (Fig. 15–7). It is open at the top. Oxygen enters the lower part of the mask and, being heavier than air, does not readily escape. The mask is removed every 2 hours and the enclosed area bathed, dried and powdered.

Nasal Catheter.   The catheter used for the administration of oxygen is flexible and has a rounded tip and several holes in the distal 1 to 2 inches. The tube is moistened and passed through a nostril into the nasopharynx. The length of the catheter to be passed may be estimated by measuring the distance between the tip of the nose and the ear lobe. The tip of the catheter should be visible just below the soft palate.

The catheter is secured and the patient advised to breathe through his nose. The catheter is changed every 8 to 10 hours; the nostrils are used alternately to minimize irritation of the mucous membrane. This method of administration interferes less with treatments and nursing care, and patients are usually more tolerant of it than of the mask.

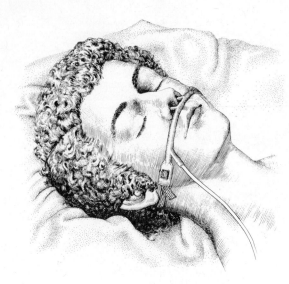

FIGURE 15–8 Plastic cannulae or prongs inserted into the nostrils to deliver oxygen.

It is also useful with comatose and restless patients. A flow rate of 4 to 8 liters per minute provides oxygen concentrations of 25 to 45 per cent.

Nasal Prongs. These are two fine, plastic tubes that stem from a common tube that connects with the oxygen source (Fig. 15–8). Each prong or cannula is inserted about ½ inch into each nostril. The nasal prongs are more acceptable to patients but are difficult to keep in place, especially if the patient is restless. They are not satisfactory for maintaining a constant or high oxygen concentration. The prongs are most useful with patients who have an increased $paCO_2$ and require a low concentration of oxygen, such as those with chronic obstructive lung disease. Prongs do not deliver the required concentration if the patient is a mouth breather or if he is hypoventilating. Abnormalities such as polyps and septum deviation impede the entrance of oxygen and reduce the concentration received. A flow rate of 5 to 10 liters per minute may deliver a concentration of 25 to 35 per cent. If the administration of oxygen by prongs is prolonged, the nasal and sinus mucous membranes may become dry and irritated.

Tent. The oxygen tent is used rarely for adults, since it is difficult to maintain a satisfactory concentration because of the repeated opening of the canopy and the fact that the oxygen, being heavier, settles to the bottom and tends to escape from the tent readily. With a high inflow of 12 to 15 liters per minute, the highest concentration inspired is about 40 per cent. However, the tent method of administration does have some advantages. The patient is more comfortable and has more freedom than when a catheter or mask is used; it is cool within the tent, and the air-oxygen mixture is adequately humidified. The patient may experience fear because of being closed in. If a tent must be used, an oxygen analyzer is used frequently to monitor the oxygen concentration within the tent.

CLOSED METHOD. If adequate oxygenation cannot be achieved by an open method of oxygen administration, the closed method is used. This involves tracheal intubation or tracheostomy to which a mechanical ventilator is connected (see p. 424).

TOXICITY OF OXYGEN. It was mentioned previously that oxygen should not be used indiscriminately. Hyperoxia may occur as the result of the administration of a high concentration of oxygen or the administration of oxygen under excessively high pressure. Very serious pathologic effects are likely to develop with exposure to 70 to 90 per cent oxygen for more than 24 hours. The lungs and the central nervous system are the primary areas of sensitivity to hyperoxia. The patient experiences chest tightness and coughing. The alveolar-capillary membrane is damaged, resulting in increased permeability and ensuing edema of the interstitial tissues and alveoli. Oxygen and carbon dioxide diffusion is impaired. Some alveoli collapse. The paO_2 falls and causes what is referred to as "refractory hypoxemia." Retention of carbon dioxide and acidosis develop.

Neurological manifestations include muscular irritability that may progress to convulsions and impaired vision. Premature infants exposed to a high oxygen concentration develop vascular changes in their eyes that lead to blindness.

HYPERCAPNIA

Hypercapnia or hypercarbia is the retention of carbon dioxide in excess of the normal range (normal $paCO_2$, 35 to 45 mm. Hg). It develops more slowly than hypoxia because it is more soluble and diffuses more readily than oxygen.

Causes of Hypercapnia

Normally, the individual eliminates excess carbon dioxide by increasing the volume and rate of respirations. The respiratory centers and chemoreceptors are sensitive to the blood tension of carbon dioxide, which provides what may be referred to as the "respiratory drive."

The causes of retention of carbon dioxide are hypoventilation, mismatching of alveolar ventilation and perfusion, circulatory failure and, rarely, increased metabolic production of carbon dioxide.

Effects and Manifestations of Hypercapnia

Initially the retention of an excess of carbon dioxide increases the respiratory drive and the respiratory rate and volume show a notable increase. If prolonged, the associated effort and energy expenditure cause the patient to experience dyspnea and exhaustion.

If the hypercapnia becomes chronic there is a decreased respiratory response as the respiratory centers and chemoreceptors become accustomed to the higher pCO_2 of the blood. Breathing becomes more dependent upon the hypoxic drive.

The retained carbon dioxide is hydrated to form carbonic acid ($H_2O + CO_2 \rightarrow H_2CO_3$), the pH is decreased and the patient develops respiratory acidosis. The normal bicarbonate-carbonic acid ratio of 20:1 is altered. The kidneys adjust to compensate for the decreased alkalinity by eliminating more chloride and hydrogen ions and by forming more bicarbonate ions. Renal compensation takes several days. Serum bicarbonate levels rise (normal: approximately 24 mEq./L.) and the urine becomes more acidic.

Circulatory changes include dilation of peripheral and cerebral vessels. The skin is warm and flushed; the patient complains of headache and manifests apathy, reduced mental ability which may progress to confusion, and loss of muscle coordination. The cerebral vascular dilation causes increased intracranial pressure, cerebral edema and papilledema.

Acidemia impairs myocardial function; the cardiac output is decreased, arrhythmias may develop and, unless cardiac dysfunction is reversed, circulatory failure occurs. The pulse becomes weak and the blood pressure falls. This promotes hypoxia, which reduces metabolism and leads to metabolic acidosis; the pH decreases even further.

Treatment of Hypercapnia

Care of the patient with carbon dioxide retention is directed towards increasing ventilation and avoiding any measure that may depress respirations. For example, sedation is not given and, if the patient has chronic obstructive lung disease and oxygen is necessary, it is used at a very low concentration to prevent removal of the hypoxic drive. The patient is encouraged to inhale and exhale fully several times at frequent intervals. A bronchodilator (e.g., salbutamol) may be prescribed to improve ventilation. If severe carbon dioxide retention is present, a mechanical ventilator may be used to provide intermittent positive pressure breathing

(IPPB) to improve alveolar ventilation. Frequent determinations of the blood gases and pH are necessary.

HYPOCAPNIA

Hypocapnia or hypocarbia occurs when the carbon dioxide content of the blood falls below the normal range.

Causes of Hypocapnia

The excessive loss of carbon dioxide is due to hyperventilation resulting from overstimulation of the respiratory center. The latter may be caused by an intracranial disorder (e.g., cerebrovascular accident), salicylate poisoning, hypermetabolism, as in thyrotoxicosis, or extreme apprehension or emotional disturbance.

Effects and Manifestations of Hypocapnia

The ventilating off of too much carbon dioxide alters the normal bicarbonate-carbonic acid ratio 20:1. The base ions are increased in proportion to the acid ions, the pH increases to above normal and respiratory alkalosis develops. The kidneys excrete more base ions and conserve hydrogen and chloride ions, but the ratio of bicarbonate to carbonic acid still remains too high. The patient complains of vertigo, blurred vision and palpitation. The cerebral disturbance causes neuromuscular irritability, reflexes are exaggerated, skeletal muscles manifest twitching and tetany may develop.

Treatment of Hypocapnia

The patient is given the necessary electrolytes to restore normal blood levels; a solution of normal saline with potassium chloride or Ringer's solution are examples of the electrolytes prescribed. Treatment is directed towards relieving the initial cause of the hyperventilation. Rebreathing of expired air may be used to increase the alveolar concentration of carbon dioxide and lower the pH.

NURSING MEASURES COMMON TO VARIOUS RESPIRATORY DISORDERS

Nursing in many respiratory disorders includes measures that are directed towards the promotion of adequate ventilation to oxygenate the blood and prevent carbon dioxide retention, removal of pulmonary secretions, and the provision of supportive care. These objectives may involve the following procedures.

Deep Breathing

Frequently, the ill patient's respirations are shallow because of weakness, pain, or depression of the respiratory center. As a result alveolar ventilation is reduced and the amount of dead air is increased. The nurse encourages the patient to take at least five deep breaths at regular frequent intervals. Instruction is given to inhale deeply, relaxing the abdominal muscles, and to exhale completely. The latter is more effective if the abdominal muscles are contracted.

If the patient has a chronic obstructive lung disease, breathing exercises are instituted. Instruction is given to inhale slowly and deeply while relaxing and "protruding" the abdomen, and then to lean forward slightly and exhale as much as is possible through pursed lips, with the abdominal muscles contracted. The patient may exert pressure on the lower abdomen with his hands to promote abdominal compression and elevation of the diaphragm in exhalation, or the nurse may assist by pressing a folded bath towel against the patient's abdomen. The breathing exercises are usually carried out two or three times daily for patients with obstructive or restrictive lung disease and may be preceded by a prescribed nebulized bronchodilator to increase their effectiveness.

Coughing

Coughing is necessary to remove secretions from the trachea and lungs. The retention of pulmonary secretions predisposes to infection, atelectasis and reduced alveolar ventilation and gas exchange. Coughing should not be suppressed unless it is nonproductive, excessive and exhausting. The patient with a pulmonary disorder usually benefits from coughing every 2 to 3 hours. The purpose of the cough maneuver is explained to the patient and instruction is given as to how to cough effectively. The patient assumes the sitting position, if possible, and a deep breath is taken, followed by three short coughs. Short coughs use less energy and are less likely to cause wheezing or airway collapse than a single large forceful exhalation. This procedure is repeated several times. The nurse provides the necessary assistance and support.

Liquefaction and raising of the secretions are facilitated by a generous fluid intake as well as by humidification of the air. A fluid intake of 3000 to 4000 ml. is recommended unless contraindicated by cardiac or renal insufficiency.

If the patient has difficulty in producing a cough, stimulation of the pharynx with the tip of a suction catheter may precipitate the desired response. It is also suggested that the application of digital pressure over the trachea just above the medial clavicular prominences may cause the patient to cough. The index finger is moved up and down over the area.[8] Another maneuver recommended is to have the patient prolong exhalations. The increased flow of air has a drying, irritating effect on the trachea.

During breathing exercises and coughing the patient is observed for signs of fatigue and allowed to rest when indicated.

The physician is advised if symptoms and chest auscultation indicate the presence of secretions that the patient is unable to raise. Deep suctioning may be necessary.

Suctioning

This is a very important procedure used to remove secretions from the oropharynx, trachea and bronchi. A sterile disposable catheter, connected to a wall source of negative pressure or to a suction machine, may be gently passed directly into the oropharynx or trachea or through an endotracheal or tracheostomy tube into the trachea or proximal portion of either bronchus.

SUCTIONING THE OROPHARYNX. This involves the use of a sterile catheter with a whistle tip which is attached to a Y connecting tube (Fig. 15–9). One arm of the Y is connected to a tube leading to the source of negative pressure. The open arm of the connecting tube serves as a vent. The patient is advised of what is to be done and its purpose. The catheter may be passed through the mouth or a nostril to the pharyngeal re-

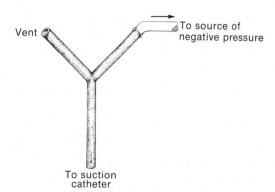

FIGURE 15–9 Y connecting tube attached to a suction catheter and source of negative pressure used in suctioning.

gion. When the tip of the catheter is in position, a finger or thumb is placed over the vent to establish suction. The catheter is gently rotated and withdrawn.

A suction catheter is available with a "built-in" vent (thumb valve) that is normally open until a thumb or finger is placed over the opening. This model eliminates the need for the Y connecting tube.

The introduction of the catheter frequently initiates the cough reflex, resulting in the removal of deeper secretions in addition to those in the pharynx.

INTRATRACHEAL SUCTIONING. Deeper suctioning is used to remove pulmonary secretions or aspirated material (food or vomitus). The procedure and its purpose are explained to the patient and any dentures are removed. A self-inflated (Ambu) mask and oxygen are brought to the bedside in the event of the patient developing cardiac dysfunction and acute respiratory insufficiency.

The nurse wears sterile gloves and introduces a sterile suction catheter moistened with sterile water or normal saline through a nostril. The diameter of the catheter must be less than half that of the trachea. When it reaches the nasopharynx, which can be noted by looking through the mouth, the tongue is grasped and drawn forward, using a square of gauze. The patient is then asked to take several deep breaths and the catheter is advanced. When it enters the larynx, coughing is initiated and, as the glottis opens widely, the catheter is readily moved into the trachea. It is attached to a Y connecting tube with one arm leading by a tube to the source

[8]Peter Ungvarski: "Mechanical Stimulation of Coughing." Am. J. Nurs., Vol. 71, No. 12 (Dec. 1971), p. 2359.

of suction. The other arm serves as a vent which is left open during the passing of the catheter. The vent is occluded to establish suction.

The catheter is gently rotated and suction is maintained while it is being withdrawn. The aspiration must be brief since it removes air as well as secretions and may deplete the patient's oxygen supply. Suction is not applied for longer than 5 to 10 consecutive seconds. If the aspiration was not sufficiently effective, allow ventilation for a few minutes before reapplying the negative pressure.

The pulse is monitored during and following suctioning; cardiac arrhythmia may develop, especially if the patient's paO_2 was below normal before starting. The pulse is observed for an increase in rate and irregularity that may occur as a result of hypoxemia and vagal nerve disturbance. Tachycardia may develop, followed by premature ventricular contractions due to the hypoxia and ensuing acidosis. The disturbance may progress to bradycardia and asystole. It may be necessary to increase the patient's paO_2 before and after each suctioning by administering oxygen; for example, the practice may be to provide 100 per cent oxygen for 5 minutes for some patients. Intratracheal suctioning is contraindicated unless absolutely necessary in patients with cardiac arrhythmia or failure, hypotension or acidosis.

Aspiration of the bronchi necessitates the use of a coudé (bent) tip catheter; its tip is introduced into the bronchus to be suctioned. Entry into the left bronchus is facilitated by having the patient turned partially on his left side with his head turned to the right and his chin up. To suction the opposite bronchus the position is reversed.

The frequency of suctioning is determined by the accumulation of secretions; unnecessary aspiration increases the risk of trauma to the mucosa by the tube. On the other hand, if secretions are profuse, frequent suctioning is necessary to promote adequate ventilation.

Note and record the characteristics of the secretions (color, consistency, composition). If they are very tenacious and difficult to remove, the physician may prescribe the instillation of 5 to 10 ml. of sterile normal saline. It is introduced into the catheter as the patient inhales, and then suction is applied.

If the patient has an endotracheal tube or a tracheostomy, suctioning is an important part of the patient's care (discussed in the sections on intubation, p. 418, and tracheostomy, p. 421.

Physical Therapy and Postural Drainage

Physical therapy is used to loosen secretions so that they can be coughed up. Percussion or clapping and vibration are the manual procedures used. The nurse or physiotherapist determines which affected lung segments require drainage. This information may be obtained by auscultation or may be indicated by the physician. Chest percussion may be used routinely over the lung bases or the complete chest during the postoperative period, or if the patient is immobilized over a long period, especially when there is a history of obstructive pulmonary disease or repeated chest infections.

Chest percussion is applied by clapping the chest with cupped hands. The chest wall is struck sharply, using both hands rapidly and alternately with uniform force for 1 or 2 minutes. Obviously, surgical or injured areas are avoided, as are the spine, abdomen and lumbar region. It is also contraindicated in patients with a pulmonary embolism. Percussion is not performed below the lower ribs.

Chest vibration may be used with clapping or as an alternative in the patient's pulmonary physical therapy. The procedure is performed by placing one hand over the other on the chest area to be vibrated and, while exerting moderate pressure, uniform vibratory movements are made to dislodge and mobilize secretions. The vibration is done to coincide with an exhalation, and pressure is relieved during inhalation.

Chest physiotherapy is usually used in conjunction with deep breathing and coughing. Postural drainage may also be used as an adjunct.

Postural drainage requires placing the patient in certain positions to promote the elimination of pulmonary secretions. The position assumed initiates gravitational movement of fluid and mucus to a level of the tracheobronchial tree that favors its removal by coughing or suctioning. As cited above, postural drainage may be used as part of a physical therapy program in which the special positioning is preceded by clapping and/or vibration to dislodge the secretions. A bronchodilator (e.g., salbutamol) may be ad-

TABLE 15–3 POSTURAL DRAINAGE POSITIONS

Area to Be Drained	Posture
Apical lobes	
Apical segment	Sitting position; patient alternately leans forward and to each side
Anterior segment	Supine position
Posterior segment	Right/left lateral, about 45° angle
Lingula	
Superior and inferior segments	Foot of bed elevated 14 to 16 inches; turned slightly to right
Middle lobe	
Medial and lateral segments	Foot of bed elevated 14 to 16 inches; turned slightly to left
Lower lobes	
Superior segment	Prone position with hips elevated on a pillow
Medial basal segment	Right lateral with hips elevated or foot of bed elevated 16 inches
Anterior basal segment	Supine position with hips elevated or foot of bed elevated 16 inches
Lateral basal segment	Lateral right/left with hips elevated or foot of bed elevated 16 inches
Posterior basal segment	Prone position with hips elevated or foot of bed elevated 16 inches

ministered by inhalation or orally to increase the effectiveness of the positioning and coughing.

The position assumed depends upon the lung segment or particular area to be drained. To promote the movement of secretions out of *upper lobes*, the patient is placed in a sitting position and alternately leans forward and to each side to drain different segments. For drainage of the *middle lobe, lower lobes* and lingula,[9] various side-lying, prone and supine positions are used. The patient may be horizontal or, to remove accumulations in lower segments, he may be tilted so that his head and chest are lower (see Table 15–3). An ambulatory patient may be positioned prone and crosswise on the bed so that his head and thorax are leaning over one side. This position especially facilitates drainage of larger bronchial tubes and, if used, precautions are necessary to insure safety and to prevent a fall and possible injury. The nurse remains with the patient each time until assured that he can safely handle the situation.

An explanation is made to the patient before commencing physical therapy and/or postural drainage so that he will know what to expect. He is advised that he will be re-

quired to cough. The patient's condition and the treatments being used (e.g., intravenous infusion) may necessitate modification of some positions, but the nurse should be familiar with the one appropriate to the drainage of various lung segments. The patient is made as comfortable as possible in whatever position is used; for example, in the lateral positions at a 45° angle a pillow is placed in front of the patient to provide support.

Each position is maintained for a minimum of 5 minutes, if possible. The patient is then encouraged to cough, and suctioning may also be necessary to assist in elimination of the dislodged secretions.

Humidification

An important consideration in the care of a patient with a respiratory disorder is the need for supplemental humidification of inspired air or oxygen.

Normally the inspired air is adequately moistened within the respiratory tract by moisture evaporated from the mucosal surface and the cilia. In a disorder the process is impaired and the mucosa is irritated and depleted of water, the mucus becomes viscous and crusted, and ciliary activity is depressed. The ensuing retention of the tenacious secretions increases airway resistance and promotes infection.

Various methods are used to humidify the

---

[9]The *lingula* is the small projection from the lower portion of the upper lobe of the left lung.

air or gas to be inspired. The method used depends mainly upon: (1) whether or not the upper airway is bypassed; (2) the degree of dehydration of the mucosa and secretions; and (3) the equipment available. A steam kettle, vaporizer or room humidifier is probably the simplest means of increasing the moisture in the inspired air.

A method commonly used to humidify inspired gas is to bubble it through water (or a prescribed diluent) to increase the water vapor content of the inhaled gas. Water vapor molecules are absorbed into the gas bubbles. The amount absorbed may be increased by heating the water. The water vapor in inspired gas also may be increased by passing the gas slowly over a large surface of water.

A more efficient method of humidification is to deliver the water in an aerosol or nebulized form. The more sophisticated humidifiers include electrically operated jet nebulizers, ultrasonic nebulizers and centrifugal aerosol generators.

The jet-type nebulizer produces a coarse spray of fluid which is directed into a stream of rapidly moving gas. Before the gas with the fluid leaves the nebulizer, it may be directed onto a baffle or the walls of the container to reduce the size of the water particles carried into the respiratory tract.

In ultrasonic nebulization, ultrahigh frequency sound waves are transmitted into water, resulting in a very fine particulate spray. The gas to be inspired is directed across the surface of the water so that the fine spray is carried with it into the respiratory tract. This humidifying technique is considered one of the most efficient means of delivering an aerosol of high density.

The centrifugal aerosol generator has a rapidly spinning disk that throws the water against a baffle or container wall, breaking it into small aerosol particles.

The cascade humidifier, in which the inspired gas is bubbled through heated water, is used frequently for humidification of the inspired gas during continuous mechanical ventilation.

The diluent used in humidifiers may be sterile distilled water, normal (0.9 per cent) saline, half-strength normal (0.45 per cent) saline or hypertonic saline.

Unless specified by the physician, water is used. It must be remembered that it is hypotonic and, with prolonged humidification,

may cause mucosal edema in high density delivery. Half-strength saline is usually the choice for prolonged administration and when the ultrasonic or heated aerosol methods are used. Hypertonic saline promotes liquefaction and elimination of secretions.

Medications, principally bronchodilators, may be administered in the aerosol or nebulized form. This method is frequently used for patients with chronic obstructive pulmonary disease. The advantage is that it avoids systemic administration and the possible associated side effects.

Endotracheal Intubation

This procedure involves the passage of a tube through the mouth or nose and larynx into the trachea. Intubation is used to establish an airway to improve ventilation or facilitate ventilatory assistance and to aspirate secretions. The passing of an endotracheal tube is a rapid means of establishing an airway in an emergency as compared with the surgical procedure of tracheotomy.

If the patient is sufficiently alert he is advised of what the procedure involves, its purpose and the ensuing interference with communication and swallowing. He is told that he will be under constant surveillance, the treatment is of a temporary nature, and a slate and pencil will be available by which he can communicate, and his fluid and nutritional needs will be met by parenteral solutions. The family receives a similar explanation of the purpose, procedure and interference with communication.

If the patient has dentures they are removed, and he is then positioned on his back with the head extended and supported on a small pillow to align the mouth, pharynx and larynx.

Using the laryngoscope, the physician introduces the endotracheal tube, and the proximal portion of the tube is secured to the patient's face. The tube, made of soft plastic, is more pliable and less traumatizing to tissue than a rubber tube (Fig. 15–10). The tube is equipped with an inflatable cuff a short distance above the distal end. When inflated, it prevents the aspiration of vomitus and oral secretions. It also permits more effective ventilation by preventing the escape of gases being delivered under pressure.

When the tube is in position the cuff is inflated with air (2 to 10 ml.) if the patient is

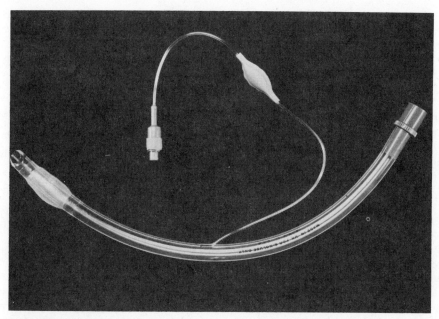

FIGURE 15–10 An endotracheal tube with an inflatable cuff which provides a seal between the trachea and tube. After the tube is inserted, the cuff is inflated by the introduction of a specified volume of air through the fine, attached tube, which is then clamped. (Courtesy of the New Mount Sinai Hospital, Toronto.)

to receive mechanical ventilatory assistance. A slight leak around the cuff is advisable to prevent pressure necrosis of the tracheal wall by the cuff. The air leak is detected by a stethoscope placed over the lateral surface of the trachea just above the area of the cuff. Near the proximal end of the fine tube leading to the cuff, and through which the air is introduced, there is a small balloon-like dilation which remains inflated when the tube is clamped. It is observed frequently and as long as it remains inflated the cuff is also inflated. The newer endotracheal tubes have softer high volume, low-pressure cuffs which reduce the possibility of tissue ischemia and trauma.

Immediately following insertion of the tube, and then at regular intervals, the chest is auscultated to determine if air is entering both lungs. If the tube is too low, the inflated cuff could completely block off a bronchus and cause atelectasis of the respective lung. An x-ray may be made to check the position of the tube; if the end rests against the carina, the terminal opening will be blocked and air entry into the bronchi will be cut off.

The endotracheal tube is distressing and a source of discomfort to the conscious patient. Prolonged use may cause damage to the vocal cords and ulceration in the trachea. If an artificial airway is necessary for longer than 48 or 72 hours, a tracheostomy is done and the endotracheal tube removed. In the case of children, the tube may be left for a longer period if passed through the nose. This is to avoid tracheostomy, if possible; more serious complications are more likely to be associated with tracheostomy in children.

The cuff is deflated for 2 to 5 minutes every hour to prevent ischemia and ensuing ulceration of the tracheal mucosa. The inspired gas is humidified before entering the endotracheal tube to liquefy secretions and prevent encrusting within the tract and tube. Frequent deep suctioning through the endotracheal tube is necessary; this is usually done during the cuff deflation. The procedure involves hyperoxygenation, oropharyngeal suctioning, deflation of the cuff, tracheal suctioning, reinflation of the cuff, and hyperoxygenation.

Suctioning may deplete the amount of oxygen reaching the alveoli. The patient is given oxygen with a self-inflating (Ambu) bag and mask (100 per cent for 5 minutes) prior to cuff deflation and suctioning, and again when the cuff is reinflated. The patient's pulse is monitored for possible cardiac dysfunction and arrhythmias (due to hypoxia) during and after the suctioning. If any irregularity occurs, suctioning is immediately discontinued and oxygen is administered with the self-inflating bag and mask.

Using a sterile glove and sterile suction catheter, the nurse removes the oropharyngeal secretions to prevent aspiration when the cuff is deflated.

The cuff is then deflated and, using sterile gloves, the nurse passes another sterile catheter, moistened in sterile water or normal saline, through the tube into the trachea. Suction is not applied while the catheter is being introduced. When in position, suction is applied and the catheter is rotated and withdrawn. If the airway is not clear of secretions, the catheter is not allowed to become contaminated and may be reintroduced into the trachea. It will likely be necessary to ventilate the patient with the self-inflating bag before passing the catheter again. If the secretions are tenacious, the physician may suggest the introduction of 5 to 10 ml. of a sterile saline solution into the tube, followed by immediate suctioning. Following suctioning the cuff is then reinflated and the patient hyperoxygenated.

Frequent mouth care is necessary, and suctioning of the oropharyngeal area at frequent intervals is done to remove the secretions that may be a response to the presence of the tube.

When the patient is to be *extubated*, equipment that should be brought to the bedside includes a self-inflating (Ambu) bag, mask, and oxygen in case the patient requires immediate ventilatory assistance. A laryngoscope, sterile endotracheal tube and sterile gloves should also be assembled so the patient can be quickly reintubated if necessary.

Before the cuff is deflated and the physician removes the tube, secretions are suctioned from the oropharynx to prevent aspiration. Following the removal of the tube, the patient is observed for respiratory distress and insufficiency. A nurse remains in attendance, constantly monitoring the patient's respirations, pulse and color. The patient is usually apprehensive and needs the nurse's presence and reassurance.

Tracheostomy

This is a surgical procedure in which an incision is made in the anterior wall of the trachea and a special tube is inserted. An airway is established which bypasses the larynx and air passages above.

INDICATIONS FOR A TRACHEOSTOMY. These are:

1. An upper airway obstruction (e.g., laryngeal newgrowth).
2. Prolonged, mechanically assisted ventilation where a seal is necessary to prevent loss of ventilatory gas that is under pressure.
3. The need for more efficient access to retained pulmonary secretions which, unless removed, may cause serious respiratory problems such as atelectasis and pneumonia.
4. The prevention of recurrent aspiration of oral secretions and vomitus.

A tracheostomy may be done in primary respiratory disorders, but it is frequently necessary with patients whose respiratory difficulty or insufficiency is secondary to disease elsewhere or to trauma. For example, it may be necessary following cerebral injury or cardiac surgery or for the patient with myasthenia gravis who has developed dysfunction of the respiratory muscles. A tracheostomy reduces the work of breathing by eliminating the resistance offered by the upper airway. It also reduces the dead space by almost 50 per cent (the normal is approximately 150 ml.).

Since endotracheal intubation has been more commonly used and can be performed very quickly, tracheostomy is rarely used in an emergency situation. The current procedure is generally elective, and is performed with an endotracheal tube in position and under aseptic conditions in an operating room. It may be necessary as an emergency measure if the patient cannot be intubated because of facial injuries or burns, laryngeal edema or severe upper airway infection. If the tracheostomy is associated with laryngectomy, it becomes permanent.

The *operative procedure* is undertaken with the patient in the dorsal position, head and neck hyperextended. A pillow or folded sheet is placed under the shoulders. A vertical or horizontal incision is made about 2 cm. above the suprasternal notch to expose the upper part of the trachea. This is then opened, usually at the level of the second and third cartilaginous rings, and a tracheostomy tube is introduced. The tube is held in

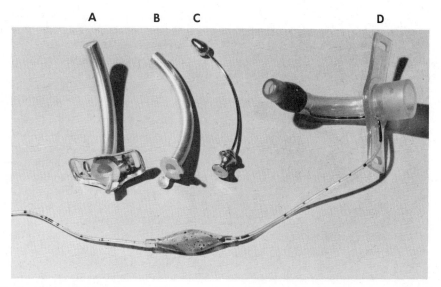

FIGURE 15–11 Tracheostomy tubes. *A,* Outer part of metal tracheostomy tube. *B,* Inner part of metal tracheostomy tube. *C,* Obturator used during insertion of the outer metal tube. *D,* Polyethylene cuffed tube.

position by laterally attached tapes which are tied securely around the patient's neck.

TRACHEOSTOMY TUBES. These are available in various sizes.[10] The diameter and length of the tube selected depends upon the size of the trachea, and is slightly smaller in diameter than the trachea. This necessitates having several sizes sterile and available at the time of the tracheostomy.

The tracheostomy tubes most commonly in use are of plastic (plastic and polyethylene) and may be single or consist of two parts, an inner and outer cannula (see Fig. 15–11). A silver double cannulated tube is also available but is rarely used. The plastic tubes are less traumatic to the patient's tissues, tend to become more pliable as they approach body temperature and are less subject to accumulating secretion encrustations. When the metal tube is used, the outer cannula is fitted with an obturator that extends beyond the distal end of the tube. Its end is blunt and smooth which facilitates the introduction of the tube. As soon as the tube is in position, the obturator is removed and the inner tube is inserted and secured.

The tube with an inner cannula provides a more efficient means of clearing the airway of secretions, since the inner tube can be removed and readily cleansed without the risk of compromising the patient's airway. The single tube (without an inner cannula) must be changed about every 3 days or more often if secretions accumulate within the tube. The tube with an inner cannula may be left for a longer period.

Most synthetic tubes now in use have a high-volume, low-pressure cuff which encircles the lower part of the outer tubes (Fig. 15–12). After the tube is in position, the cuff is inflated by introducing a small amount of air via a fine tube that leads into it. The cuff creates a seal between the trachea and the tube and prevents air from entering or escaping around the tube, in addition to preventing the aspiration of secretions or fluid into the tract below. This type of tube is used most frequently in patients who require mechanical assistance in breathing. A disadvantage of the cuff is possible ulceration of the tracheal mucosa due to pressure at the site. The cuff must be deflated at frequent, regular intervals and must remain deflated for a stated period of time.

The amount of air required to produce a seal without unnecessary pressure on tracheal tissue varies from 2 to 10 ml. While introducing the air, the nurse listens and tests for the escape of air from around the

---

[10]The size of the tubes may be indicated in the Jackson scale of sizes, which goes from No. 00 to 10, the external diameter scale, which goes from 4.5 mm. to 14 mm., or the French gauge, which goes from 13 to 42.

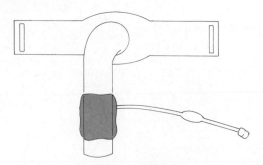

FIGURE 15–12 A cuffed tracheostomy tube.

tube. The tracheostomy tube may be blocked off momentarily while testing for leakage around the tube. A slight leak is desirable to prevent pressure ischemia of the tracheal mucosa. When the inflation is completed, the end of the fine tube is clamped with a small hemostat. The amount of air used in inflating the cuff is recorded each time; any significant change observed from one time to another is reported. A decreased amount of air used may indicate swelling and edema in the "air passage" tissues.

Near the proximal end of the fine inflating tube is a small balloon-like dilation. This is inflated and, since it is visible, may be checked frequently to determine if the tube and the cuff below remain inflated. Obviously, if the small pilot balloon becomes deflated, a leak in the system is indicated and the cuff will be deflated, thus losing the intratracheal seal.

TRACHEOSTOMY CARE. It is important for the nurse to appreciate that the patient is dependent upon the patency of the tracheostomy tube for getting air in and out. Constant attention and meticulous care are necessary to prevent serious complications and to reduce the patient's fear of "choking." Sensitivity to the patient's fears and needs is important, since he cannot communicate verbally.

PREPARATION FOR THE TRACHEOSTOMY. If the patient is sufficiently alert, and if the delay does not invoke any risk, he is advised about the need for a tracheostomy and what it involves. An explanation is made of his breathing and removal of secretions through the tube and of his temporary loss of voice. He is then reassured that someone will be in constant, close attendance and that provision will be made for him to communi-

cate by writing if he wishes. A similar explanation is given to the family. Opportunities are provided for the patient and family members to ask questions and to receive further clarification.

PREPARATION TO RECEIVE THE PATIENT. This includes assembling sterile suctioning equipment, self-inflating bag with tracheal mask, respirator if indicated, adapter to fit tracheostomy tube, oxygen, sterile tracheostomy tray with various sizes of tracheostomy tubes in case the one inserted becomes dislodged, sterile tape for securing the tube in place, gauze squares, tracheal dilator and hemostat, sterile syringe to inflate the cuff and a hemostat to clamp the fine tube leading to the cuff, humidifier (the type will depend upon whether or not the patient is to receive mechanical ventilatory assistance; if not, a nebulizer may be available which fits over the opening of the tube), equipment for frequent mouth cleansing, and a pencil and slate or pad.

POSITION. The head of the bed is usually elevated to approximately a 45° angle if the patient is conscious and the blood pressure and pulse are stable.

ASSESSMENT. Frequent monitoring of the patient's blood pressure, respiratory rate and sounds, pulse and color is necessary. An increase in the respiratory rate, rales and rhonchi and an increased pulse rate may indicate the need for suctioning. The patient may still experience respiratory insufficiency due to obstruction in the tract below the tracheostomy. This could be evidenced by marked respiratory effort, unequal movement of the sides of the chest and retraction of the soft tissues in the intercostal and supraclavicular spaces. Cyanosis and distress not relieved by suctioning are reported promptly. Increasing restlessness, especially if accompanied by a rapid pulse rate, may indicate hypoxia or bleeding.

The neck and area around the incision are inspected for possible interstitial emphysema due to air leaking into the subcutaneous tissue. The wound is observed for bleeding in the immediate postoperative period and then checked daily for signs of infection and sloughing.

The tube is checked frequently for patency and the characteristics (consistency, color, amount) of the tracheobronchial secretions are noted. Increased secretion occurs in response to the tracheal trauma and is usually colored by blood at first, but the blood content should gradually diminish and disappear. A daily specimen of the secretions for staining and culture may be requested.

If the patient is receiving mechanical ventilatory assistance, both sides of the chest are observed for movement or are auscultated for air entry. The tidal volume and minute volume are recorded hourly.

SUCTIONING. The patient's cough is less effective in clearing the airway, so suctioning is necessary. It is done hourly, or more often if necessary. The frequency may be gradually decreased as the secretions become less. One has to be sure they are less and not thick and tenacious and retained because of lack of fluids and humidification. The physician may suggest the instillation of 5 to 10 ml. of sterile saline followed immediately by suctioning.

If the patient is receiving mechanical ventilatory assistance or oxygen, he is hyperoxygenated before suctioning (O_2, 100 per cent for 3 to 5 minutes). Suctioning removes air and oxygen from the respiratory tract, as well as removing secretions, and may cause hypoxemia and ensuing cardiac arrhythmia.

The cuff on the tube is deflated and then, with sterile glove and a sterile suction catheter moistened in sterile water or normal saline, the trachea is suctioned. The negative pressure is not applied during the insertion of the catheter but is applied when it is in position and during withdrawal. Suctioning must be brief, not longer than 10 to 15 seconds. If it must be repeated, the patient is allowed several breaths or is given oxygen again.

Secretions and suctioning may initiate coughing. Secretions escaping from the tracheostomy tube are gently wiped away with sterile unfrayed gauze (free of lint and absorbent). The mucus and exudate must be cleaned away quickly before being drawn back into the tract with a breath.

TUBE AND WOUND CARE. The wound and surrounding skin are kept as dry and free of secretions as possible; moisture predisposes to infection and maceration of the tissues. The physician may indicate the antiseptic solution to be used in cleansing; hydrogen peroxide 3 per cent is frequently the solution of choice. The wound and area under the tube are protected with sterile dry gauze, folded to fit around the tube. The gauze should be unfrayed and free of lint and absorbent to prevent possible aspiration of a loose thread or particle. If the tapes securing

the tube become soiled they are replaced with fresh sterile tapes.

The inner cannula of the tracheostomy tube is carefully removed and cleansed every 3 to 6 hours, or as often as necessary (perhaps even hourly). The cannula is cleansed thoroughly using a small tube brush with detergent and cold water or hydrogen peroxide. It is then rinsed, sterilized, reinserted into the outer tube and locked in position. Any delay is avoided to prevent the drying and adherence of secretions in the lumen of the outer tube. It may be necessary to suction the outer tube to remove secretions before replacing the inner cannula. Precautions must be taken not to displace the outer tube; the tapes which secure it are checked frequently.

Single tubes are usually changed by the surgeon every 3 days; the tube with an inner cannula may be changed weekly. A tray with sterile replacement tubes and the necessary equipment is kept at the bedside.

If a mechanical ventilator is being used, the tube leading to the tracheostomy tube should be supported so it does not pull on the tracheostomy tube and cause pressure on the wound. A flexible swivel connector is used to attach the ventilatory tube of the machine to the tracheostomy tube. This permits movement and turning of the patient with minimal risk of moving or dislodging the tracheostomy tube. An irrational patient or a child may require elbow splints or arm restraints to prevent removal or interference with the tube.

The cuff on the tube is deflated hourly for 5 minutes. When reinflating, the exact prescribed amount of air is injected and recorded. The intracuff pressure may be checked on a manometer. If a seal is not necessary to prevent the escape of inspired gas, the cuff remains deflated. The newer soft, compliant "floppy" cuffs occlude the trachea sufficiently at a lower pressure and thus minimize the risk of pressure necrosis of the tracheal mucosa.

Should the tube come out of the trachea because of vigorous coughing or carelessly tied tapes, the tracheal opening closes and the patient is threatened with asphyxia. Prompt action is necessary. The tracheal wound is quickly reopened with the sterile tracheal dilator or a hemostat which is always kept at the bedside in the event of such an emergency. The opening is held open until the doctor arrives and inserts the sterile tracheostomy tube.

HUMIDIFICATION. Adequate humidification of the inspired gas is very important to prevent encrustations forming within the trachea and the tube, which increase airway resistance. As cited above, the method used will depend upon whether or not mechanical ventilation is necessary. Equipment which provides a nebulized solution is more efficient (see p. 416).

FLUIDS AND NUTRITION. A minimum fluid intake of 3000 ml. is recommended to help liquefy pulmonary secretions, unless contraindicated by cardiac insufficiency and edema. An accurate record is kept of the intake and output. The patient is not usually permitted any fluids or food by mouth; they are administered intravenously. Some patients receive feedings via a nasogastric tube. The food is in liquid form, adequately nutritious, and a prescribed volume is administered every 4 to 6 hours. The solution is warmed and allowed to flow into the stomach by gravity. When all the solution has run through, approximately 30 ml. of water is introduced to rinse the tube to keep it clean. The nostril through which the tube is passed is cleansed with a moist swab twice daily to prevent mucosal irritation. The tube is secured to the patient's face or behind an ear.

If ventilatory assistance is necessary for a prolonged period, the physician may feed the patient by total parenteral nutrition (hyperalimentation) instead of by nasogastric feedings (see p. 504).

If the tracheostomy is going to be permanent, or if the patient is not on a respirator, oral fluids are introduced gradually; if tolerated, a soft diet is given and increased gradually to a regular diet. The patient is at first fed by the nurse, and then he is encouraged to feed himself as he overcomes his apprehension about choking. The nurse remains with him until he gains sufficient confidence.

MOUTH CARE. Oral hygiene is important for the patient's comfort and to reduce the possibility of infection. The mouth is cleansed and rinsed every 2 hours until the patient is taking normal meals, at which time regular cleansing of the teeth and rinsing of the mouth after each meal and at bedtime suffice.

PSYCHOLOGICAL SUPPORT. The patient is fearful of choking and concerned about his inability to cough up the secretions and to communicate. When the nurse leaves the bedside the patient is advised of the errand and how long it will take. A signal light is given to the patient; he will be more secure if he knows he can call someone if necessary.

The nurse talks to the patient, advises him of his progress and what is going to be done, and endeavors to anticipate information the patient might want to have but cannot ask for verbally. He especially wants information about how long he is likely to be unable to breathe and communicate normally. A slate or pad and pencil are kept readily within his reach, and he is encouraged to communicate his feelings and needs. Family members are encouraged to talk to him.

A mild sedative or tranquilizer may be prescribed if the patient is fearful and emotionally disturbed. Analgesics and sedatives that may depress the respiratory center and the cough reflex are avoided.

EXTUBATION. If the patient has been receiving mechanical ventilatory assistance, removal of the tracheostomy tube is not considered until he is successfully weaned from the ventilator (see p. 429). When the tracheostomy is a temporary measure, the patient is gradually returned to breathing through the upper tract. In order to lessen tracheal injury and scarring the tube is removed as soon as possible, but without compromising adequate ventilation. The protective reflexes should be responsive; the epiglottis and glottis should close to prevent aspiration, the gag reflex should be present and the patient should be able to swallow fluids and food without risk of aspiration.

If a cuffed tube has been used, the cuff is deflated for 24 to 48 hours before the tube is removed and the patient's ability to keep upper tract secretions out of the lower tract is observed. Until the protective reflexes have been demonstrated the cuff is reinflated during and for 20 minutes after meals. A methylene blue test may be done to determine the effectiveness of the reflexes. The test involves giving the patient about 100 to 120 ml. of water containing 1 ml. of methylene blue. The trachea is then suctioned every 15 minutes for 1 hour. If the suctioned secretions do not show the presence of the methylene blue solution, the protective reflexes are considered effective.

Some physicians may suggest the insertion of a special tube with a smaller opening into the tracheostomy tube for a period of time. If this smaller opening is tolerated by the patient, then the tubes are removed.

A sterile tracheostomy tray with tubes of several sizes is kept at the bedside in case a tube may have to be reinserted after extubation. Sterile suction equipment should also be available.

When the tracheostomy tube is removed, the wound is cleansed, the wound edges are approximated and taped and a firm dressing is applied. Healing occurs spontaneously; sutures are not considered necessary. The patient is advised to place his hand over the area and exert some pressure when he coughs. He may be fearful of not being able to breathe when the tube is removed, so he is assured beforehand that his breathing is adequate via the normal route. A nurse remains with him following removal to be certain that he experiences no difficulty. Blood specimens may be taken for a day or two to determine the paO_2 and $paCO_2$ levels. Following discharge, the physician or clinic keeps track of the patient who has had a tracheostomy for at least a year. He is checked for possible scarring and tracheal stricture resulting from irritation and trauma.

HOME TRACHEOSTOMY CARE. If the tracheostomy is permanent, the patient is instructed about the care of the tube and the stoma (an artificial opening to the surface). This is done as soon as he is well enough to undertake the care in the hospital so he will develop confidence. A member of the family also receives instruction about the necessary care and precautions.

The patient may continue to have excessive secretions and may require suction equipment at home. In this case, a family member is advised where such equipment may be obtained (e.g., the National Cancer Society) and, with the patient, is instructed in the use and care of the equipment.

The patient and family are advised how to conceal the site of the tracheostomy. The shirt will cover the stoma in a man; a woman may wear a scarf or high-necked blouse or dress.

An explanation is made of the danger of aspirating water through the tracheostomy tube; this precludes swimming or immersion in water to a high level. Precautions must also be used when taking a shower.

The patient is advised to return to the clinic or to his physician at regular intervals, as directed, for changing the tube and examination of the stoma. Eventually, when the stoma is firmly healed and the tracheal opening remains patent, the physician may permit the patient or a member of the family to change the outer cannula or he may remove the tube permanently. Precautions should be used to avoid close contact with those in the environment with respiratory infection.

Self-inflating Hand Ventilator (Ambu Bag)

This is a portable ventilator that is operated manually (Fig. 15–13). It consists of a self-inflating bag which connects with a source of 100 per cent oxygen and has a short tube to which a mask is attached. A connecting adapter replaces the mask when the bag is used for a patient with an endotracheal or tracheostomy tube.

After applying the mask so that there is as tight a seal as possible, or after connecting the tube to the patient's artificial airway, the bag is squeezed with both hands. Collapse of

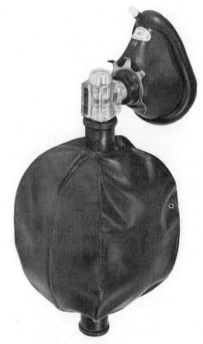

FIGURE 15–13 An Ambu resuscitator, a self-inflating, hand-compressible breathing bag with mask. (Courtesy of the Harris Calorific Co., Cleveland, Ohio; from Secor, J., Patient Care in Respiratory Problems, W. B. Saunders Co., 1969, p. 131.)

the bag delivers an adequate tidal volume of oxygen into the patient's airway.

The self-inflating hand ventilator is useful for resuscitation in an emergency. It is kept at the bedside of a patient who is receiving mechanical ventilatory assistance so it is readily available to ventilate the patient in case of malfunction of the respirator. It is also used to support the patient's ventilation when the mechanical respirator is disconnected so that the patient's airway can be suctioned.

Mechanical Ventilators

When a patient is unable to ventilate his lungs effectively and maintain adequate alveolar/blood gas exchange, a mechanical ventilator (respirator) may be used to inflate the lungs or assist the individual's inspiratory effort. The ventilator introduces air or a mixture of air and oxygen intermittently into the patients's airway by producing a positive pressure.[11] Expiration is passive when the

---

[11]Positive pressure implies a gas pressure greater than that of the atmosphere.

inflow regulating valve closes. The indications for respirator use are ventilatory insufficiency, hypoxemia and hypercapnia.

An artificial airway is necessary when a respirator is being used so that a seal is produced by a cuffed tube to prevent escape of the inspiratory gas. Initially, an endotracheal tube is generally used, but if mechanical respiratory support is necessary for longer than 48 to 72 hours a tracheostomy is done and the ventilator is connected to a cuffed tracheostomy tube.

TYPES OF VENTILATORS. Three types of positive-pressure ventilators are available: (1) pressure-regulated; (2) volume-regulated; and (3) time-regulated (Fig. 15–14).

PRESSURE-REGULATED (PRESSURE-CYCLED) MACHINE. This is designed to deliver the prescribed inspiratory gas until a predetermined pressure is achieved, regardless of the volume of gas delivered to the patient's lungs. When the preset pressure is reached, the valve for stopping the gas flow closes and exhalation occurs passively (comparable to normal exhalation). The machine is operated by compressed oxygen and the pressure setting is usually that of 15 to 20 cm. of

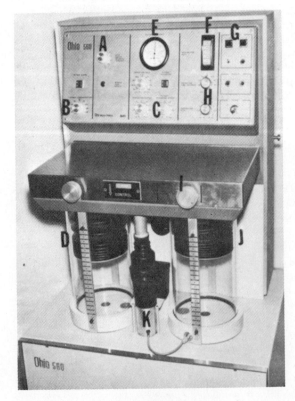

FIGURE 15–14 Volume-controlled respirator (the Ohio 560 model). A, sigh timer; B, oxygen control; C, sensitivity control; D, sigh bellows; E, delivery pressure gauge; F, rate meter; G, warning lights and audible alarm; H, flow rate control; I, bellows control; J, tidal volume bellows; K, ultrasonic nebulizer.

water; the upper limit is 30 cm. of water. A disadvantage of the pressure-cycled ventilator is that an adequate tidal volume may not always be delivered. Certain positions assumed by the patient or regressive changes within his respiratory system may reduce the lung compliance. This reduces lung capacity and the predetermined pressure is achieved with a lesser volume of gas. The pressure-cycled respirator is designed so that the patient's exhalation volume can be measured to determine tidal volume. (A small respirometer, such as a Wright respirometer, may be attached to an expiratory outlet.) If the tidal volume is deficient, the pressure setting may have to be adjusted as a result of changes in the patient's compliance.

VOLUME-REGULATED (VOLUME-CYCLED) VENTILATOR. This type delivers a prescribed volume of gas with each inspiratory phase using electrical power. Changes in the patient's position and lung compliance do not alter the lung capacity and ventilatory volume. When the predetermined volume of inspiratory gas is delivered, a valve closes off the gas flow and the passive exhalation phase is initiated by the natural recoil of the lungs. If airway resistance increases, the pressure required to deliver the preset volume will increase. Since this could be dangerous, volume-cycled ventilators have a safety pressure release valve. If an excessively high inspiratory pressure is reached, the valve interrupts the flow of gas into the airway.

TIME-CYCLED VENTILATOR. This delivers the prescribed inspiratory gas for a preset unit of time. The inspiratory pressure may become excessively high if compliance or resistance is increased, so these machines also have a safety pressure release valve.

OPERATIONAL FACTORS. Respirators may be used to provide controlled ventilation or assisted ventilation. In *controlled ventilation* the machine is set for automatic operation and for producing a set number of cycles per minute at a predetermined flow rate, regardless of the patient's respiratory effort.

In assisted ventilation the inspiratory phase of the respirator's cycle is triggered by the patient's spontaneous inspiration, complementing his ventilatory volume. Most respirators that can be set for assisted ventilation are equipped with a safety control, so that if the patient's respiratory function fails

to trigger the ventilator by a preset interval of time, controlled ventilation automatically takes over.

When mechanical ventilation is necessary, the physician indicates if the ventilatory support is to be controlled or assisted ventilation and whether the ventilator to be used is to be pressure-, volume-, or time-cycled. The oxygen/air mixture, volume or pressure setting for the delivery of the inspiratory gas, flow rate and sigh frequency are adjusted to the clinical condition of the patient (blood gases and pH, lung compliance and general condition).

The decision as to whether controlled ventilation or assisted ventilation is used is influenced by the individual's level of consciousness, spontaneous respiratory rate and severity of the respiratory insufficiency. If the controlled ventilator is used, it is important that the patient's respirations be synchronized with the respirator. If the patient is sufficiently alert he may be instructed to relax and breathe with the ventilator. Some patients find this difficult; assistance may be provided by first reducing the respiratory drive through brief overbreathing or a high gas flow rate.

The prescribed tidal volume of ventilation is set on the volume-cycled respirator. If the patient is on a pressure-cycled machine, the tidal volume is measured on a respirometer. As mentioned previously, if the tidal volume is not adequate, the pressure may have to be adjusted.

Some respirators have a built-in mechanism by which the inspiratory volume can be increased at stated intervals to produce a sigh. Periodic sighing insures more effective alveolar inflation, preventing collapse and diffuse atelectasis. The sigh frequency may be one every 10 to 15 minutes.

The oxygen concentration of the inspired gas will be prescribed on the basis of the patient's paO_2. It does not usually exceed 40 to 50 per cent. The concentration is kept as low as possible without the patient experiencing hypoxia so as to prevent oxygen toxicity (see p. 410).

Some patients have considerable tracheal irritation from the artificial airway tube and, as a result, experience continuous coughing. The physician may prescribe a small dose of a sedative or analgesic intravenously to suppress the cough reflex, or intravenous curare may be administered to produce relaxation.

The ventilators currently in use have built-in humidifiers or nebulizers and a thermostatically controlled heating element which warms the inhaled mixture. The solution container is checked frequently so that an adequate fluid level is maintained to insure continuous moistening of the inspired gas. The tube leading to the patient's airway is disconnected periodically to empty it quickly of the condensation. The tube is changed daily to prevent the colonization of organisms within it which predisposes the patient to infection.

Ventilators may malfunction, or a problem may arise within the connecting tube or the patient's airway. Unless the disturbance is recognized promptly and corrected, the patient's life is threatened. Most respirators are equipped with an audible alarm system to alert the staff when there is a malfunction within the system. Disturbances such as failure to cycle, failure to release excessive pressure, failure to reach the required pressure in a given time, and accidental disconnection of tubing trigger the alarm.

NURSING RESPONSIBILITIES. The nursing care plan for the patient who requires mechanical ventilatory assistance will vary according to the cause of the respiratory insufficiency and general condition.

Most hospitals now have a staff of inhalation therapy technicians who are available to operate the respirators. However, it is the nurse who is constantly at the patient's bedside; this necessitates understanding the underlying principles of mechanical ventilation. The nurse should be familiar with the operation of the particular machine being used and the prescribed inspiratory gas composition (percentage of air and oxygen). It is also necessary to know whether the ventilation is controlled or assisted and volume-or pressure-cycled, the prescribed volume or pressure setting for the delivery of the inspiratory gas, the flow rate and cycles per minute, and the sigh frequency. A very important nursing responsibility is the immediate recognition of the indications of ventilator malfunction and untoward reactions in the patient, as well as the initiation of prompt appropriate action.

It is essential that any nurse assuming responsibility for the care of a patient requiring mechanical ventilatory assistance has received adequate instruction and supervision in order to provide safe and effective care.

The nursing care plan will include the following considerations:

CONSTANT ATTENDANCE. The patient who is receiving mechanical ventilation must not be left unattended. If malfunction of the respirator or unfavorable changes in the patient are not immediately recognized and prompt action taken, the patient's life is threatened.

EMOTIONAL SUPPORT. The patient who requires mechanical ventilation, if sufficiently alert, finds the situation very frightening and threatening. A brief explanation of the respirator and what it is expected to achieve will allay some fear. Reassurance that someone will always be close to the bedside also helps.

The nurse must guard against becoming so preoccupied with the machine and technical procedures that the patient as a person is forgotten. It is important to address the patient by name. Being unable to communicate verbally, the patient is dependent upon signs and facial and eye expressions to convey feelings and needs unless he is able to write and provision is made for this. Recognizing the nature of the situation and its implications for the patient, the nurse acknowledges the individual's fears and concerns, talks to the patient and provides information. Touching the patient (laying one's hands on the patient's shoulder, arm or hand) also conveys empathy.

ASSESSMENT. When mechanical ventilation is first established, it is necessary to note the patient's blood pressure, pulse rate and volume, color, level of consciousness, and blood pH, gases ($paCO_2$, paO_2) and electrolyte levels to establish baselines for ongoing assessment. A chest x-ray may have been done and the findings are reviewed.

Arterial blood samples are collected at frequent intervals for pH, blood gas and electrolyte (especially bicarbonate, sodium, and potassium) determinations. Hypoxemia is a common problem and threat with these patients (normal paO_2: 70 to 100 mm. Hg). The patient may have developed respiratory acidosis due to retention of carbon dioxide, manifested by an increase in the $paCO_2$ (normal: 40 to 45 mm. Hg), a decrease in the pH (normal: pH 7.35 to 7.4) and normal or increased (compensated) level of bicarbonate (HCO_3^-). If the respirator settings are such that the patient is being hyperventilated, respiratory alkalosis may develop; the $paCO_2$

level falls below normal, the pH is increased above the normal and the HCO_3^- ions decrease. Elimination of bicarbonate by the kidneys is increased in an effort to compensate for acid/base imbalance. (See pp. 99–100 for symptoms of acidosis and alkalosis.)

The pH and blood gas levels may indicate necessary adjustments in the machine settings. For example, the concentration of oxygen and flow rate may have to be increased to increase the paO_2. If the $paCO_2$ is below normal, the dead space may be increased by lengthening the tube between the respirator and the patient, or the number of cycles per minute may be reduced. Lengthening the tube results in rebreathing the exhaled CO_2.

The blood pressure and radial and apical pulses are recorded every ½ to 1 hour, and the patient's color is noted. The interval is lengthened to every 1 to 2 hours as the condition improves. Frequent evaluation of these vital functions is very important throughout the complete period that the patient is on the respirator because of the physiological effects of the positive pressure on the thoracic structures. Normally, on inspiration, the chest expansion results in a decrease in the intrapleural pressure which favors the return of venous blood to the right side of the heart. This promotes the blood supply to the lungs as well as a greater flow to the left side of the heart. When a respirator is used, the lungs are expanded passively by internal pressure exerted by the gas "driven" into the airway. The positive pressure may also be exerted on the blood vessels and heart, producing the reverse effect to that discussed above in normal inspiration. The intrathoracic pressure is increased; there is a decreased return of venous blood to the heart, and a subsequent decrease in the pulmonary blood supply and left cardiac output. As a result of these changes, the patient's blood pressure may fall and the pulse rate increase, and he may complain of headache because of increased intracranial pressure. The abdomen is examined for distention which may occur due to gastric dilation and paralytic ileus.

A record is kept of the patient's fluid balance, and the quantity and characteristics of the respiratory tract secretions are noted. If the latter become purulent and the temperature and leukocyte count are elevated, infection is suspected immediately.

The patient's level of consciousness and orientation are assessed; an improvement may indicate improved cerebral oxygenation. An unfavorable change is reported to the physician, and gas tensions of the arterial blood are checked.

If the ventilator being used is pressure-cycled, the tidal and minute volumes are determined hourly.

The central venous pressure may be monitored hourly. A catheter is passed into the superior vena cava and is kept open between readings by maintaining an intravenous infusion. Abnormal intrathoracic pressures and venous return to the heart are reflected in central venous pressure. The physician generally indicates the range within which he wishes the pressure maintained; any deviation is reported promptly. (See p. 297.)

PATIENT'S AIRWAY. It was mentioned previously that mechanical ventilation necessitates the patient having either an endotracheal or tracheostomy cuffed tube. The artificial airway eliminates the ability to cough and remove secretions. Retained secretions predispose to infection and can obstruct bronchial tubes, bronchioles and alveoli; the airway distal to the mucus plug collapses. Distal portions of the airway cannot be cleared of secretions by suctioning. To promote movement of the secretions into an area within reach of the suction, the patient is turned hourly (side to side to back to side) and positioned semiprone three or four times daily if his condition permits. Chest physical therapy is used at frequent intervals (every 4 to 6 hours) to mobilize secretions.

Tracheal suctioning is done hourly or as needed to keep the airway as clear as possible. The patient is encouraged to cough during the period in which the respirator is detached. The nurse listens for breath sounds by auscultation and notes any secretions, abnormal sounds or resistance to air entry. For nursing responsibilities associated with the endotracheal tube or tracheostomy tube, see p. 417 and p. 418.

When the respirator has been detached and the "audible alarm" turned off during suctioning or for any other reason, the nurse makes sure that the alarm is turned on again when the respirator is reconnected to the patient's airway.

Humidification of the inspired gas plays an important role in keeping the airway clear of secretions. The fluid level in the nebulizer or humidifier is checked at frequent regular intervals to prevent the possibility of the patient receiving dry inspiratory gas.

FLUIDS AND NUTRITION. The patient's fluid and electrolyte requirements are met by intravenous infusion. The fluid intake and output are accurately measured and the balance is noted. Adequate hydration is essential to the liquefaction and removal of secretions. Nutrition may be provided by nasogastric tube feedings (see p. 503). If mechanical ventilation is necessary for a prolonged period and the patient is unable to take food by mouth, he may receive total parenteral nutrition (hyperalimentation) (see p. 504).

PREVENTION OF INFECTION. The patient's normal respiratory defense mechanisms and resistance to infection are impaired; precautions are necessary to prevent this serious complication. Most important are the measures suggested above to keep the airway cleared of secretions. Other measures include: (1) protection of the patient from contact with those (family and staff) having an infection, especially respiratory; (2) changing the tube between the patient and respirator at least once daily; (3) frequent clearing of condensation from the tube; (4) frequent washing of the nurse's hands, and always when going from one patient to another; (5) antiseptic care of the tracheostomy area, keeping it as clean and as dry as possible; and (6) frequent mouth care. Purulent secretions and elevated temperature and leukocyte count are brought to the physician's attention promptly, as they are probably signs of infection.

COMFORT MEASURES Routine physical care measures are as important to the patient as the ventilator. The nurse must be alert to possible sources of discomfort and promote relief and comfort for the patient. Frequent mouth care, back rubs, repositioning, turning pillows, and controlling lights to avoid constant glare for the patient are examples of simple nursing measures that contribute to comfort. Mouth care is especially important if the patient has an endotracheal tube. The tube may cause increased oral secretions, which are removed by suctioning as often as necessary if the patient cannot swallow them. The teeth and mouth can be cleaned with a soft toothbrush and swabs. The respirator tube is attached to the patient's airway by a swivel connecting tube so that

movement of the tube does not disturb the airway and traumatize tissues.

Care is planned so that the patient may have undisturbed rest periods. The environment is temperature-controlled and as quiet and free of confusion as possible. Conversation is guarded within the patient's hearing so as to avoid arousing fear and apprehension.

Since the patient cannot communicate his distress or discomforts verbally, it is the nurse's responsibility to anticipate them. In addition to the physical discomforts, it is necessary to keep in mind the emotional distress that is experienced (see the section above on emotional support).

COMPLICATIONS.[12, 13] Complications that may develop in the patient receiving mechanical ventilatory assistance include the following.

Atelectasis and pneumonia are two problems that may develop. Keeping the air passages free of secretions and observing the precautionary measures mentioned to prevent infection are significant factors in preventing these complications.

Cardiac insufficiency and hypotension may develop as a result of the positive pressure created within the airway and thoracic cavity which has an adverse effect on the venous return to the heart.

Petty's study[14] indicates that hyperventilation occurs in some instances as a result of the right bronchus being intubated. Following the introduction of an endotracheal tube, the physician may request an x-ray to determine the exact position of the tube to avoid possible intubation or blocking of a bronchus.

The positive pressure within the airways may cause a pneumothorax. The pressure causes an opening to form on the surface of the lung (probably as a result of the rupture of an alveolus) which permits entry of the inspired gas into the pleural cavity. The gas, under pressure, collapses the lung. Unless recognized promptly, tension pneumothorax may develop quickly. Gas enters the pleural

---

[12]Linda M. Fitzgerald: "Mechanical Ventilation." Heart Lung, Vol. 5, No. 6 (Nov-Dec.) 1976, p. 947-948.
[13]Thomas L. Petty: "Complications Occurring During Mechanical Ventilation." Heart Lung, Vol. 5. No. 1 (Jan.-Feb.) 1976, p. 112-118.
[14]Ibid., p. 113.

cavity with each inspiratory phase but does not escape with the expiratory phase. Intrapleural pressure progressively increases; mediastinal structures are displaced to the opposite side of the chest, compromising ventilation of the lung on that side. The ventilator should indicate the resistance to air entry. Unless corrected quickly, hypotension and cardiac failure occur. The emergency treatment is the insertion of a large-bore needle or tube into the affected pleural cavity to allow escape of the gas.

Some patients receiving mechanical ventilation develop gastrointestinal complications. Stress ulcers and bleeding are not uncommon. Some physicians require routine analysis of stool and gastric drainage for occult blood. Gastric dilation and paralytic ileus have also been reported in these patients. The abdomen is checked for distention several times daily; distention and vomiting are reported promptly to the physician. A nasogastric or duodenal tube may be introduced to promote drainage and relieve the distention.

FAMILY. It is only natural that the family will be very concerned about the patient who is ill enough to require ventilatory assistance. The care and treatments that the patient is receiving are likely to restrict the amount of time a relative may spend with the patient. Frequently, family members remain for hours in the hospital visiting room hoping for some information and to be told that they may see the patient. The nurse may become so involved with the responsibility of patient care that thought for the family's concern is neglected. Part of total patient care is insuring some consideration for the family; members should be informed at intervals about what is being done for the patient and what his progress is. They are told that someone will talk with them periodically and will let them know when they may see the patient.

A family member is permitted to visit briefly at frequent intervals. Such visits are important to the family and are also supportive and reassuring to the patient. In some instances a relative may be of assistance in turning the patient or in performing some similar comfort measure. This participation in care is helpful to the worried person who is probably thinking "if I could only help or do something."

Family members remaining close by are advised of the location of a telephone, washroom and restaurant.

EMERGENCY CARE. If there is a disturbance in the mechanical ventilation, it may be due to an obstruction in the airway or to malfunctioning of the ventilator. It may be that the latter can be immediately recognized and corrected; if not, help is summoned and the respirator is disconnected from the patient's airway. The cuff on the endotracheal or tracheostomy tube is deflated and the airway is suctioned. The patient is ventilated with a self-inflating resuscitation bag. If the problem is in the patient's airway and is not relieved by suctioning, it may be necessary to remove the tube. It is possible that air may enter the patient's airway but exhalation may be blocked by a mucus plug being drawn against the end of the tube. Air is trapped and the lung becomes overdistended.

WEANING. If prolonged mechanical ventilation is necessary, the patient becomes very dependent upon the respirator and is fearful of its use being discontinued. He is advised that he will be observed closely and that his respirations and blood gases will be monitored frequently. Gradual weaning from the machine is introduced as soon as the tidal volume and blood gases reach satisfactory levels. *It is important that use of the respiratory muscles be reestablished as soon as possible to prevent loss of tone and slowness of response.* The patient is taken off the machine for brief periods, which are progressively increased. A nurse remains with the patient during these periods and the patient's physiological responses, as well as emotional reaction, are noted. The blood gas tensions, tidal volume, minute ventilation and vital capacity are assessed at frequent intervals for several days.

Oxygen may be administered by mask during the initial independent respirations. Humidification of the inspired air is necessary for a few days while the respiratory mucosa readapts. The nurse remaining with the patient during the "off periods" prompts the patient to breathe deeply and encourages periodic coughing. Suctioning may still be necessary to clear the airway.

Thoracentesis (Chest Aspiration)

This procedure involves the introduction of a needle into a pleural cavity. It may be done for the purpose of aspirating fluid that has accumulated in the cavity and is compressing the lung, or it may be done to obtain a specimen of fluid for diagnostic purposes. Aseptic technique is used in withdrawing the fluid. The patient is advised of what is to be done, and the purpose, and is placed in a sitting position, leaning forward with head and arms resting on a table over the bed or several pillows. Following the cleansing of the skin and sterile draping, the physician uses a local anesthetic before introducing the needle.

The amount and characteristics of the aspirate are noted, and a sterile specimen is labelled and sent to the laboratory for examination. When the needle is withdrawn, the puncture wound is tightly sealed and covered with a sterile dressing. The patient's pulse and respirations are checked frequently for at least 2 hours. Any unfavorable changes in respirations, and color, rapid pulse rate, excessive coughing or blood-tinged sputum are reported to the physician promptly.

ACUTE RESPIRATORY FAILURE

Respiratory failure or insufficiency is present when a person is unable to maintain adequate arterial blood levels of oxygen and carbon dioxide. Acute respiratory failure develops rapidly and is characterized by an arterial pO_2 of approximately 50 mm. Hg or less. The hypoxia may or may not be accompanied by excessive retention of carbon dioxide (hypercapnia).

ETIOLOGY. Respiratory failure may be encountered in any clinical area and may be associated with a variety of disorders. The causes include: (1) trauma and surgery that incur shock; (2) intrapulmonary disorders, such as airway obstruction, pneumonia (especially viral and aspiration pneumonia) and pulmonary embolism; (3) central nervous system disorders such as drug overdose, brain tumor, cerebral injury or hemorrhage; (4) neuromoscular disease that involves respiratory muscle innervation, (e.g., myasthenia gravis and Guillain-Barré syndrome); and (5) sepsis, especially if the organisms are gram-negative.

Patients with a history of chronic obstructive pulmonary disease (asthma, emphyse-

ma) and cardiac or kidney disease, and those who are obese or debilitated are predisposed to develop acute respiratory failure when illness occurs.

Acute respiratory failure may be the result of alveolar hypoventilation (ventilatory failure) or inadequate oxygenation of the blood (oxygenation failure); in some instances both problems are present. Ventilatory failure is characterized by the retention of an excessive volume of carbon dioxide (hypercarbia) accompanied by hypoxemia. The patient develops respiratory acidosis because of the elevated $paCO_2$. It is frequently associated with general hypoventilation due to neuromuscular disturbances, chest wall injury, and chronic obstructive lung disease. The difference between ventilatory failure and oxygenation failure is that, in the latter, the carbon dioxide retention is initially slight. Examples of disorders in which oxygenation failure may be a complication are shock, pulmonary embolism, sepsis, pneumonia and renal failure. Respiratory alkalosis may be present if the individual's respirations are increased as a result of hypoxia (an excess of carbon dioxide is ventilated off).

Failure to oxygenate the blood adequately may be due to abnormal distribution of the inspired gas or ventilation-perfusion inequality. The alveoli may be filled with fluid, or the alveoli are not ventilated because of an airway obstruction or atelectasis. As a result, the blood may flow through the capillaries around the alveoli without gas exchange taking place. In other instances the alveoli may be ventilated but the respective capillaries do not receive an adequate blood supply or are occluded.

When acute oxygenation failure is severe pulmonary capillary epithelium is damaged, which leads to hemorrhage and interstitial edema. The edema decreases diffusion because fluid lies between the alveoli and capillaries. Fluid infiltrates the alveoli; surfactant secretion is decreased and there are progressively increasing patches of atelectasis. Defective gas diffusion becomes extensive and very serious. This severe form of respiratory oxygenation failure may be referred to as *shock lung, wet lung, adult respiratory distress syndrome* or *stiff lung*. The latter term (stiff lung) is attributed to the reduced lung compliance; the interstitial edema compresses the lungs. There is increased resistance to air entry in the airways and alveo-li.[15, 16]

MANIFESTATIONS. The patient may manifest the effects of hypoxemia or hypercarbia, or both. Dyspnea or tachypnea may be present, or in ventilatory failure respirations may be depressed and are slow, irregular and shallow. Cyanosis may not be present at the onset. The pulse rate increases and arrhythmias may develop. The patient may be restless and complain of headache or dizziness. Disorientation, apathy and slow responses develop as a result of the cerebral hypoxia, and may progress to unconsciousness. Periodic sustained contraction of a group of skeletal muscles (asterixis) may occur if there is marked retention of carbon dioxide. The tidal and minute volumes are usually reduced.

Auscultation and an x-ray of the chest reveal patchy consolidated areas (no air entry). Measurement of the arterial blood gases may show levels as: paO_2, 50 mm. Hg or less; and $paCO_2$, 50 to 60 mm. Hg or more. The pH is always checked to determine the presence and degree of acidosis or alkalosis.

Respiratory failure may develop quickly in a few hours after the initial insult, or the onset may be insidious over 2 or 3 days. Serial monitoring of the patient's blood gases and tidal volume and close observation of the characteristics of the respirations in circumstances where respiratory insufficiency may occur are important in early recognition of the problem.

TREATMENT AND NURSING CARE. The underlying disorder which initiated the respiratory failure is treated and therapy is immediately directed toward improving ventilation and oxygenation of the blood. Intensive, constant nursing care is required; this involves the following considerations.

VENTILATORY SUPPORT. The mode and amount of ventilatory support will depend upon the assessment made of the patient's respiratory status and general condition, and the recognition of signs and symptoms of respiratory insufficiency. Early recognition may indicate more simple support measures

such as chest physical therapy and oxygen inhalation by mask. Hypoventilation, hypoxemia and/or hypercarbia require more extreme measures

The airway is kept clear of secretions by suctioning (see p. 413), having the patient cough at regular intervals, chest physical therapy, and turning the patient hourly (side→side→back). The patient is encouraged to breathe deeply at regular frequent intervals to improve alveolar ventilation.

The patient's blood gases and tidal volume may indicate the need for mechanical ventilatory assistance. This necessitates tracheal intubation or trachesotomy and the use of a cuffed tube. The care of the patient on a mechanical ventilator is outlined on pp. 424–429.

The physician may prescribe a relatively large tidal volume to be delivered by the ventilator or the use of positive end-expiratory pressure (PEEP) in order to overcome the resistance of air entry and prevent atelectasis. In PEEP, the ventilator is set to maintain a positive pressure within the lungs during the expiratory phase. The ventilator is adapted to keep end-expiratory pressure from falling to zero. Residual capacity is increased which improves alveolar expansion and gas exchange. The pressure used is generally within the range of 5 to 20 cm. of water. If the ventilator does not have a built-in mechanism for providing positive end-expiratory pressure, it may be established by connecting the ventilator's expiratory outlet to a length of tubing. The opposite end of the tube is submerged under water for a distance equal to the prescribed pressure (5 to 20 cm. of water).

ASSESSMENT. Constant assessment of the patient with acute respiratory failure is necessary. It requires that the nurse be informed of the patient's condition and the rationale for the therapeutic program. The nurse is constantly alert to the patient's responses and for changes in his condition. It is necessary to be familiar with the laboratory reports and to appreciate their significance. Appropriate action following the recognition of clinical changes may involve promptly modifying or altering the therapy as well as informing the physician.

Nursing is concerned with frequent monitoring of the vital signs; tidal and minute

---

[15]Thomas, L. Petty: Intensive and Rehabilitative Respiratory Care, 2nd ed. Philadelphia, Lea and Febiger, 1974, pp. 182–183.

[16]Paul B. Beeson and Walsh McDermott (Eds.): Textbook of Medicine, 14th ed. Philadelphia, W.B. Saunders, 1975, pp. 836–837.

volumes are recorded hourly, and the chest is observed for the expansion of both sides and intercostal ballooning or retraction. The chest is auscultated to determine air entry and presence of secretions and to locate areas of collapsed alveoli. Continuous monitoring of cardiac function by an electrocardiogram may be established so that any irregularity may be detected immediately. Since an arrhythmia may develop during suctioning, it is helpful to be able to observe the electrocardiographic tracing during and immediately following the procedure. The blood pressure is recorded frequently; the intervals may be ½, 1, 2 or 3 hours, depending upon the patient's condition. The color of the lips, nails and skin are observed and the warmth of the skin, especially that of the limbs, is noted. Good peripheral perfusion is evidenced by warm pink skin.

Serial arterial blood specimens are obtained for paO_2, $paCO_2$, pH and serum electrolyte (K^+, Na^+, Cl^-, HCO_3^-) determinations. These reports are followed closely and adjustments made in the ventilatory support and fluid administration, when indicated by changes. For example, if the $paCO_2$ level falls below normal limits (hypocarbia) and the pH has risen above 7.5 in the patient receiving mechanical respiratory assistance, and there is a corresponding rise in blood pressure, the dead space is increased by lengthening the tube between the respirator and the patient. This increases the "rebreathing" of carbon dioxide for the purposes of increasing the $paCO_2$.

If there has been retention of carbon dioxide and respiratory acidosis has developed, there may be an increase above normal in the serum HCO_3^- and a decrease below normal in the chlorides (hypochloremia). The latter is due to a compensated retention of bicarbonate and an excessive output of chloride ions by the kidneys. Potassium may also be depleted in acidosis: hypokalemia reduces muscle response and tone and may lead to cardiac dysfunction. Such changes may necessitate the administration of potassium chloride solution intravenously.

Other parameters by which the patient is assessed include observation of the patient's orientation and level of consciousness, muscle strength (hand grasp and flexion-extension of limbs), volume and characteristics of secretions and urinary output. Cerebral hypoxia is quickly manifested in the patient's responses and muscular strength. If the secretions are scant and tenacious, humidification of the inspired gas and probably the fluid intake are increased. In order to measure the volume of urine excreted by the kidneys hourly, an indwelling catheter is passed and a calibrated collector is attached to the tubing. The urinary output reflects cardiovascular status; an hourly output of 30 ml. or less is unfavorable.

Central venous pressure may be measured regularly; this pressure provides information about the intravascular volume and the right side of the heart (see p. 297 for details of CVP). Hourly readings are made; it is important that the same zero reference point be used for each reading.

A Swan-Ganz catheter may be introduced into the pulmonary artery to obtain pressures and specimens of mixed venous blood. This is a long (100 cm.) flexible, cardiac catheter with at least two lumens and an inflatable balloon at the tip. Using aseptic technique, it is passed via an arm vein into the superior vena cava and through the right side of the heart into the pulmonary artery. It is then advanced through the main pulmonary artery into progressively smaller branches as far as it will go. It is then in the "wedge" position. The proximal end is attached to a pressure gauge by a stopcock. The balloon is inflated to record the "wedge pressure"; this reflects the filling pressure of the left atrium. Inflation of the balloon is maintained for no more than a minute. The pulmonary artery pressure is recorded with the balloon deflated. The latter provides an indication of the intravascular volume and information about pulmonary vascular resistance. The pressures are recorded hourly. The catheter is kept patent by periodic flushing with a solution of heparin or by a continuous slow infusion of saline or dextrose with heparin. A specimen of blood may be taken for pO_2 evaluation and comparison made with a simultaneous paO_2 determination. A chest x-ray is usually done to check the position of the cathether.

Before the catheter is inserted, an explanation of its purpose and what is involved is given the patient and the family. A signed consent is obtained.

FLUIDS AND NUTRITION   The fluid intake is individualized; with some patients the fluid intake may be restricted to a specific volume because of pulmonary interstitial and alveolar edema or reduced renal output. With others, a minimum of 3000 ml. of fluid daily may be recommended to help liquefy pulmonary secretions. If the patient is unable to take sufficient fluids orally because of intubation or a tracheostomy, intravenous solutions are given. An accurate record of the total daily fluid intake and output is kept and the balance determined. The choice of intravenous solution(s) used is based on the serum electrolyte concentrations and directed toward reestablishing and maintaining homeostasis.

If the illness is prolonged the patient's loss of strength and muscle wasting may be severe. The diaphragm and other respiratory muscles become weak due to mechanical ventilatory assistance as well as lack of nutrients. This attendant weakness makes the patient more dependent upon the respirator. To prevent severe weakness and to increase the individual's resistance to infection and improve his healing of wounds total parenteral nutrition (hyperalimentation) may be administered (see p. 504).

POSITIONING AND ACTIVITY. The patient is turned every 1 or 2 hours, if at all possible, to promote the drainage of pulmonary secretions and better air distribution and to prevent pressure sores. Changes of position also contribute to the patient's comfort.

Although the patient may be attached to several tubes or a monitor, the maintenance of joint movement and the prevention of contractures remain an important part of the care. The upper and lower extremities are moved actively or passively through their range of movement at least two or three times daily.

MEDICATIONS. A diuretic such as furosemide (Lasix) may be administered intravenously if pulmonary edema is present or if there has been fluid overload. The latter may occur if shock associated with the primary disorder was treated with generous amounts of fluid intravenously. The effectiveness of the diuretic is noted by accurate measurement of the urinary output. The blood pressure and central venous pressure are followed closely in case rapid loss of fluid excessively depletes the intravascular volume.

Sedatives and analgesics are used sparingly to prevent respiratory depression. A tranquilizer may be necessary when a mechanical ventilator is first used to help the patient relax and "breathe with" the respirator.

A corticosteroid preparation (e.g., hydrocortisone) may be prescribed and given intravenously to some patients with the respiratory distress syndrome. It must be remembered that steroids may suppress the patient's immune responses, increasing the hazard of infection. The nurse is alert for possible symptoms of infection such as purulent secretions, elevation of temperature and increased chest rales.

Cardiac arrhythmias and reduced cardiac output are common complications encountered in respiratory failure, especially if the patient is receiving mechanical ventilation. Medications may include an antiarrhythmia drug such as procainamide (Pronestyl) or lidocaine (Xylocaine).

If infection is present, a broad-spectrum antimicrobial preparation is administered until the causative organism and its sensitivity are determined by culturing a specimen of the secretions.

COMFORT MEASURES. Frequent mouth care contributes to the patient's comfort, in addition to preventing ulcers and infection developing in the mouth. The inability to take fluids and food orally predisposes to the accumulation of secretions and the development of sordes. The presence of an endotracheal or nasogastric tube does not preclude mouth care; swabs and applicators can be used.

Since communication is difficult for the patient, the nurse assesses the situation for possible sources of discomfort. Simple nursing measures such as turning and/or repositioning the pillow, determining if the patient is too cold or too warm, and adjusting the covers, bathing, gentle massage, combing the hair and adjusting lights so they are not shining directly into the patient's eyes are important to his well-being and should not be overlooked because of the major complex therapeutic procedures.

PSYCHOLOGICAL CARE. The need for an appreciation of the fear and concern experienced by the patient with respiratory insufficiency is imperative, and is basic to providing the necessary empathy and support. The family wants information about the patient and should not be forgotten. It is supportive to both patient and family in an intensive care situation if a relative can visit the patient, if only very briefly. If it is possible shared care, even if only in a very small way, may reduce the family members' anxiety. Both patient and family are observed for unspoken cues as to their needs.

CONVALESCENCE. The patient has a prolonged convalescence and is followed closely in the event of permanent lung damage. The lungs may undergo degenerative changes due to pulmonary fibrosis, with a resulting decrease in compliance, vital capacity and alveolar-blood gas exchange. A program of breathing exercises and gradually increased physical exercises with assessment of tolerance is instituted before the patient is discharged. The patient is advised of the required visits for follow-up, or a referral to a visiting nurse organization may be made so that necessary home guidance and supervision are provided.

If the patient has residual chronic pulmonary insufficiency, it may not be possible for him to return to his former occupation. A rehabilitation program may be planned that will provide retraining for work within his respiratory capacity.

COMMON COLD

This is an upper respiratory tract infection that has a high incidence, especially during cold weather. Although considered to be a minor disorder and self-limiting, it is distressing and uncomfortable for the individual.

The infection of the nasal cavities and nasopharynx is caused by a variety of viruses. When the viral infection is established subsequent bacterial infection may develop.

SIGNS AND SYMPTOMS. The individual experiences some general malaise, dryness and soreness of the throat; the nose feels full and blocked, necessitating mouth breathing, and then develops a watery discharge. The secondary bacterial infection develops in 2 or 3 days and the nasal discharge becomes purulent. Persons with lowered resistance and those exposed to crowds are more susceptible.

There is no specific treatment; certain measures may lessen the individual's discomfort and minimize the course of the disorder. These include rest, increased fluid intake and humidification of the air.

Acetylsalicylic acid (aspirin) may be used to provide some relief of the discomfort.

If the infection persists, a physician should be consulted. Complications that may develop are otitis media (middle ear infection), sinusitis, bronchitis and pneumonia.

The nurse's role in relation to the common cold is mainly that of health teaching. Methods of promoting resistance include a well balanced diet, adequate rest, the avoidance of chilling and fatigue and the avoidance of contact with those having a respiratory infection. Persons with an infection are advised of their responsibility and how to prevent spreading the infection.

DISORDERS OF THE LARYNX

Disease of the larynx can present serious respiratory disturbance, since the glottis normally narrows the air passageway. Inflammation or edema of the tissues may make it difficult to get air through it. Children are particularly susceptible because their glottis and laryngeal space are much smaller.

Laryngitis

Inflammation of the mucous membrane of the larynx may be acute or chronic. The acute form is usually caused by infection but may occur by inhaling irritant gases. It is frequently associated with infection in the tract above (e.g., nasopharyngitis) or tracheitis. Chronic laryngitis may develop as a result of excessive smoking, chronic inhalation of irritants (dust, chemicals), overuse of the voice or repeated acute attacks. The mucous membrane is swollen and congested and the voice is hoarse or may be reduced to a whisper.

TREATMENT. Laryngitis is treated by general rest and voice rest, the inhalation of warm moist air and restricted smoking. If the cause is infection, a specific antimicrobial drug may be prescribed.

Obstruction of the Larynx

Edema, laryngeal spasm, or aspiration of a foreign body may cause obstruction in the larynx. Any constriction or obstruction in the larynx is manifested quickly by hoarseness, dyspnea, stridor (high-pitched crowing breath sound), cyanosis and increased but ineffective inspiratory effort, evidenced by the retraction of the intercostal spaces. Prompt emergency measures are necessary or death may ensue as a result of asphyxia.

Severe *edema* and swelling of the larynx may develop rapidly and close off the glottis, completely obstructing the airway. It may occur as a result of serious inflammation, as in diphtheria and scarlet fever, or be caused by an allergic response to a drug or foreign protein in hypersensitive individuals. Edema sometimes follows trauma that unavoidably may accompany examination by a laryngoscope or bronchoscope.

A *spasm* of the muscle tissue within the walls of the larynx may occur occasionally following some types of general anesthesia and may seriously restrict the air passage; or it may be seen rarely in persons with a low calcium blood level. The latter is usually accompanied by other skeletal muscle hyperirritability and spasm, and the condition is known as tetany.

A *foreign body* that is aspirated may lodge above the narrow opening of the glottis, interfering with movement of air in and out of the tract and with vibration of the vocal cords.

TREATMENT. If a foreign body is known to be the cause, the patient should be slapped vigorously between the scapulae, or someone standing behind the individual places his arms around the victim's trunk just below the diaphragm, clasping the hands in front. Pressure is applied with the arms and hands (Fig. 15–15). The compression (Heimlich hug) forces air under pressure through the airway and may dislodge the aspirated mass. If these procedures do not dislodge the object, a laryngoscope may be quickly introduced by the physician through which the offending object may be retrieved. If the patient's breathing is completely obstructed, an emergency cricothyroidotomy[17] or tracheostomy may have to be performed to establish an airway before the foreign body can be removed.

For *edema or spasm*, intubation may be performed in which a tube is passed beyond the obstruction into the trachea to establish an airway or the physician may do a tracheostomy (see p. 418). If edema of the larynx is due to an allergic response, the patient is given epinephrine (Adrenalin) 1:1000 subcutaneously. An adrenal corticosteroid preparation such as prednisone may be prescribed for a brief period to reduce tissue sensivity. Local applications of ice to the neck may also be suggested.

When laryngeal muscle spasm is the cause of the obstruction, intravenous calcium chloride or calcium gluconate may be prescribed.

Newgrowth

A *benign papilloma or polyp* may develop within the larynx, the most frequent source being the vocal cords. Hoarseness and coughing are generally the initial symptoms,

---

[17] *Cricothryoidotomy* is an incision through the cricoid and thyroid cartilages.

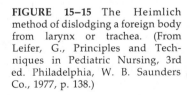

FIGURE 15–15 The Heimlich method of dislodging a foreign body from larynx or trachea. (From Leifer, G., Principles and Techniques in Pediatric Nursing, 3rd ed. Philadelphia, W. B. Saunders Co., 1977, p. 138.)

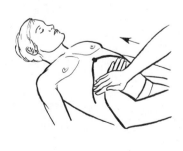

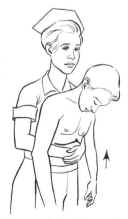

A

B

but gradually, as the tumor enlarges, breathing may become difficult. The tumor may be removed through the laryngoscope or by open surgery. Rarely is there any permanent voice impairment with this type of neoplasm.

The more serious newgrowth, *cancer*, has a higher incidence in males in the later years of life. Symptoms include hoarseness, dyspnea, cough, expectoration of blood, pain, enlargement of cervical lymph nodes and possibly dysphagia (difficulty in swallowing) as the mass encroaches on the esophagus.

Early recognition by laryngoscopy and biopsy is important. A few cases may be treated by radiation alone, but the majority of patients undergo surgical treatment. A partial laryngectomy may be done if the newgrowth appears localized. Some residual impairment of voice is likely, necessitating speech therapy following recovery from the surgery.

Many patients have a total laryngectomy, which means they will be left voiceless and with a permanent tracheostomy through which they will breathe. The tracheostomy tube used for this type of operation is shorter than the tube used when the opening is temporary to facilitate ventilation and suctioning (i.e., it does not extend as far into the trachea). The tube remains until the tissues have healed and the stoma is well established. Following recovery from surgery, the patient is helped to develop esophageal speech or to use an artificial larynx.

Nursing care of the patient who requires a total laryngectomy includes the following considerations.

PREOPERATIVE PREPARATION. The physician advises the patient and family of the need for the operation which will result in loss of the voice and a permanent opening for breathing. The nurse is prepared to answer the patient's and family's questions. They are reassured that provision will be made for the patient to communicate by writing if he wishes and that, as soon as he is well enough, instruction in esophageal speech will begin. It may be helpful to have someone who has had a laryngectomy and achieved free communication by esophageal speech visit the patient. Such an individual may be located through the local Cancer Society, or there may be an association (Lost Chord Club) of persons in the community who have had a laryngectomy. The patient and family

are advised that instruction will also be given as to the care of the tracheal stoma and that it can be concealed by a high collar or scarf.

POSTOPERATIVE CARE. The initial care is similar to that cited in the section on tracheostomy, pp. 420–423.

When the patient regains consciousness following surgery, and the pulse and blood pressure are stable, the head and shoulders are elevated to facilitate breathing and reduce the development of edema in the wound area.

The patient is observed closely for breathing difficulty, cyanosis and hemorrhage. The tissues in the resection area may be drained by tubes attached to low suction (Hemovac).

NUTRITION AND FLUIDS. A nasogastric tube may be inserted through which the patient is fed at regular intervals for a few days. This avoids possible contamination of the wound. Fluids are given intravenously.

When the nasogastric tube is removed, the patient is given sips of fluid to test the swallowing reflex. If he can swallow without difficulty, fluids and soft foods are gradually increased and, if progress is satisfactory, a normal diet is resumed.

INSTRUCTION AND REHABILITATION. The patient is instructed about the removal of secretions and the care of the stoma and tube. This is done as soon as he is well enough to undertake the care in the hospital and to develop confidence. A member of the family also is taught the necessary care and precautions. Suctioning, removal and cleansing of the *inner* laryngectomy tube, cleansing of the stoma and surrounding skin, the checking and protection of the tapes which secure the outer tube and the application of a dressing, if one is used, are components of the teaching program. The importance of an adequate fluid intake to liquefy respiratory tract secretions is explained. The discussion about wearing a scarf or high loose collar to conceal the stoma emphasizes the use of smooth, lightweight material that must be free of lint and loose threads to avoid foreign particles being drawn in on inhalation. It is also pointed out that a cover reduces the possible entry of airborne dust or other particles into the respiratory tract.

A patient may continue to have excessive secretions and may require suction equipment at home. In this case, a family member or the patient is advised where such equip-

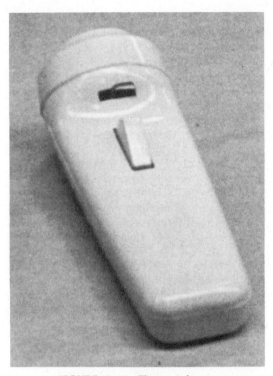

FIGURE 15–16   Electronic larynx.

the production of speech by this means is difficult and requires much patience, persistence and practice on the patient's part. He experiences periods of frustration and despair, and requires the support and encouragement of the nurse, family and physician as well as the therapist.

If the patient is unable to learn esophageal speech, the use of an artificial larynx may be introduced. This is an electronic, battery-operated instrument with a vibrating surface which the individual holds against the neck (Fig. 15–16). Vibrations are transmitted into the pharynx and mouth, where they are used to form words. The volume can be controlled by adjusting the "larynx."

The loss of voice and the permanent tracheal stoma will probably have a serious effect on the individual's socioeconomic situation. He may not be able to return to his former occupation and will require financial assistance. Retraining for another vocation may be undertaken if the patient makes satisfactory progress. A referral may be made by the nurse to a social worker or a rehabilitation officer.

ment may be obtained (e.g., the Cancer Society or the Red Cross) and is instructed in the use and care of the equipment.

An explanation is made of the danger of aspirating water through the laryngectomy tube or tracheal stoma. This precludes swimming or immersion in water to a high level. Precautions are also necessary when taking a shower; shields are available that may be used and the spray of water is directed below the neck.

The patient is advised to return to the clinic or physician at regular intervals, as directed, for the changing of the outer tube, examination of the stoma and assessment of his general physical and psychological condition. Eventually, when the stoma is firmly healed and the opening remains patent, the physician may permit the patient or a family member to change the outer cannula. In many instances patency of the stoma allows the tube to be removed permanently.

Speech therapy is commenced as soon as possible. The teaching of esophageal speech is carried out in a clinic by a speech therapist. The patient learns to swallow air and then regurgitate it, using the current of air to produce sounds and form words. Achieving

DISORDERS OF THE TRACHEA

Tracheitis

Inflammation of the trachea rarely occurs independently of laryngitis or bronchitis. Because of the size of the lumen of the trachea and its noncollapsible structure, it rarely causes any serious interference with breathing but does cause considerable discomfort and a burning, raw retrosternal pain. The discomfort may be reduced by the inhalation of warm moist air.

Compression of the Trachea

Pressure from an aortic aneurysm or new growth of neighboring structures (e.g., esophagus, lymph nodes of the mediastinum) may narrow the tracheal lumen and offer resistance to the passage of air through the trachea. Treatment is directed toward the primary disease.

ACUTE BRONCHITIS

This is an inflammation of the bronchial tubes and is frequently a sequela of an upper respiratory tract infection or influenza. The trachea is generally involved first and then the infection extends into the bronchial tubes.

SIGNS AND SYMPTOMS. The illness varies greatly from a mild indisposition, lasting 2 to 3 days, to severe symptoms and eventual pneumonia. At the onset, the patient may complain of substernal tightness and discomfort and may experience an unproductive, irritating cough. In a day or two, the cough becomes less distressing and the secretions more profuse and mucopurulent with flecks or streaks of blood. Fever, general malaise and wheezing respirations accompany the disorder. Dyspnea is common and is due to bronchospasm that develops as a reflex response to the irritation. In some instances bronchial constriction may be severe enough to result in hypoventilation and hypoxemia.

TREATMENT AND NURSING CARE

REST. The patient is confined to bed in a room in which the temperature is kept relatively constant and the air humidified. If the patient smokes, the need to refrain from it is emphasized.

COUGHING AND POSITIONING. When the cough becomes productive, the patient is encouraged to cough at regular intervals. His position is changed frequently to promote movement of secretions from distal portions of the bronchial tree to a level from which they may be more readily raised by coughing.

MEDICATIONS. An antimicrobial drug may be prescribed to shorten the course of the disease and prevent its extension to the bronchioles and alveoli. A sputum specimen may be required for identifying the causative organism and for determining antibiotic sensitivity. An expectorant such as an ammonium chloride or glycerol guiacolate preparation may be ordered. If signs of bronchospasm are present, the patient is given a bronchodilator which may be inhaled in aerosol form. Examples are isoproterenol (Isuprel), salbutamol (Ventolin), and beclomethasone (Beclovent), a corticosteroid preparation. Acetylsalicylic acid (aspirin) may be given to keep the patient more comfortable and help reduce the fever.

FLUIDS AND NUTRITION. An increased fluid intake up to 3000 to 4000 ml. daily (unless contraindicated by cardiac or renal failure) is recommended to promote liquefaction of the bronchial secretions. A soft or light nutritious diet is encouraged to maintain the patient's resistance.

CONVALESCENCE. Bronchitis can be debilitating and, although it may clear up in 7 to 10 days, the patient may find the need to resume his former activities gradually and to take extra rest. Older persons who develop the disorder recover more slowly and are more predisposed to the disease extending to bronchial pneumonia. They may not have sufficient muscular strength to cough up the secretions and, if these are retained, they predispose to complications. A longer period of convalence with plenty of rest, nutritious foods and the prevention of chilling is necessary for these elderly persons.

Chronic Obstructive Pulmonary Diseases (COPD)

Chronic bronchitis, emphysema and asthma make up a group of chronic respiratory disorders that are designated as *chronic obstructive pulmonary disease* (COPD), *chronic obstructive lung disease* (COLD) or *chronic airway obstruction*. These have varying pathologic features and each may present as a distinct disease entity, but all have the common characteristic of some narrowing of the airway that results in obstruction to the flow of air in and out of the lung. The work of breathing is markedly increased, there is increased resistance to air entry, resulting in impaired ventilation, and air is trapped in the bronchioles and alveoli, preventing normal gas exchange between the blood in the capillaries and pulmonary air as well as causing overdistention of alveoli.

Each of the chronic obstructive pulmonary diseases may occur alone or with one or both of the others. Patients are seen with COPD in varying degrees of severity. The disorder may be relatively mild, static and reversible in some; in others, the disease may be persistently progressive to severe, incapacitating respiratory insufficiency.

Chronic Bronchitis

This disease is characterized by hyperactivity of the mucus-secreting glands of the bronchial mucosa in response to prolonged or frequently recurring irritation, a chronic productive cough and recurrent infection.

The bronchial mucosa undergoes a chronic inflammatory process along with hypertrophy and an increase in the number of mucus-secreting glands. The mucus predisposes to infection. Destruction of the normal epithelial lining and the cilia occurs. The mucosa becomes edematous, thickened and scarred, leading to distortion and narrowing of the lumina of the air passages. The excessive mucus is retained, blocking bronchioles and reducing ventilation further. Some bronchospasm may be present. The obstruction to the flow of air is greater during expiration, resulting in air being trapped in the bronchioles and alveoli. Eventually the air sacs become permanently overdistended and may rupture. Pulmonary circulation may be affected; the underventilated areas produce a deficiency of oxygen that may initiate a vasoconstrictive response in the local pulmonary vessels. If this persists, the individual is likely to develop pulmonary hypertension, resulting in resistance to the output of the right side of the heart into the pulmonary artery. The patient may develop right-sided heart failure.

The disease has an insidious onset and, unless reversed, the disease process is gradually progressive. Ventilation is impaired by progressive airway obstruction, the work of breathing is increased and hypoxemia and hypercapnia develop.

ETIOLOGIC FACTORS. Prolonged inhalation of various irritants is the principal causative factor of chronic bronchitis. The common irritants are tobacco smoke, infection, and atmospheric pollutants such as dust, industrial fumes and smoke; the most frequent offender is tobacco smoke. A higher incidence is seen in older persons and in persons of poor socioeconomic circumstances. Dampness and winter cold are considered to be aggravating factors. Heredity is also thought to be a factor, since there is some evidence that members of the same family may show a predisposition to develop the disease.

MANIFESTATIONS. The respirations are continually wheezy, the patient becomes progressively more dyspneic and short of breath on exertion, and the increasing respiratory insufficiency leads to restricted physical activity. A persistent, hard, productive cough is troublesome. The sputum is tenacious, mucoid and copious. The cough is more troublesome first thing in the morning due to the accumulation of secretions during the night. Symptoms of hypoxia and hypercapnia appear along with the reduction in alveolar ventilation and diffusion.

Laboratory reports show that the $paCO_2$ is above normal, the paO_2 is below normal and the hematocrit may be above normal. The latter is a compensatory response to the hypoxia.

Pulmonary function tests indicate a reduction in the forced expiratory volume in 1 second (FEV_1), tidal volume, forced vital capacity (FVC), and forced expiratory flow rate (FEF). The residual volume is increased.

Auscultation of the chest reveals inspiratory and expiratory rhonchi.

TREATMENT AND CARE. In the initial stage of chronic bronchitis, care is directed toward avoidance of provoking irritants and the prevention of respiratory infection and further bronchial and bronchiolar deterioration.

AVOIDANCE OF PROVOKING IRRITANTS. Since chronic bronchitis is most often associated with cigarette smoking, the individual is urged and given support to give up the habit. A history of his environment and occupation is obtained and, if air pollution or industrial air contamination is considered to be a factor, the person may be advised to move or change his occupation. Since the latter involves his socioeconomic situation, it may not be easy for him to move or change his job; a consultation with the employer or rehabilitation officer may provide some solution.

PREVENTION OF INFECTION. The patient is advised to avoid contact with persons with respiratory infection and influenza at home and in public. The importance of reporting promptly to his physician or the chest clinic at the onset of a respiratory infection is emphasized. A broad-spectrum antimicrobial drug (e.g., tetracycline) is usually prescribed. If the infection is not treated it may progress to bronchopneumonia, further tissue damage and serious ventilatory impairment.

If the patient experiences chronic brochospasm with his disease, a bronchodilator (e.g., isoproterenol, salbutamol) may be prescribed to improve ventilation, prevent the trapping of air and facilitate the removal of secretions.

The patient is instructed about coughing.

The purpose of the cough is explained as is the importance of not suppressing it. Measures to make it effective are discussed (see p. 412). If the cough is troublesome during the night, warm, humidified room air may provide relief.

GENERAL HEALTH MEASURES. It is important that the person with chronic bronchitis have a nutritious diet to improve general health and resistance to infection. Obesity should be avoided, as this increases the work of breathing and the demand on the heart.

Regular physical activity that does not cause fatigue and dyspnea is encouraged to promote adequate ventilation and physical tolerance.

MORE SEVERE CHRONIC BRONCHITIS. The treatment and care of the patient with progressive, irreversible chronic bronchitis is similar to that for the patient with chronic obstructive pulmonary disease.

Pulmonary Emphysema

Pulmonary emphysema[18] is a chronic obstructive airway disease in which the alveoli are overdistended by entrapped air, leading to increased lung capacity, loss of elasticity of the lungs and destruction of intra-alveolar septal tissue. Several alveoli coalesce into one larger space. The distention of alveoli compresses capillaries, resulting in an imbalance in ventilation and perfusion and reducing essential gas exchange.

The onset is insidious but, once initiated, is progressive and nonreversible. The lung damage cannot be repaired but the patient can be helped to breathe more effectively and live with less disability. Both emphysema and chronic bronchitis frequently are present in the same patient. There is usually a long history of chronic bronchitis in which the blocking of the small terminal bronchioles with mucoid secretions leads to the entrapping of air in the alveoli and the eventual emphysema. Rarely, emphysema is primary. Heredity is suspected as having a role in some cases, since a deficiency of an enzyme (an antitrypsin) is present in some persons with emphysema.

---

[18] *Emphysema* is the Greek word meaning inflation. In medicine, it implies a swelling or distention due to an accumulation of air. It may occur in any tissue. Pulmonary emphysema indicates overdistention of air sacs in the lungs.

The disorder leads to serious disability. The incidence is higher in middle-aged and older males. Older persons are more susceptible because of the loss of natural elasticity. In recent years there has been a sharp increase in the number of persons with emphysema, and the disease accounts for a large number of deaths annually. The increase in incidence may be attributed to the number of heavy cigarette smokers in the last three or four decades, the increase in air pollution and the survival of more patients with chronic bronchitis.

SIGNS AND SYMPTOMS. The presenting manifestations vary with the extent of alveolar damage and severity of airway obstruction. Severe dyspnea is experienced, especially on exertion, and more and more energy is used in breathing. The individual may or may not have a troublesome cough; if there has been a long period of chronic bronchitis, the cough mechanism may be inefficient. The respirations are continually wheezy and the expiratory phase is notably prolonged. The patient purses his lips in an effort to increase pressure within his air passages to oppose their tendency to narrowing and collapse of bronchioles.

The chest contour changes over a period of time; it enlarges and takes on a barrel-like shape. The chest wall and diaphragm assume a relatively fixed position, with little or no movement during respirations. The use of accessory respiratory muscles is observed in the neck and shoulder girdle (sternocleidomastoid, scaleni, pectorals).

Clubbing of the fingers may be present due to the prolonged hypoxia. A bulbous enlargement develops in the distal portion of the fingers and longitudinal ridges may appear on the nails.

Laboratory reports indicate that the paO_2 and the pH are below normal and the $paCO_2$ is elevated. Respiratory acidosis develops, and an electrolyte imbalance is reflected in an increase above normal in the serum bicarbonate (HCO_3^-) and sodium (Na^+), and a decrease below normal in serum chloride (Cl^-). This imbalance is a compensatory response to the lower alkalinity resulting from the retention of CO_2 and the excess carbonic acid, H_2CO_3.

The patient's color may be normal or even flushed in comparison to the cyanosis of the patient with severe chronic bronchitis. The emphysema patient's arteries dilate in reaction to the hypercapnia.

Pulmonary function tests produce similar results as those cited under chronic bronchitis (p. 439), except that the total lung capacity generally shows a marked increase due to the loss of elastic recoil in the lungs and the distended alveoli.

The patient's pulse is weak during inspiration owing to the abnormal change in intrathoracic pressure. This is referred to as *pulsus paradoxus*. Pulmonary hypertension develops and leads to right ventricular failure. This is also aggravated by polycythemia that occurs in response to the hypoxia; the increased blood viscosity increases the work of the heart. Venous congestion develops and jugular congestion and pulsation may be observed.

Chronic obstructive lung disease has psychological as well as serious socioeconomic effects. During episodes of severe dyspnea, the patient fears suffocation. He becomes exhausted and discouraged because of the continuous conscious effort he must make to breathe, and the enforced inactivity and unemployment with resulting dependency and feeling of uselessness lead to loss of self-esteem and despondency. The individual withdraws and may become quite depressed.

The *treatment and nursing care* of the patient with emphysema are discussed later in the section on treatment and care in chronic obstructive pulmonary disease.

Asthma

Asthma is a bronchial disorder characterized by episodic narrowing of the airways and increased viscid mucus secretion. The disorder is attributed to hyperreactivity of the tracheobronchial tree to various stimuli and antigens. The narrowing of the lumina of the airways is generalized and usually reversible; it may be relieved spontaneously or by therapeutic measures.

The reaction of the overresponsive airway to stimuli is edema and thickening of the mucosa, hypersecretion by the mucous glands and contraction of bronchial and bronchiolar muscle tissue. The tissue changes are initiated by the release of endogenous chemical mediators (e.g., histamine) in response to the stimulus.

Stimuli which may precipitate the asthmatic response include allergens (see p. 53), infection, irritating inhalants (chemicals, air pollutants), cold air, acetylsalicyclic acid (aspirin), emotional stress, physical exercise, and laughing. Frequently, there is usually a personal and/or family history of one or more allergies.

Asthma may be classified as extrinsic or intrinsic. *Extrinsic asthma* develops as a result of an allergen-antibody reaction. The antibodies involved in asthma "belong to a distinct class of immunoglobulins known as IgE."[19] Increased amounts of this particular type of antibody are present in those with extrinsic or allergic asthma (atopic asthma[20]). Heredity is considered to be a factor in this type of asthma.

Intrinsic asthma is due to endogenous chemicals released directly in response to various stimuli (nonimmunologic; no antibodies are involved). These stimuli include infection, cold air, irritating inhalants, exercise, laughing and emotional stress.

MANIFESTATIONS. It is important to obtain a personal and family health history and a detailed account of the patient's condition, activities and situation at the onset of the episode. This may provide information as to the cause and influence the success of the therapeutic program.

Asthma usually has a sudden onset, with the patient experiencing a sense of suffocation, tightness in the chest, wheezing and expiratory dyspnea. Inspiration is short but expiration is a prolonged, conscious effort, using accessory muscles. The patient appears distraught, assumes an upright sitting position, has a frequent hard cough and raises a thick, viscous mucus with difficulty. Microscopic examination of the sputum reveals numerous eosinophils and gelatinous casts of the smaller bronchial tubes (Laennec's pearls). In infective asthma, the sputum will be mucopurulent. A differential leukocyte count usually reveals a marked increase in the eosinophils in allergic (extrinsic) asthma. The attacks are episodic and may end abruptly.

---

[19] Reuben M. Cherniack, et al.: Respiration in Health and Disease, 2nd ed. Philadelphia, W. B. Saunders, 1972, p. 330.

[20] *Atopic* implies a hypersensitive state attributed to hereditary factors.

Auscultation of the chest reveals rhonchi unless the airway is severely obstructed. Overinflation of the lungs due to trapping of air may make it difficult to hear breath sounds and produces a hyperresonant sound on percussion.

Pulmonary function tests show a decrease in the forced expiratory volume of 1 second (FEV_1) and maximal breathing capacity; the vital capacity is reduced.

Assessment of the arterial blood gases may indicate hypoxia, depending upon the severity and duration of the episode. In prolonged asthma and severe bronchial constriction hypercapnia will also be present. In severe and prolonged asthma the patient becomes cyanosed, and the developing respiratory insufficiency and hypoxemia may threaten his life. When severe asthma becomes prolonged and intractable, it is classified as *status asthmaticus*.

Treatment and care are discussed under the treatment and care of the patient with chronic obstructive pulmonary disease that follows.

Nursing in Chronic Obstructive Pulmonary Diseases (COPD)

The severity of chronic respiratory insufficiency varies considerably among patients. It may range from a cough, shortness of breath with some physical activities, and reversible impairment to progressive, irreversible, pulmonary dysfunction and total incapacity. Therapy and care of the patient with COPD are directed toward preserving existing lung function and preventing further irreversible tissue damage. Consideration is given to the prevention of acute exacerbations, improving the patient's ventilation, having him adapt his activities to his respiratory tolerance and, at the same time, providing as great a degree of independence, usefulness and satisfaction as possible.

Nurses have an important *preventive role* in relation to these serious incapacitating pulmonary diseases. Persons are advised of causative factors and made aware of possible respiratory irritants (e.g., household and cosmetic aerosol preparations). Because smoking is the causative factor of these diseases in a very large number of patients, nurses should discourage smoking and help those individuals who have developed the habit to give it up before irreparable damage

to their airways occurs. In relation to the nurse's preventive role, Lagerson says: "The time spent weaning a person from his cigarettes is a far better investment than the time spent 30 years later trying to wean him from a ventilator in an intensive care unit."[21] Recognizing early symptoms in individuals and urging them to seek prompt medical care are important preventive measures.

Planning care for the patient with a chronic obstructive lung disease includes the following considerations.

ASSESSMENT. A detailed history is taken of the patient's past illnesses, sociological and economic situation, life style, whether he smokes or not, and if so how much, and his family's health history.[22]

The type of pulmonary disease is determined and an assessment made of its severity. The investigation includes pulmonary function tests, chest x-ray, cardiac function evaluation, and determinations of blood gases, pH, hemoglobin and erythrocytes. Studies may be made of ventilatory function and blood gases at rest, and during and after physical exercise to establish the individual's activity tolerance. Walking, action on the treadmill and the climbing of stairs may be used in activity evaluation, but the nurse also notes the effect of personal care activities (activities of daily living) on the patient.

Assessment continues at regular frequent intervals after the diagnosis and therapeutic regimen are established to determine the effectiveness of treatment as well as the state of the disease process.

EXPLANATION. An explanation of the nature of the illness and the necessary treatment and care is made to the patient and the family. They are more likely to cooperate in implementing the prescribed therapeutic care plan if they understand the implications and that certain measures and adaptations will contribute to improvement and control of the disease and prevent exacerbations. It is usually necessary to precede the discussion of the disorder with a brief review of the

---

[21] Joanne Lagerson: "Nursing Care of Patients with Chronic Pulmonary Insufficiency." Nurs. Clin. North Am., Vol. 9, No. 1 (March 1974), p. 167.

[22] Hereditary factors are thought to have a role in the development of COPD in some persons. For example, an inherited deficiency of a particular enzyme (an antitrypsin) has been recognized as a factor in the development of emphysema in *some* patients.

normal breathing structures and mechanism.

Simple, written descriptive material may be appropriate. Useful pamphlets are available from the National Tuberculosis and Respiratory Disease Association.

PSYCHOLOGICAL SUPPORT. The psychological impact is great when the patient is told he has a chronic respiratory disorder and the implications. The long, progressively disabling disorder may mean loss of work, income, independence and socialization. In the case of a male patient, it may result in a reversal of family roles, with the wife becoming the sole source of income. The patient develops feelings of worthlessness, becomes depressed, withdraws and is reluctant to cooperate in therapeutic measures. He tends to become anxious, which aggravates his dyspnea.

The nurse conveys a willingness to listen, encouraging the individual to verbalize his fears and concerns. He is advised that he will be carefully assessed and, although it may be necessary for him to change his occupation and some forms of activity, those activities within his respiratory tolerance will be indicated. The patient is told that he will be taught to improve his breathing and that other measures will be used so that he may obtain more air and oxygen. These are expected to increase his ability to do more than he is capable of at that time. The nurse guards against fostering feelings of hopelessness and dependence; a positive attitude that manifests expected improvement should be developed. Emphasis is placed on what he may do; unless hope is conveyed, the patient will make little effort to follow the prescribed program. He should be involved in his own care and should be aware of the plans for maximum rehabilitation. Expressions which indicate that his disease is reversible or curable are avoided, since most of the patients currently seen have irreparable respiratory impairment.

Detailed information about the individual's former practices will often reveal a problem for which a solution may then be found. For example, if the nurse learns that the person must walk a considerable distance from his residence to obtain transportation to work or to a shopping area, the suggestion may be made that he should move to eliminate this. It might be suggested that he leave earlier and walk at a slow pace or, with the help of a social worker or the family, an arrangement may be made for a ride to make it possible for him to continue in his job.

IMPROVING VENTILATION AND GAS EXCHANGE. Several measures are used to relieve the patient's dyspnea and improve his ventilation and gas exchange.

CHANGE IN BREATHING PATTERN. The COPD patient usually adopts an abnormal pattern of breathing as the disease develops, characterized by dyspnea, wheezing, use of thoracic and neck accessory respiratory muscles (sternocleidomastoid and scalene) in inspiration, and evident active effort in expiration. He is advised of the need for correcting his faulty breathing in order to lessen his dyspnea, improve his ventilation and increase the exchange of oxygen and carbon dioxide between his lungs and blood.

Instruction is to breathe quietly and unhurriedly and to use the diaphragm and abdominal muscles effectively. The procedure involves the following. First, the patient is placed in the supine position with head and shoulders elevated. Sufficient support is provided if necessary to insure relaxation. The shoulders are down, the arms are at the sides and the knees are flexed so that the abdominal muscles are relaxed to reduce resistance to the descent of the contracting diaphragm. The patient is instructed to inhale slowly through his nose, allowing ballooning out of his abdomen. It may be helpful if he places a hand on his upper abdomen so he becomes aware of outward abdominal movement. He may have to make a conscious effort to refrain from using upper chest and neck muscles and concentrate on inspiration involving the abdomen and diaphragm.

The patient is instructed to exhale through loosely pursed lips and to continue breathing out after he has reached his passive expiratory level by contracting the abdominal muscles. The pursed lips increase the resistance to air flow, reducing the collapse of small airways and the trapping of air. The cycle is repeated for 5 to 10 minutes and, when he begins to master this breathing pattern, the patient is urged to exhale more completely and faster. If the pulmonary· function tests indicate that the patient's expiratory volume is below normal, the physician may suggest that he be instructed to extend exhalation time to three times that of inspiration (e.g., inspiration, a count of 2 and expiration, a count of 6). This breathing technique is usually learned first in the supine position, and then in the sitting and standing positions. When the patient demonstrates sufficient control, he then undertakes coordination of this pattern of breathing with walking and other activities. The diaphragmatic-abdominal breathing practice is carried out for 5- to 10-minute periods at the beginning and gradually extended to longer periods. The "exercise" is repeated four or five times daily. The nurse observes the patient closely at first; the period is terminated if fatigue and/or frustration are manifested.

MOBILIZATION AND REMOVAL OF SECRETIONS. It is important that the COPD patient's air passages be cleared of the secretions that tend to accumulate. Retained secretions occupy intrapulmonary space, reducing the ventilatory capacity and gas exchange, increase the resistance to air flow in the tracheobronchial tree and predispose the patient to pulmonary infection which causes further tissue damage. Removal of secretions permits ventilation of atelectatic areas.

The patient may require instruction as to how to cough effectively. He is encouraged to cough at regular intervals in the sitting position and to bend the head and trunk forward if possible while exhaling and actually coughing. If the patient becomes red in the face or distention of the neck veins is noted (due to collapse of small airways and resulting increased intrathoracic pressure), the patient is advised to take a series of short, slow coughs with his mouth open. A pillow may be pressed in against the abdomen to help elevate the diaphragm. The amount of sputum raised is noted, as are the color and consistency. (See p. 396 for further details regarding cough.)

Humidification of the room air, especially during cold weather, and a fluid intake of 2500 to 3000 ml. daily (unless contraindicated by heart failure and retention of fluid) are important to keep the pulmonary secretions liquefied. The patient is helped to establish a regular routine or time for taking fluids to insure an adequate intake. The physician may suggest that saline 2 to 5 per cent in a nebulizer be used to moisten the mucosa and liquefy secretions. An expectorant preparation may occasionally be prescribed for oral administration to promote liquefaction and removal of secretions (see section on medications, below).

Postural drainage may be necessary to move secretions by gravity from the small airways in the different lung segments to major bronchial tubes, from which they may be eliminated by coughing or suctioning (see p. 414). Postural drainage is usually only a part of a physical therapy program. Before assuming the initial posture, the patient is required to breathe deeply several times (deep, diaphragmatic breathing promotes movement of secretions along tubes) or he may receive intermittent positive pressure by means of a respirator to ensure "open airways." The inhalation of a nebulized bronchodilator may also precede postural drainage. The patient remains in each posture for 5 to 15 minutes, and percussion and vibration are applied during this period to dislodge secretions.

Postural drainage is generally used two to four times daily, depending upon the amount of secretions, and is not done within 1½ to 2 hours following a meal. It is contraindicated if the patient's vital signs are unstable or if the patient is very weak.

The retention of secretions by the COPD patient is frequently due to bronchospasm. The relief of airway obstruction caused by bronchospasm is an important measure in promoting the removal of secretions. A bronchodilating preparation is prescribed (see below).

AVOIDANCE OF RESPIRATORY IRRITANTS. The person with asthma, chronic bronchitis or emphysema should not smoke. Convincing him of the importance of this and providing necessary assistance in breaking the habit may present quite a challenge to the nurse. The patient and family are advised of the hazards of cigarette smoking and that if discontinued, the infection, cough and secretions will be less troublesome. Pamphlets and booklets published by the Tuberculosis and Respiratory Disease Association that discuss the harmful effects of smoking may be made available. The nurse tries to be persuasive and supportive without being judgmental, and praises the patient for his success in restraint.

Bronchial irritation may be reduced by avoiding the inhalation of smoke, chemical fumes and dust. This may necessitate a change of occupation and/or moving. Very cold air frequently precipitates bronchospasm, coughing and dyspnea in the person with a chronic respiratory disorder. If he must go out when the temperature is low, a scarf worn over the nose and mouth may reduce distress.

MEDICATIONS. The drugs prescribed most often for COPD patients are bronchodilators, expectorants and antibiotics. Drugs which relieve bronchospasm and reduce mucosal edema may be administered by inhalation for local effect or they may be given via the conventional routes.

BRONCHODILATORS. Examples of those commonly used are:

Salbutamol (Ventolin). This drug is available in nebulized form in a small cartridge-type dispenser for inhalation. The valve is metered to deliver a specific amount of the drug each time it is released by pressure. The dosage usually prescribed is two puffs three or four times daily. The inhalation is not repeated within 3 to 4 hours of the last dose.

Ventolin may also be administered orally. If given by this route the patient may experience palpitation and muscle tremor.

Isoproterenol (Isuprel). This is usually inhaled in aerosol or nebulized form. It may be given in conjunction with intermittent positive-pressure breathing (IPPB) and air, or a prescribed percentage of oxygen may be given to transport the drug. The patient is observed for side effects, which may be flushing of the face, rapid pulse and/or palpitation.

Aminophylline. This is an effective bronchodilator that may be administered orally or intravenously, or by rectal suppository. It is used less frequently since salbutamol and beclomethasone became available because it may cause headache, cardiac arrythmia or palpitation. Bladder irritation or nausea may develop following its intravenous or oral administration.

Epinephrine (Adrenalin). This drug is usually given subcutaneously but a preparation is also available for inhalation. It is a powerful and quick-acting bronchodilator, but its adverse cardiac side effects limit its use. If it is given the patient is observed closely for a rapid, irregular, weak pulse. Tremors, anxiety and restlessness are commonly manifested.

CORTICOSTEROIDS. A corticoid preparation may be prescribed in conjunction with another bronchodilator to enhance the effect of the latter and to reduce bronchial reactivity. It may be administered intravenously or orally if the patient has severe respiratory insufficiency, but is gradually tapered off and terminated as the condition improves. The preparation beclomethasone dipropionate (Beclovent) for inhalation is available in nebulized form in a small pressurized dispenser. Applied locally, it reduces the bronchial response of spasm without producing the side effects characteristic of long-term general administration of corticosteroids.

EXPECTORANTS. An expectorant such as a solution of ammonium chloride or potassium iodide may be prescribed to assist in liquefaction of the pulmonary secretions.

ANTIBIOTICS. A broad-spectrum antibiotic (e.g., tetracycline) is given when the earliest signs of infection appear. These may be purulent sputum, general malaise, fever and increased shortness of breath. A sputum specimen may first be collected so that the organism may be identified and sensitivity tests made in order for a specific antimicrobial drug to be prescribed and administered.

Rarely, an antibiotic is administered by aerosol. If the infection is unresponsive to antibiotics that may be given safely by the oral or parenteral routes, or the required antimicrobial drug is toxic, the administration may be by inhalation.

OTHER DRUGS. Sedatives, analgesics and tranquilizers are generally contraindicated in the patient with chronic respiratory insufficiency. These drugs depress respirations and suppress the cough reflex, predisposing the individual to hypoxia, retention of carbon dioxide and infection.

PREVENTION OF INFECTION. The most effective measure in the prevention of pulmonary infection in the patient with chronic pulmonary insufficiency is to keep the tract as free of secretions as possible. Pooling of secretions serves as an excellent medium for organisms; an acute infection may seriously impair ventilation and gas exchange and precipitate respiratory failure. The patient may receive an antimicrobial drug as a preventive measure throughout the autumn and winter months. The avoidance of close contact with those who have infection is stressed. Family members should be made aware of their responsibility to avoid transmission of infection to the patient. General debilitation and loss of weight are commonly associated with the disease. A well balanced, nutritious diet, high in vitamin C, and plenty of rest help to maintain the patient's resistance.

The patient is advised that if the sputum increases in volume or becomes purulent, or if he has a fever, general malaise or increased shortness of breath, he should seek prompt medical treatment. He may be given an antibiotic to keep on hand so that treatment can be initiated with the earliest symptoms of a respiratory infection.

INTERMITTENT POSITIVE-PRESSURE BREATHING THERAPY. IPPB may be used in chronic obstructive disease to: (1) improve air distribution throughout the airways; (2) ventilate small tubes and alveoli that are collapsed; (3) deliver nebulized or aerosol medication (the preparation reaches areas that are not medicated without the increased pressure); and (4) mobilize secretions. Some emphysema patients do not receive IPPB, since it may cause further distention of alveoli and produce the added risk of rupture of alveoli and pneumothorax.

The treatment and the reasons for it are explained to the patient. He is advised to concentrate on breathing through his mouth; at first, he may need a clip on his nose. As he inhales, he triggers the respirator and then becomes passive, allowing the machine to take over. When the preset pressure is achieved, the respirator shuts off and exhalation is passive. The patient is urged to breathe slowly; the tendency is to increase the respiratory rate. The patient's pulse and color are checked during and following treatment. The IPPB treatment is discontinued if tachycardia, arrhythmia or pallor develops.[23]

The treatment is administered daily over a period of 10 to 15 minutes. At intervals during the treatment and following it the patient is encouraged to cough and clear out the mobilized secretions. The inhalation gas may be air or a prescribed combination of oxygen and air.

OXYGEN THERAPY. The patient with COPD may develop severe hypoxia as a result of the mismatching of ventilation and perfusion (uneven distribution of inhaled air and the blood flow in the pulmonary capillaries). Some patients, especially those with emphysema, constantly have a relatively high $paCO_2$. Carbon dioxide is normally a stimulant to the respiratory center but, in the case of chronic hypercarbia, the center adapts and

is less responsive to the higher level. As a result hypoxia becomes the principal respiratory drive. The administration of a high concentration of oxygen may depress respirations and cause the retention of dangerously high amounts of carbon dioxide.

Arterial blood gas and oxygen saturation determinations may reveal that the patient has hypoxemia severe enough to cause tissue hypoxia and impaired functioning, manifested by restlessness, weakness, confusion and cardiac arrhythmias. Oxygen is administered by mask (Venturi type) in a *controlled low concentration* of 25 to 28 per cent or by nasal prongs with an oxygen flow rate of 2 liters per minute. Arterial blood gases and oxygen saturation determinations are made frequently; an increase in the carbon dioxide level is reported promptly because of the risk of carbon dioxide narcosis.

Oxygen therapy may have to be continued after the patient leaves the hospital. He and his family are advised of the necessary equipment and source of supply. Specific instructions about the oxygen administration and the necessary precautions must be clearly given verbally and in writing (see p. 408). Supervision by frequent visits from a visiting nurse or inhalation technician is important, especially during the first 2 or 3 weeks. Portable, light-weight oxygen equipment is now available which permits greater freedom of movement and more varied activities for the patient with chronic respiratory insufficiency.

GENERAL CARE MEASURES. General care, as with all patients, must be adapted to the individual as a person (his personality, life style, occupation, etc.), the severity of his pulmonary disease and associated disorder(s) and his reaction to his problems and treatment. Planning and implementing care includes consideration of the following factors.

REST AND ACTIVITY. Prolonged bed rest is discouraged, since it favors hypoventilation, depression of the cough reflex, retention of secretions and muscle wasting. Physical exercise and activity commensurate with the cardiopulmonary status are promoted as the patient achieves an improved pattern of breathing. Activity improves the appetite, helps to relieve tension and promote normal sleep, and increases muscular strength and ventilatory capacity. The patient is fearful of becoming breathless when first introduced to

---

[23]The increased intrapulmonic pressure associated with IPPB raises intrathoracic pressure, compressing the thoracic blood vessels which reduces the volume of blood entering the heart.

an exercise program. Brief periods on the treadmill and/or a stationary bicycle in the respiratory therapy unit and a graduated activity program gradually provide the necessary reassurance.

The patient's usual total daily activities are reviewed; some may be simplified to reduce energy demands, while others may have to be eliminated. Shorter work hours and more rest may be necessary. An effective physical therapy program, breathing exercises, and improvement of his general condition may increase tolerance and eventually permit resumption of some former activities. In some cases the patient may not be able to continue in any form of employment, and may even require continuing care. The patient and family may face serious socioeconomic problems. The nurse, who is familiar with the resources, makes an appropriate referral so that prompt planning for the necessary assistance is initiated. A social service worker or a rehabilitation officer may arrange for the required assistance.

DIET. A well balanced nutritious diet is provided to support the patient's resistance to infection and provide the energy utilized in coughing, controlled breathing and physical activity. It may be necessary for the patient to eat small amounts at more frequent intervals rather than have the conventional three meals. The effort of eating a full-sized meal and the shortness of breath may discourage the person from taking an adequate amount.

If the patient is overweight the caloric intake is reduced. Excess weight reduces the diaphragmatic excursion and places an increased demand on cardiopulmonary functioning.

ENVIRONMENTAL FACTORS. In order to avoid bronchial irritants, the patient may have to change his occupation. This recommendation may be rejected. It is important to point out that remaining in a situation which exposes him to irritants promotes acute exacerbations and increasing respiratory insufficiency which, in all probability, will lead to the inability to work at all. A referral may be made to a rehabilitation officer to provide assistance in finding a suitable job.

The living accommodations should be assessed and adjustments made to decrease the energy expenditure, if necessary. Factors to be considered include stairs, distance to transportation and other facilities, means of humidifying the air in his room and who is available to provide assistance for the patient.

In some instances, moving from his present residence to another locality may be helpful. For example, some patients have less bronchospasm, dyspnea and acute exacerbations in a warm, dry climate. High altitudes (4000 feet or more above sea level) are avoided; persons with COPD do not tolerate the reduced oxygen tension.

THE ASTHMA PATIENT. If the chronic obstructive lung disease is due to asthma, the aim is to relieve the bronchial spasm and prevent its recurrence.

The disorder is investigated to determine if it is extrinsic or intrinsic asthma (see p. 441). Skin tests are made when extrinsic asthma is suspected in an effort to identify the specific allergen(s) to which the patient is sensitive. This is done by the intracutaneous injection of various allergens on the back or arm. Sensitivity is indicated if an urticarial lesion (hive) develops at the site of injection. If the allergen is identified, consideration is given to its avoidance by the patient. A series of subcutaneous injections of a solution of the particular antigen(s) may be used to desensitize the individual. The prescribed dosage is at first very small and is increased very gradually. The patient is observed for at least ½ to 1 hour following each injection. An emergency cart with epinephrine (Adrenalin) 1:1000 solution and an intravenous corticoid preparation, as well as the necessary equipment for administration, should be available immediately in case a reaction is precipitated.

If the allergen is a food, it is eliminated from the patient's diet. If the antigen is a drug, the patient and family are told that any physician treating the patient should be advised of the allergy. It may also be helpful if the individual indicates the allergen on his identification card and wears a Medic Alert bracelet or tag.

Emotional stress is frequently a precipitating factor in asthma. An attempt is made to determine whether the patient is worried or disturbed about something. The nurse is alert for emotional stresses that may be aggravating the condition. These may be revealed in conversation with the patient and family or through observing their interactions. Discussion and bringing the problem out into the open may lead to elimination of the stress.

When the acute attack has abated, the necessary care for preventing another attack is discussed with the patient and family. Appropriate instruction is given in relation to the control of the environment to avoid irritants (and the allergen if the asthma is extrinsic), the prevention of respiratory infection, the importance of prompt medical treatment if an infection is imminent, and keeping emotional strain to a minimum. Medications and their administration are reviewed in detail; continued inhalation of a bronchodilator such as salbutamol (Ventolin) and/or a preparation to reduce the sensitivity of the bronchial tubes (e.g., a corticoid preparation such as Beclovent) may be prescribed.

TEACHING AND SUPERVISION. An important part of the nursing care plan for the patient with chronic bronchitis or emphysema is preparation for continuing care at home. Instruction begins with the provision of a simple, clear explanation of the disorder with emphasis on the role of continued care, much of which is the patient's responsibility. The points of care discussed above are presented to the patient and family.

A referral is made to a visiting nurse agency early enough to allow a satisfactory assessment of the home situation and the necessary adjustments to be made. Regular visits are made when the patient is home in order to counsel, coordinate and assist with his care. Careful observations are made at each visit for signs of hypoxia, infection, impaired cardiac function, general condition, nutritional status and the patient's emotional reaction to his condition. Transportation may have to be arranged for visits to the physician or clinic. Arrangements may also have to be made for a physical therapist to continue treatment and exercises. Gradually the patient and family may be able to follow the suggested program with fewer supervisory visits by the therapist and visiting nurse. If the patient can return to his former employment, the occupational nurse in the health service there is informed of the patient's condition, therapeutic regimen, and necessary restrictions.

The program of instruction includes a review of the importance of regular, effective coughing, breathing "exercises," humidification of the atmosphere, postural drainage and how these may be done. The need for activity is explained; the patient is encouraged to do as much for himself as possible. He may have to learn to walk at a slower pace and rest at frequent intervals to avoid dyspnea and fatigue. A routine of exercises for physical reconditioning may be outlined. If dyspnea develops, he should rest and concentrate on exhaling slowly and completely. Panic and fear only increase the distress. If unable to return to employment, an effort should be made to involve the patient in a hobby or activity within his cardiopulmonary capacity and in which he is interested.

Maintaining his normal weight is emphasized; if obesity is a problem, an adequate low-calorie diet guide may be provided by the dietary department. If the patient's weight is normal, the role of a well balanced nutritious diet in the prevention of infection is stressed. The need and reasons for an intake of a minimum of 3000 ml. of fluid daily are explained.

The importance of preventing infection and the necessary precautions and early signs are stressed.

Detailed verbal and written instructions are provided regarding prescribed medications or oxygen administration. Frequent visits and close surveillance by a visiting nurse are needed if the patient is using portable or intermittent oxygen.

COMPLICATIONS. The most common complications that develop in chronic obstructive airway diseases are pulmonary infection (bronchitis, pneumonia), acute respiratory failure and right-sided heart failure (cor pulmonale).

The significance and early signs of infection were mentioned earlier.

Cor pulmonale develops as a result of the pulmonary hypertension associated with respiratory insufficiency. The vasoconstriction that causes hypertension is attributed to hypoxia. The manifestations may be weakness, restlessness, increasing dyspnea, tachycardia, headache, disorientation, epigastric and precordial distress, distended neck and peripheral veins and edema. (See p. 333 for a discussion of congestive heart failure.)

Respiratory failure may have a gradual or sudden onset. The latter is most often precipitated by an acute infection; the inflammation and edema of the mucosa and the increased secretions produce further narrowing of the airways. Hypoxemia develops and carbon dioxide retention increases quickly, raising the $paCO_2$ to dangerous levels. Prompt treatment is necessary to establish an adequate airway and provide mechanical ventilatory assistance to correct the hypercarbia and hypoxia. (See p. 430 for a discussion of acute respiratory failure.)

INFLUENZA

DEFINITION AND ETIOLOGY. Influenza is an acute respiratory infection that is caused by a group of viruses. Three major types of influenza viruses have been identified, designated as A, B, and C. They are antigenic (stimulate formation of antibodies), but the antibodies are specific for each type; infection by one does not confer immunity to infection by either of the other two.

The disease may be sporadic or occur in epidemic[24] or pandemic[25] form. The influenza A virus, of which there are several strains (e.g., Asian virus, swine virus), appears to be more virulent and has been responsible for pandemics that have occurred at intervals of several years (e.g., the pandemic of 1918). A less virulent form of the disease is caused by the B virus; it may occur sporadically or as a small, localized epidemic. Infection due to the influenza C virus is mild and as a result frequently is undetected, although it may be fairly widespread.

Influenza has a higher incidence in the winter and is highly infectious. The principal mode of spread is by inhalation of infected droplets. The incubation period is 1 to 3 days and immunity is brief, as well as being type-specific.

MANIFESTATIONS. The virus invades the respiratory mucosa and the onset is usually abrupt. The patient with influenza A or B experiences general malaise, chilliness, fever, headache, aching in back and limbs and anorexia. Nausea and vomiting may occur. The patient may appear to have a head cold or complain of a sore throat, and an unproductive cough is common. Blood work may reveal leucopenia (abnormally low white blood cell count), especially in the more virulent types of infection.

The patient usually recovers from an uncomplicated illness in 7 to 10 days. Close observations are made throughout the illness for complications, especially secondary respiratory infections which are not uncommon. The viruses attack the mucosa throughout the airways; inflammation and necrosis of the epithelial tissue occur, predisposing to secondary infection by any airborne organisms (e.g., streptococcus, staphylococcus, pneumococcus). The complication may be tracheitis, bronchitis or pneumonia. Repeated attacks may lead to severe chronic respiratory insufficiency (chronic obstructive lung disease) due to the necrosis and scarring in the airways.

NURSING CARE. The patient with influenza is observed closely for early symptoms of the complications mentioned. The temperature may return to normal and the patient feel better when, several days after the onset, the temperature again rises and the individual is prostrated by secondary infection. Wheezing, chest pain, cough, purulent or blood-purulent sputum, and rapid respirations and pulse may indicate secondary infection.

Bed rest is provided until the temperature returns to normal. Activity is resumed gradually.

It is important to prevent transmission of the patient's infection; otherwise it can spread very rapidly through a family or members of an institution.

Fluid intake is increased because of the fever and to promote liquefaction and removal of any pulmonary secretions (see nursing in fever, p. 108). Mild analgesics are prescribed for relief of muscular aching and headache. A cough suppressant may also be prescribed if a dry unproductive cough is troublesome. Antibiotics are usually reserved for the treatment of bacterial infections.

PNEUMONIA

Pneumonia is the term generally used to indicate infection and inflammation of lung tissue. Pneumonitis is a synonymous term but is used less frequently than pneumonia. Guyton defines pneumonia as "any lung condition in which the alveoli become filled with a fluid and/or blood cells."[26] In the latter the fluid may be a transudate, as in pulmonary edema,

---

[24]*Epidemic* means the widespread occurrence of a disease in a community at the same time.

[25]*Pandemic* means the high incidence of a disease through one or more countries.

[26]Arthur C. Guyton: Textbook of Medical Physiology, 5th ed. Philadelphia, W. B. Saunders, 1976, p. 577.

or it may be an inflammatory exudate, as in infective pneumonia. However, fluid in the alveoli rarely remains uninfected for long since it provides a warm, moist culture medium for common airborne organisms.

TYPES AND CAUSES. Pneumonia is most often classified according to its cause. It may be bacterial or viral, or it may be categorized according to the specific causative organism; for example, the disease may be referred to as pneumococcal, streptococcal, staphylococcal, Friedländer's bacillus *(Klebsiella),* or influenzal viral pneumonia. Primary atypical pneumonia and virus pneumonia are terms used to indicate the pneumonia caused by the organism *Mycoplasma pneumoniae.*[27] The *classification by organism* is now commonly used, since identification of the specific microbe is considered important in determining the appropriate anti-infective drug to be used.

Aspiration pneumonia results from the aspiration of food, fluid or gastric contents. Lipoid pneumonia is also an aspiration pneumonia; it results from repeated use of oily medications (e.g., mineral oil, oily nose drops).

Chemical pneumonia develops following the inhalation of irritating fumes or gases.

Hypostatic pneumonia is seen most often in elderly or debilitated patients or in those immobilized for prolonged periods. Retained secretions or alveolar transudate tend to collect and become infected. The congestion begins initially in the bases of the lungs.

Still another classification which may be applied is according to the structural distribution of the disease. The pneumonia is *lobar* if a complete lobe is affected, *segmental* if it involves a segment, and *bronchial* or *lobular* if the disease is patchy throughout one or both lungs.

INCIDENCE AND PREDISPOSING FACTORS. Pneumonia has a higher incidence during colder weather and is probably related to overcrowding, hot, dry, indoor air and increased air pollution by fuel smoke. Predisposing factors also include malnutrition, chronic respiratory infection (e.g., chronic bronchitis), smoking, alcoholism which depresses reflexes (e.g., cough) and the production of antibodies, and fibrocystic disease

(mucoviscidosis). All ages are susceptible, but pneumonia is especially serious in the aged and debilitated.

MANIFESTATIONS. The onset, symptoms and course vary with different types of pneumonia. Infection of the alveoli results in their filling with inflammatory exudate (plasma, blood cells, pathologic organisms and cellular debris) that readily overflows into other alveoli, extending the infection. A whole lobe of lung tissue may become consolidated or the consolidation may be patchy; pulmonary ventilation and diffusion are impaired, and the oxygen tension of the blood is reduced to below normal. The pCO_2 level generally remains normal; the increased respiratory rate caused by the initial increase in the pCO_2 results in increased amounts of CO_2 being excreted by the normal areas of the lung. In a few days the exudate becomes more liquid and may be gradually eliminated from the alveoli by expectoration and absorption. This process is referred to as *resolution.* The disease may clear up with dramatic rapidity when specific antibacterial drugs are administered. It may run a course of 5 to 10 days; untreated, it may rapidly prove terminal (especially pneumococcal, Friedländer's and streptococcal pneumonias).

The onset of some infective pneumonias may be very sudden and frequently begins with a chill followed by fever (e.g., pneumococcal and Friedländer's). Hypostatic, staphylococcal and atypical (virus) pneumonias have a gradual onset, less abrupt than the pneumococcal type. The latter two may be associated at the onset with upper respiratory infection.

The pulse rate and respirations increase. The latter may be shallow and accompanied by an audible grunt and pain. The nostrils flare on inspiration and the face may be flushed. Cyanosis of the lips and nail beds may develop. The patient's cough may be hacking, painful and unproductive at first; later, it becomes less painful and is productive. In bronchopneumonia the sputum is tenacious, blood-streaked and mucopurulent. In pneumococcal pneumonia, the sputum is usually rust-colored, becoming purulent as resolution takes place. In Friedländer's pneumonia the pulmonary secretions are dark, reddish-brown and very tenacious.

The patient experiences general malaise, weakness, headache and aching pains. The leukocyte count is elevated in some types

---

[27]The *Mycoplasma pneumoniae* is a very small bacterium capable of passing through a filter.

(e.g., pneumococcal, staphylococcal) and normal or below normal in others (e.g., atypical, hypostatic).

Herpes simplex (cold sore or fever blister) frequently appears on the lips or around the nose and mouth. These lesions are attributed to activation of a virus that may have been dormant in the tissues. They appear as blisters first, and then rupture and become encrusted.

TREATMENT AND NURSING CARE. The pneumonia patient requires prompt anti-infective treatment and supportive care to combat his acute communicable infection and correct the interference with pulmonary ventilation and diffusion. Nursing care includes the following considerations:

OBSERVATIONS. The vital signs are recorded at frequent intervals. A sudden fall in the temperature while the pulse and respirations remain rapid is reported, especially if the blood pressure also falls. These unfavorable signs may indicate shock or a serious spread of the infection. Respiratory movements of both sides of the chest are noted and the presence or absence of air entry and abnormal breath sounds are determined by auscultation. The patient's color is checked for pallor or cyanosis. The characteristics and amount of sputum are recorded. The fluid intake and output are measured and the balance recorded. The abdomen is examined for possible distention, which is not uncommon in pneumonia. The distention may interfere with normal diaphragmatic excursions, further embarrassing the patient's respirations.

The physician is informed of marked restlessness, cyanosis, disorientation and rising pulse rate, as they may indicate increasing hypoxemia. A sputum specimen is generally requested for culture and identification of the offending organism. If possible this is collected before the patient receives any antimicrobial drugs. A leukocyte count and differential are done, and blood specimens may be obtained for paO_2 $paCO_2$ and electrolyte determinations. The chest is x-rayed to identify the areas of involvement.

REST. Physical and mental rest are important to reduce the patient's oxygen demands to a minimum. Care and treatments are organized to provide undisturbed periods. The diagnosis of pneumonia is generally very ominous and threatening to the patient; he requires reassurance and explanations of what is being done. Persisting anxiety and apprehension which are interfering with the patient's relaxation and rest are brought to the physician's attention.

MEDICATIONS. If the patient is cyanosed or dyspneic or the paO_2 is reduced to 70 mm. Hg or less, oxygen inhalation may be prescribed. It is usually administered by nasal catheter or cannulae (prongs) since the frequent coughing and expectoration tend to preclude the use of a mask. The oxygen is moistened by bubbling it through water, and the rate of flow indicated by the doctor generally ranges from 4 to 8 liters per minute.

An antibiotic is prescribed immediately; a broad-spectrum preparation (e.g., tetracycline) may be given as soon as a sputum specimen is obtained for bacteriologic study. When the causative organism is identified, the antibiotic may be changed to a specific preparation. Antimicrobial drugs must be given regularly and promptly as prescribed in order to maintain an effective blood concentration. Since some persons may be hypersensitive to penicillin and could develop a serious reaction, such as anaphylaxis, the patient is questioned about ever having had asthma, hay fever, eczema or hives and is asked if he has ever had penicillin. A sensitivity test may be done before administering the first dose. A small test dose of penicillin is given intracutaneously; hypersensitivity is manifested by a wheal or urticaria developing at the site. If hypersensitivity is known or suspected, another antibiotic is substituted for penicillin.

A cough suppressant may be prescribed during the initial unproductive, painful phase. Later, this is likely to be replaced by an expectorant such as an ammonium chloride or potassium iodide preparation to facilitate elimination of exudate and secretions.

Pleural pain may be very distressing and may interfere with the patient's rest. Acetylsalicyclic acid (aspirin) or dextropropoxyphene (Darvon) may provide relief, or a small dose of codeine may be prescribed if the pain is particularly severe. Repeated and prolonged use of any narcotic is avoided as it tends to depress the cough reflex and the respiratory center. If the patient is disoriented, he is observed closely and protected from excessive physical activity and self-injury. Side rails are used and it may be necessary to have someone in constant attendance.

CLEARANCE OF SECRETIONS. It is important to keep the airways as clear as possible to facilitate ventilation and gas exchange.

When the cough becomes productive it is encouraged at regular intervals. The patient may require instruction and support to make it effective (see p. 396). Mobilization of the secretions is promoted by physical therapy (percussion and vibration; see p. 414) and frequent change of the patient's position (he is turned side to side to back to side) at least every 2 hours. The pain generally worsens with moving and coughing; the patient needs encouragement and support in these activities and is spared as much effort as possible. The nurse may splint his chest during coughing by placing her hands over the painful area. If spontaneous coughing does not occur at least hourly, the patient is prompted to initiate it. Humidification of the inspired air (and oxygen if used) and a generous fluid intake help to liquefy the secretions, thus making it easier to clear the airways.

If the cough is ineffective, it may be necessary to use suctioning (see p. 413).

FLUIDS AND NUTRITION. The high fever, rapid respirations and increased pulmonary secretions necessitate a fluid intake of 3000 to 4000 ml. daily. This amount contributes to liquefaction of the secretions, facilitating their expectoration as well as helping to relieve the dry uncomfortable mouth. The patient perspires freely and incurs a loss of sodium as well as water. The addition of salt to broth or soup may be suggested unless contraindicated by a positive fluid balance. Because cellular activity (metabolism) is accelerated to produce the elevated temperature and there is a loss of plasma and cells in the exudate, the patient should receive a minimum of 1200 to 1500 calories daily. If he cannot tolerate solid foods, nourishing fluids and soft foods such as eggnogs, milk, junkets and custards are encouraged. Food concentrates added to fluids are useful in providing the necessary calories. The diet is increased to a full complement as soon as it can be tolerated.

POSITIONING AND EXERCISE. The patient is generally more comfortable if his head and chest are elevated. Active exercises of the lower limbs are carried out every 4 hours to reduce the possibility of venous thrombosis. The patient is confined to bed until his temperature returns to normal. Depending on the severity of his disease, he may be allowed to use a commode at the bedside rather than expend the greater amount of energy in using a bedpan. When he is allowed up, activities are gradually increased.

MOUTH AND SKIN CARE. The fever and perspiration necessitate frequent changes of gown and bedding to prevent chilling and skin irritation and to provide comfort. Flannelette sheets are more satisfactory than cotton ones. Bathing at least once daily is necessary because of the fever and perspiration.

Frequent cleansing and moistening of the mouth are necessary because of the fever, mouth breathing and infected sputum. If herpes simplex develops, the doctor may suggest an application of spirits of camphor in the vesicular stage, and then an ointment to be applied when the lesion becomes encrusted.

ELIMINATION. A mild laxative or a cleansing enema may be used if necessary for bowel elimination. As cited previously, abdominal distention may become a problem and should be relieved to prevent further respiratory difficulty. The application of heat to the abdomen may be useful in distention.

MEDICAL ASEPSIS. Bacterial and viral pneumonia are communicable diseases which may be transmitted to others by the dissemination of contaminated droplets when the patient coughs or by contact with the sputum. It may be necessary to instruct the patient to cover his mouth when he coughs, turn his head away from anyone at his bedside and promptly dispose of his used tissues into a paper bag kept within his reach. If a sputum cup is used, the disposable inner container is changed at least three times daily and the outer one is disinfected.

Visitors are restricted to the family during the acute phase and are advised of the necessary precautions for their protection. A gown is worn over the uniform while the nurse is caring for the patient and in contact with the bedding. Thorough washing of the hands follows any contact with or care for the patient. A single room provides more rest for the patient and lessens the possibility of his disease being conveyed to others. If this is not possible, he should not be placed near very ill, elderly or debilitated patients.

DISORIENTATION. The combination of fever, toxins and hypoxemia may cause disorientation. Precautions are taken to prevent self-injury and overexertion. Side rails are placed on the bed, and someone may have to remain with the patient. A sedative which is least likely to depress the respiratory center and cough reflex may be ordered.

COMPLICATIONS. The nurse must be alert for possible complications even though these rarely occur if the pneumonia has been treated in the early stage with an antimicrobial preparation. This preparation usually arrests the pneumonic process in a few days, and resolution relieves the consolidation in a relatively short period. Lack of prompt treatment of infection by a very virulent or resistant organism may result in delayed resolution or one of the following complications.

Atelectasis, or collapse of a part or of a whole lobe of the lung, ensues with the obstruction of a bronchial tube by a mucus plug. The lung tissue distal to the obstruction collapses as its residual air is absorbed into the blood. This complication frequently may be prevented by encouraging the patient to cough deeply and effectively, giving copious fluids to thin the secretions, administering chest physical therapy and turning him regularly.

A patient with pneumonia caused by resistant or very virulent organisms or whose treatment has been delayed may develop a peripheral vascular collapse, leading to *shock.* The prognosis in this complication is grave. Early signs are a fall in temperature and blood pressure while the pulse remains rapid but of lesser volume. The skin becomes cold and clammy, and the patient is less responsive. Oxygen inhalation is given; a vasopressor drug such as isoproterenol (Isuprel) or levarterenol bitartrate (Levophed) may be given in normal saline or glucose 5 per cent by intravenous infusion. The rate of flow is indicated by the physician and adjusted to the blood pressure response.

A dread complication of pneumonia is *septicemia,* in which the causative organisms may enter the blood stream and may be deposited in other tissues or organs quite remote from the lungs. Pericarditis, endocarditis, meningitis and arthritis are examples of what may be incurred by septicemia.

Empyema is a collection of pus in the pleural cavity resulting from involvement of the pleurae in the pneumonic infection. Indications include persisting high fever, chest pain and increasing dyspnea as the lung becomes compressed by the accumulation of fluid. Surgical drainage of the cavity may have to be performed if the condition fails to respond to specific chemotherapy.

CONVALESCENCE. Pneumonia can be a very debilitating disease, especially in the elderly. The duration of bed rest and of convalescence varies from one patient to another, being influenced by the severity of the disease and complications as well as by age.

Even if the acute illness is brief, the patient is advised to resume activities gradually. He may find that he tires quickly and that extra rest is necessary for several weeks. His resistance is lower for a period of time, so he is instructed to avoid contact with those with an infection as much as possible and to seek prompt treatment if he develops early symptoms of a recurrence. A high-calorie, high-protein, high-vitamin diet is recommended unless the patient is overweight. The nature of his occupation will largely determine how soon he may return to work.

It is recommended that the patient continue deep breathing exercises four times daily for 6 to 8 weeks to counteract the possible development of reduced compliance and vital capacity. These are commenced in the hospital when the temperature is normal.

BRONCHIECTASIS

Bronchiectasis is a chronic dilatation of bronchial tubes resulting from destruction of elastic and muscular tissue of the walls. It may involve any part of the lung, but the lower dependent segments are the areas affected most often.

ETIOLOGY AND PREDISPOSING FACTORS. The cause of bronchiectasis is a pulmonary infection or bronchial obstruction by extrinsic pressure, a mucus plug or an aspirated foreign body. The dilatation occurs above the obstruction.

Dilatation of the tubes results in the retention and pooling of secretions which readily become infected. The infection is perpetuated and extends, causing further tissue damage. The degree of impairment of pulmonary ventilation and oxygen uptake depends upon the amount of chronic infection and lung damage.

The onset of bronchiectasis has a higher incidence in childhood. A congenital malformation of the affected bronchial tubes and debilitation are considered to be predisposing factors in the development of the disease.

SYMPTOMS. The symptoms of bronchiectasis include a persisting cough, profuse purulent sputum with an offensive odor, periodic hemoptysis due to erosion of a blood vessel by the infective process, shortness of breath on exertion, loss of weight and reduced work capacity. A severe paroxysm of coughing is common in the morning as a result of the overnight accumulation of secretions. A change of position may also precipitate coughing when the secretions flow from the dilated saccular area into healthier tubes which are capable of initiating the cough reflex. Clubbing of the fingers and toes may develop when the disease is of long standing. Episodes of acute respiratory infection (such as pneumonia) with chest pain, fever and dyspnea occur.

The diagnosis is confirmed and the extent of the disease is determined by a bronchogram of both lungs (see p. 402).

TREATMENT AND CARE. The patient may be treated conservatively by the prolonged administration of an antimicrobial drug. The choice of the anti-infective drug will depend on the organisms present in the sputum and their sensitivity. Postural drainage is used to empty the bronchiectatic cavities of their purulent secretions and reduce the frequent coughing (see p. 414). Bronchoscopic suctioning may be used if the cavity is accessible and the secretions are viscous and difficult to raise. Deep breathing exercises are encouraged to improve alveolar ventilation; the fuller inflation of the lungs also helps to move the secretions out.

Inhalation of irritating fumes and dust, chilling, fatigue and contact with those with acute respiratory infection are avoided.

A high-calorie, high-vitamin, well-balanced diet and extra rest contribute to the patient's resistance and the prevention of pneumonia. A daily fluid intake of at least 3000 ml. is recommended to promote liquefaction and mobilization of the pulmonary secretions.

The patient is not usually hospitalized except during bronchoscopic investigation and when an acute pulmonary infection develops. The extent of his disease determines if he is able to continue at school or in his employment.

The initial period in the hospital during diagnosis usually provides an opportunity for the nurse to instruct the patient and his family about the management regimen (postural drainage, coughing, breathing exercises, diet and fluids). A referral to a clinic or to a visiting nurse agency is desirable so that the patient is supervised and teaching is reinforced at intervals.

Surgical excision of the affected segment or lobe is considered to be the most effective treatment if the bronchiectatic cavity and infection persist. Occasionally, if more than one lobe of a lung is involved, an entire lung is removed. For nursing care, see p. 460.

PLEURAL EFFUSION

A pleural effusion is an accumulation of an abnormal quantity of fluid in the interpleural space and is a symptom associated with a variety of conditions. The fluid may be a transudate or an exudate. A *transudate* may collect in the pleural space as a result of increased venous pressure incurred by congestive heart failure or an intrathoracic tumor which interferes with venous drainage in the area. Cirrhosis of the liver may cause a pleural effusion, as well as ascites. An accumulation of *exudate* in the pleural space indicates irritation and inflammation of the pleura.

SIGNS AND SYMPTOMS. The patient with an effusion may experience some pleuritic pain, which is stabbing and is worse on inspiration before the excess fluid collects. The condition may develop insidiously and may go unrecognized until the increasing volume of fluid commences to compress the lung, causing dyspnea and impaired pulmonary ventilation.

TREATMENT. A chest aspiration (thoracentesis) is done to relieve the pressure on the lung and to obtain a specimen of fluid for examination. Treatment is directed toward the disease causing the effusion.

If the exudative fluid in the pleural space becomes purulent, the condition is referred to as *thoracic empyema*. Its occurrence is rare since the advent of the improved antimicrobial drugs, but it is generally a complication of pneumonia or, less often, of tuberculosis. A culture is made of the aspirated fluid for identification of the causative organisms and their antibiotic sensitivity. The patient receives antibiotics parenterally or orally, and the drug may also be injected into the thoracic cavity following aspiration. Surgical drainage may be necessary, especially if the pus is thick. Early breathing exercises to promote reexpansion of the lung are important, since the visceral pleura tends to become thick, fibrous and resistant to stretching, reducing lung compliance and the vital capacity.

PULMONARY TUBERCULOSIS

Tuberculosis is a reportable infectious disease that is caused by the tubercle bacillus. The organism may attack other tissues in the body, but the lungs are most frequently the primary site of invasion.

INCIDENCE. The incidence of pulmonary tuberculosis has diminished in many countries where the standard of living is relatively higher (e.g., North America and European countries), but it still remains a major health problem in countries and areas that are less well developed economically and socially.

Up until the last three to four decades, the disease was seen more often in children, adolescents and young adults. In recent years, fewer younger persons become infected, but a considerable number of the older age group are infected. Most of them have controlled their disease throughout their life; with poorer health and lowered resistance in the later years, some of them develop active disease. The lower incidence in younger persons is attributed to improved socioeconomic conditions and effective chemotherapy.

Two types of tubercle bacilli may cause disease in man. One is the bovine, which is most often found in cattle and may be transmitted to man by the ingestion of infected dairy products. Fortunately, this is relatively well controlled now by the inspection and testing of herds and the pasteurization of milk. The second type of tubercle bacillus is classified as the human variety and may invade any body tissue, but has a predilection for lungs.

Infection is usually by inhalation of droplets bearing tubercle bacilli. The droplets have been expelled into the air by the sneezing or coughing of a person with active disease.

DISEASE PROCESS. Small, rounded nodules with a tendency toward central necrosis develop at the site of tissue invasion by the bacilli. These are referred to as *tubercles* and are composed of lung tissue cells, leukocytes, other phagocytic cells, fibroblasts and

tubercle bacilli. If the body defenses are strong enough to destroy the organisms, the lesion heals and may calcify.

In some instances, the reproduction of the tubercle bacilli may be minimal; a few continue to survive within the tubercle but remain confined and dormant. This person, having been infected and still harboring live bacilli, will show a positive tuberculin test in approximately 2 to 10 weeks after the initial infection; defensive cells have become sensitized and tend to inhibit or slow up the growth of tubercle bacilli. At a later date, if his resistance is lowered, the reproduction of the tubercle bacilli may be accelerated and he develops active disease. When the bacilli continue to multiply, the tubercle necroses centrally, producing soft, caseous material that may eventually be discharged from the tubercle, leaving a cavity. This caseous discharge is highly infective.

RESISTANCE AND SUSCEPTIBILITY. Susceptibility to tuberculosis appears to vary somewhat from one race of people to another, which suggests that some may have a natural resistance. The North American Indians and African Negroes show a high incidence and increased susceptibility.

Macleod indicates that some persons who have been infected and who have controlled their primary lesion are more resistant to the disease on subsequent exposure; this suggests some protection comparable to acquired immunity.[28]

Factors which lower the resistance and the ability to control the primary infection include nutritional deficiency, debilitating disease, chronic respiratory disease (e.g., asthma), excessive fatigue, overcrowding and prolonged dust inhalation such as that to which miners are subjected.

Persons receiving adrenocorticoid preparations (e.g., asthmatic and arthritic patients) over a long period also run a greater risk of developing tuberculosis because of the depressing effect of the drug on inflammation and lymphocyte and antibody production.

SIGNS AND SYMPTOMS. The onset of pulmonary tuberculosis tends to be insidious. A person may be active and may be leading his usual pattern of life over a long period during which the disease may be

---

[28]John Macleod (Ed.): Davidson's Principles and Practice of Medicine, 11th ed. Edinburgh, Churchill Livingstone, 1974, p. 355.

slowly progressing with the very gradual appearance of symptoms. The symptoms include those produced by the systemic effects of the disease and those due to the local effects of the tubercles.

The constitutional symptoms are vague and nonspecific, including lassitude, easy fatigue, malaise, loss of appetite and weight, fever (usually low grade) in the latter part of the day, tachycardia and night sweats. Those produced by the local disease process at the site of the lesion in the lungs are cough, sputum, hemoptysis, dyspnea and chest pain if the pleura is involved.

DIAGNOSTIC INVESTIGATION. The investigation of a patient for pulmonary tuberculosis involves tuberculin testing, chest x-ray and bacteriologic examination of sputum.

In tuberculin testing, a small amount of tuberculin may be injected intradermally at one site (Mantoux test) or by multiple punctures (Heaf and tine tests). One of two preparations of tuberculin may be used — namely, pure protein derivative (PPD) or old tuberculin (OT). The Mantoux test generally uses PPD, and the site is examined for induration or swelling in 48 to 72 hours. The exact size of the area of induration is recorded in millimeters. An area of 10 mm. or over is considered positive. The Heaf test uses PPD and the site is examined on the fourth to seventh day after administration. Palpable induration around at least four puncture points indicates a positive reaction. The tine test uses a multiple-puncture device and a concentrated solution of old tuberculin; the four-puncture site is examined in 48 to 72 hours. Induration of 2 mm. or more is generally considered to be a positive reaction.

If the tuberculin test is positive, this is followed by roentgenograms of the chest and a sputum examination. Even very small lesions are likely to be detected in a chest x-ray because of the natural air contrast available in the lungs. Healed lesions may be recognized by the contracted scar tissue and deposits of calcium. A sputum specimen, which is obtained in the morning when the patient first awakens, is cultured and examined for gram-positive, acid-fast bacilli. It is necessary to demonstrate the presence of tubercle bacilli, and at least three specimens produced by deep coughing are examined to confirm the diagnosis. If it is difficult to obtain a satisfactory sputum specimen, gastric contents or washings aspirated before breakfast or laryngeal swabs may be cultured. Rarely, a bronchoscopy may be done and a specimen of secretions obtained by suction.

TREATMENT AND NURSING CARE. The treatment and care of tuberculosis has undergone dynamic changes in recent years. Patients are no longer isolated in special hospitals for months and years. They remain at home, continue to work and live a normal, useful life without endangering others. The principal factors in the plan of patient care are prolonged chemotherapy, rest, and patient and family education.

CHEMOTHERAPY. The administration of specific antimicrobial drugs over a long period of time has proved very successful in the treatment of tuberculous patients. Drugs currently in use include the following:

Isoniazid (INH). This is taken orally in one or two prescribed doses daily. This drug is usually well tolerated; sensitivity or toxic reaction is uncommon. Rarely, the patient may develop general malaise, anorexia, nausea, vomiting, fever or a rash. Polyneuritis, apathy and anemia may occur.

Ethambutol. This is given orally in a single daily dose in combination with another antibacterial drug. It inhibits the synthesis of RNA and cellular phosphate, destroying and arresting reproduction of the tubercle bacilli. A side effect that may occur is reduced visual acuity.

Rifampin. This is given orally with one or two other antitubercular agents (usually ethambutol and/or isoniazid). The patient is observed for possible hepatitis.

Streptomycin. This antibiotic may be administered intramuscularly for a shorter period than the other antitubercular preparations, usually not longer than 4 or 6 months. Serious side effects of this drug are damage of the auditory nerves and consequent loss of hearing.

Para-aminosalicylic acid (PAS). This drug was one of the earliest antitubercular preparations used in conjunction with INH and streptomycin. It is given orally but is poorly tolerated for prolonged administration. It is used less often now because the patients frequently experienced anorexia, nausea, vomiting and diarrhea; chills, fever and skin rash may also occur.

Initially the patient may receive a combination of two or three of the drugs for a period of time. Later a change to one or two may be made. Isoniazid is the only preparation used singly. An example regimen is INH and rifampin daily for 4 to 6 months, and then INH and ethambutol; eventually INH only may be prescribed.

Drug therapy is continued for at least 2 years. It is important for the nurse to be familiar with the possible toxic and side effects of the drugs so that early reactions may be recognized. For example, the patient's visual acuity is determined before ethambutol is administered. An assessment of the patient's vision is made every 6 or 7 weeks as long as the patient is receiving the drug.

HOSPITALIZATION AND REST. A period of hospitalization may be necessary during sensitivity studies and initial chemotherapy, until the acute symptoms have subsided and the infectiousness of the patient is reversed. This provides an excellent opportunity to help the patient understand his disease and the required therapy and to assist him in planning his care regimen as an outpatient.

Bed rest may be recommended until acute symptoms subside and the local lesion(s) manifests a favorable response to the chemotherapy. Activity is gradually resumed, and its effect on the patient is carefully assessed. He is encouraged to take a well balanced, nutritious diet.

PATIENT AND FAMILY SUPPORT AND EDUCATION. The patient and family may be very emotionally disturbed when advised of the diagnosis. Their reactions may be very pessimistic, since they may recall that not so long ago such a diagnosis meant an incurable disease, prolonged invalidism and death. The nurse encourages them to express their concerns, and then helps them to obtain a more realistic and positive understanding of the nature of the infection.

The drug therapy program is discussed and the importance of strict adherence to it is emphasized. The patient and family are warned that if any side effects such as nausea, vomiting, diarrhea, skin rash, pain or disturbance of vision or hearing develop, the physician or clinic should be contacted.

An important part of the teaching provided by the nurse is that related to preventing the spread of the patient's infection to others. He and his family are advised of the modes of transmission and the significance of covering the nose and mouth with tissues when coughing, sneezing or raising sputum; and of the need for adequate, prompt disposal of used tissues, washing of hands, and avoidance of close contact with people. While the sputum is positive for tubercle bacilli, the patient may be required to wear a mask when close to others. In the hospital, the nurse wears the mask if the patient refuses to wear one or is careless about it. The patient is helped to appreciate his responsibility to protect others as well as to care for himself.

CONTACTS AND FOLLOW-UP. An important nursing responsibility is the identification and follow-up of patient contacts. These are members of the patient's immediate household, those in relatively close contact at school or at his place of employment, and those who are known to have been closely or frequently associated with the patient socially.

The patient with pulmonary tuberculosis requires long-term care; he and his family need long-term guidance and the support of interested, informed nurses.

In a few instances, a patient may develop a cavity which is difficult to heal by chemotherapy because of the respiratory movements. Pneumothorax may be used to place the lung at rest and bring the surfaces of the cavity together to promote healing. Rarely, surgical excision of an affected lobe or lung is undertaken if the disease is localized to one lung.

CARCINOMA OF THE LUNG

Only a small percentage of tumors of the lung are nonmalignant. The majority of newgrowths arise from the bronchial epithelium and prove to be bronchogenic carcinoma. Alveolar cell cancer is seen less often. The bronchogenic tumor may be classified as squamous cell or epidermoid cancer, adenocarcinoma, or undifferentiated or oat cell cancer. The latter is considered the most unfavorable since it grows rapidly and metastasizes very early.

The incidence is higher in males but within the last decade it has occurred with greater frequency in females. There has been an alarmingly progressive overall increase in lung cancer in the last three or four decades, and chronic irritation of the bronchial tissues is considered to be an important etiologic factor in cancer. Irritating inhalants such as cigarette smoke, air pollutants, dust and chemical gases are thought to play a significant role. Statistical surveys indicate a much higher incidence in cigarette smokers.

MANIFESTATIONS. The symptoms depend somewhat on the location of the lesion and tend to resemble those of other pulmonary disorders. They may result from encroachment of the tumor on the bronchial lumen and/or its pressure on structures in the mediastinum, base of the neck or chest wall. A persistent cough, wheezing and hemoptysis are common and, as the tumor encroaches on the bronchial lumen, increasing respiratory distress is experienced. Eventually, the tube may be obstructed, causing atelectasis of the segment distal to the lesion. Recurring attacks of bronchitis and/or pneumonia may develop as a result of retained secretions. If the carcinoma is in a small bronchial tube in a peripheral area of the lung, the patient may be asymptomatic in the early stage. His disease may progress to a relatively advanced stage before it is discovered which, in some instances, occurs on a routine physical examination or routine chest x-ray. Pain may be present if the disease invades the chest wall, causing pressure on intercostal and brachial nerve fibers. Systemic effects of the malignant disease, such as anemia, loss of weight and progressive fatigue and weakness, develop gradually.

Cancer of the lungs may be primary or secondary (metastatic). The latter may develop from carcinoma anywhere in the body, since all blood is circulated through the lungs.

DIAGNOSTIC PROCEDURES. These include chest roentgenograms, cytologic examination of sputum and bronchoscopic examination (see p. 402), which may provide a direct view of the lesion as well as a biopsy and the collection of secretions for cytologic examination. A mediastinoscopy may be performed to determine if there is involvement in this region. This procedure involves a general anesthetic and a small, midline incision, usually in the suprasternal notch. A mediastinoscope is introduced and the mediastinum explored for lesions and enlarged nodes.

TREATMENT. Early diagnosis and treatment of lung cancer, as with all cancer, produce more favorable results.

When the diagnosis of carcinoma has been confirmed, and an assessment made of the extent of involvement and severity of the disease, the physician makes a decision as to whether the treatment will be surgery, radiation, chemotherapy or a combination of these.

Surgery is generally undertaken if no metastases have been located, and as soon as the patient's general condition and pulmonary and cardiac function are carefully investigated. It may entail the excision of the affected lobe or the removal of the lung (pneumonectomy) and affected contiguous structures, such as the mediastinal nodes. Postoperative radiation therapy may be used if there is suspicion of metastases in adjacent structures, such as the large blood vessels or the chest wall. If the patient's disease has advanced to an inoperable stage when it is discovered, radiation therapy may be undertaken in an effort to arrest the growth of the neoplasm and metastasization. Chemotherapy is used when the newgrowth has metastasized beyond local invasion. (See Chapter 8 for the nursing care of the patient with a malignant disease.) If surgical treatment is used, the reader is referred to p. 460 for the care of the patient having chest surgery.

The prognosis is more favorable (1) in those who at the time of operation have no evidence of metastases or spread to contiguous structures, (2) in younger patients and in females, and (3) if the lesion is epidermoid carcinoma rather than adenocarcinoma and is located in the central or upper lobe. Early recognition and resection play a significant role. The nurse has a responsibility to urge persons to seek investigation of a chronic cough or recurring infections, discourage smoking and recommend frequent checkups and chest x-rays for those who have smoked for 15 to 20 years.

CHEST INJURIES

The commonest form of chest injury is a *fracture of the ribs* but, unless the fragments penetrate or injure the pleura and lung, it is not considered serious. However, the pain interferes with normal respiratory function, since the patient tends to immobilize the chest and take shallow respirations to minimize the pain. The hypoventilation predisposes to retention of secretions, atelectasis and pulmonary infection.

An analgesic is prescribed to relieve the pain and the patient is encouraged to breathe deeply during the period in which the analge-

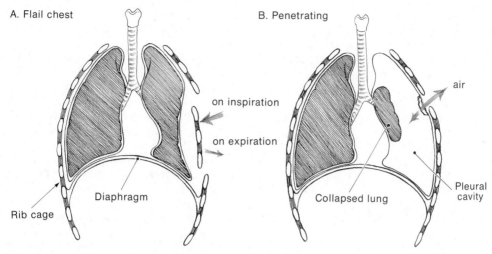

A. Flail chest

B. Penetrating

on inspiration

on expiration

air

Diaphragm

Rib cage

Collapsed lung

Pleural cavity

FIGURE 15–17 *A,* Flail chest caused by a crushing injury and multiple rib fractures. *B,* A penetrating chest injury which produces a sucking wound.

sic is effective. If the pain cannot be controlled by analgesics, an intercostal nerve block may be done to provide relief. The patient is usually more comfortable in an elevated position. Sudden, sharp chest pain, dyspnea and blood-streaked sputum are promptly brought to the physician's attention.

A *crushing injury* of the chest is frequently sustained by an automobile driver in an accident. His chest is crushed by the steering wheel and several ribs may receive multiple fractures. A portion of the rib cage is detached and displaced inward, producing a *flail chest* which is serious. (See Figure 15–17A.) On inspiration, the flail section of the chest wall is pulled in, and on expiration it moves out. This is referred to as *paradoxical respiration.* Obviously, the patient suffers respiratory insufficiency, leading to hypoxia and retention of carbon dioxide which further stimulate respirations. Secretions are also retained, predisposing to infection. Treatment is aimed at immobilizing the chest wall to reduce the paradoxical respirations. Pressure dressings may be used, or some form of traction to the chest wall may be employed by means of the application of towel clips or wires to the affected area and their connection to weights suspended by ropes over pulleys. If the sternum is fractured surgical fixation of the fragments by wiring may be undertaken.

Currently, most patients are treated by mechanical ventilatory support and no attempt is made to apply external immobilization of the chest. A tracheostomy is done and a volume-controlled respirator is used; internal stabilization of the chest is achieved by the use of a large tidal volume at a slow respiratory rate. Initially, 100 per cent oxygen may be used to reduce the patient's spontaneous respirations. Sedation or a muscle relaxant may be necessary if the patient's respiratory efforts cannot be coordinated with the respirator. If pleural leaks are suspected, air loss may be assessed by monitoring the outflow with a Wright respirometer.

Injury to the pleura or lung frequently complicates the condition, causing pneumothorax (collapse of the lung) or hemothorax (collection of blood in the thoracic cavity). Chest aspiration will probably be necessary to remove serum and blood, and a catheter may be left in the pleural cavity to allow for a continuous escape of air and fluid. An effort may be made to reduce the patient's pain with an intercostal nerve block. Narcotics are used sparingly, since they depress respirations and the cough reflex. The condition is usually complicated by severe shock and probably by other injuries.

Penetrating chest wounds produce what is commonly referred to as a *sucking wound.* Air passes freely in and out of the pleural cavity, and the lung of the affected side collapses. The air may accumulate to displace the mediastinum to the unaffected side, interfering with the normal respiratory capacity of the lung on that side by compression.

An immediate effort to seal off the opening into the chest wall is mandatory. In the emergency situation, a towel, handkerchief or any clean material at hand is used until surgical treatment is available. A thoracotomy may be done to control the bleeding and repair damaged tissues. The intrapleural cavity has been entered and the nursing care of the patient following the surgery is similar to that of any patient who has chest surgery.

NURSING THE THORACIC SURGICAL PATIENT

In pulmonary disorders, the thoracic operative procedures performed include pneumonectomy, lobectomy, segmental resection and decortication.

Pneumonectomy, in which an entire lung is removed, involves the ligation of a large pulmonary artery, two large pulmonary veins and a bronchus. The phrenic nerve on the operative side is crushed or severed to permit the diaphragm to rise to reduce the size of the cavity that remains. Pneumonectomy is used in cancer of the lung or for widespread unilateral bronchiectasis, tuberculosis or abscesses.

A *lobectomy* is the removal of a lobe of a lung and is used when the disease is confined to that particular lobe.

Segmental resection is used when the person's disease is localized to a segment of a lung, making it possible to conserve functional tissue and lessen the degree of overdistention in the other lung by removing only the affected segment.

Decortication is a surgical procedure in which a thick fibrous membrane that has replaced the visceral pleura is removed. The membrane, which causes restrictive respiratory insufficiency, may develop with empyema (a collection of pus in the pleural cavity), pleural effusion or prolonged hemothorax (blood in the pleural cavity).

Preoperative Nursing Care

The patient who is to have chest surgery usually undergoes a period in which evaluation studies are made and care is given to improve his general condition.

PSYCHOLOGICAL PREPARATION. The patient facing chest surgery is likely to be quite apprehensive. He needs emotional support and some understanding of what is being done and what is going to take place. The physician describes the condition and the proposed surgery to the patient and his family. Following this, the nurse is usually required to answer questions and reinforce what the doctor has said. The patient is encouraged to express his fears and concerns, with the nurse manifesting interest and a willingness to listen. Questions should not be evaded but answered knowledgeably. Home problems may be revealed and should be referred to the appropriate sources for assistance (e.g., Social Service or Welfare Department or a visiting nurse agency), thus relieving the patient's concerns to some extent.

A brief description of what to expect when he arrives in the operating room and after surgery proves helpful. Since the frequent postoperative monitoring and recording of blood pressure, pulse and respirations might cause him some concern for his condition, he is advised before the operation that these observations are made to inform the attendant staff as to his progress.

OBSERVATIONS. During the preoperative period, vital signs, hydration and nutritional status are noted, and the patient is observed for indications of any condition such as an acute respiratory or skin infection that may predispose to postoperative complications.

NUTRITION AND FLUIDS. The general nutritional status and resistance may be improved by a high-calorie diet with an increase in the protein and vitamin content. If the patient's appetite is poor and increased intake poses a problem, the calorie and protein intake may be provided for in commercial concentrates that can be added to a glass of milk or fruit juice. The fluid intake is generally increased to provide optimum hydration and to promote effective removal of pulmonary secretions.

SECRETIONS. The amount and characteristics (consistency, color, purulent or nonpurulent) of the patient's sputum are carefully noted and recorded. If he has retained secretions, postural drainage and physical therapy may be used to clear the lung of as much infective material as possible (see pp. 413–414).

ANTIBIOTICS. If the condition is infectious, a broad-spectrum antibiotic will probably be prescribed to reduce the infection. It may be administered orally or parenterally.

MOUTH CARE. Frequent antiseptic mouthwashes contribute to reducing infective organisms as well as to the comfort of the patient. Frequent expectoration of purulent sputum and the objectionable taste which may develop tend to depress the appetite. Keeping the mouth clean may encourage the patient to take necessary food.

INSTRUCTION AS TO POSTOPERATIVE ROLE. Much attention is given to preparing the patient for what will take place after the operation. Oxygen administration, the use of a respirator to reduce the patient's work of breathing, the frequent use of the suction to remove secretions, the drainage tubes in his chest, the frequent turning and early ambulation are judiciously explained.

The patient is advised that he will be expected to cough at least every 1 to 2 hours to promote reexpansion of the lung in the case of partial resection and to promote drainage from the thoracic cavity and the removal of intrapulmonary secretions. He is taught to inhale deeply and cough with the mouth and throat open and is encouraged to practice this during the preoperative period. The importance of regular periods of deep breathing which he will be expected to carry out is emphasized. The nurse or a physiotherapist explains and demonstrates the leg exercises which he will be required to do to prevent circulatory stasis and thrombus formation, and the posture training and arm exercises to preserve good posture and normal range of motion. The patient is advised if he is to be transferred to an intensive care unit following surgery and should, if possible, have some contact with the nurse who will care for him.

EVALUATION TESTS. Pulmonary function tests and complete blood studies are done. A chest x-ray will likely have been taken during the initial investigation but may be repeated to determine if there is any change. An electrocardiogram is usually requested by the anesthetist. Blood work will include arterial blood gas determinations and typing, with arrangements for compatible blood to be available at the time of surgery. The procedures and their purpose are explained to the patient.

IMMEDIATE PREOPERATIVE CARE. The immediate preparation beginning the day before operation is similar to that suggested for most major surgery in Chapter 10. A large skin area is shaved and cleaned, since the exact site of incision varies. The doctor may not consider an enema necessary if early ambulation is anticipated. Postural drainage may be required before the patient goes to operation. If atropine is ordered as preoperative medication, the postural drainage should be done before the atropine is administered. A final check is made to see that the operative consent has been signed, that the urinalysis and vital signs are normal and that the patient's urinary bladder is empty. A close relative may be allowed to visit briefly with the patient before the preoperative sedative is administered and then is shown to a sitting room where the family may wait during the operation.

Postoperative Nursing Care

During the operation certain pieces of equipment are assembled in the patient's unit and are checked for functioning. These include the following, as well as those prepared for all patients having major surgery (see p. 176):

1. Respiratory suction equipment
2. Equipment for closed chest (water-seal) drainage
3. Two large hemostats
4. Equipment for oxygen administration: mask, catheter or cannulae, tubing and bottle for humidification
5. Equipment for measuring central venous pressure
6. Thoracentesis (chest aspiration) tray

OBSERVATIONS. The arterial blood pressure, pulse and respirations are noted every 15 minutes for the first 2 to 3 hours and then the interval is increased to ½ to 1 hour for the succeeding 8 to 10 hours if the vital signs are stabilized. Since venous return to the right atrium is influenced by respiratory movements, and intrathoracic pressure changes, hourly recording of the central venous pressure may be required. This pressure also reflects the ability of the right side of the heart to forward the blood. The reduction in the pulmonary vascular bed following lung resection may offer resistance to the outflow of the right side of the heart, causing an elevation of venous blood pressure. The pressure is obtained by the installation of a fine venous catheter threaded through an antecubital vein (basilic or cephalic vein) into the superior vena cava (see p. 297). The surgeon usually indicates the level of elevation of venous pressure at which he is to be notified and at which the fluid intake is restricted.

The rise and fall of both sides of the chest in respiration should be noted. Dyspnea, decreased movement of one side of the chest on inspiration (except in pneumonectomy), cyanosis or chest pain may manifest a pneumothorax and should be reported promptly to the physician. This may develop as a result of air or fluid collecting in the pleural cavity and compressing the lung. It must be treated quickly by chest aspiration (thoracentesis), or the patient may die of respiratory insufficiency. Respirations are also observed for audible moist sounds. A portable chest x-ray may be done daily for 2 to 3 days to determine lung expansion and detect the presence of fluid and air in the pleural cavity.

The wound area and chest drainage are examined frequently for any indications of bleeding. The sealed drainage system is checked frequently for functioning (see p. 465), and the tubing connections are examined for security. The volume of drainage is measured at regular 8–hour intervals. The intake and output are recorded, and the fluid balance is estimated.

The nurse may also be required to measure the patient's tidal and minute volumes (see p. 393). Arterial blood specimens may be necessary for blood gas determinations which indicate possible respiratory insufficiency and the need for mechanical assistance and/or increased oxygen inhalation.

POSITIONING. With the return of consciousness and stabilization of the blood pressure and pulse, the head of the bed is raised gradually to a 30° to 45° angle. This facilitates the patient's breathing by lowering the diaphragm. The patient is turned every 1 to 2 hours, and the physician usually specifies whether he may be turned on either side or to one side only. In the case of a pneumonectomy, turning is from the back to the affected side only so that there is no restriction placed on the remaining lung, which is carrying the full respiratory load. With partial resection, the patient usually may be turned from back to left side to back to right side, and so on. If a sternum-splitting incision is used the patient is generally most

comfortable on his back, but is encouraged to assume a lateral position for at least brief periods. During any moving or turning of the patient, precautions are necessary to prevent dislodging the chest drainage tubes. As the patient turns, the tubes are firmly clamped near the chest with forceps, and are lifted to prevent dragging or pulling. When he is positioned, the clamps are removed and a final check is made to be sure that the closed drainage system is patent.

OXYGEN ADMINISTRATION. The patient usually receives oxygen by mask, catheter or nasal prongs for at least the first 24 to 36 hours (see p. 408). The administration is not prolonged unless the patient is experiencing some respiratory insufficiency. Most patients seem to adapt fairly quickly to the remaining lung capacity. Occasionally a patient becomes dependent on the oxygen therapy and is fearful of having it discontinued. In such instances a gradual withdrawal is necessary.

MOBILIZATION OF PULMONARY SECRETIONS. As soon as the blood pressure is stabilized, the patient is asked to cough every 1 to 2 hours or more often if there is evidence of retained secretions. Removal of secretions may prevent atelectasis and infection and will improve ventilation of the lung. It is sufficiently important that the patient be wakened to cough at regular intervals throughout the night. Even with preoperative instruction and practice, the patient is usually fearful and may find the procedure difficult. Suctioning is used to clear the pharyngeal part of the tract and will also precipitate coughing. The latter loosens secretions in the lower tracheobronchial passages and raises them to the upper tract from which the patient may cough them up, or they may be reached by suction. The nurse assists the patient to a sitting position for coughing and, standing at the side of the bed which is opposite to the patient's incision, supports the operative side of the chest, back and front, with her hands. The patient is asked to take several deep breaths and to cough with each expiration. If the cough and suctioning are not productive, it is brought to the physician's attention. An expectorant or nebulized solution may be prescribed to liquefy the secretions, making them easier to raise.

Physical therapy (vibration and percussion) may be used to dislodge secretions from peripheral bronchial tubes and bronchioles (see p. 414). A humidifier in the room may also be helpful. Endotracheal suctioning may have to be done by the physician if the secretions continue to be retained. For this a number 14 or 16 Fr catheter is attached to the suction and, with the patient in an upright sitting position, his tongue is gently pulled forward, and the catheter is passed via the nose into the larynx. The patient is asked to inhale deeply or cough, which opens the glottis, and the doctor quickly forwards the catheter into the trachea. Violent coughing ensues, dislodging secretions to within reach of the suction.

DEEP BREATHING. The patient's respirations tend to be shallow, since deep breaths are likely to cause some discomfort. He is encouraged to take five to ten deep breaths hourly and is given an explanation of the need to promote full expansion of the remaining lung tissue and the drainage of air and fluid from the thoracic cavity. As the lung expands to occupy more space, the pressure increases within the pleural cavity, forcing air and fluid through the drainage tube.

FLUIDS AND NUTRITION. The blood loss at operation is replaced by a blood transfusion, and fluids are usually given intravenously for the first 24 to 48 hours. The rate at which the fluid is given must be carefully controlled to prevent too rapid filling of the reduced vascular compartment and subsequent pulmonary edema, which is manifested by dyspnea, bubbling sounds and frothy sputum. The physician may indicate the rate at which the intravenous fluid may be administered, which usually does not exceed 40 drops per minute. The rate of flow is also regulated according to the central venous pressure.

Clear fluids may be given as soon as there is no nausea and vomiting and gradually are increased in volume as tolerated. The patient may have a soft diet the first postoperative day, if he can take it, and a regular diet the following day. Extra fluids are provided, unless contraindicated by increased venous pressure, to reduce the tenaciousness of the respiratory secretions.

RELIEF OF PAIN. When closing the chest wall, the surgeon may inject the intercostal nerves with a novocaine preparation to reduce the pain. Narcotic drugs are used sparingly since they generally depress respirations and the cough reflex. A small dose of morphine or meperidine hydrochloride (Demerol) may be prescribed for pain, but judgment must be used in administering it. The patient should not be allowed to suffer unnecessarily, but it is also important that he cough to remove secretions and breathe deeply to ventilate the remaining lung tissue adequately.

EXERCISE AND MOBILITY. Passive extension and flexion movements of the lower limbs are carried out by the nurse every 3 to 4 hours until the physician indicates that the patient may begin active exercises. The latter may be limited or delayed by the chest drainage but, if his progress is satisfactory, postural and arm exercises will probably be started the third postoperative day. If his condition is satisfactory, he may be assisted out of bed on the second or third day. The exercises and early ambulation stimulate circulation and respirations, prevent venous stasis and thrombus formation and promote normal posture. They also tend to assure the patient of a favorable progress and bolster his morale.

CLOSED CHEST DRAINAGE. Following intrathoracic surgery, fluid and air may collect in the space between the lungs and chest wall. If allowed to remain, the accumulation may prevent reexpansion of the lung on the operative side and may also cause pressure on the large blood vessels, heart and unaffected lung, interfering with circulation and reducing ventilation. A collection of serosanguineous fluid predisposes to infection because it is a good culture medium. It may also cause pleural thickening that could reduce the ventilatory and diffusion capacity of the lung.

When the surgery is completed, a closed or water-seal drainage system is established to allow the escape of air and fluid from the pleural cavity and reestablish the normal negative pressure, while preventing any reflux. Two tubes are generally placed in the operative area and are secured by a suture to the chest wall. One tube is placed in the anterior upper part of the operative area and mainly serves in the escape of air; the second tube is usually placed in the posterior base of the cavity for fluid drainage.

METHODS. Various methods are used to achieve closed drainage, but the principle is the same with all — that is, to allow air and fluid to pass in one direction only. The difference in the methods is generally in the number of bottles used, whether or not suction is applied and whether or not a flutter valve is introduced into the system.

Water-seal drainage may be established with one bottle fitted with a two-holed rubber stopper through which two glass or plastic tubes pass (Fig. 15–18A). The chest tubes are connected to a fairly long tube leading to the drainage bottle, where it is connected to a glass or plastic tube which has its distal end submerged at all times in sterile water or sterile normal saline to a designated depth (usually 3 to 5 cm.). The depth of tube submersion determines the pressure exerted by the water — hence the term "water-seal drainage." A small, short glass tube, serving as an air vent, passes through the second hole of the tight-fitting, two-holed rubber stopper. The water level must be marked clearly on the bottle so that the amount of drainage can be determined accurately. When preparing the setup, a strip of adhesive may be placed lengthwise on the drainage bottle and marked off at calibrations of 100 ml., 200 ml., 300 ml., etc.

With each expiration, the respiratory muscles relax, the intrapleural space is diminished and the pressure within the space is increased, exceeding that exerted by the water at the end of the tube, so fluid and air are forced from the cavity into the water in the bottle. The air may be seen bubbling through the water, from which it passes, escaping from the bottle through the vent. With inspiration the pleural space enlarges and the pressure within it decreases, causing water to rise a few inches in the distal end of the tube. The evacuation of fluid and air from the intrapleural space results in greater space and less pressure. As a result, lung expansion is increased.

The alternating changes in pressure in the pleural cavity result in repeated fluctuations in the water level in the distal end of the drainage tube; these fluctuations correspond to the patient's breathing in and out and indicate a patent system, serving as a guide to the nurse. If the water level does not oscillate, it may be suspected that the tube is blocked by a blood clot or fibrin. If this occurs, the tube is "milked" toward the drainage bottle in an effort to relieve the blockage and, if this is not successful, the physician is notified at once. In order to prevent blocking the tube is usually "milked" at least hourly. Fluctuation of the fluid level in the tube ceases when the lung has fully reex-

panded. The physician confirms this by an x-ray of the chest before removing the drainage tube.

Coughing and deep breathing alter the intrapleural space and pressure to a greater degree than normal respirations and, as a result, are important in promoting drainage of the cavity, removal of air and fluid and the reexpansion of remaining lung tissue.

To prevent water from being sucked into the chest, the drainage bottle must be kept at floor level or well below the level of the bed (2 to 3 feet below the patient's chest). The negative chest pressure is equivalent to 10 to 20 cm. of water and sucks the water up into the tube only to that level. If the bottle must be lifted or moved, the drainage tube is securely clamped near the chest wall by *two strong hemostats which must always be available at the bedside.*

A safer method for preventing the possibility of water accidentally entering the chest cavity, and which also keeps the drainage separated from the water, is to use *two bottles.* The second one contains the water, leaving the drainage bottle dry (Fig. 15–18B). When only one bottle is used, fluid drainage from the chest raises the level of the fluid, increasing the pressure at the distal end of the tube. More pressure is then required to force the fluid down on expiration and allow the escape of air and fluid. Blood and serum are more likely to collect and clot in the tube. In the two-bottle system, the first bottle is sealed and does not contain water; the shorter of the glass tubes is connected to the second bottle, which also has two glass tubes. The first (drainage) bottle is connected to the longer tube in the second bottle. The distal end of this tube is submerged in sterile water to a designated depth (3 to 5 cm.). The second tube in bottle 2 is short and acts as an air vent.

If there is a considerable amount of air leaking into the pleural cavity from the intrapulmonary space, or if the patient's cough and respirations are not sufficiently strong to facilitate the clearance of fluid and air from the chest cavity, *continuous gentle suction* may be applied. This necessitates a two-bottle system; the first bottle serves as a drainage bottle and *waterseal.* The short air-vent tube in bottle 1 is connected to the second bottle which has a three-holed stopper through which two short tubes and one longer tube pass (see Fig. 15–18C). The lower end

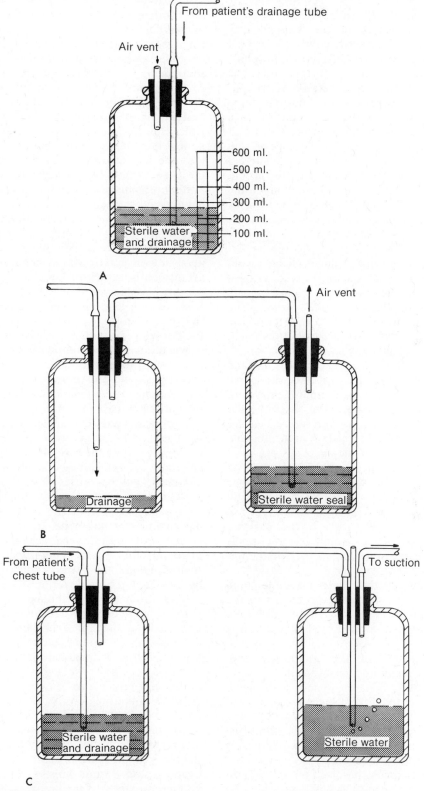

FIGURE 15–18 *A,* Water-seal chest drainage system using one bottle. *B,* Water-seal chest drainage system using two bottles. *C,* Water-seal chest drainage system using two bottles and suction.

of the longer tube is submerged in water to a designated depth. The upper end is open to the air. This tube controls the degree of suction applied to the pleural cavity. One short tube is connected to bottle 1; the second short tube is connected to a suction apparatus. The usual suction machine creates too strong a negative pressure to be applied directly to the pleural cavity. This may be reduced by a valve and meter (such as is used in "wall suction") inserted between the suction and the water-seal bottle. If the portable suction machine is used, the negative pressure is controlled by the depth of submersion of the lower end of the open glass tube in bottle 2. A continuous bubbling in the control bottle (bottle 2) indicates that the suction is being maintained.

Recently disposable closed drainage receptacles have become available. These are used with suction and have two compartments comparable to the two-bottle system. The receptacle is suspended from the side of the bed to eliminate the danger of bottles being knocked over and broken.

The water-seal system is cumbersome and also restricts patient mobility. The nurse and patient are continuously apprehensive of such things as tubes becoming disconnected and bottles being broken. As a safety measure and to permit greater freedom in turning and earlier ambulation, some surgeons prefer to introduce a plastic flutter valve into the system. It is placed between the chest drainage tube and the drainage bottle. Suction may still be applied.

RESPONSIBILITIES AND PRECAUTIONS. When any method of waterseal drainage is used, nursing responsibilities include the following considerations.

It is important that the nurse understand the purpose and operating principles of the system, as well as the precautions to be observed to prevent air and fluid from entering the chest cavity which could cause a pneumothorax (collapse of the lung) and life-threatening respiratory insufficiency.

If the bottle system is used, a directive should be received from the physician as to the depth to which the underwater tube should be submerged. The bottle should be calibrated so that the volume of water used is known and the drainage may be measured.

The system must be checked at frequent intervals for patency. This is determined by noting the oscillating water level in the sub-

merged tube; this rises with inspiration and falls with expiration. When suction is employed fluctuations of the water level do not occur because the continuous suction holds the water level in the tube at a fixed level. The suction may be interrupted briefly and the column of water observed for fluctuations. If the water level does not fluctuate in a closed system, the tube should be examined for possible kinks or compression caused by the patient lying on it. A clot may be obstructing the tube and may be dislodged by "milking" the tube toward the drainage bottle. If the system remains nonfunctional, the physician is informed at once.

As a precaution, all connections between the rubber and glass tubes are taped with adhesive to prevent their separation and to keep air from entering the system. The bottles are placed in a rack or taped to the floor to prevent accidental moving or knocking over. Visitors and ward personnel are warned not to disturb them, and a warning sign placed by the bottles is helpful.

The drainage tube is supported and lies free in a trough formed by pinning a fold in the sheet. It should not be looped but should be long enough to avoid marked restriction of the patient's moving and turning.

The characteristics and volume of the drainage are noted and recorded frequently, especially during the first 24 to 48 hours. It is generally colored by blood at first, but gradually clears and decreases in amount.

Changing the drainage bottle may be done by the physician or is the responsibility of designated persons who fully understand closed drainage. Each drainage tube is clamped close to the chest wall with two hemostats, and the bottle is quickly replaced by a clean, calibrated sterile bottle.

If an interruption or break in the closed system should occur as a result of the disconnection of a tube or a broken bottle, the drainage tube(s) should be clamped off close to the chest wall immediately to prevent air from entering the chest cavity. An accumulation of air in the pleural cavity could cause a collapse of the lung on the affected side and produce compression of the unaffected lung, heart and large blood vessels. Associated symptoms are a complaint by the patient of tightness or pressure in the chest, dyspnea, cyanosis and a rapid pulse. The surgeon is notified promptly of the break in the system, and arrangements are made to reestablish drainage quickly. As a precaution, an extra set of sterile bottles and connections is always available. A thoracentesis may be necessary to remove air from the cavity.

Regular frequent coughing and deep breathing are important since they increase the intrapulmonic and intrapleural pressures, forcing air and fluid out of the cavity and promoting lung expansion.

When turning the patient, or when giving any care, precautions are taken not to dislodge or disconnect the drainage tubes. A final check is made to make sure the patient is not lying on a portion of the tube and that there are no loops or kinks present to interfere with drainage.

Even if the system appears to be functioning satisfactorily, any patient complaint of pressure or pain in the chest, dyspnea, cyanosis or a rapid, weak pulse is brought promptly to the physician's attention

. When the lung is fully expanded and no fluid remains in the pleural cavity, the tubes are removed. The water in the closed drainage bottle will have stopped fluctuating, and the lung expansion is confirmed by the physician by percussion, auscultation and a chest x-ray.

When the tube is withdrawn from the chest cavity, the wound is sealed by the application of petroleum jelly gauze and adhesive. The patient is observed closely for the next 24 hours for possible leakage of air into the chest and ensuing pneumothorax.

CONVALESCENCE AND REHABILITATION. The convalescence and rehabilitation must be adapted to each individual patient. Generally, the patient requires a fairly long period of convalescence during which he is encouraged to continue his exercises and deep breathing. Activity is gradually increased, and the patient's reaction to it is noted. The doctor is informed if there is persisting dyspnea or shortness of breath, and the activity is restricted until a greater exercise tolerance is developed. The body has to adjust to a reduced respiratory capacity, and the patient who has had a pneumonectomy will require a greater period of adjustment. The patient may not be able to resume his former occupation and may need help to find lighter work within his respiratory capacity.

In preparation for going home, the patient receives instructions about the exercises, deep breathing and coughing which are to be continued. The recommended amounts of rest and activity are explained. If distance and travel do not present too great a problem, the patient may be requested to return to the physiotherapy department for exercise supervision once or twice weekly or arrangements may be made to have a physiotherapist or a nurse visit him at home to counsel and assess his progress. He may experience some numbness, pain, or heaviness in the operative area due to interruption of the intercostal nerves but may be reassured that this is generally temporary.

PULMONARY EMBOLISM

Pulmonary embolism is a life-threatening condition that is secondary to a variety of medical and surgical disorders. A pulmonary artery is blocked by a foreign mass (embolus) that has been carried along in the blood stream from its source until it reaches an artery through which it cannot pass. Most often the embolus is a thrombus, but it may consist of fat, air, atherosclerotic plaques or small masses of tissue or cancer cells.

Even though it is suggested that many cases go unrecognized, the incidence of pulmonary embolism is considered to have increased in recent years.[29, 30] This increase is attributed to the advances in therapeutic measures which permit the survival of many very ill persons. Previously they did not live long enough to develop the complication of pulmonary embolism. Older persons make up a larger proportion of this group than they did a few decades ago. More of them have surgery and are hospitalized.

A fat embolus may follow bone surgery or fracture or may be associated with burns, nephritis or liver disease. An air embolus may be the result of air entering a venous or arterial line. An embolus of tissue or tumor cells may arise from primary lesions or metastases. The source of the thromboembolus is most often the deep veins of the lower limbs.

Patients predisposed to embolism include those who are subjected to long-term bed rest and immobility, have varicosities, have had

[29]Joan B. Fitzmaurice and A. A. Sasahara: "Current Concepts of Pulmonary Embolism: Implications for Nursing Practice." Heart Lung, Vol. 3, No. 2 (March-April 1974), p. 209.

[30]Mary Wyper: "Pulmonary Embolism: Fighting the Silent Killer." Nurs. '75, Vol. 5, No. 10 (Oct. 1975), p. 31.

surgery, an injury or a fracture, and are elderly.

As mentioned, a greater number of pulmonary emboli are thrombi. Factors that contribute to the formation of thrombi are stasis or pooling of blood, disruption of the endothelial lining (intima) of the vessel, and hypercoagulability of the blood. The thrombus may be dislodged by a mechanical force such as strong, sudden muscle contraction, trauma or pressure, or by spontaneous separation of the clot or a part of it. It is carried by the blood through the right side of the heart into the pulmonary artery, increasing in size as it is bloodborne. Eventually it becomes lodged in an artery, impeding flow of blood beyond that point in that branch of the pulmonary artery. Infarction of an area of the lung tissue may occur. (Pulmonary infarction is the necrosis of an area of lung tissue.) In some instances the thrombus fragments before it is lodged and forms multiple emboli. The branches of the artery beyond an embolism in the lung are not perfused and gas exchange is reduced. The occlusion reduces the volume of blood delivered by the pulmonary veins to the left side of the heart. As a result, cardiac output is decreased, coronary and cerebral blood flow and pulse volume are reduced and the blood pressure falls. Due to the obstruction to the blood flow, pressure builds up in the pulmonary artery and its other branches and gradually is reflected in other systemic veins (jugular, hepatic).

SIGNS AND SYMPTOMS. Manifestations of a pulmonary embolism depend upon the size of the vessel occluded. The onset may be dramatic and present as an immediate crisis. In some instances the embolism may be manifested by subtle changes.

It is important that nurses be aware of the conditions that predispose patients to pulmonary embolism and that they be alert for clinical signs and symptoms that may signal impending embolism. For example, if a patient complains of tenderness or pain in the calf of a leg or if redness, edema or swelling is observed in a lower limb, which may indicate phlebitis or venous thrombus formation, the limb is handled gently and the patient is advised to rest and keep the affected leg extended and relaxed. He is cautioned to avoid moving it quickly and forcefully. The physician is notified promptly of the manifestations.

The patient with a pulmonary embolism complains of pain and probably a sensation of pressure in the chest, develops rapid respirations, dyspnea, a cough and tachycardia and may expectorate bright blood and blood-streaked mucus. His pulse becomes rapid and weak, apprehension and restlessness are manifested, and some degree of shock very quickly becomes apparent. If infarction is present, the temperature gradually becomes elevated and a leukocytosis is likely to be present. Rales may be heard in the area of involvement.

DIAGNOSTIC PROCEDURES. A chest x-ray may be done, since an embolism produces an area of opacity and an absence of the normal vascular outline in the area beyond the occlusion.

A lung scan may be done to identify the nonperfused area(s) of the lung. This involves an intravenous injection of a radioactive substance such as a combination of radioactive iodine (I^{131}) and serum albumin; the particles are large enough to be trapped in the small pulmonary arterioles and capillaries. A scanner is passed back and forth over the patient's chest, recording areas of the lung perfused by blood containing the radioisotope. Nonperfused areas do not show up on the scan.

A pulmonary angiogram may be used to confirm and locate the embolism. A radiopaque dye preparation is given intravenously and then an x-ray is taken. The pulmonary arteries are outlined and an embolus can be confirmed and located.

Blood specimens are obtained and examined for the leukocyte count and sedimentation rate, which are usually elevated, especially if there is an infarcted area. Serum enzyme levels may be determined: lactic acid dehydrogenase (LDH) is elevated if there is a pulmonary infarction, and serum glutamic-oxaloacetic transaminase (SGOT) is normal unless the pulmonary hypertension is severe enough to have caused right-sided heart failure and ensuing liver congestion. Blood gases, paO_2, $paCO_2$ and the pH are ascertained to provide information about the extent of impairment to gas exchange. The oxygen level is frequently below normal, but the carbon dioxide usually remains normal or may even be decreased as a result of the tachypnea which the patient develops.

An electrocardiogram is done to assess cardiac functioning because of the possible pulmonary hypertension and hypoxia that could result in cardiac insufficiency.

TREATMENT AND NURSING CARE. The care of a patient with a pulmonary embolism involves supportive measures and the prevention of heart failure and further emboli formation. If the patient is in severe shock and the condition is serious, he is cared for in the intensive care unit where a nurse is constantly at the bedside and continuous monitoring of cardiac functioning and blood pressure are possible.

REST AND ACTIVITY. The patient is kept at absolute rest for 5 to 7 days to prevent further embolization; during that period thrombi should become organized and firmly attached to the vessel wall. Reducing mobility also decreases the demands on the cardiopulmonary system. If the patient survives the first week, activity is resumed very gradually.

OXYGEN. Oxygen may be given by mask or nasal prongs to relieve the hypoxia and shortness of breath. (See p. 408 for a discussion of the administration of oxygen.)

MEDICATIONS. An intravenous line is established immediately and the anticoagulant heparin is administered. The initial dose is followed by continuous slow infusion or regular intermittent doses of heparin by intravenous infusion, so as to maintain a clotting time of 20 to 30 minutes or a prothrombin time twice that of the normal. After a few days an oral anticoagulant may be prescribed, and the administration of heparin is gradually tapered off.

An analgesic such as meperidine hydrochloride (Demerol) is usually given to relieve the patient's pain and anxiety.

OBSERVATIONS. Continuous cardiac monitoring is usually established. An intravenous line is used to measure the central venous pressure hourly. It was indicated above that the occlusion results in pulmonary artery hypertension, placing an excessive demand on the right side of the heart and producing systemic venous congestion (see p. 297 for a discussion of the central venous pressure procedure). The blood pressure, respirations and color are recorded every $1/2$ to 1 hour; the frequency is decreased as the condition becomes stabilized. The temperature is recorded every 3 to 4 hours; a high fever usually denotes a large infarction. Laboratory reports are noted by the nurse and correlated with other responses in order to make decisions (e.g., to notify the physician of change) and plan nursing care. The patient's orientation, level of consciousness and general strength are also noted.

PSYCHOLOGICAL CARE. Apprehension and fear of impending disaster are common to these patients. The sudden onset and prompt emergency response of personnel are alarming to the patient and family. The physician or nurse explains the situation and the nurse reassures both that everything possible is being done. An explanation is made of the enforced immobility, continuous intravenous infusion and repeated monitoring of vital signs. An informed patient, knowing what to expect, is less tense and anxious. Someone remains in constant attendance or very close by until the person's condition is stabilized. Having someone with him provides reassurance for the patient.

SURGICAL INTERVENTION. If the patient does not improve with supportive and anticoagulant therapy, surgical intervention may be undertaken. A cardiopulmonary bypass is used and the operative procedure is embolectomy. If there is a high risk of repeated thromboemboli, an inferior vena cava plication may be done. This procedure involves making folds in the walls of the vessel to narrow its lumen so that emboli remain at that point without blocking the blood flow. Other procedures which are used are partial ligation of the inferior vena cava (same principle as the plication) and the introduction of an intracaval umbrella filter.

INSTRUCTION. Once a patient has had a pulmonary thromboembolism there is a high risk of recurrence. Anticoagulant therapy may be continued for a period of time. If it is, the following points are discussed with the patient and family:

1. The need to take the drug exactly as prescribed and indicated in the written instructions.
2. The importance of continued medical surveillance and keeping laboratory appointments for blood clotting assessment.
3. The signs of overanticoagulation that would prompt the need for immediate contact with the physician or clinic. These include blood in the stool or urine, excessive menstrual flow, continuous bleeding

from a small laceration, bleeding gums and epistaxis.

4. Some physicians may request the patient to avoid foods high in vitamin K. These include dark green leafy vegetables, cauliflower, liver and egg yolk.

The patient is advised to avoid all self-prescribed medication because of the possible untoward interaction with the anticoagulant.

The role of venous stasis in the problem and the important measures to prevent circulatory stasis are reviewed. This discussion emphasizes the avoidance of positions which cause prolonged compression on the calves of the legs, long periods of immobility and prolonged flexion of the legs. If the patient has varicosities, the wearing of support hose is recommended. Sitting should be alternated with periods of walking around or lying flat; venous blood pools in the pelvic region as well as in the lower limbs. The patient is also advised to avoid sitting with his legs crossed.

PULMONARY FIBROSIS

Pulmonary fibrosis refers to diffuse tissue changes in the interstitial tissues of the lung. The latter form the supporting framework for the airways, blood vessels and lymphatics of the lungs. Pulmonary fibrosis causes ventilatory and diffusion dysfunction. Lung compliance is markedly decreased, so the respiratory disorder may be classified as restrictive pulmonary disease.

The tissue changes may be caused by a variety of disorders, such as collagen disease, infection, silicosis, asbestosis, cystic fibrosis, prolonged or repeated pulmonary edema, and heavy smoking.

The care of the patient is similar to that outlined for the patient with chronic obstructive pulmonary disease (see p. 442).

OCCUPATIONAL LUNG DISEASE

The inhalation of dust particles or irritating gases may cause pulmonary disease and respiratory insufficiency. The most common problem is *pneumoconiosis,* which refers to disease produced by the inhalation of dust. Pulmonary disease caused by the inhalation of irritating gases has a lesser incidence. There has been a greater awareness of the latter and precautions have been observed to a greater extent. When an individual develops a respiratory disorder due to irritating fumes it is usually due to accidental exposure.

Pneumoconiosis may be associated with mineral or organic dusts. The more common pneumoconioses due to mineral dusts are encountered in industry or mining. These include *asbestosis,* produced by the inhalation of asbestos dust which causes pulmonary interstitial fibrosis, *silicosis,* caused by the inhalation of silicon dioxide particles which results in nodular pulmonary fibrosis, and *coal workers' pneumoconiosis,* which develops in coal miners due to the inhalation of coal dust and is characterized by interstitial fibrosis.

Pneumoconiosis caused by organic dust is seen most often in agricultural workers and may be referred to as *farmer's lung.* Fungal spores may be inhaled by those handling moldy hay or mushroom compost. Cotton or hemp dust may damage the pulmonary tracts of textile industrial workers. Chronic inflammation and fibrosis occur in the disorders caused by organic dusts.

Pneumoconioses cause progressive tissue changes that result in respiratory disease of a restrictive nature. The patient's lung compliance is markedly reduced, and chronic respiratory insufficiency develops. Some of these conditions (e.g., silicosis and asbestosis) are considered to be possible predisposing causes of cancer of the lung and tuberculosis.

The treatment of these patients is similar to that of patients with chronic obstructive pulmonary disease (see p. 442). If the condition is complicated by tuberculosis, the patient receives the care cited on p. 456.

Prophylaxis is the important measure in relation to these disorders. Every effort should be made to prevent inhalation of the etiologic dusts. More rigid regulations for the protection of workers are slowly being established and enforced in industry. Protection is achieved by damping systems, improved exhaust and ventilation systems, and the use of masks or respirators by employees. Employers are encouraged to establish an industrial health program that includes frequent routine medical and radiologic examination and employee education. Employees are encouraged to report promptly symptoms of respiratory disorders such as repeated colds, sputum, cough, loss of weight and strength, tendency to fatigue easily and shortness of breath on exertion.

With early signs of pulmonary changes, the individual is advised to change his occupation. In later stages of the disease, the patient may be very limited in what he can do because of the restrictive respiratory insufficiency. Respiratory failure and cor pulmonale may develop.

References

Books

Bryan, Clifford D., and Taylor, Joan P.: Manual of Respiratory Therapy. St. Louis, C. V. Mosby, 1973.
Cherniack, Reuben M., Cherniack, Louis, and Naimark, Arnold: Respiration in Health and Disease, 2nd ed. Philadelphia, W. B. Saunders, 1972.
Crews, Eli Rush, and Lapuerta, Leopoldo: A Manual of Respiratory Failure. Springfield, Ill., Charles C Thomas, 1972.
Egan, Donald F.: Fundamentals of Respiratory Therapy, 2nd ed. St. Louis, C. V. Mosby, 1973.
Ganong, William F.: Review of Medical Physiology, 7th ed. Los Altos, Cal. Lange, 1975. Chapters 34–37.
Harper, Harold A.: Review of Physiological Chemistry, 15th ed. Los Altos, Cal., Lange, 1975, Chapter 11.
Kyle, Helena Dutton, and Ennis, Ella Gray W.: Manual for the Nursing Care of Patients with Respiratory Diseases. Chapel Hill, University of North Carolina, 1973.
MacBryde, Cyril M., and Blacklow, Robert S.: Signs and Symptoms, 5th ed. Philadelphia, J. B. Lippincott, 1970, Chapters 17, 19.
Macleod, John (Ed.): Davidson's Principles and Practice of Medicine, 11th ed. Edinburgh, Churchill Livingstone, 1974, pp. 312–427.
Murray, John F.: The Normal Lung, Philadelphia, W. B. Saunders, 1976.
Petty, Thomas L.: Intensive and Rehabilitative Respiratory Care, 2nd ed. Philadelphia, Lea and Febiger, 1974.
Sabiston, David C., Jr. (Ed.): Davis-Christopher Textbook of Surgery, 11th ed. Philadelphia, W. B. Saunders, 1977.
Thorn, G. W., et al. (Eds.): Principles of Internal Medicine, 8th ed. New York, McGraw-Hill, 1977.

Periodicals

Abraham, S.: "The Management of Patients with Chronic Bronchitis and Cor Pulmonale." Heart Lung, Vol. 6, No. 1 (Jan.-Feb. 1977), pp. 104–108.
Alexander, Mary, and Brown, Marie Scott: "Physical Examination: Part 12, Examining Chest and Lungs." Nurs.'75, Vol. 5, No. 1 (Jan. 1975), pp. 44–48.
Allen, Carol B.: "Just Breathing." Nurs. '74, Vol. 4, No.11 (Nov. 1974), pp. 22–23.
Baldwin, Linda (Ed.): "Symposium: Pulmonary Embolism." Heart Lung, Vol. 3, No. 2 (March-April 1974), pp. 207–235.
Bobear, John B.: "Obstructive Airways Disease." Postgrad. Med., Vol. 60, No. 3 (Sept. 1976), pp. 177–185.
Bone, Roger C.: "Treatment of Adult Respiratory Distress Syndrome with Diuretics, Dialysis and Positive End-Expiratory Pressure." Crit. Care Med., Vol. 6, No. 3 (May-June 1978), pp. 136–139.
Burrows, Benjamin (Ed.): "Symposium on Chronic Respiratory Disease." Med. Clin. North Am., Vol. 57, No. 3 (May 1973).
Butler, Ellen K.: "Symptom Assessment in Critical Care." Heart Lung, Vol. 4, No. 4 (July-Aug. 1975), pp. 599–606.
Chrisman, Marilyn: "Dyspnea." Am. J. Nurs., Vol. 74, No. 4 (April 1974), pp. 643–646.
Chusid, E. Leslie, and Bryan, Hewitt: "Application of Ventilators in Acute Respiratory Failure." Med. Clin. North Am., Vol. 57, No. 6 (Nov. 1973), pp. 1551–1557.
Ciuca, Rudy: "Cor Pulmonale." Nurs. '73, Vol. 3, No. 1 (Jan. 1973), pp. 10–14.
Cohen, Stephen, et al.: "Blood-Gas and Acid-Base Concepts in Respiratory Care." Am. J. Nurs., Vol. 76, No. 6 (June 1976), pp. 963–993.
Connor, George, et al.: "Tracheostomy. When it is Needed — How it is Done — Details of Care." Am. J. Nurs., Vol. 72, No. 1 (Jan. 1972), pp. 68–75.
Copland, G. M., et al.: "Respiratory Failure: What Is It and How Do I Treat It?" Can. Family Physician, Vol. 22, No. 3 (March 1976), pp. 53–57.
————: "Directions to the Patient for Correct Use of an Aerosol Nebulizer." Can. Family Physician, Vol. 22, No. 3 (March 1976), p. 66.

DeKornfield, Thomas J.: "The Adult Respiratory Distress Syndrome." Resp. Technol., Vol. 12, No. 1 (Spring 1976), pp. 6–7.

Delaney, Mary T.: "Examining the Chest, Part 1: The Lungs." Nurs. '75, Vol. 5, No. 8 (Aug. 1975), pp. 12–14.

Dewey, Jackie: "18 Ways to Live With Asthma." Nurs. '75, Vol. 5, No. 4 (April 1975), pp. 48–51.

Durkin, Deborah: "Pulmonary Fat Embolism: A Complication of Fracture." Heart Lung, Vol. 5, No. 3 (May-June 1976), pp. 477–481.

Fitzgerald, Linda M.: "Weaning the Patient from Mechanical Ventilation." Heart Lung, Vol 5, No. 2 (March-April 1976), pp. 228–234.

———: "Mechanical Ventilation." Heart Lung, Vol. 5, No. 6 (Nov.-Dec. 1976), pp. 939–949.

Foss, Georgia: "Postural Drainage." Am. J. Nurs., Vol. 73, No. 4 (April 1973), pp. 666–669.

Fuhs, Margaret, and Stein, Alice M.: "Better Ways to Cope with COPD." Nurs. '76, Vol. 6, No. 2 (Feb. 1976), pp. 28–38.

Gracey, Douglas R.: "Adult Respiratory Distress Syndrome." Heart Lung, Vol. 4, No. 2 (March-April 1975), pp. 280–283.

Griffith, Elizabeth Welk: "Nursing Process: A Patient with Respiratory Dysfunction." Nurs. Clin. North Am., Vol. 6, No. 1 (March 1971), pp. 145–154.

Hirschberg, Gerald: "Promoting Patient Mobility and Preventing Secondary Disabilities." Nurs. '77, Vol. 7, No. 5 (May 1977), pp. 42–47.

Ingram, Roland H., Jr. (Ed.): "Symposium on Chronic Obstructive Pulmonary Disease." Postgrad. Med., Vol. 54, No. 3 (Sept. 1973).

Keyes, Jack L.: "Blood-Gas Analysis and the Assessment of Acid-Base Status." Heart Lung, Vol. 5, No. 2 (March-April 1976), pp. 247–255.

Kudla, Mary Susan: "The Care of the Patient with Respiratory Insufficiency." Nurs. Clin. North Am., Vol. 8, No. 1 (March 1973), pp. 183–190.

Laycock, Joan: "Nursing the Patient on the Ventilator." Nurs. Clin. North Am., Vol. 10, No. 1 (March 1975), pp. 17–25.

McCallum, Helen: "How I Live With Emphysema." Can. Nurse, Vol. 68, No. 2 (Feb. 1972), pp. 34–36.

McFadyen, Carol: "The Respiratory Nurse in Action." Can. Nurse, Vol. 74, No. 1 (Jan. 1978), p. 31.

Moody, Linda: "Asthma: Physiology and Patient Care." Am. J. Nurs., Vol. 73, No. 7 (July 1973), pp. 1212–1217.

———: "Primer for Pulmonary Hygiene." Am. J. Nurs., Vol. 77, No. 1 (Jan. 1977), pp. 104–106.

Nett, Louise, and Petty, Thomas L.: "Why Emphysema Patients Are the Way They Are." Am. J. Nurs., Vol. 70, No. 6 (June 1970), pp. 1251–1253.

———: "Oxygen Toxicity." Am. J. Nurs., Vol. 73, No. 9 (Sept. 1973), pp. 1556–1558.

O'Dell, Ardis J.: "Emergency Care in Establishing an Effective Airway." Nurs. Clin. North Am., Vol. 8, No. 3 (Sept. 1973) pp. 413–424.

Petty, Thomas L.: "Complications Occurring During Mechanical Ventilation." Heart Lung, Vol. 5, No. 1 (Jan.-Feb. 1976), pp. 112–118.

Robertson, K. Joy, and Guzzetta, Cathleen E.: "Arterial Blood-Gas Interpretations in the Respiratory Intensive-Care Unit." Heart Lung, Vol. 5, No. 2 (March-April 1976), pp. 256–260.

Seriff, Nathan S., et al.: "Acute Respiratory Failure." Med. Clin. North Am., Vol. 57, No. 6 (Nov. 1973), pp. 1539–1550.

Slessor, Gail: "Auscultation of the Chest — A Clinical Nursing Skill." Can. Nurse, Vol. 69, No. 4 (April 1973), pp. 40–43.

Stead, William W.: "Modern Therapy of Tuberculosis." Primary Care, Vol. 1, No. 1 (March 1974), pp. 11–22.

———, and Dutt, Asim K.: "Diagnosis of Tuberculosis." Primary Care, Vol. 2, No. 4 (Dec. 1975), pp. 621–626.

Sweetwood, Hannelore: "Emphysema: Incidence Still Climbing, Nursing Care Vital." Nurs. '72, Vol. 2, No. 11 (Nov. 1972), pp. 8–12.

Taylor, Carol M.: "Pneumococcal Pneumonia: Your Patient's Second Threat." Nurs. '76, Vol. 6, No. 3 (March 1976), pp. 30–38.

Tinker, John H., and Wehner, Robert: "The Nurse and the Ventilator." Am. J. Nurs., Vol. 74, No. 7 (July 1974), pp. 1276–1278.

Traver, Gayle (Ed.): "Symposium on Care in Respiratory Disease." Nurs. Clin. North Amer., Vol. 9, No. 1 (March 1974), pp. 97–207.

Tyler, Martha L., and Synnestvedt, Norwin: "Artificial Airways." Nurs. '73, Vol. 3, No. 2 (Feb. 1973), pp. 21–36.

Van Meter, Margaret: "Chest Tubes — Basic Techniques for Better Care." Nurs. '74, Vol. 4, No. 12 (Dec. 1974), pp. 48–55.

Waterson, Marian: "Teaching Your Patients Postural Drainage." Nurs. '78, Vol. 8, No. 3 (March 1978), pp. 51–52.

White, Helen A.: "Tracheostomy. Care With a Cuffed Tube." Am. J. Nurs., Vol. 72, No. 1 (Jan. 1972), pp. 75–77.

Wright. M. G., and Nemetz, E.: "Tuberculosis in the '70s." Can. Nurse, Vol. 68, No. 6 (June 1972), pp. 27–29.

Zeluff, George W., Jenkins, Daniel, and Greenbery, S. Donald: "Asbestos — Useful and Dangerous." Heart Lung, Vol. 5, No. 3 (May-June 1976), pp. 482–484.

16

Nursing in Disorders of the Alimentary Canal

THE ALIMENTARY CANAL

The alimentary canal, or what is frequently referred to as the gastrointestinal tract, consists of a long hollow tube extending from the lips to the anus. It is divided into the mouth, pharynx, esophagus, stomach (Greek, *gaster*) and intestines (Greek, *enteron*). Modifications in structure occur in different parts of the tract, and are correlated with the particular functions featured in the respective area and the likely condition of the content when it reaches that part. The primary function of the gastrointestinal tract is to provide the body cells with a continual supply of nutrients, electrolytes and water. To do so it performs the functions of digestion, absorption of food and fluid into the blood and elimination of residue and waste products.

Food sustains life and determines an individual's nutritional status, as reflected in his state of health, activities, levels of achievement and resistance to and ability to handle disease. It supplies the body with the energy required for all its activities (e.g., respiration, circulation of the blood, muscular activity and work). Food provides the materials for tissue growth and repair and those essential for the production of substances by the body cells (e.g., hormones and enzymes). Essential regulatory substances such as vitamins are also obtained from foods. Most foods are complex compounds; chemical and mechanical processes occur in the gastrointestinal tract to break them down into absorbable forms.

If food is withheld or a disorder within the tract interrupts the essential processing of the nutrients, the individual's survival is threatened.

Structural Divisions of the Gastrointestinal Tract (See Figure 16–1.)

MOUTH. The mouth, or oral cavity, the initial part of the tract, is lined by a mucous membrane which secretes mucus to mix with the food, facilitating its movement through the pharynx and esophagus. Although the mouth is primarily concerned with the ingestion of food, it also plays an important role in speech.

The tongue, teeth and salivary glands are contained within the mouth. The *tongue* is comprised of muscular tissue enclosed in mucous membrane, The upper surface is studded with numerous papillae and contains taste buds. The tongue functions in swallowing and speech as well as in taste.

Early in life, the human organism develops 20 primary deciduous *teeth* — 10 upper and 10 lower. Beginning in the fifth or sixth year and continuing over a period of several years, the deciduous teeth are replaced by a permanent set of 16 in the upper jaw and 16 in the lower jaw. The front teeth are shaped for biting and tearing, and the remainder for grinding and masticating food.

473

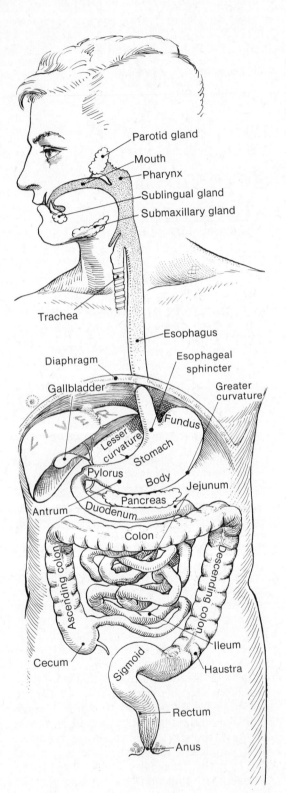

FIGURE 16–1 Structural divisions of the alimentary canal.

Hence, loss of teeth, or defects in them, can lead to indigestion or malnutrition.

Each tooth consists of a crown and root. The crown is the exposed portion which has a hard external covering of enamel and an internal substance called dentine. The root is the part buried in the jaw bone and has a covering of cementum, a substance softer and less smooth than the enamel. A central cavity running the length of the tooth contains nerves and blood vessels.

There are three pairs of *salivary glands* whose ducts open onto the surface of the mouth. The parotid glands lie in front of and below the ear and produce a thin, watery secretion that includes an important digestive enzyme, ptyalin. The submaxillary and sublingual glands are located in the floor of the mouth. The sublingual glands secrete only mucus; the submaxillary glands produce both a watery and mucous secretion. The secretions of the salivary glands and the oral mucosa collectively form the saliva. For the composition and functions of saliva see page 478.

PHARYNX. The second segment of the tract is the pharynx, which is a muscular tube lined with mucous membrane continuous with that of the mouth, respiratory tract and esophagus. It serves as a common pathway for food and air. When its muscular tissue contracts, it directs food and fluid into the esophagus simultaneously closing off the entrances to the larynx and nasal cavities.

ESOPHAGUS. The esophagus is a narrow muscular tube, approximately 10 inches long, that passes down behind the trachea and heart, through the mediastinum and diaphragm to the stomach. It is lined with mucous membrane and has an outer protective coat of fibrous tissue.

STOMACH. The stomach and the intestines, the remaining portions of the digestive tract, lie within the abdominal cavity. The stomach is located just below the diaphragm and is the widest part of the alimentary canal which makes possible its retention of a considerable amount of food while it undergoes certain changes. The stomach is divided into three segments: the fundus, body and pylorus (Fig. 16–1).

The gastric walls have three layers of muscle tissue; one in which the fibers run longitudinally, a second one in which they are circular, and a third in which they run obliquely to the others (Fig. 16–2). The circular muscle layer is thickened at the opening of the esophagus into the stomach to form the *cardiac* or *esophageal sphincter.* Similarly, the opening into the small intestine is guarded by the *pyloric sphincter.*

The mucous membrane lining is thick and lies in folds to allow for distensibility as the stomach fills. It contains numerous minute glands made up of three types of secreting cells: the chief, or zymogen, cells secrete the gastric enzymes, the parietal cells produce hydrochloric acid, and mucous glands provide mucus. The glandular secretions are poured out into the stomach to form collectively the gastric juice.

SMALL INTESTINE. The small intestine is the longest portion of the alimentary canal, being approximately 18 to 20 feet, and is divided into the *duodenum, jejunum* and *ileum.* The duodenum is the short, proximal portion which originates with the gastric pylorus. It receives the bile and the pancreatic enzymes through a sphincter (sphincter of Oddi) at the junction of the common bile duct and the duodenum. The long jejunum and ileum lie in loops and fill the greater part of the abdominal cavity.

The mucosal surface of the small intestine is covered with many finger-like processes called villi, each of which contains a central lymph channel, called a lacteal, and a network of capillaries. Most digestion and absorption take place in the small intestine where circular folds increase the surface area and somewhat retard the passage of the food, thus favoring absorption. The molecules of digested food are picked up by the blood in the capillaries and the lymph in the lacteals.

The small intestine contains many glands which secrete digestive enzymes (see p. 482), hormones and mucus into the lumen of the tube. Lymph nodes appear in clusters throughout the small intestine and are referred to as Peyer's patches.

LARGE INTESTINE. The large intestine has a greater diameter than that of the small intestine and is divided into the *cecum, colon, rectum* and *anal canal.* The ileum opens into a pouch-like structure, the cecum, in the right lower abdominal quadrant. The *appendix,* a slender blind tube, is attached to the cecum and is a frequent site

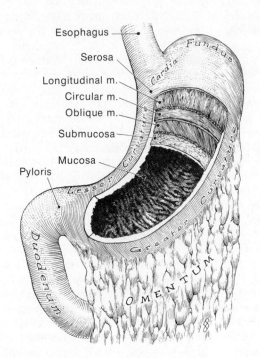

Esophagus
Serosa
Longitudinal m.
Circular m.
Oblique m.
Submucosa
Mucosa
Pyloris
Fundus
Cardia
Lesser Curvature
Greater Curvature
Duodenum
OMENTUM

FIGURE 16–2 The stomach.

of inflammation and infection (appendicitis). At the junction of the ileum and cecum, an *ileocecal valve* functions to allow contents to pass in one direction only — from the ileum to the cecum.

The large intestine ascends the right side of the abdominal cavity from the cecum as the ascending colon and flexes at the undersurface of the liver to form the transverse colon. The descending colon passes down the left side of the abdomen and, since it takes an S-shaped course through the pelvis, becomes the sigmoid colon.

The mucosa of the large intestine has no villi but has many goblet cells which secrete mucus. The longitudinal muscle tissue is arranged in three strips that are shorter than the other tissues, resulting in small

sacs along the wall of the tube called *haustra* (Fig. 16–1).

The rectum is a continuation of the sigmoid along the anterior surface of the sacrum and coccyx. It is about 6 to 7 inches long and contains vertical folds referred to as rectal columns. Each column contains an artery and vein. The veins frequently become varicosed, forming hemorrhoids.

The short terminal portion of the alimentary tube, the anal canal, opens onto the body surface at the anus. The opening between the rectum and the anal canal is controlled by the *internal anal sphincter,* which is not under the control of the will. The anus is controlled by the *external anal sphincter* which, after infancy, is under voluntary control.

PERITONEUM. The outer protective coat of the stomach and intestines is serous membrane and is known as the *visceral peritoneum*. The abdominal cavity is lined with serous membrane called the *parietal peritoneum*. A fan-like expanse is reflected off the posterior abdominal wall and extends to the intestine where it becomes continuous with the visceral peritoneum. This portion of serous membrane is known as the *mesentery*; it supports the intestine and transmits blood vessels, lymphatics and nerves. A sheet of peritoneum, the *great omentum,* is reflected off the stomach to lie like an apron in front of the intestines. The great omentum protects the intestines and, when infection or inflammation of the peritoneum (peritonitis) occurs, it makes an effort to wall off the affected area by surrounding it to prevent a spread of the infection. The *lesser omentum* is a fold of peritoneum extending from the liver to the stomach.

BLOOD SUPPLY TO THE ALIMENTARY CANAL. The mouth, tongue and pharynx derive their blood supply from the external carotid arteries via the lingual and external maxillary arteries. The esophageal artery arises from the thoracic aorta. Three main arteries supply the stomach, the left, right and short gastric arteries. The left gastric is a branch of the celiac which is a large, short artery arising from the abdominal aorta. The other two gastrics originate from the other main branches of the celiac, the hepatic and splenic arteries.

The remainder of the tract is nourished by the superior and inferior mesenteric arteries, direct branches of the abdominal aorta.

The blood into which the digested food products are absorbed is carried by the superior and inferior mesenteric veins into the portal vein, which transmits it to the liver. This makes the food products immediately available to the liver for its functions.

Accessory Structures of Digestion

THE BILE SYSTEM AND PANCREAS. The bile system and pancreas are discussed in separate chapters. See Chapter 17 for the biliary system and Chapter 18 for the pancreas.

DIGESTION

Digestion consists of mechanical and chemical processes. The mechanical processes involve the neuromuscular tissues of the alimentary tract and have as their purposes the movement of food through the tract, the mixing of it with digestive secretions, and the repeated breaking up of the food mass to bring more of it in contact with the absorptive surface. These processes include mastication, deglutition (swallowing) and movements of the stomach, intestines, and defecation. The chemical processes are chemical reactions catalyzed by enzymes to reduce the food to simpler compounds.

The digestive enzymes are substances secreted by mucosal cells of the alimentary tract and by the associated digestive organs (pancreas and liver). Like all enzymes in the body they act as catalysts (i.e, they promote and speed up chemical reactions without becoming a part of them). All enzymes are specific and, in the case of the digestive enzymes, each is secreted only by cells in a certain area of the digestive system. They are classified according to the food they act upon. An enzyme which promotes the breakdown of protein is called a *proteinase*, one that acts upon starches is an *amylase*, and a fat splitting enzyme is known as a *lipase*.

The principal reaction in chemical digestion is hydrolysis, which is the breaking up of a large molecule of a substance into smaller molecules by combining it with water. For example, in the digestion of cane sugar, one molecule of the sugar and one molecule of water yields two molecules of simple diffusible glucose that can be absorbed:

$$C_{12}H_{22}O_{11} + H_2O \xrightarrow{\text{enzyme}} 2(C_6H_{12}O_6)$$

Most food undergoes several chemical reactions before it is reduced to a form that can be absorbed. The steps in the digestive breakdown of protein, carbohydrate and fat follow.

Protein → proteoses → peptones → polypeptides → amino acids

Carbohydrate
Starch (polysaccharide) → maltose → glucose
Disaccharides
    maltose → glucose
    sucrose → glucose and fructose
    lactose → glucose and galactose
Fat → glycerol and fatty acids

Digestion takes place entirely within the alimentary canal, and the motility and secretions vary from one area of the digestive tract to another. In the following section, digestion is discussed as it occurs in each of the different parts of the alimentary tract.

Motility, Secretion and Digestion in the Mouth, Pharynx and Esophagus

MOTILITY IN THE MOUTH, PHARYNX AND ESOPHAGUS. The mouth performs mastication and the initial part of swallowing. The pharynx and esophagus are concerned only with swallowing.

MASTICATION. Most of the food entering the mouth undergoes biting and grinding by the teeth to reduce its size for swallowing and mixing with the saliva to produce a moist pulpy mass, called a bolus. Mastication is achieved by the contractions of the muscles of the lower jaw, lips, cheeks, and tongue. Movement of the lower jaw is responsible for the biting and grinding done by the teeth.

DEGLUTITION. Deglutition is the term applied to the transmission of food and fluid from the mouth to the stomach and is commonly referred to as swallowing. When mastication is completed, the food is moved to the posterior oral cavity by the tongue and cheeks and is then forced into the pharynx. Certain reflexes then occur in rapid succession. Muscles in the walls of the pharynx contract, drawing the soft palate up and back and closing off the entrance to the nasal cavities. The larynx is raised, bringing its opening against the epiglottis and the base of the tongue, thus preventing the food from entering the respiratory tract. The food cannot reenter the mouth, for the back of the tongue is raised to block the opening. The pressure exerted on the bolus by the tongue and pharyngeal constriction forces the food into the only open route, the esophagus.

The reflex responses of the pharynx to the entrance of food or fluid may be depressed by local anesthetic. To prevent aspiration following anesthetization of the pharynx, food and fluid are withheld until the swallowing reflexes have returned. This applies following laryngoscopy, bronchoscopy, esophagoscopy, gastroscopy and surgery on the mouth or throat.

When the bolus enters the esophagus, it stimulates the circular muscle of the section it is in and inhibits that of the portion immediately ahead. Thus, the food is squeezed out of the first section into the relaxed portion. The process is repeated, producing a wave of alternating contractions and relaxations along the esophagus. The wave of inhibition which precedes the bolus reaches the cardiac sphincter, causing it to open, and the bolus enters the stomach.

The more liquid the bolus, the more rapidly it travels through the esophagus.

SECRETION AND DIGESTION IN THE MOUTH, PHARYNX AND ESOPHAGUS. Saliva is secreted by the salivary glands; added to it is a small amount of mucus produced by the mucous membrane of the oral cavity. The amount of saliva secreted varies from approximately 1 to 1.5 liters per day, depending on the quantity and quality of food taken. A greater volume of food requires an increased output of saliva, and appetizing foods also stimulate the output. The saliva is swallowed and much of the fluid is reclaimed by absorption. Any interference with swallowing or any condition that provokes loss of saliva from the mouth results in a considerable loss of body fluid, contributing to dehydration.

Saliva is usually slightly acidic with a pH of 6.6 to 6.9 and consists of:
Water (97 to 99 per cent)
Mucin
Sodium, potassium, bicarbonate and chloride
(The bicarbonate salts of saliva are responsible for the formation of most of the tartar on the teeth. The salts, when exposed to air, release CO_2 and the bicarbonate is transformed to an insoluble carbonate.)
Enzyme ptyalin
Organisms
Epithelial cells from the mucosa

FUNCTIONS OF SALIVA. One of the

functions of saliva is to moisten the food and lubricate the oral cavity in order to facilitate swallowing. Dry food is put into solution by saliva, making possible the taste sensation, since only food in solution reaches the taste buds which are recessed in small pits in the tongue. Speech is made more articulate when the oral structures are moist.

The enzyme ptyalin acts on starches, reducing them to maltose. This is the only chemical digestive function performed by the saliva. The action of ptyalin may be continued for a brief period in the stomach, as the saliva is swallowed with the food. Ptyalin is only effective in an alkaline or very mild acid medium; in the stomach it is inactivated by the presence of the hydrochloric acid.

Saliva has a cleansing effect; it washes away food particles and other debris. If these are allowed to accumulate, they could act as a culture medium for organisms. Patients who are not secreting the normal amount of saliva require frequent cleansing mouth care.

The salivary glands excrete certain substances from the blood into the saliva. Lead, sulfur and potassium iodide may be transferred to the saliva. Similarly, urea may be noticeable in the saliva of persons whose kidneys fail to excrete the normal amount of urea.

Finally, saliva has a role in relation to the water balance. The moisture of the mouth largely determines the sense of thirst. A reduction in salivary output occurs with dehydration and a sense of thirst accompanies the dry mouth. When the fluids are replenished, the mouth again becomes moistened by saliva and the sense of thirst is alleviated.

REGULATION OF SALIVARY SECRETION. Control of the salivary glands is by the autonomic nervous system; each gland has both a parasympathetic and sympathetic nerve supply which deliver impulses from a salivary center in the medulla of the brain stem. Sensory nerves conduct impulses from the mouth to the salivary center to influence its action. The sensory impulses arise from taste and from pressure created by the presence of food or some instrument in the mouth. One is familiar with the experience of increased salivation when the dentist is working in the mouth.

An increased output of saliva may be a conditioned response to the sight, smell or thought of food. It implies previous experience with food and impulses are transmitted from higher centers of the brain to the salivary center in the medulla.

Parasympathetic innervation results in an increased volume of a watery secretion containing the enzyme ptyalin; sympathetic innervation causes a scanty flow of a thick, viscous saliva. The generalized sympathetic innervation associated with fright or nervousness and stress frequently produces a dry, "sticky" mouth.

No enzymes are secreted by the pharynx and esophagus; therefore, no chemical digestion is attributed to these areas. The mucous membrane produces mucus that facilitates the movement of food in swallowing. The mucus also protects the mucosa from any abrasive effect the food might have upon it and from tissue digestion by gastric juice that might escape into the esophagus.

There is an esophagosalivary reflex that increases salivation. A mass or bolus pressing on the walls of the esophagus for any length of time gives rise to sensory impulses, resulting in stimulation of the salivary glands. The increased volume of saliva which is swallowed is an effort to "wash down" the mass. One sees this in the patient with cancer of the esophagus who experiences the problem of excessive salivation.

Motility, Secretion and Digestion in the Stomach

GASTRIC MOTILITY. The stomach retains the food and churns it about for a period of time until it undergoes certain chemical and physical changes. It ejects its content in frequent small spurts into the duodenum. When the content has become mixed with the gastric secretions, its consistency changes to a thick fluid. This fluid is referred to as *chyme*.

When the stomach is empty it produces periodic contractions that give the sensation of hunger. The contractions may gradually increase in intensity and be referred to as hunger pains. With the entrance of food, the gastric muscle tissue relaxes and the stomach dilates to accommodate the food (receptive relaxation). Small waves of contraction are gradually resumed, mixing and liquefying the food. The contractions progressively become more vigorous, especially in the distal half of the stomach. Pressure in the pyloric antrum results in a portion of the gastric content being ejected into the duodenum with each strong peristaltic wave.

Fluid substances pass through the stomach quickly; solid food may take 3 to 5 hours, depending on the type of food. Fat remains in the stomach longer than protein, and protein longer than carbohydrate.

Gastric motility and emptying are influenced by mechanical and chemical factors in the duodenum. A volume of chyme filling the duodenum initiates an enterogastric reflex; sensory impulses arise in the walls of the duodenum that result in inhibitory reflex responses by the gastric muscle. The fat content of chyme stimulates the duodenal mucosa to secrete the hormone enterogastrone into the blood. On reaching the stomach, enterogastrone depresses gastric contractions.

To summarize, gastric motility is increased as the stomach becomes empty and as the content becomes fluid. It decreases when the gastric content is semisolid, high in fat and when the duodenum is full.

GASTRIC SECRETION AND DIGESTION. The gastric glands secrete a clear, colorless, slimy fluid of high acidity (pH 0.9 to 1.5) that contributes to chemical digestion and changes the food to a more fluid consistency.

The constituents of gastric juice are:

Water (97 to 99 per cent)

Hydrochloric acid (0.2 to 0.5 per cent)

Enzymes:

  pepsinogen (inactive pepsin)

  rennin

  gastric lipase

Inorganic salts of sodium, potassium and magnesium.

Hematopoietic or intrinsic factor (promotes absorption of Vitamin B_{12})

  Mucus

The hydrochloric acid and enzymes are the substances concerned with chemical digestion. Pepsinogen is activated to pepsin by the hydrochloric acid and the initial breakdown of proteins occurs. Pepsin reduces proteins to proteoses and peptones. Rennin is a specific proteolytic enzyme that converts the soluble caseinogen of milk to insoluble paracasein. The paracasein, with the calcium of the milk, produces a curd, a more solid form that results in its retention in the stomach while it is digested by pepsin. Gastric lipase is produced in small amounts. Emulsified fats may undergo some reduction but fat digestion in the stomach is relatively insignificant.

The hydrochloric acid secreted by the parietal cells destroys many bacteria which are ingested with food. The acidity of chyme, due to the hydrochloric acid secretion, stimulates the secretion of the hormone secretin (prosecretin) by the duodenal mucosa. Secretin influences the pancreatic cells to release a fluid high in sodium bicarbonate.

REGULATION OF GASTRIC SECRETION. The amount of gastric juice produced varies somewhat with the types of food taken, but with average meals, it is about 2 liters per day. With fasting, and during the night, the volume is reduced.

Secretion is influenced by mechanical, nervous and hormonal factors, and it is customary to describe gastric secretion as occuring in certain phases—the psychic or cephalic, gastric and intestinal phases. The *psychic phase* of gastric secretion occurs before the food reaches the stomach. When food is tasted and chewed, sensory impulses from the mouth enter the central nervous system and result in parasympathetic innervation via vagus nerve fibers, stimulating the gastric glands to pour out their secretions. The more appetizing the food is, the greater will be the vagal innervation and the response of the gastric glands. Psychic stimulation by the thought, smell or sight of appetizing food may produce the same effect. Conversely, sympathetic innervation depresses the gastric glands and secretion is reduced. Emotional disturbances such as worry, fear and grief result in a decrease in gastric secretion.

Food reaching the stomach further stimulates its secretion, producing what is known as the *gastric phase*. The food causes a direct mechanical stimulation of the gastric glands and initiates sensory nerve impulses that are delivered via vagus nerve fibers to the medulla, resulting in return impulses, via vagal motor fibers that increase the activity of the gastric glands. Chemical stimulation is by a hormone, gastrin, that is released by the gastric mucosa into the blood. Distention of the stomach, particularly in the pyloric region, and certain foods, referred to as secretogogues, evoke the release of gastrin. Proteins, particularly meats, are high in secretogogues, which are soluble in water. Meat soups and broths increase gastric secretion and therefore are used at the beginning of a meal in preparation for the food to follow. Such preparations are excluded from the diet of peptic ulcer patients, since an increased output of the highly acid juice further irritates and erodes their lesion.

The question has always arisen as to why the pepsinogen activated by the hydrochloric acid (pepsin) does not digest the gastric tissue. The mucus secreted by the mucosal glands plays an important role in protecting the surface. Schottelius and Schottelius indicate that the stomach is also protected by the fusion of the columnar epithelial cells which comprise the mucosal surface. This arrangement provides a barrier which may be broken down by some substances, such as ethyl alcohol and acetylsalicylic acid.[1]

Histamine has been found to stimulate the parietal cells of the gastric glands, resulting in an increased output of hydrochloric acid. The gastric mucosal cells have a high histamine content. It is suggested that two types of histamine receptors, H_1 and H_2, are present, and the H_2 receptors initiate the release of histamine which stimules the secretion of hydrochloric acid.[2] If the physician finds it necessary to determine if the patient's cells are producing acid, or if he is lacking hydrochloric acid (achlorhydric), a histamine-like substance is injected and the gastric juice aspirated for analysis.

The *intestinal phase* of gastric secretion involves an increase in the concentration of the hormone gastrin, which is associated with the passage of chyme from the stomach into the duodenum. The increased concentration of gastrin stimulates pepsinogen and hydrochloric acid secretion.

Motility, secretions and digestion in the small intestine

MOTILITY OF THE SMALL INTESTINE. Food moves slowly through the small intestine so that digestion may be completed

and the simpler molecules absorbed. The motor activities perform three functions: food is mixed with bile and with pancreatic and intestinal secretions, the mass is broken up to bring it into contact with the absorptive surfaces, and the unabsorbed content is moved into the large intestine.

Rhythmicity and automaticity are two notable features of the muscle tissue of this division of the alimentary canal; waves of contractions move down the tract at an orderly rate, appropriate to the stage of digestion and absorption. Contractions of the longitudinal and circular layers of muscle tissue produce two major types of movement, namely, *segmentation* and *peristalsis*. Segmentation occurs with areas of the circular muscle contracting and dividing the intestine into a series of alternating constricted and relaxed areas, giving the tube the appearance of a string of sausages. The mass of food stimulates the circular muscle of the section it is in, while those areas behind and ahead remain relaxed. The content in the contracted area is divided into two segments; one is squeezed into the relaxed portion of the intestine ahead and the other is forced back into the relaxed area behind the constriction. The area of contracted circular muscle relaxes and contraction occurs in the previously relaxed areas. Segmentation serves to break up the mass of content so it is mixed with the digestive juice and so more of it is brought into contact with the absorptive surfaces.

Mixing of the chyme and intestinal juice and absorption are facilitated by oscillations of the villi of the mucosa.

Peristalsis is a wave-like muscular activity consisting of a wave of inhibition followed by a wave of contraction. The advancing portion of the wave involves relaxation of an area of the circular muscle and contraction of the longitudinal muscle, producing a sac-like dilatation. The posterior part of the wave consists of contraction of the circular muscle, producing a constricted area in the tube. The peristaltic waves vary in intensity and in the distance they travel. Some go only a short distance while others pass over a long section, pushing the content much further along the tract. Those that traverse a considerable length of the tract may be referred to as peristaltic rushes.

The small intestine terminates with the ileocecal valve, which guards the opening into the

[1]Byron A. Schottelius and Dorothy D. Schottelius: Physiology, 7th ed. S. Louis, C.V.Mosby, 1973, p. 391.

[2]Wm. F. Ganong: Medical Physiology, 7th ed. Los Altos, Cal., Lange, 1975, p. 360.

cecum. The pressure in the small intestine forces open the valve and the fluid passes through into the large bowel.

Muscular and villi activity of the small intestine is regulated by both an intrinsic and extrinsic mechanism. The intrinsic control is by two neural plexuses (networks). One, the myenteric or Auerbach's plexus, is located between the longitudinal and circular layers of muscle tissue. The second intrinsic plexus lies between the circular muscular tissue and the submucosa. The receptors associated with the plexuses are sensitive to stretch or irritation of the mucosa. The reflex response is contraction of the muscle tissues which initiates segmentation, peristalsis and movements of the villi.

The extrinsic mechanism concerned with the motility of the small intestine is parasympathetic innervation via vagal nerve fibers and sympathetic innervation through splanchnic nerves. Parasympathetic impulses stimulate the muscle tissue and conversely sympathetic innervation tends to slow motility. Autonomic nerve impulses are not essential to intestinal motility but do influence it.

SECRETION IN THE SMALL INTESTINE. The digestive juice in the small intestine includes external pancreatic secretions and bile as well as the secretions of the intestinal mucosal glands.

PANCREATIC JUICE AND BILE. Approximately 700 to 1200 ml. of pancreatic secretions enter the duodenum daily and consist of:

Water (97 to 98 per cent)
Enzymes:
  amylase (amylolytic)
  amylopsin
  proteinases (proteolytic)
    trypsinogen (inactive trypsin)
    chymotrypsinogan (inactive chymotrypsin)
    procarboxypeptidase (inactive carboxypeptidase)
  lipase (lipolytic)
    steapsin
Salts: principal ones are sodium and potassium bicarbonate and sodium alkaline phosphate.

Because of the salts, the pancreatic secretion is alkaline, with a pH of 7.5 to 8.4, and neutralizes the acid chyme.

For the secretion and composition of bile, see page 578. Bile does not contain a digestive enzyme, but the bile salts do facilitate the digestion of fat by the pancreatic lipase.

Regulation of Pancreatic Enzyme and Bile Secretion. Pancreatic secretion into the intestine is regulated mainly by hormones secreted by the intestinal mucosa. The entrance of the acid solution chyme into the duodenum causes the release of secretin (prosecretin) into the blood. When secretin reaches the pancreas, it activates the cells to secrete a fluid high in sodium bicarbonate. Failure to produce this alkaline solution may result in damage to the duodenum by the chyme, which is strongly acid and contains pepsin. The duodenal mucosa is not as well protected by mucus as the gastric mucosa.

A second hormone cholecystokinin-pancreozymin (CCK), is also produced by the duodenal mucosa when food enters from the stomach. It is carried to the pancreas where it causes the cells to produce a thicker solution rich in enzymes. CCK also produces contractions of the gallbladder and enhances the action of secretin stimulating the alkaline pancreatic fluid. Secretion of CCK by the duodenal mucosa is stimulated by the presence of fatty acids and amino acids in the chyme.

Some control of pancreatic secretion is also exerted via the vagus nerve. It is suggested that this is part of the gastric reflex. Sensory impulses are initiated by food in the stomach and result in vagal stimulation of the pancreatic cells to produce enzymes.

The liver cells secrete bile continuously, but the amount is increased when food is taken, especially fat and protein. It is thought that the hormone secretin, which excites the pancreas, may also cause an increased output of bile. Probably the most effective mechanism is stimulation of the liver cells by bile salts. The bile salts are absorbed from the intestine and activate the liver cells to form bile. As noted above, CCK causes the gallbladder to contract and bile flows into the common bile duct. It also causes relaxation of the sphincter of Oddi, and bile that has been stored in the gallbladder enters the intestine. Bile salts are then available to be absorbed to stimulate the liver cells. In a fasting state, bile does not enter the duodenum and the secretion of bile is decreased.

INTESTINAL JUICE (SUCCUS ENTERICUS). The mucosa of the small intestine produces 2 to 3 liters of fluid per day. The solution, called succus entericus, is rich in bicarbonate, and the pH varies from 7.0 to 9.0, depending on the region of the intestine. The composition of succus entericus is:

Water
Salts
Mucin
Epithelial cells
Enzymes:
    enterokinase, which activates the trypsinogen and probably procarboxypeptidase
    erepsin
    lipase
    sucrase
    maltase
    lactase

Regulation of Small Intestinal Secretion. Several factors are said to influence intestinal secretion. The pressure of its content produces a direct effect on the mucosa which results in an increased amount of intestinal juice. A substance called gastric inhibitory peptide (GIP) that has been isolated from intestinal mucosa stimulates intestinal secretion, depresses gastric secretion and increases insulin secretion.[3] Secretion may also be influenced by the autonomic nervous system; parasympathetic innervation increases secretions, and sympathetic innervation decreases the output.

DIGESTION IN THE SMALL INTESTINE. Most chemical digestion takes place in the small intestine.

Any polysaccharides which have not been reduced by ptyalin to maltose are acted upon by the pancreatic enzyme amylase (amylopsin). Disaccharidases (enzymes) reduce disaccharides to monosaccharides by hydrolysis, producing the simple absorbable sugars glucose, galactose and fructose. The intestinal enzyme maltase hydrolyzes maltose, lactase splits lactose, and sucrase breaks down sucrose.

Protein digestion initiated in the stomach by pepsin is completed by several pancreatic and intestinal enzymes. Trypsinogen is activated in the intestine by enterokinase and is then known as trypsin. Chymotrypsinogen is converted to the active form chymotrypsin by trypsin, and procarboxypeptidase becomes active carboxypeptidase. The proteolytic enzymes trypsin, chymotrypsin, carboxypeptidase and intestinal erepsin reduce proteins (polypeptides) to simpler forms of peptides and then to absorbable amino acids.

The breakdown of fats into glycerol and fatty acids is done mainly by the pancreatic lipase, steapsin. The intestinal lipase is less effective. Fat digestion is greatly facilitated by bile which emulsifies the fat.

Motility, Secretion and Digestion in the Large Intestine

MOTILITY OF THE LARGE INTESTINE. Contractions of the muscular tissue in the large intestine mix and knead the content as well as move it through the large intestine toward the terminal portion. The mixing and kneading movements are performed in the ascending and transverse colons and facilitate the absorption of water.

Peristalsis in the colon occurs as a mass movement three or four times a day, moving the content toward the rectum. When the content reaches the distal portion of the colon, it is then moved into the rectum. As the food proceeded through the mouth, stomach and small intestine, a large amount of water was added to it. Much of this water is reclaimed by absorption in the colon which changes the consistency of the remaining content. The latter becomes a soft, solid mass referred to as feces.[4]

Peristaltic movements in the large intestine are reflexly stimulated by the entrance of food into the stomach. This gastrocolic reflex, as it is termed, is usually most evident after breakfast when the stomach has been empty for a longer period of time. It results in the feces being moved into the rectum, giving rise to the desire to defecate. Reflex stimulation originating with emotion, and distention or irritation of the colon, will also initiate movement.

Defecation is the term applied to the expulsion of feces from the rectum and has both an involuntary and voluntary phase. Normally, the rectum remains empty until just before defecation. When feces enter the rectum, the local distention and pressure give rise to sen-

---

[3]Ibid., p. 362.

[4]*Feces* is the Latin word for dregs.

sory impulses that initiate reflex impulses to the internal anal sphincter and to the muscle tissue of the sigmoid colon and the rectum. The sphincter relaxes and the muscle tissue contracts, moving the feces into the anal canal. The external anal sphincter is under voluntary control and must also relax for evacuation of the rectum. Defecation may be assisted voluntarily by contracting the abdominal muscles and by forceful expiration with the glottis closed to increase the intra-abdominal pressure.

If the defecation reflex is ignored and the external sphincter is kept closed, the defecation desire soon wanes. Eventually, with repeated ignoring of the defecation reflex, local stimulation by distention and pressure is lost. Feces accumulate in the rectum and lower colon, causing constipation.

Normally 8 to 10 hours are required for the chyme to pass through the small intestine and to reach the distal portion of the colon, where it accumulates until defecation. The content of the alimentary canal that is not absorbed may take 24 hours or longer to pass through the entire canal.

Fecal matter consists of unabsorbed food residue, mucus, digestive secretions (gastric, intestinal, pancreatic and liver), water and microorganisms. The water content is progressively reduced by absorption as the feces move through the large intestine so that, normally, on elimination the stool is a formed mass. If the feces are moved rapidly through the large intestine, less water is absorbed and the stool is unformed and liquid. If movement of the feces and elimination are delayed, an excessive amount of water is absorbed and the stool becomes hard and dry.

SECRETION AND DIGESTION IN THE LARGE INTESTINE. The large intestine has no role in digestion. It secretes a large amount of viscous alkaline mucus that lubricates the feces, facilitating their movement through the large bowel. The mucus also protects the mucosa from mechanical and chemical injury, and its alkalinity neutralizes acids formed by bacterial action, which is considerable in the colon.

Irritation of an area of the large intestine results in an increased output of mucus as well as an outpouring by the mucosa of large amounts of water and electrolytes in an effort to dilute and wash away the irritant. This causes the condition known as diarrhea (fre-quent liquid stools). The loss of fluid and electrolytes may cause dehydration and an electrolyte imbalance.

INTESTINAL MICROORGANISMS. Many microorganisms inhabit the intestine, and colon bacilli are present in large numbers. The tract is sterile at birth, but in a short time organisms which have been ingested with food are present in the intestine. These organisms are useful in that they synthesize vitamin K, which is essential to the production of prothrombin. A deficiency of vitamin K can result in uncontrollable hemorrhage. Intestinal bacteria also synthesize thiamine, riboflavin, and folic acid. The organisms normally found in the intestine are non-pathogenic to the tract but may cause disease if they are carried into other tissues.

Bacteria cause some fermentation and putrefaction of the intestinal content. The fermentation process breaks the content down into still simpler components and at the same time produces gas. The organisms may cause a breakdown of unabsorbed amino acids which may release poisonous substances such as histamine, indole, choline, ammonia, skatole and hydrogen sulfide. However, since this usually takes place in the large bowel, little of these toxic products are absorbed. If they are absorbed, the liver detoxifies them.

Absorption

Absorption is the movement of food, water, or drugs from the alimentary canal into the blood to make them available to the cells throughout the body. It is performed passively by the physicochemical processes of diffusion, osmosis and filtration or by active transport by the cells.

There are two channels by which food may be absorbed, the capillaries of the mucosa and the lacteals. Water, salts, glucose, amino acids and some fatty acids and glycerol are absorbed into the capillaries. The larger proportion of the products of fat digestion is absorbed into the lacteals.

Like digestion, most absorption takes place in the small intestine. Its surface is especially adapted by the many circular folds in the mucous membrane to increase the surface area. The whole surface is also studded with millions of villi which are the most important structures of absorption. The network of capillaries and the central lymph channel of each villus take up much of the digested food. Special epithelial cells of the villi are responsible for the active transport of materials across the membrane.

ABSORPTION IN THE MOUTH. No food is absorbed from the mouth, but a few drugs may be taken into the blood through the buccal mucosa. Examples of these are nitroglycerine and epinephrine.

ABSORPTION IN THE STOMACH. Absorption in the stomach is relatively negligible. The gastric mucosa does not actively transport food molecules across it but, if the concentration is high in the stomach (creating a considerable gradient between the blood and the stomach), glucose, water and electrolytes may be absorbed. Alcohol and some drugs are also absorbed from the stomach.

ABSORPTION IN THE SMALL INTESTINE. Minerals, vitamins, water, drugs, amino acids, simple sugars, fatty acids and glycerol are freely absorbed from the small intestine. Most absorption takes place in the upper part of the small intestine.

ABSORPTION IN THE COLON. Large amounts of water are absorbed in the colon. Approximately 500 ml. of fluid pass from the small intestine into the colon daily. About 400 ml. of water are absorbed from this, leaving 100 ml. to be excreted in the feces. Small amounts of glucose and salts are also absorbed by the large intestine, and a number of drugs may be administered by this channel.

ABSORPTION OF VITAMINS. The water-soluble vitamins B complex and C are generally readily absorbed from the small intestine. The exception is vitamin B_{12}. For absorption of B_{12}, a substance called the intrinsic factor is necessary and is secreted by the mucosa of the stomach. A deficiency of the intrinsic factor or of vitamin B_{12} causes a deficiency in the production of mature red blood cells.

The fat-soluble vitamins A, D, E and K are absorbed from the small intestine if bile salts and pancreatic lipase are present.

Fate of Foods in the Body

When food is absorbed it is taken from the blood by tissue cells. Some of it is used by the cells to meet the material requirements for the construction of tissue for growth and maintenance or for the production of substances such as hormones and enzymes. Much of the food is broken down to produce the energy required by the body to carry out its many functions. All cells require substances that furnish energy but, since those of different tissues vary in composition and function, the cells select materials to meet their special needs in respect to such differences. Glucose and fat are used mainly to supply energy, while requirements for cellular structure and chemical products are met principally by the amino acids and minerals.

When the foods are taken into the cells they undergo physical and chemical changes which comprise *metabolism*. When the cellular activity results in the synthesis of tissue substance, the process is referred to as *anabolism*, or anabolic metabolism. The processes that break down the materials into simpler forms and release energy are called *catabolism*, or catabolic metabolism.

FATE OF CARBOHYDRATES IN THE BODY. Carbohydrates are absorbed as glucose, fructose and galactose and are the main energy source. Fructose and most of the galactose are converted to glucose by the liver. Some galactose remains as such and is one of the components of the myelin sheath found around many nerve fibers. The sheath is a fatty, insulating membrane that prevents the loss of the nerve impulse.

Glucose may be oxidized by the cells to provide energy; it is temporarily stored as glycogen in the liver or muscles or converted to fat and stored as such. It is also used in small amounts in the synthesis of tissue substances and secretions and is circulated in the blood for a period of time, providing what is known as the blood sugar. If it is in excess, some may be excreted in the urine.

OXIDATION OF GLUCOSE. The oxidation of glucose by the cells to acquire energy is a complex process involving a series of many chemical reactions. Each reaction is catalyzed by a specific enzyme with the final end products being energy, water and carbon dioxide.

It is not the intent to give the details here of the biochemical reactions that take place in the oxidation of glucose. If such information is desired, the reader should consult a textbook of biochemistry or medical physiology. The catabolism of glucose involves two main processes, glycolysis and the citric acid cycle (Kreb's cycle or tricarboxylic acid cycle).

Glycolysis splits the glucose molecule into

two pyruvic acid molecules, at the same time releasing some energy. Ten successive chemical reactions are necessary to achieve glycolysis. The pyruvic acid molecules then embark on a series of chemical reactions which compose the citric acid cycle. Each of the ten chemical changes occurring in the citric acid cycle also requires a specific enzyme. The net result of the metabolism of one molecule of glucose is energy plus six molecules of carbon dioxide plus six molecules of water ($C_6H_{12}O_6 + 6O_2 \rightarrow E + 6CO_2 + 6H_2O$). Some of the energy that is released by the chemical reactions forms heat energy, and the remainder is stored in the cell as adenosine triphosphate (ATP). ATP is a compound with three phosphoric acid radicals; two of these radicals are connected to the compound by high energy bonds which can be split off readily when energy is needed by the cell to promote other chemical changes. If one phosphate radical is released, the compound is changed to adenosine diphosphate (ADP). As energy is released by other chemical reactions, the energy is used to bond the free phosphate radical to ADP and then to regenerate ATP. These energy changes go on continually with the chemical processes that constitute metabolism.

The glucose that is not needed to maintain a normal concentration in the blood or for immediate oxidation is converted by several chemical reactions and enzymes to glycogen and stored as such. Most of the glycogen is found in the muscle and liver cells. The muscle cells store it for their own use for contraction. The liver stores it and, as the blood concentration falls, converts the glycogen back to glucose and releases it into the blood. The process by which the glucose is converted to glycogen is known as *glycogenesis;* the reconversion of the glycogen to glucose is called *glycogenolysis*.

BLOOD SUGAR. The blood sugar concentration is relatively constant, the normal being 80 to 120 mg. per 100 ml. of blood. It may rise to 130 to 140 mg. per cent after a meal, but falls to normal within 2 or 3 hours. Maintenance of the blood sugar level within normal limits is especially important for normal functioning and survival of the brain cells. A concentration of at least 80 mg. per cent of glucose in the blood is necessary in order to meet the needs of the cells.

A deficiency in the blood sugar concentration is quickly manifested by central nervous system disturbances. The person may become confused and lose muscle coordination and strength. If the deficiency is severe, loss of consciousness may occur and unless corrected, death may ensue. If the brain cells are deprived of glucose for even a very few hours they may suffer permanent damage.

Hypoglycemia is the term given to a blood sugar concentration below the normal. If the concentration is above the normal, the condition is known as *hyperglcemia*.

Regulation of the Blood Sugar Concentration. Maintenance of the blood glucose within normal limits is done mainly by hormones. When the blood sugar concentration falls, the liver cells may be activated by two hormones, glucagon and epinephrine, to convert glycogen to glucose and release it into the blood. Glucagon is secreted by the pancreas when the blood sugar falls below the normal level. Epinephrine is secreted by the medulla of the adrenal glands. Sympathetic innervation to the adrenal glands is excited by a low blood sugar concentration, resulting in a release of epinephrine into the blood.

Insulin, a hormone secreted by cells in the islands of Langerhans of the pancreas, brings about a decrease in the blood sugar concentration by promoting the transport of glucose into the tissue cells. If the blood sugar level decreases toward or below the lower normal limits, there is a corresponding decrease in the secretion of insulin.

The adrenal cortex also secretes the hormones, glucocorticoids, that increase the blood sugar concentration. A decrease in the blood sugar stimulates the adenohypophysis (anterior pituitary gland) to release the adrenocorticotropic (ACTH) hormone which brings about the release of glucocorticoids. The increase in blood sugar is brought about by the glucocorticoids stimulating the liver cells to form glucose from noncarbohydrate substances. Protein and fats may be broken down and glycogen or glucose formed. This process may be referred to as glyconeogenesis or, if glucose is produced, as *gluconeogenesis*.

Similarly, the lowered blood sugar may cause the release of the thyroid-stimulating hormone (TSH) by the adenohypophysis and a resulting increase in the output of thyroxin, which promotes gluconeogenesis.

LIPOGENESIS. When the absorbed glucose exceeds what the cells use and what can be stored as glycogen, it may be converted to fat and stored in the fat depots of the body.

EXCRETION OF GLUCOSE BY THE KIDNEYS. As the blood flows through the kidney, much of the plasma and its solutes escape into the kidney tubules. Normally, all of the glucose that escapes is reabsorbed and the urine is sugar-free. If the blood sugar becomes abnormally high, not all the glucose is reabsorbed from the kidney tubule back into the blood; that rejected by the renal cells passes out into the urine. The level of blood sugar at which glucose is excreted in the urine is referred to as the *renal glucose threshold* and is approximately 160 to 165 mg. per cent, but this may vary with individuals. This excretion of the sugar, rather than its usual reabsorption, does reduce the blood sugar to some extent and is considered as a mechanism active in the regulation of the blood sugar.

FATE OF FATS IN THE BODY. Fatty acids and glycerol are absorbed into the lacteals of the villi and are combined in the process to form neutral fat. The absorbed fat is carried into the major lymph channels and reaches the blood through the thoracic lymphatic duct. Fats may be used by the body cells to provide energy, synthesize fat compounds or be stored as fatty tissue.

In the use of fats to provide energy, the neutral fat is first broken down by the liver into glycerol and fatty acids. The glycerol is converted to glycogen which is then converted to glucose.

The fatty acids are split by a series of chemical changes, mainly occurring in the liver. In each reaction, two carbon atoms and energy are freed in an oxidation process, finally ending up with acetoacetic acid and smaller amounts of beta-hydroxybutyric acid and acetone. These acids, because of their chemical structure, may be referred to as ketone acids or ketone bodies and the process by which they are formed is called *ketogenesis*. The ketones move out of the liver into the blood and are transported to the cells in need of energy where they are metabolized via the citric acid cycle, releasing energy and ending up as carbon dioxide and water. Although 1 gram of fat has more than twice as much energy value (9.3 calories) as does 1 gram of glucose (4.1 calories), as long as glucose is available to the cells, it is used in preference to fats.

The amount of ketones in the blood normally is very low and depends on a balance between the production by the liver and the assimilation by the tissue cells. Occasionally the rate of ketogenesis may exceed the rate at which the cells complete the metabolism, resulting in an accumulation of ketone acids in the blood and ketonuria. The condition is called ketosis and may occur when there is an increased use of endogenous fat for energy, as in starvation, or if there is a deficiency of glucose or a disturbance in the metabolism of glucose, as in diabetes mellitus. Ketosis may also develop with a diet high in fats (ketogenic diet).

Fat is necessary in the body for the formation of some essential fatty compounds such as phospholipids, lecithin, steroids and cholesterol. These compounds are built into other tissues. For example, phospholipids and cholesterol are necessary components of cell membranes,

The fat that is not used for energy or for the synthesis of certain tissue substances is stored as fatty tissue in areas of the body called the fat depots. Most of the fat is deposited in the subcutaneous tissue, in the abdomen, especially on the mesentery and omentum, around the kidneys and between the muscle fibers.

A certain amount of stored fat is of value. The subcutaneous fatty tissue insulates the body against an excessive heat loss and against the cold of the external environment. Fatty tissue also provides a protective cushion for the body against trauma.

Following a meal not all the absorbed fat may enter the liver. Some of it moves directly into the fat depots so that the concentration of fat in the blood is quickly lowered. The fat in the tissues is mobilized when it is needed for energy. There is a constant movement of fat in and out of the fatty tissue.

As with carbohydrate metabolism, certain hormones produced in the body may influence fat metabolism. Most of them increase fat mobilization and fat utilization by the cells. These hormones include the growth or somatotropic hormone secreted by the adenohypophysis, thyroxine, cortisone secreted by the adrenal cortices, and epinephrine released by the medulla of the adrenals. Insulin increases lipid synthesis and utilization. Estrogen secreted by the ovaries increases the deposition of fats in the tissues.

FATE OF PROTEIN IN THE BODY. The absorbed amino acids may be built into body tissue or used in the synthesis of cell products, such as enzymes and hormones, or the formation of protein compounds, such as plasma proteins. They may be converted to nonnitrogenous substances, such as carbohydrate or fat, which may be stored or oxidized to produce energy. From the large number of different amino acids, the cells select only those that they need to produce their particular type of protoplasm and cell products. Amino acids are very important to the child, whose protein requirement is more than twice that of the adult as he grows and amasses more tissue.

The amino acids that are not used by the cells for structure or cell products are taken into the liver where they may be stored or converted to a nonnitrogenous compound. By this means the liver prevents an excessive concentration of amino acids in the blood. Only a small amount can be stored but, when the blood concentration of amino acids falls, the liver releases the reserve.

Amino acids may be converted to glucose by the liver cells by a process called *deamination*. The amino radical is removed from the amino acid, forming ammonia. Since the ammonia would be toxic to tissue cells, it is combined with carbon dioxide to form urea. The urea is released from the liver into the general circulation and excreted by the kidneys.

The residual molecular elements of the amino acid are converted to glucose or fat and are oxidized to meet energy requirements. Normally, carbohydrate and fat provide the energy required by the cells. If these become deficient, protein is moved into the liver and is deaminized to meet the cells' energy needs. In starvation, this involves the use of blood proteins and tissue protein and deprives the cells of structural and functional amino acids. The cells' normal activities are disrupted and survival is threatened.

Some amino acids may be synthesized by the liver cells. The amino radical is removed from one amino acid and is attached to the molecule of a carbohydrate or a fatty acid. This process is called *transamination*.

Protein metabolism is influenced by certain hormones. The somatotropic (growth) hormone, thyroxine, and testosterone (male hormone) stimulate the use of protein in the synthesis of tissue and cell products. The glucocorticoids promote mobilization of amino acids into the blood from the cells and their conversion to glucose.

DISORDERS OF THE DIGESTIVE SYSTEM

Disorders of the digestive system are many and varied; they may interfere with the ingestion, digestion and/or absorption of food and fluids or with the elimination of residue. Any dysfunction threatens the well-being, functional capacity, and perhaps the survival of the person. The manifestations depend largely on the location of the disorder in the system as well as the nature of the etiologic factor. Different diseases may cause similar disorders of function — that is, several manifestation that develop are nonspecific.

Modern health education places much emphasis on nutrition, and any interference with the ability to take and retain food creates anxiety in the individual. The common knowledge of the high incidence of malignant disease in the gastrointestinal tract may cause considerable concern in anyone with any digestive upset. Fortunately, the digestive system has considerable reserve; parts of it may be removed and the patient, with some necessary adjustments in diet and living habits, may continue to live a useful life.

Frequently a disturbance of function in the alimentary tract is secondary to disease in another part of the body. For example, some disorders of the brain may be manifested first by vomiting or difficulty in swallowing. It may be a complaint of indigestion that brings the patient with primary anemia to the physician. Fatigue or emotional stress may be the basis of malfunctioning of the gastrointestinal tract and most of us at some time have experienced functional disturbance in the stomach or bowel during a period of anxiety or grief. Some persons have an autonomic nervous system that appears to be more sensitive than that of others and, as a result, readily experience some malfunctioning of the digestive system coincidental with some form of stress. The patient may worry about the symptoms, creating a nervous stress that contributes to perpetuating the dysfunction.

The patient whose medical investigation rules out organic and structural disease still requires the nurse's understanding sympathy and must be observed for emotional stress that may be the basis of his illness.

MANIFESTATIONS OF DISORDERS OF THE ALIMENTARY CANAL

Pain

Pain caused by a digestive disorder may be due to strong contractions of muscle tissue, stretching of a viscus, chemical or mechanical irritation of the mucosa, inflammation of the peritoneum, or direct irritation or pressure on associated nerves. It may occur in any part of the abdomen or in some instance is referred to a site remote from its origin. For example, pain arising from a peptic ulcer or from the biliary tract may be referred to an upper area of the back.

Heartburn is a form of pain that is described as a burning sensation felt behind the sternum. It is usually attributed to irritation of the esophageal mucosa by reflux of gastric acid fluid into the esophagus and may be accompanied by regurgitation of some stomach content into the mouth.

A patient may complain of a sense of fullness, especially after eating. Normally, the stomach relaxes and distends to accommodate food without increasing the intragastric pressure. This accommodation may not occur if there is a disease, such as carcinoma, or if the patient is in an anxious state.

Significant characteristics of the pain must be noted and recorded. Meaningful clues include the duration, location (see Fig. 16–3), and the nature and onset of the pain as described by the patient. Aggravating factors such as activity, the taking of food or medicine, or some specific experience or emotional stress may exist. Nausea, vomiting, flatulence and defecation associated with the pain are pertinent observations. The effect of pain on each individual varies and also varies with the cause and nature of the pain. For example, the patient experiencing gallstone or kidney stone colic writhes in agony while the patient with peritonitis or paralytic ileus tends to remain immobile. The patient is observed for such changes as restlessness, pallor, perspiration, weakness and changes in the vital signs.

Anorexia

Loss of appetite is a common complaint of patients with a digestive disorder but is also associated with disorders in practically all parts of the body. The individual may even express a revulsion to the odors of food. It may be functional in origin, resulting from an emotional upset. Persistent refusal of food due to psychological disturbance is referred to as anorexia nervosa.

Nausea and Vomiting

Nausea is an unpleasant sensation in which one has a feeling of discomfort in the region of the stomach and the inclination to vomit.

Vomiting is the ejection of the gastric contents through the mouth and is usually preceded by nausea and hypersalivation. There may be nausea without vomiting, and vomiting may occasionally occur without being preceded by nausea. The involuntary muscular activity that precedes or accompanies vomiting is referred to as retching.

Nausea and vomiting are very common symptoms and are seen in a great variety of conditions. They can be manifestations of a digestive dysfunction or they may accompany practically any acute illness or stress situation. The nurse is frequently called upon to comfort and support a patient who is vomiting and to make pertinent observations which may prove significant to the physician in making a diagnosis and planning treatment.

The vomiting process is initiated by a vomiting or emetic center in the medulla oblongata. This center may be excited by sensory impulses originating in the stomach or intestines, by impulses of psychic origin when fright, unpleasant sights, odors or severe pain are experienced, or by impulses from a group of neurons referred to as the chemoreceptor trigger zone in the floor of the fourth ventricle. The cells in the trigger zone are sensitive to certain chemicals in the blood and to impulses from the portion of the internal ear concerned with equilibrium. Vomiting in motion sickness, radiation therapy, toxemia and with the taking of certain drugs such as apomorphine and digitalis results from impulses that arise from the chemoreceptor trigger

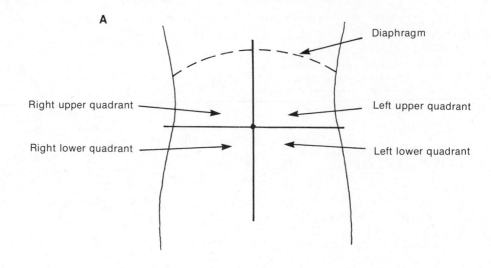

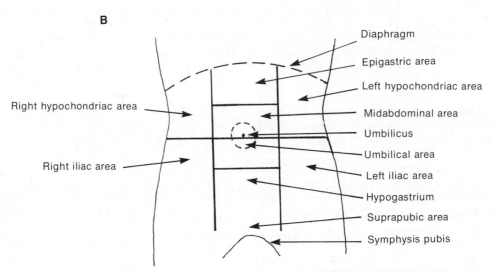

FIGURE 16–3 *A* and *B,* Abdominal areas. *C,* Abdominal structures located in each abdominal quadrant.

zone. The sensitivity of the vomiting center varies in different individuals; some vomit very readily and with little effort while others are not affected even though the stimulus may be similar and of equal intensity.

The impulses discharged by the vomiting center result in a quick, deep inspiration followed by closure of the glottis and epiglottis, closure of the nasopharynx by elevation of the soft palate, and relaxation of the esophagus, cardiac sphincter and stomach. Vigorous contraction of the diaphragm and abdominal muscles increases intra-abdominal pressure which forces the gastric content up through the relaxed esophagus and the mouth. The stomach plays a passive role.

One should be alert to the possible effects of vomiting, regardless of its cause. Considerable muscular energy can be expended in frequent vomiting and may result in exhaustion.

Obviously, nausea and vomiting interfere with normal nutrition and, if prolonged, malnutrition and loss of weight and strength occur. The reduced intake and loss of fluid may rapidly lead to dehydration. Loss of gastric secretion may deplete the body electrolytes and cause acid-base imbalance. Acidosis may develop as the patient becomes dependent on his body fat as a source of energy. The patient may complain of abdominal soreness from the retching and muscular

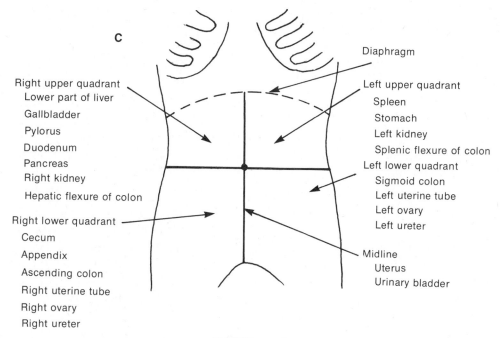

C

Right upper quadrant
  Lower part of liver
  Gallbladder
  Pylorus
  Duodenum
  Pancreas
  Right kidney
  Hepatic flexure of colon

Right lower quadrant
  Cecum
  Appendix
  Ascending colon
  Right uterine tube
  Right ovary
  Right ureter

Diaphragm

Left upper quadrant
  Spleen
  Stomach
  Left kidney
  Splenic flexure of colon
Left lower quadrant
  Sigmoid colon
  Left uterine tube
  Left ovary
  Left ureter

Midline
  Uterus
  Urinary bladder

FIGURE 16–3C.

effort and may become extremely worried about his condition, which may further aggravate the disturbance.

The patient who is nauseated and is vomiting, regardless of the cause, requires the following *nursing considerations*.

SUPPORTIVE MEASURES. Sympathetic attention and understanding can mean a great deal to the patient. Remaining with him to hold his head or a painful site, holding the basin, cleansing his mouth and lips, and making sincere efforts to relieve the discomfort provide some support. Positioning should facilitate drainage of the vomitus from the mouth to prevent possible aspiration. Encouraging the patient to take several deep breaths may help to reduce nausea and offset vomiting.

OBSERVATIONS. The following factors should be noted: (1) whether the vomiting was preceded by nausea; (2) whether there was retching or the vomitus was regurgitated without effort; (3) the quantity, consistency, color, content and frequency of the emesis; (4) the time of day; (5) any association with the ingestion of food or drugs; and (6) the effect on the patient (e.g., fluid balance, exhaustion).

FOOD AND FLUIDS. Oral intake is usually withheld for a period of time and is resumed gradually in small amounts. If the vomiting is due to local irritation, it may be helpful to have the patient take a whole glass of water to "wash out" the stomach. If vomiting is prolonged, an intravenous infusion of fluids may be necessary to prevent or correct dehydration and replace electrolytes.

HYGIENIC MEASURES. The mouth is rinsed after each emesis and the basin emptied promptly. Soiled bedding and clothing should be changed and the room ventilated. The odor or sight of vomitus may contribute to the patient's discomfort and may cause repetitive vomiting. The patient may be reassured by having a clean basin always within reach, but it is less suggestive if covered with a clean towel.

ENVIRONMENT. Rest, quiet and a minimum of disturbance may reduce the incidence of vomiting. Nausea tends to increase with motion; any change of position should be made slowly. Subdued lighting may reduce external stimuli and be conducive to rest.

PSYCHOLOGICAL CARE. Since worry or fear can perpetuate nausea and vomiting, the patient is encouraged to verbalize his concerns. Problems may come to light which may be explained or solved. For example, he may be anxious about a home situation that could be cared for by the social or welfare service. The care must be individualized; what may prove helpful with one person may not be tolerated by another.

MEDICATION. An antiemetic or a sedative may be prescribed. Diazepam (Valium) or flurazepam (Dalmane) may be administered orally or parenterally for sedation. Dimenhydrinate (Dramamine or Gravol) and meclizine hydrochloride (Novicalm) are examples of antiemetics which may be used.

If the vomiting continues, gastric drainage by means of a nasogastric tube may be established (see p. 499).

Regurgitation

Ejection of small amounts of chyme or gastric secretion through the esophagus into the mouth without the vomiting mechanism being employed is referred to as regurgitation. It may occur owing to some incompetency of the esophageal-gastric (cardiac) sphicter, as seen in infants, or it may be a symptom of organic disease.

Bleeding from the Gastrointestinal Tract

Bleeding in the alimentary canal may be manifested by the vomiting of blood (hematemesis), by melena, which is the passage of a black, tarry stool containing blood pigments, or by the passage of frank blood from the bowel. Hematemesis and melena occur as a result of bleeding in the upper digestive tract. The characteristic black tarry appearance of the stool is due to the effect of the digestive enzymes on the blood. Frank blood in the stool usually originates with bleeding in the colon, rectum or anal canal.

It may be necessary in some instances to examine the blood that has been ejected through the mouth to determine whether it has been coughed up (hemoptysis) or vomited. Blood from the respiratory tract is a brighter red and frothy because of the contained air; that from the stomach is usually darker and may contain small clots and food particles.

Melena may be so slight that it goes unrec-

ognized unless a stool specimen is submitted for laboratory examination for occult blood.

The most frequent cause of hematemesis and melena is peptic ulcer, but esophageal varices, carcinoma, injuries or a blood dyscrasia may account for the bleeding in other cases. Any evidence of bleeding should be promptly reported to the physician. The patient who has hematemesis or tarry stool is put at rest and his blood pressure, pulse, respirations, color and general state (e.g., strength and consciousness) are checked.

Bleeding from the lower part of the tract may be due to a newgrowth, ulcerative colitis, hemorrhoids or an anorectal fissure. The patient is advised to see a physician immediately for early diagnosis and treatment.

Dysphagia and Odynophagia

Dysphagia is defined as difficulty in swallowing. The patient may be able to swallow soft foods and liquids but may be unable to take firmer, more solid foods. Others may be able to swallow but complain of pain on doing so which may be referred to as odynophagia.

Dysphagia may be due to mechanical obstruction, dysfunction in the neuromuscular structures involved in swallowing or to diseases of the mouth, pharynx or larynx. Pain associated with swallowing frequently indicates an organic lesion such as an ulcer due to acid reflux from the stomach.

Loss of Weight and Strength

Obviously, if food cannot be taken, digested or absorbed, body tissue cells are deprived of their requirements for normal functioning. Body stores and actual tissue are mobilized to meet the needs, but eventually these may be depleted. The patient manifests loss of weight, strength and efficiency.

If the problem is related to a specific food, symptoms characteristic of a lack of that particular food will appear. For example, effects of a protein deficiency include muscle wasting, weakness, hypoalbuminemia, edema, anemia and, in the child, retarded growth and development. If there is a disturbance in the absorption of vitamin K due to a lack of bile salts in the intestine, the deficiency may be manifested by bleeding, since prothrombin, necessary for blood coagulation, will not be produced by the liver.

Changes in the Mouth

Changes in the mouth may be of local origin or may be associated with digestive or general disorders. Disturbances may take the form of a coated or furry tongue, dryness, soreness, small ulcers (aphthous ulcers) and halitosis. Changes due to local conditions may be caused by inflammation, infection, neoplastic disease or injury of the tongue, buccal mucosa or lips. Any sore that does not heal in 2 weeks should be investigated.

Flatulence

Flatulence is an excessive amount of gas in the gastrointestinal tract. The patient may complain of a "full, bloated feeling," pressure or actual pain. The abdomen may be distended and the patient may eructate gas from the stomach through the mouth or may expel gas (flatus) from the bowel. Excessive gas in the stomach or bowel is frequently due to swallowed air. Aerophagia, or the unconscious swallowing of air, may be seen in nervous persons and in patients who are nauseated or experiencing some digestive stress. It is sometimes helpful to advise patients to make a conscious effort to avoid the swallowing or to hold something such as a wooden or plastic applicator between their teeth.

Excessive gas in the intestines may result from the ingestion of excessive amounts of gas-forming foods (cabbage, turnips, onions, etc.) or from abnormal fermentation of the food due to bacterial action. Flatulence and distention occur with any obstruction in the tract and with paralysis of peristalsis.

Borborygmi (singular, borborygmus) is a term applied to the sounds made by the movement of a gas and fluid mixture in the intestines that are loud enough to be heard by the patient and others close by. The sound can be a significant observation, especially where there is some question of obstruction. The sounds do occur in the normal alimentary tract on occasion.

Abdominal Rigidity

Rigidity of any area of the abdominal wall due to excessively tense muscle tone may be evident in patients with disease of the gastrointestinal tract. The muscle contraction is usually a response to irritation of an underlying structure. This symptom is usually noted by palpation of the abdomen when examining the patient.

Change in the Normal Pattern of Bowel Elimination

A disorder of the intestine may cause a retarded or an accelerated movement of contents through the intestine. Delayed movement may cause *constipation* characterized by infrequent, hard, dry stools or may result in a complete failure of the passage of feces which is referred to as *obstipation.* Acceleration of the content causes *diarrhea,* which is frequent liquid or unformed stools. The person who experiences any persistent change in his normal pattern of bowel elimination should consult a physician.

For a discussion on constipation and diarrhea see page 538.

Hiccup (Hiccough, Singultus)

Persisting hiccups or frequent attacks of hiccups may be associated with organic disease of the digestive system. They are caused by intermittent spasms of the diaphragm due to gastric distention, irritation of the phrenic nerve or a metabolic disorder such as uremia or toxemia which affects the central nervous system. The frequency of the attacks and the effect of the hiccups on the patient should be noted. Dehydration, acid-base imbalance and malnutrition may develop, since hiccups may interfere with the taking of fluids and food. Disturbed rest and the expenditure of muscular energy may cause exhaustion. In many instances, the patient becomes fearful because of the persistence of the condition.

Jaundice

An excessive concentration of bilirubin in the blood causes a yellow discoloration of the sclerae, skin and mucous membranes. It is commonly associated with liver disease (liver cell jaundice), obstruction to the flow of bile through the biliary ducts (obstructive jaundice), and a rapid increase in the destruction of red blood cells which frees bilirubin more rapidly than the liver cells can excrete it in bile (hemolytic jaundice). In obstructive jaundice, the flow of bile may be impeded in the intrahepatic ducts, as in hepatitis (inflammation of the liver) or the obstruction may be in the extrahepatic ducts. The latter is most frequently caused by gallstones in the duct or by a neoplasm which constricts the biliary tract and may be situated in the upper gastrointestinal tract (e.g., duodenum).

ASSESSMENT AND DIAGNOSTIC PROCEDURES IN DISORDERS OF THE DIGESTIVE SYSTEM

Physical Examination

Examination of the patient with a disorder of the alimentary canal includes *inspection* and *palpation,* and *auscultation* and *percussion* if an abdominal area is involved.

ORAL CAVITY AND LIPS. A tongue depressor and light are needed to examine the oral cavity and tongue for lesions, sordes, dehydration, bleeding and discolored areas (e.g., leukoplakia; see p. 509). Whether or not the tongue is coated or is abnormally smooth is noted. The condition of the teeth and gums (gingivae) are also checked. The odor of the breath is noted to determine if it is offensive or is characteristic of that associated with a specific condition. For example, the odor of acetone may be associated with acidosis or starvation, that of urea with renal insufficiency and that of alcohol with alcoholism.

The lips are scrutinized for lesions (e.g., lumps, cracks, blisters, ulcers), dryness and abnormal color and palpated if necessary to determine the presence and extent of a mass.

ABDOMEN. Examination of the abdomen requires the patient to lie on his back with arms at his sides, a pillow under his head and knees flexed. The latter promote relaxation of the abdominal muscles. The patient is protected from unnecessary exposure and chilling and is advised of what is to take place.

The surface is inspected for contour, distention, discolored areas or unusual pigmentation, masses, striae, and symmetry. The umbilicus is observed for eversion or displacement from the midline. The abdomen is examined for movement; peristaltic waves are not normally visible and, if seen, usually indicate intestinal obstruction, especially if

associated with some distention. Prominent, dilated veins which may indicate obstruction of the portal circulation as a result of liver disease and pulsation of an artery are recorded. The latter might be due to an aortic aneurysm. Rarely, an excessive amount of hair may be encountered and is usually associated with an adrenocortical disturbance.

In palpation of the abdomen, a very light pressure is used at first using the palmar surfaces of the fingers which are extended and together. A superficial mass, which may be distended viscera, areas of tenderness and resistance offered by abdominal muscles may be detected. If tenderness is elicited by gentle palpation over McBurney's point,[5] appendicitis is suspected (Fig. 16–2A). Rebound tenderness following the abrupt release of palpation pressure on the abdominal wall is associated with peritoneal inflammation.

When the entire abdomen has been palpated superficially, deep palpation may be used to identify deeper-lying tenderness and to obtain information as to the size and mobility of a mass and the enlargement or position of an organ (e.g., locating the lower border of the liver and determining if the spleen is enlarged). Normally, the lower edge of the liver lies just above the lower right costal margin. If it extends below, it is enlarged. Normally, only the lower tip of the spleen is palpable but if it is enlarged it is readily identified by deep palpation.

Auscultation of the abdomen is used to assess peristalsis by listening for bowel sounds. One should listen for a period of 5 minutes, since normal peristaltic activity occurs at intervals of 5 to 15 seconds in the small intestine. An absence of bowel sounds occurs in peritonitis and paralytic ileus (see p. 545). Excessive activity may occur in an area in an effort to overcome an obstruction. Palpation or movement of a part may produce a splashing sound (succussion), indicating fluid and air within.

Abnormal vascular sounds (bruits) may also be detected by abdominal auscultation. For example, an aortic aneurysm or a tortuous vessel compressed by a tumor or enlarged viscus produces a bruit.

Percussion is most often used to determine

---

[5]*McBurney's point* lies in the lower right quadrant approximately two inches from the right anterior spine of the ilium and corresponds to the area in which the appendix is usually located.

the presence of gas or air in the intestine, detect urinary bladder distention or identify the location and size of solid viscera. The fingers of one hand are placed on the abdomen while the fingers of the other hand are used to tap the second finger. A hollow resonant sound (tympany) is heard if there is gas; a dull, flat sound reflects density or solid tissue such as liver, spleen or newgrowth.

Except for the mouth, which is readily accessible to viewing and palpation, diagnosis of disorders of the digestive system are rarely made without the assistance of various investigative procedures. These include the following tests.

Blood Studies

LEUKOCYTE COUNT. An increase in the number of white blood cells (leukocytosis), particularly neutrophils, may indicate infection and an acute inflammatory process. This test is of significance in conditions such as appendicitis, acute enteritis, colitis and acute gallbladder disease (cholecystitis). Normal: 5000 to 10,000 per cu. mm.

ERYTHROCYTE COUNT, HEMOGLOBIN CONCENTRATION AND HEMATOCRIT. A deficiency in the number of red blood cells and in the amount of hemoglobin may indicate the loss of blood or nutritional deficiency and provide information as to the patient's condition. Normal: erythrocytes, $4\frac{1}{2}$ to 5 million per cu. mm.; hemoglobin, 12 to 16 Gm. per 100 ml.

The hematocrit may be determined to indicate the volume percentage of erythrocytes. Normal: hematocrit, males, 45 to 50 per cent; females, 40 to 45 per cent.

BLEEDING TIME AND PROTHROMBIN TIME. These are especially important if there are indications of hemorrhage. An increase in either predisposes the individual to a greater loss of blood. Normal: bleeding time, 2 to 5 minutes; prothrombin time, 12 to 20 seconds.

Roentgenography and Fluoroscopy

Radiologic examination is a very valuable procedure in diagnosing disorders of the digestive system, particularly those of the alimentary canal. A radiopaque substance, barium sulfate, may be given by mouth ("barium swallow or barium meal"), and flu-oroscopic studies are made and x-ray pictures taken as it passes through the esophagus, stomach and intestines. The rate at which it moves through the tract and outlines of the various parts are studied. When the barium is followed by a series of x-rays taken at intervals of several hours the procedure may be referred to as a gastrointestinal x-ray series.

The patient who is to have a barium swallow usually has a light evening meal and then nothing but sips of water until several hours after he has received the barium the next morning. As soon as the radiologist indicates that the patient may have a meal, it should be served promptly. The patient may be very tired and may be experiencing weakness and discomfort because of the lack of food.

Following the taking of the barium, and when the first studies of the series are completed, the patient is offered a mouthwash, since the barium is chalky and clings to the oral mucosa. When the series is completed, which may be the day after the barium was administered, the physician should be consulted as to whether a cleansing enema or a laxative is to be given to clear the tract of the barium. Otherwise it tends to cause constipation, fecal impaction and considerable discomfort.

X-ray examination of the large intestine and rectum is done by giving an enema of the barium solution. The lower bowel has been emptied previously by the administration of a laxative and a cleansing enema. Specific directions as to which laxative and enema solution are to be used and the time they are to be administered should be received from the x-ray department or the attending physician. Food will probably be withheld for 18 to 24 hours preceding the barium enema, but the patient is allowed fluids.

The patient receives an explanation as to why the food is withheld. Also, he is advised as to what will happen when he goes to the x-ray department and the importance of his retaining the barium until the necessary studies and films are made.

The barium enema is given in the x-ray room, and its progress through the rectum and colon are observed by fluoroscopy. X-ray films are also made to be studied later. Provision is made for the expelling of the enema, and then more films are made. A mild laxative is usually prescribed to insure complete elimination of residual barium.

Endoscopy

The recent introduction of the fiberoptic endoscopes has made it possible to view the esophagus, stomach, duodenum, colon and rectum more thoroughly. Their flexibility facilitates passage of the endoscope and more efficient examination, with much less trauma and discomfort for the patient. Two bundles of flexible, very fine glass fibers are carried in the shaft. One bundle transmits light which illuminates the organ being viewed, and the second transmits an image back to the operator. A tube in the shaft makes it possible to inflate the area being viewed, eradicating folds so that the complete surface may be seen. A camera may be attached for taking pictures of a lesion or of an area that requires further study.

ESOPHAGOSCOPY AND GASTROSCOPY. The esophagus may be examined and a biopsy specimen obtained by *esophagoscopy* if the patient has complained of dysphagia, gastric reflux or regurgitation, or hematemesis. Esophagoscopy is useful in localizing bleeding and is also used to remove a foreign body or a bolus that has lodged in the esophagus.

Gastroscopy is usually used to obtain more detailed information about a lesion (e.g., ulcer) that has been identified as being present by previous barium x-ray. A biopsy is taken and pictures may be made of the lesion. It may also be used to assess the healing of an ulcer.

The improvement in endoscopic instruments has made it possible in some instances to arrest hemorrhage by the direct application of electrocautery or a hemostatic preparation to the bleeding site.

The gastroscope may be passed through the pylorus to examine the duodenum. The ampulla of Vater may be cannulated and viewed, and a radiopaque dye injected to demonstrate the pancreatic and common bile ducts (cholangiopancreatograph). Endoscopic examination may also be extended into the jejunum.

NURSING CARE IN ESOPHAGOSCOPY AND GASTROSCOPY. Preparation for either of these diagnostic procedures should begin with an explanation to the patient of what to expect. The physician may have described the examination and its values, but the patient will most likely still have questions. The nurse should have sufficient understanding of the procedure to be able to answer the patient's questions judiciously.

The patient is advised that he will be taken to the special treatment room or to the operating room for the examination. A written consent for the procedure is obtained. The esophagus and the stomach must be completely empty. No food or fluid is given for 6 to 8 hours before the procedure. In gastroscopy, the physician may request a gastric lavage to be done several hours before the examination in patients in whom some pyloric obstruction is suspected. Dentures and jewelry are removed and, in the case of the female, the hair is confined under a turban, or if it is long, it should be braided. Adults usually receive a sedative such as meperidine (Demerol), morphine or a barbiturate preparation 30 minutes to 1 hour before the scheduled time. Atropine may also be ordered. The patient empties his bladder before leaving his room to avoid such need during the examination.

The pharyngeal area is sprayed with a local anesthetic before the gastroscope or esophagoscope is introduced. A general anesthetic may be given in the case of a child or, rarely, it may be used for a nervous adult in order to get better relaxation. A nurse remains beside the patient to give reassurance and support during the procedure and to assist with positioning. In esophagoscopy, the patient's head and shoulders are extended over the head of the table. In gastroscopy, a lateral position is used.

Following the examination, the patient is allowed to rest. All food and fluids are withheld until the effect of the local anesthetic has worn off and the gag reflex returns (usually 4 to 6 hours). Before giving any fluid, the reflex may be tested by genty touching the back of the throat with an applicator or spoon. The patient may complain of a sore throat or soreness in midchest. Warm fluids may be soothing and may provide some relief. Any expectoration or vomiting of blood or severe pain should be reported promptly to the physician.

COLONOSCOPY. The flexible fiberoptic colonoscope has made possible the visualization of the complete colon, the taking of a biopsy and pictures of a lesion and the removal of polyps.

NURSING CARE IN COLONOSCOPY. The patient is advised of the purpose of the examination and what to expect and is asked to sign a statement giving consent. The bowel must be absolutely clean. The patient is usually admitted 3 days before the colonoscopy and kept on clear fluids. Castor oil is given the day before and tap water enemas given early on the day of the examination until the return flow is clear.

An alternative method of cleansing the gastrointestinal tract that may be prescribed is the giving of a saline lavage.[6] The day before the colonoscopy, a duodenal tube is passed and 1 liter of a specially prepared solution of potassium chloride, sodium chloride and sodium bicarbonate is given (via the duodenal tube) every 4 hours until 4 to 5 liters are given. No food is taken after 4 hours before the lavage is begun. The patient may have water to drink if he wishes. The physicians who prescribe this method of cleansing the bowel before a colonoscopy consider it efficient and less distressing for the patient than castor oil purgation. The patient does not have to be hospitalized for as long a preexamination period, and food is restricted for a shorter period.

The patient is told that it will be helpful during the examination to take deep breaths with his mouth slightly open and to relax the abdominal muscles. Sedation (meperidine hydrochloride or diazepam) is given 30 minutes to 1 hour before the scheduled colonoscopy; a general anesthetic is not given because the patient is requested to indicate pain during the examination. The patient is usually placed in the recumbent position on his left side and the nurse remains at the patient's head, providing necessary support.

Following the colonoscopy, the patient is allowed to rest and receives food and fluids. The patient is observed for signs of bleeding, pain and abdominal tenderness and rigidity. If polyps were removed, a specific directive is received from the physician as to the patient's diet. The intake may be restricted to fluids for a period of time, and then a low-residue diet is gradually introduced.

SIGMOIDOSCOPY AND PROCTOSCOPY. A direct examination of the anal canal, the rec-

tum and the sigmoid colon may be made by means of a sigmoidoscope. Proctoscopy is direct viewing of the rectum and anal canal by means of a proctoscope.

NURSING CARE IN SIGMOIDOSCOPY AND PROCTOSCOPY. These examinations may be performed in the doctor's office or in the ward treatment room of the hospital. A tissue specimen (biopsy) may also be obtained at the same time.

An explanation of the procedure is given to the patient in which he is advised of the position that he will be required to assume. The knee-chest and the left lateral are the positions commonly used. The lower bowel should be empty; cleansing enemas are usually given 2 to 3 hours before the scheduled time. A low-residue diet may be prescribed for the preceding day. The patient is usually required to provide a written consent.

A nurse remains with the patient to assist with the positioning and provide support. Unnecessary exposure should be avoided by adequate drapes. In the knee-chest position the patient lies face down and draws his knees up so that his weight is borne by the chest and knees. The feet are extended over the end of the table, arms at the sides or at sides of the head, and the head is turned to one side. In the left lateral or Sims' position the lower limbs are flexed, with the right one being drawn up further than the left. Suction is made available to remove any secretion or fluid feces that interfere with visualization of the bowel mucosa.

After the examination, the anal region is cleansed and the patient is allowed to rest. The nurse may be responsible for seeing that the tissue specimen is placed in the appropriate container, correctly labelled and delivered to the pathology laboratory.

CHOLECYSTOGRAPHY. Radiography is also used in the diagnosis of gallbladder disease and may be referred to as cholecystography. A radiopaque organic iodine compound (e.g., Telepaque or Cholografin) that is eliminated in the bile is given orally or intravenously. The patient is allowed a fat-free evening meal which is followed by the administration of the "dye" the night before the x-ray examination. Then, only water is allowed until after the first x-ray. The iodine compound is absorbed, secreted by the liver cells in the bile and, normally, concentrated in the gallbladder, since there was no fat in

[6]Arnold G. Levy, et al.: "Saline Lavage: A Rapid, Effective and Acceptable Method for Cleansing the Gastrointestinal Tract." Gastroenterology, Vol. 70, No. 2 (Feb. 1976), pp. 157–161.

the meal to stimulate the emptying of the gallbladder.

An x-ray film is taken in the morning (approximately 12 hours after the "dye" was given) to determine if the gallbladder has filled. Calculi may be observed if present.

Following this first film, the patient is given a meal containing fat. A rich eggnog or thickly buttered toast and an egg may be used. After 1 hour, a final roentgenogram is taken. Normally, after a fatty meal, the gallbladder contracts and empties bile into the small intestine via the common bile duct.

To summarize, cholecystography provides information as to whether the gallbladder fills and empties and whether it contains gallstones.

Gastric Secretory Tests

Common gastric function tests used in the investigation of patients with symptoms of gastrointestinal disease include the measurement of the volume of secretions over a stated period and the determination of hydrochloric acid (HCl) secretion under basal conditions and then in response to a gastric stimulant. Gastric analysis in which a quantitative estimation is required involves the use of a nasogastric tube to aspirate the gastric contents. If the test is done only to determine whether HCl is being secreted or not, aspiration of the gastric contents is unnecessary.

ANALYSIS OF GASTRIC CONTENTS. A fasting period of 8 to 10 hours precedes the test. A tube is passed into the stomach and the gastric content is aspirated by a syringe. The volume of this aspirate is noted, recorded and labelled for determination of the acid concentration.

Following this initial specimen, the directions may be to aspirate the gastric secretion at intervals of 15 minutes for 1 hour. Each specimen is placed in a separate tube and numbered according to the order in which it is collected. These specimens provide information about the *basal secretory activity*[7] of the stomach.

Usually, this fractional analysis procedure to evaluate secretory function includes the parenteral administration of a secretory stimulant such as histamine phosphate (subcutaneously), betazole hydrochloride (Histalog, subcutaneously), pentagastrin (intramuscularly), or insulin (subcutaneously). The drug is administered after the initial aspiration. Aspiration specimens are then collected at intervals of 15 minutes for one hour.

If histamine is the choice of the physician, an antihistamine preparation may be administered ½ hour before the histamine is given to offset the undesirable effects of the drug. Histamine is not used if there is a history of allergy or asthma. The patient is observed closely for possible toxic effects. If he complains of dizziness or weakness, or manifests local irritation at the site of the injection, flushing of the face or pallor, sweating, dyspnea or a rapid weak pulse, the physician is notified at once. A severe drop in blood pressure may occur and the patient may develop shock. Epinephrine should be readily available for prompt administration in case of a reaction.

If insulin is used as a secretory stimulant, the patient is observed closely for signs of hypoglycemia (insulin shock). Complaints of nervousness, hunger pains, weakness or faintness or signs of cold, clammy perspiration should be reported promptly. The physician may start an intravenous infusion of normal saline before the insulin is given so that 50 per cent glucose may be given without delay if hypoglycemia develops.

The normal basal gastric secretion is 30 to 70 ml. per hour and the HCl production 1 to 2.5 mEq. per hour. The normal maximum acid output in response to a secretory stimulant is 15 to 25 mEq. per hour.[8]

Achlorhydria indicates a deficiency in the gastric secretion of HCl. The term is applied when the pH of the gastric content is less than 6 following the administration of a secretory stimulant. Achlorhydria may be associated with cancer of the stomach, chronic gastritis, gastric ulcer or pernicious anemia.

Hyperchlorhydria is a term used to describe an excessive secretion of HCl. An increase in acid secretion is seen in duodenal ulcer and the Zollinger-Ellison syndrome.

DIAGNEX BLUE TEST (TUBELESS GASTRIC TEST). A simpler test than that using

---

[7]*Basal secretion* is the secretion produced during a fasting period and in which the patient has received no secretory stimulant.

[8]P. B. Beeson and W. McDermott: Textbook of Medicine, 14th ed. Philadelphia, W. B. Saunders, 1975, p. 1889.

aspirated specimens may be used to determine if the patient is achlorhydric. Neither volume nor acidity of the secretions is quantified in this test.

After a fasting period of 8 to 10 hours, the patient receives caffeine sodium benzoate and carbacrylic resin with azure A dye (Diagnex Blue, azuresin) and water. The patient voids just before the drugs are given and then again in 2 hours to provide a urine specimen to be examined for the azure dye.

The caffeine sodium benzoate stimulates the gastric parietal cells to secrete hydrochloric acid. The acid frees the dye from the resin, allowing it to be absorbed. It is then excreted from the blood in the urine. Unless there is acid to react with the carbacrylic resin compound, the dye remains bound to the resin which is nonabsorbable from the digestive tract. The presence of dye in the urine indicates the secretion of hydrochloric acid in the stomach. The concentration of the dye corresponds to the amount of acid released. If the urine is negative for the dye, it is attributed to achlorhydria.

NIGHTLY GASTRIC ASPIRATION. When the patient has some pyloric obstruction, the doctor may order a nightly aspiration. The patient receives his prescribed diet during the day; then, at about 10 P.M. his stomach content is aspirated and measured. The amount of food residue and secretions in the stomach at this time gives the physician information as to the severity of the obstruction. It also relieves the patient of the sense of fullness, pain and discomfort resulting from the over-distended stomach and prevents vomiting.

ANALYSIS OF GASTRIC CONTENT OR VOMITUS. Examination of a specimen of vomitus or aspirated gastric content may be made to detect the presence of blood, bile or organisms (e.g., tubercle bacillus).

Stool Examination

A stool specimen may be examined in the investigation of disorders of the digestive system for blood, urobilinogen, parasites, organisms or specific food residue. A small amount of stool is removed on a tongue depressor to the appropriate container (a waxed cardboard container with a lid). If the examination is for parasites, the specimen is kept warm and must be delivered to the laboratory promptly. If it is to determine the presence of occult

blood, red meat is not included in the patient's diet for the 24 hours preceding the stool collection. If an enema is necessary to obtain a stool specimen, the solution used is clear water or normal saline.

When anything unusual is noted about a patient's stool, such as the presence of blood, excessive mucus or parasites, the stool should be kept until it is seen by the doctor.

Peritoneoscopy (Laparoscopy)

Rarely, an endoscope is introduced into the peritoneal cavity to examine its contents. A small area of the abdominal wall is surgically prepared as for any surgery, a local anesthetic is introduced into the abdominal tissue and a small incision is then made through which the laparoscope is passed. The procedure is performed under strict surgical asepsis. A biopsy or a specimen of fluid may be obtained.

Following the examination, the wound is surgically dressed and the patient is observed for signs of bleeding or visceral trauma.

Exfoliative Cytology

In this test cells shed from the gastric mucosa are examined to determine if they are normal or manifest malignant changes. The cells are obtained by lavaging the stomach through a gastric tube (e.g., Levin tube) with normal saline. The patient is required to fast for the 6 to 8 hours preceding the lavage. The volume of lavage solution is indicated by the physician or laboratory. All the aspirate is sent for analysis.

NURSING IN DISORDERS OF THE DIGESTIVE SYSTEM

Gastric and Intestinal Intubation

The investigation or treatment of many medical and surgical patients may include the passage of a tube into the stomach or small intestine via the nose or mouth and the esophagus. The purpose may be to withdraw fluid from the stomach or intestine for analysis, to remove fluid and gas (decompression of the stomach or intestine), to wash out the stomach (gastric lavage), to apply cold or pressure to the walls of the esophagus, stomach or small intestine, or to administer feedings or drugs.

TYPES OF TUBES. Many different tubes are encountered and the type used varies with the purpose. The composition varies and the tube may have one or two lumens and may have a small inflatable bag attached at the distal end. Longer tubes are necessary for intestinal intubation. The following are commonly used (see Fig. 16–4).

LEVIN TUBE. This tube has a single lumen with several openings at the distal end and is used for gastric intubation.

REHFUSS TUBE. The Rehfuss tube has only one lumen which terminates in a small metal bulb with vertical slits. It is used for the aspiration of gastric or duodenal secretions.

STOMACH PUMP OR EWALD TUBE. This large tube has a bulb incorporated into the proximal portion for the purpose of producing suction. It is introduced through the mouth into the stomach and is used to withdraw larger volumes of gastric content quickly and to wash out the stomach. See Fig. 16–5.

MILLER-ABBOTT TUBE. The Miller-Abbott tube used for intestinal intubation is quite long and has two lumens. One lumen serves to aspirate intestinal fluid and gas, and the other opens into a small rubber bag which is inflated after the tube is passed. The balloon causes pressure which stimulates intestinal motility. In some instances, mercury is used in the balloon instead of air; its weight facilitates the movement of the tube through the pylorus and along the intestine.

The inlets at the proximal end must be clearly marked to indicate which lumen is for drainage and which is kept clamped off to maintain the inflation of the balloon. The tube is marked off in centimeters so the distance it has passed may be determined.

CANTOR TUBE. The Cantor tube is used for intestinal aspiration. It has a small rubber bag at its distal end which contains 5 to 10 cc. of Hg. The lumen of the tube is sealed off at its junction with the bag, and the openings that permit aspiration are above the bag.

HARRIS TUBE. This tube is smaller than the Cantor tube but resembles it in that it has a single lumen and a bag containing mercury attached below the holes. In both the Cantor and Harris tubes the mercury is introduced into the balloons before intubation by a syringe and needle. The mercury will not escape through the fine needle hole.

SALEM TUBE. This is a double lumen sump tube. One lumen is for drainage and is connected to suction; the second lumen is open to the air and serves to prevent the negative pressure from becoming excessive when the gastric mucosa is sucked into the drainage openings of the primary lumen. This offsets possible traumatic effects to the mucosa.

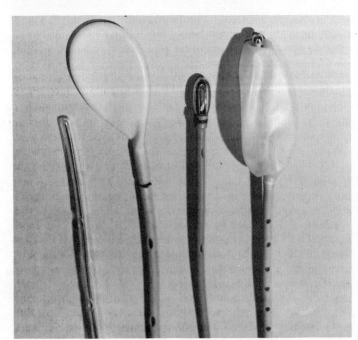

FIGURE 16–4 Tubes that are used in gastric and intestinal intubation. From left to right: Levin tube, Cantor tube, Rehfuss tube, and Miller-Abbott tube. (Courtesy of the New Sinai Hospital, Toronto.)

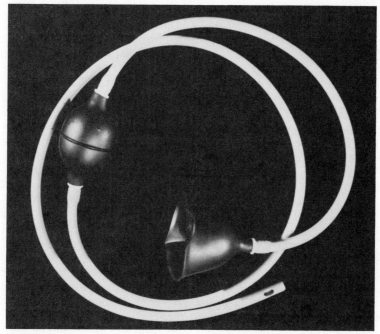

FIGURE 16–5   The stomach pump or Ewald tube. (Courtesy of the New Mount Sinai Hospital, Toronto.)

NURSING RESPONSIBILITIES. Suction may be applied intermittently or continuously for aspiration of gastric or intestinal contents. The suction may be provided by a syringe for the purpose of collecting specimens or for occasional aspiration of a small amount. More frequent or continuous suction may be provided by the Wangensteen setup in which suction is created by water displacement or by a small electric pump at the patient's bedside. The electric suction apparatus may be set for intermittent or continuous suctioning. Piped suction from a central source may be available through a wall outlet with a valve and gauge by which the amount of suction is controlled.

Gastrointestinal suctioning must be gentle; the amount of suction or pull exerted is kept low to avoid drawing the soft tissue structures to the openings which would obstruct drainage and possibly damage the tissues.

Following gastric surgery, aspiration may be achieved by applying suction to a gastrostomy tube. A catheter with several side openings is inserted into the stomach through an abdominal incision and secured by sutures. This method of aspiration eliminates the discomfort and irritation associated with a na-sogastric tube that is necessary for several days.

ASSISTING WITH THE INSERTION OF THE TUBE.   An explanation of the treatment is made to the patient. This includes the purpose and what may be expected both during and following the insertion of the tube. He is advised that the insertion will be easier and quicker if he relaxes, breathes deeply through his mouth and swallows when instructed to do so to advance the tube.

The tube, if rubber, is chilled in a bowl of ice chips so it is stiffer and less likely to curl up; it is lubricated with a water-soluble jelly. If the tube is too stiff it is immersed in warm water.

The distance from the patient's ear lobe to the bridge of his nose and from this point to the xiphoid process provides a fairly close estimate of the length of tube required to reach the stomach.

The head of the bed is elevated, and the patient's head is hyperextended during the initial introduction of the tube through a naris or the mouth. When the patient is asked to swallow, the head is slightly flexed to the more natural position for swallowing. The tube is gently pushed downward as the patient swallows, but it should not be advanced faster than the swallowing or it will curl up in the pharynx and cause gagging. The patient may be allowed sips of water to make the swallowing easier.

To make sure the tube is in the esophagus and not in the trachea, the proximal end may be submerged in water; bubbles will appear as the patient exhales if the tube is in the trachea. Or the patient may be asked to speak or hum, which is not possible if the tube is in the larynx.

In intestinal intubation, when the tube reaches the stomach the patient is required to assume various positions to promote its passage through the pylorus and the duodenum. The usual procedure is to place the patient on his right side for 1 to 2 hours, and then on his back with the head of the bed elevated for 1 to 2 hours. Advancement of the tube may be followed by fluoroscopy, and suggestions are made as to the desirable positioning of the patient. When the Miller-Abbott tube is used, the physician may inflate the balloon when it reaches the stomach on the basis that it simulates a food mass and stimulates motility to carry it through the pylorus. In other instances, the balloon may not be inflated until the tube has passed into the duodenum.

SECURING THE TUBE. The tube is secured to the face with narrow strips of nonallergenic adhesive when it has been advanced to the desired position if it is to be left in place for several hours or days. It must be checked several times daily for security, and the skin is examined for possible irritation from the adhesive.

If the tube is attached to a drainage bottle, it should be supported in a "trough" made in the bottom sheet or by a tape or towel pinned to the bedding to prevent tension on the nasogastric tube. The connecting tube should be long enough to prevent displacement of the gastrointestinal tube and to permit free movement of the patient in bed.

MOUTH AND NOSE CARE. The patient usually experiences considerable discomfort from the tube being in the nose and throat and from the dryness due to mouth breathing and restricted oral intake. The mouth should be cleansed and rinsed frequently. Normal cleansing of the teeth is encouraged and need not interfere with the nasogastric tube. Petroleum jelly, face cream or oil may be applied to the lips. Chewing gum may be permitted to stimulate salivary secretion and small sips of water may be allowed in some instances.

The nostril may become irritated and secretions accumulate and encrust. It should be gently cleansed with a swab moistened in water or normal saline and a light application of water-soluble jelly or mineral oil made.

Turning the patient hourly helps to shift the tube sufficiently to relieve constant pressure on one area of the throat. Throat lozenges may be ordered to lessen throat irritation.

MAINTENANCE OF DRAINAGE. After the tube is in place and connected to the suction apparatus, it is necessary to check the system at frequent intervals for functioning. Mechanical failure of the apparatus might occur, or drainage may be interrupted by a blocking of the tube by mucus or a blood clot and could result in pain, vomiting, or serious distention of the stomach or intestine. The surgeon may order the tube to be irrigated by syringe at regular intervals or only if it is blocked. The solution and volume to be used for irrigating are specifically stated. After injection of the solution, some of the fluid may be aspirated using the syringe to determine if the tube is clear. The amounts of solution injected and aspirated are accurately measured and recorded on the fluid balance sheet.

The characteristics of the drainage fluid are noted and the total volume is recorded every 8 to 12 hours. The volume is an important factor in determining the fluid and electrolyte replacement needed. Loss of gastric secretions incurs a loss of hydrogen and chlorine ions (HCl) that may result in alkalosis. Loss of intestinal fluid may result in a severe loss of bicarbonate (HCO_3^-) and potassium and cause acidosis. The bottle is washed each time it is emptied as well as the connecting tubing.

REMOVAL OF THE TUBE. Before removal, the tube may be clamped and left in place while oral fluid is introduced. If the fluid is tolerated, an order may then be given to remove the tube. The gastric tube is withdrawn gently and quickly. The patient is instructed to hold his breath to avoid possible aspiration of fluid or mucus that may escape from the tube into the oropharynx during removal.

The intestinal tube is removed slowly, a few inches at a time. The lumen into the air-inflated balloon is opened, and the air is allowed to escape. When slight resistance is encountered owing to the intestinal peristalsis, the tube is left for a few minutes and then withdrawal is resumed. The physician should be notified if resistance to removal persists; force should not be used. If the tube has a mercury-filled bag at its distal end, the latter is brought out through the mouth and the bag removed. The remainder of the tube may then be pulled through the nostril. As with the removal of the gastric tube, the patient is asked to hold his breath as the terminal portion of the tube is drawn from the esophagus.

The mouth should be cleansed and rinsed immediately following the removal of the tube. The patient may complain of some soreness in the throat and nose which usually subsides in a day or two.

Gastric Gavage

When a patient is unable to take fluid and foods by mouth, a nasogastric tube (usually the Levin) may be passed through which a specially prepared solution of essential nutrients is introduced directly into the stomach. This method of feeding a patient may be referred to as gastric gavage or tube feeding. The nurse assists with the intubation as described on page 501. The tube may be left in place, but should be removed every 5 to 6 days, thoroughly cleaned and reinserted through the other naris. With infants and young children the tube is inserted prior to each feeding. When the tube is to be left in place, it is secured to the patient's face with narrow strips of adhesive.

The physician indicates the specific feeding to be used to meet the patient's nutritional needs. Various feedings are used. The foods of a normal diet may be liquefied in a blender and given, or a protein supplement and vitamins may be added to a mixture of eggs, milk and orange juice. For information as to the component, nutrients, amounts and preparation of feedings, the reader is referred to recent publications on diet therapy.[9]

The prescribed amount of solution is warmed (100 to 105° F., 38 to 40° C.) in a water bath and brought to the bedside on a clean tray with a container of approximately 70 to 80 ml. of water and the barrel of an Asepto

syringe. If this is the initial feeding, an explanation of the procedure is given to the patient. The head of the bed is elevated and 30 to 40 ml. of water is introduced into the tube to determine its patency.

The feeding is administered slowly and allowed to flow into the stomach by gravity. To avoid air entering the stomach, the funnel is not allowed to empty completely until all the fluid is given. When the feeding is completed, the tube is cleansed by rinsing it with 30 to 40 ml. of water and is then clamped. If regurgitation or vomiting occurs, it may be that the prescribed volume is too great. A smaller amount given more frequently may be tolerated.

Frequent mouth care is necessary and the nostril through which the tube passes requires attention.

For removal of the tube see page 502.

Gastrostomy

This is the surgical establishment of an opening into the stomach through the abdominal wall and the insertion of a tube through which fluids and liquefied food may be introduced directly into the stomach.

Before the gastrostomy, the procedure is discussed with the patient so he understands the purpose of the surgery and what is entailed postoperatively. The patient's written consent and the usual preoperative preparation for abdominal surgery are necessary. General or local anesthesia is used and a small incision made in the abdominal wall and stomach. A large catheter (No. 20 or 22F) is inserted into the stomach and secured by sutures put through the tissues and the tube. In some instances, a Foley catheter is used and a purse string suture used around it. The layers of tissue are then closed around the tube.

A gastrostomy may be a temporary procedure during a period of corrective surgery or it may be permanent when an esophageal obstruction is considered inoperable or there has been an esophagectomy.

The patient generally finds it difficult to accept a gastrostomy. He is denied the natural process of eating and its associated pleasures such as taste and sociability. Personnel caring for the patient, the family and friends should acknowledge to the patient that they understand his concern and tendency to withdraw. An effort is made to find interests for

[9]Sue Rodwell Williams: Nutrition and Diet Therapy, 3rd ed. St. Louis, C. V. Mosby, 1977.

the patient and to treat him as normally as possible.

For the first day or two postoperatively, water or a glucose solution in prescribed amounts is given through the tube; then, regular feedings are given according to the physician's orders. The food preparations used in gastrostomy are similar to those cited above for gastric gavage or are regular foods put through a blender. The required amount of feeding is warmed and given through a funnel or the barrel of a syringe attached to the gastric tube. The patient's head and shoulders are elevated and he remains in this position for ½ hour after the feeding to prevent regurgitation into the esophagus and leakage around the tube. The tube is cleansed following the feeding by rinsing it with 30 to 40 ml. of water and is then clamped.

A gauze dressing is applied to the wound following inspection of the skin for excoriation. The escape of even a small amount of gastric juice from around the tube may irritate the skin because of its acid-pepsin content. The dressing is changed whenever there is drainage, and the skin is cleansed thoroughly with soap and water and dried. A protective coating of petroleum jelly or a prescribed ointment or powder is then applied.

The feedings may have to be adjusted from time to time. Too much fat or carbohydrate may cause diarrhea. Complaints of a full feeling or abdominal discomfort may necessitate a decrease in the amount of feeding given. A record of the patient's weight is made which also serves as a guide in adjusting the caloric value of the feeding formula.

The tube is removed in approximately 1 to 2 weeks when the opening (stoma) and the channel through the layers of tissue are well established and healing has sealed off the peritoneal cavity. The tube is reinserted for each feeding and the stoma covered with a small dressing pad between feedings. A shorter tube with a flange that holds the tube in place is available for a permanent stoma. The tube also has a screw cap that seals the tube off between feedings.

Since the feedings correspond to the patient's meals, meticulous care should be used in relation to the equipment and to the preparation and administration. Such considerations as a clean, fresh towel covering the tray and clean equipment free of stains may lessen the patient's aversion to this unnatural method of taking his meal. When the patient receives blender feedings, he may feel more hopeful and "less different" if advised he is receiving foods included in a normal diet. Strict privacy should be provided during the feeding as the patient is sensitive.

The patient's mouth will require special attention. Frequent cleansing and rinsing are essential. Some satisfaction may be derived from the taking of various fluids (e.g., fruit juice), retaining them in the mouth for a brief period and then expectorating them. The physician may encourage the patient to take foods which he desires, masticate them and then expectorate the bolus. These measures help to keep the mouth in better condition, stimulate gastric secretion and may provide some satisfaction through taste for the patient.

If the patient is to be fed by gastrostomy over a long period while various stages of treatment are carried out or if the gastrostomy is permanent, he is taught to feed himself. Instruction is given to the patient and a member of the family in the preparation of the feeding and the care of the stoma. Financial assistance may be necessary to provide a blender or prescribed commercial feeding preparations. The nurse may direct the family to the appropriate community resources for the necessary assistance or make the contact for them.

Intravenous Alimentation (Total Parenteral Nutrition; Hyperalimentation)

Intravenous alimentation is the infusion, into a large central vein, of solutions of amino acids, glucose, electrolytes, trace amounts of essential minerals, vitamins, and lipids (fat emulsions) in sufficient concentrations to meet individual requirements for normal metabolism, tissue maintenance and energy demands.[10]

Intravenous alimentation may be used with patients who: (1) are unable or unwilling to take nutrition orally or receive it by gavage; (2) are unconscious for a prolonged period; (3)

---

[10]The *electrolytes* included in the solutions are sodium, potassium, chlorine, calcium, magnesium and phosphate. The *minerals* essential in trace amounts are iron, copper, cobalt, zinc, iodine, manganese and chromium.

have a condition such as Crohn's disease or a bowel fistula that requires that the intestinal tract be given a rest; (4) have had a massive intestinal resection which may have been necessitated by a mesenteric thrombosis or a volvulus; or (5) are in a hypercatabolic state, in which body tissue is broken down and a negative nitrogen balance results (e.g., burns). In the case of an intestinal resection, if only a part of the small intestine is removed, intravenous alimentation is used while the remaining small bowel adapts and increases its absorption of food to compensate for the section removed. If there is insufficient absorptive area left (total intestinal resection), the hyperalimentation procedure becomes the permanent means by which the individual receives nutrition.

PROCEDURE. In most hospitals in which intravenous alimentation is used, a hyperalimentation team is specially prepared to start and supervise these complex intravenous infusions. A physician of the team inserts the catheter, and only a physician or a nurse of the team changes the dressing, tubing and filters, puts up the solutions and makes certain frequent observations.

Strict surgical asepsis is mandatory throughout the insertion of the catheter, when handling the solutions and tubes, and when caring for the "wound" (site of insertion). Infection causes a serious problem; the alimentation line serves as an excellent culture medium and, since it leads directly into the blood, bacterial invasion will cause septicemia.

PREPARATION OF THE PATIENT. If the patient is conscious, and especially if total parenteral nutrition is to be prolonged or permanent, he and his family receive a detailed explanation of the procedure, its purpose and subsequent care. They are encouraged to ask questions and time is taken to answer them. They may require assurance that the patient will be able to eat normally after a period of being fed this way.

The site of insertion is shaved and cleansed first with acetone to remove fatty secretion and then with a strong antiseptic (e.g., povidone-iodine) and alcohol.

INSERTION OF CATHETER. The alimentation solution is infused into a large, valveless intrathoracic vein; a plastic vascular catheter is usually passed via an internal jugular vein or subclavian vein into the superior vena cava. It is necessary to use a large vein since highly concentrated (hypertonic) solutions are likely to cause severe phlebitis in smaller peripheral veins. When the solution is dripped into a large vein it is rapidly diluted in the large volume of blood and osmolality of the plasma is therefore not notably increased.

If the condition permits, the patient is positioned for a brief period with the head lower than the rest of his body; this distends the neck and upper intrathoracic vessels which facilitates the passage of the catheter.

A sterile field around the site of insertion is provided by the application of sterile drapes and the physician and assistants wear sterile gloves. They, as well as the patient, wear masks to prevent airborne contamination by mouth and nose organisms. A local anesthetic is used in the area to be punctured and a large needle is passed into the subclavian or internal jugular vein. Entry into the subclavian vein is made just below the clavicle (subclavicular) which provides greater freedom of movement for the patient's neck and arms. A small intravascular catheter is threaded through the needle and advanced into the superior vena cava. The needle is withdrawn and an isotonic solution attached for infusion. The physician may suture the catheter to the skin at the site of insertion to prevent dislodgement or movement of the tube in and out. The site is cleansed of any blood and dried, and an air-occlusive dressing is applied. The latter is sealed and secured by the application of tincture of benzoin to its edges. A chest x-ray is taken before infusion of the alimentation solution to determine the position of the catheter.

SOLUTIONS. The solutions used to provide total parenteral nutrition are very concentrated and are prescribed individually. They are contained in collapsible plastic bags to avoid possible air embolism.

The infusion tube which is attached to the catheter when not connected to a solution flask is sealed with a sterile cap. The frequency with which the intravenous tubing and/or filter(s) are changed is indicated by the physician. If contamination occurs or is even suspected, a physician or nurse of the hyperalimentation team is notified and the tubing is changed. All tubing changes are made quickly to reduce air entry and the risk of embolism. The patient lies flat and is asked to perform the Valsalva maneuver.[11] The infusion line may contain one or two micropore filters. Some physicians omit a filter on the basis that organisms may collect and multiply in the filter, thus increasing the risk of infection. Tubing connections are always reinforced with adhesive to insure maintenance of an intact line.

A specific directive is received from the physician as to the rate of flow of the solution. *The rate must be kept constant* for maximum benefit. If the infusion is too rapid, glucose is not metabolized rapidly enough to maintain a normal blood sugar level. The latter is likely to exceed the glucose renal threshold and glucose is excreted in the urine, taking with it essential water and electrolytes. The rate of flow (drops per minute) is checked frequently since the rate of a gravity drip may vary with changes in the patient's position.

Only the prescribed alimentation solutions are administered through the catheter into the superior vena cava. *No medications* (e.g., antibiotic, digoxin), *plasma,* or *other solutions* are given via the alimentation venous line. Also, the alimentation intravenous line must not be used for drawing blood for specimens. To maintain the patency of the tube a prescribed solution of heparin is introduced into the tube following the administration of the solutions.

DRESSING.   The dressing is changed at intervals specified by the physician; this varies from daily to every 5 days. Strict aseptic technique similar to that cited for the insertion of the catheter is observed. The "soiled" dressing is removed with forceps and the area cleansed with acetone and a strong antiseptic (e.g., povidone-iodine) and alcohol. There may be an order to apply Betadine ointment before placing the clean gauze dressing to the area. Caution is necessary to avoid dislodging the catheter. The edges of the dressing are sealed with tincture of benzoin and then an air-occlusive dressing is provided by the application of Elastoplast or adhesive tape.

If the dressing becomes moist or soiled, it is promptly reported and changed. If the patient is receiving respiratory humidification therapy (e.g., humidified oxygen), the area is sealed off and protected by plastic.

MOUTH CARE.   Regular, frequent cleaning of the teeth followed by a mouthwash is very important. The lack of oral food and fluid intake causes discomfort and favors the growth of organisms present in the mouth, producing sordes, inflammation and tooth cavities. If the intravenous alimentation is prolonged or permanent, the patient may be permitted hard candy or sugarless gum, or a small amount of food which he chews and then expectorates. Some patients may be able to take small amounts of clear fluids or specified nutrients if their gastrointestinal tract is intact.

OBSERVATIONS.   The following observations are very important.

The patient's blood pressure, pulse, respirations and color are recorded frequently following the insertion of the catheter.

Any complaint of pain or tightness in the chest or change in level of responses is reported promptly. It may be associated with an air embolism or a pneumothorax or hemothorax.

The temperature, pulse and respirations are recorded two to four times daily. An elevation of temperature and increased pulse rate may indicate infection.

A urine specimen is examined every 6 hours for sugar and acetone. Blood specimens are submitted at stated intervals for determination of glucose, urea and serum electrolyte levels. Hyperglycemia may develop, necessitating the administration of regular insulin.

Blood cultures are done and checked for fungi as well as bacteria.

The patient's weight is recorded daily. The intake and output are recorded and the fluid balance noted.

The site of insertion is examined carefully each time the dressing is changed for inflammation, edema, sloughing or purulent discharge.

PSYCHOLOGICAL SUPPORT.   The patient receiving total parenteral nutrition for a prolonged period requires psychological support; he feels "very different." Repeated explanations of the purpose and value of the feedings are necessary. As he gradually acquires an understanding of the procedure, it becomes more acceptable. When his condition permits, ambulation and "doing things"

---

[11]The *Valsalva maneuver* involves a forcible expiratory effort against a closed glottis. This increases intrathoracic pressure and reduces the possibility of air entering the circulatory system.

contribute to a reduction in concern. The patient is encouraged when advised of his weight gain.

ELIMINATION. Bowel elimination decreases and the patient may worry about this. He is advised that nothing enters the tract; a small cleansing enema may be prescribed every few days for some patients to remove mucus and secretions.

DISCONTINUING INTRAVENOUS ALIMENTATION. The solutions are reduced gradually to prevent a sudden fall in blood glucose. When the alimentation solutions are withdrawn, a solution of glucose 5% is infused over several hours before the physician removes the catheter. Oral intake is gradually increased.

INSTRUCTION FOR PERMANENT INTRAVENOUS ALIMENTATION. If this method of receiving nutrition is to be permanent, the family and patient are prepared for his discharge from the hospital. They are taught how to put up the solutions, the maintenance of asepsis, indications of problems (e.g., symptoms of infection), care of the site of catheter insertion, and how often the tube is changed and by whom. They are advised of the necessary supplies and how they are obtained. The patient is also taught to test his urine for glucose and acetone and to make a daily record of his weight.

The patient is not discharged until he has demonstrated efficient self-care. A member of the hyperalimentation team provides the instruction and follows the patient at home.

Gastric Hypothermia

A continuous internal application of cold is rarely used to treat gastric hemorrhage.

The stomach is first lavaged with ice water or saline to remove the gastric content and blood clots in order that the cold may be brought in more direct contact with the stomach wall. This is also necessary to prevent overdistention of the stomach when the cooling bag is inflated. The large Ewald tube is then removed and replaced with a double lumen tube with a large distensible bag resembling the shape of the stomach that is inflated with a cold solution. One lumen is used as an inflow tube to the bag, and the other as an outflow.

A 50 per cent mixture of alcohol and water is cooled to 0° C. and approximately 600 ml. is introduced slowly into the bag. The inflow and outflow lumens are connected to a cooling reservoir in a refrigerating machine. The solution is continually circulated through the closed system by means of a pump. The inflated bag applies pressure as well as cold to the site of the bleeding.

A nasogastric tube may be inserted along with the cooling tube to maintain gastric decompression and provide information as to the bleeding.

The treatment may be continued for as long as 48 hours. The bag is gradually deflated and the tube left in place for a period of time in case bleeding starts again.

An electric warming blanket set low is used to maintain body temperature and keep the patient comfortably warm. The rectal temperature is recorded at frequent intervals. The pulse and blood pressure will be observed closely because of the hemorrhage; pulse irregularity may develop as a result of the proximity of the cold tube to the heart and should be reported promptly.

MOUTH AND SALIVARY GLAND DISORDERS

Disorders of the mouth and contained structures are numerous and, as cited previously, may be of local origin or may be secondary to disease elsewhere in the digestive system or in some other system. Primary lesions may be due to bacterial, viral or fungal infection, chemical irritation, congenital malformation, injury or neoplastic disease. General diseases frequently accompanied by a mouth disorder include vitamin B complex or C deficiency, blood dyscrasias, metallic medication intoxication, infectious disease and any condition that interferes with the normal fluid and food intake or salivary secretion.

Predisposing factors in mouth lesions are debilitation, poor dietary habits, poor oral and dental hygiene, dehydration, emotional stress and mouth breathing.

The mouth is concerned with mastication, swallowing food and fluids and with speech production. Saliva is secreted into the mouth, changing the consistency of food and facilitating swallowing. It also expedites speech. A healthy oral mucosa is moist, intact and of a dark pink color. Healthy gums (gingivae) are a lighter pink and firm and fit closely to the teeth, forming papillae to fill the interdental spaces. The tongue, a light pink, is moist and has minute papillae on the superior surface. A slight white "fur" may be present, particularly in the morning.

Assessment and Signs of Mouth and Salivary Gland Disorders

EXAMINATION OF THE ORAL CAVITY. The condition of the mouth is checked in all patients since it provides information relating to the general condition as well as exposes any local lesions. A tongue depressor and flashlight are used to inspect: (1) the lips, tongue and oral mucosa for color, lesions and moisture; (2) the gums for excessive redness, soft puffiness and recession; (3) the teeth for jaggedness and caries; and (4) the accumulation of offensive secretions (sordes). The pharynx is also checked for inflammation and purulent secretions.

Observation of the mouth may elicit significant information as to the patient's state of hydration and nutrition as well as manifestations of systemic disease and local disorders. The tongue and mouth are the first sites to reflect dehydration; the mouth and tongue become dry and the latter becomes furred. Bleeding of the gums may indicate a deficiency of vitamin C or an infection. Excessive salivation (sialorrhea) may be associated with a vitamin B deficiency, certain medications or a newgrowth in the mouth or esophagus.

MANIFESTATIONS OF A MOUTH DISORDER. The patient may complain of discomfort, especially when taking food, and as a result rejects adequate nutrition. There may be a palpable mass or a swollen area evident within the oral cavity or on the external surface. Bleeding of the gums or from a lesion may be present. An offensive breath may indicate sordes or infection. Excessive salivation or dryness and/or disagreeable taste may be present. The individual may experience difficulty with clear speech or with swallowing.

Only a few of the more common disorders are presented here.

Stomatitis

This is a term applied to inflammation of the oral mucosa. In some instances, it may involve the gums, angles of the mouth or the lips.

The *causes* are numerous, and include excessive smoking, dental sepsis, dehydration, vitamin deficiency, blood dyscrasia such as primary anemia and leukemia, local or systemic infection and a sensitivity to certain foods or drugs. The mucosa is very red and tender and ulcerative areas may develop.

HERPETIC STOMATITIS. This condition is also known as *aphthous stomatitis* or *ulcerative stomatitis*. The lesion may occur singly or in crops on the mucosa of the mouth or on the tongue. It is commonly referred to as a *canker sore* and appears first as a small, sore inflamed area, followed by vesicle formation. The vesicle ruptures, leaving an ulcer which usually heals in a few days. The condition is painful and the patient complains of a burning sensation.

Frequent attacks of multiple lesions can be very distressing to the patient and may interfere with food intake. Treatment is usually on an empirical basis; what may be effective for one patient may not be so with another. Since herpetic stomatitis is usually secondary to some other disorder (e.g., inflammatory intestinal disease, vitamin B_{12} deficiency), it tends to be recurrent. Various diagnostic procedures may be necessary before the primary cause is identified.

Local therapeutic measures are mainly palliative and are aimed at relief of the discomfort, prevention of infection and promotion of healing of the ulcers. Caustic agents such as silver nitrate should not be applied to the lesions as they only increase the erosion of tissue. A mild mouthwash such as sodium bicarbonate is used. Vitamin B complex and vitamin C may be prescribed. Local applications of cortisone in the form of an ointment or as a pellet may be used. A preparation commonly used is betamethasone disodium phosphate (Betnesol, Celestone) in pellet form; each tablet contains 0.1 to 0.2 mg. of cortisone. The pellet is held in the mouth as near the ulcers as possible. The physician may also suggest some form of analgesic lozenge to relieve the discomfort. Bland foods and fluids, not too hot, are taken.

In stubborn cases, typhoid and/or smallpox vaccine may be given to increase the patient's viral resistance.

Thrush (Moniliasis)

Thrush is caused by the fungus *Candida albicans* and may also be referred to as *candidiasis*. It occurs most frequently in infants and children and in the very old, but may also appear in debilitated persons. Occasionally, it follows prolonged use of certain antibacterial drugs such as tetracycline (Achromycin) and chloramphenicol (Chloromycetin). Areas of superficial ulceration occur in the oral mucosa or gums, and the membrane over the lesion becomes white and is easily detached. The lesions respond to local application of 1 per cent gentian violet or to an antifungal antibiotic solution such as nystatin (Mycostatin). Attention is also directed to the patient's diet in an effort to improve his resistance and general condition.

Herpes simplex (Herpes labialis)

This condition is commonly called *fever blisters* or *cold sores* and occurs on the lips or skin surrounding the lips. It is due to a virus that is harbored by the cells in this region in a dormant state, the primary invasion having occurred early in life. Fever and a lowered resistance predispose to the viral activity. The lesion appears as a small inflamed area which develops a vesicle that ruptures, leaving a superficial ulcer that forms a dry crust. There may be one or several lesions and they most frequently occur with acute respiratory infections or exposure to sun and temperature changes. There is no specific treatment, but an ointment may be prescribed to soften the crust to prevent cracking and bleeding.

Vincent's Angina (Trench Mouth)

This is an inflammation of the gums (gingivitis) followed by ulceration and necrosis. It is thought to be caused by proliferation of specific fusiform bacilli and spirochetes which are present in only small numbers in normal mouths.

The gums are swollen and painful and bleed readily. Excessive salivary secretion and an offensive breath are usually present. There is a loss of marginal gum tissue and of the interdental papillae by the ulceration and necrosis. Lesions may develop on the buccal and pharyngeal mucosa. A smear may be made from the affected area to confirm the diagnosis. Predisposing factors are poor oral and dental hygiene, malnutrition and debilitation. It may be associated with infections, mononucleosis, alcoholism or a blood dyscrasia.

Mouthwashes are given frequently; a solution of hydrogen peroxide, saline or sodium perborate may be used. An antibiotic by parenteral administration is prescribed and may be supplemented by topical administration. The patient will require instrumentative treatment by a dentist as soon as the acute stage is over.

The condition is infectious and can be transmitted to other persons unless precautions are taken.

Leukoplakia

This condition is characterized by patchy, yellowish-white, firm, thickened areas of the oral mucous membrane or of the tongue. The lesion results from hyperplasia of surface epithelial tissue and keratinization.

The lesions are painless and are considered serious since they may be precancerous. They occur most frequently in men after the fourth decade of life. The lesions usually develop in response to chronic irritation that may be mechanical, chemical, thermal or infective in origin. The lesions may disappear with elimination of the irritation. In many instances, the cause is unknown.

Teeth are checked and defects corrected that may be causing irritation. Smoking should be discontinued and a high-vitamin diet is prescribed. If the area is fissured or ulcerated, a biopsy is done to determine if cancer has developed. If malignant changes have taken place, surgical excision and radiation therapy are used.

Cancer of the Mouth

Carcinoma may develop on the tongue or buccal mucosa, but the most frequent site is the lower lip. It has a much higher incidence in males between the ages of 50 and 60 years. It usually appears first on the lip or mucosa as leukoplakia, as a roughened area or as a persisting ulcer.

The lesion in cancer of the tongue or buccal mucosa usually appears as a small firm lump. Later the area breaks down, leaving a painful ulcer. If the condition goes untreated, swallowing and speech become difficult, hypersalivation develops, the mucosa becomes infected and the malignant growth metastasizes to the jaw and to lymph nodes in the neck.

As with all malignant disease, early recognition and treatment are extremely important; *any sore that resists treatment and persists for 3 weeks should receive prompt medical attention.*

Treatment involves surgical excision of the cancerous tissue and radiation therapy. Irradiation may be by interstitial implantation of needles, seeds or molds containing radium (see p. 000). When metastasis to lymph nodes is suspected, more radical surgery may be performed to include dissection of the cervical lymphatics. Extension of the malignant disease into the jaw may necessitate extirpation of the jaw.

Parotitis

Inflammation of a parotid gland is the most common disturbance of the salivary glands and may be due to infection by the specific virus that causes mumps, or it may develop as a result of any nonspecific bacterial invasion of the gland. Nonspecific parotitis may occur as a complication in febrile diseases or when dehydration is present and there is a lack of attention to oral hygiene. It tends to develop more readily in older and debilitated persons. The onset is sudden, the gland becomes swollen and painful and the patient develops a fever.

It is treated by the parenteral administration of antibiotics. If suppuration develops, surgical drainage is necessary. The fluid intake is increased and frequent mouth care is necessary. The local application of an ice bag to the area may be prescribed if pus has not formed.

Obstruction to the Flow of Saliva

Obstruction of any one of the salivary glands may be due to intrinsic or extrinsic causes. Disease within the gland or duct may be infection, newgrowth or a calculus. In conditions that cause inflammation, the duct may be occluded by swelling and edema or later by the resulting scar tissue. Extrinsic causes such as a tumor or infection in neighboring structures may compress the duct, or scar tissue resulting from stomatitis may close off the duct orifice.

The obstruction is manifested by swelling of the affected gland. The swelling is most pronounced during meals because of the salivary stimulation and may subside between meals. Pain and tenderness may be due to the pressure or to the condition causing the obstruction. Fever and general malaise may accompany infection.

Constriction of the duct is treated by probing and dilatation. A calculus may be removed via the duct or, if this approach should fail, surgical removal may have to be undertaken.

A tumor in a salivary gland causes a more gradual swelling unrelated to salivary stimulation. It is treated by prompt surgical excision of the gland. The parotid gland is the most frequent site of salivary tumors; the submaxillary gland is next in order of incidence. If the physician suspects the tumor is malignant because of its firmness, fixation and involvement of the facial nerve, a biopsy may be done to confirm the diagnosis. Surgery is the therapy of choice since malignant newgrowths of the salivary glands are radiation-resistant. Carcinoma involves radical surgery. In the case of cancer of a parotid gland, removal of the mandible and dissection of the cervical lymphatics may be necessary. Surgical excision of the submaxillary gland for malignancy includes dissection of the cervical lymphatics and possibly resection of the mandible. Following such disfiguring surgery as the extirpation of the lower jaw, a prosthesis may be constructed of a synthetic material which is physically and chemically inert and is implanted in the area to restore a normal appearance.

Following any surgery on the parotid gland, the patient is observed for signs of facial paralysis because of the close proximity of the facial nerve to the operative site. In some instances the facial nerve may be involved by a malignant tumor and is removed with the gland, leaving the patient with some permanent facial paralysis.

Fracture of the Jaw

Fracture of the jaw is a relatively common injury in motor accidents, some sports and violent disagreements. Diagnosis may be made on crepitus, apparent deformity, and abnormal, painful movement of the mandible, and is confirmed by x-ray.

TREATMENT. If the fragments are displaced, they are approximated and the lower jaw is immobilized (Fig. 16–6). The latter may be achieved by wiring the lower jaw to the upper jaw or by attaching soft metal bars to the upper and lower teeth. These bars have hooks from which rubber bands extend

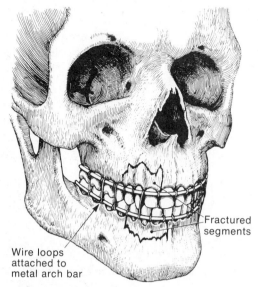

Wire loops
attached to
metal arch bar

Fractured
segments

FIGURE 16–6 Immobilization of fractured jaw by wiring the lower jaw to the upper jaw.

between the upper and lower jaws, applying traction and fixation.

NURSING CARE. Following immobilization of the lower jaw, the patient is placed in a semiprone or lateral position to promote oral drainage and prevent aspiration of secretions during recovery from anesthesia. A wire cutter is kept at the bedside; if the patient vomits, the wire or bands that immobilize the lower jaw must be released immediately so the mouth can be opened to prevent aspiration. A nasogastric tube may be passed and attached to low suction to remove gastric contents and reduce the risk of aspiration. Pharyngeal and oral suctioning with a small catheter may be necessary to remove secretions; trauma and resulting edema of pharyngeal tissues may interfere with swallowing.

The patient receives a high-calorie fluid diet. It may be given for a brief period via the nasogastric tube but as soon as possible it is taken orally through a drinking tube.

The mouth is thoroughly cleansed every 2 hours after each feeding. Normal saline or a mild antiseptic mouthwash may be used. The buccal mucosa and exposed areas of the gums are examined twice daily for lesions and sordes.

Early ambulation is encouraged and the patient may be discharged from the hospital as soon as he can care for himself. The nurse will be responsible for teaching the patient and/or a family member the importance of good oral hygiene and how to carry out the necessary cleansing and inspection. The diet, with suggestions for variation, and its preparation and ingestion, are discussed in detail. When the wires are removed, the patient is urged to see a dentist.

MOUTH CARE AND NURSING IN MOUTH DISORDERS

Oral and Dental Care

Since the mouth is open to the environment, it is a normal habitat of organisms. A healthy, intact mucous membrane, a normal flow of saliva, good hygienic care and an adequate food and fluid intake maintain sufficient resistance to keep the organisms at a safe minimum. Also, the mouth is highly vascular, which contributes to its resistance and quick healing.

A patient may require encouragement and guidance in establishing better dental and mouth care. The importance of frequent brushing of the teeth, the technique of reaching all accessible areas, the avoidance of injury to soft tissues, regular visits to the dentist, and the role of nutrition and adequate fluids should be included in discussions with patients. Ill-fitting dentures may be a source of discomfort to a patient and may interfere with his taking an adequate diet or may cause actual mouth lesions. The person should be urged to have the problem corrected.

Frequently, ill persons are not able to perform their own dental and mouth care and the nurse accepts the responsibility. Care should be taken not to injure soft tissues and to reach the less accessible regions. Removable dentures are taken out frequently and cleansed, and the mouth is cared for before they are replaced.

If the tongue is coated, the mouth dry, and thick, tenacious secretions accumulate and encrust, special nursing attention is necessary. The mouth and teeth should be gently cleansed at least every 2 to 3 hours to reduce the patient's discomfort as well as the number of mouth organisms. A tongue depressor wrapped with gauze or cotton swabs moistened with an antiseptic mouthwash may be used. Saline or a solution of sodium bicarbonate or hydrogen peroxide may also be used. Following cleansing, the mouth should be rinsed thoroughly. The rinsing may not be possible if the patient is unconscious or if there is danger of aspiration of the fluid, in which case moist applicators are used. A light application of mineral oil helps to protect the mucosa and prevent drying. A mixture of lemon juice and oil or glycerin may prove more palatable and refreshing to the patient; the lemon juice tends to increase salivation. Petroleum jelly or cold cream may be applied to the lips.

If there are ulcers or infection and inflammation, the care and treatment are prescribed by the physician. Cleansing may be by mouthwashes or irrigations, since brushing or swabbing might injure the affected tissues or be too distressing to the patient. Local applications of drugs may be made directly by swabs to the affected areas, by mouthwash or by the dissolving of lozenges or pellets in the mouth. Systemic medications may also be prescribed to treat mouth conditions. Antibiotics and vitamins B complex and C are probably the most common.

Nursing Responsibilities

When caring for a patient with a mouth disorder, it should be remembered that the mouth and associated structures are concerned with the ingestion, mastication and swallowing of food, the sense of taste and with speech. Disease in the mouth may also cause respiratory difficulty.

Factors to be considered when planning patient care will depend upon the nature and severity of the disorder, whether surgery is involved and the degree to which there is impairment of functions.

MEDICAL ASEPSIS. Strict medical asepsis should be observed in the care of patients with mouth disorders. The secretions are likely to contain organisms, and precautions are necessary to prevent their spread to other persons. Equipment used for mouth care should be individualized and is disinfected at least once daily. Special attention should be given to thorough washing of the hands after any treatment or care given the patient. If the condition is infectious and the bedding possibly contaminated by oral secretions, a gown should be worn to avoid cross infection.

At the same time, in the interest of the patient, it is important that precautions be used to prevent introducing organisms into the mouth when there is any disorder, a break in the mucosa or lowered resistance. Also, for esthetic reasons, strict cleanliness is observed; chipped items such as mouthwash cups and basins should not be used and the nurse's hands should be washed just before giving mouth care.

OBSERVATIONS. Frequent intraoral examination is made for changes in the mucosa and lesions, degree of moisture and presence of bleeding. The patient is observed for any difficulty with swallowing, talking or breathing. The temperature is checked for possible elevation that may indicate infection or a respiratory complication.

ABNORMAL SALIVARY SECRETION. Hypersalivation may pose a problem in the care of some patients. Others may experience a very dry mouth as a result of less saliva being secreted.

An excess of saliva may cause drooling or very frequent expectoration, and the lips and the skin around the mouth may become excoriated. A protective substance such as petroleum jelly may be applied to the lips and skin. A sputum cup or basin and abundant soft tissues are supplied, and a paper bag for tissue disposal is placed within the patient's reach. Drainage may be accomplished by placing one end of a gauze wick in the mouth and the other end in a basin. In some instances a dental suction tip or soft catheter attached to a source of low negative pressure is used to provide continuous drainage. A lateral or semiprone position facilitates drainage and reduces the risk of aspiration. Rarely, an antisecretory drug (e.g., belladonna or atropine preparation) is prescribed to suppress salivation.

A lack of salivary secretion may be associated with a disease process of the mouth that involves the salivary glands or with a condition in which the mouth is kept open and the individual continuously breathes through his mouth. It frequently occurs when the patient has had radiation treatment for cancer of the mouth. The fluid intake is increased unless contraindicated. Frequent oral irrigation or mouthwashes with a bland nonirritating solution followed by the application of mineral oil or glycerin and lemon juice are usually helpful. The sucking of fruit (lemon) lozenges which are sufficiently tart to stimulate salivary secretion may also provide some comfort. Humidification of the air in the patient's room may be necessary.

NUTRITION AND FLUIDS. The condition of the mouth is greatly influenced by the patient's nutrition and state of hydration. Conversely, the individual's nutritional status and hydration are affected by the condition of the mouth and associated structures. The ingestion of food and fluids stimulates salivary secretion and prevents an accumulation of secretions, cellular debris and organisms. If permitted, food and fluids should be encouraged when there are lesions and the mouth is sore to promote healing and resistance as well as salivary secretion. Soft nonirritating foods are served and hot food and fluids are avoided. Fluids may have to be taken through a tube.

Failure of the patient to take sufficient fluids and food is brought to the physician's attention. Parenteral fluids, feedings via a nasogastric tube (see p. 503) or intravenous alimentation (see p. 504) may be necessary.

SURGICAL CARE. Surgical intervention may be necessary. The procedure used depends upon the location, nature and extent of the disease. Operative procedures on the mouth and associated structures most frequently involve resection for cancer and, if radical, may necessitate reconstructive plastic surgery.

PREOPERATIVE PREPARATION. The patient facing surgery on the mouth or associated structures may be quite fearful and concerned about the results, particularly if radical surgery is to be performed. The surgery may be disfiguring and it may interfere with normal swallowing and speech. The patient is encouraged to verbalize his concerns and to ask questions. An explanation of what is entailed in the surgical treatment is given to the patient and family. They are advised as to what they may expect after the operation, how fluids and nutrients will be administered and that a means of communication by writing will be provided.

If the removal of a part of the jaw or other disfiguring surgery is planned, they may be advised of the reconstructive surgery and prostheses that are now used to provide a normal appearance.

Attention should be directed toward improving the patient's nutritional status and attaining optimal hydration during the preoperative period. Antiseptic mouthwashes or irrigations may be ordered so the mouth will be as clean as possible for the surgery. Factors cited in Chapter 10 as general preparation apply to the patient. The anesthesia may be general or local; for example, a local anesthetic is used in excision of a lip tumor but, in more extensive and radical surgery, general anesthesia is used.

POSTOPERATIVE CARE. This depends on the extent of the surgery. The patient who has intraoral or radical surgery will be more dependent and will require constant nursing attention.

Serious concern in the postoperative stage involves maintenance of an airway. The operative procedure may have necessitated a tracheostomy, and care will include that cited on p. 418. If the patient's airway remains intact, the nurse is constantly alert for interference with respirations by edematous tissues, bleeding or aspiration. To facilitate drainage and prevent aspiration, the patient is placed in a semiprone or lateral position. As soon as the vital signs are stable, the head of the bed is usually elevated. The patient will experience less difficulty with breathing in this position, and this also tends to reduce the edema in the operative area. Frequent gentle suctioning with a small catheter may be necessary.

The possibility of hemorrhage should be kept in mind, since the mouth is a very vascular area. After the first 24 hours irrigations may be ordered to remove the secretions and old blood to reduce the possibility of infection. Also, irrigation of the mouth generally contributes to the patient's comfort.

Nutrition may be provided via a nasogastric tube for the first few days and intravenous fluids are administered. When oral foods and fluids are permitted, a small amount of clear liquid is given to test the patient's ability to swallow. Any choking, coughing or difficulty in swallowing should be reported and the fluid withheld until further directions. If there is no problem the fluids are gradually increased and soft, nonirritating foods are introduced. Extremes of temperature are avoided. The mouth is cleansed before each meal to improve the sense of taste and again following the meal.

If the patient has prolonged difficulty with swallowing, or if reconstructive plastic surgery is undertaken, intravenous alimentation may be given.

Medications may include antibiotics to control infection and analgesics for the relief of pain.

Early ambulation is usually encouraged to prevent respiratory complications and to improve the patient's morale.

The patient may be very sensitive about his appearance and may withdraw. Every effort should be made to have him feel accepted. The cooperation of family and friends is necessary in this; it may be helpful to discuss the problem with them and to advise them that it is important that the patient not sense any revulsion on their part and that they treat him as normal. Cleanliness and tidiness of the patient and his immediate environment are important factors.

The surgery may have involved the tongue, interfering with communication.[12] Paper and a pencil or a slate should be kept within reach of the patient at all times. Anticipation of his needs by the thoughtful nurse will give him confidence and reduce his concern about his lack of ability to communicate. Referral to a speech therapist may be made for the provision of speech training.

In cases in which the external surface of the lips, face or neck is involved, care is taken to keep the area dry and free of contamination by vomitus and oral secretions in order to prevent infection and sloughing.

RADIATION THERAPY. When interstitial radiation implants are used, attached threads may be secured to the neighboring skin. Since this is a very accessible area to the patient, he must be cautioned not to interfere with the implants and threads. He is also advised to keep conversation to a minimum since movement of the tongue and jaw may displace or shift the implants.

PREPARATION FOR HOME CARE. Nursing care should include consideration of the necessary care after the patient goes home from the hospital. His condition may be such that modifications in his diet and activities are needed and that continuing care is necessary.

Instructions concerning the patient's care should be given to the patient and a member of his family. Before the patient leaves the hospital, he is provided with the opportunity for self-care in order to gain understanding and confidence. Appropriate referrals to a social service or a visiting nurse organization may be made by the nurse. A return to his former occupation may not be possible, and retraining for suitable work may be necessary.

Radical Neck Dissection (En Bloc Dissection)

This radical surgical procedure involves the excision of a large portion of the neck tissue on the side of a primary malignant newgrowth of the head, neck, mouth or tongue (Fig. 16–7). Metastasis of the cancer to the cervical lymph nodes occurs early in the disease, so the surgery removes all the nonvital tissues on the affected side of the neck. These include the lymphatic network, sternocleidomastoid, omohyoid and digastric muscles, internal jugular vein, and submandibular glands. The incisions are extensive; one approach may be a Y-shaped incision or two separate horizontal incisions may be made. The neck dissection may be combined with the excision of the primary lesion. If the cancer involves the midline or both sides of the affected area, a bilateral neck dissection is done. The patient's airway may be compromised by bleeding, edema, and swelling of tissues, so a tracheostomy may be necessary. It is usually done at the time of operation if a bilateral dissection is done. One or two drainage tubes with several openings are placed in the wound and portable wound suction may be applied. This arrangement serves two purposes — the removal of serum, lymph and blood, and the drawing down of the skin flaps to obliterate the space left by the extensive excision of tissue.

The *nursing care* discussed above for mouth disorders is applicable in the care of the patient who has radical neck dissection.

PREOPERATIVE CARE. This requires that the patient and family understand the extent of the surgery, the problems that are likely to be encountered and how they will be handled. Time is provided for the patient and family to express their concerns and ask questions. Honest factual answers are important. There is usually considerable apprehension and concern about disfigurement and the ability to breathe and swallow. Local

---

[12]Surgical removal of the tongue (*total glossectomy*) or the excision of a portion of it (*partial glossectomy*).

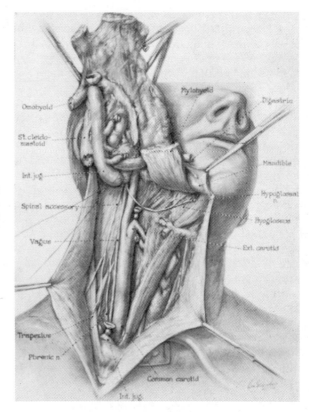

FIGURE 16–7 Drawing showing the extent of the usual radical neck dissection. (From Edgerton, M. T., and DeVito, R. T. In: Converse, J. M., ed.: Reconstructive Plastic Surgery. Volume III. Philadelphia, W. B. Saunders Company, 1964.)

skin preparation of a wide area of the neck and face is necessary.

POSTOPERATIVE CARE. In addition to the factors cited on p. 513, planning care involves the following considerations.

POSITIONING. Following recovery from anesthesia, the head of the bed is elevated to facilitate breathing and reduce edema in the operative area.

OBSERVATIONS. The patient is observed very closely for respiratory distress which may be evidenced by rapid, shallow noisy (stridor) respirations, dyspnea, increasing pulse rate and cyanosis. An accumulation of blood and/or lymph within the tissues or edema may compress the airway. Blood pressure and pulse are recorded at frequent intervals so that early changes associated with hemorrhage or shock may be recognized promptly and appropriate action taken. The rectal temperature is taken every 4 hours; an elevation may indicate local or respiratory infection and the need for an antibiotic. The dressing and drainage from the tubes are examined frequently; if there is

evidence of bleeding the physician is notified immediately.

The patient's face is checked for possible paralysis on the same side as the dissection; the facial nerve may be damaged during the surgery. Similarly, choking on secretions or fluids (when they are permitted) is brought to the physician's attention; nerve damage may impair the reflexive responses of the glottis, epiglottis and posterior pharynx that normally prevent aspiration. The lower part of the face and the neck may be edematous for a few days because of interference with lymph drainage. If this persists or becomes excessive it is noted and reported, since the pressure on the tissues and skin flaps retards healing and promotes sloughing.

DEEP BREATHING AND COUGHING. The patient is encouraged and given the necessary assistance to breathe deeply and cough at frequent intervals. The nurse assists him to assume the sitting position and then supports the patient's head and neck by placing a hand on each side. Gentle suctioning of the oropharyngeal area may be necessary.

When the patient is well enough, he is taught to support his head when he is going to sit up and while coughing.

WOUND CARE. A large pressure dressing may be applied to reduce edema and immobilize the skin flaps which tend to move easily because of the underlying space. The dressing usually requires reinforcement during the first 3 to 5 days and then is changed by the surgeon for a smaller dressing which is less cumbersome for the patient. With regular changing of the dressing, the nurse inspects the wound(s) carefully for sloughing and possible necrosis. Ischemia of the skin flaps and the underlying space predisposes the area to necrosis. Any bleeding from the wound, even if very slight, is brought to the surgeon's attention immediately. Infection and sloughing within the wound may erode the carotid artery and lead to a severe hemorrhage.

MOUTH CARE. Frequent cleansing of the mouth is necessary. The method used is influenced by the site of the primary lesion. For example, if a partial glossectomy was done, the mouth is gently irrigated with a soft catheter and prescribed solution (e.g., normal saline). The patient is turned on his side or sits up with his head over a basin, and the solution is allowed to flow in under low pressure to lessen the danger of aspiration. Precautions are taken to avoid soiling the dressing by the return flow. The patient is instructed to hold his breath or exhale while the solution is being introduced; a brief explanation of why he must guard against inhaling at this time is given. The flow is interrupted at frequent intervals to allow the patient to adjust and breathe freely. Glycerin and lemon swabs may be used and generally are very acceptable to the patient, as they give the mouth a clean fresh feeling.

EMOTIONAL SUPPORT. The patient who has had a neck dissection may become discouraged and depressed and withdraw. He is concerned about the difficulty in communicating with others, and in swallowing. He may be fearful that his breathing is threatened and is distressed because of the scarring and change in his appearance. Healing and recovery of normal speech and ingestion take considerable time. All these problems, the pain and discomfort experienced, and the fact that the diagnosis was cancer may give rise to despondency and despair.

The nurse advises the patient that his concerns and feelings are recognized. He is encouraged to communicate his fears and ask questions by using a pad or slate and pencil. He is reassured that a speech therapist will provide assistance as soon as he is well enough. Privacy is respected until he is less self-conscious of his appearance, and he may then gradually socialize with a few others. The patient's appearance is discussed with the family, and the need for them to accept the patient without hesitation or revulsion is emphasized. Encouraging and assisting the patient to pay particular attention to personal hygiene and grooming are helpful. Wearing of a soft scarf will reduce the area of scarred tissue that is exposed.

If the patient has difficulty resuming a normal eating and swallowing pattern the nurse remains with him, encouraging him and making suggestions that may help (e.g., position of the head, favorable area of the mouth in which to place food). If privacy is provided, he is more likely to persist. The need for nutrition to promote healing and the regaining of strength are stressed.

The patient has problems that are difficult to cope with; understanding, a positive attitude that matters will improve, interest and encouragement on the part of the nurse do help the patient. Such support fosters a more positive, hopeful attitude in the patient and family and assists with meeting his emotional needs.

PAIN. A mild analgesic is usually sufficient to control the patient's discomfort. Sedatives and narcotics are avoided because of their depressing effect on respirations. The patient may complain of headache for a few days owing to the interference with cerebral venous drainage by the tying off of the internal jugular vein. This gradually disappears as the circulatory system adapts.

REHABILITATION EXERCISES. The removal of muscles in neck dissection results in weakness and a drop in the shoulder of the affected side, in addition to restricted neck movement. When the wounds are firmly healed an exercise program is commenced. The number of times each prescribed exercise is done is limited to start with and gradually increased as the individual's tolerance improves.

Head exercises include turning the head to each side, alternative lateral and forward flexion, and extension (bending of the head back). The patient is cautioned to begin these exercises very gently and avoid quick jerky movements.

When doing shoulder exercises, the patient assumes the sitting position with arms flexed and hands in front, the arms and shoulders are drawn back, elevated, and then rotated.

The patient stands beside a small table or stool on which he may lean with the arm of the unaffected side and bends forward; the arm on the affected side is swung from the shoulder, forward and backward, swung in front of the body towards the opposite side and then back and out to the side, and then the arm is raised and moved down and around in circular motion.

The physician may recommend support of the arm to raise the dropped shoulder to a normal level. The support may be a sling or a padded chair arm or table while the patient is sitting.

FOLLOW-UP. The patient requires long-term supervision with frequent visits to his physician or the clinic. Some patients require home visits by a visiting nurse. These frequent contacts provide necessary support and assist the patient to make the psychological adjustment to his situation. The patient's problems are explored and suggestions or assistance given. His weight is checked at each visit, as these patients frequently neglect taking adequate nutrition.

DISORDERS OF THE ESOPHAGUS

The transmission of food and saliva from the mouth to the stomach — the only function of the esophagus — may be impaired by a disturbance in neuromuscular functioning, a decrease or obstruction in the lumen of the tube, or by inflammation and degeneration of tissue in the wall of the esophagus. Causes of these changes may be extrinsic or intrinsic.

Extrinsic Causes of Esophageal Disorders

DISEASE OF NEIGHBORING STRUCTURES. Since the mouth, tongue and pharynx are involved in directing food into the esophagus, it is obvious that disease in any one of these structures may interefere with the initial phase of swallowing. This may be seen in severe stomatitis, pharyngitis, tonsillitis, cleft palate and neoplastic disease of the mouth or tongue. The condition may actually interfere with the swallowing process or cause so much pain that the patient avoids swallowing.

Compression of the esophagus by enlargement or newgrowths of neighboring structures occurs rarely. Examples are goiter (enlargement of the thyroid), aortic aneurysm and enlargement of the mediastinal lymph glands as in Hodgkin's disease.

NEUROLOGICAL DISORDER. Dysphagia (difficulty in swallowing) may result from a nervous system disorder that affects innervation to the muscle tissue of the esophagus. Damage to the swallowing center in the medulla or to nerve fibers of the tenth cranial (vagus) nerve concerned with the swallowing mechanism may cause a partial or complete paralysis. Paralysis may occur in the pharyngeal area owing to interference with normal innervation via the ninth (glossopharyngeal) cranial nerve. Failure of the normal pharyngeal phase of swallowing may result in food passing into the trachea and the nasal cavities. The sphincter at the esophageal opening may remain relaxed, allowing air to be drawn into the esophagus during inspiration.

Conditions in which paralysis of swallowing is commonly seen include myasthenia gravis (failure of nerve impulse transmission at the neuromuscular junction), poliomyelitis that involves the motor neurons in the swallowing center, and cerebrovascular accident (stroke).

Intrinsic Causes of Esophageal Disorders

Intrinsic causes include congenital anomalies, inflammatory disease, achalasia, diverticulum and neoplasms.

CONGENITAL ANOMALIES. A congenital anomaly may occasionally be the cause of impaired swallowing in the newborn infant. The commonest malformations of the esophagus include atresia, stenosis and tracheoesophageal fistula. In atresia, the esophagus is interrupted, ending in a blind pouch. Stenosis is a constriction of the tube at one point that prevents the passage of food to the stomach. In a tracheoesophageal fistula there is an opening between the trachea and the esophagus. This may be combined with atresia, in which case the esophagus opens into and ends in the trachea. In other instances, the esophagus may be complete, but a short tube exists between it and the trachea.

Manifestations of an esophageal malformation in the newborn may be continuous drooling (since the normal amount of saliva cannot be swallowed), regurgitation of the feeding, choking and cyanosis. Prompt recognition and reporting of any indication of difficulty in swallowing may mean the infant's life. Early diagnosis and surgical treatment are necessary in the first few days of life if the infant is to survive. The infant's need for fluids and nourishment is paramount. A gastrostomy may be done in which an opening is made into the stomach through which a tube may be passed. Food is then introduced directly into the stomach. Later, surgery is undertaken to correct the anomaly.

INFLAMMATION (ESOPHAGITIS) AND ULCERATION OF THE ESOPHAGUS. Inflammation and ulceration of the mucosa and underlying tissues of the esophagus may result from injury or irritation by a rough or sharp foreign body, corrosive substances (strong acids and alkalies), retained food that undergoes decomposition, or regurgitated gastric juice. During the acute stage of trauma and inflammation, the patient experiences pain and difficulty in swallowing. As the affected area heals, fibrous scar tissue or thin membranous webs form which constrict the lumen of the tube, resulting in dysphagia. The stricture is treated by gradual dilation by the introduction of bougies. Generally, repeated treatments at intervals for a year or longer are necessary to establish a satisfactory lumen.

Gastrostomy may be necessary in severe constriction in order to provide foods and fluids for the patient. The gastrostomy may also serve for retrograde bougienage in which a very fine bougie, usually a silk cord, is passed into the esophagus. It remains in place between dilation treatments, one end protruding from the nose, the other from the gastrostomy opening. The cord is secured by tying the two ends together. During dilations, the larger bougies are attached to the lower end of the cord and pulled up through the esophagus.

If bougie therapy is not successful, surgical resection of the constricted area with end-to-end anastomosis may be performed. When the area is extensive, surgical reconstruction of the esophagus may be undertaken. A plastic tube or a segment of intestine may be implanted to provide a patent passageway.

ACHALASIA (CARDIOSPASM). This condition is failure of the esophagogastric (cardiac) sphincter to relax to allow the passage of food into the stomach accompanied by a lack of tone in the musculature and normal peristalsis, particularly in the lower part of the tube. The result is an accumulation and stagnation of food and fluids in the esophagus which may cause irritation and inflammation. The patient experiences regurgitation, heartburn (pyrosis), discomfort and dysphagia. The weak peristalsis and failure of relaxation of the sphincter are attributed to degenerative changes or malfunctioning in the nerve plexus (Auerbach's plexus) that innervates the esophageal muscle tissue.

Treatment is dilatation of the sphincter and is palliative, since the esophageal peristalsis tends to remain ineffective. A bougie with an inflatable bag at the lower end is inserted under a fluoroscope. When the bag reaches the sphincter, it is filled with water. This stretches the muscle fibers of the sphincter, and many of them may be ruptured. The sphincter remains partially open and food enters the stomach by gravity. The dilatation procedure may have to be repeated and, if the results are still unsatisfactory, surgical division of the sphincter (cardiomyotomy) may be performed.

With the loss of sphincter control due to either bougie or surgical therapy, regurgitation of gastric content into the esophagus is likely to occur and cause *reflux esophagitis*. This condition may also be associated with hiatus hernia, pregnancy or a shorter than normal esophagus. The patient is instructed to take small meals to prevent gastric distention, not to take any food within 2 hours of going to bed, to remain upright for 1 to 2 hours after a meal, to avoid activities that increase intra-abdominal pressure such as straining and stooping, and to sleep with the head of the bed elevated. These suggestions reduce the possibility of regurgitation of gastric contents into the esophagus. Frequent doses of a liquid antacid preparation may be prescribed to neutralize the gastric contents.

DIVERTICULUM OF THE ESOPHAGUS. An esophageal diverticulum is an outpouching of the wall, and may be classified as a pulsion or traction diverticulum or according to location as pharyngoesophageal, midesophageal or epiphrenic. Diagnosis is made by x-ray examination during a barium swallow or by an esophagoscopy. A *pulsion diverticulum* consists of mucosal and submucosal tissue protruding through a weakened area of the muscle tissue. The weakness of the muscle tissue is thought to be of congenital origin or due to aging in the older person. The most frequent site of this type of diverticulum is in the pharyngoesophageal area and just above the diaphragm. A *traction diverticulum* develops most frequently in the midesophagus in the region of the bifurcation of the trachea. It usually involves all the layers of tissue and is less saccular than the pulsion diverticulum. The cause is inflammatory disease in adjacent structures, such as the mediastinal lymph nodes. The inflammation extends to the esophageal wall, and adhesions may form that put traction on the wall, causing the outpouching.

The symptoms depend on the size of the sacculation and the amount of food it retains. Regurgitation of stagnant food, dysphagia, halitosis, pain in the chest and weight loss may be experienced by the patient. Food collects in the diverticulum and may undergo decomposition and cause esophagitis. Gurgling sounds may be heard in the neck in the pharyngoesophageal diverticulum. A traction diverticulum, being less saccular and having a wide-open neck, does not usually retain food and may actually go undiscovered until there is some x-ray examination.

When the symptoms of diverticulum are severe, surgical excision of the sac may be necessary. A pharyngoesophageal diverticulum is approached through a cervical incision above the clavicular level. A transthoracic approach is used for the removal of diverticula located below the pharyngoesophageal area.

NEOPLASMS OF THE ESOPHAGUS. *Benign tumors* occur rarely in the esophagus. The most common of these are leiomyomas which are tumors of nonstriated muscle tissue. Those encountered less frequently are polyps, cysts, fibromas, adenomas and fibrolipomas. As the tumor imposes itself on the lumen of the esophagus or interferes with normal muscle activity, dysphagia occurs. The patient first experiences difficulty in swallowing the more solid foods, such as meat and bread. The tumor is excised and whether the approach is transesophageal, cervical or thoracic will depend on the location and the nature of the tumor.

Cancer of the esophagus tends to develop more often in the older age group. Its incidence is mainly in males between 50 and 70 years of age, and the lower third of the esophagus is the most common site. The majority of malignant tumors of the esophagus are squamous cell cancer (epidermoid cancer). Adenocarcinoma may occur but is most frequently secondary to gastric carcinoma.

The patient complains first of dysphagia with solid foods which gradually progresses to difficulty with liquids. Substernal discomfort and pain, regurgitation and loss of weight and strength are experienced with steadily increasing severity. In advanced stages, bleeding may occur. Structures adjacent to the primary lesion may become involved; the disease may spread to the trachea, bronchi, stomach, diaphragm or associated lymph nodes, depending upon its location in the esophagus.

Diagnosis is made by x-ray examination and an esophagoscopy. A biopsy is obtained and a smear from the lesion is probably taken for cytologic study during the endoscopic examination.

Treatment may be by surgical resection and/or irradiation. Various surgical procedures are employed. The affected part of the esophagus is resected with a wide margin of normal tissue as well as the regional lymph nodes. If the lesion is in the lower part, the upper portion of the stomach is also removed (esophagogastrectomy). The remaining proximal portion of the esophagus is anastomosed to the stomach which is drawn up into the thoracic cavity (esophagogastrostomy). A nasogastric tube is passed and remains until the anastomosis is fairly well healed and peristalsis is established.

If the cancer is located in the middle or upper portions of the esophagus, or if a large area is involved, it is more difficult to treat the patient surgically. A segment of the patient's intestine (jejunum or colon) may be implanted to replace the resected esophagus. More recently, a plastic tube has been used to reestablish a passageway between the remaining esophagus and the stomach.

Following diagnosis and investigation of the patient's general condition, the surgeon may conclude that radical surgery is inadvisable. Radiation therapy may be used with some benefit. A plastic nasogastric tube may be inserted through the constricted area and left in place so the patient can be given fluids and nourishment. Complications of ulceration and bleeding may develop with this latter palliative procedure. More often, a gastrostomy is employed by which nutrition is maintained for the remainder of the patient's life (see p. 503).

ESOPHAGEAL VARICES. This serious condition is associated with cirrhosis of the liver and is discussed on pp. 590.

Nursing in Disorders of the Esophagus

EMOTIONAL PROBLEMS. A disturbance in swallowing may interfere with the patient's ability to take food and fluid and to dispose of his saliva in the normal way. He may become very self-conscious about the latter problem and consider his life is really threatened by the former. Even slight dysphagia makes the patient very apprehensive; having experienced some difficulty, he may resort to fluids and soft foods that do not provide an adequate diet. He is nervous when eating with others because he fears the embarrassment of choking and regurgitation; anxiety may only worsen his dysphagia. The patient requires sympathetic understanding and acknowledgement of his concerns.

OBSERVATIONS. An accurate recording is made of the patient's fluid and food intake. Difficulty with any one type of food should be noted and that food avoided in future feedings. The physician may request a daily record of the patient's weight but this may have to be omitted, since a loss of weight may only increase the patient's anxiety. The frequency of regurgitation is noted and the amount and nature of the regurgitated material recorded.

CARE OF THE SALIVA. The patient may not be able to swallow his saliva. Soft paper wipes, a paper bag for their disposal and a sputum cup should be within his reach at all times. Hypersalivation is common in some esophageal conditions, such as tumors. A gauze wick placed in the side of the mouth with the other end in a basin may also be used. Frequent suctioning may be necessary with the very ill and weak patient.

Frequent expectoration and wiping of the mouth may cause irritation of the lips and the skin around the mouth. Gentle bathing, drying and an application of a protective cream at frequent intervals will prevent excoriation.

Some provision should be made at night for salivary drainage. A thick towel folded over a plastic or rubber bed protector may be placed under the patient's face. He is encouraged to lie on either side to promote drainage and reduce the possibility of aspiration.

MOUTH HYGIENE. Frequent cleansing and rinsing of the mouth are necessary to decrease the number of organisms and control possible offensive odor. Normally, many of these are swallowed and destroyed by the gastric juice. The patient with esophageal disease may experience an objectionable taste. Mouth care is refreshing for the patient who is constantly aware of the saliva that he cannot dispose of in the normal way.

POSITIONING. If the patient is still able to take some fluids and food by mouth, swallowing is less difficult if he is in the sitting position. The head of the bed may be raised, and the patient is given the necessary assistance to assume an upright position. The very ill and weak patient may have to be kept in a lateral or semiprone position to facilitate salivary drainage and prevent aspiration.

HYDRATION AND NUTRITION. The esophagus may not be completely obstructed, and the patient may be able to swallow liquids and semiliquids or even soft, blended, solid food. He may, however, be very fearful of choking and regurgitation. Encouragement and reassurance from a nurse who remains with him during his meal may make the difference between his taking and rejecting the essential nutrition and fluids. The more relaxed patient is more likely to have less difficulty in swallowing.

When swallowing has become almost impossible, the physician may pass a nasogastric tube and leave it in. Tube feedings are then provided to sustain the patient (see p. 503). If the patient's esophagus is completely obstructed and a nasogastric tube cannot be passed, a gastrostomy may be done and feedings given via the tube that is inserted into the stomach through an abdominal incision (see discussion of gastrostomy, p. 503).

Intravenous fluids may also be necessary to maintain a normal fluid and electrolyte balance. The patient's fluid intake and output are measured and recorded and observations made for any deficiency.

SURGICAL CARE. Surgical intervention in esophageal disorders involves entering the thoracic cavity in most instances. In planning care, the factors cited in the section on care in chest surgery (p. 460) are considered. Since partial gastric resection or esophageal anastomosis with the stomach is frequently part of the intervention, the principles which apply to nursing in gastric surgery also apply (see p. 533).

PREOPERATIVE NURSING CARE. The care of the patient who is to have esophageal surgery is directed toward improving his nutritional status and establishing an optimal fluid and electrolyte balance. The patient is encouraged to take the maximum that he can manage orally. High-calorie, high-protein liquids or semiliquid foods may be used, but if the condition limits the oral intake and the patient is emaciated and dehydrated, tube feedings and parenteral fluids may be ordered, or a gastrostomy may even be considered necessary. Blood transfusions may be necessary to correct anemia that has resulted from nutritional deficiency.

The patient and his family look for support and understanding from the nurse. They realize the seriousness of the surgery and are usually very apprehensive. The attentive nurse who gives consideration to the patient's needs and demonstrates understanding of his concern for his future may contribute much to lessening his fears and despair.

An explanation of what may be expected in the postoperative period is made and the patient's and family's questions answered willingly.

An explanation is given of the multiple pieces of equipment that will be necessary at his bedside after the operation and of the need for the nasogastric, chest and intravenous

tubes and frequent suctioning. The importance of deep breathing, coughing, frequent turning and the simple foot and leg exercises is stressed, and instructions are given on how to cough and do the exercises. The discussion of the postoperative period should be extended over several periods and, as the patient talks about it and asks questions, his apprehension of the situation may be reduced. Any explanation should be discreet, in order to avoid arousing unnecessary anxiety, and should be in simple lay terms.

Particular attention is given to oral hygiene; rinsing frequently with antiseptic mouthwash will help to prevent mouth and respiratory infections.

The usual considerations are given to the immediate general preoperative care (see p. 178). Specific orders as to local preparation are received from the physician, since the area of skin to be prepared will probably vary with the surgical approach planned.

If reconstructive surgery is anticipated that may involve the use of a segment of the patient's intestine (jejunum or colon) to replace the resected esophagus, an oral antibiotic or sulfonamide may be ordered for several days prior to the resection to reduce the intestinal bacteria. If the patient is being tube-fed, the preparation is put into solution and given through the nasogastric or gastrostomy tube.

POSTOPERATIVE NURSING CARE. Preparation to receive the patient from the operating room includes the assembling of the following equipment:

Sphygmomanometer and stethoscope
Respiratory and gastric suctioning equipment
Infusion pole
Equipment for oxygen administration
Two large hemostats
Tray of equipment for chest aspiration
Tray of equipment for emergency tracheostomy

Following operation, the principles of care include those applicable to the care of a patient having had chest and gastric surgery.

If a nasogastric tube has been introduced in the operating room, it is usually attached to a suction apparatus for continuous removal of gastric secretions. The drainage may be colored with blood the first few hours but should gradually assume the characteristics of normal secretions. Directions will be given when the suction is to be discontinued and when nasogastric fluids and feedings are to be given. A temporary gastrostomy may be used for drainage and feedings; the nasogastric tube may simply be kept in position to maintain a patent esophagus.

The nasogastric tube may be removed in 4 to 7 days, and small amounts of water may then be given. Any difficulty in swallowing or regurgitation is promptly reported. The patient will find swallowing easier if he is sitting up. If he has no difficulty with water, the fluids are gradually varied and increased in volume. The diet gradually progresses to semiliquids, blended or soft foods and a normal diet. Parenteral fluids and gastrostomy feedings are continued until the patient is able to swallow adequate amounts of fluids and food. If the surgical procedure entailed an esophagogastric anastomosis with the stomach being drawn up into the thoracic cavity, the patient may not be able to take the ordinary amount of food or fluid at one time without experiencing pressure in his chest and some dyspnea. In this event, the patient is fed smaller amounts at more frequent intervals and should remain upright in the sitting position for 1 to 2 hours after eating.

A frequent check is made of the patient's temperature and white blood cell count for any indication of infection. If either is increased to levels above the normal, parenteral administration of an antibiotic is ordered. In some instances the surgeon may prefer to start the antibiotic administration after the operation as a prophylactic measure against infection.

A record is kept of the patient's intake and output and the balance noted until a normal intake by mouth is well established.

Frequent mouth care is necessary; it contributes to the patient's comfort as well as preventing sores, ulceration of the mucosa and offensive breath.

Since the patient's food intake has probably been limited for a period of time he may be emaciated and very weak, which predispose to pressure sores unless special preventive measures are taken. His position is changed every 2 hours, and pressure areas are kept clean and dry and are gently massaged. Alcohol is not used since it tends to dry the skin; a preparation with a creamy base is preferable. Soft resilient material such as sheepskin is placed under specific pressure areas to protect them, and an alternating pressure mattress may be used.

If the lesion was located in the proximal portion of the esophagus, a cervical approach may have been used in surgery without entry into the thoracic cavity. This eliminates the closed water-seal drainage and reduces respiratory problems.

Early ambulation is encouraged but the patient will probably require considerable assistance and support because of physical weakness and emotional despair. The convalescent period is usually prolonged, during which the patient will probably have to adjust to and learn to manage modifications in his diet and pattern of eating. Obviously, his condition will determine whether he returns to his former occupation. He and his family may be faced with socioeconomic problems that should be recognized by the nurse. Assistance may be sought from the social worker or an appropriate service or welfare organization. The visiting nurse may be contacted to assess the home situation and help the family plan for the patient's care.

Hiatus Hernia (Diaphragmatic Hernia)

The openings in the diaphragm which accommodate the esophagus and aorta are potential sites for the herniation of abdominal viscera into the thoracic cavity. The hiatus through which the esophagus passes is the most vulnerable area; normally, when esophageal content passes into the stomach it does not return to the esophagus. If it does, it is referred to as reflux (a return flow).

ETIOLOGY. The chief causes of the defect in the diaphragm are considered to be a congenital weakness and the aging process. The former probably results from a defect in the fusion of tissues around the opening. The incidence of hiatal hernia is much greater in middle-aged and elderly persons, and is probably due to weakening of the diaphragmatic muscle. The weakness or gap that occurs results in imperfect closure of the hiatus around the esophagus. Rarely, the hernia may be caused by trauma such as a fractured rib or perforating foreign object (e.g., bullet) or prolonged, extreme intra-abdominal pressure as occurs in ascites or pregnancy.

CLASSIFICATION. The hernia may be classified as sliding (esophagogastric) or rolling (paraesophageal; see Fig. 16–8). A *sliding hiatal hernia* is one in which the esophagogastric junction and a portion of the fundus of the stomach ride up into the thoracic cavity. In a sliding hernia, the cardiac sphincter at the esophagogastric opening (cardia) loses competency, resulting in reflux of the gastric contents into the esophagus. In a *rolling* or *paraesophageal hernia,* a sac-like portion of the peritoneum and stomach herniates through into the thorax alongside the esophagus. A section of omentum may also be extruded. The cardiac sphincter usually remains competent but the displaced portion of the stomach occupies space within the mediastinum and may cause respiratory distress or impaired cardiac function by direct pressure on the heart. Distention of the herniated segment or strangulation may develop, which demands emergency surgery.

MANIFESTATIONS. The symptoms depend upon the size of the hernia and the amount of displaced viscus. Intermittent mild digestive disturbances only may be experienced. The patient may complain of substernal burning pain or discomfort (heartburn), regurgitation of acid fluid, belching, a feeling of fullness and shortness of breath. The symptoms are frequently precipitated by stooping over, straining associated with increased intra-abdominal pressure or a large meal. It may also be brought on when the patient is recumbent and may be relieved when he sits up.

Frequent reflux may cause esophagitis, ulceration and bleeding. Scarring may develop that causes some constriction and probably dysphagia. Rarely, the herniated portion is so large that it becomes incarcerated and even strangulated. Respirations and cardiac function are likely to be compromised.

DIAGNOSIS. This is made by the patient's history and by a barium ingestion with fluoroscopic and roentgenographic studies. The pain of reflux esophagitis associated with hiatal hernia is frequently similar to that associated with angina pectoris and myocardial infarction. It may radiate up into the neck and down the left arm. As a result, when the patient initially presents with an acute epi-

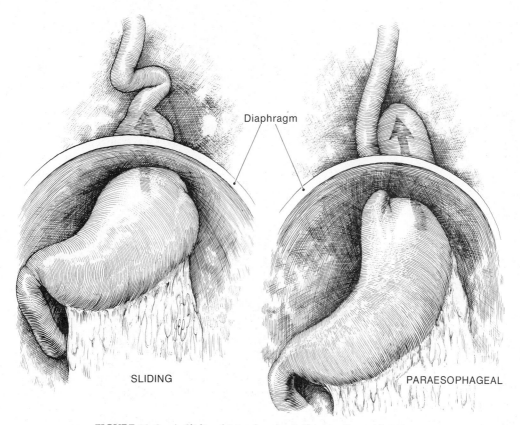

FIGURE 16–8 *A,* Sliding hiatus hernia. *B,* Paraesophageal hernia.

sode, the physician has an electrocardiogram made to differentiate.

THERAPEUTIC MANAGEMENT. A slight hernia may be controlled and the patient kept relatively asymptomatic by loss of weight (if he is obese), the avoidance of heavy lifting, and frequent, small, bland meals. Gas-forming foods, coffee and alcohol are avoided. An antacid such as an aluminum hydroxide preparation (e.g., Maalox) is usually prescribed to be taken after meals and at bedtime. The patient is advised to remain in an upright position for at least 2 hours after a meal. The head of his bed is elevated on blocks.

If a loop of the intestine or a portion of the stomach becomes confined in the thoracic cavity, surgical treatment is essential to return the viscus to the abdominal cavity. The surgical approach is usually made through the chest but occasionally may be made via the abdominal cavity. Following replacement of the viscus, the hiatus hernia is repaired. A nasogastric tube is likely to be introduced, and mild suction is applied to prevent vomiting and intestinal distention. Fluids are administered by intravenous infusion for the first day or two, and then gradually introduced by mouth when the gastric suction is discontinued. For nursing care when a thoracotomy is used, see p. 460. For nursing care when the abdominal approach is used see p. 533.

GASTRIC DISORDERS

The gastric disorders seen most frequently are pyloric stenosis, gastritis, peptic ulcer and carcinoma.

Pyloric Stenosis

This condition may be congenital, or it may be secondary to peptic ulcer or carcinoma of the stomach. Secondary pyloric stenosis is discussed as a complication with the causative condition (see p. 532).

Gastritis

The term gastritis implies inflammation of the stomach. The condition may be acute or chronic and the pathologic process is usually limited to the mucosa.

The causes of *acute inflammation* may be the ingestion of large quantities of alcohol, contaminated foods, or foods to which the person is sensitive or allergic, such as seafood, mushrooms or salicylates (e.g., aspirin). Infective gastritis is most frequently due to the ingestion of foods bearing staphylococci or salmonella organisms.

The patient with acute gastritis becomes ill suddenly and suffers severe epigastric pain, nausea, vomiting and fever. The attack may last a few hours to a few days. Dehydration develops rapidly and the patient becomes prostrate. The treatment includes nothing by mouth, bed rest and parenteral fluids. Clear fluids are given when the symptoms subside and, if tolerated, a bland diet of soft foods is introduced and progressively increased until a normal diet is resumed.

Chronic gastritis occurs with prolonged and repeated irritation of the mucosa and results in atrophic changes in the mucosa and glands. The cause may be evasive, since the condition may be associated with other diseases, such as pernicious anemia, and with the degenerative changes of aging. It may result from constant subjection of the stomach to an ingested irritant, such as alcohol, and frequently accompanies a gastric ulcer or gastric carcinoma.

The symptoms of chronic gastritis are usually ill-defined but may include anorexia, discomfort and a full feeling after meals, flatulence, heartburn, nausea and occasionally hematemesis. A bland diet is recommended with abstinence from foods and fluids that seem to aggravate the condition. Spicy and raw foods, fats and very hot foods are poorly tolerated. Alcohol, coffee and salicylates should be avoided. The patient may lose considerable weight as he tends to restrict his food intake to avoid the distress it may precipitate. Attention is directed toward improving his general nutritional status by encouraging a well-balanced diet of nonirritating foods. Milk, buttermilk and eggnogs between meals may be tolerated and are nutritious.

Peptic Ulcer

A peptic ulcer is the erosion of a circumscribed area of tissue in the wall of an area of the gastrointestinal tract that is accessible to gastric secretions. The actual erosion is caused by the digestive action of hydrochloric acid and pepsin. The most frequent sites of the ulcer are the stomach, proximal portion of the duodenum and the esophagus, as these areas are accessible to gastric secretions. It occurs more frequently in the duodenum than the stomach, less often in the esophagus and rarely in the jejunum. The ulcer penetrates the mucosa and may invade the underlying submucosal and muscular tissues. Ulcers tend to recur; some heal promptly while others become chronic.

ETIOLOGY. There is no conclusion as to the initiating cause of peptic ulcer. Normally, hydrochloric acid and pepsin are secreted but ulceration does not occur. This is attributed to the following defensive factors. The mucosa secretes sufficient mucus to dilute the secretions and provides a protective coating that prevents mucosal digestion by the acid-pepsin action. The duodenum has the additional protection of the strong alkalinity of the bile and pancreatic and intestinal secretions which neutralize the acidic chyme. Still another defense is a healthy resistant mucosa which has a good blood supply and is capable of continuous rapid regeneration of the mucosal epithelial cells.

A peptic ulcer may develop when the secretory output of hydrochloric acid and pepsin is in excess of the normal or when the protective mechanisms are inadequate in relation to the amount of acid and pepsin produced. Guyton states, "The usual cause of peptic ulceration is too much secretion of gastric juice in relation to the degree of protection afforded by the mucous secretion and the neutralization of the gastric acid by duodenal juices."[13] The problem is: what causes a hypersecretion of acid and pepsin or lowers mucosal resistance? Factors that are suspect include individual physiological differences such as greater parietal cell mass, greater sensitivity of the cells to the stimulating hormone gastrin, excessive production of gastrin and more rapid passage of gastric contents into the duodenum, resulting in more free acid and pepsin being delivered to the duodenum. The major factor is considered to be a disturbance in the autonomic nervous control of gastric secretion that results in increased vagal (parasympathetic) innervation, causing prolonged secretion of hydrochloric acid and pepsin.

The following are considered to be potential contributing factors in the development of an imbalance between the secretion of hydrochloric acid and pepsin and the defensive mechanisms of the mucosa.

EMOTIONAL FACTORS. Emotional tension, anxiety, frustration and stress may cause an imbalance in the autonomic nervous system, resulting in increased vagal stimulation of gastric secretion.

INFLAMMATION. Gastritis and trauma of the mucosa reduces the resistance of the membrane to digestion. Cell destruction is accelerated and cell reproduction, which normally renews the superficial layers quickly, may be retarded.

HEREDITY. Genetic factors appear to have a role, since studies on incidence show there is a tendency for peptic disease to occur in families and in persons of certain blood types. There is correlation between duodenal ulcer and the blood type O while gastric ulcer patients are more often of the blood group A.

TRAUMA AND SERIOUS ILLNESS. The patient with severe tissue injury such as that produced by extensive burns may develop severe peptic ulceration. It has been recognized as a complication frequently associated with any serious illness, especially if it is characterized by hypotension or respiratory insufficiency. These ulcers may be referred to as *stress ulcers.*

CERTAIN DRUGS. Some drugs, e.g., acetylsalicylic acid (aspirin), adrenal steroids (cortisone), indomethacin (Indocin) and phenylbutazone (Butazolidin), are ulcerogenic in some persons.

BILE REFLUX. The reflux of bile and pancreatic enzymes into the stomach due to an incompetent pyloric sphincter may lead to a gastric ulcer. The bile salts damage the gastric mucosa, predisposing it to ulceration.

ENDOCRINE SECRETIONS. Rarely, severe peptic ulceration is caused by marked gastric hypersecretion that occurs in response to an excessive gastrin concentration in the blood. The gastrin is produced by a tumor of the islets of the pancreas. This disorder is known as the Zollinger-Ellison syndrome.

Peptic ulceration also develops in hyperparathyroidism. The disturbance is attributed to the altered serum calcium level.

SEX. Peptic ulcer has a much higher incidence in men than in women. It has been

---

[13]Arthur C. Guyton: Textbook of Medical Physiology, 5th ed. Philadelphia, W. B. Saunders, 1976, p. 894.

suggested that estrogenic hormones in the female may account for this.

OTHER FACTORS. Poor dietary habits, particularly irregular meals, are thought to be an aggravating factor. Abnormally long periods between meals in persons with a prolonged hypersecretion of acid and pepsin leave the mucosa vulnerable. The protective mechanisms cannot withstand the acid-pepsin action without the diluting and neutralizing assistance of food. Smoking and excessive amounts of alcohol or coffee increase gastric secretion.

INCIDENCE. Peptic ulcer is a common disease and has a higher incidence in males between the ages of 40 and 55 years. Duodenal ulcer is much more common than gastric ulcer, and the incidence of gastric ulcer (not associated with cancer) is higher in females than in males. The patients frequently experience seasonal exacerbations in the spring and autumn.

MANIFESTATIONS. The prominent symptom of peptic ulcer is epigastric *pain* with definite characteristics. It may radiate to the back. The pain is usually described by the patient as gnawing or burning and of being rhythmic in its development and relief in relation to the ingestion of food. The onset of pain may be immediately or up to 4 hours after a meal, depending upon the location of the ulcer, and is relieved by taking food or an antacid. In the case of an *esophageal ulcer,* the pain develops within a few minutes after the meal. It may be intermittent and the patient usually complains of heartburn and regurgitation. Pain associated with a *gastric ulcer* usually occurs ½ to 1 hour after the ingestion of food; that of *duodenal ulcer* is delayed for approximately 2 to 4 hours. The patient's rest is frequently disturbed by nocturnal pain, especially with a duodenal ulcer. Although the ingestion of food generally provides relief, in a few instances it may be the initiating factor of the ulcer pain, particularly if the food is coarse or highly seasoned.

Vomiting is not a common incident in peptic ulcer but may occur if the ulcer pain is very severe or if the ulcer is in the pyloric region. In the case of the latter, inflammation and edema of the surrounding tissues, pyloric spasm or contracted scar tissue resulting from ulceration may narrow the lumen of the pylorus. This may delay the emptying of the stomach and may cause vomiting.

The ulcer patient usually maintains his *weight,* since he eats frequently to relieve his pain unless his condition is complicated by vomiting.

DIAGNOSIS. Investigation of the patient for peptic ulcer may include roentgenograms with a barium meal, gastric analysis to determine the hydrochloric acid secretion, gastroscopy and stool examination for occult blood. See pp. 495–496 and 498–499.

TREATMENT AND NURSING CARE. Treatment of the peptic ulcer patient is directed toward the relief of symptoms, healing of the ulcer and the prevention of complications and recurrence. A regimen of rest, nonirritating diet and various medications is designed to reduce gastric secretory and motor activity, dilute the gastric juice and neutralize much of the hydrochloric acid that is secreted in order to promote healing.

Hospitalization is not always necessary. It may be that the patient's home situation and his understanding and acceptance of the treatment are such that he may progress satisfactorily at home. If it is suspected that the patient will not adhere to the treatment regimen or if his home situation is not conducive to the preparation of his diet or to relaxation, hospitalization may be recommended until the symptoms are relieved and the patient and his family appreciate and plan for the necessary adjustments. A period in the hospital may be beneficial if the patient's usual environment is the source of incompatibilities, anxiety and frustration that aggravate his disease. Treatment and care should be individualized for all patients, but it is extremely important with the ulcer patient. This means that those concerned with his care must get to know the patient and his pattern of living.

Nursing care includes the following considerations.

ADHERENCE TO TREATMENT REGIMEN. It is important that the nurse caring for the ulcer patient understand the treatment aims and the significance of strict adherence to the prescribed therapeutic regimen. The patient's response of annoyance to delayed or irregular feedings and medications can result in hypersecretion and hypermotility that further aggravate his condition and delay healing.

OBSERVATIONS. The patient's response to the treatment and his ability and willingness to cooperate in the prescribed schedule are assessed at frequent intervals. He should be observed for evidence of mental conflicts, anxieties and emotional factors that may be influencing his disease.

Prompt recognition and reporting of early symptoms of complications which may develop are an important nursing responsibility.

REST. Mental and physical rest are necessary if reduced gastric activity is to be achieved. This is the basic principle of ulcer treatment. A brief period of bed rest may be recommended, or the patient may remain ambulatory with some restriction in activity and an increase in his hours of rest. A period away from his work situation is necessary if the symptoms are severe, but for some persons it may be considered better to let them carry on rather than impose the anxiety created by the loss of financial income or by the disorganization of their work. The need for a full "lunch hour," preferably away from the job, and for leaving the work behind when he leaves the work situation should be stressed with the patient who is continuing or resuming work.

Other factors that contribute to rest should receive attention, such as a quiet pleasant environment, physical comfort, undisturbed rest periods, the avoidance of visitors who may arouse pent-up feelings, relaxing diversions of interest to the patient and the avoidance of delays in relation to his treatments and requests. Anxiety should be relieved: psychological stress may aggravate the ulcer disease, and the symptoms in turn evoke further anxiety. The patient at home is encouraged to develop interests within his limitations.

The hospital or visiting nurse has an important role in recognizing and reducing underlying anxiety. Frequently, the ulcer patient tends to keep his concerns to himself, but if he recognizes the nurse as a sympathetic understanding person who is prepared to help and not to judge, he may confide his problems and emotional stress. The verbal expression of these in itself can be of value, for so often the problems kept to oneself tend to acquire inordinate proportions and therefore assume unrealistic importance. The nurse takes time to listen and encourages the patient to exhaust the pent-up tensions that tend to aggravate gastric hypersecretion and hypermotility. As an objective person, she may help the patient see the problems in normal perspective and may make constructive suggestions. It may be necessary for the patient to modify his lifestyle to prevent recurrence of peptic ulceration.

A sedative or tranquilizer to promote rest and relaxation may be prescribed in ulcer therapy.

DIET. Considerable controversy has arisen in recent years regarding the value or effectiveness of the restrictive bland diet that was traditional in the treatment of peptic ulcer disease. The usual practice now is to encourage a more liberal diet than that used in the past. It is suggested that important principles to be observed are that: (1) the patient receive a nutritionally adequate diet; (2) substances which stimulate gastric secretion (e.g., coffee, strong tea, highly seasoned food, citrus fruit and alcohol) be avoided; (3) meals be taken regularly; and (4) foods which the patient recognizes as actually precipitating symptoms be avoided. Dietary modifications and restrictions will vary with the severity of the patient's symptoms and with the particular physician; a very rigid dietary regimen may be prescribed for some, while others will receive a fairly liberal diet.

In the acute phase of peptic ulcer disease, it may be customary to commence with small frequent feedings which are bland, easily digested, and mechanically, chemically, and thermally nonirritating. Foods that are *avoided* in these meals include coarse grain cereals, raw fruits and vegetables, nuts, pork, gas-forming foods, fried foods, tea, coffee, carbonated beverages, meat stock soups, spices and rich pastries. Very hot and very cold foods are not served. The use of whole milk and cream is no longer considered necessary. Skim milk is used instead, since diets which include large amounts of whole milk and cream have been associated with an increased incidence of myocardial infarction in ulcer patients.[14]

As the symptoms lessen and disappear, the diet is liberalized in accord with the patient's tolerance. During the gradual progression to a regular diet, the individual identifies the foods that precipitate discomfort *for him* and should be omitted from *his* diet. The importance of a

---

[14]Marcus A. Krupp and Milton J. Chatton: Current Medical Diagnosis and Treatment. Los Altos, Cal., Lange, 1975, p. 341.

well-balanced diet should be stressed to the patient in order to avoid nutritional deficiencies. Vitamin C and iron deficiencies may develop if the patient does not have a sufficiently balanced diet. Eventually, the patient is encouraged to take as normal a diet as possible, eliminating only the foods that are found to give discomfort.

If the patient's symptoms are very severe, the physician may prescribe a very rigid dietary regimen. Initially, it may consist of small hourly feedings or may be restricted to 120 to 200 ml. of milk only every waking hour. Generally, the milk is taken only during the night if the patient wakens or if the medical directive is to waken the patient. The initial treatment may consist of a continuous intra-duodenal drip of milk or a solution of aluminum hydroxide passed through a nasogastric tube. The continuous drip provides more constant neutralization in the patient with a marked hypersecretion of acid. Its disadvantages are the discomfort of the tube to the patient and the restrictions it places on his mobility. Rarely, a gastrojejunal tube is passed, and frequent feedings are given through it which bypass the stomach and ulcer area; stimulation of gastric secretion and motility and irritation of the ulcer by direct contact with the food are eliminated.

If the patient's ulcer is esophageal, in order to prevent reflux, small meals low in fat and fluid content are recommended. The patient is also advised to avoid lying down within the 2 hours following the ingestion of food. An erect trunk, by virtue of gravity, prevents reflux. He should sleep with the head of the bed elevated at least 6 inches.

The frequency of feedings varies, as does the content. Again, the patient's tolerance is determined. Some are comfortable with three regular meals but require a snack midmorning, midafternoon and before retiring. Other individuals adjust better to more frequent (probably 4 to 6), smaller meals.

MOUTH CARE. If the patient is on frequent milk feedings, he is encouraged to rinse his mouth after each feeding, since the residue in the mouth may tend to bias him against the feedings. It also favors the growth of organisms and the accumulation of mucus. A mild antiseptic mouthwash or clear water only may be used.

MEDICATIONS. Medical treatment of the patient with a gastric or duodenal ulcer includes the administration of a liquid antacid preparation. An anticholinergic drug may also be prescribed to decrease gastric motility, as well as a sedative or tranquilizer to promote rest.

Antacids. An antacid is given to raise the pH of gastric contents. It is administered 1 hour after each meal and the dose is individualized on the basis of that required to reduce the patient's pain. For this reason it is important for the nurse to note the patient's response. Initially, the antacid may be indicated in hourly doses; then, as the pain diminishes, it is taken less frequently (probably four doses a day).

The antacids commonly used singly or in combination are aluminum hydroxide, magnesium oxide and calcium carbonate. The preparations of aluminum hydroxide and calcium carbonate (especially the latter) tend to cause constipation, whereas magnesium oxide has a laxative effect. Calcium carbonate is contraindicated for patients with fluid or electrolyte imbalance or a history of renal disease or calculi; it may cause hypercalcemia and hypercalcuria. These drugs are nonabsorbable; *absorbable antacids such as sodium bicarbonate are not used,* since they would produce alkalosis.

Anticholinergic (Parasympatholytic) Drugs. Anticholinergic drugs that depress gastric secretion and motility may be used. Stimulation of parasympathetic nerve fibers results in the release of the chemical mediator acetylcholine at the junction of the fibers with the effector structures to initiate their responses. In the case of the stomach, parasympathetic innervation increases acid-pepsin secretion and muscular activity. Anticholinergic drugs may depress the release of acetylcholine or may block the nerve impulse before it reaches the neuroeffector junction, or they may block the action of acetylcholine even if it is released. These drugs do not inhibit total gastric acid-pepsin secretion, but they are considered of value in reducing the excessive secretion and hypermotility characteristic of peptic ulcer patients. The dosage of anticholinergic drugs is individualized since the reactions are variable from one person to another.

Examples of such drugs are: atropine sulfate, tincture of belladonna, which is more often used than atropine since its liquid form permits finer regulation of the dosage; synthetic anticholinergic drugs, such as methantheline bromide (Banthine) given in tablet form, propantheline bromide (Pro-Banthine) tablets, dicyclomine hydrochloride (Bentyl) capsules, and scopolamine methylbromide (Pamine) tablets may be administered. These drugs are given several times a day; the frequency may vary slightly with different physicians and with patients' responses.

Side effects are common to anticholinergic drugs and should be familiar to the nurse. The patient should be observed for dryness of the mouth, blurring of vision, urinary retention, constipation, tachycardia, palpitation and nervous excitation. Anticholinergic drugs are not given if the patient has glaucoma, prostatic hypertrophy or a rapid pulse rate. Older persons are more susceptible to the toxic effects of these drugs.

Sedatives and Tranquilizers. Tension and emotional stress are capable of increasing gastric secretion and motility. For this reason, sedatives are frequently a part of the treatment regimen of the ulcer patient. Small doses may be ordered throughout the day, with a larger dose being given at bedtime. Small doses of phenobarbital may be used, or amobarbital (Amytal), diazepam (Valium) or flurazepam (Dalmane) may be the drug of choice.

If the patient's ulcer is located in the esophagus, a parasympathetic stimulant may be prescribed in addition to an antacid. The purpose is to tighten up the cardiac sphincter at the junction of the esophagus and stomach and reduce reflux. Examples of the parasympathetic stimulants used are benthanechol chloride (Urecholine) and metoclopramide (Maxeran). The patient is observed for side effects, which may be disturbances in vision, crampy abdominal pain or dyspnea.

Salicylate medications such as acetylsalicylic acid (aspirin) are contraindicated for the patient with a peptic or reflux ulcer or with a history of one. They are considered ulcerogenic and predispose the individual to gastrointestinal bleeding. If a mild analgesic is needed, as for a headache, acetaminophen (Tylenol or Atasol) may be ordered.

SMOKING. Ulcer patients are advised to abstain from smoking, particularly cigarettes. It is considered to increase gastric motility and secretion and delay healing of the ulcer.

INSTRUCTIONS TO THE ULCER PA-

TIENT. The nurse has an important role in helping the patient to understand and accept the treatment and adjustments recommended by the physician. His progress in the acute stage and the prevention of recurrence of the ulcer may be greatly influenced by the nurse's recognition of the patient's needs in this area and by careful planning to provide the necessary assistance.

If possible, it is helpful to include a responsible family member in some of the discussions, which should be spread out over several days. The patient and family are given sufficient opportunity to ask questions. Obviously, some patients require more help than others, but generally the factors that should receive attention are as follows:

Clarification of the Nature of the Disorder. The patient should have some understanding of the nature of his disease and the principles of the suggested therapeutic measures. With such knowledge, he is more likely to cooperate. He is advised that ulcers are prone to recur and that his respect, or lack of it, for the prescribed regimen may play an important role in whether he remains symptom-free or has a recurrence.

Diet. An outline of the prescribed diet is given to the patient, and the necessary dietary modifications and their principles are discussed with him. The importance of regular, unhurried meals in a relaxed environment, his recognition of foods that cause discomfort and the elimination of them from his diet, and the avoidance of coffee, tea, condiments, carbonated and alcoholic beverages and overeating are explained. Some directives relating to the selection and preparation of the patient's food may be necessary. For example, fried foods should be limited, and boiled or broiled meats are preferable in order the eliminate the stimulating extract (secretogogue). The process of puréeing or blending of foods, if such is prescribed, and the usefulness of commercially prepared baby foods may be suggested if roughage is a problem.

Medications. An important part of the planned instruction is information and directives related to the drugs prescribed. Their purpose, the importance of taking them at the times suggested, and possible side effects are discussed.

Avoidance of Noxious Agents. The patient is advised to continue the restrictions on smoking and alcohol. He is told of the inadvisability of taking aspirin and any medications that are not prescribed.

Rest and Diversion. The need to avoid fatigue and emotional upsets and to forget his work when he leaves his work situation are emphasized. The patient should understand the role of anxiety, worry and frustration in his disease. The importance of relaxation and some diversion is stressed, and some practical suggestions made as to how these may be achieved.

Complications. Any pain, vomiting, abdominal distention or gastric distress should be reported promptly to his physician so early treatment may be instituted.

SURGICAL TREATMENT. If the ulcer fails to heal with medical treatment and the symp-

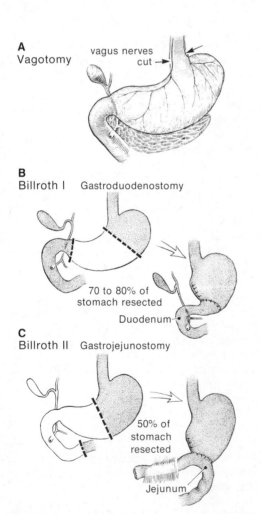

A Vagotomy — vagus nerves cut

B Billroth I — Gastroduodenostomy

70 to 80% of stomach resected

Duodenum

C Billroth II — Gastrojejunostomy

50% of stomach resected

Jejunum

FIGURE 16–9 Subtotal gastric resection. *A,* Billroth I (gastroduodenostomy). *B,* Billroth II (gastrojejunostomy).

toms persist, if there has been bleeding or if the ulcer has resulted in some obstruction in the gastric outlet, surgical treatment may be considered necessary. Various operative procedures are used in the surgical treatment of an uncomplicated ulcer in order to reduce the gastric acid secretion. Current operative approaches include the following procedures (see Fig. 16–9). Gastric resection (subtotal gastrectomy) is the removal of a portion of the stomach, including the ulcer-bearing area. An anastomosis is then made between the gastric stump and the duodenum (gastroduodenostomy; Billroth I) or jejunum (gastrojejunostomy; Billroth II) to restore gastrointestinal continuity.

Gastric resection plus vagotomy may be done. Vagotomy is a resection of the vagus nerve to reduce the stimulation of gastric secretion. It also reduces the motility of the stomach and may interfere with gastric emptying. For this reason it is rarely performed alone but is combined with a gastric resection or with a gastroenterostomy to provide effective gastric emptying.

A combined vagotomy and resection of the antrum of the stomach (antrectomy) may be performed. The vagotomy reduces the innervation that increases the gastric secretion; removal of the antrum removes the source of the chemical stimulus, gastrin.

Vagotomy with pyloroplasty involves plastic surgery of the pylorus to relieve pyloric stricture as well as interruption of the vagus nerve fibers. In some instances a gastroenterostomy may be done instead of the pyloroplasty to improve gastric drainage.

COMPLICATIONS OF PEPTIC ULCERATION. The complications that commonly occur with peptic ulcer are serious and usually account for the deaths attributed to peptic ulcer. They are hemorrhage, perforation, and pyloric obstruction.

HEMORRHAGE. Peptic ulceration is the commonest cause of hematemesis and melena. The loss of blood is due to erosion of a blood vessel at the ulcer site. Most of the patients who have a hemorrhage are known to have or to have had an ulcer but, in a few, it may be the first symptom that prompts them to seek treatment.

Vomiting of blood and the passing of black tarry stools are the prominent indications of serious ulcer bleeding. The patient experiences weakness, apprehension, dizziness and faintness which may progress rapidly to prostration and loss of consciousness. His skin becomes pale, cold and clammy, his pulse is rapid and thready and the blood pressure is abnormally low. Rapid respirations manifest air hunger and hypoxemia. If a large vessel is eroded, the signs and symptoms appear more rapidly and collapse occurs quickly.

Management.   Prompt hospital treatment is necessary and includes absolute rest, blood transfusions, parenteral fluids, oxygen administration and treatment of the ulcer.

The patient is restless and very apprehensive. Rest is promoted by the administration of a sedative, a quiet environment, reassurance and a minimum of disturbance. An effort must be made by those around the patient to avoid exhibiting apprehension. The patient may be less apprehensive if he is told something about his condition and is advised that treatment is well under control. He should not be left alone, and relatives are asked to control their emotions when in the patient's immediate environment.

The foot of the bed may be elevated to encourage the maintenance of a blood supply to the more vital areas. A constant check is made of the patient's pulse, color and respirations, and the blood pressure is recorded every 15 minutes. This interval is lengthened as the patient shows improvement. On admission, the patient's blood is typed and a transfusion started as soon as compatible blood is available. The rate of flow is kept slow and carefully controlled to avoid a rapid increase in blood pressure which would increase the bleeding.

Nothing is given by mouth at first. A nasogastric tube may be passed and gentle suction may be applied to remove the blood. A double lumen or large gastric tube may be used and intragastric lavages of iced saline or water given to retard blood flow and gastric secretion. As much as 10 liters over a period of 30 to 60 minutes may be used.

A vasopressor drug such as vasopressin (Pitressin) or norepinephrine (Levophed, levarterenol) may be instilled into the stomach and the nasogastric tube clamped for 30 minutes in order to produce local vasoconstriction to check the bleeding. After retention of the drug for the designated period, the stomach may be gently irrigated to determine if the vasopressor has been effective. The blood pressure and pulse must be monitored very closely.

In place of the local application of a vaso-

constrictor, vasopressin (Pitressin) may be administered intravenously. It is given in glucose 5 per cent in water over a period of 30 to 45 minutes. The resulting arteriolar constriction slows the bleeding.

Rarely, a gastroscopy may be done to locate the bleeding site and apply electrocautery or a topical application of a hemostatic preparation to control the bleeding.

Frequent mouth care is necessary because of the hematemesis, dehydration and the discomfort of extreme thirst. Small oral feedings or a continuous drip of cold milk may be ordered within a few hours if the patient has recovered from the shock caused by the loss of blood and has stopped vomiting. The early feedings are considered to have some advantages. The milk reduces the acidity of the gastric juice and gives the ulcer a better chance to heal and check the bleeding; it provides nutrition and helps to maintain a normal fluid and electrolyte balance. If there is blood in the stomach, it is diluted by the milk and is less likely to cause nausea and vomiting. The patient's anxiety may be lessened and his general morale improved by the fact that he is receiving food again. Antacid medication will also be prescribed.

When the bleeding has ceased, a progressive ulcer diet is ordered as cited on page 527 in the care of the peptic ulcer patient. Bed rest is continued to promote ulcer healing and until the severe anemia is corrected. Bed exercises are instituted with the physician's approval to prevent vascular complications and weakness. It may be necessary to exclude the abdominal contractions that are usually a part of bed exercises.

A preparation of iron will probably be ordered for the development of hemoglobin. Parenteral injections may be used at first; then an oral preparation may be given with feedings.

Some blood may still remain in the intestine after bleeding is controlled, but laxatives and enemas are withheld for 3 to 4 days. The physician may then order a small dose of a mild laxative such as milk of magnesia, or a cleansing enema may be given.

If the bleeding cannot be brought under control, emergency surgery may be undertaken. The ulcer area is resected, and the vessels leading to it are ligated.

PERFORATION.   A peptic ulcer may progressively erode the submucosal, muscular and serous layers of the gastrointestinal wall.

When the serous membranous layer is penetrated, some of the stomach or duodenal content escapes into the peritoneal cavity and causes a generalized peritonitis by chemical irritation and infection. Perforation has a higher incidence in duodenal ulceration and may occur in a few persons with no previous history of ulcer.

When perforation takes place, the patient immediately experiences sudden, incapacitating abdominal pain that begins in the epigastric region but spreads through the abdomen as more of the peritoneum becomes irritated by the intragastrointestinal content. The patient exhibits pallor, a cold clammy skin, rapid pulse, shallow grunting respirations and probably nausea and vomiting. The abdomen becomes rigid and board-like.

Perforation demands immediate treatment; the earlier the treatment is instituted, the greater is the patient's chance for recovery. The physician may consider emergency surgery advisable, or the patient's condition and history may be such that the perforation is treated by nonsurgical conservative methods. The surgical procedure may consist of gastric resection or simple closure of the perforation by suturing the serous layer and reinforcing the area with a patch of omentum. The peritoneal cavity is cleared of the intragastrointestinal fluid that seeped through the perforation. In addition to the usual preoperative procedures for emergency surgery, preparation will include the insertion of a nasogastric tube and an intravenous infusion of electrolytes and fluids. An explanation of the need for surgery and what it entails will be made by the surgeon, and the nurse briefly explains the necessary preparatory procedures as she proceeds with them. For postoperative nursing care, see the section on nursing care following gastric surgery, page 533.

Nonoperative treatment usually includes an analgesic such as morphine or meperidine hydrochloride (Demerol) by parenteral administration, aspiration of the stomach content using a large tube followed by the insertion of a nasogastric tube and continuous gastric suctioning, intravenous electrolytes and fluids (fluids may include whole blood) and antibiotic therapy. If the patient's condition is satisfactory, continuous gastric suctioning is replaced by intermittent aspiration after 30 to 48 hours. After 3 to 5 days, small amounts of fluid may be ordered by mouth at stated intervals and, if tolerated, the tube is removed and the oral intake is progressively increased.

PYLORIC OBSTRUCTION. The third serious complication of peptic ulcer disease is constriction of the pylorus. This may be caused by inflammation, edema and spasm when the ulcer is in the acute stage or by scar tissue which is formed as the ulcer heals. The ulcer may be gastric in the region of the pylorus, or it may be in the duodenum. The constriction causes gastric retention and dilatation.

The patient complains of a full feeling which causes greater discomfort toward the end of the day. Pain may be experienced following eating as gastric contractions increase in intensity in an effort to overcome the obstruction. The contractions gradually decline and the stomach becomes atonic and dilates. Severe anorexia develops and the patient vomits large amounts irregularly. The loss of nutrients, water and electrolytes leads to loss of weight, weakness, dehydration and acid-base imbalance (alkalosis).

If the obstruction is due to the active ulceration process, it is treated medically by gastric aspiration and intravenous fluids. The stomach may be completely emptied of its contents and first washed out with normal saline by means of a large stomach tube. Then a nasogastric tube is passed and continuous or intermittent suctioning is used for 2 to 3 days; withdrawal of gastric secretions reduces the acid-pepsin irritation of the ulcer, and the inflammation, edema and spasm that are responsible for the pyloric constriction gradually subside. The muscle tissue in the stomach walls gradually recover its tone and normal contractility.

Frequent small feedings are gradually introduced and the amount of gastric retention determined by a bedtime aspiration (4 hours after the last feeding). Normally, the volume of residue should not exceed 250 ml. When there is evidence of sufficient gastric outflow, aspirations are discontinued and the patient placed on the usual peptic ulcer dietary regimen.

The nursing care of the patient with a pyloric obstruction includes careful observations and recording of the exact amount and characteristics of all vomitus and aspirated material, the total fluid intake and output for each 12 or 24 hours, the time pain occurs in relation to food intake and the patient's weight and general condition. The upper abdomen should be examined for distention.

Obstruction due to contraction of fibrous scar tissue is treated by surgery. A gastric resection with a gastroenterostomy or pyloroplasty may be performed.

Cancer of the Stomach

Although cancer of the stomach still accounts for a large number of deaths each year, there has been a significant decline over the last three decades. The incidence is higher in males and in those 60 years of age and over.

As in the case with all cancers, the cause is unknown but certain factors are considered predisposing. Familial or hereditary tendency is thought to play a role. There is a higher incidence in persons belonging to blood group A and in persons with atrophy of the gastric mucosa, achlorhydria and chronic gastric ulceration.

Any region of the stomach may be involved, but the most frequent sites are the pylorus and antrum.

SYMPTOMS. The manifestations are vague and insidious. At first, the patient may complain of some mild discomfort after he eats but, as the disease advances, belching, regurgitation, nausea and vomiting may be experienced, and there is a progressive loss of appetite, weight and strength. Blood may appear in the vomitus and stool when there is ulceration at the cancer site. Pain is usually a late symptom. Unfortunately, because the early symptoms are mild and vague, the person tends to delay seeing a physician, and the disease becomes well advanced before there is medical intervention. Nurses should be aware of this problem and, on learning that a patient is experiencing even mild "digestive" disturbances, should urge him to seek medical advice.

DIAGNOSIS. Investigation of the patient includes x-ray examinations, analysis of gastric content for acidity, cytologic studies of gastric fluid, gastroscopy and biopsy, examination of the stool for blood, hemoglobin estimation and blood cell counts.

The gastric analysis is done to determine if there is a decrease in the secretion of hydrochloric acid as the majority of patients with cancer of the stomach demonstrate a hypochlorhydria or an achlorhydria. The blood examinations will probably show some deficiency of hemoglobin and red blood cells, as anemia is a characteristic of gastric cancer

due to the chronic bleeding, reduced production of the intrinsic factor by the gastric mucosa, reduced absorption of iron because of the hypochlorhydria and nutritional deficits.

METASTASES. Gastric carcinoma develops and metastasizes rapidly; all too often there has been a spread to some other structure(s) by the time of diagnosis. There may be direct extension to neighboring organs (e.g., esophagus, duodenum) or an indirect spread via the lymph and venous blood. The spleen, abdominal lymph nodes, peritoneum, liver, pancreas and lungs are frequent sites of metastases. The left supraclavicular and axillary nodes may also be affected.

TREATMENT AND NURSING CARE. At present, surgery is considered to be the only therapeutic approach to gastric cancer. The surgical procedure used will depend on the site of the cancer and its extension or possible course of extension. A subtotal gastrectomy or, rarely, a total gastrectomy is performed and may include resection of the duodenum, excision of the areas of lymphatic spread (omentum, spleen), resection of the pancreas or resection of the lower esophagus. In subtotal gastrectomy, the stomach is anastomosed to the jejunum (gastrojejunostomy) if it has been the lower part of the stomach that has been removed. In the case of removal of the proximal portion of the stomach the operation is completed by anastomosis of the esophagus to the remaining stomach (esophagoantrostomy). Total gastrectomy and a resection of the esophagus necessitate entrance into the thoracic cavity. Continuity of the alimentary tract is restored by an esophagojejunostomy.

The preoperative and postoperative nursing care of the gastric surgical patient is presented below. Care of the patient following a complete gastrectomy will include the care necessary for any patient who has had chest surgery (p. 460). The patient who has had his stomach or a large part of it removed will require small frequent meals of easily digested bland foods and vitamin B_{12} injections throughout the remainder of his life.

NURSING THE PATIENT WHO HAS GASTRIC SURGERY

Preoperative Nursing Care

The patient is admitted to the hospital several days prior to surgery unless a complication such as perforation of an ulcer demands an immediate operation. A general assessment is made of his condition by the surgeon and anesthetist and treatment is instituted according to their findings.

PSYCHOLOGICAL PREPARATION. The patient who is to have elective gastric surgery has considerable anxiety and apprehension, particularly if the anticipated procedure is a gastrectomy. In addition to the fears and problems that any surgery may create for the patient and his family (see Chapter 10), this patient is probably concerned about how he can survive without a portion of his stomach, and he may fear malignancy. The surgeon, in recommending and explaining the operation, may mention the possible sequelae or changes in gastrointestinal function that a few patients may experience postoperatively.

The understanding nurse encourages the patient to express his feelings and ask questions. An explanation may be necessary to reassure him that the continuity of his gastrointestinal tract will be reestablished, that he will be able to take food in the normal way, and that only a few dietary modifications may be necessary because of the diminished gastric capacity.

The postoperative care is discussed briefly so that the patient may have some idea as to what to expect and will not be alarmed by the frequent checking of his pulse and blood pressure, gastric suctioning, and intravenous administration.

PHYSICAL PREPARATION. The patient's diet and fluid intake may have been inadequate for some time because of his disease. Nutritional, electrolyte and fluid deficits are determined, and efforts are made to correct them. When his condition permits solid food, total calories and protein and vitamin content are increased and given in frequent small feedings. Foods that are normally contraindicated for patients with peptic ulcer are avoided (fried foods, spices, etc.). Fluids are provided between meals and, if well diluted citrus fruit juices are tolerated, they are encouraged, since they provide vitamin C, potassium and calories. If solid food cannot be managed, semifluids, blender feedings or liquids containing commercial protein preparations may be ordered. The patient may not be able to take sufficient quantities by mouth and may receive various intravenous solutions (glucose, electrolytes, amino acids) to improve his fluid and nutritional status. Paren-

teral preparations of vitamins B complex, C and K may also be given.

Blood studies are done to determine the needs of the patient. The findings govern the medicinal preparations ordered and if anemia is present a blood transfusion may be given.

An accurate record is made of the fluid intake and output, and the patient is weighed daily. The weight is significant in determining the patient's nutritional status and progress as well as for establishing a comparative basis for the postoperative period.

Postoperatively, the patient who has had gastric surgery tends to take very shallow breaths. The normal excursion of the diaphragm and chest walls may cause pain in the operative area which is in the upper part of the abdomen, so the patient restricts respiratory movements. Shallow respirations decrease the respiratory exchange of oxygen and carbon dioxide and promote the accumulation of respiratory secretions in the alveoli and bronchioles; this may lead to serious pulmonary complications. The importance of deep breathing, coughing, exercises and early ambulation that will be part of his postoperative care is discussed with the patient. Demonstrations of these activities by the nurse and practice by the patient should accompany the explanation to make it easier for him after the operation and to ensure greater cooperation on his part. The patient is asked to stop smoking and is given the reasons.

Any indication of a respiratory disturbance or infection, such as a nasal discharge, expectoration of sputum, cough, shortness of breath and temperature elevation, is brought to the physician's attention.

If the patient has been receiving oral feedings, these may be reduced to clear fluids the day before operation and nothing is given in the immediate 8 to 12 hours preceding operation. A nasogastric tube is inserted the night before operation, and suction is used to empty the stomach of secretions and any food residue. The tube is left in place when the patient goes to the operating room.

In addition to the foregoing considerations, preparation of the patient will include the general preoperative care cited in Chapter 10.

Postoperative Nursing Care

SPECIAL EQUIPMENT. Preparation to receive the patient from the operating room includes the assembling of equipment for gastric suctioning, intravenous infusion, and mouth care.

OBSERVATIONS. When the patient returns, the nasogastric or gastrostomy tube is connected to the suction as ordered, and the intravenous infusion checked to make sure the transfer has not displaced the needle.

Close observation is made of the patient for the first 24 to 48 hours for early signs of shock, hemorrhage and interference with the gastric drainage system. The blood pressure, pulse, respirations, color, temperature and moisture of the skin, gastric drainage, wound site and patient's response are checked frequently.

An accurate record is made of the fluid intake and output. The latter will include any emesis and gastric drainage as well as the urinary output.

OXYGEN ADMINISTRATION. Oxygen may be ordered but is not usually necessary for a prolonged period if the patient makes uncomplicated progress.

GASTRIC DRAINAGE (see p. 499). Gentle gastric suctioning and nothing by mouth are continued for the first few days to prevent the escape of gastric secretions and fluid through the stomach suture line into the peritoneal cavity and to minimize vomiting and distention. Drainage may be via a nasogastric or gastrostomy tube that is positioned in the stomach through a stab wound. The number of days the nasogastric tube is left in and oral fluids are withheld varies with each surgeon and will also depend on the patient's progress. The characteristics and exact volume of the drainage are noted. It will most likely be colored by blood at first but usually clears in a few hours. The physician is notified if large amounts of blood appear or if the drainage continues to be blood-colored. The tube may become obstructed by mucus or a small blood clot. An order may be received to clear it with a syringe and a small amount of normal saline or water (25 to 30 ml.).

The surgeon's order may be for continuous low suction, or the drainage tube may be attached to a pump which automatically applies intermittent suctioning. After 24 to 36 hours, the tube may be connected to the suctioning apparatus only for stated periods at intervals; the volume which is aspirated is recorded each time.

POSITIONING. When the patient regains consciousness and his blood pressure and pulse are stabilized, the head of the bed may be gradually elevated to promote gastric drainage and deeper breathing. The patient is turned hourly from side to side to back to side.

DEEP BREATHING AND COUGHING. The patient is reminded hourly to take five to ten deep breaths and to cough several times to prevent pulmonary complications. Necessary encouragement and support are provided by the nurse who holds a small pillow lightly over the operative site and places a hand on the patient's back during the coughing. The nurse acknowledges the patient's distress but at the same time emphasizes the importance of deep breathing and coughing in the prevention of other problems.

EXERCISES AND EARLY AMBULATION. Simple limb exercises to prevent venous stasis are started the morning after operation. If the patient is too weak or too ill for active participation, the limbs are put through a range of passive movements by the nurse. The surgeon usually suggests that the patient be assisted to a sitting position on the side of the bed the day after the operation and then to sit in a chair on the second day. Self-care activities are gradually encouraged with an explanation to the patient of their advantages. In addition to preventing pulmonary and vascular complications, early ambulation and patient activity help to reestablish normal gastrointestinal motility.

NUTRITION AND FLUIDS. Parenteral fluids are used to sustain the patient over the first few days. Different procedures are used to introduce the first fluids; the surgeon may have the nasogastric tube removed and small stated amounts of water given every half hour or every hour. The amount is gradually increased if tolerated. The directive may be to introduce a specific amount of water at intervals through the nasogastric tube which is then clamped.

If the patient tolerates the increased amounts of water without experiencing vomiting, pain or distention, feedings of clear sweetened tea, equal parts of milk and water, whole milk, creamed soups, gruel and blender preparations are progressively added over 2 to 3 days *but only on specific orders from the surgeon.*

With normal progress, the patient is usually receiving a soft bland diet by the fifth to seventh day. The volume given at any one time should remain small because of the reduced capacity of the stomach. Foods high in calories are selected and served in frequent, small amounts. The patient's weight is recorded regularly, and the physician is advised if there is a loss or a failure to gain. Inability of the patient to take the prescribed diet and any regurgitation, vomiting, distention or complaint of pain should be reported.

By the time the patient is ready to leave the hospital he will most likely be taking a light bland diet of high-calorie foods divided into six meals. Fluids may be omitted from the meals and taken in between so their volume will not prevent the patient from taking sufficient solid food. The patient is advised that he may gradually increase the amount taken at regular meals and, if no discomfort is experienced, he may eventually need only three or four meals with milk and other fluids taken between them.

MOUTH CARE. Frequent cleansing and moistening of the mouth are necessary to lessen the patient's discomfort while the nasogastric tube is in place and oral fluids are restricted. The tube may cause irritation that results in mucus secretion which, if allowed to collect, might be aspirated. The nostril through which the tube is passed should also be cleansed and moistened and receive a *very light* application of mineral oil or petroleum jelly.

ELIMINATION. The urinary output is recorded and totaled for each 24 hours. A small cleansing enema may be ordered on the third postoperative day to cleanse the lower bowel of blood that may be in the tract from the surgical procedure. The enema may be repeated every other day when oral intake is started. A mild laxative such as milk of magnesia may be prescribed after 4 or 5 days.

MEDICATIONS. Considerable pain is experienced by the patient who has had gastric surgery. An analgesic, such as meperidine hydrochloride (Demerol) by parenteral administration, is usually ordered to relieve the patient's discomfort but judicious use is necessary. Oversedation makes it difficult to promote deep breathing and coughing; on the other hand, the patient should not be allowed to suffer unnecessarily since pain may contribute to shock.

Vitamins B complex and C and iron may be ordered, since the natural food sources of these will be restricted in the diet for a period of time.

INSTRUCTIONS. Preparation of the patient for leaving the hospital includes discussions with him and a member of his family of the necessary dietary and activity modifications. The importance of frequent small meals of nonirritating foods high in calories is explained. The size of the meals may be gradually increased when they are comfortably tolerated. The remaining portion of the stomach progressively adapts to larger quantities and, after several months, the person may find that he can manage three regular meals. Suggestions are made as to food selection and preparation. Written dietary instructions and outlines may be necessary for some patients. The patient is advised to weigh himself regularly, to report to the clinic or physician at the scheduled dates and to get in touch with the physician promptly if he has pain, vomiting, progressive loss of weight or other distressing symptoms.

Considerable rest will be necessary for some time and he should lie down for at least ½ hour after each meal. Normal activities are resumed very gradually and should not be allowed to interfere with regularity of his meals.

If a total gastrectomy is done or a large section of the stomach is removed, the patient will require regular parenteral administration of a maintenance dose of cyanocobalamin (vitamin B_{12}). The patient is advised of the importance of receiving this. Arrangements are made for him to receive the vitamin B_{12} at the scheduled times; it may be given at the clinic or in the physician's office, by a visiting nurse or by a family member who is taught to give the drug subcutaneously.

The patient and family are informed of the assistance available to them from the visiting nurse agencies. Economic problems may be a concern because of the prolonged illness and convalescence, and the family may have difficulty in providing the diet and care suggested for the patient. A social worker may be asked to see them to arrange for the necessary assistance, or the nurse may refer the problem to an appropriate source.

Postgastrectomy Problems

A few patients experience some gastrointestinal dysfunction after gastric surgery, mainly because of the anatomical changes made by the surgery.

DUMPING SYNDROME. Following gastric surgery that results in a disruption or bypass of the pyloric sphincter, the patient may experience a complex of symptoms referred to as the dumping syndrome. The symptoms are related to intestinal and vasomotor disturbances and are precipitated by eating. The syndrome may appear before the meal is completed or soon after, and lasts only a few minutes to a half hour. It may not occur with every meal but is more likely to develop following a large meal or one that contained a high content of carbohydrates (especially sugar) or salt.

The patient may experience epigastric fullness, nausea, crampy abdominal pains, distention, diarrhea, muscular weakness, dizziness, fainting, palpitation and sweating. He is pale and his pulse is rapid.

Normally, the gastric content is delivered in small amounts into the intestine by the pylorus. Following a gastric resection, vagotomy or gastroenterostomy, the normal pyloric control of the volume moving from the stomach into the small intestine is absent. The dumping syndrome is caused by the precipitous passage into the small intestine of a relatively large amount of gastric content that has not undergone the usual dilution and digestive changes. The exact mechanism by which the characteristic responses are initiated is not entirely clear; it is suggested that the following factors are implicated.

First, the sudden distention of the proximal portion of the small intestine initiates sympathetic reflexes. Second, the fluid that moved quickly out of the stomach is hypertonic, having a high concentration of sugar and/or electrolytes. The hyperosmolarity of the intestinal contents results in the movement of fluid from the intravascular spaces into the jejunum. The complex of symptoms is attributed to the distention of the jejunum, the decreased intravascular volume and the reflex responses of the sympathetic nervous system. It is also suggested that serotonin is released into the blood by the intestine and plays a role in producing the symptoms. As cited above, the etiology is not clearly understood. Only a relatively small percentage of patients develop the problem. Physicians have observed that the severity of the syndrome increases with emotional instability.[15]

Treatment of the dumping syndrome is by dietary modifications. The symptoms gradually subside in most patients, and eventually a more normal dietary pattern may be resumed. Rarely, if the condition cannot be controlled by dietary and drug management and is incapacitating, surgical treatment is employed. An operation is performed to delay gastric emptying and may consist of narrowing the anastomotic opening from the stomach into the small intestine.

The necessary dietary modifications include the avoidance of large meals and a reduced intake of salty and sweet foods. No fluids are given with meals. Six small, dry meals consisting mainly of proteins and fats are planned to meet the patient's caloric requirement. Liquids are taken between meals to maintain normal hydration but should be limited during the half hour preceding and following a meal. The patient is advised to eat slowly and to lie down for a half hour following each meal.

The symptoms cause considerable emotional reaction in the patient. He should be encouraged to persevere with the suggested dietary regimen and should be reassured that as time goes on the condition will gradually subside as the gastrointestinal tract adapts to the structural changes. To avoid the distressing symptoms, the patient may tend to reduce his food intake to dangerously low amounts that result in weight loss and nutritional deficiencies.

In addition to the dietary treatment, anticholinergic drugs may be prescribed to decrease gastrointestinal motility.

NUTRITIONAL DEFICIENCY. The patient who has had a gastric resection may have a problem in maintaining his normal weight. The cause is usually a lack of sufficient food intake because the diminished gastric capacity results in quick satiety and an overfull feeling or it may be due, as cited above, to the distressing dumping syndrome precipitated by eating. Frequent high-calorie feedings that are acceptable to the patient are planned. Small amounts are given at first and are gradually increased with the patient's tolerance. Part of the problem may be the patient's psychological reaction to the need for continuing dietary modifications; he may have expected no problems or restrictions once he had surgical treatment. The need for a period of time for necessary adjustments by his digestive system should be discussed with the patient to obtain his cooperation.

[15]David C. Sabiston (Ed.): Davis-Christopher Textbook of Surgery, 11th ed. Philadelphia, W. B. Saunders, 1977, p. 933.

ANEMIA. Iron deficiency may occur as a result of decreased iron absorption. Normal absorption is facilitated by gastric acidity which has been reduced in the gastrectomy patient. The bypassing of the duodenum by a gastrojejunostomy may also reduce the amount of iron absorption in many of these patients. The deficiency may be due to a poor dietary intake of foods that provide iron (red meat, liver, leafy vegetables, whole milk, eggs and certain cereals). The diet may be corrected to contain the necessary sources and supplemented by an iron drug preparation, such as ferrous sulfate tablets.

Anemia may be present as a result of a deficiency in the secretion of the intrinsic factor (due to the loss of gastric mucosa by the gastric resection) which promotes the absorption of vitamin B_{12}. It may develop within a few months after the gastrectomy but is not common until 2 to 3 years have elapsed. The patient may be given weekly vitamin B_{12} by subcutaneous or intramuscular injections until a normal erythrocyte count is established. Then a maintenance dose is given monthly throughout the remainder of the patient's life.

HYPOGLYCEMIA. A few patients who have had a gastrectomy may exhibit the manifestations characteristic of hypoglycemia 2 to 3 hours after taking a meal. The condition is referred to as late *postprandial* or *postcibal hypoglycemia*. The patient's symptoms are weakness, tremulousness, faintness, sweating and palpitation due to a fall in the blood sugar level to 50 to 60 mg. per cent. It is explained on the basis of the rapid absorption of glucose from the intestine, causing a sudden hyperglycemia. The latter stimulates an excessive output of insulin which rapidly lowers the blood sugar concentration to an abnormally low level.

The condition is controlled by the patient's taking a high-protein diet, decreasing the carbohydrate intake, and shortening the interval between meals. Some form of sugar (candy, honey, lump sugar or orange juice) should be quickly available to the patient as soon as the early symptoms of hypoglycemia are experienced.

OSTEOMALACIA. Rarely, a patient may develop osteomalacia[16] which, in the postgas-

trectomy patient, is attributed to decreased absorption of vitamin D and calcium. The malabsorption is usually associated with diarrhea or steatorrhea. Vitamin D and calcium supplements are given.

DISORDERS OF THE INTESTINES

Disorders of the *small intestine* may cause disturbances in digestion, absorption and the movement of content along the gastrointestinal tract. A prolonged or serious dysfunction threatens the patient's nutritional status.

A disturbance in function of the *large intestine* interferes with the excretion of bowel waste and, if the right half of the colon is involved, the normal absorption of water and salts may be reduced and cause dehydration.

Constipation and Diarrhea

Intestinal dysfunction may be manifested by a retarded or accelerated movement of contents through the intestine. Delayed movement causes *constipation,* which is characterized by infrequent, hard dry stools, or may result in a complete failure of the excretion of feces, which may be referred to as *obstipation.* The prolonged retention of the feces results in the absorption of increased amounts of water which accounts for the abnormal consistency of the stools. The symptom of dysfunction may be *diarrhea,* which is characterized by frequent liquid or unformed stools.

CONSTIPATION. The majority of persons normally defecate once every 24 hours but there is considerable variance in the frequency among healthy persons. Some persons have more than one bowel movement daily, while others may have an evacuation of a normally moist stool once every 2 or 3 days. Such variances in frequency of bowel elimination may be compatible with health. An individual is considered to be constipated if bowel elimination is unexplainably delayed for several days or if the stool is so hard and dry that it is difficult to express.

Constipation may be a delay in the passage of feces through the colon, referred to as colonic constipation, or it may be a prolonged retention of the feces in the rectum, designated as *rectal constipation* or *dyschezia.*

---

[16]*Osteomalacia* is a disorder characterized by decalcification of the bones and a weakening of their structure.

CAUSES. The causes of constipation are many and varied. It may be associated with organic disease, or it may be a functional disturbance.

Disease within the colon or rectum may narrow the lumen of the bowel and offer resistance to the forward movement of content. Common examples are newgrowths of the intestine; inflammation which causes spasm, scarring and adhesions; and partial volvulus (twisting of the bowel). Severe ascites (accumulation of fluid in the peritoneal cavity) or a tumor, such as an ovarian cyst or uterine fibroid, may compress the colon and delay the movement of intestinal content.

Failure of the normal propulsive movement may occur due to some disturbance or imbalance in the innervation of the intestine. The derangement may result in excessive tone and spasm in a segment of the bowel that retards the movement of the content. The spasm may be induced by a hypersensitivity of the colon or by anxiety. Constipation may be associated with injury or degeneration of the spinal cord or cauda equina, which affects the nerve supply to the colon and rectum.

Megacolon (large colon) may account for constipation in infants. It is a congenital anomaly in which there is an absence of certain nerve structures (parasympathetic ganglia) in a segment of the colon, resulting in failure of peristalsis in the affected portion of the bowel. The most frequent site is the sigmoid and it is seen more often in males. The affected segment is constricted and does not participate in normal peristaltic activity. Fecal content accumulates in the adjacent preceding colon and dilation occurs. The condition is also known as *Hirschsprung's disease*. Surgical resection of the colon may be considered necessary and is done in two stages: a colostomy is done first, and then resection of the affected area and anastomosis are performed.

Constipation may be associated with any illness in which there is diminished intake of food and fluid or in cases in which the diet is modified and lacks fiber, resulting in less residue. The lesser amount of food does not provide sufficient bulk to stimulate peristalsis. Dehydration causes a small, dry, hard stool that may irritate the colon, causing spasm, or may fail to stimulate normal colon motility.

Constipation is frequently secondary to physical inactivity or prolonged bed rest. It is a common complaint among persons with sedentary occupations who probably ride to and from work and do not participate in any type of physical exercise.

Occasionally, drugs used in treatment may depress peristalsis and cause a delay in the excretion of feces. Common examples of such drugs are opiates (e.g., codeine) and anticholinergic drugs (e.g., Pro-Banthine).

Expulsion of the feces is aided by increasing the intra-abdominal pressure to compress the colon and rectum. This involves contraction of the muscles of the abdominal wall and of the diaphragm. Weakness of these muscles due to disease, senility, malnutrition or inactivity may contribute to constipation. Similarly, lack of tone in the intestinal musculature or weakness of the levator ani muscles may impair peristalsis and the expulsive power.

Frequent causes of constipation in persons who are not ill are faulty defecation habits, faulty diet and the habitual use of laxatives. If the urge to defecate is ignored and evacuation delayed, the reflex becomes weak as the rectal mucosa adapts to the pressure of the content. Repeated failure to respond to defecation reflex may eventually result in the rectum's becoming insensitive to the presence of a fecal mass and the reflex is not initiated. The person may delay response to the defecation urge because he does not find it convenient to interrupt what he is doing or because toilet facilities may not be available.

A deficiency of foods with cellulose and fibrous content in the diet may be the cause of constipation. Refined foods and those that leave little residue after absorption fail to produce sufficient bulk to stimulate colonic motility.

Many persons have an inordinate concern about bowel elimination and think they must have a daily bowel movement or a frequent purge and resort to unnecessary, repeated use of a laxative. Loss of intestinal tone and reduced peristaltic response to normal food residue follow the use of a laxative, and then too often the laxative is repeated. The colon is not allowed to regain its natural rhythmic response to the normal fecal mass.

Constipation may cause considerable discomfort; the person may experience abdominal pain, a full feeling and abdominal distention. There is a loss of appetite accompanied by headache and eventually nausea and vomiting. The hard dry masses of fecal matter may damage the intestinal mucosa and lead to a fissure. Hemorrhoids are frequently the result of chronic constipation.

MANAGEMENT. The person who experiences a change in his normal pattern of bowel elimination that persists beyond a few days or that recurs at frequent intervals is urged to consult a physician. The underlying cause of the constipation is then identified, and treatment may be initiated.

It may be necessary to advise the individual that daily bowel elimination is not essential to health for some persons.

Diet. Dietary modifications may be necessary. The total daily food intake may need to be increased and each meal should include one or two foods that will provide a liberal amount of fiber (roughage). Emphasis is placed on whole grain cereals and bread, fresh fruits and vegetables, and fruit juices. A minimum of eight glasses or approximately 2 liters of liquid should be taken each day. Many persons find a glass of hot water helpful when taken approximately ½ hour before breakfast.

If the constipation is due to spastic response of an irritable or hypersensitive colon, a bland diet with a minimum of roughage is recommended. Raw fruits and vegetables and large amounts of those high in fiber content are avoided. Spiced and fried foods and iced food and fluids should be restricted. For more details as to the diet for constipation, the reader is referred to a diet therapy text.

Establishing a Regular Time. It may be helpful to explain to the person in simple terms the physiological mechanism of defecation so he may grasp the significance of responding to the initial urge for defecation. The importance of establishing a regular time for bowel elimination, preferably after breakfast, is stressed. This may necessitate an increase in the amount of breakfast taken to provide sufficient food to stimulate the necessary wave of intestinal peristalsis.

Flexion of the thighs on the abdomen helps to promote bowel evacuation. A footstool placed in front of the toilet raises and supports the feet and assists in assuming the suggested flexion position.

Exercise. Some physical exercise is essential; walking is especially good. Good tone in the abdominal muscles is important; exercises to increase the strength of the abdominal muscles may be suggested. Examples of prescribed exercises are as follows: The patient lies on his back on the floor or bed with his arms folded across his chest and raises himself to the sitting position, keeping his heels on the floor. From the supine position, the patient raises his lower limbs without bending his knees. These exercises are done two or three times daily, and the patient is also encouraged to contract his abdominal muscles several times at frequent intervals through the day.

Laxatives and Enemas. Laxatives, enemas and suppositories that the patient may be accustomed to using are discontinued. If the diet and exercises are not sufficient at the beginning to establish normal bowel elimination, mild laxatives may be employed until the defecation reflex is restored and bowel irritability and spasm are reduced. The physician may suggest the use of a preparation that swells when it combines with fluid in the gastrointestinal tract and provides a stimulating bulk. Examples of bulking laxatives are agar and psyllium seed (Metamucil).

A stool softener may be ordered to prevent severe straining at stool and injury to the rectal and anal tissues. The stool softeners in use are mineral oil and preparations of dioctyl sodium sulfosuccinate (Colace, Doxinate). These latter preparations act as wetting agents, allowing water to penetrate and mix with the fecal mass. Mineral oil should not be used for prolonged periods because it may prevent normal intestinal absorption, especially of fat-soluble vitamins. Prolonged use also predisposes to lipoid pneumonia.

Milk of magnesia is a mild laxative that is commonly used. It is contraindicated in patients with any renal insufficiency.

Some persons who have been addicted to the use of laxatives may require the use of a stronger laxative at first. The dosage should be gradually decreased and the drug withdrawn completely as soon as possible.

FECAL IMPACTION. Occasionally, feces accumulate in the rectum, producing a hard dry mass that forms a partial or complete obstruction. It occurs most often in older persons and in those with central nervous system disorders. Crampy pain is experienced in the lower abdomen and liquid stools may be passed without expelling the impacted mass.

A retention enema of warm oil or a solution of dioctyl sodium sulfosuccinate (strength of solution to be ordered by the physician) may be given. This is followed in a few hours by digital breaking up and removal of the mass. A cleansing enema of saline or tap water is then given. The process of disimpaction is usually very exhausting for the patient. Following the enema, he is made comfortable and is allowed to rest.

DIARRHEA. This term implies an accelerated movement of content through the intestine, resulting in frequent liquid or unformed stools. The feces pass through the colon before the normal amount of water is absorbed.

Diarrhea is a symptom of many different disorders which may be within the bowel or may be extrinsic to the intestine. Changes characteristic of organic disease may occur in the intestine and result in diarrhea, or the bowel may be structurally normal with the hypermotility being functional. The more common causes of diarrhea are presented here as intrinsic or extrinsic, although there are many different etiologic classifications in medical literature.

INTRINSIC CAUSES. Normally the stimulus for peristalsis arises within the intestine. It may cause direct stimulation of the muscle tissue, or it may initiate sensory nerve impulses that are transmitted into the central nervous system, resulting in parasympathetic nerve impulses being carried out to the intestine that then stimulate its motility. Disease or irritations within the bowel which may increase either direct stimulation or reflex hypermotility include the following:

Infection. Food or fluid contaminated by salmonella, shigella or staphylococcal organisms is the most common cause of intestinal infection and may be referred to as bacterial food poisoning.

The shigella bacilli cause bacillary dysentery, and the primary source is usually the excreta of an infected person. This disease is rare, except under crowded and poor sanitary conditions.

The salmonella bacilli may inhabit the intestine of man, fowl and animals and may be the source of infection to others. It may be transmitted by the meat of infected animals and by food or water contaminated by the excreta of infected humans or animals. Sporadic outbreaks occur and may be due to a human carrier employed in the handling of food. Ingested salmonella or shigella organisms multiply, causing irritation and inflam-

mation of the intestine, resulting in diarrhea accompanied by crampy abdominal pain, fever, nausea and vomiting.

If the infection is by staphylococci, the irritation and inflammation of the intestine are due to the toxin produced by the organisms. Food may become contaminated by a handler who has an infected lesion on his body or who is carrying the organisms in his nose or throat. Meat, custard and cream-filled desserts allowed to remain at ordinary room temperature are common offenders and may contain considerable toxin when ingested. As a result, the manifestations of food poisoning — nausea, vomiting, fever, and diarrhea — occur within a few hours of ingestion of the contaminated food. The patient becomes very ill and quickly prostrated.

Neoplasms. Diarrhea may be a symptom of a malignant newgrowth of the colon and may be alternated with periods of constipation.

Dietary Factors. An excessive amount of coarse foods or highly seasoned irritating foods may produce hypermotility of the bowel. Occasionally, allergy to a certain food may account for diarrhea; if the intestinal mucosa is sensitive to the food, it becomes hyperemic and edematous and causes increased reflex hypermotility.

Malabsorption. Impaired absorption of foods may be due to incomplete digestion or to a defect in the absorptive process of the small intestine. Obviously, with reduced digestion and absorption, an increase in the bulk of the colon content results and is a stimulus to intestinal motility. The stools are bulky, have an offensive odor and usually contain large amounts of fats which are irritating to the bowel mucosa and initiate reflex peristalsis. General malnutrition is also evident.

Diverticulitis. A pouch or sac may occur in the wall of the intestine and is known as a diverticulum (Fig. 16–10). It may be congenital or may develop as a result of a weakening of an area of the muscle tissue in the wall. There may be several diverticula, or the defect may occur singly.

Diverticula of the large intestine are more likely to give rise to trouble, as the more solid fecal content tends to collect and be retained in the sac, setting up an inflammation that causes increased reflex peristalsis and diarrhea.

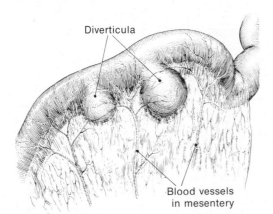

Diverticula

Blood vessels
in mesentery

FIGURE 16–10   Intestinal diverticulum.

Laxatives.   Many laxatives act by direct irritation of the intestinal mucosa, resulting in the content being hurried through the colon before the normal amount of water is absorbed.

Antibiotics.   Diarrhea sometimes accompanies the oral administration of antibiotics. They may irritate the mucosa or alter the normal bacterial flora of the intestinal tract. The most frequent offenders are the tetracycline preparations.

Idiopathic Inflammation.   Patients with ulcerative colitis or regional enteritis experience severe diarrhea. No specific cause has been recognized for either condition.

EXTRINSIC CAUSES.   Diarrhea accompanies a variety of disorders in which the stimulus that results in increased parasympathetic innervation to the bowel originates outside the intestine.

Emotional Stress.   Anxiety or underlying tension is frequently the basis of diarrhea, producing a condition which may be referred to as the irritable bowel or colon syndrome (see p. 544). On investigation, disturbances may be revealed that are secondary to the diarrhea, but there is no organic disease in the intestine or elsewhere. The intestinal hypermotility is entirely functional and is considered psychogenic. The patient is usually sensitive and has a nervous temperament; a study of the patient's total life situation may reveal a specific emotional conflict that will probably account for his diarrhea.

General or Systemic Disorders.   Frequently, diarrhea is associated with general diseases, particularly if they cause toxemia. Examples of such conditions are acute infectious disease, hyperthyroidism and uremia.

EFFECTS.   Depending on the cause, diarrhea may be self-limiting by ridding the intestine of the irritating causative factor, it may be persistent, or there may be remissions and exacerbations. Severe diarrhea may produce serious changes in the body which in some instances may become irreversible and fatal. Infants, young children, and seriously ill and elderly persons tolerate diarrhea less well, and serious effects may develop rapidly; prompt action is necessary at the onset with these persons.

Body fluids, electrolytes and nutrients are lost in the frequent liquid stools; the patient becomes dehydrated, develops nutritional deficiencies and loses weight and strength. Acidosis may develop because of the depleted sodium and bicarbonate ions. Severe crampy abdominal pain and tenesmus (painful spasm of the anus) frequently accompany the diarrhea. The patient loses sleep, becomes exhausted and may become emotionally disturbed because he is embarrassed by the frequency and urgency of the diarrheal stools and perhaps is fearful that the cause is cancer.

NURSING THE PATIENT WITH DIARRHEA.   Any person who experiences diarrhea for more than a day or two or who has recurring attacks is urged to seek medical advice. The symptom should not be ignored, since it may be an early manifestation of a serious condition. Treatment is directed toward correction of the physiological effects of the diarrhea (e.g., fluid and electrolyte imbalance), identification and elimination of the cause, control of the diarrhea, identification of nutritious foods tolerated by the patient and encouragement for him to take them, and provision of psychological support. In the case of acute diarrhea due to infection, it is important to prevent the spread of the disorder to others.

Investigation.   Investigation by the physician to determine the cause of the diarrhea may require several days during which symptomatic and supportive treatment are necessary. Diagnostic procedures may include a sigmoidoscopy or colonoscopy, stool cultures, x-rays of the bowel and blood chemistry studies to determine potassium, sodium, chloride and bicarbonate concentrations (see p. 80).

Observations.   It is important to obtain the following information: (1) the patient's previous bowel habit; (2) the number of bowel movements each day; (3) the volume and consistency of the stools; (4) whether the stools contain abnormal components, such as blood and excessive mucus; (5) whether there is exacerbation with certain foods or activities; and (6) whether the diarrhea is worse during the day or the night. Functional diarrhea tends to occur during the day, while that associated with organic disease is generally as disturbing at night as during the day.

Rest. Bed rest, with the patient remaining flat, is recommended for acute diarrhea; this may help to reduce peristalsis and decreases the energy demands. The weak patient is given the necessary assistance on and off the bedpan. Some patients are unable to relax and rest because of a constant fear of not receiving the bedpan in time; in such instances it may be helpful to make an exception and leave a clean covered bedpan at the bedside within the patient's reach.

Fluids and Nutrition. Fluids and electrolytes are replaced by intravenous infusions. If oral fluids are tolerated, water, sweetened clear tea, fat-free broth and gruel may be given. Skim milk and strained fruit juices may also be allowed by some doctors. Carbonated drinks, whole milk and iced fluids are usually avoided.

The diet is expanded as soon as possible to reduce the possibility of nutritional deficiencies. A high-calorie, high-vitamin and high-protein bland diet is gradually introduced, and the patient is observed as to the intestinal response. Roughage and gas-producing foods are restricted at first; whole grain bread and cereals, raw fruits and vegetables and highly seasoned and fried foods are not used. Concentrated sweets and fats are likely to be poorly tolerated. Fiber-containing foods and roughage are gradually introduced as tolerated. A prolonged bland diet is likely to become unpalatable, resulting in an inadequate nutritional intake. If the diarrhea is due to malabsorption, a gluten-free diet may be ordered in which foods are avoided that contain any wheat, rye, and barley grains or flour.

The first few mouthfuls of a meal may initiate a mass peristaltic wave, and the meal is interrupted. The patient's tray should be removed from the room and the hot foods kept warm. Following the necessary postdefecation care, the tray is returned. The patient may require some persuasion to complete his meal, as he is discouraged and is afraid that if he eats it will just precipitate another stool.

Esthetic and Hygienic Factors. Placement of the patient on the ward receives consideration. If ambulatory, he should be near toilet facilities; if confined to bed, privacy should be provided so the patient is less embarrassed by his frequent use of the bedpan.

The anal region should be left clean after each defecation and, if the skin around the anus is irritated, it is washed and a protective cream applied. Soiled bedding or clothing is changed promptly. Provision is made for thorough washing of the patient's hands after each defecation and the room is ventilated to avoid embarassment for him.

Diversion. Something to occupy the patient and divert his attention may prove beneficial. If the diarrhea is a reaction to stress, efforts are directed toward identifying the source of the emotional disturbance. The patient is encouraged to express his feelings and is reassured that there is no serious disease. New interests and activity in hobbies or sports may be suggested. Sedatives or tranquilizers may be ordered to relieve the emotional tension.

Medications. Various drugs may be used in the treatment of diarrhea. Drugs to reduce intestinal spasm and motility may be ordered. Examples are camphorated tincture of opium (paregoric), diphenoxylate hydrochloride (Lomotil) and tincture of belladonna. Drugs to provide a protective coating on the intestinal mucosa or to provide an adsorbent which condenses and holds irritating substances are used. Examples are aluminum silicate (Kaolin, Kaopectate), aluminum hydroxide gel (Amphojel) and bismuth subcarbonate. An anti-infective drug may be ordered if the diarrhea is of microbial origin. Sulfonamide preparations that are poorly absorbed but have a local effect are frequently used orally. Examples are succinylsulfathiazole (Sulfasuxidine) and phthalylsulfacetamide (Thalamyd).

Medical Asepsis. Cases of acute diarrhea are considered potentially infectious until otherwise indicated. Precautions are used to prevent the possible spread of infection to others. A gown is worn by all personnel when giving care, and the hands are scrubbed with soap and running water after each contact. The patient's linen is placed in a mesh laundry bag within a regular one so that it will not have to be handled by other workers. Treatment equipment and the bedpan are disinfected after each use. Depending on the causative organism, it may be considered necessary to disinfect the feces before the usual disposal by covering the stool with a 10 per cent formalin or 5 per cent cresol (Lysol) solution for 60 minutes. Visitors are restricted to members of the family who may be asked to wear a gown and to avoid contact with the patient and his bed.

Acute infectious diarrhea may readily spread throughout a family, school or neighborhood because of a common source of infected food or water or by the spread from an infected person. The nurse may play an important role in the prevention of diarrhea by alerting people to the hazards of exposed and unrefrigerated foods, particularly meat and those with cream filling or topping. Opportunities may arise to emphasize the hygienic handling of food and the importance of thorough hand washing after going to the toilet and the handling of soiled clothing.

The family in which a member develops acute diarrhea should be advised of the necessary precautions in caring for him to prevent the spread to others. If several members of a family become ill at one time, questions should be raised as to recently ingested food and its source.

If a large number of cases are found in a school or community, the local health authorities should be notified so that a systematic investigation as to the possible source may be instituted. Occasionally, acute diarrhea may spread through the patients on one ward of a hospital. The primary source of such an outbreak should be sought. Ward personnel are urged to practice rigid medical asepsis, for infection may be carried from one patient to another or from a ward worker to patients through failure to thoroughly wash the hands between patients, after handling bedpans or linen, or after going to the toilet.

Irritable Bowel Syndrome

This is a functional disorder of the colon and may be alluded to as *spastic colon, irritable bowel* or *nervous diarrhea*. The syndrome has a higher incidence in females, with the onset frequently occurring between the ages of 20 and 40 years. The individual is generally tense, anxious and ill at ease.

MANIFESTATIONS. The disorder is characterized by episodes of abdominal pain, defecation disturbance which may take the form of diarrhea or constipation, or alternating small hard stools and liquid stools. Exacerbations are frequently related to emotional stress caused by the individual's life situation. The abdominal pain tends to be colicky and may be fairly general or often may be referred to the left lower quadrant. The ingestion of food may initiate the urge to defecate which may lead to anorexia and loss of weight. Defecation may provide temporary relief of pain. Frequently abdominal distention and audible intestinal rumblings (borborygmus) are noted, and the patient complains of fatigue and weakness.

Investigation includes a barium enema and a sigmoidoscopy or colonoscopy (see p. 496). Stool specimens may be examined for organisms and parasites.

MANAGEMENT. Since this is a functional disorder usually associated with tension and psychological stress, the patient is encouraged to talk about her concerns. It may take several approaches to establish sufficient confidence to have the patient talk about that which worries her or why she is unhappy with her life situation. She has to realize that the listener appreciates her concerns and is willing to listen and help find a solution. Following the investigation, the physician's reassurance that there is no inflammation, lesion or malignant growth reduces the patient's concerns.

A mild sedative or tranquilizer such as diazepam (Valium) may be prescribed for a period of time but is not continued indefinitely. When constipation is troublesome, a bulk-producing laxative such as psyllium seed (Metamucil) is recommended. The habit of taking laxatives is discouraged. The patient is encouraged to take a well-balanced diet with an increased amount of fiber-containing foods (e.g., bran).

An anticholinergic preparation (see p. 528) may be given to reduce the colonic spasms that may occur.

Intestinal Obstruction

Obstruction to the passage of intestinal content may occur in the small or large bowel and is a serious, life-threatening condition that demands prompt attention.

CAUSES. The cause of the obstruction may be within the wall or lumen of the intestine itself, or it may be extrinsic. It may be classified as mechanical, neurogenic or vascular and may be acquired or congenital (see Table 16–1).

Causes of *mechanical obstruction* include: inflammation, edema and scarring of the intestinal wall; tumors of the bowel or of a neighboring structure; adhesions, which are bands of fibrous scar tissue formed by the peritoneal tissue following inflammation and which may cause kinking and constriction of the intestine; occlusion by a mass, such as a hard, dry fecal accumulation, a large bolus of unchewed and undigested food, a gallstone or a foreign body; and intra-abdominal abscess.

Strangulated hernia, in which a loop of the intestine escapes from the peritoneal cavity through a defect in the abdominal wall, results in constriction of the lumen of the bowel and a blockage as well as compression of the blood vessels. The constriction may lead to gangrene of the protruding segment of the intestine.

Obstruction may result from *intussusception*, a condition in which a segment of the intestine is invaginated into the segment immediately below. This telescoping results in compression of the attached mesentery between the layers of intestine in the intussusception and interference with the blood supply to the bowel. Intussusception occurs mainly in infants and young children.

Volvulus, which is a twisting of a loop of bowel on itself, interrupts the passage of intestinal contents and the blood supply to the involved segment. Older persons are more often affected, and the twisted section of bowel is usually the sigmoid colon.

Congenital malformations may be responsible for intestinal obstruction in the newborn. The anomaly may be a stenosis or atresia in an area of the small or large intestine, or it may be an imperforate anus. The infant fails to pass meconium.

In *neurogenic obstruction,* peristalsis is inhibited by a disturbance in the normal nerve supply to the intestine. Often this is an imbalance in the autonomic innervation which results in a cessation of peristalsis. It may develop with peritonitis, pancreatitis, severe toxemia as in pneumonia and uremia, shock, or spinal cord lesions, or occasionally after extensive abdominal surgery. An electrolyte imbalance in which the blood potassium is below normal also predisposes to intestinal immobility. The inhibition of peristalsis due to impaired innervation causes the condition known as *paralytic* or *adynamic ileus.* Dynamic or spastic ileus occurs rarely in some toxic conditions and is associated with intestinal hyperactivity. The spasm of a segment is severe enough to obliterate the lumen.

Obstruction of *vascular origin* is due to interference with the blood supply to a segment of the intestine and may be secondary to mechanical obstruction, or it may be primary and itself cause failure of bowel activity. Thrombosis and occlusion of a mesenteric artery may occur, blocking the blood source to a large portion of the bowel and arresting peristalsis. When the interruption in the blood supply is secondary, the condition is referred to as strangulation.

SYMPTOMS AND EFFECTS. The symptoms and effects of obstruction depend on whether it is in the small or large bowel and whether or not the blood supply to the intestine is maintained.

The first symptom of mechanical obstruction is colicky abdominal *pain* due to the bowel spasms. The crampy pains are accompanied by high-pitched bowel sounds. In paralytic ileus, the pain is steady and is due mainly to the distention. There is an absence of bowel sounds in this type of obstruction. No fecal matter or gas is passed after that which was below the obstruction is evacuated.

In small bowel obstruction, *vomiting* begins earlier and is frequent; the vomitus at first consists of stomach content and then of fluid containing bile. Eventually it becomes dark brown and fecal in character as the intes-

TABLE 16–1 CAUSES OF INTESTINAL OBSTRUCTION

Mechanical	Nonmechanical
Inflammation and edema of the intestinal wall	Neurogenic disturbances
Scarring of the intestinal wall	Paralytic or adynamic ileus
Adhesions	Dynamic ileus
Newgrowths (intramural and extramural)	Interrupted blood supply
Foreign body	Mesenteric thrombosis
Incarcerated hernia	Strangulation of blood vessels secondary to:
Volvulus	Incarcerated hernia
Intussusception	Volvulus
Congenital stenosis and atresia	Intussusception

tine becomes distended with excessive fluids and gas which overflow into the stomach.

The *abdomen becomes distended* because of the accumulation of gas and fluids in the bowel. Intestinal secretions are increased and the loss of fluid and electrolytes in vomiting leads to *severe dehydration and electrolyte imbalance*. Extravasation of plasma from the capillaries adds to the accumulation of fluid in the intestine as the veins are compressed by distention. This depletes the circulating blood volume and causes *shock*.

The patient's general condition may deteriorate rapidly. Unless the bowel is decompressed and fluid and electrolytes are replaced, a serious state of shock develops, manifested by restlessness, anxiety, a rapid weak pulse, low blood pressure, subnormal temperature, grayish pallor and cold clammy skin.

If decompression of the intestine is not established, the pressure created within the intestinal lumen may increase until it exceeds venous and capillary pressure. This causes congestion, edema and necrosis of the mural tissue and may lead to perforation of the intestine.

The colicky pain becomes continuous as peristalsis diminishes, and the intestine loses its tone because of the marked distention and strangulation. Bowel sounds diminish and the vomiting changes character; it is no longer preceded by nausea and retching; the vomitus comes up without effort (regurgitated).

Peritonitis may develop as the weakened intestinal wall becomes permeable to organisms. Generalized abdominal tenderness and rigidity become evident.

Obstruction of the large intestine is less acute, and the symptoms develop over a longer period of time. Complete constipation (obstipation) and crampy abdominal pain are the patient's first complaints. Distention of the large bowel develops more slowly since fluid is absorbed, but eventually the distention may be very marked as the segment of the bowel is closed off by the obstruction at one end and the ileocecal valve at the other. The ileocecal valve will permit the entrance of content from the ileum but not until the later stage does the content of the colon and cecum back up into the ileum. Vomiting and the attendant dehydration and electrolyte imbalance occur in this later stage.

DIAGNOSIS. Diagnostic investigation in intestinal obstruction may include an x-ray examination of the abdomen in which the presence and levels of gas and fluid may be apparent without a contrast medium. Blood studies are made to determine the leukocyte and differential counts, since a leukocytosis may develop with certain causes of obstruction. Hemoglobin and hematocrit estimations are made since they rise as dehydration and hemoconcentration develop. Serum electrolyte determinations are made so that deficiencies may be corrected. Those usually requiring attention are sodium, chloride and potassium.

Bowel content eliminated from below the obstruction may be examined for blood which may be present if the obstruction is due to intussusception or to cancer of the large intestine.

TREATMENT. Intestinal obstruction other than that due to paralytic ileus is treated surgically. In simple mechanical obstruction without strangulation, the operation may be delayed for a brief period in which medical treatment is used to improve the patient's general condition. This treatment includes intestinal intubation and suctioning to remove the accumulation of gas and fluid and to relieve the vomiting, pain and distention (see p. 500).

Fluid and electrolytes are given intravenously to replace the losses; as much as 5 to 6 liters may be ordered daily as long as there is intestinal suctioning. An accurate record of all fluid output and intake is necessary. The physician bases the electrolyte replacement as well as the amount of intravenous fluid on the volume of intestinal fluid lost in vomiting and aspiration. Glucose is included in the intravenous solution to provide calories. A blood transfusion may be used to increase the circulating blood volume and relieve shock, if present.

If there is evidence of interference with the blood supply to the obstructed intestine, emergency surgery is undertaken.

The surgical procedure used in intestinal obstruction depends upon the cause of obstruction and the patient's general condition. If the obstruction is due to adhesions, they are severed. It may involve resection of the affected area of intestine and anastomosis to restore continuity of the tract or a bypass of the lesion by anastomosing a part above the obstruction to a lower part (usually the colon). In the case of an incarcerated hernia, volvulus or intussusception, the obstruction is relieved and the intestine examined for viability. If the blood supply has been interrupted for some time or is not reestablished, a segment of the bowel may be gangrenous, necessitating resection and anastomosis. The surgery may entail an ileostomy, cecostomy, or colostomy, which may be a temporary measure while an anastomosis heals or it may be done to establish drainage above the obstruction, making it possible to delay more extensive surgery until the patient's condition improves.[17] In some instances, the enterocutaneous fistula (colostomy or ileostomy) is permanent.

For nursing care of the surgically treated patient, see p. 548.

Intestinal obstruction due to paralytic ileus, as mentioned previously, is not treated by surgery. Intestinal intubation with a long weighted tube and suctioning are used to remove gas and fluid and reduce the distention. Fluid and electrolyte deficiencies are corrected; the serum potassium level receives special attention because hypokalemia favors the peristaltic dysfunction. Paralytic ileus is most frequently a secondary condition; as the primary disorder improves and decompression occurs, peristalsis is usually reestablished gradually.

Cancer of the Intestine

The colon and rectum are leading sites of cancer and the incidence is very much higher than cancer of the small intestine. The discussion that follows relates principally to the large intestine. The most common site is the rectum; the sigmoid, cecum and ascending colon are next in order of frequency. Cancer of the colon or rectum may occur at any age but has its highest incidence in the fifth and sixth decades.

Conditions that frequently precede cancer of the bowel are ulcerative colitis that has been active for several years and multiple polyps (polyposis) in the bowel.

The malignant growth may be papillary, soft and friable, or a firm nodular mass projecting into the lumen; it may be a ring-shaped (annular) mass of firm fibrous tissue, causing a constriction of the bowel, or it may be ulcerative and necrotic, leading to bleeding and perforation.

SIGNS AND SYMPTOMS. Manifestations vary with the location of the lesion in the intestine. If the neoplasm is in the *small intestine,* the symptoms develop insidiously and are vague and less noticeable. They include anorexia, nausea and vomiting, anemia, loss of weight and strength, and occult blood in the stool. Obstructive symptoms appear gradually and the patient develops abdominal pain. If the tumor is in the duodenum, the manifestations may be similar to those of a peptic ulcer.

If the site of the neoplasm is in the *colon or rectum,* the commonest early signs are a change in bowel habit and blood in the stool. Any person manifesting either of these signs is urged to seek prompt medical attention.

There may be increasing constipation or perhaps alternating bouts of constipation and diarrhea. The stool may gradually become smaller and ribbon-like in form and may be streaked with blood, mucus and pus. A continuous defecation urge and the feeling that evacuation is incomplete after passing a stool may be experienced. The patient presents a general picture of ill health with a loss of weight and progressive anemia. Laboratory examination of the stool will probably reveal occult blood. In cancer of the large bowel, abdominal pain is usually a late symptom; at first the patient may have a vague discomfort, and later he may experience a colicky pain which gradually becomes more severe. Unfortunately, if the cancer is in the cecum or ascending (right) colon, the early symptoms are more insidious and difficult to detect until the mass is large enough to be observed by palpation. Occasionally, the first symptoms recognized are those associated with complications, such as obstruction or perforation of the bowel.

DIAGNOSIS. A neoplasm in the *small intestine* may be recognized when barium sulfate is taken by mouth and the passage of the barium through the small intestine followed. Any delay at a given section may indicate narrowing of the lumen by a mass. The intraluminal contour of the small intestine is also recorded by x-rays.

Investigation of the *large intestine* involves a colonoscopy, sigmoidoscopy or proctos-

---

[17]*Ileostomy* is an opening from the ileum onto the external surface of the abdomen. Intestinal content is eliminated through this opening.

Cecostomy is an opening through the abdominal wall into the cecum to provide elimination of the intestinal contents.

Colostomy is an opening through the abdominal wall into the colon. Feces are diverted through this opening onto the external surface of the abdomen.

copy (see p. 496–497). A biopsy of the lesion, if it is located, is done at the time of the endoscopic examination. Roentgenography is done with a barium enema providing a contrast medium. The patient's hematocrit and hemoglobin are checked for possible anemia, and stool specimens are examined for blood, parasites and pus.

TREATMENT. If the neoplasm has precipitated an obstruction, intestinal intubation and suction are used to decompress the stomach and intestine. Fluid, electrolyte and blood deficiencies are corrected. Surgical treatment of the tumor in the small intestine is undertaken and involves wide resection, removal of regional lymph nodes and anastomosis or, if the cancer is considered inoperable, a bypass may be done. If a large portion of the small intestine is removed, absorption of nutrients may be so restricted that the patient will require intravenous alimentation (see p. 504).

Cancer of the colon is treated by resection of the bowel and anastomosis. This operation may have to be preceded by an emergency colostomy or cecostomy for the relief of bowel obstruction. The resection is performed and the colostomy closed when the patient has recovered from the acute bowel obstruction. If the cancer involves the sigmoid colon and rectum, an abdominoperineal resection is done in which the entire anus, rectum and sigmoid are removed, leaving the patient with a permanent colostomy. Radiotherapy may be used postoperatively when the tissues have healed.

When the malignant disease is advanced and has metastasized to other structures, it may be considered inoperable. Treatment is then directed toward relieving the obstruction by a cecostomy or colostomy, correcting the anemia, providing relief of pain and keeping the patient as comfortable as possible (see Nursing Care of Patients with Cancer, Chapter 8).

For nursing care of the patient who has bowel resection, see below. For colostomy care, see page 551.

NURSING THE PATIENT WHO HAS INTESTINAL SURGERY

Preoperative Nursing Care

The preoperative care for a patient undergoing intestinal surgery is the same as that for any patient undergoing abdominal surgery (see p. 164) in addition to the following special considerations because the actual intestinal tract is to be entered.

The patient is hospitalized several days before the operation for assessment of his general condition and for correction of disorders secondary to his disease, such as anemia, nutritional and fluid deficiencies and infection. This may not be possible if there is an acute bowel obstruction or strangulation which demands immediate surgery.

PSYCHOLOGICAL PREPARATION. Since the patient is facing major surgery, he and his family are likely to be very anxious. There is probably fear of malignancy as well as concern for the patient's survival. The surgeon may have advised the patient that it might be necessary to divert his bowel content through an abdominal opening (colostomy or ileostomy), depending on the findings at operation. (See page 551 for information concerning an ileostomy and colostomy.)

The patient is encouraged to talk about his fears and ask questions. The nurse helps by being a willing listener and by indicating understanding and acceptance of his concerns. His questions are discreetly answered if possible without adding to his anxiety. Frequent visits to the patient and appropriate forms of diversion reduce his concentration on his condition. In talking with the patient and his family, socioeconomic or home problems may come to light for which the nurse may be able to suggest a solution or arrange for assistance from appropriate sources.

The equipment and procedures that will be used postoperatively are briefly described, and their purpose and the patient's role are explained. These procedures most likely include intestinal suctioning, intravenous therapy, frequent checking of vital signs, the withholding of oral fluids and food, frequent coughing, deep breathing, and early ambulation. Knowing something of what to expect prevents fear and unnecessary concern for his condition when these procedures are put into use postoperatively.

PHYSICAL PREPARATION. Observations are made for signs of possible dehydration. Extra fluids are given for optimal hydration; parenteral solutions may be ordered to correct electrolyte disturbances or if the patient is unable to take sufficient quantities by mouth. A high-calorie, low-residue diet that includes extra protein and vitamins is desirable if it can be taken. If sufficient solid foods cannot be taken, a protein concentrate may be given in solution, and the necessary vitamins may be ordered in medicinal form.

Usually, only clear fluids are allowed during the 24 to 36 hours preceding the operation so that the intestine will be empty. The sudden change in diet is explained to the patient if he has been receiving a more liberal one.

During the preoperative period, the patient may receive an oral antimicrobial drug to destroy intestinal organisms ("sterilization" of the bowel). Examples of drugs used for this purpose are succinylsulfathiazole (Sulfasuxidine), phthalylsulfathiazole (Sulfathalidine), and neomycin sulfate. Very little, if any, of these drugs is absorbed. If the drug used causes diarrhea, it should be reported promptly, as the patient cannot afford loss of fluid and nutrients.

Some sedation may be necessary to reduce the patient's anxiety and to promote rest. A small dose, three or four times daily, may be ordered.

Blood transfusions may be given to correct existing anemia and to improve the patient's general condition.

IMMEDIATE PREOPERATIVE CARE. A laxative may be ordered 2 nights before operation and a cleansing enema given the night before so that there will be as little intestinal content as possible at the time of operation. The surgeon may also request intestinal intubation and suctioning for the same purpose. The passage of the tube may be done 24 hours or more before operation, since it takes several hours for the tube to advance the desired distance in the intestine (see p. 502). The intestinal tube is left in place, and suctioning is resumed after surgery to remove blood, secretions and gas so that distention and leakage through the suture line of the anastomosis may be prevented.

In some instances, only nasogastric intubation may be required, in which case the tube is passed a few hours before the operation.

Postoperative Nursing Care

See section on General Postoperative Care also, page 178.

The postoperative care will vary somewhat with the different surgical procedures that may be done on the intestine and with the level of the intestine involved. The patient may have had a resection of a segment of the bowel and an end-to-end anastomosis to restore the continuity of the tract or the bowel may be retained, but an opening is made into the bowel through which the content is discharged onto the surface of the abdomen (colostomy or ileostomy). In cancer of the rectum or sigmoid colon or in ulcerative colitis, the patient may have had an abdominoperineal resection in which the lower segment of the colon, the rectum and the anus are removed, and the remaining terminal part of the intestine is brought to the abdominal surface to establish a permanent colostomy.

PREPARATION TO RECEIVE THE PATIENT. As well as that listed on p. 178, the following equipment may be necessary and should be assembled and ready for immediate use when the patient returns from operation: intestinal suctioning apparatus; equipment for intravenous infusion and blood transfusion; equipment for the administration of oxygen; urinary drainage bag and tubing to connect to the retention catheter; and equipment for mouth care.

OBSERVATIONS. A frequent check is made of the patient's vital signs, response, and wound areas for early signs of shock or hemorrhage. A sudden elevation of temperature may indicate infection. Frequent observation of the intestinal suction and drainage is necessary to make sure there is no blockage of the tube or mechanical failure of the suction apparatus.

An accurate record is made of the fluid intake and output which includes the intestinal drainage. Serum electrolyte determinations are made frequently; deficiencies commonly occur with prolonged gastrointestinal suctioning. Particular attention is given to the sodium, chloride, potassium and bicarbonate levels. Central venous pressure may be monitored to provide a guide for the rate and volume of intravenous infusion that may be used safely (see p. 297). Too rapid infusion or an excessive volume may overload the individual's circulatory system, predisposing to pulmonary edema and heart failure. The amount and types of solutions to be given intravenously may be estimated by the physician on the basis of the records of the fluid balance, central venous pressure and laboratory reports.

The abdomen is examined for distention and rigidity; the development of either condition should be brought to the surgeon's attention promptly. Using a stethoscope, the abdomen is examined for bowel sounds to determine if peristalsis is established.

INTESTINAL DRAINAGE. When a resection of the bowel has been done, decompression is continued until the anastomosis is partially healed and peristalsis is reestablished.

The characteristics, as well as the exact amount, of the drainage are noted. It may be slightly colored by blood at first but should clear in a few hours. Persistence of blood-colored drainage or the appearance of large amounts of blood should be reported.

The intestinal suction tube may become obstructed by a small clot or by mucus and may require irrigation; a specific order as to the solution and the amount to be used is necessary. The suctioning may be discontinued for stated intervals the second or third postoperative day, and the patient's reaction is noted. The volume aspirated following each period of nonsuctioning is carefully noted and recorded.

POSITIONING. With the patient's return to consciousness and stabilization of his vital signs, the head of the bed may be slightly elevated. He is encouraged to change his position hourly and is given the necessary assistance. Frequent change of position favors better ventilation and the prevention of circulatory stasis. The nasogastrointestinal tube shifts with turning, preventing prolonged pressure by the tube on one area of the mucous membrane in the throat.

The patient who has had an abdominoperineal resection usually lies on either side; moving is very difficult and painful for him at first because of the perineal wound, so the nurse helps him to change sides every hour or two. A pillow used to support the lower limb that is uppermost may help to lessen the discomfort.

DEEP BREATHING AND COUGHING. Pain and weakness may result in shallow breathing and may predispose to pulmonary complications. The patient is required to take five to ten deep breaths hourly to ventilate his alveoli fully and to cough several times to dislodge any mucus that may collect. The nurse supports the patient and may ease some distress by placing one hand lightly over the abdominal incision. A pillow held against the abdomen may help.

MOUTH AND NASAL CARE. Frequent cleansing and moistening of the mouth are necessary to lessen the patient's discomfort and prevent parotitis during the restriction of oral fluids. The nostril through which the intestinal tube is passed requires cleansing of the mucus secreted in response to the irritation. A light application of a water-soluble lubricant may be made after swabbing with water or saline.

NUTRITION AND HYDRATION. Nothing is given orally the first few days; intravenous fluids are used to sustain the patient. Oral intake is started with specific small amounts of water. If there is no untoward response, the amount is gradually increased and other fluids are introduced.

During the initial introduction of oral fluids, the intestinal suctioning may be discontinued and the tube clamped and left in place until the patient's response is determined. If the fluids are tolerated, the tube is removed, and the diet progresses through fluids to soft foods and then to a light, bland diet. Carbonated fluids and gas-forming foods must be avoided.

If a large portion of the small intestine has been resected, the patient may require intravenous alimentation (see p. 504). This may be a temporary means of providing adequate nourishment until the remaining small intestine adapts to the demand on it for increased absorption. In some instances, total parenteral nutrition becomes a permanent measure.

ELIMINATION. The patient who has an abdominoperineal resection will have a retention catheter inserted into the bladder either preoperatively or immediately on completion of the operation. This is to prevent urinary retention, since most of these patients have difficulty in voiding. In the female patient it protects the perineal wound from urine contamination. The catheter may have to be irrigated at regular intervals with an antiseptic solution.

In bowel resection and anastomosis, the passage of any gas by rectum should be recorded; this probably indicates the reestablishment of peristalsis. A small cleansing enema may be ordered on the fourth or fifth day, and a mild laxative may be prescribed when food is being taken by mouth.

Elimination via an ileostomy or colostomy and the necessary care involved are discussed on page 551.

EXERCISES AND AMBULATION. The patient who has had a resection with anastomosis is out of bed a day or two after operation. If an abdominoperineal resection has been done, the patient usually remains in bed for several days. Lower limb exercises are important to prevent circulatory stasis and thrombosis. The patient tends to lie with the thighs and knees flexed; they should be straightened out several times daily and dorsiflexion of the feet, flexion and extension of the toes and tensing of the thigh muscles carried out.

CARE OF WOUNDS. The patient who has an abdominoperineal resection has three wounds. There is a large abdominal incision through which the colon is severed above the affected segment of the colon and the distal portion is dissected and placed in the pelvic cavity outside the peritoneal cavity. A second smaller incision is in the left abdomen through which the end of the proximal colon is brought and secured to form a permanent colostomy. The colon is kept clamped until the operation is completed to prevent contamination by intestinal content. The third incision is in the perineum through which the lower severed portion of the colon, sigmoid, rectum and anal canal are removed.

The larger abdominal wound is protected from contamination from the colostomy drainage. A sheet of plastic may be used over the dressing.

The perineal wound may be packed with gauze impregnated with petrolatum jelly and may have a soft rubber tissue drain. There is likely to be free serosanguineous drainage from this area, and the dressing requires frequent reinforcing during the first 24 hours. The physician changes the dressing the first few times and, if packing has been used, it is gradually removed and the wound cavity allowed to heal by granulation. The T binder is kept snug to avoid dressings rubbing on the wound or becoming displaced. Irrigations with a solution, such as normal saline or hydrogen peroxide, by means of a small catheter inserted into the wounds are used to remove tissue debris. As soon as the patient is able to be out of bed, a sitz bath at a temperature of 37.8 to 40.6° C. (100 to 105° F.) is used once or twice daily to stimulate circulation in the perineal area and promote healing. A rubber air ring is placed under the patient during the bath so the water can readily reach the wound and to reduce the discomfort of direct pressure on the area. Someone remains with the patient during the

baths in case he becomes weak or faint.

The perineal wound may not be completely healed when the patient leaves the hospital. He is taught the management of the sitz baths and dressings at home. A referral may be made to the visiting nurse organization in his district so that he will receive the necessary assistance and reassurance when on his own. If the required dressings pose an economic problem, they can probably be obtained from the local chapter of the National Cancer Society. If necessary, this agency may also provide a means of transportation for the patient to go to the clinic or the doctor's office.

Care of the colostomy is discussed in the following section.

Ileostomy and Colostomy Care

The treatment of some intestinal disorders may necessitate surgery that establishes an opening into the bowel through which the intestinal content is discharged onto the surface of the abdomen. The opening may be temporary or permanent. A temporary diversion of the bowel content may be necessary while some abnormal condition below the level of the stoma is corrected or for quick decompression and drainage in obstruction. Later, the normal continuity of the tract is restored and the stoma is eliminated. If the opening is permanent, the portion of the bowel below is generally removed.

The operations performed are ileostomy, cecostomy and colostomy.

Ileostomy

An ileostomy involves transection of the ileum and bringing the proximal end out to the abdominal surface to form a stoma. An ileal stoma usually protrudes ½ to ¾ of an inch which makes the management easier than with a stoma that is level with the abdominal surface. The latter predisposes to seepage around the ileostomy appliance and excoriation of the skin. The removal of the distal severed portion of the bowel may be done at the same operation or may be postponed until the patient's condition is improved. If the lower part of the intestine is to be retained for a period of time, it is closed or, in some instances, the severed end may also be brought out to the abdominal surface.

An ileostomy is most frequently performed for Crohn's disease, or for colitis that does not respond to medical treatment and is incapacitating. It may also be necessary for patients with multiple polyposis of the colon or an intestinal obstruction in the upper portion of the colon.

Recently, some surgeons have been performing an ileostomy that eliminates the need for the patient to wear an external pouch or bag over the stoma. It is referred to as the *pouch ileostomy* or *continent ileostomy* (Fig. 16–11).[18, 19] This type of ileostomy is reserved for patients with chronic ulcerative colitis or multiple polyposis. It is not performed on those with regional enteritis (Crohn's disease) since the pouch may become affected.

The surgical procedure involves the formation of an internal pouch in the distal segment of the ileum. The pouch serves as a reservoir for the intestinal content. The pouch is drained at regular intervals by the insertion of a catheter through the stoma. The capacity of the reservoir gradually increases, and may reach 500 to 1000 ml. over several months to a year. As the capacity increases, there is a corresponding decrease in the frequency of drainage required. Continuous discharge and leakage of the fluid or semifluid between evacuations of the pouch is prevented by the formation of a valve-like structure at the internal end of the ileum that leads from the stoma to the ileal pouch. Pressure of the contents of the pouch closes the valve, but it is structured so that it opens when the gentle pressure of a catheter is exerted against it on the stomal side.

The postoperative period for the pouch ileostomy is longer than that for the patient who has had the conventional ileostomy. It involves gastrointestinal drainage via a nasogastric tube, intravenous fluids and continuous catheter drainage of the pouch for several days while the pouch heals. In addition, the patient will probably have had a colectomy or an abdominoperineal resection of colon, rectum and anal canal. However, the advantages associated with an ileal pouch, such as the

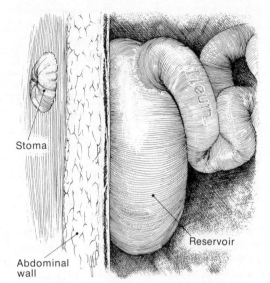

Stoma

Reservoir

Abdominal wall

FIGURE 16–11 Pouch (continent) ileostomy.

elimination of continuous drainage and the wearing of a bag, make the more involved procedure acceptable to the patient.

Colostomy

A colostomy is an opening of the colon onto the surface of the abdomen. It may be in the transverse or descending colon. If the colostomy is a temporary measure, the transverse colon is usually the segment used. A loop of the colon is brought to the abdominal surface, secured and left unopened until the peritoneum heals sufficiently to prevent fecal matter escaping into the peritoneal cavity. The bowel becomes adherent to the wound edges and an incision is then made into it in 2 to 4 days.

When the sigmoid colon, rectum and anal canal are removed, as in cancer of the sigmoid and rectum, the terminal end of the descending colon is brought to the abdominal surface to form a permanent colostomy.

Cecostomy

Rarely, in large bowel obstruction, decompression of the distended bowel is achieved by a cecostomy. A small opening is made in the cecum through a small lower right abdominal incision and a fairly large tube is inserted through which the bowel content escapes to the exterior. The tube is attached to a drainage receptacle and remains in place until the

[18]Arlene Wentworth and Barbara Cox: "Nursing the Patient with a Continent Ileostomy." Am. J. Nurs., Vol. 76, No. 9 (Sept. 1976), pp. 1424–1428.

[19]Eleanor Hyman, et al.: "The Pouch Ileostomy: New Applications of Time-Tested Techniques." Nurs. '77, Vol. 7, No. 9 (Sept. 1977), pp. 44–47.

patient's condition is such that he can withstand the more extensive surgery necessary to relieve the obstruction.

Nursing Considerations in Ileostomy and Colostomy

DIFFERENCES BETWEEN ILEOSTOMY AND COLOSTOMY. Certain differences exist between an ileostomy and colostomy that result in different problems and necessitate different types of care. For example, control of the discharge is determined by the location of the stoma; drainage from the ileum is of liquid consistency and is rich in enzymes that cause excoriation and erosion of the skin. It flows almost continuously, requiring the constant wearing of a receptive appliance unless an ileal pouch is constructed. There may be quiescent periods but they are not predictable and cannot be controlled. Complications are a more common occurrence with an ileostomy than with a colostomy, and odor presents a greater problem if there is continuous drainage. Irrigations are not used with the conventional ileostomy; the introduction of anything into the ileal stoma is discouraged for fear of injury to the intestine.

Colostomy drainage is usually more manageable and less irritating to the skin unless the opening is into the ascending colon; the drainage then is similar to that from an ileostomy. The colostomy is more often in the transverse or descending colon and much of the fluid and electrolytes have been absorbed from the fecal content, leaving it semisolid or solid by the time it reaches the stoma. Irrigations may be necessary but, in some instances, the sigmoid colostomy may be so well controlled that it resembles normal bowel movement, and the patient does not have to wear a receptive bag continuously.

Intestinal activity in the individual with a colostomy or ileostomy may be influenced by diet, fluid intake and emotions, just as in the normal person.

PSYCHOLOGICAL PREOPERATIVE PREPARATION. When the physician advises the patient preoperatively that a colostomy or ileostomy may or will be necessary, the patient is emotionally disturbed. Obviously, if the colostomy is a temporary measure it will be accepted more readily but, if it is likely to be permanent, the patient may be more concerned abut this than about the operation or his primary condition. His immediate response may be "it would be better to die than have that." He may become resentful or show marked depression, withdrawal and despair. He perceives this change in his body as making him unclean and unacceptable to society. There are fears because of odor and soiling. It is best to let the patient and his family express their feelings before attempting explanations. The nurse can help by being a willing listener, answering their questions and using every opportunity available to assure the patient that the "ostomy" can be cared for without interfering with his work and social life. When the patient recovers from the initial blow, discussions may then be held as to how he will care for his ileostomy or colostomy.

It is very helpful if he is visited by an ostomate — a person who has had an ileostomy or colostomy and who has learned to manage his care and live an active, independent life. The request for such a person to visit may be made to the local Ileostomy Association; the members of the association see this service as one of their functions. If there is no local association, the physician or the visiting nurse organization may know of someone. Seeing this person, who is cheerful and appears quite normal, makes a tremendous impression on the patient; his attitude may change and result in his acceptance of the situation. Following this, the patient is likely to manifest an interest in learning about postoperative management. The nurse capitalizes on this and plans the appropriate instruction. He is advised that for the first few postoperative days the drainage may be fairly free and erratic but will gradually become more regular. This may offset some of the discouragement experienced when the patient is actually faced with the discharge of his bowel content onto the surface of the abdomen.

The nurse needs to know the patient's concerns and he (the patient) needs to recognize that the nurse wants to listen to him, has time to listen to him and really wants to help him.

The type of equipment used is shown to the patient, and an explanation is made of the immediate postoperative period and how he will be helped to take over his care gradually. Information brochures relating to ostomy care and the life style of the ostomate are provided.

CARE OF THE PATIENT WITH AN ILEOSTOMY OR A COLOSTOMY. The care of the patient who has an ileostomy or a colostomy is directed toward: (1) providing comfort for the patient; (2) preventing peristomal skin excoriation; (3) controlling offensive odors; (4) providing psychological support that will help the patient to accept the change in his body function; and (5) teaching and helping the patient to undertake effective self-care.

General preoperative and postoperative care are similar to that for the pateint who has intestinal surgery (p. 548).

CARE OF THE CONVENTIONAL ILEOSTOMY OR COLOSTOMY. During the first few days following surgery, the stoma is swollen and edematous and the volume of drainage is usually small. When the patient is permitted to take fluids and foods by mouth, peristalsis and secretion are stimulated and drainage increases.

Following surgery the skin is washed with warm water and dried. A washer of karaya gum, slightly moistened, is fitted snugly around the stoma to protect the skin and an open-ended, transparent, disposable plastic bag is applied. The transparency of the bag makes it possible to observe the stoma and the color of the drainage at frequent intervals during the postoperative period. The bag is attached to an adhesive-backed square which secures the bag over the stoma. A hole is cut in the adhesive to fit the stoma and is sized to leave a margin of not more than ⅛ inch. Too large an opening exposes the skin to irritating drainage; too small an opening may traumatize or constrict the stoma. The size of the stoma is determined by a stoma-measuring card. Nonallergenic adhesive or micropore tape is applied over the edges of the adhesive square to maintain a seal. Several folds and a clamp or elastic bands are used to close the lower end of the bag securely.

During this initial period the bag is applied so that the lower end is at the patient's side, making emptying and rinsing possible while the patient is in bed. When the patient is allowed up, the bag is positioned so that it is suspended down over the lower abdomen toward his feet.

If there is a large volume of drainage, which may occur if the ileostomy or colostomy was an emergency measure, it may be necessary to attach a drainage tube to the bag. Elastic bands and adhesive are used to secure the bag around the tube. The latter drains into a closed drainage receptacle similar to that used for urinary drainage.

The disposable bag is emptied when it is one-third to one-half full; if allowed to fill it becomes too heavy and the pull on the bag may break the seal and cause leakage. The lower end of the bag is opened and the contents allowed to drain into a receptacle. Using a syringe, the bag is then rinsed with lukewarm water. The volume and characteristics (color, consistency and composition) of the drainage are noted and recorded. The appliance is changed daily until replaced by reusable equipment. A special solvent is available that enables the adhesive to be removed without damage to the skin. It may be applied with an eye dropper or an absorbent wipe. When the bag is removed, the skin is *gently* cleansed with warm water and thoroughly dried before reapplication of the karaya washer and a clean disposable pouch. In addition to karaya, which comes in the form of washers, powder and ointment, several preparations are available that may be used as a protective skin barrier (e.g., Stomahesive wafers, Desitin ointment). A patient's skin may be sensitive to one, necessitating the use of another.

Each time the pouch is changed the condition of the skin and stoma is noted. The latter should be bright red and moist; if it is bluish or gray and dry the physician is notified, as the change may indicate impaired circulation or strangulation. The skin is examined carefully for possible excoriation or any break. Skin irritation is treated promptly and a more effective protective barrier is provided. Fewer skin problems are encountered by the colostomy patient than by the ileostomy patient.

Ongoing Care. The patient is fitted for a reuseable appliance as soon as possible so that he can become familiar with its use and care before leaving the hospital. A well-fitting comfortable appliance means a great deal; the patient is likely to have more confidence and develop a more positive outlook. Several types of appliances are available from surgical supply companies; the surgeon or enterostomal therapist recommends the appliance most suited to the individual patient. The location and size of the stoma and the contour and firmness of the patient's abdomen are factors that must be considered in the selection and fitting of a reusable appliance. It should be simple and fit closely to prevent leakage without causing injury to the stoma or skin. The prevention of leaking is especially important for the patient with an ileostomy since the fecal drainage is liquid and cannot be controlled. With the colostomy patient, the drainage may be semiliquid and controlled by irrigations. The appliance should be inconspicuous, allow freedom of activity and be odor-proof. The essential parts include (Fig. 16–12)

1. A stoma-measuring card. The opening in the karaya washer (if used) and the double-faced adhesive disc must fit snugly to protect the skin; a margin of no more than approximately $1/16$ to $1/8$ inch is desirable.
2. A product to protect the skin. Examples of common preparations are karaya washers, karaya powder or ointment, Stomahesive wafers, Resifilm spray.
3. A double-faced adhesive disc to secure the pouch to the skin. One side of the disc adheres to the skin and the other side attaches to the mounting ring (face plate).
4. A lightweight mounting ring (which may also be called face plate) made of plastic or rubber. One side of the ring has a rim around a center hole. The side without the rim is secured to one adhesive surface of the double-faced adhesive disc. The pouch or rim side of the ring may have "hooks" to which a belt may be attached.
5. A lightweight open-ended pouch that may be washed when removed and reused several times. The upper opening of the pouch is stretched over the rim of the mounting ring and secured by special rubber rings that are provided with the appliance. The lower end is tapered to form a narrower outlet. A clamp is also provided for closing the distal end of the bag. Until the colostomy patient develops control of the drainage by irrigation, an open-ended pouch is used. When control is developed a closed pouch is recommended.
6. A narrow, lightweight elasticized belt which attaches to the mounting ring or pouch may be worn.
7. Micropore or nonallergenic tape. This is applied over the edges of the ring for security and to prevent leakage.
8. A deodorizing agent. Examples are Banish and Ostobon. A tissue or absorbent wipe may be soaked with the agent and placed in the ileostomy pouch.

The reusable bag usually requires emptying several times daily, especially with an ileostomy. The lower end of the bag is opened and the contents drained directly into the toilet. Using a syringe the bag is then rinsed and closed. As noted with the use of the disposable bag, the bag should be emptied when one-third to one-half full to avoid loosening the disc by the weight.

The pouch may be removed daily from the rim of the mounting ring by some patients and replaced with a clean one. This must be done very carefully to maintain the seal by the disc. If the seal is broken or if the patient complains of any burning or itching, the complete appliance is changed immediately; otherwise, the appliance is changed once or twice weekly by the ileostomy patient. A regular schedule should be arranged for emptying and changing the equipment; it should be at a time of day when drainage is at a minimum. This is determined by observation.

The colostomy appliance is changed when the bowel is irrigated. When control develops and irrigation is used less frequently, the pouch is changed daily and, if adhesive rings or squares are used, they are changed once or twice weekly. They are changed more often if they become soiled or if the patient experiences burning, itching or discomfort of the underlying skin.

In preparation for *application* of the reuseable appliance, the hole in the karaya washer (if used) is sized to fit the stoma and the washer is then lightly moistened with water. The pouch is placed over the rim of the mounting ring and secured. The pouch outlet is closed and clamped. The paper is peeled from one side of the double-faced adhesive disc and is then placed smoothly on the face of the mounting ring. The hole of the disc must be the same size as the hole in the ring and be directly over it.

When *removing* the appliance, a solvent is used sparingly on an absorbent wipe or with an eyedropper to remove the adhesive. The skin is washed *gently* and dried thoroughly. The skin and stoma are carefully inspected. If the skin is irritated or excoriated a product such as karaya powder, Stomahesive or Colley-Seal may be applied. When the skin is dry, the karaya washer is applied and the paper is peeled from the other surface of the double-faced adhesive disc. The latter is then centered over the stoma and applied with the outlet end of the pouch directed toward the patient's feet. Nonallergenic or micropore

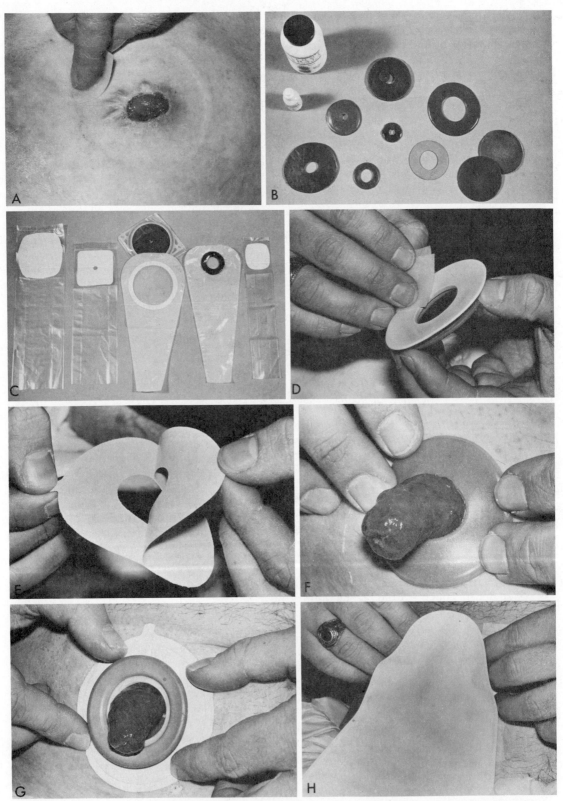

FIGURE 16–12 *A,* Stoma (sigmoid colostomy). *B,* Skin protectors. *C,* Examples of disposable temporary colostomy or ileostomy pouches. *D,* Mounting ring. *E,* Double-faced adhesive ring. *F,* Karaya washer in position around stoma. *G,* Mounting ring in position. *H,* Pouch being attached to mounting ring. (Courtesy of Enid Wilson, R. N., B.S.N., Stomal Therapist and Medical Photography Department, Sunnybrook Medical Center, Toronto.)

tape is then applied to the edges of the mounting ring to insure a seal and for security. If the patient finds a belt necessary it is applied then, and is secured to the mounting ring or pouch.

The reusable ileostomy or colostomy appliance that was removed is cleansed immediately after application of the clean unit has been completed. The adhesive disc is removed from the mounting ring (face plate) and discarded. The ring is cleansed first with an adhesive remover and then with a brush under cool running water.

If the pouch is to be used again it is left attached to the mounting ring and flushed out with cool running water. The appliance is then left to soak for 30 minutes in a detergent solution, after which it is rinsed well and hung up to dry. A paper towel placed within the bag will keep the surfaces separated and facilitate airing of the pouch. When the appliance is dry, powder the pouch inside and out with talcum powder or cornstarch.

Odor is a constant source of concern to the ileostomy or colostomy patient and his family. It may be controlled by a clean, odor-free, well-fitting appliance, efficient emptying and flushing of the bag, and the use of a commercial deodorant. The deodorant (e.g., Banish, Ostobon) is placed on a tissue or absorbent wipe and dropped into the pouch. Deodorant tablets of bismuth subgallate or chlorophyll are also available for oral administration but *should only be taken if prescribed by the physician*. Bags should not be kept in use too long; eventually they absorb odors that are impossible to remove entirely. The bags now available make it possible to change more often and prevent odor.

COLOSTOMY IRRIGATION. A colostomy may be controlled entirely by diet, especially if the colostomy is in the descending colon or sigmoid; others may require an irrigation daily or every second day. The purposes of irrigating the colostomy are to remove feces, gas and mucus from the intestine and establish a regular time of emptying the lower tract so that spontaneous, irregular drainage is less likely to occur and interfere with the person's activities and usual life style. During the initial postoperative recovery stage, the irrigation is done at the patient's bedside. When the patient is able, it is done in the bathroom.

The equipment for an irrigation includes the following:

1. Two quart enema can or bag with tubing (approximately 40 to 44 inches), connecting tube and clamp.
2. Catheter, number 18 or 20 French, or special colostomy irrigating tip which has a rubber or metal cup that fits over the stoma to prevent continual outflow while the solution is being introduced into the intestine.
3. Lubricating jelly.
4. Toilet tissue or cellucotton for cleaning and absorbing any leakage around the stoma.
5. Basin and small rubber sheet to receive the drainage, or an irrigating cup that is fitted over the stoma and held in place by a belt. The catheter is inserted through the cup and a tubular sheath or irrigating sleeve is also attached to the cup for drainage.
6. Basin of water for cleansing.
7. Paper bag or newspaper for discard.
8. Dressings or clean colostomy bag.

Five hundred to 2000 ml of tap water at 40.5° C. (105° F.) may be used, and the container is elevated 18 to 24 inches above the colostomy. The head of the bed may be raised or, if the patient is ambulatory, he may sit on a chair or on the toilet. The toilet should be used as soon as the patient is able; it has a beneficial psychological effect because of the association with normal defecation. If the rubber irrigating cup and tubular sheath are not available, a trough leading into the basin or toilet may be formed with a rubber or plastic sheet to receive the discharge. The catheter is lubricated and, after the air is expelled from the tubing, is inserted gently 4 to 8 inches. The water is introduced slowly. The rate of flow and pressure are regulated according to the patient's reaction. If he experiences cramps, the solution container should be lowered and the rate of flow decreased. Cramping indicates excessive contraction of the bowel which may actually retard the elimination of the bowel content. At first 500 ml. of fluid is given, and this is increased as the need is determined. The amount required to stimulate peristalsis and satisfactory elimination varies with patients; some may require 1500 to 2000 ml. The actual irrigation and elimination process takes approximately 30 to 40 minutes. Some form of diversion for the patient, such as reading or listening to the radio, may be helpful.

When evacuation is complete, the patient is

left clean and dry, the skin is protected with powder and a clean colostomy bag is applied. Drainage between irrigations may indicate that insufficient irrigating fluid was given or the fluid was given too quickly, or may be the result of constipation. If there is evidence of the latter, diet adjustment and increased fluid intake may be necessary.

A regular schedule should be set up for colostomy irrigation and for changing the colostomy appliance. The irrigation is most effective early in the morning, since this approximates the normal time of defecation. If bowel regularity is developed, irrigation every other day may be sufficient.

CARE OF A POUCH ILEOSTOMY. General preoperative preparation is similar to that cited for intestinal surgery (p. 548). The procedure of tube drainage of the ileal pouch, the nasogastric drainage and the withholding of food and fluids by mouth that follow the operation are discussed with the patient and family, and opportunities are provided for them to ask questions.

The patient is returned from the operation with a catheter inserted through the stoma and valve into the pouch. The catheter is connected to a closed drainage system. It is important to maintain continuous drainage and prevent an accumulation of secretions, gas and fecal matter in the pouch in order to promote healing and prevent complications. If the pouch becomes distended, ileal contents may seep through the suture lines and cause peritonitis. Regular, frequent irrigation of the tube may be required to promote drainage. Sterile normal saline or water may be used, and a directive is received regarding the exact volume that is to be introduced very gently with a syringe. Suction is not applied to withdraw the fluid; the return flow should drain by gravity through the catheter. If it is retained, the physician is notified.

The color of the drainage is checked frequently; it may be colored by blood at first but the blood content progressively decreases over the first 2 days. If it does not, it is reported. The volume of the ileal discharge is also recorded. The fecal drainage eventually may become semiliquid as the diet is increased and the capacity and retention of the pouch increase. Thicker pouch content may cause a drainage problem since "solid" particles may obstruct the drainage tube, necessitating irrigation, increased fluid intake and adjustment in the diet.

A lightweight dressing with a hole in the center for the catheter covers the stoma and surgical wound. This is changed daily and the stoma inspected for color, swelling and edema.

The nasogastric tube is attached to low negative pressure to prevent the possibility of gastric secretions and gas accumulating and distending the gastrointestinal tract. The patient is not allowed anything by mouth until the tube is removed. He is sustained by the administration of intravenous fluids. The fluid balance and serum electrolyte levels are followed closely; the volume and composition of the intravenous fluids are based on these reports.

The catheter into the pouch is disconnected from the closed drainage system in approximately 10 to 12 days and is corked. The stopper is removed hourly for drainage of the pouch. During the night the catheter is reconnected to the drainage system. The period between the drainages is gradually increased by 15-minute intervals and eventually, when the interval has been lengthened to approximately 3 hours, the catheter is removed. The pouch is then drained every 3 hours by reinsertion of the catheter.

The capacity of the pouch gradually increases and, in 6 months to a year, a capacity of 500 to 1000 ml. is achieved. As the pouch progressively accommodates more and more, the frequency of the catheter insertion for drainage decreases, the objective being three or four times daily. Twenty-four-hour drainage is measured and recorded for many weeks. If the pouch does not drain freely when the tube is introduced, gentle irrigation with a prescribed volume is used.

When the nasogastric tube is removed, the patient receives small amounts of clear fluid exclusive of carbonated drinks. If these are tolerated without distention or vomiting the amounts are increased, followed by a progressive increase from more nourishing fluids through soft to a light normal diet. Food tolerance tends to be an individual matter; the introduction of "new" foods one at a time makes it possible to identify those that are troublesome. Gas-forming foods, raw fruits and vegetables, foods with a high cellulose or fiber content, corn, celery, lettuce, beans, peas and cabbage are frequently among those not tolerated.

PSYCHOLOGICAL SUPPORT. As soon as the patient has recovered sufficiently from the operation, the nurse concentrates on helping him to accept his "ostomy" and on teaching him the necessary care and management. Although there may have been considerable discussion of the modified method of elimination preoperatively, when the patient is actually faced with it he may be filled with revulsion and become discouraged and depressed. The patient is again concerned about his future social acceptance. Acceptance comes first from the nurse, who willingly makes every effort to keep the patient clean and comfortable without any hesitation or aversion. Personal contact by touch as in the bathing of the patient and positioning and cleansing around the stoma in a perfectly natural and matter-of-fact manner tells the patient that he is not unacceptable. The nurse encourages and gradually introduces self-care with an understanding of the patient's reactions to the adjustments he must make. The patient may find it helpful to have the interest of and another visit from the ostomate who visited before.

FLUIDS AND NUTRITION. The ileostomy or colostomy patient usually starts out on a light, low-residue diet to which foods of a regular, normal diet are added gradually. Tolerance varies with patients but, by careful personal experimentation with foods, each person will recognize what he can and cannot take. The foods that most often have to be eliminated are those with a high-fiber or high-cellulose content. Nuts, prunes, celery, corn, pineapple, turnips, beans, cabbage and onions tend to be troublesome.

A well-balanced diet is encouraged and the person's weight followed. Patients are advised to eat slowly and to chew their foods well, which reduces the risk of a fecal bolus blocking the stoma. Emptying the pouch or changing the appliance just before mealtime should be avoided.

Considerable water and salts are lost in ileostomy drainage, especially during the first 2 or 3 months. Gradually, the small intestine adapts to the lack of colonic function and absorbs more water and salts. Until then extra water and foods rich in sodium and potassium should be taken. The patient may erroneously think that limiting his fluid intake will cause the intestinal drainage to be less fluid.

COMPLICATIONS. Potential complications with an ileostomy or colostomy include prolapse or retraction of the stoma, obstruction of the stoma, fluid and electrolyte imbalance, renal calculus and fistula.

In *prolapse of the stoma,* the mesentery of the remaining intestine is not secured sufficiently to the abdominal wall and/or the opening in the abdominal wall is too large. Increased intra-abdominal pressure results in a segment of the ileum or colon being forced out onto the abdomen. If several inches of the bowel is extruded, the patient assumes the dorsal recumbent position with the head and shoulders slightly raised and the knees flexed. A sterile towel or dressing moistened in sterile water or normal saline is placed over the area. The physician may attempt manual replacement of the extruded segment or recommend surgical repair.

Retraction of the stoma occurs as the result of shrinking scar tissue in the supporting tissues of the abdominal wall. The opening becomes flush with the abdominal surface, making it difficult to protect the skin from the irritating effluent. Correction is by surgery.

Obstruction of the stoma may be caused by a fecal bolus formed as a result of insufficient mastication of food or the ingestion of fibrous or cellulose foods that are too bulky to pass through the stoma. Examples of such foods are corn, celery, bran, coconut and nuts. The blockage may be relieved by an irrigation given by the physician. An obstruction may also be caused by a volvulus of the ileum near the stoma. If there is no ileal or colostomy discharge, the physician is notified. Unless the obstruction is relieved, the patient will develop nausea, vomiting, crampy pain and abdominal distention.

Ileostomy dysfunction sometimes occurs, and is characterized by sporadic free liquid drainage with a very offensive odor. It is associated with peristomal scarring and stenosis which causes trapping of the intestinal contents until pressure and irritation result in the discharge. Dilation of the stoma may be necessary.

Normally, much of the water and electrolytes contained in the small intestinal content is reabsorbed in the colon. The person with an ileostomy loses considerable water, sodium and potassium in the ileal drainage and may develop *fluid and electrolyte imbalance.* The patient is encouraged to drink a minimum of 1500 to 2000 ml. of fluid daily, add salt to his foods and include potassium-containing foods (e.g., orange juice, banana, meat) in his diet. If the ileal drainage becomes excessive, fluids containing potassium and sodium are increased to compensate for the loss. Tomato juice, orange juice, tea with sugar and bouillon are fluids that may be used. If the excessive drainage cannot be controlled the physician is notified. An antidiarrheal drug may be prescribed, serum electrolyte levels determined and intravenous fluids administered to correct dehydration and electrolyte imbalance.

The ileostomy patient is predisposed to the formation of a *renal calculus* (kidney stone) because of the water and sodium loss in drainage. This further emphasizes the importance of a greater fluid and electrolyte intake for the person with an ileostomy or colostomy, especially if the latter is on the right side.

Rarely, an ileostomy or colostomy is complicated by a *fistula.* An opening develops in the ileum and the drainage forms a tract to the surface. This may be the result of a poorly fitting appliance or the recurrence of the primary disease. The drainage causes tissue irritation and erosion. Surgical intervention may be used to resect the tract and may include reconstruction of the stoma. Healing may necessitate complete rest of the intestine; the patient may receive total intravenous nutrition (hyperalimentation) until the area is healed.

Herniation of the intestine due to a weakness of the muscular tissue at the site of the stoma may occur. It is recognized as a bulging area. Support may be provided by the ileostomy or colostomy appliance.

PREPARATION FOR DISCHARGE FROM HOSPITAL. A plan of instruction is developed to prepare the patient for assuming care of his ileostomy or colostomy and for living a healthy, active life. During the first few days after the operation, the patient's experience with pain and discomfort generally precludes concern about the stoma and his future care and activity. Gradually an awareness of the situation develops and the patient's reaction must be assessed. There may be a brief period of depression and withdrawal. Obviously, while reacting in this way, the patient is not receptive to any formal instruction. The nurse encourages verbalization of his concern by being a good listener and accepting his reactions and anxiety. The nurse's attitude is extremely important; any sign of distaste when caring for the patient or indication of haste to cut short the contact is likely to be interpreted by the patient that he is unacceptable. To him,

this reflects what will happen in his future, and fosters feelings of depression and resentment, making rehabilitation difficult.

The preparation for the patient's discharge from the hospital should include a member of the family. Participation by the person with an ileostomy or colostomy who visited the patient may be very helpful in reinforcing the information. Teaching includes explanations, discussions and demonstrations related to the following factors

Management of the Ileostomy and Colostomy. Active patient participation in stomal and appliance care is introduced gradually but as early as possible. By the time he leaves the hospital, the patient should be engaged in self-care and be confident in the fact that support and assistance are available to him in the hospital and at home.

At first, as the nurse cares for the ileostomy or colostomy, each step of the procedure is clearly described without minute details. Then, gradually, the patient is given the opportunity to perform part of the care. His participation is increased from day to day until eventually he is prepared to undertake complete care. This progressive, step-by-step approach takes time and patience but is less frustrating and discouraging for the patient. As he learns to assume self-care in the hospital, the nurse offers suggestions as to how he may manage the same procedure at home.

More formalized and detailed instruction includes directions for and demonstrations of:

1. The necessary equipment and supplies. In addition to discussing and demonstrating the various parts of the appliance, a written list is provided and information given as to how and where the products may be obtained.

2. Emptying of the pouch, care of the stoma and changing of the appliance. Planned discussions reinforce the learning that took place as the patient undertook, step-by-step, the daily care. It also gives him and the members of the family an opportunity to ask questions.

Additional directions for care and use usually accompany the appliance and should be read by the patient. Several useful booklets about ileostomy and colostomy care are usually available from the local branch of the Ostomy Association and may be given to the patient by a visiting ostomate. Each hospital also has printed directions which serve as a guide for the patient. The importance of establishing a regular schedule for care is emphasized.

3. Irrigation of the colostomy. In addition to demonstrating and explaining the procedure and having the patient do it himself, written directions are given to him. Assistance may be necessary in deciding how the irrigation can be fitted in with his daily routine.

4. Care of the skin. The need for thorough but gentle cleansing of the skin is stressed, as is the use of a protective skin barrier because of the irritating effect of the enzyme-containing discharge. Inspection for redness and excoriation is described and advice given as to what should be done if either is present.

5. Care of the appliance. Cleansing of the mounting ring and reusable pouches is demonstrated and a written directive given.

6. Control of odor. The role of regular emptying, changing and thorough cleansing of the appliance in controlling odor is discussed. The use of a deodorant in the bag is encouraged.

7. Problems or complications. Problems such as excessive drainage, blockage of the stoma, excoriation, burning sensation or itching of the skin are discussed as to possible causes, how they are recognized and the appropriate action.

Nutrition and Fluids. The patient is advised that foods high in cellulose and fiber and some raw vegetables and fruits may be troublesome. A list of foods known to lead to a problem, and therefore to be avoided, is provided. The importance of a well-balanced diet and the taking of additional amounts of sodium, potassium and water is explained. It is suggested that one new food be added at a time so those that cannot be tolerated may be identified.

. *Bathing.* The patient may take a shower or tub bath with the appliance in place or, if the discharge is at a minimum, the appliance may be removed and the stoma covered with a soft dressing and waterproof adhesive. Showering without the appliance is good for the skin. The patient must be sure that no soap residue remains, since this interferes with the seal provided by the adhesive disc. Bathing is usually done before applying a fresh appliance because the moisture is likely to loosen the adhesive disc.

Some ostomates may have sufficient confidence to go swimming, since their appliance is concealed by a bathing suit.

Activity. Activity for the ileostomy and colostomy patient is normal except for heavy lifting, which predisposes to prolapse of the stoma and hernia, and body contact sports, which could result in injury to the stoma. The patient is encouraged to return to his occupation and recreational activities. Many ostomates find that their general health is so much better than previously that they enjoy being able to participate in so much.

The patient may be concerned about sexual relationships; he is advised that the change in body image need not be a deterrent to satisfactory sex relations. If an abdominoperineal resection has been done, injury to parasympathetic nerves may very occasionally result in impotency. The female may experience some discomfort during intercourse for a period of time because of the perineal wound. Brochures dealing with "sex and the ostomate" are available from the Ostomy Association. Copies should be kept at the hospital so one is available to the patient. This matter of sexual relationships is something the individual may wish to discuss freely with the ostomate who visits.

Medications. Laxatives or other drugs should not be taken unless prescribed. If a medicine is ordered by a physician other than the gastroenterologist, the patient reminds him of his ileostomy. Some preparations should be only in powder or liquid form to insure absorption.

Sources of Assistance. The ostomate is likely to be very apprehensive about leaving the protective hospital environment. A list of persons or associations from whom advice or assistance may be sought is provided with their telephone numbers. This list may include the hospital nurse or clinical nurse specialist who has cared for the patient, enterostomal therapist, physician or hospital resident, visiting ostomate, visiting nurse association, and local branch of the Ostomy Association.

Care of the Ileal Pouch. As soon as the tube is removed, plans are made to teach the patient how to insert the catheter to empty the pouch. As cited earlier, the catheter is passed every 2 hours at first, and then the interval is gradually lengthened over the next 4 to 6 months. The patient is advised that if he experiences discomfort or a full sensation in the pouch, the pouch should be intubated to avoid distention and excessive pressure on the valve. The patient observes the passing of the catheter by the nurse, who explains the procedure as she does it and gives the patient the opportunity to ask questions. The patient then undertakes the passing of the catheter through the stoma and valve. The nurse remains during the procedure until assured that the patient is competent and sufficiently confident. He learns the details of carrying out the procedure, and may use a basin to receive the projectile drainage or may prefer to let it flow directly into the toilet. If the ileal outflow is slow, the patient is advised that he may bear down. Instructions are given as to the frequency and volume of drainage that would be considered inadequate, and what to do if this occurs. The physician may want the patient to be taught to irrigate the pouch in the event of insufficient drainage.

Cleansing of the stoma and the skin and covering it with a small dressing (e.g., 2-inch square Band-Aid or a piece of disposable diaper) are reviewed in preparation for discharge.

The necessary supplies are obtained for the patient and include a small case with two catheters, water-soluble lubricant for the catheter, a syringe, dressings and micropore tape. The sources for supplies are given and instructions supplied as to their care. The patient is instructed to wash the catheter in detergent solution thoroughly and rinse well.

It is important for the person with an ileal pouch to carry a card or wear a Medic Alert bracelet or pendant indicating his "condition" and the need for drainage of the pouch. If he loses consciousness or is injured, this would be necessary to avoid excessive and dangerous distention of the pouch.

OTHER INTESTINAL DISORDERS

Appendicitis

The appendix, a narrow blind tube extending from the inferior part of the cecum, is a common site of inflammation which may necessitate its surgical removal. The appendix has no essential function in the human, and there is no change in body function with its removal.

The commonest cause of appendicitis is obstruction of the lumen by a fecolith (a small, hard mass of accumulated feces) or a solid foreign body, or by disease or scar tissue in the walls of the appendix. Secretion collects in the tube, causing distention that results in pressure on the intramural blood vessels. The mucosa ulcerates and readily becomes infected; the walls may become gangrenous because of the interference with the blood supply, and perforation is likely to occur. A ruptured appendix is serious; it allows the escape of organisms into the peritoneal cavity and may cause an abscess in the appendiceal region or a generalized peritonitis.

The disease may occur at any age but is more common in children over 4 years of age, adolescents and young adults. Early diagnosis and treatment of appendicitis is important to prevent serious complications.

Manifestations of appendicitis are abdominal pain, nausea and vomiting, a moderate elevation in temperature and a leukocytosis with the increase being in the polymorphonuclear cells. At the onset, the pain may be diffuse or referred to the central portion of the abdomen or the lower epigastric region, and is described as crampy. As the inflammation involves the walls of the appendix, the pain becomes localized to the lower right quadrant or McBurney's point.[20] The area is tender on palpation, and rigidity gradually develops in the muscles (muscle guarding). Rebound tenderness may be present which is determined by palpation of the left lower quadrant. With the sudden release of the pressure, the patient experiences pain or discomfort in the appendix region. The patient moves slowly and carefully to avoid jolting and movement that increase the pain, and tends to keep his right thigh flexed.

The omentum and adjacent bowel may become adherent to the inflamed appendix, walling off the area. If the appendix ruptures, an abscess will most likely form in the walled-off cavity. But, if perforation occurs before the area is walled off, a generalized peritonitis develops; the patient complains of pain and tenderness over the whole abdomen which

---

[20]*McBurney's point* refers to the area about 2 inches from the anterior superior iliac spine on a line with the umbilicus. It corresponds with the normal position of the appendix.

becomes rigid (board-like) and distended. The distention is due to inhibited bowel motility, which may be referred to as paralytic or adynamic ileus.

Examination of the patient includes palpation of the abdomen and a differential leukocyte determination. The physician may also do a rectal examination, and a vaginal pelvic examination may be done on the female.

The *treatment* of appendicitis depends on the stage to which the disease has advanced. If it is still localized to the appendix, an appendectomy is done as soon as the diagnosis is established. If the appendix has ruptured and there is an abscess or peritonitis, the patient may be treated conservatively with antibiotics and parenteral fluids and given very little or nothing by mouth to reduce gastrointestinal activity. Gastrointestinal decompression is used if there are generalized peritonitis and a paralytic ileus. Surgery may be undertaken later to remove the appendix.

NURSING IN APPENDICITIS. The person with abdominal pain is urged to seek medical advice and self-treatment is discouraged, particularly the taking of a laxative or an enema which could be serious, since either could cause perforation of the appendix through stimulation of peristalsis. The patient is also advised not to take food or fluid until seen by the doctor. This is in case immediate surgery is necessary. In most instances, surgery is performed as soon as the diagnosis is established unless perforation is suspected. For preparation for emergency surgery, see page 171. If the appendix was intact at the time of removal, the patient usually makes a rapid, uneventful recovery with a short period of hospitalization (5 to 7 days). For postoperative nursing care, see page 000.

If an abscess is present, a drainage tube is placed in the abscess cavity at the time of operation. This necessitates cleansing of the wound and changing of the dressing at intervals. The patient's head and shoulders are elevated; this may help to keep the infection localized to the appendiceal region. Large doses of an antibiotic are ordered, and the patient should receive plenty of fluids. An accurate record of the intake should be kept and, if the patient cannot take sufficient quantities by mouth, parenteral supplements may be ordered. Close observations are made for possible extension of the infection and generalized peritonitis. Abdominal distention, nausea and vomiting, lack of bowel activity, an elevated temperature and rapid pulse are brought promptly to the surgeon's attention.

Peritonitis

Peritonitis is a localized or generalized inflammation of the peritoneum and is most often a secondary condition. It is usually acute but may be chronic. The inflammatory response may be due to bacterial invasion or chemical irritation caused by bile, pancreatic, gastric or intestinal secretions, urine or blood escaping into the peritoneal cavity. A common infectious agent is *Escherichia coli* which has escaped from the intestinal lumen.

Intestinal motility is depressed and the intestine becomes distended with gas and fluid. The peritoneal serous membrane becomes hyperemic and edematous and there is an outpouring of fluid into the cavity that incurs serious fluid, electrolyte and protein imbalances.

The patient experiences abdominal pain, nausea, vomiting and distention. The abdomen becomes rigid (muscle guarding) and progressively more distended. A leukocytosis and fever may develop. The pulse becomes rapid and there is a decrease in blood volume due to loss of intravascular volume. The respirations may be shallow and rapid as a result of ventilatory interference by extreme abdominal distention. Unless quickly reversed, the patient shows signs of shock. He is pale and prostrate; the skin is cool and moist. Bowel sounds are absent as peristalsis is arrested.

Treatment is directed toward the primary condition (e.g., surgery to close a perforated ulcer), relieving the distention and reestablishing peristalsis, combating infection and shock, and replacing fluids and electrolytes.

Gastric and intestinal intubation and continuous suctioning are established. Nothing is given orally. An intravenous infusion is administered and the solutions used may be based upon laboratory determinations of serum electrolyte levels. A blood transfusion may be given to counteract shock and replace protein lost in the inflammatory exudate. An antibiotic is administered if organisms are the causative factor of the peritonitis.

The patient is very ill and requires constant supportive nursing care. He is nursed in a medium Fowler's position.

Regional Enteritis (Regional Ileitis, Crohn's Disease)

This is a chronic inflammatory disease of unknown cause that may develop in *any part of the gastrointestinal tract* but has a predilection for the terminal portion of the ileum. The intestinal walls in the affected area are swollen and edematous, and the lumen is narrowed. Patchy areas of granulomatous inflammation and ulceration develop and extend throughout the entire wall. The bowel may perforate and form an internal or external fistula (an abnormal passage) into another loop of the intestine or onto the skin. As the inflammation subsides there is scarring and stenosis, which may lead to a partial obstruction of the bowel. More than one area of the intestine may be involved, while the intervening segments remain unaffected.

The incidence of the disease has increased in the Western world in the last two decades and, although it may develop at any age, the onset is most often between the ages of 20 and 40 years. Both sexes are affected equally. Heredity is thought to play a role because of the familial incidence. Impaired cellular immunity or an autoimmune reaction to an unidentified antigen has been suggested as a possible etiologic factor.

MANIFESTATIONS. The patient experiences abdominal pain and tenderness, a low-grade fever and frequent watery stools that may contain pus and particles of undigested food. Some abdominal rigidity due to peritoneal irritation may be seen, and there is usually a slight leukocytosis. As the disease progresses malnutrition, loss of weight and strength, dehydration, and anemia develop because of loss of appetite and interference with normal intestinal absorption. The condition may persist, or there may be remissions and exacerbations. The course is very unpredictable, varying considerably with the individual. Some patients develop serious complications such as fistula, obstruction and perforation. In others the disease may become progressively less severe over a lengthy period.

TREATMENT AND CARE. Care of the patient with Crohn's disease is principally supportive and symptomatic. Efforts are directed toward relief of pain, control of diarrhea, correction of fluid, electrolyte and nutritional deficiencies, treatment of secondary infection, and reduction of the patient's emotional distress. The physical condition and emotional state of the patient have important roles in the progress of the disease and in preventing an exacerbation.

SUPPORTIVE CARE. The amount of assistance and the extent of modification in life pattern required by the patient depends upon the severity of the disease and his strength and nutritional status. Much of the nursing care discussed in the section on diarrhea (p. 541) is applicable to the patient with Crohn's disease.

Rest and Psychological Support. Physical and mental rest are important for the person with regional enteritis. In severe attacks, bed rest is recommended. A reduction in energy expenditure and extra hours of rest during the day may be suggested for less debilitated patients whose disease is less active. In addition to advising the patient that he can contribute to favorable progress by getting adequate rest, the avoidance of emotional disturbance is stressed. This is difficult, since the patient has been advised of the nature of his disease and the limited success of current treatment. He should know that the course and severity vary, and that many patients do lead relatively normal lives. The nurse may help by being a willing listener when patient and family express their concerns and despair. Acceptance of their feelings, working through problems and providing realistic encouragement contribute to support. Realization that his problems are recognized and that his reactions are understood and accepted assists the patient to cope with circumstances and reality. Some type of diversion should be provided; constant worry about the condition may increase intestinal motility.

Fluids and Nutrition. An excessive loss of fluid in diarrhea and a probable reduced intake by the patient because of abdominal pain and "feeling sick" may lead to dehydration. The daily intake and output are recorded and the fluid balance is noted. The patient is encouraged and, if necessary, given assistance to take adequate amounts of fluid. Intravenous infusion may be necessary to correct dehydration and maintain sufficient intake.

Serum electrolyte levels, especially potassium and sodium, are determined, as an abnormal amount may be lost in the stools or through fistula drainage. Replacement is made by intravenous fluids. A blood transfusion may be necessary to correct anemia that has resulted from nutritional deficiencies. These develop due to insufficient food intake and/or impaired intestinal absorption. Currently, special therapeutic diets (e.g., low-residue) receive less consideration than formerly. The patient is encouraged to take a well-balanced, nutritious diet. He is advised to eliminate only those foods which he cannot tolerate or digest. These vary among patients but usually raw vegetables, raw fruits and fats are common problems. Fat intolerance is attributed to the loss of bile salts (failure of the intestine to reabsorb the salts). Some patients may find that they have to keep the roughage content low and that vitamin supplements may be necessary.

As part of the treatment of an acute attack, the physician may have the patient sustained by total parenteral nutrition. Nothing is given orally and the intestine is "placed at rest." If a patient is not taking or absorbing enough to support even limited body activity, his dietary intake may be supplemented by intravenous nutrition (see p. 504 for total parenteral nutrition).

MEDICATIONS. Several types of drugs are used in the treatment of regional enteritis. Those commonly administered include:

Corticosteroid Preparations. These (e.g., prednisone) are prescribed for their anti-inflammatory action. The patient receives large doses for 1 to 2 weeks and the dose is then progressively decreased to a maintenance level. Observations are necessary for side effects such as retention of sodium and water, hypokalemia and hypertension.

Azathioprine (Imuran). This is anti-inflammatory and immunosuppressive. Although the prescribed dosage in regional enteritis is smaller (1.5 to 3 mg. per kg. body weight) than that used for the prevention of transplant rejection (1.5 to 5 mg. per kg. body weight), the patient's resistance to infection is lowered. The nurse and patient observe the necessary measures to prevent infection.

Salicylazosulfapyridine (Azulfidine). This is an anti-infective drug. When prescribed, it is important that the patient take a minimum of 2500 ml. of fluid daily, as with any sulfonamide preparation. This is to prevent possible crystallization of the sulfonamide in the renal tubules.

Antibiotics. A fistula complicated by infection or a stagnant area or loop of intestine in which there is an overgrowth of bacteria may be treated with an antimicrobial agent (e.g., tetracycline).

Codeine. This may be prescribed in small doses to relieve abdominal pain and help control the diarrhea.

Mild Sedatives. One of these, such as diazepam (Valium), in small doses may be ordered to reduce the patient's anxiety and emotional stress.

Nutritional Supplements. Due to malabsorption the patient may require various supplements such as iron, cyanacobalamin (vitamin B_{12}), folic acid and multiple vitamins. Fat-soluble vitamins may have to be given parenterally because of malabsorption.

COMPLICATIONS. These are common in regional enteritis. The ensuing scar tissue of the inflammatory process narrows the lumen of the intestine and may cause partial or complete bowel obstruction. Damaged areas of intestine result in impaired absorption which may lead to various nutritional abnormalities.

An abscess may develop at the site of active disease; inflamed loops of intestine may be bound together to form blind loops. The inflammation involves all layers of the intestinal wall which predisposes to perforation, leading to generalized peritonitis or the development of a fistula. The latter may form between the intestine and another abdominal organ or may form a passage to the skin surface.

SURGICAL INTERVENTION. This is usually reserved for the patient with complications or where the disease is intractable and incapacitating. The surgical procedures used may be a resection and end-to-end anastomosis, resection and ileostomy, bypass of the diseased area by anastomosis, or bypass with closure of the proximal end of the bypassed portion. Unfortunately, following surgery, the disease tends to recur. If an extensive resection is done, the absorptive surface is so diminished that malnutrition is a very serious problem. Massive resection may necessitate permanent total parenteral nutrition (see p. 504).

Idiopathic Ulcerative Colitis

Ulcerative colitis is characterized by severe inflammation and ulceration of the mucosa of the rectum and of a part or all of the colon. The process usually begins in the rectosigmoid area and spreads up the descending colon. There is marked hyperemia and edema in the affected area, followed by ulceration. The denuded areas result in infection, abscesses and a loss of fluid, electrolytes and blood.

ETIOLOGY. The cause of this disease remains obscure. There is at present support for the theory that it is due to an autoimmune reaction in which the body forms antibodies that destroy the normal protective mucus which coats the bowel. A genetic factor is thought to be involved because of the familial incidence of the disease. Infection, hypersensitivity to a particular food, insecurity and emotional stress have been considered to be implicated in the development of colitis but none has been proven conclusively to be an etiologic factor. The personality characteristics of excessive dependence, immaturity, hostility and depression frequently manifested by the patient with colitis are probably the result of the disorder rather than the cause; they are common to persons with any chronic disease characterized by exacerbations and remissions. Frequently arthritis, skin lesions or iritis is associated with ulcerative colitis and is considered to be a response to the same causative factor responsible for the disease in the colon.

Ulcerative colitis affects both sexes equally and, although it may occur at any age, the onset occurs most frequently during the second and third decades.

MANIFESTATIONS AND COURSE. The onset is usually insidious; rarely it may develop suddenly with intense severity. The patient has frequent diarrheal stools containing blood, mucus and pus, accompanied by colicky abdominal pain. There is abdominal tenderness, especially on the left side, and rectal involvement causes tenesmus (painful, ineffective straining). Dehydration, anemia and loss of weight and strength develop, and the patient may have a low-grade fever. The prolonged and distressing symptoms and incapacitation cause emotional stress, and the patient may become very discouraged and depressed.

Diagnostic investigation includes a sigmoidoscopy or colonoscopy (see p. 496). The examination reveals a friable mucosa that bleeds readily, ulcers and sloughing areas and probably loss of haustra, which are the normal pouch-like structures of the colon. A biopsy is carried out during the endoscopic examination. A barium enema may be used with an x-ray examination but is not given in severe, acute colitis because of the danger of perforation of the bowel. Laboratory tests include determinations of hemoglobin, hematocrit, leukocyte count and sedimentation rate. The latter two are elevated with colitis. Electrolyte level and blood protein determinations are necessary, since there may be dysfunction in absorption in the proximal portion of the colon and excessive losses in the frequent, diarrheal stools.

The course of ulcerative colitis is unpredictable. The patient may have a complete recovery but, more often, there are relapses in subsequent months or years. An acute exacerbation may be precipitated by nervous or physical strain. The patient's history may reveal a recent bereavement, a home or job conflict, an acute infection or probably dietary indiscretions or bowel irritation by laxatives.

Persisting and frequent recurrences are likely to cause serious *complications*. Severe hemorrhage may occur if a large vessel is eroded, necessitating emergency surgical treatment in which a colectomy is usually done. Perforation of an ulcerated area of the bowel, leading to generalized peritonitis, is a less common complication but very serious. Perforation of the rectum frequently causes an abscess and fistula in the perirectal or perianal regions. When the disease is prolonged, the affected colon tends to become a smooth, narrow, inflexible tube. The mucosa becomes thin and the walls are infiltrated by scar tissue that causes a stenosis that may result in obstruction. Occasionally, polyps develop in the ulcerated colon and may give rise to bleeding. The incidence of cancer of the colon is higher in persons who have had ulcerative colitis for several years than in the general population.

TREATMENT AND NURSING CARE. The patient is usually hospitalized during an acute attack of ulcerative colitis so that a more intensive therapeutic and supportive program may be provided. Also, hospitalization may remove the patient from an environment that has stress factors which aggravate his disease. Treatment and care are directed toward reducing colonic activity, combating secondary infection, improving the patient's general condition by correcting the malnutrition and anemia, and alleviating emotional stress.

EMOTIONAL SUPPORT. It should be understood by all those caring for the ulcerative colitis patient that sensitivity, dependence and insecurity are common characteristics of these patients and that they tend to have inner tensions and bottled-up feelings which are not expressed. Every appropriate means possible should be considered to make the patient mentally and physically comfortable. It is important that the nurse convey to the patient by thoughtful attention and words that she knows and cares about what he is experiencing and how he feels about his total situation.

Understanding sympathetic care is extremely important in gradually establishing confidence and a relationship that is conducive to more effective treatment. The patient is tactfully encouraged to talk about himself and his life activities while the nurse listens carefully for problems that may be responsible for aggravating his disorder. He may actually feel better after talking to the nurse because someone has been interested enough to listen.

Orientation to the environment and an explanation of care and treatments are necessary. The best timing for certain activities and the beneficial effects of such may be discussed; for example, it may be advisable to leave the patient undisturbed following a meal and to delay the bath or other care procedures to avoid movement and activities that may stimulate bowel activity. If the sensitive patient is not advised of the purpose of the delay, he may feel neglected.

Some form of appropriate diversion should be provided to reduce the patient's preoccupation with his disease. Visitors are screened to avoid those who may worry the patient or stir up inner conflicts. Mild sedation may be necessary to promote rest and reduce his level of anxiety.

OBSERVATIONS. The number, volume, consistency and content of the stools are noted and recorded. A close check is made of the patient's hydration and nutritional status from day to day. His weight is recorded daily unless it proves a source of concern to the patient, in which case it is discontinued and only noted once or twice weekly.

The nurse is alert to the possibility of perforation and hemorrhage and should promptly report any changes in the patient that might be early indications of these complications.

The foods taken by the patient are noted and observations made as to whether the patient's diarrhea increases after any one particular food is taken.

REST. Bed rest, quiet and relaxation tend to reduce intestinal motility and are recommended during the acute phase. Activity is gradually resumed as the severe diarrhea and fever subside. Nursing care is planned to permit undisturbed periods of rest. Assistance is given the weak and debilitated patient in turning and in getting on and off the bedpan or getting in and out of bed to go to the bathroom, which can be exhausting to him.

POSITIONING AND SKIN CARE. The patient with ulcerative colitis may become emaciated, which necessitates special attention to the bony prominences to prevent decubitus ulcers. The areas are kept clean and dry and are gently and frequently massaged. Pressure on the bony prominences may be relieved by using an alternating air mattress or pieces of sponge rubber or sheepskin. The rim of the bedpan or commode should be padded to protect the skin. The anal region is washed after each defecation, and a protective ointment or cream such as petrolatum jelly or zinc oxide is applied. If severe tenesmus is experienced, warm compresses or an ointment such as dibucaine hydrochloride (Nupercaine) may be applied to the anus for relief.

The patient tends to lie curled up in one position with the legs and thighs continuously flexed, which predisposes to contractures. There is a reluctance to move about in bed or turn for fear of stimulating peristalsis and another bowel movement. He must be encouraged to turn and change his position every 1 to 2 hours. Full extension of the lower limbs should be required at frequent intervals and, if possible, the prone position should be assumed for a few minutes two or three times daily.

NUTRITION AND HYDRATION. In serious acute attacks, oral food and fluids may be withdrawn for a brief period in an effort to reduce intestinal activity to a minimum while the patient is maintained on parenteral fluids or total parenteral nutrition.

When food is permitted, a high-calorie,

high-protein, nonirritating low-residue diet is given. Milk is usually poorly tolerated. Iced fluids, carbonated drinks, raw fruits and vegetables and all foods suspected of stimulating bowel activity are avoided. Recently, some physicians have suggested a more liberal diet with elimination of only those foods that the patient recognizes as increasing the diarrhea.

Nutrition of the patient requires a great deal of attention. The patient may develop serious nutritional deficiencies. Anorexia presents a problem, and there are serious losses of essential nutrients, fluid and electrolytes in the frequent stools. In many instances, the nurse must work at getting the patient to take sufficient nourishment; it may be necessary to provide frequent small meals. An effort is made to serve foods the patient likes, to provide variety, and to have the tray attractively arranged. A discouraging factor commonly encountered is that, as soon as the patient starts to eat, peristalsis is stimulated and he must have the bedpan. When this happens the tray should be removed from the room and returned after the patient has used the pan and received the necessary hygienic care, and the room is ventilated. Hot foods should be kept warm or reheated. Encouragement and praise are given as the patient manages to take larger amounts of food.

Even though a fair amount may be taken orally, fluid and electrolyte losses may have to be replaced by intravenous infusions. Blood transfusions may be given to correct anemia and to restore a normal blood volume. Impaired absorption of the foods and vitamins, as well as restriction of certain foods, contributes to the need for vitamin supplements, particularly ascorbic acid and the vitamin B complex.

ENVIRONMENT. Preferably, the ulcerative colitis patient should be in a room by himself so he will be less embarrassed by his frequent use of the bedpan and the odor involved. If this is not possible, he should be placed in an area that can be screened to provide privacy and can be readily ventilated. If he has bathroom privileges, he should be placed near the bathroom.

It may be necessary to keep a clean, covered bedpan at the bedside because of the patient's urgency and to prevent concern about getting it in time. The bed linen is kept clean and fresh. Extra covers may be needed for the patient for warmth; chilling should be avoided because of his lowered resistance.

MEDICATIONS. Various drugs are used in treating the patient with colitis. Nearly all patients receive small, regular doses of a sedative to promote rest and relaxation and to alleviate some of the emotional stress so common to this disorder. Examples of sedatives that may be prescribed are amobarbital (Amytal), diazepam (Valium) and flurazepam (Dalmane).

Secondary infection of the raw ulcerated areas of the bowel is treated by the oral administration of an anti-infective drug. A compound of sulfapyridine and acetylsalicylic acid (salicylazosulfapyridine, Azulfidine) or an antibiotic may be administered orally. The patient receiving a sulfonamide preparation is observed for side effects such as skin rash, leukopenia, anemia, nausea, vomiting and headache and requires a minimum of 2500 ml. of fluid daily. If the infection extends deeply into the colonic wall, a parenteral antibiotic may be prescribed.

Anticholinergic drugs to reduce peristalsis may be used in some instances. Examples are propantheline (Pro-Banthine) and methantheline bromide (Banthine).

A corticosteroid such as prednisone is considered an effective anti-inflammatory drug in inducing a remission of severe colitis. Initially, the dosage is high (e.g., 40 to 60 mg. daily) and is given in divided doses. As the diarrhea and melena decrease, the dose is gradually reduced. The physician may keep the patient on a maintenance dose for 2 to 3 months or may discontinue it much earlier. If the patient is too ill to take the corticosteroid by mouth, an intravenous preparation (e.g., corticotropin) may be used during the initial acute stage.

The patient who is receiving any corticoid preparation, particularly over a long period, must be observed for possible undesirable effects. He may develop sodium and fluid retention and ensuing edema, hypokalemia, hypertension, a false sense of well-being, lowered resistance to infection, a moon face and hirsutism.

Azathioprine (Imuran) may be prescribed for patients who do not respond favorably to salicylazosulfapyridine (Azulfidine) and corticosteroids. The patient who is receiving it must be observed closely for signs of infection because of the drug's immunosuppressive effect.

Hematinics such as iron may be prescribed to aid in correcting the anemia, and vitamin supplements may be necessary, as cited earlier.

SURGICAL TREATMENT. A colectomy with a permanent ileostomy may be considered advisable in persisting colitis that fails to respond to medical treatment, or when there are frequent severe exacerbations which cause physical and psychological disability to the extent that the patient cannot lead a useful and independent life. Longstanding ulcerative colitis predisposes to malignant changes in the bowel. For pre- and post-operative care in intestinal surgery see page 548.

Complications, such as hemorrhage and perforation of the bowel, are usually indications for emergency surgery.

For nursing care of the patient who has a colectomy and ileostomy see page 553.

Anorectal complications are common in patients with ulcerative colitis. Infection passes through the wall of the rectum and causes perirectal or perianal abscesses and fistulas that open onto the perineal area, discharging blood and pus. These complications require surgical treatment; the abscesses are drained, the fistula is excised and the area is left open to heal by granulation from within out to the surface.

INSTRUCTIONS. The possibility of a recurrence of the ulcerative colitis is reduced if the patient understands and respects certain care and precautions. The patient is encouraged to return to his occupation and to live as normal and useful a life as possible. A balance between rest, work and recreation is advisable. Assistance is given the patient in solving home or socioeconomic problems, since a relapse can frequently be attributed to a psychosocial disturbance. A social worker may be asked to see the patient or family to help solve existing problems, or a referral may be made to a welfare department or service organization from which help may be obtained. The family should be advised as to their role in supporting the patient.

Emphasis is placed on the importance of a nourishing diet with the elimination of certain foods that are found to be irritating to the colon. Chilling, exhaustion and contact with persons having a cold or infection are to be avoided, since a relapse may follow.

RECTAL AND ANAL DISORDERS

Hemorrhoids

Hemorrhoids are basically varicose dilatations of the veins lying under the mucous membranous lining of the anal canal. Accompanying the dilatation of the venous plexuses is an enlargement of the supporting tissues. This tissue and the dilated vein form the mass referred to as a hemorrhoid (Fig. 16–13). They are a very common distressing condition and may be classified as internal or external. *Internal hemorrhoids* underlie the upper portion of the anal canal which is lined by mucous membrane similar to that of the intestine. *External hemorrhoids* occur in veins in the lower portion of the canal, which is lined by smooth skin. The external hemorrhoids cause more pain and pruritus because the skin in that area contains pain receptors.

ETIOLOGY. The cause of hemorrhoids is basically an increased back pressure of the blood in the rectal and anal veins, leading to dilatation. In many instances no cause of the increased pressure and dilatation is identified. They have a high incidence in persons with varicosities in the legs and seem to be influenced by heredity, for several members

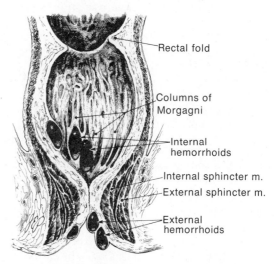

FIGURE 16–13 Internal and external hemorrhoids.

of the same family may be affected. Predisposing factors are chronic constipation, pregnancy, intra-abdominal tumors, portal hypertension and long periods of standing.

SYMPTOMS. Manifestations of hemorrhoids are bleeding with defecation, protrusion of a small mass through the anus, pain (especially with and following defecation), itching, and a feeling of a mass or pressure in the anal canal. Protrusion of hemorrhoids usually occurs with defecation and, for a period of time, the individual may be able to replace them manually within the canal. The hemorrhoid may become so large that it may be strangulated on prolapse through the anus and become thrombosed by constriction of the anal sphincter. Edema, inflammation and swelling ensue, and severe pain is experienced.

TREATMENT AND CARE. Anyone who has pain or bleeding in the anorectal area is urged to see a physician promptly, for these may be indications of a more ominous condition. Temporary relief in hemorrhoids may be obtained by the application of hot, moist compresses or the use of a sitz bath. An analgesic ointment such as dibucaine hydrochloride (Nupercaine) or suppositories containing an analgesic and astringent may be prescribed. Constipation should be avoided; mineral oil or dioctyl sodium sulfosuccinate (Colace) may be prescribed to keep the stool soft.

Hemorrhoids may be treated by surgical excision (hemorrhoidectomy), injection with a sclerosing agent or ligation. Injection treatment is not used if there is an infection, severe prolapse or thrombosis of the hemorrhoids. The sclerosing agent may be phenol 5 per cent in oil or a combined solution of quinine and urea. It is injected into the submucosal tissue, not into the vein, causing a fibrosing and shrinking of the supporting tissues. Ligation of a hemorrhoid is achieved by the application of a special surgical rubber band. The tissue distal to the band becomes necrotic and separates.

Preparation for surgery includes cleansing of the lower bowel by enemas and cleansing and shaving of the anal and perianal area. At the completion of the excision of the hemorrhoids, a small rubber tube or vaseline gauze packing may be inserted into the rectum to permit the escape of flatus and the drainage of blood should bleeding occur. Hemorrhage is the most common complication following hemorrhoidectomy; the dressing, vital signs and patient's reaction should be checked frequently during the first 12 hours. Considerable pain and discomfort are experienced and an analgesic is usually necessary to provide relief and ensure rest. The patient may find the prone and lateral positions more comfortable. When on his back, pressure on the operative area may be relieved by a sponge rubber cushion.

If a tube or packing has been used, it is usually removed the first or second postoperative day, and a sitz bath is ordered twice daily which generally provides considerable comfort. A rubber air ring should be provided for the patient during the bath and someone should remain with him in case of weakness and fainting. The patient is encouraged to be active and may be out of bed and walking the day after operation.

Urinary retention is a common problem, especially during the first 24 hours, and catheterization may be necessary.

A light diet is usually permitted as soon as the patient can tolerate it. In some instances, a low-residue diet is ordered until the patient's bowels move.

A mild, stool-softening laxative, such as mineral oil or dioctyl sodium sulfosuccinate (Colace), is usually given once or twice daily, starting on the second postoperative day. If there is no bowel action on the third day, an oil retention enema followed by a gentle cleansing water or saline enema may be ordered.

The patient may be permitted to leave the hospital once defecation is established and there is no abnormal rectal discharge. He is advised to continue the sitz baths, avoid constipation by taking plenty of fluids and including fresh fruits and roughage in his diet, and to resume a moderate amount of activity. The doctor may suggest that the laxative should be continued with a gradual decrease in the dosage until it can be omitted. The patient is given an appointment to see his surgeon or visit the clinic in 2 or 3 weeks for an examination. Occasionally anal stricture develops, and dilatation at regular intervals may be necessary.

Perianal Abscess

Infection and abscess formation may occur in the tissues around the rectum and anus. The most frequent site is the fatty tissue in the space between the rectum and the ischial tuberosity. The infection may originate in the anal glands, which normally drain into the canal. A gland may become blocked and infected and may rupture into the ischiorectal tissue, causing infection and abscess formation. It may also be caused by organisms escaping from the anal canal through a fissure into the surrounding tissue. A fissure is an ulcerated linear area in the lining of the anal canal.

The patient complains of pain in and around the rectum and anus and develops a fever, leukocytosis and local tenderness and swelling near the anus.

The affected area is incised and drained as soon as possible to prevent rupture into the intestine. The incision is packed with gauze impregnated with petrolatum jelly, and the area is allowed to heal and fill in by granulation — that is, from the inside out. The packing is changed daily and moist hot compresses or petrolatum jelly dressings are used over the area. Sitz baths may be ordered twice daily. Precautions are taken to prevent soiling of the dressing during voiding and defecation; a square of plastic material or oiled silk may be placed over the dressing. The female bed patient may lie in the prone positon while voiding into a basin. A low-residue diet is given for several days, and laxatives that produce liquid stools are avoided.

The wound may still be open when the patient leaves hospital; instruction is necessary as to the wound care, the taking of sitz baths, the need for thorough cleansing after voiding and defecation, and the importance of follow-up visits to the clinic or the surgeon.

Fistula in Ano

This is an abnormal tract extending from the lumen of the anal canal through the perianal tissue to the skin surface beside the anus. It is usually the result of a perianal or ischiorectal abscess and may be associated with ulcerative colitis or a tubercular infection. There is a persistent bloodstained purulent discharge.

Surgical treatment may consist of dissection of the tract or of simply opening it up widely for adequate drainage. Gauze packing is inserted, and the wound is left to heal by granulation. This usually requires several weeks, and the patient is taught to care for the wound so that he may convalesce at home.

Pilonidal Sinus

A pilonidal (hair-bearing) sinus is a small tract underneath the skin that develops in the cleft between the buttocks in the sacrococcygeal region. It may have several openings onto the surface and occurs most frequently in persons with a deep cleft and a generous growth of hair on the skin. The sinus is thought to be of congenital origin. The moist, soft skin of the area and the movement of the buttocks contribute to the penetration of the skin by short stiff hairs. The area is constantly irritated and readily becomes infected, forming a pilonidal abscess. The person may not know of the sinus until infection becomes manifested by local pain, redness, swelling and purulent drainage.

The condition is treated by incision and drainage. The sinus is laid open and cleansed of hair and pus. A soft rubber drain or gauze packing is inserted and the wound heals by granulation. Daily sitz baths may be prescribed to promote drainage and healing. If there is no infection, the sinus tract is excised and the wound is closed.

Precautions are necessary to avoid contamination of the dressings and wound when the patient voids or defecates. Bowel movements are delayed for the first few days, and straining at stool is avoided. A stool-softening laxative may be used and an oil retention enema given before the first bowel movement.

The patient may be confined to bed for several days and is required to lie in the prone or lateral position. When moving or when allowed up, strain on the incision is avoided and, when walking is permitted, short steps should be taken.

HERNIA

A hernia is a defect in the normal continuity of the wall of a cavity through which a structure contained in the cavity may protrude. It applies most frequently to a defect in the abdominal wall, the respiratory diaphragm or the pelvic floor. A pelvic hernia, or weakness of the muscle and fascia that support the pelvic structures, may result in prolapse of the pelvic organs—the bladder, rectum and uterus. Pelvic herniation frequently occurs in the female following delivery of a child. Prolapse of the bladder is referred to as a cystocele, prolapse of the rectum as rectocele and that of the uterus is known simply as uterine prolapse.

Herniation of the diaphragm is discussed in the section on hiatus hernia (see p. 522).

Abdominal Hernia

Unless qualified by diaphragmatic or pelvic, the term hernia refers to abdominal hernia. Various classifications and descriptive terms are used in relation to abdominal hernias (Fig. 16–14).

CONGENITAL OR ACQUIRED HERNIAS. A hernia may be congenital, which implies that the defect in the abdominal wall was present at birth. The acquired hernia develops later in life and is most often due to heavy lifting and excessive strain on the abdominal wall or to a weakening due to surgery.

INGUINAL, FEMORAL AND UMBILICAL HERNIAS. These terms denote the location of the hernia. The inguinal hernia may occur at the site at which either the left or right spermatic cord or the round ligament emerges from the abdominal cavity and enters the respective inguinal canal. Each

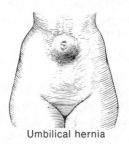

Umbilical hernia

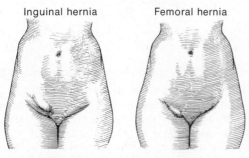

Inguinal hernia   Femoral hernia

FIGURE 16–14   Types of abdominal hernia.

canal proceeds obliquely through the abdominal muscles and terminates in the aponeurosis of the external oblique muscle. The spermatic cord passes from the canal and descends into the scrotum; the round ligament of the female emerges and inserts in the labium majus. The opening through which the cord or ligament enters the canal is referred to as the *internal* or *deep inguinal ring;* the point of exit is called the *external* or *superficial inguinal* ring. These inguinal rings are weak areas and may become the site of a hernia when intra-abdominal pressure is increased. During fetal development, when the cord or ligament enters the canal, it pushes ahead of it a portion of the peritoneum (processus vaginalis) that normally becomes obliterated. In some instances it may persist and predisposes to the protrusion of a segment of intestine or omentum into the canal.

An inguinal hernia may be classified as indirect or direct. The term indirect is applied when there is a herniation of a portion of the peritoneum and a segment of bowel through the internal ring and inguinal canal. The hernia contents may continue into the scrotum or labium. The indirect hernia is considered to be basically congenital.

A direct inguinal hernia is usually acquired and is a herniation of peritoneum and bowel through a weakened area in the abdominal wall in the inguinal region. It develops as a result of continuous or frequent increased intra-abdominal pressure.

A *femoral hernia* occurs in the area of the abdominal wall through which the femoral artery passes from the abdominal cavity into the thigh. The femoral ring of each side is located in the groin. A portion of bowel or omentum may escape through the femoral ring, producing a swelling and mass in the groin.

An *umbilical hernia* is due to a failure of the fascia in the area of the umbilicus to close completely or heal firmly. It is usually recognized with the increased intra-abdominal pressure associated with crying, straining and coughing.

REDUCIBLE OR IRREDUCIBLE (INCARCERATED) HERNIA. A reducible hernia is one in which the contents of the hernia can be manually replaced in the abdominal cavity. If the bowel or omentum cannot be returned to the cavity, it is referred to as an irreducible or incarcerated hernia. The irreducibility is determined by the size of the inguinal ring through which the viscera escaped and by the amount of intra-abdominal pressure.

STRANGULATED HERNIA. When a hernia is irreducible there may be compression at the internal ring of the blood vessels supplying the viscus within the hernia. Unless relieved promptly, the strangulated viscus becomes gangrenous.

INCISIONAL OR VENTRAL HERNIA. Protrusion of a segment of intestine or omentum through an old incision may occur if there is incomplete or poor healing of the abdominal muscle and fascia.

DOUBLE HERNIA. If herniation occurs in both inguinal canals or both femoral rings it is said to be double, or bilateral.

Causes and Incidence of Hernia

Most abdominal hernias other than incisional are thought to occur primarily as the result of a congenital weakness at the site. The hernia may be evident early in life, or it may not develop until later when the weakened area is subjected to increased intra-abdominal pressure or to an increased relaxation or weakening of the abdominal muscles and fascial tissues. The increased intra-abdominal pressure may be due to severe coughing, straining at stool, vomiting, heavy lifting, obesity, pregnancy or a tumor. Loss of muscular tone and weakening of the fascial tissues may develop as the result of sedentary habits, prolonged illness or malnutrition.

Incisional hernia occurs most frequently following wound infection and drainage and is more likely to develop in patients who were very debilitated or obese at the time of operation.

Inguinal hernia has a much higher incidence in males, and femoral hernia is more common in females. Umbilical hernia that becomes manifest after infancy is seen more often in females.

An abdominal hernia is usually recognized first as a swelling at the site involved when the patient is upright or when he coughs. The swelling disappears when the person lies down and the hernia contents return to the abdominal cavity. Pain may be present due to traction on the viscus or local irritation of

the peritoneum, and is relieved when the hernia is reduced. If the hernia cannot be reduced, impairment of the blood supply to the herniated bowel is likely to develop, causing strangulation, increasingly severe pain and symptoms of bowel obstruction. A strangulated hernia presents an acute surgical emergency.

Treatment and Nursing Care of Hernia

The desirable and most effective treatment of hernia is surgical repair (herniorrhaphy). The hernia contents are replaced into the peritoneal cavity, the hernial sac is removed, and the weakened defective area in the abdominal wall is repaired by firm suturing of the muscular and fascial tissues over or around the openings. Precautions are taken in the repair of an inguinal hernia to avoid trauma of the spermatic cord or round ligament.

More conservative treatment may be necessary in some instances in which surgery would be too great a risk or the patient simply refuses operation. The hernia is reduced, and the patient is fitted with a truss, which is a firm pad that is placed directly to the skin against the hernia opening and held in place by a belt. It is fitted and applied while the patient is in the dorsal recumbent position. The truss is worn only during the day unless there is frequent coughing or vomiting that increases intra-abdominal pressure. The skin under the truss and belt should be bathed daily and lightly powdered to prevent irritation.

The truss is applied only if the hernia is reduced; otherwise, serious damage could be done to the hernia contents. The physician advises the patient that he can probably reduce the hernia by lying flat with feet elevated and gently pushing the contents through the hernia orifice. If at any time he cannot readily reduce the hernia, prompt medical assistance should be sought. Overmanipulation in attempting reduction traumatizes the herniated viscera, causing swelling and edema that further predispose to strangulation.

The nurse has an important role in encouraging persons with a hernia to accept the physician's advice of surgical repair. The patient may find it difficult to submit to surgery when not experiencing any discomfort or disability. Left unrepaired, the hernia may become larger and restrict certain activities which could affect his employment. The repair becomes more difficult as the defect in the abdominal wall becomes larger, and there is an increasing risk of the hernia becoming irreducible and strangulated, which would necessitate emergency surgery.

Preparation for herniorrhaphy includes the usual considerations cited in the discussion of preoperative nursing care on page 164. Close observation should be made to detect any signs of respiratory infection, since the increased intra-abdominal pressure associated with coughing could weaken or break down the repair postoperatively. Local skin preparation includes the abdomen, the pubis and the upper part of the thigh on the affected side.

If the hernia is irreducible and strangulated, demanding surgical intervention as quickly as possible, the preparation is the same as that for any emergency surgery (see p. 171) and will most likely include gastric or intestinal intubation and suctioning to relieve the vomiting and distention. Intravenous fluids may be given during the brief preparation and continued during the operation, as the patient may have lost much fluid. If signs of shock are present, a blood transfusion may be given to increase the circulating volume.

Postoperatively, the patient usually makes a rapid, uneventful recovery if the hernia was uncomplicated by strangulation at the time of repair. The male patient who has an inguinal herniorrhaphy may require a scrotal support in the form of a suspensory or elastic athletic support to reduce tension on the spermatic cord and possible edema and swelling. The scrotum should be examined frequently during the first 2 or 3 postoperative days. Rarely, bleeding into the scrotum and the formation of a hematoma may occur, and swelling or discoloration should be reported. Application of ice bags to the scrotum may be suggested to relieve swelling and pain.

Urinary retention is a common postoperative problem and may necessitate catheterization. Excessive distention of the bladder is to be avoided because of pressure on the repair. In the case of a male, and if the patient's condition permits and the surgeon approves, he may be able to void more easily if he stands.

The patient who has had an inguinal or femoral herniorrhaphy is usually allowed out of bed the day after operation unless there is swelling of the scrotum, and is encouraged to move about. Before leaving the hospital, the patient is advised of the needed restriction in strenuous activities, such as lifting or pushing, and the importance of avoiding constipation and straining at stool. The physician discusses the patient's return to his occupation; the length of time needed before he returns to work is influenced by the type of work he does, his age and the size of the hernia that was repaired. If his job involves heavy lifting and straining that might predispose a recurrence of the hernia, the surgeon may recommend a change of job. This may be a problem for the patient, and the assistance of a social or rehabilitation worker may be necessary to place the patient in less strenuous work. There could be a period of unemployment that creates hardships for his family; it may be necessary to arrange for financial assistance or welfare service.

The *surgical* treatment of the *irreducible hernia* involves the release of the hernial contents and reestablishment of the blood supply to the bowel segment; the latter is encouraged by the application of warm moist towels. If the released bowel remains devoid of circulation and is gangrenous, it is resected and an end-to-end anastomosis is done. The hernia is repaired as quickly as possible. The nursing care involves the same considerations as for a regular herniorrhaphy as well as those necessary because of the bowel resection. For a discussion of care involved with a bowel resection, see page 548.

The repair of an *incisional hernia* involves the excision of the old scar, opening of the peritoneal sac, replacement of the protruding viscus into the abdominal cavity and firm closure of the peritoneum and fascia. Preparation of the patient for surgery may include the insertion of a nasogastric tube which is left in place for 1 to 2 days postoperatively to prevent vomiting and distention which would put a strain on the repaired area.

Treatment of an *umbilical hernia* in an infant will depend on the size of the fascial defect. The hernia may be treated by the continuous application of gentle pressure by means of elastic tape or a girdle-type of band made of crepe or elastic bandage. The mother should be instructed as to its purpose, and she is told to examine the area frequently to note any change. If the protruded area appears to be enlarging, the infant should be seen by the physician. The child's increasing activity, sitting up, standing and walking strengthen the abdominal wall and a small hernia may close without surgical intervention. If the defect is relatively large and protrusion of the intestine is readily apparent under the skin, the surgeon may consider early surgical repair necessary to prevent the possibility of rupture of the hernial sac (peritoneum) and ensuing peritonitis.

References

Books

Bockus, Henry L. (Ed.): Gastroenterology, 3rd ed. Volume II: The Small Intestine and Colon. Philadelphia, W. B. Saunders, 1976.

Davenport, Horace W.: Physiology of the Digestive Tract, 4th ed. Chicago, Year Book, 1977.

Ganong, William F.: Medical Physiology, 7th ed. Los Altos, Cal., Lange, 1975. Chapters 25 and 26.

Harper, Harold A.: Review of Physiological Chemistry, 15th ed. Los Altos, Cal., Lange, 1975. Chapter 12.

Krupp, Marcus A., and Chatton, Milton J.: Current Medical Diagnosis and Treatment. Los Altos, Cal., Lange, 1975, pp. 319–369.

MacBryde, Cyril M., and Blacklow, Robert S.: Signs and Symptoms, 5th ed. Philadelphia, J. B. Lippincott, 1970.

Macleod, John (Ed.): Davidson's Principles and Practice of Medicine, 11th ed. Edinburgh, Churchill Livingstone, 1974, pp. 428–528.

Sabiston, David C. (Ed.): Davis-Christopher Textbook of Surgery, 11th ed. Philadelphia, W. B. Saunders, 1976. Chapters 28–34.

Schottelius, Byron A., and Schottelius, Dorothy D.: Physiology, 17th ed. St. Louis, C. V. Mosby, 1973. Chapters 19, 20, 22.

Spiro, Howard M.: Clinical Gastroenterology, 2nd ed. New York, Macmillan, 1977.

Thorn, G. W., et al. (Ed.): Harrison's Principles of Internal Medicine, 8th ed. New York, McGraw-Hill, 1977.

Periodicals

Abrams, Jerome S., and Willard, Carolyn J.: "Aftercare of the Patient with an Ileostomy." Primary Care, Vol. 1, No. 4 (Dec. 1974), pp. 691–706.

Altshuler, Anne: "Esophageal Varices in Children." Am. J. Nurs., Vol. 72, No. 4 (April 1972), pp. 687–693.

Ball, Barbara (Ed.): "Caring Makes the Difference." Nurs. '75, Vol. 5, No. 11 (Nov. 1975), pp. 34–39.

Bass, Linda: "More Fiber—Less Constipation." Am. J. Nurs., Vol. 77, No. 2 (Feb. 1977), pp. 254–255.

Bean, Helen A.: "Cancer of the Mouth and Lip." Can. Fam. Physician, Vol. 22, No. 5 (May 1976), pp. 74–76.

Beardall, P. J.: "Laparoscopy." Can. Nurse, Vol. 69, No. 4 (April 1973), pp. 34–36.

Bericks, Virginia C.: "The Psychological Hurdle of New Ostomates: Helping Them Up . . . and Over." Nurs. '74, Vol. 4, No. 10 (Oct. 1974), pp. 52–55.

Borgen, Linda: "Total Parenteral Nutrition in Adults." Am. J. Nurs., Vol. 78, No. 2 (Feb. 1978), pp. 224–228.

Boucher, Margaret: "Broken Jaw Guide and Cookbook." Am. J. Nurs., Vol. 77, No. 5 (May 1977), pp. 831–833.

Braasch, John W., and Brooke-Conden, G. L.: "Disability after Gastric Surgery." Surg. Clin. North Am., Vol. 56, No. 3 (June 1976), pp. 607–613.

Brandborg, Lloyd L.: "Peptic Ulcer Disease." Primary Care, Vol. 2, No. 1 (March 1975), pp. 109–119.

Brunner, Lillian S.: "What to Do (and What to Teach Your Patient) about Peptic Ulcer." Nurs. '76, Vol. 6, No. 11 (Nov. 1976), pp. 27–34.

Buchan, D. J.: "Mind-Body Relationships in Gastrointestinal Disease." Can. Nurse, Vol. 67, No. 3 (March 1971), pp. 35–37.

————:"Diagnosis and Management of Inflammatory Bowel Disease." Can. Fam. Physician, Vol. 22, No. 8 (Aug. 1976), pp. 47–51.

Buckley, J. E., et al.: "Feeding Patients with Dysphagia." Nurs. Forum, Vol. XV, No. 1 (1976), pp. 69–85.

Cady, Blake, et al.: "Treatment of Gastric Cancer." Surg. Clin. North Am., Vol. 56, No. 3 (June 1976), pp. 599–605.

Colley, Rita, and Phillips, Karen: "Helping with Hyperalimentation." Nurs. '73, Vol. 3, No. 7 (July 1973), pp. 6–17.

Connors, Melba: "Ostomy Care: A Personal Approach." Am. J. Nurs., Vol. 74, No. 8 (Aug. 1974), pp. 1422–25.

Conway, Alice, and Williams, Tamara: "Parenteral Alimentation." Am. J. Nurs., Vol., 76, No. 4 (April 1976), pp. 574–577.

Cooperman, Avram (Ed.): "Symposium on Peptic Ulcer Disease." Surg. Clin. North Am., Vol. 56, No. 6 (Dec. 1976).

———, and Hoerr, Stanley O.: "Pyloroplasty." Surg. Clin. North Am., Vol. 55, No. 5 (Oct. 1975), pp. 1019–1024.

Copeland, Lucia: "Chronic Diarrhea in Infancy." Am. J. Nurs., Vol. 77, No. 3 (March 1977), pp. 461–463.

Cosper, Bonnie: "Physiological Colostomy." Am. J. Nurs., Vol. 75, No. 11 (Nov. 1975), pp. 2014–2016.

Curtis, Christine: "Colonoscopy. The Nurse's Role." Am. J. Nurs., Vol. 75, No. 3 (March 1975), pp. 430–432.

Deitel, Mervyn: "Intravenous Hyperalimentation." Can. Nurse, Vol. 69, No. 1 (Jan. 1973), pp. 38–43.

DeLuca, Joanne C.: "The Ulcerative Colitis Personality." Nurs. Clin. North Am., Vol. 5, No. 1 (March 1970), pp. 23–34.

Dudas, Susan (Ed.): "Symposium on Care of the Ostomy Patient." Nurs. Clin. North Am., Vol. 11, No. 3 (Sept. 1976).

Dudrick, S. J., et al.: "Parenteral Hyperalimentation, Metabolic Problems and Solutions." Ann. Surg., Vol. 176 (1972), pp. 259–64.

Gaffney, Terry Weiler, and Campbell, Rosemary Peterson: "Feeding Techniques for Dysphagic Patients." Am. J. Nurs., Vol. 74, No. 12 (Dec. 1974), pp. 2194–95.

Gallagher, Ann M.: "Body Image Changes in the Patient with a Colostomy." Nurs. Clin. North Am., Vol. 7, No. 4 (Dec. 1972), pp. 669–76.

Given, Barbara, and Simmons, Sandra: "Care of a Patient with a Gastric Ulcer." Am. J. Nurs., Vol. 70, No. 7 (July 1970), pp. 1472–75.

Habeeb, Marjorie C., and Kallstrom, Mina D.: "Bowel Program for Institutionalized Adults." Am. J. Nurs., Vol. 76, No. 4 (April 1976), pp. 606–608.

Herman, Robert E.: "Shunt Operations for Portal Hypertension." Surg. Clin. North Am., Vol. 55, No. 5 (Oct. 1975), pp. 1073–1087.

Hyman, Eleanor, et al.: "The Pouch Ileostomy: New Applications of Time-tested Techniques." Nurs. '77, Vol. 7, No. 9 (Sept. 1977), pp. 44–47.

Jackson, Bettie S.: "Ulcerative Colitis from an Etiological Perspective." Am. J. Nurs., Vol. 73, No. 2 (Feb. 1973), pp. 258–261.

Jensen, Vicki: "Better Techniques for Stoma Bagging. Part 2, Colostomies." Nurs. '74, Vol. 4, No. 8 (Aug. 1974), pp. 30–35.

Keaveny, Mary E. (Moderator): "Helping Patients Live with Colostomy." Nurs. '72, Vol. 2, No. 7 (July 1972), pp. 4–10.

Keusch, Gerald: "Bacterial Diarrheas." Am. J. Nurs., Vol. 73, No. 6 (June 1973), pp. 1028–32.

Lamanske, Jacqueline: "Helping the Ileostomy Patient to Help Himself." Nurs. '77, Vol. 7, No. 1 (Jan. 1977), pp. 34–39.

Levy, Arnold G., et al.: "Saline Lavage: A Rapid, Effective and Acceptable Method for Cleansing the Gastrointestinal Tract." Gastroenterology, Vol. 70, No. 2 (Feb. 1976), pp. 157–161.

Literte, Jean Willacker: "Nursing Care of Patients with Intestinal Obstruction." Am. J. Nurs., Vol. 77, No. 6 (June 1977), pp. 1003–06.

Magee, D. F. (Ed.): "Symposium on Gastrointestinal Physiology." Med. Clin. North Am., Vol. 58, No. 6 (Nov. 1974).

Mansell, Ellen, et al.: "Patient Assessment: Examination of the Abdomen." Am. J. Nurs., Vol. 74, No. 9 (Sept. 1974), pp. 1679–1702.

McConnell, Edwina A.: "How to Truly Help the Patient with a Radical Neck Dissection." Nurs. '76, Vol. 6, No. 11 (Nov. 1976), pp. 58–65.

———: "All About Gastrointestinal Intubation." Nurs. '75, Vol. 7, No. 1 (Jan. 1977), pp. 34–39.

Mowchenko, Gloria: "Care of Patients with G.I. Diseases That Have a Psychological Component." Can. Nurse, Vol. 67, No. 3 (March 1971), pp. 38–40.

Niebel, Harold H., and Keough, Gertrude: "Oral Cancer Detection." Am. J. Nurs., Vol. 73, No. 4 (April 1973), pp. 684–86.

Prout, Brian J.: "The Irritable Colon Syndrome—Very Common but Often Missed." Mod. Med., Vol. 45, No. 13 (July 15, 1977), pp. 36–40.

Reif, Laura: "Managing a Life with Chronic Disease." Am. J. Nurs., Vol. 73, No. 2 (Feb. 1973), pp. 261–264.

Schauder, Marilyn R.: "Ostomy Care. Cone Irrigations." Am. J. Nurs., Vol. 74, No. 8 (Aug. 1974), pp. 1424–1425.

Secor, Sophia M.: "Colostomy Rehabilitation." Am. J. Nurs., Vol. 70, No. 11 (Nov. 1970), pp. 2400–2401.

Sheridan, Jane Law: "Obstructions of the Intestinal Tract." Nurs. Clin. North Am., Vol. 10, No. 1 (March 1975), pp. 147–155.

Shrock, Theodore R., et al.: "Forum on Surgery for Duodenal Ulcer: How to Pick the Patient and the Procedure." Mod. Med., Vol. 45, No. 7 (April 1977), pp. 78–81.

Stahlgren, Leroy H., and Morris, Nicholas W.: "Intestinal Obstruction." Am. J. Nurs., Vol. 77, No. 6 (June 1977), pp. 999–1002.

Sweet, Karen: "Hiatal Hernia: What to Guard Against Most in Postop Patients." Nurs. '77, Vol. 7, No. 8 (Aug. 1977), pp. 36–43.

Watt, Rosemary C.: "Colostomy Irrigation—Yes or No?" Am. J Nurs., Vol. 77, No. 3 (March 1977), pp. 442–444.

Wentworth, Arlene, and Cox, Barbara: "Nursing the Patient with a Continent Ileostomy." Am. J. Nurs., Vol. 76, No. 9 (Sept. 1976), pp. 1424–1428.

Wiley, Loy (Ed.): "Hyperalimentation. Its Help and Risk." Nurs. '72, Vol. 2, No. 4 (April 1972), pp. 26–31.

_____: "The G.I. Bleeder." Nurs. '75, Vol. 5, No. 9 (Sept. 1975), pp. 48–54.

Williams, Lester F., Jr.: "An Acute Abdomen." Am. J. Nurs., Vol. 71, No. 2 (Feb. 1971), pp. 299–303.

17

Nursing in Disorders of the Liver and Biliary Tract

PHYSIOLOGY OF THE BILIARY SYSTEM

The biliary system consists of the liver, gallbladder and bile ducts.

LIVER

The liver is the largest organ of the body and is situated in the upper abdominal cavity immediately below the diaphragm. It is divided into four lobes and is highly vascular, receiving its blood supply from two sources. The portal vein carries blood from the stomach, intestines, spleen and pancreas into the liver. The hepatic[1] artery delivers blood from the aorta. The blood from both sources leaves the liver by a common pathway, the hepatic vein, which joins the inferior vena cava.

The liver tissue is organized in functional units called lobules. Each lobule consists of rows of cells radiating out from a central vein. Subdivisions of the hepatic artery and portal vein deliver blood into small spaces called sinusoids between the rows of cells, bringing the blood in direct contact with the hepatic cells. From the sinusoids it enters the central vein. Large phagocytic, reticuloendothelial cells called Kupffer cells lie scattered within the sinusoids to ingest

---

[1]From *hepar*, the Latin word meaning liver.

and destroy organisms and other foreign material within the blood. The central veins from the lobules empty into sublobular collecting veins, which unite to form the hepatic vein. Minute ducts into which bile is discharged are also formed between the rows of hepatic cells. The small lobular bile ducts are directed toward the surface of the lobules where they unite to form larger ducts. Eventually, the bile from the lobules is transmitted in one main channel, the hepatic duct, which joins the bile duct from the gallbladder (cystic duct) to form the common bile duct (Fig. 17–1).

Functions of the Liver

The liver performs a variety of very important complex functions. It is a vital organ, performing a major role in total body metabolism. The liver synthesizes, processes and/or stores many of the substances that are essential to normal body functioning. It also processes and excretes some substances that would be harmful if left in their original form or retained.

BILE PRODUCTION AND EXCRETION. The liver cells secrete 500 to 1000 ml. of bile daily into the hepatic ducts. It is a yellow-green or brownish fluid that is strongly alkaline and bitter to the taste. The constituents of bile are:

WATER (90 TO 97 PER CENT). The water content is reduced when the bile is stored

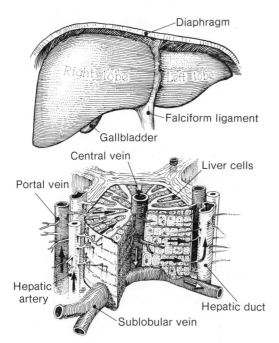

FIGURE 17–1 The liver and an enlarged section of a lobule.

in the gallbladder where it is concentrated six to ten times.

BILE PIGMENTS. The pigments resulting from the breakdown of red blood cells and from foods are excreted as the bile pigments *bilirubin* and *biliverdin*. Bilirubin is orange-red and is in greater concentration in man; biliverdin is green and predominates in those persons or species whose diet is mainly vegetable.

In the intestine, bile pigments are acted upon by bacteria and reduced to urobilinogen. Part of the urobilinogen is excreted in the feces, giving them the normal brown color. The remainder is absorbed into the blood. A small amount is excreted in the urine and the rest is returned to the liver where it is reconverted to bilirubin and again is secreted in the bile.

BILE SALTS. These are sodium and potassium salts of certain amino acids that function in digestion and absorption. The bile salts emulsify fats, increase the digestive action of the fat-splitting enzyme, and promote absorption of fats, fat-soluble vitamins and calcium salts. The bile salts are reclaimed from the intestine and returned to the liver by the portal circulation where they stimulate the hepatic cells to secrete bile. They are reused in the secretion.

OTHER CONSTITUENTS. Sodium and calcium salts, cholesterol, fatty acids and mucin are other substances in bile.

Bile is discharged by the common bile duct into the duodenum through the sphincter of Oddi. The functions of bile may be summarized as follows:

Bile promotes the digestion and absorption of fats in the small intestine. Because it is alkaline, it neutralizes the acidic chyme when it moves into the small intestine. It stimulates peristalsis of the large intestine, which is the basis of the use of bile salts in preparations of laxatives. The reabsorbed bile salts stimulate hepatic cells to secrete bile. Bile is an excretory medium for some drugs, toxins, excess minerals (e.g., copper and zinc), pigments and cholesterol.

METABOLIC FUNCTIONS. The liver has a role in the metabolism of *carbohydrates, proteins and fats*. Briefly, it converts glucose to glycogen and stores it (glycogenesis), reconverting it to glucose and releasing it into the blood when required in order to maintain an adequate blood sugar concentration. Glucose in excess of what can be converted to glycogen is converted to fat (lipogenesis) in the liver. The simple sugars, or monosaccharides, fructose and galactose cannot be utilized by the cells, so the liver changes the molecules to glucose.

Fats may be both synthesized and catabolized by the liver. Cholesterol, lecithin, phospholipids and lipoproteins are examples of substances that may be formed by the liver. Fats are desaturated or may be broken down into ketone acids or acetate.

Protein may be deaminized, a process in which the amine radical is removed and the remaining elements are used to form glycogen or other compounds to meet tissue needs. The amine radical is converted to urea and released into the blood for elimination by the kidneys. Amino acids are also used in the liver to form blood proteins, enzymes and structural compounds. Amino acids may be converted to carbohydrates to provide a source of energy.

STORAGE. The liver stores glycogen, vitamins A, D, E, K and B$_{12}$, iron, phospholipids, cholesterol, and a small amount of protein and fat.

FORMATION OF CERTAIN BLOOD COMPONENTS. In the fetus, the liver produces the erythrocytes. This activity gradually diminishes after midterm when erythropoiesis in the bone marrow increases. After birth, the liver stores vitamin B_{12} and releases it as necessary to promote the production of erythrocytes.

Heparin, and the blood proteins serum albumin, fibrinogen and alpha and beta globulins are formed by the hepatic cells. The liver also synthesizes most of the blood-clotting factors; it is the primary source of prothrombin, fibrinogen and Factors V, VII, VIII, IX, XI and XII.

DESTRUCTION OF ERYTHROCYTES. The Kupffer cells break down the worn-out erythrocytes. The hemoglobin is released, the iron and globin are split off, and bilirubin is formed from the waste products and is excreted in bile. The iron is reclaimed, combined with a protein to form ferritin and stored until it is needed for the formation of hemoglobin.

DETOXIFICATION OF HARMFUL SUBSTANCES. Certain drugs and chemicals that could be harmful to tissue cells are changed by the liver and rendered harmless before being circulated and excreted by the kidneys. The liver detoxifies by conjugation, oxidation or hydrolysis. In conjugation, it combines the toxic substance with some other material to produce an inoffensive compound (e.g., benzoic acid is changed to hippuric acid). Barbiturates, nicotine and strychnine are drugs that are oxidized and completely destroyed by the liver.

The body itself produces certain chemicals (hormones) that, unless destroyed, would reach too high a concentration. Examples of physiological products that are destroyed in the liver are the antidiuretic hormone (ADH), progesterone and adrenocorticoid secretions.

The Kupffer cells also protect the body by destroying organisms that may have been absorbed from the intestine.

HEAT PRODUCTION. The liver is second only to muscle tissue in the production of heat by its continuous cell activity. Under basal (resting) conditions, the liver is responsible for most of the body heat.

GALLBLADDER AND BILE DUCTS

The gallbladder is a sac on the undersurface of the liver with an average capacity of 40 to 50 ml. The cystic duct leading from the gallbladder merges with the hepatic duct to form the common bile duct. The latter unites with the pancreatic duct to form the ampulla of Vater, which opens into the duodenum. This opening is controlled by the sphincter of Oddi (Fig. 17–2).

Smooth muscle, connective tissue and a mucous membranous lining compose the walls of the gallbladder and ducts.

The functions of the gallbladder are to concentrate and store the bile. When the stomach and duodenum are empty of food, the sphincter of Oddi remains contracted. During this period, the bile that is continuously secreted accumulates in the gallbladder. Contraction of the sac to eject the bile is dependent upon hormonal stimulation. When food enters the duodenum, a hormone called cholecystokinin-pancreozymin (CCK-PZ or CCK) is secreted by cells of the duodenal mucosa. It is carried in the

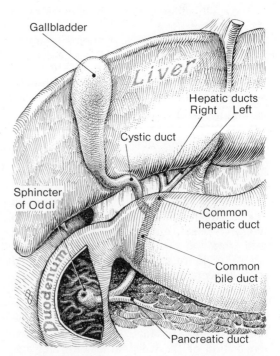

FIGURE 17–2. The gallbladder and extrahepatic biliary tract.

blood and, on reaching the gallbladder, stimulates the smooth muscle tissue to contract and eject bile. CCK also produces relaxation of the sphincter of Oddi, which allows the flow of bile into the duodenum.

LIVER DISORDERS

Liver function is essential to life and, fortunately, this large organ has exceptional functional ability and regenerative capacity. If liver disease is limited and tissue damage is localized to one area of the organ, the body is not likely to suffer serious impairment of function. If there is diffuse disease and parenchymal damage, dysfunction is more marked. Liver disease may be acute or chronic, and disturbed function may be reversible or irreversible, depending on the amount of tissue involved and the nature of the cause.

INDICATIONS AND ASSESSMENT OF LIVER DISORDERS

Manifestations of Impaired Liver Function

JAUNDICE (ICTERUS). This is an indication of an excess of bilirubin in the blood, resulting in a yellowish staining of the tissues that may be seen in the sclerae, mucous membranes and skin. The cause may be intrahepatic or extrahepatic disease, and according to the cause, the jaundice may be classified as hepatocellular, obstructive or hemolytic.

The *hepatocellular type of jaundice* is associated with intrinsic liver disease and is due to failure of the hepatic cells to take up the bilirubin resulting from the breakdown of red blood cells and excrete it as bile. Jaundice may not be present in chronic liver disease (e.g., cirrhosis), especially in the early stages, since regeneration of the hepatic cells may parallel the damage.

Obstructive jaundice is caused by an interference with the flow of bile in the extrahepatic ducts. It is most often due to the impaction of gallstones in the common bile duct, but may occur as the result of a stricture in the duct or neoplastic disease in neighboring structures (e.g., pancreas)

compressing the duct. *Hemolytic jaundice* occurs when there is an inordinate destruction of red blood cells, resulting in excessive bilirubin formation.

The jaundiced patient's urine is likely to be dark because of the bilirubin or urobilinogen content. Urobilinogen is not present in obstructive jaundice, since it is formed in the intestine. The stools are pale gray in obstructive and severe hepatocellular jaundice.

PRURITUS. The itching of the skin experienced by many patients with jaundice is attributed to irritation of the cutaneous sensory nerves by the retained bile salts.

GENERAL CONSTITUTIONAL SYMPTOMS. The patient complains of a poor appetite, vague digestive discomfort and flatulence, and loses weight. Lassitude, weakness and muscle wasting develop as a result of the impaired storage of carbohydrates and protein metabolism. A low-grade fever may be present.

PAIN. Dull, aching pain in the right upper abdominal quadrant is a common complaint, especially in acute liver disease. Tenderness is manifested on palpation.

BLEEDING TENDENCY. Inadequate production of prothrombin and other blood-clotting factors results in failure of the normal clotting process. Spontaneous bleeding may occur, manifested by purpura, epistaxis, bleeding of the oral mucous membrane, and/or melena.

ASCITES AND EDEMA. An accumulation of fluid in the peritoneal cavity develops with progressive liver disease, such as cirrhosis. The hepatic tissue damage, obliteration of blood vessels, and compression by the fibrous tissue (scar) replacement produce a resistance to the inflow and outflow of blood from the portal vein. The resulting increase in the blood pressure within the portal vein and its contributaries promotes the escape of fluid into the peritoneal cavity.

Some patients also develop a generalized edema because of the failure of the liver to produce sufficient serum albumin to maintain the normal colloidal osmotic pressure of the blood (see p. 75). Some blood protein is also lost in the transudate in ascites. Reduced liver activity results in increased concentrations of antidiuretic hormone and aldosterone (an adrenocorticoid secretion), further contributing to edema. These secretions, normally destroyed by the liver, promote reabsorption of water and sodium by the kidneys.

DILATED VEINS AND VARICOSITIES. The portal hypertension associated with liver disease is reflected in changes within the veins that drain into the portal vein. They become dilated and varicosities develop. The esophageal and gastric veins are commonly affected and, because they are close to the surface, one may rupture, resulting in massive hemorrhage manifested by hematemesis or melena or both. Hemorrhoids develop because of the pressure and resistance to blood flow within the rectal veins.

SPLENOMEGALY. The spleen enlarges because of the hyperplasia of the reticuloendothelial tissue and congestion, causing considerable discomfort for the patient.

SKIN CHANGES. In progressive chronic liver failure, several changes are likely to appear in the skin. Arterial spiders (spider angiomas or nevi) may develop in which a superficial arteriole gives rise to a series of fine, radiating branches readily visible on the surface. These lesions are seen predominantly on the face, neck, arms and chest, and are attributed to high estrogen levels in the blood. Gynecomastia and atrophy of the testicles may occur in males for the same reason. Normally, estrogen is destroyed in the liver.

The palms of the hands are frequently mottled, bright red and warm because of capillary dilatation (palmar erythema). There is a loss of axillary and pubic hair in both sexes, and facial hair grows more slowly than usual in the male.

NEUROLOGICAL DISTURBANCES. Severe hepatic insufficiency leads to various mental changes. The patient may manifest irritability and behavior not previously characteristic. He may become inactive, apathetic and forgetful. These symptoms may progress to confusion, lack of cooperation, stupor and eventually coma.

Twitching and a peculiar coarse tremor, referred to as flapping tremor, develop. Flapping tremor consists of a series of rapid, irregular alternating flexion and extension movements at the wrist and finger joints. The tremor may be referred to as *asterixis*. It occurs when the arms and hands are extended.

Ammonia toxicity is considered to be an important factor in producing the mental changes, coma and other abnormal central nervous system responses. The liver is unable to convert the ammonia that results from a breakdown of amino acids to urea.

FETOR HEPATICUS. In advanced liver disease, the breath has a fecal odor and the patient complains of a bad taste in the mouth. It is attributed to disturbed amino acid metabolism and abnormal bacterial action in the intestine.

Diagnostic and Liver Function Tests

PLASMA PROTEIN ELECTROPHORESIS (SERUM ALBUMIN AND GLOBULIN CONCENTRATIONS). Serum albumin is produced by the liver and, normally, is of greater concentration than globulin, most of which is produced by the lymphoid tissues. In disease of the liver cells, the amount of albumin decreases, and the ratio of albumin to globulin is reversed.

Normal: Total serum proteins, 6.5 to 7.9 Gm. per 100 ml. Albumin, 4.7 to 5.7 Gm. per 100 ml. Globulin, 1.5 to 2.5 Gm. per 100 ml. A/G ratio, 3:1.

SERUM BILIRUBIN (VAN DEN BERGH'S TEST). This test gives an estimation of the concentration of bilirubin in the blood and indicates whether it is conjugated or unconjugated. Normally, the liver cells extract the pigment from the blood and convert it to a water-soluble compound (bilirubin diglucuronide) before excreting it in bile. Unconjugated bilirubin is usually reported as "indirect bilirubin" and the conjugated form as "direct bilirubin." In obstructive jaundice, the conjugate (direct) bilirubin level is increased. In hemolytic jaundice, unconjugated (indirect) bilirubin is the predominant pigment in the blood.

Normal: Conjugated (direct) bilirubin, 0.2 mg. or less per cent. Unconjugated (indirect) bilirubin, 0.2 to 0.7 mg. per cent. Total serum bilirubin, 0.4 to 1.1 mg. per cent.

ICTERUS INDEX. This test is a rough estimate of the concentration of bilirubin in the blood. The intensity of the yellowness of the serum is observed. It may be used to determine the decrease or increase of jaundice.

Normal: 4 to 6 units.

SERUM ALKALINE PHOSPHATASE. Normally this enzyme is excreted in the bile by the hepatic cells. The blood concentration may be increased when there is liver disease or obstruction in the bile ducts.

Normal: 2.0 to 4.5 Bodansky units; 5.0 to 13.0 King-Armstrong units.

SERUM TRANSAMINASES. The liver cells contain the enzymes serum glutamic-oxaloacetic transaminase (SGOT) and serum glutamic-pyruvic transaminase (SGPT). Since they are released into the blood when the cells are damaged, their concentration may be used to estimate liver damage.

Normal: SGOT, 5 to 40 units; SGPT, 5 to 35 units.

PROTHROMBIN TIME. The liver is responsible for the synthesis of several clotting factors. The prothrombin time or activity reflects the effects of liver dysfunction on blood coagulation.

Normal: 13 to 17 seconds, or 75 to 100 per cent activity.

GALACTOSE TOLERANCE TEST. Normally, most of the galactose is quickly taken from the blood and converted to glycogen by the liver cells. An abnormal concentration in the blood 1 to 2 hours following the administration of 100 ml. of a 25 per cent solution of galactose flavored with lemon juice indicates impaired function of the liver. This may be used to assist in differentiating between hepatocellular jaundice and obstructive jaundice. The galactose is given after an 8- to 10-hour fast, and a blood sample is collected 1, 1½ and 2 hours following the administration.

BROMSULPHALEIN (BSP) TEST. Bromsulphalein is a dye normally excreted by the liver cells in the bile. The test is used to detect liver cell damage and impaired function. It is not used if obstruction in the bile ducts is suspected, because the dye would be retained in the body. Five mg. of bromsulphalein for each kilogram of the patient's body weight is given intravenously, and a venous blood specimen is collected from another vein in 45 minutes. Normally, only 5 per cent or less of the dye given remains in the blood.

HIPPURIC ACID TEST. Benzoic acid is detoxified by the liver cells by its combination with glycine to form hippuric acid, which is then circulated in the blood and eliminated in the urine. To test hepatic function, sodium benzoate is given either by mouth or by intravenous injection. Urine is then collected and examined for the hippuric acid concentration.

The procedure is as follows: 6 Gm. of sodium benzoate is dissolved in 250 ml. of water and given orally. The urine is collected over the next 1 to 4 hours. An alternative method is by giving 1.77 Gm. of sodium benzoate slowly by intravenous, and collecting a urine specimen in 1 hour.

Normally, with the oral administration of the sodium benzoate, 2 to 3.5 Gm. of hippuric acid will be excreted in the urine in 4 hours. Following the intravenous administration, 0.7 Gm. of hippuric acid should appear in the urine in 1 hour.

SERUM CHOLESTEROL. The concentration of cholesterol in the blood falls in liver disease when cell function is impaired and rises in obstructive jaundice.

Normal: 150 to 250 mg. per cent.

URINARY BILIRUBIN. A urinalysis may be requested for bilirubin. Normally, this bile pigment is not present in urine. It is present in the urine in obstructive jaundice and hepatocellular jaundice but is absent in hemolytic jaundice.

URINARY UROBILINOGEN. Conjugated bilirubin is changed to urobilinogen by bacterial action when the bile reaches the small intestine. Most of the urobilinogen is then excreted in the feces, and the remainder is absorbed. A small amount of the absorbed urobilinogen is excreted in the urine, but the larger portion is claimed by the liver to be excreted in the bile. If the liver cells are damaged they may not perform this latter function, and the amount of urobilinogen excreted by the kidneys is increased. The amount of the pigment in the urine may be decreased below the normal amount in obstructive jaundice when bile is not reaching the intestine or if the bacterial content of the intestine is reduced, as it is in oral administration of antibiotics.

Normal: Less than 4 mg. in the urine per 24 hours, or less than 1.0 Ehrlich units in 2 hours.

BLOOD AMMONIA. In severe impairment of liver function, the ammonia concentration in the blood is elevated and may lead to hepatic coma.

Normal: 30 to 70 μg. (mcg.) per cent.

PERCUTANEOUS LIVER BIOPSY. A small specimen of liver tissue may be examined microscopically to assist in the diagnosis of liver disease. The specimen is obtained by aspiration with a special liver biopsy needle. Using a lateral approach, the needle is passed through the right eighth, ninth or tenth intercostal space, or may be introduced below the costal margin if the liver is enlarged.

Previous to the procedure, the patient's bleeding, coagulation and prothrombin times are checked. The biopsy is not done if there is a prolongation of these. An explanation is made to the patient of the purpose of the biopsy and what will be expected of him during and after the procedure. He is required to sign a consent. His pulse, respirations and blood pressure are noted by the nurse for comparison following the biopsy.

The patient is placed in the supine position close to the right side of the bed. The area is cleansed, and an antiseptic and sterile drape are applied. A local anesthetic is then injected at the puncture site. The patient is instructed to take two or three deep breaths, and then to stop breathing following exhalation. The physician quickly introduces the biopsy needle, aspirates and withdraws, taking only a few seconds.

Following the biopsy, absolute bed rest is necessary for 24 hours. The patient is required to lie on his right side with a small pillow under the costal margin. This position places pressure against the biopsy site, preventing the escape of blood and bile. Close observation is made of the patient for hemorrhage for 24 hours. The pulse, respirations, blood pressure, color and general condition are noted and recorded every 30 minutes for 2 to 3 hours. The interval is then gradually increased if there are no significant changes. Abdominal pain, tenderness and any rigidity are reported, since they may indicate irritation and inflammation of the peritoneum due to the leakage of bile from the liver.

RADIOISOTOPE LIVER SCAN. A radioactive isotope known to be taken up normally by the liver may be given intravenously, and an estimation is then made of its uptake by means of a special external radioactivity detector. Rose bengal tagged with radioactive iodine (I^{131}), gold (Au^{198}) or vitamin B_{12} tagged with radioactive cobalt (Co^{60}) may be used. The photoscan made by the detector indicates nonfunctioning and functioning areas of the liver tissue. Areas or lesions which do not take up the radioactive material appear as blanks or as much lighter areas in the recording of the scan.

FLOCCULATION AND TURBIDITY TESTS. The *cephalin-cholesterol flocculation* and *thymol turbidity tests* may be done to determine any quantitative changes in serum proteins. In the cephalin-cholesterol test, a specimen of the patient's serum is added to a cephalin-cholesterol suspension. Flocculation occurs if there is a decrease in the albumin or globulin fractions of the proteins.

In the thymol turbidity test, serum is added to a solution of thymol. Turbidity occurs if there is an increase in the globulin or a decrease in the albumin fraction.

These tests are used only occasionally; other evaluation procedures are considered more reliable and definitive.

OTHER STUDIES. A *barium swallow* under fluoroscopic examination (see p. 495) or an *esophagoscopy* (see p. 496) may be done. The latter is used to detect venous dilation and varicosities in the esophagus resulting from portal hypertension. A *splenoportogram* may be undertaken in which an opaque dye is injected into the spleen and an x-ray taken of the upper abdomen and lower chest. The dilated portal vein and its branches show up, and gastroesophageal varices may be recognized.

LIVER DISORDERS

Viral Hepatitis

The commonest inflammatory disease of the liver is due to viruses. Two types of these are currently recognized: one is referred to as the IH or A virus; the other is known as the SH or B virus. Hepatitis due to the former organism is classified as infectious (or epidemic) hepatitis; that caused by the SH virus is known as homologous serum hepatitis. The principal differences are in their mode of infection, incubation period and severity.

HEPATITIS A (INFECTIOUS HEPATI-

TIS). This type of hepatitis accounts for the greater number of cases of hepatitis. The disease can be epidemic and has a higher incidence in children and young adults. It has an incubation period of 10 to 50 days and is included in the *reportable* diseases. The virus A is present in the blood and feces and may be transmitted by contaminated food or water, parenteral injections of infected plasma or blood, or parenteral injections with contaminated syringes or needles. It may spread rapidly among children, especially in overcrowded and poor sanitary conditions.

MANIFESTATIONS. The virus attacks the hepatic cells, and inflammation and necrosis follow. The swelling and congestion interfere with normal bile formation and flow, resulting in intrahepatic obstructive jaundice and elevated blood bilirubin levels. Transaminase levels (SGOT and SGPT) rise sharply because of the necrosis, and the protein electrophoresis and serum albumin-globulin ratio may indicate a reduced formation of albumin and an increase in the gamma globulin. The latter points to the acute infectious nature of the disorder. Urinalysis reveals an excess of urobilinogen, especially in the initial stage. The blood is examined for the presence of a hepatitis antigen that has been identified and called hepatitis B antigen (HBAg, or the Australia antigen). It is characteristic of hepatitis B and is not found in the blood of the patient with hepatitis A unless he has had a previous attack of hepatitis B. Fortunately, in most cases complete regeneration of the liver cells occurs on recovery with a minimum of fibrous tissue formation and scarring. Very few patients experience residual impairment of liver function.

The signs and symptoms may vary in intensity from one individual to another. The onset is usually manifested by vague symptoms such as fatigue, loss of appetite, nausea, vomiting, headache, fleeting abdominal and joint pains, and fever. After several days, abdominal tenderness and pain in the right upper quadrant are more predominant, the urine becomes dark, either constipation or diarrhea may be troublesome, the stools may be abnormally light in color and jaundice becomes evident.

DIAGNOSTIC PROCEDURES. Urine specimens are submitted for assessment of uro-bilinogen content. In viral hepatitis there is an excess of this substance in the initial stage of the disease. If the inflammatory process is widespread, intrahepatic biliary obstruction may result in the appearance of bilirubin in the urine and the disappearance of the urobilinogen.

The serum bilirubin level is elevated, serum flocculation tests are positive and the serum enzymes SGPT and SGOT are elevated. A blood specimen is examined for the hepatitis B antigen (HBAg, Australia antigen) to rule out serum hepatitis.

HEPATITIS B (SERUM HEPATITIS). Hepatitis B is caused by the virus B, and has an insidious onset. The principal mode of transmission is by the injection of infected blood and blood products. Syringes, needles and tubing used in parenteral administrations or for the withdrawal of blood or body fluids may provide the means of transmission if reused and not disinfected adequately. Because of this, hepatitis B is a common problem among drug addicts. The disease may also be spread by the fecal-oral route. The incubation period ranges from 6 weeks to 6 months. It is more common in adults than children; hepatitis A tends to have a high frequency in children and young adults.

SIGNS AND SYMPTOMS. The clinical features are similar to those of hepatitis A (see above). The onset is less abrupt, and hepatitis B is usually more prolonged and debilitating. Following recovery, the individual may be a carrier of the virus in his blood and obviously should not be a blood donor. In hepatitis B, blood examination reveals the presence of the hepatitis B antigen, the factor that differentiates hepatitis B from hepatitis A.

TREATMENT AND NURSING CARE IN VIRAL HEPATITIS. Since there is no specific treatment for viral hepatitis, supportive therapy and attention to the patient's discomforts constitute the principal care.

REST. The patient is kept on bed rest during the active stage of the disease. With subsidence of fever, there is a decrease in the tenderness of the liver and a lowering of the serum bilirubin and transaminase levels. Activity is resumed slowly, and the patient is observed for reactions. Some persons regain their strength slowly and should not be encouraged to resume full activity until they feel equal to it.

MEDICATIONS. Many drugs (such as barbiturates, acetaminophen, oral contraceptives and morphine) which are normally inactivated by the liver are not prescribed. The patient is advised that he should not take any drug that has not been prescribed by the physician during this illness.

NUTRITION AND FLUIDS. In the acute stage, it is difficult for the patient to take sufficient fluids and food because of the nausea, vomiting and aversion to food. An increased fluid intake of at least 3000 ml. is necessary because of the fever and to promote urinary elimination of the serum bilirubin. If the patient cannot tolerate fluids orally, glucose 5 or 10 per cent may be given intravenously to sustain the patient.

A high-calorie diet of 3000 calories is recommended; nutritional deficiency retards the liver's ability to overcome the infection and regenerate functional tissue. As soon as the nausea and vomiting are controlled, the patient is offered small amounts of high-calorie foods frequently. These are gradually increased until the ultimate goal of 3000 calories is achieved. The diet consists principally of protein and carbohydrate. The fat content may be restricted while there is jaundice but is increased, as tolerated, by the addition of whole milk, eggs and butter, which make the diet more palatable. Fried foods, fat meat and rich foods, such as pastries, usually are avoided for several weeks or months after recovery. The patient is advised not to take alcohol for at least 6 months.

The patient's weight is checked at regular intervals, since there may have been a considerable loss in the early phase of the disease.

SKIN CARE. Frequent bathing and changes of linen during the period of fever are necessary. The use of soap is avoided if the patient is jaundiced, and the bath water should be warm but not hot. The heat and the alkali in the soap tend to increase the pruritus frequently associated with jaundice. Starch or sodium bicarbonate added to the bath water or oatmeal tied in a bag and squeezed through the water may provide some relief from the itching. Calamine lotion applied following the bath may also be used. The fingernails are kept short and clean to prevent injury and infection of the skin in case of scratching

PREVENTION OF THE SPREAD OF INFEC-TION. All patients with viral hepatitis are treated as potentially infectious and are isolated. Personnel caring for the patient are informed of the possible sources of the infective organisms (feces, vomitus, urine and blood) and of the fact that they are usually resistant to heat, antiseptics, and prolonged exposure to cold and freezing.

The patient occupies a single room, and a gown is worn by those giving contact care. The hands are scrubbed under running water with liquid soap after each contact. The bed linen is placed in a clean bag at the bedside, labeled "Isolation" and is disinfected before being laundered. Disposable dishes, glasses and treatment equipment are used as much as possible. If disposable supplies are unavailable, dishes and other contaminated articles are kept separate for the patient's individual use and disinfected. The use of disposable equipment for procedures involving penetration of the skin (e.g., needles and syringes) is recommended, and gloves should be worn by those handling them. Before discarding used syringes and needles, the tips are broken off and the articles securely wrapped and placed in an "isolation" disposal container. If nondisposable syringes and needles must be used, they are disinfected after use by high dry heat or by autoclave. If such facilities are not available, the equipment is boiled for at least 30 minutes. Blood specimens should be clearly labeled "Hepatitis" to protect laboratory personnel.

If it is necessary to take the temperature by rectum, the nurse wears gloves while handling the thermometer, which is kept immersed in a strong disinfectant and thoroughly rinsed before use. Some institutions recommend discarding the thermometer when the patient is discharged since it cannot be sterilized by heat.

The patient is advised of the importance of thorough hand washing after going to the toilet. Gloves are worn when handling the patient's bedpan; excreta should be flushed promptly down the toilet, or the policy in the particular situation may require that stools be disinfected before the usual disposal. The feces may be covered with a disinfectant such as cresol (Lysol) 5 per cent or formalin 10 per cent for at least 1 hour before disposal.

The period of isolation is determined by

the physician according to the patient's progress. At the most, it is of 3 weeks' duration.

CONTACTS. Known contacts of infectious hepatitis A are advised to consult a physician as soon as possible. An intramuscular injection of human serum gamma globulin may be given to provide protection. It is effective against the virus A but not against the virus B organism. The gamma globulin may not always provide immunity, but is found to lessen the severity of the disease should the person develop it.

FOLLOW-UP. The patient is encouraged to continue medical supervision; laboratory and physical examinations are done to detect possible progressive or residual impairment of liver function. Supervision is usually continued for 1 year. The intervals between visits to clinic or physician are gradually increased if the findings are favorable. The patient who has had hepatitis B is advised that he should not serve as a blood donor.

Toxic Hepatitis

Rarely, inflammation and degenerative changes in the liver occur as a result of a chemical. Carbon tetrachloride, phosphorus, sulfonamides, arsenical preparations and chloroform are examples of suggested offenders. The patient is treated by prompt withdrawal of the causative chemical, rest and supportive care.

Cirrhosis of the Liver

The term cirrhosis denotes chronic degenerative tissue changes occurring in the liver. There is destruction of parenchymal cells and formation of excessive dense fibrous scar tissue. Blood, lymph and bile channels within the liver become distorted, compressed and effaced, with subsequent intrahepatic congestion, portal hypertension and impaired liver function. (For functions, see p. 578.) The fibrous tissue changes result in the liver becoming smaller and firmer. The surface is usually rough because of small projecting nodules of regenerated hepatic cells, and is frequently described as a "hobnail surface."

ETIOLOGIC FACTORS

DIETARY DEFICIENCY. Many cases of cirrhosis of the liver are thought to be the result of malnutrition and a deficiency of protein. An accumulation of fat in the liver has been produced experimentally in animals by the restriction of protein. This dietary constituent is necessary for the provision of substances essential for normal fat metabolism in the liver, one of which is choline. Methionine, an amino acid, is necessary for the synthesis of choline by the body.

ALCOHOLISM. Cirrhosis of the liver is a common sequel to chronic alcoholism. It is suggested that the degenerative liver changes develop as a result of interference with normal nutrition over a relatively long period. Persons who become dependent on alcohol are often indifferent to food and consume less. The calories provided by the alcoholic beverages[2] suppress the appetite for food, resulting in a lack of essential food factors. Many persons show a marked improvement in the earlier stages of cirrhosis when alcohol ingestion is discontinued and a high-protein, high-vitamin diet is taken. Such evidence supports the theory that the liver changes in the alcoholic are secondary to the associated malnutrition.

It is also thought that liver damage in the alcoholic may be related to an increased choline requirement incurred by the alcohol.

HEPATITIS. Severe hepatitis in which there has been extensive necrosis followed by considerable scarring may lead to cirrhosis.

CHRONIC CHOLESTASIS. Degenerative changes characteristic of cirrhosis may also occur with prolonged cholestasis (obstruction to the flow of bile). The cause is usually partial obstruction by a stone or stricture within the extrahepatic bile ducts, but may be intrahepatic as a result of infection or inflammation and subsequent stricture of the small ducts within the liver.

HEPATIC INFILTRATION. Fibrotic changes in the liver may be associated with the infiltration of certain substances. Examples

---

[2]One ounce of alcohol provides approximately 75 to 90 calories.

include excessive glycogen which accumulates in the liver in the individual with von Gierke's disease,[3] enlargement and fibrosis develop. Similarly, Gaucher's disease[4] results from an abnormal reticuloendothelial cell content that incurs liver fibrosis and dysfunction.

CLASSIFICATION. Certain terms may be used to classify cirrhosis according to the cause and changes that occur. Cirrhosis due to nutritional deficiency and alcoholism may be referred to as *Laennec's, portal* or *atrophic cirrhosis*. When cirrhotic changes are a result of massive hepatic necrosis and subsequent fibrous scarring, the condition is known as *postnecrotic cirrhosis*. The term *biliary cirrhosis* is used to denote cirrhosis associated with cholestasis.

SIGNS AND SYMPTOMS. The liver has considerable reserves; early cirrhotic changes generally go unrecognized without apparent manifestations. With the characteristic insidious progress, signs and symptoms of impaired liver function appear gradually over a period of years. In the early stages the symptoms are vague digestive disturbances; the patient experiences anorexia, flatulence, nausea and loss of weight. Later, jaundice, dependent edema, spider angiomas, anemia and increased abdominal girth develop. Splenomegaly, neurological involvement (hepatic coma) and hemorrhage from esophageal varices are characteristic of advanced cirrhosis and serious liver dysfunction.

The severity of liver dysfunction is determined by various liver function tests (see p. 582) as well as by history, symptoms and physical examination. Palpation of the liver and spleen provides significant information. The liver is enlarged and firm and may have a rough surface; the spleen is enlarged owing to the resistance by the liver to the flow of blood from the portal vein.

---

[3]*Von Gierke's disease* is a congenital disorder characterized by excessive storage of glycogen in the liver which results in hypoglycemia. The disorder is due to an enzyme deficiency.

[4]*Gaucher's disease* is an inherited disorder characterized by a deficiency of an enzyme that results in abnormal metabolism of glucocerebroside. Normally, this compound is broken down by the enzyme to useable glucose. When it is not, it accumulates in reticuloendothelial cells.

TREATMENT AND NURSING CARE. The care required by the patient with cirrhosis depends upon the extent of the liver damage.

NUTRITION. Since the progress of the disease is influenced by nutrition, a diet of 2500 to 3000 calories, high in protein (110 to 150 Gm.), carbohydrates and vitamins is recommended. Sufficient fat to make the diet palatable is added if the patient can tolerate it and is not jaundiced. Three small meals with in-between snacks will probably be more acceptable than three large meals. Sodium intake is restricted because of the tendency to develop edema and ascites. Low-sodium protein concentrate and low-sodium milk are available and may be used to assist with the protein intake. Total abstinence from alcohol is very important.

If the liver insufficiency is serious, and the patient is exhibiting neurological disturbances (e.g., depressed awareness, dulled mentation, confusion, asterixis and hyperreflexia) and an elevation in blood ammonia, protein is eliminated from the diet. The patient is sustained on carbohydrates. The disturbance of the nervous system is attributed to failure of the liver to metabolize the nitrogenous wastes; the ammonia level rises because it is not deaminized to form urea. If coma develops, intravenous infusions are used to support the patient.

MEDICATIONS. Multivitamin preparations are prescribed. Parenteral vitamin K may be given if the prothrombin level is below normal and if a tendency to bleeding is manifested by petechiae, ecchymosis, epistaxis, melena or hematemesis. Vitamin B_{12} injections may be necessary to correct anemia.

Although the patient with cirrhosis usually develops edema and ascites due to portal hypertension and decreased plasma oncotic pressure because of reduced liver production of blood proteins, the physician is usually reluctant to prescribe a diuretic because of the possible electrolyte imbalance and excessive reduction of intravascular volume. If a diuretic is given, the patient is observed closely for indications of hypokalemia and shock. Serum levels of potassium, sodium, chloride and ammonia are determined frequently.

Potentially toxic drugs normally inactivated by the liver are avoided. Examples of these are barbiturates, amobarbital, diazepam, acetaminophen, oral contraceptives and opiates.

REST AND ACTIVITY.   If there is no ascites or signs of impending hepatic coma, the patient remains ambulatory, and a limited amount of activity that does not produce excessive fatigue is encouraged to promote appetite as well as circulation.

In more advanced liver impairment, bed rest is recommended. The patient's lassitude necessitates thoughtful nursing measures such as frequent change of position, special skin care and passive exercises to combat the effects of prolonged inactivity.

OBSERVATIONS.   The patient is weighed at the same time each day with the same amount of clothing and is observed for signs of edema. The exact amount of nutrition taken daily is noted; resourcefulness on the part of the nurse is needed frequently to have the patient take nourishment. Physical weakness and lethargy may necessitate feeding the patient.

The daily fluid intake and output are measured and recorded. The abdomen is examined daily for evidence of developing ascites, and the girth is measured and recorded.

The nurse notes the patient's responses, orientation and level of awareness. Any indication of nervous system dysfunction is brought to the physician's attention. Side rails are placed on the bed to protect the very lethargic, confused or comatose patient.

PREVENTION OF INFECTION.   Resistance to infection is lowered in the patient with cirrhosis of the liver. Precautions are taken to prevent possible exposure to any source of infection.

ABDOMINAL PARACENTESIS.   An abdominal paracentesis may be necessary if the fluid in the peritoneal cavity reaches a volume that is causing respiratory distress, compression of abdominal viscera and blood vessels, and considerable pain and discomfort. The nurse explains the aspiration procedure to the patient, and makes sure his bladder is empty. The head of the bed is elevated and the patient is supported with pillows. The physician may wish to have the patient sitting on the side of the bed with a support to his back and feet. A sphygmomanometer is placed in readiness on one arm so that the blood pressure may be checked during and after the paracentesis.

The necessary sterile equipment and fluid receptacle are brought to the bedside. Following the application of an antiseptic and sterile drapes, the physician injects the site with a local anesthetic before introducing the trocar and cannula. A tube is attached to the cannula to drain the fluid into the receptacle.

During the procedure, the nurse checks the patient's pulse, color and blood pressure and provides necessary support. The physician is promptly alerted if the pulse becomes rapid and weak, pallor is noted, or there is a fall in blood pressure. Not more than 1 or 2 liters is withdrawn at one time. Removal of the fluid results in the loss of considerable plasma protein, especially serum albumin. Also, the sudden reduction of intra-abdominal pressure results in a dilatation of the abdominal blood vessels and a pooling of a large volume of blood that may lead to circulatory collapse and shock.

A sterile dressing is applied to the site of the paracentesis when the cannula is withdrawn, and an abdominal binder is applied snugly. The patient is returned to the dorsal recumbent position, and the head of the bed is lowered. The amount and character of the fluid are recorded. The abdominal site is kept clean and dry to prevent infection and discomfort. The pulse, color and blood pressure are checked at frequent intervals for several hours. A plasma or whole blood infusion may follow the paracentesis to replace the lost protein. Increased diuresis may be observed with the decreased pressure on the renal blood vessels.

INSTRUCTION.   The patient who improves sufficiently to go home is advised as to what extent he must restrict his usual activity. Strict adherence to his diet, total abstinence from alcohol, and the avoidance of infection and physical strain are stressed when interpreting the regimen prescribed by the physician to the patient and family. He will be required to visit his doctor or a clinic at regular intervals. A referral to a visiting nursing agency may be necessary so that consistent supervision is insured. The agency is advised of the recommended regimen and of the changes that may indicate regression, necessitating prompt medical care.

The prognosis for patients with cirrhosis depends on the degree of liver insufficiency. If treatment is instituted in the early stages and the patient is sufficiently motivated to adhere to the suggested care, he is likely to live a normal life span. If portal hypertension has developed with resultant ascites and esophageal varices, the prognosis is grave.

COMPLICATIONS OF CIRRHOSIS AND THEIR MANAGEMENT. Hepatic encephalopathy and coma, and esophagogastric varices are common complications.

HEPATIC COMA. Before the patient with cirrhosis of the liver develops coma, neurological disturbances are manifested. These include mental dullness, slow responses, forgetfulness and disorientation. Muscle reflexes are exaggerated, and muscular rigidity and asterixis (flapping tremor) are also present. The cause of the neurological involvement is failure of the liver to metabolize and detoxify nitrogenous substances; the toxic materials such as ammonia remain in the blood and are carried into the cerebral circulation. The failure may be due to hepatocellular necrosis or because portal blood bypasses the liver and reaches the central nervous system by being shunted directly into the systemic circulation.

Nursing measures used in the care of any unconscious person are applicable to the patient in hepatic coma (see p. 159).

PORTAL HYPERTENSION. The flow of blood from the portal vein through the liver may meet with resistance due to disease and cirrhotic changes in the liver. Pressure rises within the portal venous system, causing portal hypertension. The latter is defined as a portal pressure in excess of 25 to 30 cm. of saline.[5] The increased pressure in the portal vein produces a back-up in the veins that normally empty into the portal system. Collateral circulatory channels develop between the portal vein and the systemic circulatory system to bypass the liver.

The veins most seriously affected by portal hypertension are those in the gastric cardia region and the lower part of the esophagus. The veins become engorged and tortuous; the walls are weakened, predisposing them to rupture. These varicosed veins appear as large bulbous protrusions under the mucosa. The congestion in the mesenteric veins causes hemorrhoids and is also reflected in the apparent congested cutaneous veins around the umbilicus (caput medusae). In addition to varices, problems associated with portal hypertension include congestive splenomegaly and ascites.

The severity of portal hypertension may be assessed by manometry and angiography. The manometry procedure requires the patient's written consent. A sedative may be ordered for the patient before he is transported to the operating room or radiology department. Under aseptic conditions, a needle is introduced into the spleen and then attached to a manometer. The pressure is recorded as the *splenic pulp pressure* in cm. of saline. Normal splenic pulp pressure is 20 to 25 cm. of saline. The spleen is used since it reflects portal vein pressure, is more readily located for introduction of the needle, and reduces the risk of injury to other viscera. Following measurement of the pressure, a *splenoportogram* may be done. A radiopaque dye may be injected into the spleen. This is carried into the portal venous system and roentgenograms are made to visualize the portal veins, associated vessels and collateral channels.

BLEEDING ESOPHAGOGASTRIC VARICES. The esophagogastric varices are frequently the site of rupture of the vascular wall and severe hemorrhage. The perforation and bleeding may be caused by mechanical trauma from "rough" food passing over a varicosity, erosion and ulceration of the mucosa and venous wall by gastric acid secretion, or sudden increased intra-abdominal pressure associated with coughing, vomiting, straining at stool or physical exertion. Severe hematemesis occurs: some blood will enter the intestine and eventually the person passes tarry stools.

Prompt emergency treatment and care of bleeding esophagogastric varices are necessary; the excessive loss of blood is life-threatening.

Control of Bleeding. Various measures are used to control bleeding and include the following:

Balloon Tamponade. A Sengstaken-Blakemore tube, a nasogastric tube with three lumens, may be inserted. One lumen ends in an elongated balloon that is inflated to exert pressure against the esophageal wall; another ends in a small balloon that is positioned just within the stomach and, when inflated, com-

[5]Thorn, G. W., et al. (Eds.): Harrison's Principles of Internal Medicine. 8th ed. New York, McGraw-Hill, 1977, p. 1547.

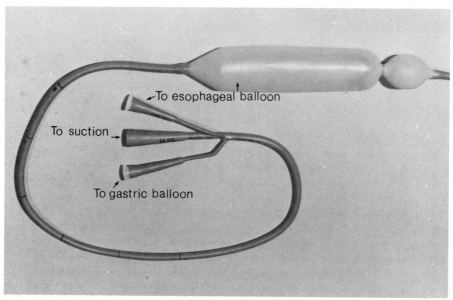

FIGURE 17–3   A Sengstaken-Blakemore tube which is used in the treatment of bleeding esophageal varices. The tube has three lumens. One leads to the longer inflatable balloon that is positioned in the esophagus to provide pressure. A second lumen ends in the smaller balloon that lies just within the stomach. The third lumen opens into the stomach to permit gastric drainage. (Courtesy of the New Mount Sinai Hospital, Toronto.)

presses varices in the cardia and anchors the tube in place (Fig. 17–3); and the third lumen opens into the stomach, extending well beyond the balloon in the cardia. The third lumen permits drainage or aspiration of the gastric content; its proximal end is usually attached to suction. Removal of gastric contents reduces the amount of blood entering the intestine. Digestion of blood in the intestine produces nitrogenous wastes that, when absorbed, predispose the patient to hepatic coma. Before the tube is inserted, the tube and balloons are tested for leaks. The nurse makes sure that the proximal end of each lumen is identified and clearly labeled to prevent possible error in inflation or deflation of tubes after insertion. The pressures to be maintained within the balloons are indicated by the physician and are usually 25 to 30 mm. Hg; excessive pressure can cause tissue ulceration (Fig. 17–4). Inadequate inflation is ineffective in checking bleeding and may also permit shifting of the tube. The gastric drainage is checked frequently for blood content which should progressively decrease following the insertion of the tube. In some instances, when the tube is in place and the balloons inflated, the physician may lavage the stomach with ice water until the return flow is clear.

A nurse remains in constant attendance; the patient is observed closely for any indication of respiratory distress. Saliva or blood escaping around the tube into the oropharynx may be aspirated. The patient is unable to

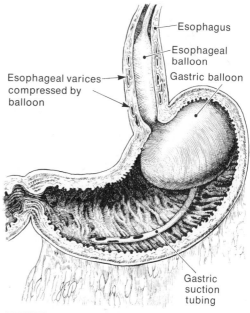

FIGURE 17–4   A Sengstaken-Blakemore tube in position with the esophageal and gastric balloons inflated.

swallow his saliva, so provision is made for suctioning or for expectoration into tissues or a basin.

The tube is positioned within the nostrils to exert a minimum of pull and pressure, and then secured. Frequent moistening and a very light application of a lubricant to the nasal mucosa may reduce the irritation.

Compression by the inflated balloons is not usually continued longer than 48 hours. Pressure for a longer period could cause edema, ulceration and perforation. The tube is left in position for continued gastric drainage and for the balloons to be reinflated readily if bleeding resumes. In some instances, the physician may order deflation of the balloons for 5 to 10 minutes every 8 hours to reduce the risk of tissue damage.

Gastric cooling. Rarely, a continuous application of cold to the esophagus and cardia of the stomach may be used in an attempt to arrest variceal bleeding. A special double-lumen tube with balloons is inserted. By means of a mechanical pump, there is a steady circulation of a cold solution through the balloons and a refrigeration unit.

Vasopressin infusion. Vasopressin (Pitressin) may be administered by a usual intravenous route or, with the assistance of angiography, may be given directly into the superior mesenteric artery. The Pitressin produces arterial vasoconstriction which reduces portal venous pressure by decreasing the volume of blood entering the portal system. The patient may experience crampy abdominal pain and be incontinent of stool.

Surgical treatment. If the measures cited above are not effective in checking the hemorrhage, emergency surgery may be performed to relieve portal hypertension. Different surgical procedures are used. A portocaval shunt in which an anastomosis is made between the portal vein and the inferior vena cava (Fig. 17–5B), a splenorenal venous shunt (Fig. 17–5C), an anastomosis between the superior mesenteric vein and the inferior vena cava (mesocaval shunt, Fig. 17–5D) or a transesophageal ligation of the varices may be done. As an emergency measure, there is considerable risk. It is preferable if the patient's condition can be stabilized and surgery undertaken when bleeding is arrested.

Care following a surgical shunt is similar to that of patients undergoing any abdominal surgery. Close observation for hemorrhage and abdominal distention is important. If a nasogastric tube is passed to control vomiting and distention, a soft rubber tube is selected and is introduced very gently to avoid precipitating hemorrhage by rupturing a varicosity. Specific orders are received from the surgeon as to how much the patient may move and whether deep breathing, coughing, and leg exercises are to be carried out. Similarly, the patient receives nothing by mouth until specifically ordered.

In the case of a splenorenal shunt, a retention catheter is inserted, and a close check is kept on the urinary output.

Vitamin K. Parenteral injections of vitamin K are prescribed to increase the patient's blood-clotting power.

Observations. The patient requires continuous attention and ongoing assessment.

The blood pressure and pulse are recorded every 15 to 30 minutes until the bleeding is controlled. The intervals are gradually increased as the patient's condition shows improvement and stabilization. The patient's respirations, color and responses are noted; persisting gray pallor, rapid shallow respirations and dulling of awareness and responses are unfavorable signs.

The pressures in the balloons are checked at frequent intervals and corrected if necessary to the prescribed pressure. The gastric drainage is observed for amount and blood content. Persisting bright blood in the drainage is brought to the physician's attention. The fluid intake and output are recorded, and the balance determined daily. Stools are examined for blood content.

Supportive Measures. The patient with bleeding esophagogastric varices is critically ill and needs physical and psychological support.

Blood Transfusion. Replacement of the blood lost is imperative. Fresh blood rather than stored is preferable in order to replace the thrombocytes lost.

Nutrition and Fluids. The patient is sustained for several days by intravenous infusion. Glucose in distilled water and plasma are solutions that may be used. An intravenous line is maintained until the patient is able to take fluids by mouth.

Fluids may be introduced via the tube in the stomach before it is removed. When the tube is removed, small amounts of nutritious fluids

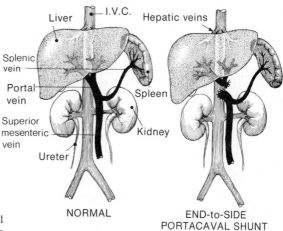

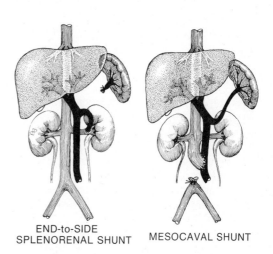

NORMAL

END-to-SIDE PORTACAVAL SHUNT

END-to-SIDE SPLENORENAL SHUNT

MESOCAVAL SHUNT

FIGURE 17–5 Portal shunts used to relieve portal hypertension. *A,* normal portal system. *B,* Anastomosis of the portal vein and the inferior vena cava. *C,* Anastomosis of the splenic vein and the renal vein. *D,* Anastomosis of the superior mesenteric vein and the inferior vena cava.

are given. The diet is progressively increased to a light diet as tolerated. Roughage and raw fruits and vegetables are avoided. The patient is advised to chew his food well in small amounts so that the bolus is small and less likely to traumatize a vulnerable area in the esophagus or cardia of the stomach.

Rest and Positioning.   The patient is kept absolutely at rest. A directive is received from the physician as to whether the patient may or may not be turned. He may have to remain stationary to avoid displacing the balloons. Passive movements of the lower limbs are usually permitted to prevent circulatory stasis. The head of the bed is elevated, unless contraindicated by shock. This position may reduce the flow of blood into the portal system.

Psychological Support.   The hemateme-sis, emergency measures and rapid loss of strength are very frightening to the patient. His fears and concerns should be acknowledged, and reassurance provided that everything possible is being done and that someone will remain with him. Some explanation is calmly made as to what is happening and what is going to be done. Sedation may be necessary to allay the patient's tension and anxiety and provide rest. The patient may be less apprehensive and more relaxed if a family member is permitted to be with him when it does not interfere with treatments. The family is naturally concerned and should be kept informed about the patient's progress and what is being done.

Mouth Care.   The inability to swallow saliva and to receive anything by mouth necessitates special mouth care. Suctioning may be necessary to remove secretions. Tissues or a basin are provided into which the patient may expectorate. The mouth is cleansed with moist applicators and petroleum jelly, or cold cream is applied to the lips to prevent irritation that may develop with the repeated use of tissues.

Elimination. As cited previously, the blood that escapes into the intestine becomes a source of nitrogenous substances, especially ammonia. Intestinal bacteria and enzymes promote the breakdown of the protein in the blood. The substances are absorbed into the blood but are not detoxified by the diseased liver. The elevated blood level of ammonia causes hepatic coma.

To remove the blood before it can be broken down, enemas may be ordered and a laxative may be administered via the gastric tube.

Accidental Injury to the Liver

Rupture of the liver in accidents is not uncommon. Any interruption of the capsule enclosing the hepatic tissue carries the risk of severe internal hemorrhage that may prove fatal before surgical intervention is possible. A blood transfusion is given, and surgical repair undertaken. Control of the bleeding is of prime importance. The area may be sutured or packed, or Oxycel gauze (Gelfoam) may be applied. The latter supplies fibers on which the clot may form more easily. A drainage tube into the abdominal cavity or a sump drain attached to low suction may be used. In addition to the loss of blood incurred in injury, peritonitis may develop as a result of the chemical irritation caused by the bile that may escape from the liver. Destruction of liver cells may also follow the injury, resulting in impaired liver function.

Neoplastic Disease

Benign and primary malignant newgrowths are rare in the liver, but it is a frequent site of metastasis, especially if the primary malignant neoplasm is in the abdominal cavity. The malignant cells may be transported to the liver via the portal venous or hepatic arterial blood or via the lymph. In many instances, secondaries in the liver are discovered before the primary source. The liver enlarges and signs of liver insufficiency develop. The patient experiences pain, food intolerance, anemia, emaciation and ascites.

If a primary newgrowth is confined to one lobe of the liver, a hepatic lobectomy may be done. Following the operation, the patient is observed closely for possible hemorrhage and biliary peritonitis. More often, chemotherapy is used (see p. 143). The drug may be administered by direct hepatic arterial infusion.

Liver Abscess

Infection with subsequent abscess formation occurs rarely and is most often associated with amoebic dysentery. The causative organisms (*Entamoeba histolytica*) are carried by the portal blood stream from the bowel. The pyogenic infection may also be caused by staphylococcus, streptococcus or *Escherichia coli*. Along with manifestations of impaired liver function, the patient has chills and a high fever. There may be one or multiple small abscesses which frequently coalesce, forming one large cavity.

The patient is treated with antibiotics and also receives chloroquine or emetine hydrochloride (antiamebic drugs) if the abscess is a complication of amebiasis. The abscess is drained by aspiration followed by the injection of an antibiotic into the cavity. Open surgical drainage is avoided if possible because of the danger of dissemination of the infection within the peritoneal cavity and resultant peritonitis.

DISORDERS OF THE GALLBLADDER AND BILE DUCTS

Calculi formation, inflammation or neoplastic disease may occur in the extrahepatic biliary system (gallbladder and ducts). These disease processes interfere with the normal flow of bile into the duodenum.

Manifestations

Disease of the extrahepatic biliary system may be acute or chronic, and the intensity of the signs and symptoms parallels the severity of the condition.

PAIN. The pain associated with gallbladder or biliary duct disease may be felt in the right upper abdomen or midepigastric region or is referred to the right scapular area. It may be a persistent, dull ache or very severe and disabling. The onset may follow a meal containing fatty foods. When it is very severe and prostrating, the pain is described as biliary colic.

DIGESTIVE DISTURBANCES. The patient may experience flatulence and an uncomfortable full feeling or nausea, especially after the ingestion of fatty or fried foods. Vomiting is usual if the patient has biliary colic or develops obstructive jaundice.

JAUNDICE. Obstruction of the hepatic or common bile duct as a result of a calculus, edema, stricture or neoplasm causes absorption of bile into the blood, and the patient develops obstructive jaundice.

FEVER. Chills and an elevation of temperature frequently accompany infection and inflammation within the gallbladder or bile ducts.

LEUKOCYTOSIS. An elevation in the white blood cell count develops with cholecystitis.

BLEEDING TENDENCY. An obstruction to the flow of bile into the intestine decreases the absorption of vitamin K, resulting in a reduced prothrombin level and failure of the normal blood-clotting process.

Cholelithiasis

This is the term used for stones in the gallbladder (Table 17–1). Their formation is not understood. They vary in shape and size and consist mainly of cholesterol and bile pigments. There may be one stone or many and, although they may develop in both sexes, they occur more often in middle-aged females. The incidence is high in individuals with regional enteritis.

SIGNS AND SYMPTOMS. Cholelithiasis may not give rise to any disturbance in many persons; in others, the stones cause signs and symptoms ranging from mild digestive disturbances following fat ingestion to all those previously cited under manifestations. Gallstones may cause acute or chronic inflammation of the gallbladder (cholecystitis), or cholestasis (stasis of the bile) within the liver leading to impaired function of that organ. Small stones tend to cause more acute problems, since they may escape into the ducts. If this happens, the patient suffers intense, inca-

TABLE 17–1 NOMENCLATURE IN DISORDERS OF THE EXTRAHEPATIC BILIARY SYSTEM

Cholelithiasis	Gallstones or calculi in the gallbladder.
Cholecystitis	Inflammation of the gallbladder.
Cholecystectomy	Surgical removal of the gallbladder.
Cholestasis	Stoppage or suppression of the flow of bile.
Cholecystostomy	Incision into the gallbladder and the insertion of a tube for drainage.
Choledocholithiasis	Gallstone(s) in the common bile duct.
Choledochitis	Inflammation of the common bile duct.
Choledocholithotomy	Surgical removal of stone from the common bile duct.
Choledochotomy	Incision and exploration of the common bile duct.
Choledochoduodenostomy	Anastomosis of the common bile duct to the duodenum.

be passed into the duodenum, or it may lodge in the cystic or common bile duct or the ampulla of Vater. Impaction of a stone in the common bile duct leads to obstructive jaundice.

TREATMENT AND NURSING CARE. Cholelithiasis is treated surgically by removal of the gallbladder (*cholecystectomy*) and exploration of the common bile duct for a stone or stricture. The surgery is not usually done during an acute attack unless obstruction of the common bile duct persists.

During an episode of biliary colic, the patient remains in bed. An antispasmodic drug such as atropine, propantheline (Pro-Banthine) or nitroglycerin may be ordered to relieve the painful reflex spasm that occurs in response to the stone in a duct. Morphine or meperidine hydrochloride (Demerol) may also be prescribed in conjunction with one of the above drugs, but some physicians avoid their use because they oppose relaxation of the sphincter of Oddi.

Food and fluids by mouth are withheld, and the patient is given intravenous fluids. If vomiting and abdominal distention occur, a nasogastric tube is passed and suction drainage established. Local applications of heat to the upper abdomen may be ordered; precautions to guard against burning are necessary, since the excruciating colic pain and the analgesics may dull the patient's awareness of the heat.

Following the acute episode and removal of the nasogastric tube, clear fluids are given and gradually increased to a light, low-fat diet as tolerated.

The patient is observed for signs of jaundice, and the color of all stools is noted. The nurse may be requested to save the stools for examination for the presence of the stone that may have passed from the biliary tract into the intestine.

If the patient is jaundiced, and the stools are a pale gray, indicating an absence of bile in the intestine, a daily dose of vitamin K (Synkayvite, Mephyton, Hykinone) is given parenterally to maintain prothrombin formation and prevent bleeding.

Cholecystitis

Inflammation of the gallbladder may be acute or chronic. Acute cholecystitis is most often associated with gallstones but may occur as a result of infection. The patient manifests pain and tenderness in the right upper abdominal quadrant or midepigastrium, fever, nausea and vomiting and leukocytosis. The severity of the symptoms varies with the degree of inflammation. Jaundice may develop if the inflammation involves the biliary ducts.

MANAGEMENT. The treatment includes bed rest, intravenous fluids, analgesics and antibiotics. If the condition persists or worsens, it may indicate suppuration (empyema of the gallbladder), necessitating prompt surgery. A *cholecystostomy* (drainage of the gallbladder) or a *cholecystectomy* (removal of the gallbladder) may be done.

Chronic cholecystitis is characterized by a long history of vague digestive complaints. The patient experiences abdominal discomfort and flatulence after a large rich meal or one high in fats. A dull, aching pain and nausea and vomiting may occur at times. The intensity and probably the frequency of the symptoms insidiously increase over months or years.

The chronic inflammation results in scarring and thickening of the wall of the gallbladder and cholestasis. If calculi are present, they progressively increase in size or number. The patient may have subacute or acute exacerbations in which he becomes incapacitated by nausea and vomiting, moderate fever and probably mild colic. The condition is usually treated surgically by removal of the gallbladder.

Carcinoma of the Gallbladder

Cancer of the gallbladder is rare and is usually associated with calculi. It is usually recognized when a cholecystectomy is done because of stones. The symptoms may be similar to those of chronic cholecystitis, gradually increasing in severity with persisting pain. Obstructive jaundice frequently develops with compression of the biliary ducts by the enlarging gallbladder. Obstructive jaundice may also result from extension of the malignant disease to the common bile duct.

Bile Duct Disorders

Obstruction of the common bile duct may occur as a result of a gallstone that has escaped from the gallbladder (*choledocholithiasis*), inflammation (*choledochitis* or *cholangitis*), neoplasm or a stricture formed by scar tissue following trauma and inflammation. The duct above the obstruction dilates and obstructive jaundice develops.

In the case of an impacted stone, the duct is opened and the calculus is removed. When a stricture is present and the area is sufficiently small, it is resected and an end-to-end anastomosis performed. If the obstruction is due to primary carcinoma, excision may be undertaken and the duct stump anastomosed to the duodenum (*choledochoduodenostomy*) or the jejunum (*choledochojejunostomy*).

Extrinsic pressure on the bile ducts obstructing the flow of bile may occur with cancer of the pancreas or duodenum.

When surgery involves an extrahepatic bile duct, a T tube is inserted at the site of entry into the duct to maintain bile drainage during recovery of the tissues (choledochostomy). The stem portion of the tube is brought out on the abdominal surface through a stab wound or the incision and is attached to a drainage bottle. Surgery on a bile duct is usually accompanied by a cholecystectomy, since the gallbladder is frequently the origin of the problem.

Nursing Care of Patients with Extrahepatic Disorders

Surgery is not usually done during an acute attack of cholecystitis or cholelithiasis unless the signs and symptoms are unremitting or progressive. The patient is kept at rest, and food is withheld. If there is vomiting, a nasogastric tube is passed and suction-siphonage is established (see p. 500). The temperature, pulse and respirations are recorded every 3 or 4 hours; a sudden elevation is reported promptly. The patient is checked for signs of obstructive jaundice and abdominal distention.

When the vomiting is controlled and the nasogastric tube removed, oral fluids are given and graduated, as tolerated, to a light, bland, low-fat diet. If the patient is obese, the caloric intake is limited to approximately 1000 calories daily.

PREOPERATIVE CARE. Preoperative preparation (see p. 164) for surgery on the extrahepatic biliary system includes close observation for jaundice and the administration of vitamin K to raise the prothrombin level. Special attention is given to having the patient understand the importance of the frequent coughing and deep breathing that he will be required to carry out after the operation. Because of the site of the surgery, the patient tends to take very shallow breaths to prevent pain and discomfort, predisposing to respiratory complications. A nasogastric tube may be passed before the patient is taken to the operating room.

POSTOPERATIVE CARE. General postoperative care as outlined in Chapter 10 is applicable. Close observation for bleeding is necessary, since low prothrombin levels may still exist.

The drainage tube that is inserted in a cholecystostomy or choledochostomy is generally clamped during the transfer from the operating room; after the patient is transferred, it is immediately attached to a drainage receptacle which is placed at the level specified by the surgeon. The tubing leading to the receptacle is secured to the dressing and lower bed linen and should have sufficient slack to prevent traction and dislodgment. The patient is advised as to how to turn to avoid a pull on the tube and of the need to be sure that it is not kinked or compressed. The drainage is observed frequently during the first 24 hours in case of hemorrhage. There may be a small amount of blood mixed with bile in the first few hours, but persistent bleeding is reported to the surgeon. The character and daily amount of bile drainage are recorded. If there is a prolonged loss of bile, it may be given back to the patient through a nasogastric tube for the purpose of promoting more normal digestion and absorption in the intestine. For esthetic reasons, the patient is not usually told of this procedure.

The dressing is checked frequently for possible bleeding or bile leakage. After a few days, the drainage tube is clamped for stated intervals and is removed when the surgeon considers the common bile duct is patent. Following removal of the tube, the dressing is observed for bile seepage. If the dressing is soiled with bile, it is changed frequently, the skin and wound are cleansed, and petroleum jelly gauze, an ointment or powder is applied to prevent excoriation and maceration of the skin by the strongly alkaline bile. The patient is also observed for signs of peritonitis; an elevation of temperature, abdominal pain, distention and rigidity are reported at once.

Until the procedures become less painful and the patient is less fearful, the nurse's assistance and support are required during the frequent, regular coughing, deep breathing and change of position.

Early ambulation is generally urged, and provision is made for a small drainage receptacle that may be attached to the patient's dressing gown if there is a tube in the common bile duct.

The urine, stools, sclerae and skin are checked for any indication of obstructive jaundice.

The patient receives intravenous solutions of glucose and electrolytes until the nasogastric tube is removed and oral fluids and food are tolerated. The fat content of the diet is limited.

In preparation for discharge, the patient's diet is discussed. Generally, the surgeon will suggest that the patient gradually increase the fat intake over a period of 4 to 6 months and find his own level of tolerance.

References

Books

Beeson, Paul B., and McDermott, Walsh (Eds.): Textbook of Medicine, 15th ed. Philadelphia, W. B. Saunders, 1979.

Bockus, Henry L. (Ed.): Gastroenterology, 3rd ed. Vol. III, The Liver, Gallbladder, Bile Ducts, Pancreas. Philadelphia, W. B. Saunders, 1976. Sections 7 and 8.

Ganong, William F.: Review of Medical Physiology, 7th ed. Los Altos, Cal., Lange, 1975.

Krupp, Marcus A, and Chatton, Milton J.: Current Medical Diagnosis and Treatment. Los Altos, Cal., Lange, 1975, pp. 369–391.

Macleod, John (Ed.): Davidson's Principles and Practice of Medicine, 11th ed. Edinburgh, Churchill Livingstone, 1974, pp. 529–578.

Sabiston, David C. (Ed.): Textbook of Surgery, 11th ed. Philadelphia, W. B. Saunders, 1977.

Spiro, Howard M.: Clinical Gastroenterology, 2nd ed. New York, Macmillan, 1977. Chapters 41–46, 53.

Thorn, G. W., et al. (Eds.): Harrison's Principles of Internal Medicine, 8th ed. New York, McGraw-Hill, 1977.

Periodicals

Altshuler, Anne: "Esophageal Varices in Children." Am. J. Nurs., Vol. 72, No. 4 (April 1972), pp. 687–693.

Baranowski, Karen, and Greene, Harry L., III: "Viral Hepatitis." Nurs. '76, Vol. 6, No. 5 (May 1976), pp. 31–39.

Bartlett, M. K., et al.: "The Removal of Biliary Duct Stones." Surg. Clin. North Am., Vol. 54, No. 3 (June 1974), pp. 599–611.

Blumberg, Baruch S.: "The Hepatitis B Virus — New Routes for an Old Traveler." Mod. Med., Vol. 45, No. 15 (Sept. 15, 1977), pp. 34–39.

Boyer, Carol A., and Ochlberg, Susan M. (Eds.): "Symposium on Diseases of the Liver." Nurs. Clin. North Am., Vol. 12, No. 2 (June 1977), pp. 257–356.

Carey, Larry C. (Ed.): "Symposium on Surgery of the Liver, Spleen and Pancreas." Surg. Clin. North Am., Vol. 55, No. 2 (April 1975).

Coyne, Martin J., and Schoenfield, Leslie J.: "Gallstone Disease." Postgrad. Med., Vol. 57, No. 1 (Jan. 1975), pp. 153–158.

Dolan, Patricia O'Connor, and Greene, Harry L., III: "Conquering Cirrhosis of the Liver and a Dangerous Complication." Nurs. '76, Vol. 6, No. 11 (Nov. 1976), pp. 44–53.

Gillies, Dee Ann, and Alyn, Irene Barrett: "How Well Do You Understand Cirrhosis?" Nurs. '75, Vol. 5, No. 1 (Jan. 1975), pp. 38–43.

Ginsberg, Allen L.: "The Use of Standard Gamma Globulin for the Prevention of Hepatitis B." Dig. Dis., Vol. 21, No. 5 (May 1976), pp. 404–407.

Iber, Frank L.: "Putting the Liver in Clear Focus (Blood Tests, Scans, X-rays, Biopsies)." Mod. Med., Vol. 42, No. 22 (Oct. 28, 1974), pp. 36–40.

Kreps, Edward, et al.: "Hepatic Crisis." Nurs. '74, Vol. 4, No. 2 (Feb. 1974), pp. 15–19.

Lim, Robert C., et al.: "Postoperative Treatment of Patients after Liver Resection for Trauma." Arch. Surg., Vol. 112, No. 4 (April 1977), pp. 429–433.

Malt, Ronald A.: "Emergency and Elective Operations for Bleeding Esophageal Varices." Surg. Clin. North Am., Vol. 54, No. 3 (June 1974), pp. 561–571.

McConnell, Edwina A.: "All About Gastrointestinal Intubation." Nurs. '75, Vol. 5, No. 9 (Sept. 1975), pp. 31–37.

McInnis, W. D., et al.: "Hepatic Trauma." Arch. Surg., Vol. 112, No. 2 (Feb. 1977), pp. 157–161.

Nusbaum, Morene: "Bleeding Esophageal Varices." Mod. Med., Vol. 44, No. 12 (June 15, 1976), pp. 36–40.

Rains, A. J. Harding: "Gall-Stones." Practitioner, Vol. 214, No. 1284 (June 1975), pp. 749–762.

Zimmerman, Hyman J. (Ed.): "Symposium on Diseases of the Liver." Med. Clin. North Am., Vol. 59, No. 4 (July 1975).

18

Nursing in Disorders of the Pancreas

PHYSIOLOGY OF THE PANCREAS

The pancreas is a fish-shaped gland; the thicker portion, referred to as the head, lies in the curve of the duodenum, and the remainder extends to the left directly behind the stomach (Fig. 18–1). It has two distinct types of essential functional cells. Groups of one type secrete into small ducts which drain into a main channel running the length of the gland. This collecting channel is called the *pancreatic duct,* or the duct of Wirsung, and passes out of the head of the pancreas to unite with the common bile duct to form the ampulla of Vater. In a few persons, the duct may have a direct entrance to the duodenum via the duct of Santorini. Because the secretion of this type of cell flows through ducts, it is classified as an *external or exocrine secretion.*

The other type of parenchymal cell is scattered in insular groups, forming what are known as the islets of Langerhans. These cells produce secretions which are classified as *internal or endocrine secretions* because they are absorbed into the blood and are not secreted into ducts.

Exocrine Functions

The external secretion passes through the ampulla of Vater and sphincter of Oddi into the duodenum. It is strongly aklaline, owing to a high bicarbonate content. Several important digestive enzymes (trypsinogen, chymotrypsin, procarboxypeptidase, amy-lopsin and lipase) involved in the breakdown of proteins, carbohydrates and fats are contained in the exocrine secretion. Regulation of the secretion of these enzymes and their role in digestion is discussed under Digestion in the Small Intestine on page 482.

Endocrine Functions

The endocrine functions of the pancreas are the production of insulin and glucagon.

Insulin is secreted by the beta cells of the islets of Langerhans. It has a major role in the metabolism of glucose and regulation of the blood sugar level. The transfer of glucose from the blood into most body cells is facilitated by insulin, but neurons and erythrocytes are not dependent upon it for the uptake of glucose. Insulin promotes utilization of glucose by the cells and the storage of glucose as glycogen in the liver. It also influences fatty acid synthesis (esterification) in fatty tissue and the uptake and conversion of amino acids into body proteins.

Glucagon is formed by the alpha cells of the islets of Langerhans. It is suggested that it is "also secreted by the gastrointestinal tract,"[1] although Harper states that the glucagon produced by the gastric and duodenal mucosa is not chemically identical with pancreatic glucagon and does not carry out the same actions.[2] Its primary

[1]William F. Ganong: Review of Medical Physiology, 7th ed. Los Altos, Cal., Lange, 1975, p. 248.
[2]Harold A. Harper: Review of Physiological Chemistry, 15th ed. Los Altos, Cal., Lange, 1975, p. 469.

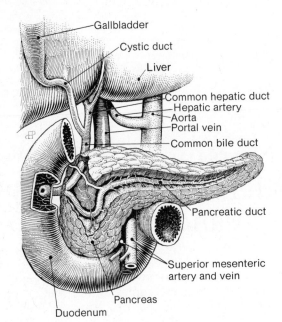

- Gallbladder
- Cystic duct
- Liver
- Common hepatic duct
- Hepatic artery
- Aorta
- Portal vein
- Common bile duct
- Pancreatic duct
- Superior mesenteric artery and vein
- Pancreas
- Duodenum

FIGURE 18–1 Diagram of the pancreas and central pancreatic duct in relationship to the duodenum and the common bile duct.

function is the mobilization of metabolic substances from storage depots. It stimulates the conversion of liver glycogen to glucose and its release into the blood when the blood sugar falls below the normal level. It also promotes the breakdown of fats to fatty acids and glycerol and the release of potassium from the liver.

The two hormones, insulin and glucagon, secreted by the islets of Langerhans are opposite in effect.

DISORDERS OF THE PANCREAS

Inflammation and neoplastic disease are the pathologic conditions seen most frequently in the pancreas. Like the liver, the pancreas has a large reserve capacity; a portion of the gland may be destroyed or become nonfunctional and the remainder will compensate sufficiently to maintain normal physiology.

PANCREATITIS

Inflammation of the pancreas may be acute or chronic with recurrent acute episodes.

Acute Pancreatitis

Acute pancreatitis is a potentially serious disorder; the severity of the inflammation varies. In the mild form the pancreas becomes swollen and edematous and, with treatment, the patient is likely to recover within a few days. If the process is severe and persists, necrosis and hemorrhage ensue. Necrosis results from intrapancreatic activation of the proteinases and lipase, initiating autodigestion of the pancreatic tissue and blood vessels. Enzymes and blood may escape into the surrounding tissue and peritoneal cavity; peritonitis, paralytic ileus or ascites may develop.

Etiology

Pancreatitis is considered to be the result of some factor or change within the pancreas that effects activation of the proteinases and lipase of the exocrine secretion, with subsequent breakdown of the ducts, parenchymal tissue and blood vessels. The causative factor may be an obstruction to the flow of the pancreatic secretion within the ducts. Continued secretion produces dilatation and back pressure, resulting in duct disruption and the escape of enzymes into the parenchyma. The obstruction may be due to a calculus in the pancreatic duct, a newgrowth, or fibrosis following some irritation within the pancreas.

A gallstone in the ampulla of Vater, compression of the ampulla by an extrinsic newgrowth, or spasm or edema of the sphincter of Oddi may be the initiating factor. It is suggested that such an obstruction causes a reflux of bile into the pancreas, promoting activation of the enzymes and ensuing autodigestion.

Other possible etiologic factors are considered to be infection and injury of the pancreas. Pancreatitis is most frequently associated with biliary tract disease and alcoholism and has a higher incidence in middle-aged individuals.

Manifestations

Acute pancreatitis has a sudden onset, being preceded usually by only mild, vague digestive disturbances. The principal signs and symptoms are pain, gastrointestinal disturbances, obstructive jaundice, shock and hyperglycemia.

PAIN. At first, constant severe incapacitating pain occurs in the upper abdomen, penetrating through to the back. It may be described as burning or boring. Later, with progression of the disease, the pain becomes more generalized in the abdomen.

GASTROINTESTINAL DISTURBANCES. Nausea and vomiting occur and persist. Constipation may be a problem. Abdominal distention and rigidity appear as a result of the development of peritonitis. The latter is caused by chemical irritation of the viscera and peritoneum by the enzymes that escape from the pancreas. Peristalsis diminishes, and eventually paralytic ileus and intestinal obstruction may complicate the patient's condition further.

SHOCK. The patient has the appearance of being very ill; he becomes anxious and prostrated. Severe shock develops; the skin is pale, cold and clammy, the pulse is rapid and thready, and the temperature, which may have been elevated, falls to subnormal. Shock is attributed to the severity of the constant pain, the exudation of plasma into the peritoneal cavity that occurs with the peritonitis, and the loss of blood resulting from the erosion of vessels within the pancreas associated with necrotizing and hemorrhagic pancreatitis.

VITAL SIGNS. The temperature may be elevated in the early stage but may become subnormal if peritonitis and shock develop. The pulse is rapid, and the blood pressure falls with the decrease in the intravascular volume due to dehydration and the concomitant shock. The patient is flushed at first, and then usually becomes pale. If peritonitis develops, he is likely to become a dusky or cyanotic color.

OBSTRUCTIVE JAUNDICE. If the head of the pancreas is involved, it may compress the common bile duct and cause obstructive jaundice.

BLOOD CHANGES. With the escape of enzymes into the pancreatic parenchyma and peritoneal cavity, fatty tissue is broken down into glycerol and fatty acids. The latter combine with calcium to form insoluble calcium compounds. The serum calcium level falls and may be severe enough to produce tetany and affect heart action (prolonged diastole). The serum bilirubin level may be elevated after 2 to 3 days.

Hemoconcentration develops as a result of the loss of plasma. The prothrombin level falls because of the lack of absorption of vitamin K. Serum amylase and lipase levels are elevated.

DISTURBANCE IN GLUCOSE METABOLISM. A deficiency of insulin may develop when the islets of Langerhans are involved in the pathologic process, and hyperglycemia and glucosuria (sugar in the urine) may be present.

Diagnostic Procedures

The following diagnostic tests may be carried out on the patient suspected of having pancreatitis.

LABORATORY ANALYSES. Various blood, urine and stool examinations may be used in diagnosing pancreatitis and in assessing the patient's progress.

BLOOD TESTS. These include the following:

Concentration of Pancreatic Enzymes. Some of the enzymes secreted by the pancreas are normally absorbed into the blood and eventually are excreted in the urine. An elevation of the serum amylase and lipase levels occurs when there is an obstruction of the pancreatic ducts and necrosis of the cells.

Normal: Serum amylase, 60 to 180 units per cent (Somogyi method). Serum lipase, 1.5 units or less.

Serum Calcium Level. As cited in manifestations of pancreatitis, the disease causes a decrease in the blood calcium level.

Normal: 4.5 to 6.0 mEq. per liter or 9 to 11 mg. per cent.

Blood Sugar Concentration. Damage to the islets of Langerhans may cause a reduction in insulin secretion and hyperglycemia.

Normal: Fasting, 80 to 120 mg. per cent.

Serum Bilirubin Level. The serum bilirubin is elevated if the pancreatitis is associated with biliary tract disease or edema of the organ which causes compression of the common bile duct or ampulla of Vater.

Normal: 0.3 to 100 mg. per cent.

Leukocyte Count. The white blood cell count is elevated; the increase is in the polymorphonuclear leukocytes and is quite marked in necrotizing and hemorrhagic pancreatitis.

Normal: 5000 to 7000 per cu. mm.

Prothrombin Time. As indicated previously, less prothrombin is produced because of interference with the absorption of vitamin K.

Normal: 13 to 17 seconds, or 75 to 100 per cent activity.

URINALYSES. These tests include the following:

Urinary Amylase Excretion. Urinalysis may indicate an increase in the excretion of the enzyme amylase in pancreatitis.

Normal: 260 to 950 units in a 24-hour specimen.

Glucosuria. Dysfunction of the pancreas may incur a deficiency of insulin, resulting in hyperglycemia and the excretion of excess glucose in the urine.

STOOL EXAMINATION. Analysis of stool specimens made over a specified number of hours may be done to determine the quantitative fat content. Failure of the pancreatic lipase to reach the intestine results in undigested and unabsorbed fat.

Normal: 3 to 5 Gm. in 24 hours.

ROENTGENOGRAPHY. A radiologic examination is made of the abdomen. It may reveal gallstones, accumulation of gas in the duodenum or calcification in the pancreas.

PANCREAS SCAN. A scan may be done if tumors of the pancreas are suspected, or to assess the extent of fibrosed, nonfunctional tissue. The patient receives selenium-75 (Se^{75}) tagged with methionine by intravenous injection. The radioactive substance is taken up by the pancreas; methionine is used in the formation of enzymes. The pancreas is then scanned with a scintillation counter and a graph indicates the amount of the radioactive tracer uptake and by which internal areas of the pancreas. Abnormal areas of tissue do not take up the radioactive selenium and leave voids in the scan.

Treatment and Nursing Care

The patient with acute pancreatitis is critically ill. Care is directed toward the reduction of pancreatic secretion to a minimum, relief of pain, prevention of shock or correction if it has developed, correction of electrolyte and fluid imbalances and prevention of infection. Nursing responsibilities involve the following considerations.

RELIEF OF PAIN. Meperidine hydrochloride (Demerol) is used parenterally to relieve the patient's pain in preference to opiate preparations (morphine, codeine) since the latter tend to stimulate the contraction of the sphincter of Oddi. The patient is assisted in turning and moving and in finding the least painful position. Frequent attendance and verbal and nonverbal conveyance of an appreciation of the patient's suffering may contribute to making the pain less intolerable.

OBSERVATIONS. The patient's condition may change rapidly with progressive necrosis and resulting hemorrhage. The *vital signs* and the *general response and appearance of the patient* are observed frequently. A rapid weak pulse, a fall in blood pressure, pallor and increasing weakness may manifest hemorrhage or shock and are immediately brought to the physician's attention. Frequent *hemoglobin* and *hematocrit estimations* may be requested to detect hemoconcentration which would indicate the loss of plasma into the peritoneal cavity. An accurate record is kept of the *fluid intake and output.*

The *intensity and location of the pain* are noted, and the abdomen is examined for distention and rigidity. All *stools* are examined and, if they are bulky, greasy and foul-smelling or show other abnormalities, they are saved until seen by the physician.

The *sclerae and skin* are observed for any yellow tinge that would indicate the development of jaundice.

GASTRIC DRAINAGE. A nasogastric tube is passed and continuous suction drainage is established. This relieves vomiting and distention and prevents the acid gastric secretion from entering the duodenum, which would stimulate the release of the hormones secretin and cholecystokinin-pancreozymin. The color, consistency and 24-hour volume of the drainage are recorded.

FLUIDS AND NUTRITION. The patient receives nothing by mouth to avoid stimulating the secretion of the pancreatic enzymes. The restoration and maintenance of normal blood volume is very important to prevent or correct shock. Plasma or whole blood may be given intravenously, in addition to electrolyte and glucose solutions. A close check is kept on the blood chemistry, volume of gastrointestinal drainage, urinary output and amount of perspiration to determine the specific electrolyte and fluid needs.

When oral intake is permitted, fluids are introduced in small amounts. The principal nutrient given at first is carbohydrate; protein is added gradually, according to the patient's tolerance. Fats are avoided. The diet is progressively increased to a high-protein, high-carbohydrate, low-fat, light diet. Four or five small meals are recommended. A preparation of extract of pancreas (pancreatin) may be prescribed orally with meals to assist in digestion. Large meals are avoided, and total abstinence from alcohol is stressed.

MOUTH AND NASAL CARE. Frequent cleansing and rinsing of the mouth are necessary during the period in which oral intake is restricted because the anticholinergic drug which the patient may be receiving suppresses salivary secretion. Oil, petroleum jelly or a cream is used on the lips to prevent cracking. The nostrils are cleansed with an applicator which has been slightly moistened with normal saline, and a light application of petroleum jelly or water-soluble lubricant is made to the nostril through which the tube passes to prevent irritation and excoriation.

MEDICATIONS. As well as analgesics, the patient may receive an anticholinergic drug such as propantheline bromide (Pro-Banthine) and atropine sulfate by intramuscular or subcutaneous injection. These drugs inhibit vagal nerve stimulation of the pancreatic enzymes and promote relaxation of the sphincter of Oddi. If an anticholinergic drug is prescribed, the patient will experience a very dry mouth and close observations are made for the possible side effects of urinary retention and paralytic ileus.

An antibiotic is usually ordered as a prophylactic measure since inflammation and necrosis make the pancreas very vulnerable to infection.

When the gastric drainage is discontinued, an antacid such as aluminum hydroxide gel (Amphojel) or a combination of aluminum hydroxide and magnesium hydroxide (Maalox) may be given orally at frequent intervals to reduce the acidity of the chyme entering the duodenum.

Parenteral administration of vitamin K may be necessary to maintain normal prothrombin production and prevent bleeding.

COMPLICATIONS. If *paralytic ileus* and intestinal obstruction develop, a Miller-Abbott tube may be passed into the intestine and decompression suction established (see p. 500). *Obstruction of the duodenum* may develop because of the swollen edematous pancreas. Escaping pancreatic enzymes may digest an area of the gastric or duodenal wall, causing *severe hemorrhage* as well as perforation of the eroded organ.

Another complication that rarely develops in pancreatitis is the formation of one or more *pseudocysts*. Accumulations of inflammatory exudate, liquefied necrotic tissue and secretions become walled off by a capsule of fibrous tissue. The cyst is atypical in that there is no epithelial lining characteristic of true cysts. This accounts for the term pseudocyst. A pseudocyst may form within or on the surface of the pancreas or in a neighboring area into which pancreatic secretions have escaped. It may enlarge and impose on surrounding structures. The common bile duct may be blocked, the duodenum or stomach may be displaced, or the diaphragm may be elevated. The deviation and location are usually recognized in an x-ray.

The symptoms depend on the size and location of the cyst(s). In some instances resolution takes place spontaneously, or the cysts may produce persisting pain, digestive disturbances, anorexia, loss of weight and mechanical interference with other organs. Surgical drainage may be necessary and may be internal or external, depending on the location of the cyst. Internal drainage is achieved by anastomosing the cyst to the small intestine. If drainage is established through the skin, petroleum jelly gauze or a protective ointment or powder is essential to prevent excoriation of the skin by the enzyme content of the drainage.

PREPARATION FOR LEAVING HOSPITAL. A long convalescence follows recovery from an acute episode of pancreatitis. The necessary care to avert an exacerbation is discussed with the patient and his family. The importance of strict adherence to the prescribed diet, total abstinence from alcohol and the avoidance of large meals are explained. Verbal and written instructions are given about the content and preparation of the recommended low-fat, high-protein, high-carbohydrate diet.

If anticholinergic drugs or antacids are to be continued, verbal and written directions are given which include advice as to early side effects that should be reported to the physician. To assist with digestion, the patient with chronic pancreatitis may need to continue to take extract of pancreas (pancreatin) orally with each meal.

The patient is encouraged to develop a special interest or hobby within his activity tolerance to help him through the convalescent period. Activities are gradually resumed and the individual may return to his former occupation in 1 to 2 months. A referral to a visiting nurse agency may be advisable to provide necessary supervision.

SURGICAL INTERVENTION. Surgery is not usually undertaken during an acute attack of pancreatitis unless there is increasing obstructive jaundice due to an impacted stone. The various operative procedures that may be used to treat the patient may be performed on the biliary tract or directly on the pancreas. They include exploration of the common bile duct and ampulla of Vater and the insertion of a T-tube for drainage, cholecystostomy, cholecystec-tomy, sphincterotomy to relieve obstruction caused by spasm of the sphincter of Oddi, anastomosis between the common bile duct and duodenum, or anastomosis between the gallbladder and the jejunum. Surgery on the pancreas may involve the removal of calculi in the pancreatic duct, drainage of a pseudocyst, or partial or complete pancreatectomy. Rarely, in severe chronic pancreatitis, sensory nerves (splanchnic nerves) which transmit pain impulses from the pancreas may be interrupted to relieve intractable pain.

The nursing care of patients having surgical treatment is similar to that required by patients having biliary tract surgery (see p. 597).

Chronic Pancreatitis

Chronic pancreatitis may develop following an initial acute episode or may develop insidiously. Recurrent acute exacerbations are likely to occur. It is frequently associated with alcoholism, chronic biliary tract disease, or hypercalcemia due to hyperparathyroidism.

The chronic form of the disease is characterized by progressive fibrosing and calcification of areas in the pancreas following inflammation and necrosis. The degree of impaired function and the intensity of its signs and symptoms are proportionate to the amount of continuing inflammation or frequency of acute episodes and ensuing tissue damage.

Manifestations

The patient with chronic pancreatitis experiences recurrent attacks of pain in the epigastric region and right upper quadrant which progressively becomes persistent. Anorexia, nausea, flatulence and constipation are common problems. Episodes are frequently precipitated by the ingestion of alcohol or a large meal with considerable fatty content.

As more and more of the pancreatic parenchyma becomes nonfunctional, a deficiency of enzyme secretion occurs in the intestine. Less fat and protein are digested; the patient's stools become bulky, greasy and offensive (steatorrhea) and there is a progressive weight loss. A deficiency of insulin secretion may result in diabetes.

Investigative Procedures

The tests cited for the investigation of the patient for acute pancreatitis may be used to assess the severity of chronic pancreatitis. The secretin-pancreozymin test may also be used, in which pancreatic exocrine function is evaluated by analyzing aspirated duodenal content following stimulation first by an intravenous injection of secretin and then by an injection of pancreozymin.

The dosage of the hormones is calculated by the physician on the basis of the patient's weight. A double-lumen duodenal tube is passed; one lumen permits aspiration of the gastric content, and the duodenal content is withdrawn through the other at stated intervals over a period of 80 minutes. The total volume is estimated, and the bicarbonate and amylase concentrations are determined.

Normal: Total secretion, at least 2.0 ml. per kg. of body weight. Bicarbonate, 90 mEq. per liter. Amylase, 6.0 units per kg. of body weight.

In chronic pancreatitis, exocrine function of the pancreas may also be assessed by analyzing the duodenal content for the enzyme trypsin following a test meal of food that causes the release of the hormones secretin and cholecystokinin-pancreozymin which stimulate pancreatic exocrine function. A single-lumen duodenal tube is passed and the test meal, consisting of skim milk powder and dextrose dissolved in water, is given. Aspirations are made at stated intervals over 2 hours, and the specimens are analyzed for trypsin content.[3]

Endoscopic examination of pancreatic and biliary ducts (cholangiopancreatography) may also be done. Using a fiberoptic duodenoscope, the ampulla of Vater is cannulated and a radiopaque dye is introduced under fluoroscopic viewing. If the biliary and pancreatic ducts are patent,

they are visualized on the x-ray films that are taken. This test is not used if acute pancreatitis is suspected.

The procedure is explained to the patient so he will have some idea of what to expect (passing of the tube, positions to be assumed, etc.). He receives nothing by mouth for 6 to 8 hours preceding the test, and dentures are removed before being transported to the examination room. Sedation and atropine sulfate may be administered parenterally.

Following the examination, the patient is observed for possible pancreatitis and cholangitis. These complications are manifested by chill, fever, abdominal pain, elevated serum amylase level, nausea and vomiting.

Treatment and Care

In some instances, slight impairment by chronic pancreatitis may be controlled by dietary adjustments and the avoidance of emotional stress, fatigue and infection.

A low-fat diet and four or five small meals rather than the usual three larger ones are recommended. The patient's fear of precipitating more severe pain may lead to a reluctance to eat and a resulting serious weight loss. He must be encouraged to take nourishing foods that he can tolerate. Impaired digestion due to insufficient quantities of enzymes in the intestine may be corrected by the administration of pancreatic enzyme supplements (preparation of pancreatic extract). Total alcohol abstinence must be respected to avoid precipitation of an acute episode.

Decreased insulin secretion may necessitate the giving of insulin to control glucose metabolism.

As the disease becomes more advanced, the pain experienced by the patient may indicate frequent doses of an analgesic. Not infrequently, this becomes complicated by the person's development of a tolerance for the drug, necessitating progressively larger doses; actual addiction may become a problem.

Rarely, surgical intervention may be used to drain pseudocysts or to relieve intractable pain. Partial pancreatectomy or anastomosis of the pancreatic duct with the jejunum may be undertaken.

[3]D. H. Hanscom: "Diagnostic Tests in Pancreatic Disease." Med. Clin. North Am., Vol. 52, No. 6 (Nov. 1968), pp. 1483–1492.

NEOPLASMS OF THE PANCREAS

Carcinoma

Cancer of the pancreas usually arises from the ducts and, although it may occur in any part of the organ, it is most commonly seen in the head.

The patient experiences pain, progressive weakness and loss of weight. Jaundice develops if the newgrowth encroaches on the ampulla of Vater or common bile duct. The cancer may spread by direct invasion to adjacent structures and by metastasis to the liver.

TREATMENT. The condition is treated surgically if recognized sufficiently early and if it is the head of the pancreas that is involved. Newgrowths in the body and tail have usually metastasized by the time they are identified. Rarely, a pancreatoduodenal resection may be done; this procedure involves resection of the head of the pancreas, ampulla of Vater, duodenum and pylorus with anastomosis between the common bile duct and jejunum, anastomosis between the pancreas and jejunum, and a gastrojejunostomy. Palliative operations that may be used include a cholecystojejunostomy to relieve obstructive jaundice and a side-to-side anastomosis of the main pancreatic duct (duct of Wirsung) to the jejunum. Radiation therapy and/or chemotherapy may be used but have not been found to be very effective.

Preparation for surgery includes a high-calorie, low-fat diet if tolerated by the patient, intravenous infusion of glucose and electrolyte solutions, blood transfusions, and parenteral vitamin K if there is jaundice. Postoperative care includes gastrointestinal decompression to prevent distention of the jejunum and pressure on the sites of the anastomoses. The patient is supported by blood transfusions and intravenous electrolytes and glucose. Vitamin K administration may be continued.

Tumors of Islet Cells

A benign tumor may develop in non-beta islet cells and may become malignant. The tumor cells secrete gastrin freely, causing the Zollinger-Ellison syndrome, which is characterized by gastric hypersecretion and persisting peptic ulceration. The treatment is surgical removal of the tumors or total gastrectomy. Nursing care of the patient is similar to that cited under gastric surgery, page 533.

Occasionally an adenoma develops from beta cells of the islets of Langerhans, causing an excessive secretion of insulin (hyperinsulinism) and hypoglycemia. The adenoma is usually benign but, rarely, may be adenocarcinoma.

The symptoms presented by the patient are mainly due to the effect of the abnormally low blood sugar (50 mg. or less per cent) on the brain cells. Brain cells are more sensitive to glucose deficiency than other body cells. The initial symptoms are hunger, restlessness and apprehension. These progress to weakness, loss of coordination, tremors, diaphoresis, disorientation, convulsions and coma. The manifestations appear during a fasting period (early morning) or following extreme exertion. Prompt administration of some form of glucose is necessary to raise the blood sugar. If the hypoglycemia remains untreated, the glucose deficiency may result in permanent brain cell damage or death. When early signs are recognized, the patient is given sugar or orange juice with sugar. In the more advanced stage of hypoglycemia, glucose 50 per cent is given intravenously.

Surgical treatment may consist of excision of the adenoma or subtotal or total pancreatectomy. Preparation for the surgery includes a high-carbohydrate, high-protein diet and intravenous infusions of glucose solution to restore glycogen reserves. The glucose infusion is continued during the operation. Following surgery, close observation is made for a recurrence of hypoglycemia. If a total pancreatectomy is done, the patient will receive supplemental insulin and pancreatic extract for the remainder of his life.

Diabetes mellitus is discussed in Chapter 22.

CYSTIC FIBROSIS

Cystic fibrosis is a congenital disease characterized by impaired functioning of the exocrine and mucus-secreting glands throughout the body. The secretions, especially those of the respiratory tract, are abnormally viscous. The sweat and saliva of affected persons have inordinate concentrations of sodium and chloride.

This disease is usually recognized in infancy because of the serious respiratory problems incurred by the thick, tenacious mucus. The secretions are retained, blocking bronchioles and alveoli, and the patient's vital capacity is reduced. As a result, he is very vulnerable to infection.

The viscous nature of the exocrine secretions of the pancreas causes a stasis and obstruction in ducts, which may result in cyst-like dilatations and degeneration of tissue and ensuing fibrosis. A deficiency of pancreatic enzymes in the intestine produces incomplete digestion and absorption as well as steatorrhea. The islets of Làngerhans are not usually affected. In severe disease, the newborn may fail to pass meconium because of intestinal obstruction, and an ileostomy may have to be done.

Cystic fibrosis is currently considered to be a hereditary disease (recessive trait) that is transmitted by a defective gene received from each parent. It is thought that the defect may result in the lack of a specific enzyme, causing interference with the cells' production of their secretions.

The child requires constant, intensive care and supervision. Special measures such as humidifiers and mist tents are used to keep the air in the patient's environment moist to help liquefy the respiratory secretions. Postural drainage, chest percussion and vibration, regular coughing and breathing exercises are also employed. Antimicrobial preparations may be prescribed to prevent infection. Obviously, any contact with persons who have an infection must be avoided.

The patient receives a high-calorie, high-carbohydrate, high-protein, low-fat diet. A preparation of pancreatic extract (pancreatin) is given to promote digestion and absorption. In warm weather, sodium and chloride depletion may occur as a result of increased sweating and may necessitate an increased intake of these electrolytes either orally or by intravenous infusion.

The family is referred to a visiting nursing organization and to a branch of the National Cystic Fibrosis Foundation. The parents generally need considerable assistance in establishing a plan of care for the patient; the socioeconomic demands are great. The medications and therapeutic equipment are expensive, and there is a continuous demand on the parents' time in providing the necessary observation and care. Frequent visits to the clinic or physician's office are necessary.

References

Books

Beeson, Paul B., and McDermott, Walsh (Eds.): Textbook of Medicine, 15th ed. Philadelphia, W. B. Saunders, 1979.

Bockus, Henry L. (Ed.): Gastroenterology, 3rd ed. Vol. III: The Liver, Gallbladder, Bile Ducts, Pancreas. Philadelphia, W. B. Saunders, 1976. Section 9.

Ganong, William F.: Review of Medical Physiology, 7th ed. Los Altos, Cal., Lange, 1975, pp. 248–264 and 368–370.

Krupp, Marcus A., and Chatton, Milton J.: Current Medical Diagnosis and Treatment. Los Altos, Cal., Lange, 1975, pp. 392–395.

Macleod, John (Ed.): Davidson's Principles and Practice of Medicine, 11th ed. Edinburgh, Churchill Livingstone, 1974, pp. 480–487.

Sabiston, David C. (Ed.): Textbook of Surgery, 11th ed. Philadelphia, W. B. Saunders, 1977. Chapter 37.

Schottelius, Byron, A., and Schottelius, Dorothy D.: Physiology, 17th ed. St. Louis, C. V. Mosby, 1973, pp. 394 and 496–498.

Spiro, Howard M.: Clinical Gastroenterology, 2nd ed. New York, Macmillan, 1977. Chapters 47–52.

Thorn, G. W., et al. (Eds.): Harrison's Principles of Internal Medicine, 8th ed. New York, McGraw-Hill, 1977.

Periodicals

Belinsky, Irmgard: "Fiberoptic Advances: Visualizing the Pancreatic and Biliary Ducts." Am. J. Nurs., Vol. 76, No. 6 (June 1976), pp. 936–937.

Bloom, S. R.: "Glucagon." J. Hosp. Med., Vol. 13, No. 2 (Feb. 1975), pp. 150–158.

Burnette, Betty Anne: "Family Adjustment to Cystic Fibrosis." Am. J. Nurs., Vol. 75, No. 11 (Nov. 1975), pp. 1986–1989.

Campbell, Graeme: "Pancreatic Cysts." Practitioner, Vol. 214, No. 1284 (June 1975), pp. 786–794.

Graham, N. G.: "Acute Pancreatitis." Practitioner, Vol. 214, No. 1284 (June 1975), pp. 763–775.

Holzel, A.: "Cystic Fibrosis." Practitioner, Vol. 214, No. 1284 (June 1975), pp. 776–785.

Kafka, Eugene C., and Kalser, Martin H.: "Pancreatic Disease." Postgrad. Med., Vol. 57, No. 1 (Jan. 1975), pp. 140–145.

Marcotte, Ange-Aimée: "Cystic Fibrosis." Can. Nurse, Vol. 71, No. 7 (July 1975), pp. 32–37.

Nardi, George L.: "Remediable Pancreatitis." Surg. Clin. North Am., Vol. 54, No. 3 (June 1974), pp. 613–620.

Simmons, Sandra, and Given, Barbara: "Acute Pancreatitis." Am. J. Nurs., Vol. 71, No. 5 (May 1971), pp. 934–939.

19

Nursing in Disorders of the Urinary System

THE URINARY SYSTEM

The urinary system consists of two kidneys, two ureters, the bladder and urethra. The kidneys are the primary functional structures in which urine is formed. The ureters are drainage tubes which transmit the urine from the kidneys to the bladder where it is temporarily stored. The urethra is a duct that carries the urine to the exterior surface of the body.

Structure of the Kidneys

The kidneys are paired, bean-shaped organs that lie retroperitoneally against the dorsal abdominal wall. Each kidney is enclosed in a fibrous capsule and is embedded in fatty tissue. It consists of approximately 1,000,000 nephrons, many blood vessels and collecting tubules, and a pelvis. The kidney is anatomically divided into an outer, dark red portion called the *cortex* and an inner, lighter-colored section lying between the cortex and the pelvis called the *medulla* (Fig. 19–1). The medullary tissue is arranged in *conical or pyramidal masses* separated by *renal columns* formed by projections of cortical tissue. The blood vessels, nerves and ureter enter or leave the kidney at the hilum, the indentation on the medial surface.

NEPHRON. The nephron is the functional unit of the kidney. It consists of a narrow, convoluted tubule and a tuft of capillaries referred to as a *glomerulus*. The upper end of the tubule is dilated and invaginated to envelop the glomerulus and is called *Bowman's capsule*. According to their position, the nephrons may be classified as superficial cortical or juxtamedullary nephrons. The latter lie deep in the cortex with their glomeruli and capsules close to the medulla and their tubules extending deep into the medulla.

The tubule is divided into three segments — the *proximal convoluted tubule,* the hairpin-like *loop of Henle* and the *distal convoluted tubule* (Fig. 19–2). A major function of the tubules is to convey water and solutes in either direction across the tubular cells between the interstitial fluid and the tubular content. The thickness and structure of the walls differ from one segment to another: this arrangement accounts for different substances being reabsorbed and secreted in different sections of the tubule.[1] Movement across the tubular membrane may be active (using cellular energy) or passive.

---

[1]In relation to kidney function, *reabsorbed* means the movement of substances from the tubular content to the interstitial fluid. *Secreted* implies the transport of substances from the interstitial fluid to the tubular lumen. *Endocrine secretion* indicates the cellular production of a substance and its release directly into the blood stream.

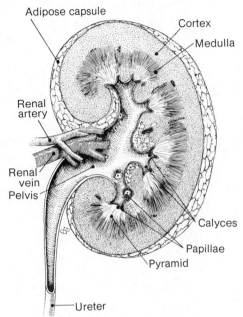

FIGURE 19-1 Cross section of kidney.

The proximal convoluted tubule is the longest portion of the nephron and has thin walls consisting of a single layer of cells. The intraluminal surface of the cells has minute finger-like extensions known as *microvilli*, forming what is called a brush border layer. The villi are thought to play an important role in reabsorption of glucose and amino acids.

The loops of Henle vary in length and lie mainly in the medulla. The walls in the descending limb become thinner as they approach the loop. Modifications in the cells result in the walls of the ascending limb of the loop being thicker. Its terminal portion approximates the glomerulus of the nephron, of which it is a part, and its afferent arteriole.

The distal convoluted tubule is shorter than the other portions of the tubule. In the area of the tubule where the distal tubule commences, the epithelial cells differ and form an area referred to as the *macula densa*. The cells in the remainder of the tubule are sensitive to the concentration of antidiuretic hormone (ADH) and adrenocortical steroids which influence reabsorption of substances by the distal tubule

COLLECTING TUBULES. The distal tubules coalesce to form straight collecting tubules which unite to form progressively larger collecting tubules. Groups of the larger tubes come together to form a pyramid-like structure in the medulla. The apex of each pyramid is known as the *papilla* and contains the terminations of collecting tubules through which the urine passes into a cup-like pouch (calyx) of the renal pelvis.

KIDNEY PELVIS. When the ureter joins the kidney, it expands to form a funnel-shaped receiving basin for the urine delivered by the collecting tubules. It has numerous projecting pouches (calyces), each of which encases a renal papilla and is called a *calyx*.

BLOOD SUPPLY. The renal artery to each kidney arises from the abdominal aorta. When the artery enters the kidney, it progressively subdivides to become afferent arterioles. Each *afferent arteriole* enters a nephron to form a glomerulus. The glomerular capillaries unite to form the *efferent arteriole*, which terminates in a second capillary network in which the tubule is invested. The blood pressure in this second set of capillaries is much lower than that in the glomerulus. The blood is then collected into venules and eventually into a renal vein that carries it to the inferior vena cava.

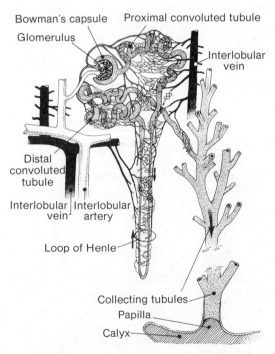

FIGURE 19-2 A renal unit or nephron of the cortex of the kidney is shown with its blood supply and a collecting tubule.

A large volume of blood is continuously circulated through the kidneys. It is estimated that the renal blood flow averages about 1000 to 1200 ml. per minute in an adult, approximately 23 to 24 per cent of the cardiac output.

Just before the afferent arteriole becomes the glomerulus, the cells change and increase in the middle tissue layer of the vascular wall. These special cells are known as *juxtaglomerular cells*. They are responsible for the production of the chemical *renin*.

INNERVATION. Sympathetic nerve fibers from the thoracolumbar autonomic nervous system transmit impulses to the afferent and efferent arterioles, causing vasoconstriction.

Renal Functions

Normal functioning of the body cells is greatly dependent upon a relative constancy of the internal environment. The kidneys play a major role in maintaining this constancy by regulating the water and electrolyte content and the acid-base balance of the body; they *conserve* appropriate amounts of essential substances vital to normal cellular function (e.g., glucose) and *excrete* excesses, the waste products of metabolism, toxic substances and drugs in the urine. The kidneys also have an important *endocrine role* — the production of renin and erythropoietin, and their release into the blood when needed. The processes involved in these functions performed by the kidneys are filtration, selective reabsorption, the transport of substances from the interstitial fluid to the tubule and endocrine secretion (Table 19–1).

FILTRATION. The permeability of the glomerular capillaries is comparable to that

TABLE 19–1 RENAL FUNCTIONS

Overall Function: Homeostasis — the maintenance of a suitable environment for optimum cellular function.
1. Conservation of appropriate amounts of essential substances.
2. Excretion of end products of metabolism, excesses, toxic substances and drugs.
3. Regulation of the pH of body fluids by the elimination of nonvolatile acids.
4. Endocrine secretion of renin and erythropoietin.

of the capillaries elsewhere in the body, and the same principles that govern the movement of fluid out of the arteriolar ends of the capillaries throughout the body are applicable to the filtration process in the glomeruli. The hydrostatic pressure of the blood in the glomerular capillaries is approximately 70 mm. Hg, which is considerably higher than that in the other capillaries of the body. This hydrostatic pressure is opposed by the osmotic pressure of the blood proteins (approximately 30 mm. Hg) plus the hydrostatic pressure in Bowman's capsule (about 20 mm. Hg). The net filtration force is 20 mm. Hg (hydrostatic blood pressure [70] — colloidal osmotic pressure [30] — capsular hydrostatic pressure [20] = 20 mm. Hg).

The average volume of filtrate in both kidneys is estimated to be about 180 liters each day. The glomerular filtration rate (GFR) is directly proportional to the filtration force; the normal rate is approximately 125 ml. per minute. Factors which may alter the glomerular filtration rate are:

1. Change in glomerular capillary hydrostatic pressure, which may be incurred by an increase or decrease in systemic blood pressure or by constriction or dilation of the afferent and efferent arterioles.
2. Increase or decrease in renal artery blood volume.
3. Increase or decrease in the hydrostatic pressure within Bowman's capsule due to compression by ureteral obstruction or disease within the kidney, causing swelling confined within the renal capsule.
4. Decrease or increase in the oncotic pressure (concentration of plasma proteins).
5. Increased glomerular permeability due to disease, such as nephrotic syndrome.
6. Decrease in glomeruli incurred by pathologic destruction.

The glomerular filtration rate can be measured by determining the excretion volume and plasma concentration of a substance which is readily filtered through the glomeruli but not secreted or reabsorbed by the renal tubules.

Many solutes escape from the blood in the glomerular filtrate, but small amounts of only a few of them appear in urine. The formed elements and plasma proteins of the blood do not normally pass out of the glomeruli; the composition of the filtrate is the same as plasma minus the plasma proteins.

TUBULAR REABSORPTION. Reabsorption and secretion are complex renal activities. The composition and volume of the filtrate which enters Bowman's capsule differ markedly from those of urine. Of the 180 liters of filtrate produced in 24 hours, only about 1.5 liters are excreted as urine. Most of the water and many of the solid constituents of the filtrate are needed by the body to maintain homeostasis and normal cell metabolism. Other substances, such as urea, creatinine, uric acid, sulfates and phosphates are waste products of metabolism and are excreted in the urine. The tubule cells selectively reabsorb according to the body's needs. Certain substances, such as glucose and amino acids, are completely reabsorbed when their plasma concentrations are within normal range but appear in the urine when the normal is exceeded. About 99 per cent of the water in the filtrate is reclaimed. Reabsorption of the inorganic salts (e.g., sodium, chloride, calcium, potassium, bicarbonate) is variable, depending mainly on their plasma levels. Reabsorption and secretion are carried out very discriminatively, based on the preceding factors.

Some constituents of the filtrate are passively reabsorbed by diffusion and osmosis through the tubular membrane. Others are reabsorbed by active cellular transport, which entails energy expenditure on the part of the tubular cells and the presence of certain enzymes. The location of reabsorption and secretion in the tubules varies with different filtrate constituents. The *proximal convoluted tubule* is responsible for the greatest amount of reabsorption. All of the glucose and amino acids and a large proportion of the water and other essential substances are reabsorbed here. Only about 20 to 25 per cent of the total volume of filtrate enters the loop of Henle.

In the medulla there are branches of the efferent arterioles of juxtamedullary nephrons that form hairpin loops which approximate the loops of Henle. Each vascular loop of capillaries is called a *vasa recta*. The flow in the ascending limb of the vascular loop is sluggish, so ions diffuse out of the blood readily.

The vasa recta and the loop of Henle play an important role in concentrating the urine and conserving water by means of the countercurrent mechanism and determination of the peritubular osmolality. The countercurrent mechanism implies a ∪ arrangement in which the fluid flows in opposite directions in the two limbs (ascending and descending) and there are interactions between them that alter the osmolality of the fluid along its course in the tube, with the modification being greatest at the base of the loop (Fig. 19–3).

The *loop of Henle* seems to be concerned principally with the transport of sodium chloride ions and water. The ascending limb (the thicker segment) is impermeable to water. It actively transports sodium and chloride ions out into the interstitial fluid, and the tubular fluid becomes hypotonic. The descending limb of the loop of Henle is permeable to water; water moves out to the interstitial fluid which has become hypertonic. At the same time sodium and chloride ions diffuse into the descending limb. The osmolality of the fluid within the descending limb progressively becomes more hypertonic as it approaches the base of the loop. The osmolality of the medullary interstitial fluid is increased, and sodium chloride diffuses into the blood in the descending limb of the vasa recta. But, as the blood flows in the opposite direction in the ascending limb, sodium chloride readily diffuses out again into the medullary interstitium; the osmolality of the blood as it leaves the medulla

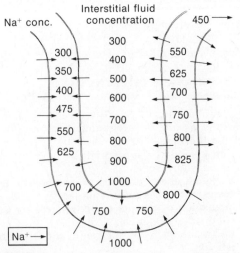

FIGURE 19–3 Sodium concentrations in the loop of Henle.

is only slightly higher than when it entered the vasa recta.

The maintenance of the volume and concentration of body fluids within a narrow normal range is largely controlled by the ability of the kidney tubules to concentrate or dilute the urine. When body fluids are diluted by an excess of water or diminished solute intake (especially sodium), the urine becomes dilute and the volume is increased. Conversely, if the concentration of body fluids is raised to above the normal level by an excessive intake of solutes or an extrarenal loss of water, water reabsorption from the filtrate is increased, concentrating the urine and decreasing the output volume.

The dilution and concentration of urine depend principally on two factors: first, the osmotic pressure of the peritubular fluid, which in turn is mainly dependent on the normal functioning of the loop of Henle and the distal convoluted tubules; and secondly, on the concentration of the antidiuretic hormone in the blood.

The fluid entering the distal tubule is hypotonic, but the volume and osmolality are modified very selectively as it proceeds through the distal and collecting tubules.

Reabsorption of water from the hypotonic filtrate in the distal convoluted and collecting tubules is regulated by the *antidiuretic hormone* (ADH), which increases the permeability of their membranous walls. It is produced by the hypothalamus in the brain, and is stored and released into the blood by the neurohypophysis (posterior pituitary gland). Receptors in the hypothalamus are sensitive to changes in the osmotic pressure of the blood. When the pressure is increased to above normal (for example, by additional sodium), impulses are delivered to the neurohypophysis, resulting in the release of ADH which increases water reabsorption in the tubules. Conversely, if the osmotic pressure falls below the homeostatic level, the release of ADH is inhibited. The tubular membrane becomes relatively impermeable, restricting the reabsorption of water, and the urine is dilute.

The reabsorption of sodium by active cellular transport in the distal and collecting tubules is influenced by the adrenocortical hormone *aldosterone*. A high concentration of aldosterone stimulates the distal tubular cells to reabsorb increasing amounts of sodium. A deficiency of the hormone, such as occurs in Addison's disease, reduces the amount of sodium reclaimed, resulting in an excessive loss in urine. Aldosterone also affects the amount of potassium reclaimed and excreted. Increased concentrations of the hormone promote excretion of the electrolyte, and a deficient amount of aldosterone produces excessive retention of potassium.

TUBULAR SECRETION AND EXCRETION. Tubular cells are capable of actively transporting some substances from the blood into the filtrate — a reverse process to that of reabsorption. The potassium concentration of plasma is regulated by this process. Practically all of the potassium that escapes from the plasma into the filtrate is reabsorbed in the proximal tubule. Any excess in the blood is then actively secreted by the distal tubules and is excreted in exchange for sodium ions.

Cells of the distal tubules play an important role in maintaining a normal acid-base balance. They do this by secreting hydrogen ions into the lumen of the tubules in exchange for sodium ions and by forming ammonium radicals that combine with chlorine ions to form ammonium chloride, which is excreted in the urine (see p. 95 for a discussion of the role of the kidney in pH regulation).

Some drugs are also excreted by active tubular removal from the blood into the tubules. These include Diodrast, para-aminohippuric acid and phenolsulfonphthalein, which may be used to investigate renal function.

ENDOCRINE RENAL SECRETIONS. The kidney produces two endocrine secretions, renin and erythropoietin.

Renin is a proteolytic enzyme that reacts with a fraction of the plasma globulin (angiotensinogen), producing a substance called angiotensin I which is converted to angiotensin II by another enzyme in the lungs. As angiotensin II circulates it causes vasoconstriction of the systemic arterioles and stimulates the secretion of aldosterone and, to a lesser degree, glucocorticoids (Fig. 19–4).

Three factors are suggested as influencing the production and release of renin. The juxtaglomerular cells release renin in response to decreased arteriolar blood vol-

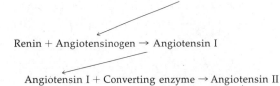

$$\text{Renin} + \text{Angiotensinogen} \rightarrow \text{Angiotensin I}$$

$$\text{Angiotensin I} + \text{Converting enzyme} \rightarrow \text{Angiotensin II}$$
$$\downarrow$$
Constriction of arterioles
Secretion of aldosterone

FIGURE 19–4 Decrease in intravascular volume and/or fall in blood pressure, or stimulation of the macula densa by decreased sodium content in tubular fluid entering the distal tubule.

ume and pressure. The macula densa is sensitive to sodium concentration; a decrease in the sodium content of the tubular fluid entering the distal tubule brings about the release of renin. The release of renin and the ensuing formation of angiotensin II stimulates the release of aldosterone which promotes the retention of sodium ions. Sympathetic stimulation of the juxtaglomerular cells may be associated with the production of renin. The stimulation may be mediated by the release of catecholamines (e.g., adrenalin) by the adrenal medulla or by renal sympathetic innervation.[2, 3]

A second hormone produced by the kidneys is the *renal erythropoietic factor* (REF, erythrogenin). It is produced and secreted into the blood in response to hypoxia, and functions in the maintenance of normal erythrocyte production by the bone marrow. Erythrogenin reacts with a plasma globulin to produce erythropoietin which stimulates the bone marrow to produce and release red blood cells.

Characteristics and Composition of Urine

When the filtrate flows into the main collecting tubules and renal pelvis, it becomes urine. The average volume excreted in 24 hours is approximately 1.5 liters but varies with fluid losses through other channels (e.g., perspiration) and fluid intake. The reaction of urine is usually acid, with a pH of about 6.0, but may range from 4.8 to 8.0 with a varied dietary intake. The acidity increases with high protein ingestion and tis-

sue catabolism, while a vegetable diet produces an alkaline urine.

The specific gravity, which gives a rough estimate of the concentration of solids, ranges from 1.003 to 1.040. The composition of urine varies with dietary intake and metabolic wastes produced. Normally, about 90 to 95 per cent of urine is water. An average of 60 Gm. of organic and inorganic solid wastes are eliminated daily. The chief solutes are urea, creatinine, uric acid and the chlorides, phosphates and sulfates of sodium, potassium, calcium, magnesium and ammonia.

Ureters, Bladder and Urethra

URETERS. Each of the two ureters is a tube 10 to 12 inches in length, extending from a kidney to the bladder. They are situated behind the parietal peritoneum and enter the posterior wall of the lower half of the bladder obliquely. The slanted entrance forms a flap in the bladder wall that serves as a valve to prevent a reflux of urine as the bladder fills or contracts. Each ureter consists of an outer fibrous covering, a middle layer of muscle tissue, and a mucous membrane lining which is continuous with that of the bladder and the renal pelvis.

The function of these tubes is simply to convey urine from the kidneys to the bladder. Contraction of the ureteral muscular tissue produces peristaltic waves which move the urine along the tube and into the bladder in spurts.

BLADDER. The urinary bladder serves as a temporary reservoir for the urine, which it expels at intervals from the body. It is a collapsible muscular sac that lies behind the symphysis pubis. Three layers of plain muscle tissue form the bladder walls. The fibers are arranged in longitudinal, circular and spiral layers. Collectively, these layers are referred to as the *detrusor muscle*. The ureteral orifices in the posterior wall and the urethral opening outline a triangular area called the *trigone*. When the bladder is empty, the mucous membrane lining falls into folds (rugae) except in the area of the trigone (Fig. 9–5).

URETHRA. The *urethra* is a slender tube that conveys urine from the bladder to the exterior. It has a thin layer of plain muscle tissue and is lined with a mucous membrane which is continuous with that of the bladder. The opening from the bladder is controlled by two sphincters: an internal

[2]William F. Ganong: Review of Medical Physiology, 7th ed. Los Altos, Cal., Lange, 1975, pp. 342–343.

[3]Warren H. Chapman, et al.: The Urinary System. Philadelphia, W. B. Saunders, 1973, p. 61.

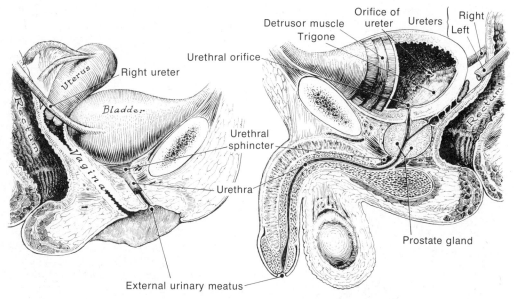

FIGURE 19-5 The bladder, ureters, urethra and prostate.

one which is under autonomic (involuntary) nervous system control, and an external one which is voluntarily controlled by the cerebral cortex. The external urethral orifice is known as the urinary meatus.

In the female, the urethra is about 1.5 inches long and lies anterior to the vagina. The male urethra is approximately 8 inches in length and, on leaving the bladder, passes through the prostate gland. As well as conveying the urine, the male urethra receives the semen from the ejaculatory ducts of the reproductive system, transmitting it through the meatus (Fig. 19–5).

Micturition

This is a term used for the elimination of urine from the bladder. The process involves both autonomic (involuntary) and voluntary nervous impulses. When 300 to 400 ml. of urine collect in the bladder, receptors that are sensitive to stretching initiate impulses which are transmitted by afferent nerve fibers into the lower part of the spinal cord (Fig. 19–6). A reflex response via parasympathetic nerves to the bladder results in contractions of the detrusor muscle and relaxation of the internal sphincter.

The initial impulses from the stretch receptors are also relayed via a spinocortical tract to the cerebral cortex, producing an awareness of the need to void. When a person is prepared to empty the bladder, voluntary impulses are initiated which descend the cord and are carried out to the external

sphincter, causing it to relax. With both sphincters relaxed, urine drains from the bladder through the urethra. Infants and very young children empty their bladder whenever the micturition reflex is initiated, as they have not yet developed voluntary control over the external sphincter. Obviously, any interruption of the spinocortical impulse pathway interferes with control

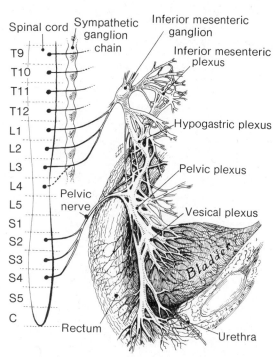

FIGURE 19-6 A diagram showing innervation of the bladder.

of the external sphincter, resulting in involuntary voiding.

IMPAIRED RENAL FUNCTION

Impaired renal function may be due to primary disease in the kidneys or may be secondary to a disorder in an area or areas of the body outside of the kidneys (e.g., cardiac failure, shock, hemorrhage, trauma, respiratory failure, newgrowth compression, urinary bladder infection).

MANIFESTATIONS AND DIAGNOSIS OF IMPAIRED RENAL FUNCTION

Manifestations

In impaired kidney function, the constancy of the internal environment (homeostasis), which is essential for the normal functioning of all body cells, is disrupted. The normal volume, composition and reaction of the body fluids may be altered by the inability of the kidneys to conserve essential substances and excrete excesses, metabolic wastes and toxic substances; disturbances in the functioning of other organs readily develop. Consequently, the signs and symptoms of renal insufficiency are varied, and many are not directly referable to the urinary system. Whether the disease is acute or chronic and whether it affects the glomeruli or the tubules will also vary the manifestations.

ABNORMAL URINARY VOLUME. Oliguria or anuria may develop, especially in acute and advanced renal failure. *Oliguria* means that less than 500 ml. of urine is formed in 24 hours. *Anuria* implies a urinary output of less than 250 ml. in 24 hours and is sometimes referred to as a renal shutdown. The diminished urine formation may be associated with decreased glomerular filtration due to renal disease (e.g., glomerulonephritis), hypotension as in shock and dehydration, decreased renal blood flow or an obstruction within the tubules.

Polyuria, a volume of urine in excess of the normal (over 2000 ml. in 24 hours), may also indicate renal disturbance in which the ability of the tubules to reabsorb water and concentrate the solid wastes is limited. It is most often seen in chronic kidney disease or it may be secondary to diabetes insipidus as a result of a deficiency in the secretion of vasopressin (antidiuretic hormone). Polyuria may not be a manifestation of renal disease but may indicate a disorder elsewhere. Frequently, polyuria is the symptom that may cause an individual to go to a physician where, on investigation, he is found to have diabetes mellitus.

Nocturia (voiding during the night) usually accompanies polyuria and the person becomes desperate for undisturbed rest. Inability of the kidneys to reabsorb the normal amount of water and to concentrate the wastes may be referred to as *hyposthenuria*. As well as the excessive volume, a low specific gravity of approximately 1.010 of the urine persists because the impaired tubules cannot concentrate or vary the amount of solids.

ABNORMAL CONSTITUENTS IN THE URINE. Abnormal constituents revealed in urinalysis vary with the underlying renal disease. They include protein (usually albumin), blood, casts, pus and organisms.

The large molecular structure of serum albumin inhibits its filtration through normal glomeruli. *Albuminuria* usually indicates inflammation and almost always indicates damage to the glomeruli. *Hematuria* denotes blood in the urine and may be macroscopic or recognized only by microscopic examination. It indicates some pathologic process within the kidneys or postrenal structures.

Urinary casts are microscopic cylindrical structures formed in the distal and collecting tubules by the agglutination of cells and cellular debris in a protein matrix. They are molded or cast in the shape of the tubule. Depending on their composition, casts are usually classified as red blood cell, epithelial, hyaline, granular or fatty. They point to the presence of some inflammatory or degenerative process within the tubules. Obviously, *pus and bacteria* in the urine indicate infection in the kidneys or urinary tract.

ABNORMAL URINE COLOR. Abnormal discoloration of urine may be associated with infection within the urinary tract, but more often occurs with a disorder extrinsic to the kidneys and urinary tract. Examples of disorders in which the urine is discolored are: myoglobinuria, in which there has been a release of myoglobin from muscle cells, as occurs in a crushing injury; hemoglobinuria, which may develop following a blood transfusion reaction in which there is a breakdown of erythrocytes and the release of hemoglobin; porphyria, a genetic disorder in which normal use of porphyrin in the formation of hemoglobin does not occur, resulting in porphyrins being eliminated in the urine; and melanoma, a skin newgrowth characterized by excessive pigmentation.

AZOTEMIA. Metabolic wastes accumulate in the blood. Urea, creatinine and uric acid levels are elevated. In acute failure and anuria, the levels rise rapidly. In chronic kidney disease, even though there may be polyuria, the blood urea progressively rises.

FLUID, ELECTROLYTE AND pH IMBALANCES. Generalized *edema* may be one of the early symptoms of renal insufficiency and usually becomes apparent first around the eyes. It may be due to decreased glomerular filtration and the retention of water and sodium, or to an abnormal permeability of the glomeruli to plasma proteins, especially serum albumin. The latter defect is associated with a condition known as nephrosis that occurs more often in children. The loss of plasma protein causes a decrease in the colloidal osmotic pressure of the blood, and an excess of water remains in the interstitial spaces. The urine is high in albumin, and the plasma protein is abnormally low.

In some instances of chronic renal failure due to impaired tubular function, the excessive volume of urine excreted (polyuria) may lead to *dehydration* unless there is a corresponding increase in the water intake.

Deficiencies or excesses of electrolytes may occur, depending on the nature of the renal disturbance and the degree of tissue damage. Failure of impaired tubules to secrete potassium ions is a serious development in renal insufficiency. Abnormal concentrations of sodium and calcium as well as hyperkalemia may also develop, and may seriously affect cardiac function and threaten the patient's life.

Failure of the kidneys' capacity to excrete hydrogen ions by the formation and excretion of acid sodium phosphate and ammonia results in their accumulation in the blood and *acidosis* (see p. 98).

VITAL SIGNS. An elevation of blood pressure occurs in most patients with renal insufficiency associated with parenchymal disease of the kidneys. It is attributed to an increase in the blood volume as a result of the retention of sodium and water or a decrease in the renal blood flow and consequent secretion of renin by the juxtaglomerular cells. The renin results in the formation of angiotensin II which causes vasoconstriction of the arterioles and increased aldosterone release.

The pulse may become weak because of heart failure which may result from hypertension, excessive fluid load or disturbed electrolyte concentrations. Of the electrolyte disturbances, hyperkalemia (elevated serum potassium) is the most serious (see p. 89).

The patient may experience dyspnea due to pulmonary edema. Kussmaul's breathing (deep rapid respirations), characteristic of acidosis, may be manifested. In advanced renal failure, the breath has an ammoniacal or "uremic" odor.

Fever is associated with infection in the kidneys or secondary infection, such as pneumonia, that may develop readily if pulmonary edema is present.

GASTROINTESTINAL DISTURBANCES. The patient experiences anorexia and, in the later stages of renal dysfunction, nausea and vomiting. Diarrhea may also be troublesome in the acute stage. Hiccups may develop in advanced failure, and the oral mucosa may become sore and ulcerated.

HEADACHE AND PAIN. Headache is an early complaint as a result of the hypertension and cerebral edema. Pain and tenderness in the back between the lower ribs and iliac crest occur in acute kidney disease because of the stretching of the renal capsule.

VISUAL DISTURBANCES. The patient may complain of "spots before his eyes" or blurred vision which are attributed to edema of the optic papillae (papilledema). Loss of vision may actually occur as a result of a retinal hemorrhage.

NEUROLOGICAL MANIFESTATIONS. Signs of both irritation and depression of the nervous system appear in renal failure. The patient becomes irritable, lethargic and drowsy. He may become disoriented and progress to a comatose state. Muscular twitching may be noticeable and, in advanced kidney disease, may be an indication of ensuing convulsions.

SKIN CHANGES. In progressive renal insufficiency, the skin may take on a yellowish-brown discoloration. Dryness and scaliness are common with chronic disease and polyuria. The patient may complain of pruritus, and excoriated lesions may appear from scratching. In advanced failure, urea frost may be manifested, formed by deposits of small white crystals of urea excreted by the sweat glands. The frost is usually first seen around the mouth.

HEMATOLOGIC CHANGES. Most patients with prolonged renal disease show a reduction in the production of red blood cells and a resultant anemia. Normal kidneys, as well as the liver, contribute erythropoietin which stimulates erythropoiesis. In the diseased kidney, this activity may be decreased.

With uremia, the patient develops a bleeding tendency; the thrombocytes are defective and the bleeding time increases. Petechiae, purpura or bleeding from mucous membranes may be manifested.

Diagnostic Procedures

The investigation of renal dysfunction may include examination of urine specimens which may be voided or obtained by bladder or urethral catheterization, blood chemistry determinations, renal function tests, roentgenographic studies and ultrasound procedures.

URINE EXAMINATIONS. The specimen of urine submitted for analysis is *voided* unless the physician requests that it be a *midstream* sample or collected by *catheter*. The voided specimen should be of the first voiding in the morning, if possible, since it provides some information about the kidneys' ability to concentrate wastes. Midstream and catheter samples are collected in sterile containers. All specimens are labelled clearly with the patient's name, time collected, method of collection and the examination required.

The color and clarity of the urine are noted, the reaction and specific gravity are determined, and tests are made for the presence and amounts of protein, sugar, ketone bodies (acetone, acetoacetic acid and hydroxybutyric acid), urea, creatinine, sodium, potassium, chloride, bicarbonate, sulfates and phosphates. Microscopic examination of the urinary sediment, which is obtained by centrifuging the urine, may reveal abnormal constituents such as blood cells, casts, pus and bacteria.

If the urine is to be cultured, a midstream or catheter specimen is collected. Catheterization is avoided, if possible, because of the danger of introducing infection into the urethra or bladder. To obtain a midstream sample from a female, the perineum and meatus are cleansed the same as for catheterization to prevent possible contamination from the perineum and vaginal secretion. In the case of the male, the external meatus is cleansed before voiding. Following the cleansing, the patient is instructed to void, and the first 50 ml. of urine are discarded to eliminate possible contamination by organisms that may be in the urethra.

A *24-hour collection* of urine may be requested for quantitative determination of the total solid content or of specific substances such as protein, glucose, certain electrolytes and hormones. When the collection is started, the patient voids and that urine is discarded. At the end of the 24 hours he voids and the urine is included in the specimen. The urine is refrigerated or kept in a cool place. If the patient is ambulatory, it is made clear to him that all his urine is to be saved during the designated period.

BLOOD CHEMISTRY DETERMINATIONS. Impaired glomerular filtration and loss of tubular ability to reabsorb and excrete discriminately lead to alterations in plasma composition. Blood specimens may be requested to determine the concentration of the following substances:

Protein Metabolic Nitrogenous Wastes
    Urea nitrogen (BUN) — Normal: 10 to 20 mg. per cent
    Creatinine — Normal: 0.5 to 1.5 mg. per cent
    Uric acid — Normal: 3 to 7 mg. per cent

Electrolytes
    Serum sodium — Normal: 135 to 145 mEq./liter
    Serum potassium — Normal: 3.5 to 5.0 mEq./liter
    Serum calcium — Normal: 4.5 to 6.0 mEq./liter
    Serum chloride — Normal: 96 to 106 mEq./liter
    Total serum base — Normal: 145 to 160 mEq./liter
    Serum phosphorus (inorganic) — Normal: 1.0 to 1.5 mEq./liter or 2.4 to 4.5 mg. per cent

Plasma Proteins — Normal: 6 to 8 Gm. per cent
    Albumin — Normal: 3.5 to 5.5 Gm. per cent
    Globulin — Normal: 1.5 to 3.5 Gm. per cent

HEMATOLOGIC EVALUATION. The hemoglobin concentration and hematocrit are determined, since anemia is a common problem. If infection is suspected a leukocyte count is done, and a thrombocyte count and prothrombin time may be needed in advanced chronic renal failure.

RENAL FUNCTION TESTS. Renal function tests may be classified according to the kidney function being evaluated. In renal function, the removal or clearance of substances from the blood is achieved by glomerular filtration and tubular cell activity. If a substance passes freely through the glomeruli, and is neither reabsorbed or secreted by the tubules, the quantity appearing in the urine is the same as that filtered by the glomeruli. By measuring the amount excreted in the urine in a specified period of time, information is obtained about the efficiency of glomerular filtration. The substances used for this evaluation may be creatinine or urea, which are naturally occurring metabolites, or inulin.

GLOMERULAR FILTRATION RATE. For determining the glomerular filtration rate, the urea, creatinine or inulin clearance test may be used.

The *urea clearance test* involves the following procedure: Breakfast may be withheld until the test is completed or a light breakfast without protein is taken; tea and coffee may be given. The patient is given a minimum of 500 to 1000 ml. of water to drink to promote urine formation. He is asked to void and this urine is discarded. The time is noted. A venous blood specimen is obtained for determination of the blood urea nitrogen. The patient is asked to void 1 and 2 hours after the discarded urine was voided. These specimens are kept separate and sent to the laboratory. The specimen labels indicate the exact time the urine was collected. A venous blood sample is collected about ½ hour before each urine specimen is collected. From the BUN and the concentration of urea in the urine formed in 1 and 2 hours the laboratory calculates the volume of blood cleared of urea per minute. The formula used in the calculation is $GFR = \frac{U \times V}{P}$, in which GFR is the glomerular filtration rate, U represents the concentration of the "clearance substance" in the urine, V is the volume of urine secreted per minute, and P indicates the plasma concentration of the clearance substance. Normally, 75 to 120 ml. of plasma are cleared of urea per minute.

In the *creatinine clearance test,* the patient is kept at rest during the test, since endogenous creatinine is produced in muscular activity. Meat should be eliminated from the diet for a period of 48 hours before the test. A 24-hour specimen of urine and a venous blood specimen are collected for creatinine concentration determinations. The rate of urinary excretion per minute is calculated. The normal amount of creatinine excreted in 24 hours varies with age; in an adult the normal is about 1.2 to 1.7 Gm., and in a child it is approximately 0.36 Gm. Calculations are made to determine the volume of plasma cleared of creatinine per minute, which is the glomerular filtration rate.

Inulin, a polysaccharide, is given intravenously and, normally, is readily filtered through the glomeruli but is neither secreted nor reabsorbed by tubular cells. The patient is encouraged to drink 500 to 1000 ml. of water 1 to 2 hours preceding the administration of the inulin. A directive is received from the physician as to the time urine specimens are to be collected and a blood sample taken. The formula given above is used to calculate the GFR. The inulin clearance test is considered to be the most accurate method for measuring the GFR.

TUBULAR FUNCTION. Assessment of tubular function involves testing the kidneys' ability to concentrate or dilute solid wastes, excrete phenolsulfonphthalein (PSP) and acidify the urine.

In order to maintain homeostasis, normal kidney function is able to vary the concentration of solid wastes and the volume of urine according to the volume of body fluids. When there is an excessive loss of body fluid by other channels or a restricted intake, more water is reabsorbed by the renal tubules; the solid wastes are excreted in a smaller volume of urine and the specific gravity is high. Conversely, with a large fluid intake, less water is reabsorbed by the tubules, the volume of urine is greater and the specific gravity is lower than usual. This ability to vary the volume and concentration of the urine appropriately is impaired in tubular damage and may be tested by a concentration or dilution test.

The *concentration test* is designed to determine the kidney's ability to concentrate urine when the fluid intake is restricted. Fluids are restricted over a specified period. Then, two or three urine specimens are collected, and the specific gravity of each is determined. If the kidneys are normal, the specific gravity is not less than 1.024. The procedure regarding the period of fluid restriction and the number of specimens collected varies in different institutions. The commonly used Fishberg concentration test involves restricted fluids with the evening meal (approximately 200 ml.) and then no food or fluid until the test is completed the next morning. Three hourly urine specimens are collected in the morning (e.g., at 6, 7 and 8 A.M.). The time of voiding each specimen is indicated on the labels. *All the urine voided each time must be submitted to the laboratory.* Before the test is begun, the patient receives an explanation so he will understand the reasons for the fluid restriction and collection of specimens.

The *dilution test* evaluates the ability of the kidneys to dilute the urine following a relatively large fluid intake. The procedure is as follows: The patient remains in bed. Upon awakening in the morning he voids, and that urine is discarded. The test is explained to the patient, and he is then given 1 liter of fluid over a period of 30 to 45 minutes. The fluid may be water, lemonade or clear weak tea. The patient voids in 1, 2, 3 and 4 hours, and *all the urine voided each time is submitted to the laboratory.* The time of voiding is indicated on each specimen. With normal kidney functioning, the specific gravity of the first specimen should be about 1.002, with a gradual increase occurring in the others.

The *phenolsulfonphthalein (PSP)* test indicates the secretory ability of the renal tubules. PSP is a red dye that is given intravenously and is completely excreted in a short time by normal kidneys. Less than total excretion of that given may indicate tubular damage and inefficiency or an obstruction of urinary flow through the renal pelves or lower urinary tract.

The procedure entails giving the patient approximately 400 to 500 ml. of water and having him empty his bladder. This urine is discarded. The physician gives the prescribed amount (usually 1 ml.) of PSP intravenously, and the exact time is noted. The patient is kept at rest during the test. Urine specimens are then collected 15, 30, 60 and 120 minutes after the dye is administered. *All the urine voided each time is included in the specimens,* and the time each was voided is clearly indicated on the labels. The intervals for the collection of urine specimens may vary in different situations; the nurse should receive a specific directive. Normally, about 25 per cent is eliminated in the first 15 minutes, 40 to 50 per cent of the dye is excreted over 1 hour and 75 per cent over 2 hours.

Normal renal tubules are able to excrete acid ions and conserve base ions to maintain the normal pH of body fluids. Urinalysis includes testing the urine for acidity.

RENAL SCAN. The condition of the kidneys may also be studied by administering radioactive iodohippurate (Hippuran-I^{131}) intravenously and observing its distribution in the kidney and its elimination. As the Hippuran-I^{131} passes through the kidneys, scintillation probes or counters are placed over the kidneys to record the renal concentration of the radioactive substance in the form of a tracing called a renogram. A tracing is obtained for each kidney. From the renograms the physician is able to assess the vascularization of the kidneys.

Voided urine specimens may also be collected following the injection, and are tested for the content of radioactive iodohippurate. Normally, about 75 per cent is excreted within 30 to 40 minutes.

INTRAVENOUS PYELOGRAM. A radiopaque substance that is eliminated by the kidneys is given intravenously, and a series of x-ray films are made at intervals to note the concentration of the contrast medium in the renal pelves, ureters and bladder.

Preparation for an intravenous pyelogram includes an explanation of the procedure to the patient and questioning as to whether he has any allergies or has ever had asthma, eczema or a reaction to iodine. The physician is advised if any sensitivity or allergy is indicated by the patient. No fluids are given for 8 to 10 hours preceding the examination to provide a better concentration of the radiopaque substance. Castor oil or another laxative may be ordered the day before, and an enema given 2 to 3 hours before the test to cleanse the intestines of gas and feces which produce shadows on the film. The vigorous catharsis may be quite exhausting to the patient; he should be allowed to rest undisturbed as much as possible. If the patient is weak or elderly, he is advised to signal for the nurse so that assistance can be given when he goes to the bathroom. The laxative is contraindicated if the patient has a gastrointestinal condition, such as peptic ulcer or colitis.

The contrast medium which is given intravenously is an iodide preparation to which the patient may be sensitive. An emergency tray or cart should be readily available in the event of a reaction. The cart should have epinephrine (adrenalin), intravenous antihistamine and adrenocorticosteroid preparations, and a vasopressor agent such as norepinephrine (Levophed) or metaraminol (Aramine). Oxygen and a self-inflating resuscitation bag and mask should also be available. The patient is advised that he is likely to experience a salty taste and a sudden flush of warmth during the slow injection of the dye. He is observed closely for signs of respiratory distress, cold, clammy perspiration and urticaria. These and any complaints of unusual sensations are promptly reported to the physician.

Following the x-ray series, the patient is encouraged to take additional fluids to correct the dehydration incurred by the restriction of fluids and cleansing of the bowel.

CYSTOSCOPY AND RETROGRADE PYELOGRAM. Cystoscopy involves the passage of a cystoscope through the urethra into the bladder. The instrument is equipped with a light which permits direct visualization of the internal surface of the bladder. A long, fine catheter may also be introduced into each renal pelvis through the cystoscope (ureteral catheterization), and a urine specimen collected from each kidney. Ureteral catheterization may be used to obtain specimens from one or both kidneys for microscopic examination and culture, or in renal function tests when the function of each kidney is to be determined. For example, during cystoscopy and ureteral catheterization, phenosulfonphthalein (PSP) may be given intravenously, and its appearance in the urine from each kidney noted and timed. Normally, it appears in 4 to 6 minutes following the administration. The specimens must be labelled as to right or left ureter.

A radiopaque iodide preparation may then be introduced into the catheters, and x-rays are taken which outline the renal pelves and ureters. This procedure is referred to as a *retrograde pyelogram,* and may be used in place of intravenous pyelography because the patient is sensitive to the intravenous contrast medium.

Preparation of the patient for a cystoscopy includes an explanation of the procedure. The well prepared patient who knows what to expect is more relaxed, which lessens the spasms of the urethral sphincters and the associated discomfort. When the lithotomy position is described, he is assured that he will be draped so there will be minimal exposure. If there is an existing problem that interferes with comfortable flexion of the lower limbs, it is brought to the attention of the cystoscopy room staff so the positioning may be modified accordingly. The patient's signature indicating his consent for the examination is usually required. He is given extra fluids for several hours preceding the examination to insure a satisfactory flow of urine for specimens.

He may also receive a sedative such as sodium pentobarbital (Nembutal) or meperidine hydrochloride (Demerol) ½ hour before the cystoscopy to promote relaxation. Children usually receive a general anesthetic, so food and fluid are restricted for 6 to 8 hours preceding and intravenous fluid is administered to insure urinary flow.

Upon completion of the examination, the patient rests in bed for a few hours. Discomfort in the back or bladder region may be relieved by local heat application (hot water bottle or electric heating pad) or a warm tub bath if the patient's condition permits. Additional fluids are encouraged. Any severe pain or persisting bright blood in the urine is reported to the physician.

RENAL ANGIOGRAPHY. Renal blood vessels may be outlined on an x-ray film following the administration of a radiopaque substance into the vascular system. The contrast medium may be injected directly into the aorta through a small catheter introduced into a femoral artery, and passed retrogradely into the aorta to just above the origin of the renal arteries. Since the patient may be sensitive to the radiopaque iodide preparation, the same precautions as cited for intravenous pyelography should be followed. Preparation of the patient is similar to that noted for the patient having intravenous pyelography. The site of catheter introduction into the femoral artery is observed frequently for bleeding for several hours. The site is also inspected for local swelling, redness and tenderness. The temperature of the lower limbs is noted and the popliteal and pedal pulses are checked. Any indication of impaired circulation is reported promptly.

PERCUTANEOUS RENAL BIOPSY. A biopsy is a valuable test in diagnosis and assessment of the effects of treatment but carries with it the risk of hemorrhage. It is contraindicated if the patient has hypertension, a bleeding tendency, only one kidney, or suspected perirenal abscess. Before a patient is posted for renal biopsy, coagulation, bleeding and prothrombin times are determined. If these are satisfactory, the patient's blood is typed and compatible blood is kept available in the event of hemorrhage. An explanation is made to the patient of what he may expect. He is advised that he will be in the prone position over a firm pillow (kidney elevator) for a brief period. A written consent is required for the procedure.

The exact location of the kidney is identified by x-ray which may include an intravenous pyelogram and the position indicated on the skin surface. The skin is cleansed and local anesthesia is used. The patient is instructed to hold his breath during the insertion of the needle and the actual taking of the specimen. Following the removal of the biopsy needle, pressure is applied to the site for 15 minutes, and then a pressure dressing is applied.

The blood pressure and pulse are recorded every 15 minutes for 1 hour, then every 30 minutes for a period of 1 to 2 hours, and then every 4 hours for 24 hours. A specimen of urine is sent to the laboratory daily for 3 to 4 days for examination for blood. The patient is kept on bed rest in the dorsal recumbent position for 36 to 48 hours, or until the urine is cleared of blood.

RETROGRADE RENAL BRUSH BIOPSY.[4] Recently, a diagnostic procedure has been introduced that involves brushing the tissue surface to obtain cells for cytologic examination.

The patient receives a general anesthetic and an intravenous infusion is started so that a contrast dye can be given to facilitate the movement of the brush. A cystoscopic examination is done to rule out abnormalities at bladder and urethral levels. A special ureteral catheter is introduced through which the biopsy brush is passed into the pelvis. The urologist manipulates the brush into appropriate areas and moves the brush back and forth several times to pick up cells which become entrapped in the bristles.

When the brush is withdrawn, the ureteral catheter is irrigated and the washings and brush tip are retained for cytology examination. A 24-hour collection of urine may be requested; it also undergoes cytologic examination.

When the patient recovers from the anes-

thetic, he is encouraged to take fluids freely. The patient may experience colicky renal pain and require an analgesic.

DISORDERS INVOLVING RENAL DYSFUNCTION

Uremia

Uremia may be defined as a symptomatic blood elevation of metabolic products normally excreted in the urine. It is not a disease entity but rather a state or complex of symptoms reflecting failure of the kidneys to excrete the metabolic wastes and excess substances. The uremic state may develop rapidly with acute renal failure or gradually over a period of months or years in chronic renal insufficiency.

The onset of uremia is usually marked by an increase in the patient's hypertension, nausea and vomiting, persisting severe headache, visual disturbances and weakness. Muscular twitching, disorientation, convulsions and coma are ominous signs. The volume of urinary output may be reduced, body chemistry, fluid volume and pH are abnormal, and generalized edema, cardiac failure and pulmonary edema are likely to ensue as a result of the sodium, potassium and fluid retention.

Uremia may be corrected by treatment of the cause of impaired renal function. During this period, the blood level of wastes may be reduced by dialysis (see p. 631). In the case of chronic renal failure due to permanent kidney damage, the patient may be maintained on regular hemodialysis once or twice weekly and controlled dietary and fluid intake.

Hydronephrosis

Hydronephrosis implies distention of the renal tubules, calyces and pelvis by the accumulation of fluid secondary to defective urinary drainage. The cause of the obstruction may be an intrinsic or extrinsic newgrowth, stricture of the ureter due to inflammation or fibrous scar tissue, or a calculus. In infants, it may develop as the result of a congenital developmental error in the form of a stricture or aberrant structure.

Hydronephrosis produces a palpable mass, pain, and renal tissue damage by compression. The cause is sought and treated.

If infection is the initiating factor or is su-

---

[4]Rita R. Gittes: "Retrograde Renal and Ureteral Brush Biopsy." Am. J. Nurs., Vol. 78, No. 3 (March 1978), pp. 410–412.

perimposed, the accumulated fluid may be purulent. The condition may then be referred to as *pyonephrosis*.

Acute Renal Failure

Acute renal failure is a sudden, severe interruption of kidney function that in most instances is a complication of another disorder and is reversible. It is generally characterized by a urinary output of 400 ml. or less in 24 hours.

ETIOLOGY. The primary or initiating causes of acute renal failure are many, but the basic mechanisms causing the failure in most instances are tubular necrosis due to inadequate tissue perfusion and hypoxia, or acute inflammation of glomeruli. Possible causes include the following.

Inadequate renal perfusion, which may be associated with shock (traumatic, surgical, septic), cardiac failure, hemorrhage, dehydration, renal artery occlusion, or sequestration of plasma as occurs in burns, may be a factor.

Nephrotoxic agents that are possible causes of a renal shutdown may be endogenous or exogenous in origin. Epithelial cells are destroyed; the tubular lumens are obliterated by swelling and edema of the tissues as well as by casts formed from the sloughed cells. Examples of endogenous nephrotoxins are hemoglobin, released in hemolysis of erythrocytes following incompatible blood transfusion, and myoglobin, released from muscle cells in crushing injuries. The molecules of hemoglobin pass through the glomeruli and become concentrated in the tubules, obstructing the flow of filtrate. Similarly, the tubular necrosis that follows a crushing injury is attributed to the myoglobin accumulating in the tubules and causing an obstruction, as well as to shock. The individual who has been "pinned down under a weight" for a period of time or who has been subjected to limb ischemia may appear in satisfactory condition when released, but should be put to bed under close observation. He is likely to develop severe shock, acute renal failure and gross edema of the injured part hours later.

Exogenous nephrotoxins may be poisons or drugs. Poisons, which may be taken accidentally or with suicidal intent, include carbon tetrachloride, ethylene glycol (a constituent of antifreeze), bichloride of mercury,

chloroform and lead. Common pharmaceuticals which may prove toxic and damaging to the tubules include sulfonamide preparations (e.g., sulfadiazine), salicylates, phenacetin, kanamycin and amphotericin B. Generally, these have been administered in excessive dosage or the patient has a hypersensitivity.

A third factor implicated in acute renal failure is *obstruction to urinary outflow,* especially if the obstruction is prolonged. Calculi, a newgrowth or prostatic hypertrophy may obstruct collecting tubules, the pelvis, a ureter or the bladder; the accumulation of fluid within the kidney compresses blood vessels and nephrons, seriously reducing kidney function.

Glomerulonephritis associated with posthemolytic streptococcal infection may precipitate acute renal failure (see p. 648).

SIGNS AND SYMPTOMS. Acute renal failure is reflected in a marked decrease in urinary output, the effects produced by the retention of an excess of certain biochemical substances in the blood and a decrease in the pH of body fluids. Blood urea and serum creatinine, potassium and sodium chloride concentrations are elevated; the pH is decreased and bicarbonate, hematocrit and hemoglobin levels are below normal.

The first sign of acute renal failure is oliguria which may progress rapidly to anuria. In conditions in which renal insufficiency frequently occurs the physician may request an indwelling catheter so that the hourly production of urine may be determined. If the patient is anuric, a retention catheter is not used in order to reduce the possibility of high-risk infection. An output of less than 30 ml. per hour is an indication for concern and is reported immediately. If oliguria or anuria persists for a few days, manifestations of water retention and disturbances of blood chemistry are likely to develop. Sodium and water retention cause edema and, unless the fluid intake is controlled, overhydration may lead to cardiac failure and pulmonary edema. The serum sodium and chloride levels may not appear abnormal because of the dilution by the retained fluid.

The elevation in serum potassium becomes a serious threat to heart action. In addition to the fact that potassium is not being eliminated by the kidneys, hemolysis and the breakdown of tissue cells by the primary condition (trauma, burns, sepsis, etc.) increase the concentration of potassium ions in the blood. Metabolic acidosis which also develops in acute renal failure promotes the movement of potassium out of the cells. Hyperkalemia may be manifested by depression of tendon reflexes, numbness, muscular weakness, flaccid paralysis and decreased respiratory rate and volume. Cardiac arrhythmias are common, and arrest may occur.[5]

The rate of the accumulation of nitrogenous wastes (urea and creatinine) in the blood varies with the cause of the renal insufficiency. If there is rapid catabolism, as in infection, fever, and pathologic destruction of tissue, the blood concentration of nitrogenous wastes may rise more quickly. The onset of the uremic state is usually marked by mental changes, nausea and vomiting, and probably hiccups. The patient complains of pruritus.

Metabolic acidosis develops because the hydrogen ions produced in metabolism are not being eliminated by the renal tubules. Respirations are increased in rate and depth, and an acidotic odor of the breath becomes noticeable.

Leukocytosis may be present; anemia is likely to develop fairly quickly, and is manifested by a decrease in the hematocrit and hemoglobin. If the renal failure persists, the patient may develop a bleeding tendency. Ulcerated areas in the mouth are common and may bleed. Vomitus and stools may contain blood, and petechiae, and ecchymoses may appear. As the condition worsens, disseminated intravascular coagulation (DIC) may develop (see p. 262).

The patient becomes drowsy and may progress to a comatose state. Muscle twitching and convulsions may also develop.

NURSING CARE. The outcome in acute renal failure is unpredictable. Many patients do recover; tubular healing and repair occur, and there is no serious residual impairment. Those who do not recover are not necessarily terminated by renal failure alone; frequently, the cause is the seriousness of the underlying cause or the combination of several associated disorders and complications. The patient with renal insufficiency is very susceptible to infection, especially pulmonary. Fluid in the alveoli (pulmonary edema) and the retention of secretions due to inability to cough because

of weakness predispose to pneumonia. Early recognition of renal insufficiency and prompt treatment are important. The nurse may play an important role in early recognition by being familiar with the possible causes of renal failure and by being alert to any significant decrease in a patient's urinary output.

If the renal failure is reversible, the patient experiences a period of diuresis following the oliguric period; large volumes of urine are excreted. The patient's fluid balance and electrolyte levels are observed closely, since excessive losses may occur due to tubular inability to concentrate the urine at this time. A diuretic phase may not be observed if the patient has been treated by dialysis.

The following discussion focuses on care related to the renal failure. Efforts are directed toward the maintenance of electrolyte concentrations within a range compatible with life, the prevention of overhydration and minimal production of nitrogenous wastes.

OBSERVATIONS. The patient with acute renal failure is seriously ill and requires constant nursing care and close observation for changes which may occur suddenly. An accurate record of the fluid intake and output is essential. An indwelling catheter may be used so that the hourly production of urine may be determined. As cited previously, an output of less than 30 ml. hourly or 500 ml. daily is ominous. Any evident perspiration is recorded, as this will be taken into consideration when estimating the volume of fluid the patient should have.

The *pulse, respirations* and *blood pressure* are checked frequently. Cardiac function may be impaired by the retention of potassium and fluid or by hypertension which may accompany renal parenchymal disease. Frequent electrocardiograms may be done to detect changes in the waves indicative of an elevated serum potassium level (hyperkalemia) or continuous monitoring is established, if available.

Any edema is noted, and the patient's weight is recorded daily if he is on a weighing bed. A loss each day of approximately 0.2 to 0.3 kg. may be expected as a result of catabolism and the restricted intake. No loss or a gain usually indicates fluid retention. The respirations are observed for signs of developing pulmonary edema, which may result from overhydration and cardiac failure. A noticeable increase in the volume and depth of respirations may point to acidosis.

---

[5]In hyperkalemia, the electrocardiogram shows a prolonged Q R S complex and increased amplitude and peaking of T waves.

The blood pressure is taken at frequent regular intervals to provide information on the patient's progress. A progressive rise in excess of normal levels is reported to the physician; it may point to increasing uremia. The temperature is taken every 4 hours, even if normal, since a sudden elevation may occur and indicate complicating infection.

Muscular twitching, increasing drowsiness and disorientation are reported, since they may be manifestations of uremia, cerebral edema and approaching convulsions and coma.

Frequent laboratory determinations of blood urea and serum creatinine and electrolytes are followed closely. The sodium and potassium levels are especially important in decisions relating to the types of solutions to be administered, and the patient's fluid balance and weight are used in determining the daily volume of fluid to be given.

The hematocrit and hemoglobin are noted; a transfusion of packed cells may be necessary as treatment for anemia.

FLUIDS AND NUTRITION. The daily fluid intake is limited to 500 ml. plus an amount equal to the urinary output of the preceding 24 hours. The 500 ml. replaces the obligatory loss through the skin and lungs. The fluid that may be given will depend on the laboratory findings. An explanation of the fluid restriction is made to the patient so he will understand why he may have only a limited amount distributed over 24 hours.

A minimum of 100 to 200 Gm. of potassium-free carbohydrate is given daily to reduce the amount of tissue protein and fat broken down for energy. Protein is restricted to avoid a further rise in blood urea. If the patient is not vomiting, it may be taken orally. A part of the carbohydrate may be administered as glucose dissolved in part of the allotted volume of water. A few drops of lemon juice may be added to make the solution less insipid. The physician may prefer to administer the carbohydrate by intravenous infusion of glucose in water, reserving only a small volume of water to be given orally. If hyperkalemia is present, 50 ml. glucose 50 per cent may be given intravenously with a dose of regular insulin. This promotes the movement of potassium into the cells as well as providing calories.

Some physicians provide essential amino acids as well as hypertonic glucose by infusion into a central vein (parenteral alimenta-

tion; see p. 504) on the basis that the protein is necessary for synthesis of body tissue, enzymes, antibodies, etc.[6] The delivery of these nutrients requires the administration of a considerable volume of fluid, so parenteral administration of nutrients is used only if the patient is treated by hemodialysis to remove the excess fluid and prevent overloading the heart.

REST. The patient's activity is restricted to minimize the production of metabolic wastes. The nurse explains the need for rest to the patient, bathes him and provides assistance in order to conserve his energy during necessary movement.

MOUTH AND SKIN CARE. In renal failure, the mouth requires special care. The tongue becomes coated, salivary secretion is reduced, and the mucosa and lips are dry and frequently encrusted. Ulcerative lesions may develop, and the patient may be distressed by the disagreeable taste frequently associated with uremia. Sordes predisposes him to respiratory infection, local mouth infections and parotitis. Frequent cleansing of the mouth with hydrogen peroxide and rinsing with an antiseptic mouthwash are necessary, followed by a light application of mineral oil to which a few drops of lemon juice may be added. Petroleum jelly or cold cream is applied to the lips. The limited fluid intake and dry mouth frequently are a great source of distress to the patient. Resourcefulness on the part of the nurse may reduce the discomfort. Rinsing the mouth with ice-cold mouthwash or water is more acceptable than using lukewarm solutions. Occasional rinsing of the mouth with ice-cold fruit juice or ginger ale provides a change. Tart fruit candies such as "lemon drops" are helpful to stimulate secretions, reduce thirst and, at the same time, supply a little sugar.

The patient is bathed daily to remove the increased wastes that may be excreted in perspiration and to provide comfort. His position is changed frequently, and pressure areas are gently massaged and protected by squares of skeepskin to prevent pressure sores.

PREVENTION OF INFECTION. Infection is extremely hazardous in renal failure; the patient is more susceptible and handles it poorly. When it is possible, the patient is placed in

---

[6]W. Peter Geis and S. Iwatsuki: "Acute and Chronic Renal Failure." Surg. Clin. North Am., Vol. 57, No. 6 (Dec. 1977), p. 1269.

a single room, and no one with an infection is permitted to care for or visit him. Frequent change of position, deep breathing and coughing are instituted to prevent pulmonary stasis and complications. The nurse who is also caring for other patients may be required to wear a mask and gown when giving care to the person with renal failure.

If infection develops, an antibiotic is administered. Tetracycline is not used because it has a marked catabolic effect and increases the creatinine level.

EMOTIONAL SUPPORT. Acute renal failure that is secondary to some serious disorder certainly heightens the patient's fear and anxiety. He requires an explanation of what is wrong and what is being done for him, as well as reassurance that someone will remain with him. If the patient is sufficiently alert, questions may be asked and should be answered.

PRECAUTIONS. Side rails are kept in position since the uremic patient may become drowsy and disoriented. High nitrogenous waste retention frequently leads to convulsions and coma.

MEDICATIONS. Furosemide (Lasix) may be given intravenously for two or three doses, but, if the urinary output is not satisfactorily reestablished, the drug is not usually repeated.

Administering a drug to a patient in renal failure requires knowledge of the metabolic and excretory course of the drug — that is, what happens to it within the body. Those drugs with which renal cells normally react or which are excreted by the kidneys are not given or, if used, are administered in smaller dosages than usually prescribed. Drugs containing potassium or sodium must also not be given.

DIURETIC PHASE. Improvement in renal function is manifested by a steady increase in the volume of urine. The latter may rise rapidly to as much as 3000 to 3500 ml. in 24 hours. The diuresis is accompanied by marked losses of potassium, sodium and water because the tubules have not yet regained their ability to regulate the volume and composition of urine. Frequent serum electrolyte determinations continue, and necessary replacements are made either orally or intravenously. The fluid intake is increased to cover the volume lost. The nitrogenous waste concentration (BUN) decreases more slowly.

The patient receives a soft diet and then a light diet with limited protein content, which is increased gradually as the blood urea level falls. The nurse continues to record the intake and output, and renal concentration tests may be done to determine if there is some residual insufficiency due to tubular necrosis.

PREPARATION FOR DISCHARGE. Before being discharged from the hospital, the patient and family are advised that activity should be resumed gradually and that extra rest will be necessary for several weeks. Dietary instructions are given; the importance of avoiding infection is stressed, and suggestions are made as to protective measures to be used. The patient is advised of the date he is to see his physician or go to the clinic for a checkup, and is told that he will be expected to take with him a specimen of the urine voided on rising that morning. The prolonged convalescence frequently causes socioeconomic problems for the patient and family. The nurse may be able to assist by a referral to a social service or welfare organization.

DIALYSIS. If conservative measures are not effective in correcting the renal insufficiency, hemodialysis or peritoneal dialysis may be instituted. Indications for dialysis are hyperkalemia, increasing blood urea and serum creatinine levels and pulmonary edema. Hemodialysis is considered preferable for the patient with acute renal failure; there is greater patient tolerance of daily short periods of dialysis as opposed to lengthy dialyses every 2 to 3 days (see discussions of hemodialysis, p. 634; peritoneal dialysis, p. 632).

COMPLICATIONS. Complications which commonly develop in renal failure include hyperkalemia, cardiac insufficiency, convulsions and coma.

Hyperkalemia. Since potassium is liberated from the cells in tissue breakdown and cannot be eliminated in renal failure, the extracellular concentration may reach toxic levels. Cardiac function becomes impaired, and failure or sudden cardiac arrest may occur. The nurse should be alert to possible clinical symptoms of potassium intoxication which include generalized muscular weakness, shallow respirations, complaints of tingling sensation or numbness in the limbs and around the mouth, a slow irregular pulse, and a fall in blood pressure.

As well as insuring that no potassium is ingested in fluid or food, preventive measures may include the oral or rectal administration of a cation exchange resin, such as sodium polystyrene sulfonate (Kayexalate). The resin preparation combines with the potassium in the gastrointestinal secretions, preventing its absorption. As cited earlier, if hyperkalemia develops, an intravenous infusion of glucose with a dose of regular insulin may be given. This is to promote the deposition of the glucose as glycogen, a process which utilizes potassium. A solution of sodium bicarbonate or sodium lactate and probably calcium may be administered to counteract the effect of the excess potassium on the heart. An antiarrhythmic drug may also be prescribed.

Cardiac Insufficiency. Heart failure may occur as the result of the retention of sodium and water. The pulse may become weak and pulmonary edema may develop, causing dyspnea and moist respirations. If hypertension is associated with the renal failure, it may also be a factor in heart failure. Digitalis may be prescribed to strengthen the heart. A phlebotomy may be done and 300 to 500 ml. of blood withdrawn to reduce the intravascular volume and venous return.

Convulsions. Convulsions may occur and are usually preceded by muscular twitching, persisting severe headache, severe hypertension, increasing edema and rising blood urea level. Padded side rails are placed on the bed to prevent self-injury of the patient. During a seizure only sufficient restraint is used to protect the patient from injury. Magnesium sulfate may be ordered intramuscularly or amobarbital sodium (Amytal sodium) intravenously.

Coma. Increasing drowsiness may indicate increasing uremia and may progress to disorientation and coma. The delirious patient requires constant attendance, and a sedative such as amobarbital sodium may be prescribed. If the patient becomes comatose, the care appropriate for any unconscious patient is applicable (see p. 159).

Chronic Renal Failure

Chronic renal insufficiency is due to progressive disease of both kidneys. Irreversible damage to nephrons occurs that eventually leads to the retention of many waste and toxic products of metabolism, fluid and electrolyte imbalances, metabolic acidosis, anemia, hypertension and decalcification of bone tissue (renal osteodystrophy).

ETIOLOGY. The most frequent causes of progressive renal failure are the following.

CHRONIC PYELONEPHRITIS. This is a chronic infectious, inflammatory process that results in progressive fibrosing and destruction of nephrons.

CHRONIC OR PROLIFERATIVE GLOMERULO-NEPHRITIS. This involves chronic inflammation, fibrosing and destruction of glomeruli and ensuing degeneration of the respective tubules.

POLYCYSTIC KIDNEY DISEASE. Progressive enlargement of the cysts compresses functional renal parenchyma increasing renal insufficiency.

NEPHROSCLEROSIS. This is secondary to hypertension and atherosclerosis.

Other diseases which may cause chronic renal failure include systemic lupus erythematosus, obstructive postrenal disease (e.g., calculi and neoplasms) and hyperparathyroidism.

MANIFESTATIONS. The patient may pass through the early stage of chronic kidney impairment without the renal disease being recognized. It may first be discovered in a routine physical examination, revealed by an elevation in blood pressure and by albuminuria. The rate of destruction of functional tissue varies among individuals and with the primary etiologic factor. Some persons live a normal active life for many years because the functioning nephrons compensate to some extent for those destroyed. Others, whose disease progresses rapidly, may enter the advanced uremic phase in a matter of a few months. In compensation the glomerular filtration rate per nephron is increased as are the reabsorption and secretory functions of the tubules. However, a deficit still exists which progressively increases.

Gradually, with increasing nephron destruction, the patient enters the phase in which renal compensation can no longer maintain homeostasis, and symptoms become apparent. Filtration is impaired, and there is a loss of tubular ability to vary the composition and volume of urine according to the need to conserve or eliminate urinary solutes and water.

The signs and symptoms vary considerably in patients in the early stage of uncompensated insufficiency but tend to become similar in the more advanced stage. An elevation in blood pressure, lassitude, headache and loss of weight may be the earliest manifestations. Urinalysis reveals albumin due to increased permeability of glomeruli. The loss of plasma protein as the disease progresses may be severe enough to produce the nephrotic syndrome (see p. 650). As more and more nephrons are destroyed, decreased filtration results in the retention of metabolic wastes. The blood urea and serum creatinine levels rise. Creatinine and urea clearance tests show a decrease in ml. per minute, and the severity of failure may be categorized as mild, moderate, severe or terminal on the basis of the clearance test findings. For example, if the creatinine clearance test is used, 100 to 50 ml. per minute may be interpreted as mild failure, 50 to 15 ml. per minute as moderate failure, 15 to 5 ml. per minute as severe failure, and less than 5 ml. per minute as terminal stage.

With a progressive decrease in glomerular filtration and the development of hypertension, the patient experiences increasing fatigue and lassitude, more severe headaches and loss of weight. Nausea, especially in the mornings, and anorexia become troublesome.

Initially, in chronic renal failure the 24-hour urinary volume is increased and the patient experiences nocturia as a result of tubular inability to concentrate the glomerular filtrate. The concentration of solutes in the urine is invariable, producing a fixed specific gravity. If the fluid intake does not cover the increased fluid loss, the patient develops a negative fluid balance and the retention of solid wastes is increased.

Tubular destruction causes electrolyte imbalances. There is usually an excessive loss of sodium which may produce hyponatremia unless there is adequate replacement. Potassium retention is not usually a problem until the terminal oliguric phase. In moderately severe failure, metabolic acidosis develops and hypocalcemia may also be a problem, contributing to muscular twitching and general weakness.

Eventually, the urinary output is reduced, hypertension becomes severe, and the nitrogenous waste and potassium blood concentrations rise sharply. The patient is pale, and the hematocrit and hemoglobin determinations indicate anemia which accounts in part for the fatigue and reduced efficiency. In chronic renal failure a bleeding tendency is also manifested; the thrombocyte count is low and the prothrombin time is abnormal. Petechiae, ecchymoses and bleeding of mucous membranes may be observed.

The central nervous system is affected by the retained wastes; the person is irritable, memory, reasoning and judgment are impaired and the attention span is shortened. In the advanced uremic stage, the patient manifests confusion, disorientation, drowsiness and stupor. Restlessness and twitching may be observed and frequently precede convulsive seizures.

Pruritus is a source of irritation for the renal failure patient, attributed to the precipitation of retained phosphates into the skin.

A cessation of ovulation and menstruation in the female with chronic renal failure is common, and the male patient may experience loss of libido and impotence.

Late symptoms are anuria, generalized edema, persistent headache of increasing severity, nausea and vomiting, hiccups, diarrhea, muscular twitching, convulsions, ulceration of the mouth, fetid breath, rapid deep respirations indicating acidosis, drowsiness, disorientation and coma. As a result of the severe hypertension and water retention, a cerebrovascular accident or cardiac failure and pulmonary edema may supervene.

TREATMENT AND NURSING CARE. The physician advises the patient and his family of the diagnosis, but it is frequently the nurse who must answer many of their questions, provide emotional support, and help them to understand and accept the prescribed regimen. The patient is usually in the hospital when the diagnosis of chronic renal disease is made, having probably had a series of kidney function tests. At first, he may be resentful and unable to accept the fact that he has a progressive chronic disease. Instruction is likely to fall on deaf ears until he works through his immediate reactions. The nurse provides opportunities for him to verbalize his feelings and is alert for signs of his acceptance of his condition and readiness to learn how he may help himself.

Care is directed toward having the patient live as useful, comfortable and satisfying life as possible within the limitations imposed by his disease. The primary cause of the renal failure is treated to retard the progression of his disease (e.g. hypertension, pyelonephritis). The therapeutic plan includes measures to correct the body biochemistry and modify symptoms.

Conservative treatment is reserved for

those patients who can be maintained without dialysis or transplantation, and includes the following considerations.

ASSESSMENT. The nurse obtains a history of the patient. Information about his life situation and previous health problems and practices is taken into consideration in planning how his needs may be met, and in helping the individual and his family solve their problems.

The plan of care in any stage of renal failure includes frequent ongoing assessment. Obviously, the evaluation becomes more frequent as the disease advances and when the patient is hospitalized. Significant clinical factors that are observed include:

1. Vital Signs. The blood pressure is especially important, and is usually checked in both the lying and sitting positions. Since cardiac arrhythmias and failure are common complications, the heart rate, volume and sounds are carefully noted. An electrocardiogram is done, and in advanced stages continuous EKG monitoring may be established. An elevation in temperature may indicate infection to which the patient is predisposed.

2. Renal function tests and frequent urinalysis are necessary. (See p. 619.)

3. Blood Urea and pH, Serum Creatinine and Electrolyte, Hemoglobin, and Hematocrit Levels. These are followed closely. Diet, fluid intake and activity are regulated on these findings.

4. Fluid Balance, Weight and Edema. An accurate record of the intake and output is kept. Skin turgor is noted, and the periorbital and sacral areas and ankles are examined frequently for evidence of fluid retention. Loss of weight may indicate an excessive breakdown of tissue which increases the production of creatinine. A weight gain may be due to the retention of sodium and water.

5. Chest Auscultation. In addition to observing the patient for dyspnea and audible moist respirations, the chest is auscultated for possible rales.

6. How the Patient Feels. In assessing the renal failure patient, it is important that the nurse avoid basing assessment entirely on laboratory reports and objective manifestations. Subjective symptoms are significant and varied. For example, increasingly severe headache or extreme fatigue may indicate an increase in blood pressure and retained nitrogenous wastes. Twitching and restlessness of lower limbs, blurred vision,

"inability to think" or "can't remember" may point to central nervous system involvement and impending terminal phase.

7. The Patient's Emotional Reaction to the Disease. If the nurse is to provide support for the patient, it is necessary to assess his perspective; observe the patient closely and listen for innuendoes that convey feelings.

DIET AND FLUIDS. The goal in dietary and fluid intake is to balance the intake with the output. The prescribed diet varies with the severity of the disease. Restrictions are based on serum electrolyte and urea levels, urinary volume and composition and presenting symptoms. A diet of 2000 calories is desirable to provide sufficient energy that will permit activity without the breakdown of tissue protein and fat. In the early stage of the disease, protein is limited to 30 to 50 Gm. daily to minimize the production of nitrogenous wastes. The prescribed amount is adjusted according to the blood urea (BUN). Carbohydrate and fat provide the remaining calories. Anorexia may be a problem; it may be helpful to offer small amounts at more frequent intervals. The patient may be encouraged to make a greater effort to take nourishment if he receives an explanation of its significance in preventing an increase in the breakdown of body tissue which results in an elevation in serum creatinine.

If the patient is experiencing nausea, an antiemetic such as prochlorperazine (Compazine) or dimenhydrinate (Gravol) may be prescribed. In the case of the patient who develops the nephrotic syndrome, protein is not restricted but, instead, is probably increased above the average dietary intake (see p. 651). Since the impaired tubular reabsorption usually results in an excessive loss of sodium, salt is not restricted in the diet unless there is edema or severe hypertension. A determination is made of the 24-hour excretion of sodium in the urine. The patient may actually develop hyponatremia which may be manifested by muscular cramps.

The fluid intake should cover the fluid loss. Tubular reabsorption of water is decreased in chronic renal failure, so the intake should be increased accordingly. Generally in the early stage, a minimum of 2000 ml. is required to prevent dehydration from the increased urinary output. A record is made of the 24-hour intake and output. The patient is advised that he should not take more than 500 ml. in excess of his urinary output; as well as incurring edema, excessive water in the presence of the abnormal sodium loss may precipitate hyponatremia. Any significant decrease in the urinary output, indicating a positive fluid balance, is reported to the doctor, as it may signal more advanced failure. When oliguria supervenes, the fluid intake is adjusted according to the urinary output. The daily intake is 400 to 500 ml. plus the measurable loss (e.g., urine and emesis). A diuretic such as furosemide (Lasix) may be prescribed to promote diuresis and reduce blood pressure.

ACTIVITY. Although the patient's renal reserve is diminished, in the early stage of the disease his kidney function may be adequate as long as the prescribed diet and fluid intake are followed and metabolic extremes are avoided. The patient is encouraged to remain active within the limits of his strength but is advised to avoid undue fatigue; physical activity should be moderate to avoid excessive catabolism, which increases serum creatinine. He requires more rest than the normal person. While still active, it is suggested that he should have 10 hours of sleep at night and should rest 1 hour during the morning and afternoon. The person at work may plan for 1 hour at noon and for 1 hour at the completion of his workday before his evening meal. Whether he is able to resume his former occupation or not depends on its demands. Certainly the ability to continue to be a useful, independent member of society provides self-esteem and emotional well-being. Suitable recreation and diversion in which the patient is interested should receive consideration. It lessens the focus on his disease and provides a more normal, balanced life.

HYPERTENSION AND ANEMIA. These are common concomitant problems of chronic renal insufficiency. The patient will probably be required to take an antihypertensive drug such as methyldopa (Aldomet), hydralazine (Apresoline) or guanethidine (Ismelin). The anemia is not responsive to the usual hematinic drugs; periodic blood transfusions of packed cells may be necessary.

SKIN CARE. As the patient's blood urea accumulates, pruritus may become troublesome. Bathing with *warm* water, avoiding the use of soap and an application of calamine lotion may be used to provide relief of the itching.

MOUTH CARE. The patient is encouraged to use a mild antiseptic mouthwash at least three or four times daily. Sour fruit candy or gum may help to relieve dryness. In moderately severe and in advanced renal insufficiency, the patient develops sordes and is predisposed to ulceration and infection in the mouth. A disagreeable taste and offensive breath become troublesome. Cleansing with an antiseptic solution or hydrogen peroxide every 2 hours becomes necessary. Lemon juice and glycerin may be applied. Ice-cold mouthwash or liquids used in mouth care are refreshing and more acceptable to the patient.

HEADACHE. The patient may experience severe headaches. He is kept at rest with the head and shoulders elevated. A mild analgesic is administered; cold compresses or an ice bag is applied and the environment kept as free of stimuli as possible. The blood pressure and blood urea levels are checked.

SAFETY. Side rails may be necessary if the patient is confined to bed. Confusion and restlessness or stupor may develop and result in the patient falling out of bed.

If a calcium and phosphorus imbalance develops it may indicate bone tissue disease which involves decalcification. The disorder is referred to as *renal osteodystrophy*. Osteomalacia and osteitis fibrosa develop in the bones, causing tenderness and predisposing to fractures. This disorder is attributed to failure of the kidneys to activate vitamin D which normally promotes absorption of calcium and to the hyperphosphatemia resulting from decreased nephron function. The decreased serum calcium stimulates the release of the parathyroid hormone which causes the movement of calcium out of bones. The complication of osteodystrophy is treated by the administration of a preparation of vitamin D.

INSTRUCTION AND SUPERVISION. Since the patient and his family must assume the responsibility for following the prescribed regimen, the nurse plans a program of instruction. A simple explanation of the role of the kidneys in eliminating body wastes is helpful before attempting to explain the importance of avoiding extra demands on the kidneys and how this is achieved.

Diet outlines are reviewed, indicating food selection and preparation to meet the protein restriction and the daily calorie requirement. The measurement and distribution of the required fluid intake over the 24 hours are discussed. The patient is instructed to record his weight daily and to do this at the same time each day with the same amount of clothing. Any increase in weight, puffiness around the eyes, swelling of the feet or hands, frequent headaches and increasing fatigue should be brought to the physician's attention. Measurement of his urinary output is recommended, and the patient is advised that an output of less than two-thirds of his intake must be reported.

Infection increases the production of metabolic wastes, especially if accompanied by fever and a reduced fluid intake. The importance of avoiding chilling and exposure to persons with an infection is stressed. Practical suggestions are made as to how the possibility of exposure may be minimized. If the patient does develop a respiratory infection or any other disturbance, it is advisable for him to get in touch with the physician.

Frequent visits to the doctor or a clinic are necessary, and the patient is advised to take a urine specimen and his weight and intake and output records with him each time. His blood pressure and weight are checked, and the patient is questioned about his appetite and urinary volume. Blood specimens are taken to determine the hematocrit, hemoglobin level, and electrolyte and nitrogenous waste concentrations.

In some instances, the patient and his family may be able to follow the therapeutic program, make necessary observations and recognize significant changes. Other patients may require a referral to a visiting nurse organization. The visiting nurse may assist with diet planning, check the patient's blood pressure and weight, counsel him as to activity and note any signs of deterioration. If the patient is returning to work, the occupational nurse at his place of employment is advised of the situation so she may provide the necessary assistance and follow the patient's progress.

It is very helpful if the patient and his family have the opportunity to discuss their problems and express their concerns with someone who shows an interest in them and will take the time to listen. Frequently problems are revealed to the nurse that she may be able to help solve, or significant information may be received that requires immediate referral to the physician.

ADVANCED RENAL FAILURE. In the oliguric and uremic phase of chronic renal disease, the care is similar to that cited for the patient with acute renal failure. Rest, more stringent dietary and fluid restrictions, special skin and mouth care and close observation for disorientation, convulsions, coma, cardiac failure and pulmonary edema are necessary. A dialysis program is established and kidney transplantation may be considered.

DIALYSIS AND KIDNEY TRANSPLANTATION

When conservative treatment will no longer adequately control the blood concentration of wastes and the fluid and electrolyte balance within limits compatible with life, regular *dialysis* may be employed to maintain the patient. If both kidneys are severely damaged by infection, polycystic disease or newgrowths, or if there is severe hypertension that cannot be controlled by conservative treatment, bilateral nephrectomy may be done, and the patient maintained entirely on hemodialysis two or three times weekly. Such a patient is a likely candidate for a *kidney transplant.*

Dialysis

When the renal failure patient who is being cared for on a conservative therapeutic regimen manifests a steadily increasing blood urea level while on a restricted protein diet, a serum creatinine level of 12 to 15 mg. per cent or over, progressive hypertension, metabolic acidosis, hyperkalemia or a threat to cardiac and respiratory sufficiency by the retention of sodium and water, dialysis may be instituted.

Dialysis is a physicochemical process and refers to the separation of two solutions by a semi-permeable membrane through which water and some solutes may pass. Molecules and ions of solutes which are small enough to permeate the membrane pass through along a concentration gradient from higher to lower until an equilibrium is established on either side. The size of the pores of the dialysis membrane permits only the transfer of small molecular solutes. Larger molecular substances such as proteins and blood cells do not pass through the membrane. The movement of water through the dialyzing membrane is governed by the osmolality of the solutions; it passes from the solution of lower osmotic pressure to that of greater osmotic pressure. These physicochemical processes, diffusion and osmosis, always proceed toward a zero concentration gradient.

Dialysis is a therapeutic procedure used in acute and chronic renal failure to lower the blood level of metabolic waste products (urea, creatinine, uric acid) and toxic substances and to correct abnormal electrolyte and fluid imbalances. Two methods currently in use are *peritoneal dialysis* and *extracorporeal hemodialysis*. The latter dialysis occurs outside of the body using a dialyzing machine that may be referred to as an "artificial kidney."

Although the procedures in the two types of dialysis differ, the purposes and principles are the same. In hemodialysis a semipermeable membrane separates the patient's circulating blood from a specially prepared solution known as the *dialysate*. In peritoneal dialysis, the peritoneum is the membrane which separates the dialysate from the patient's interstitial fluid; the dialysate is introduced into the peritoneal cavity.

The dialysate is generally a specially prepared aqueous solution of sodium, calcium, magnesium, potassium chloride, lactate or acetate and glucose. The composition of the solution varies according to the patient's serum electrolyte concentrations; for example, potassium may be omitted if the patient has hyperkalemia. The glucose is added to provide a hypertonicity and osmotic pressure that moves water from the patient into the dialysate to relieve overhydration and hypertension. Lactate or acetate is included to raise the pH; it is converted to bicarbonate ions within the body.

Urea, creatinine and uric acid are removed from the patient by dialysis because they are not present in the dialyzing solution. Water is removed if there is overhydration, since the osmolality of the dialysate is greater than that of body fluids which are dilute because there is an excess. If the serum potassium is elevated, diffusion occurs in the direction of the dialysate until there is an equilibrium on both sides of the dialyzing membrane.

A regular dialysis regimen has prolonged the life of many patients with chronic renal failure. It has permitted many of them to continue in their jobs and be independent, useful members of society. Although hospital dialysis units have increased in number in recent years, particularly in larger medical centers, the number of patients that can be treated is still limited. The hospital-based unit usually necessitates the patient being away from his work at least 2 days a week. Because of this, the units' limitations, and the distance of many patients from a center, dialysis at home has been made possible for some patients. At present, the number being treated at home is small but is increasing steadily.

PERITONEAL DIALYSIS. In this method of dialysis, the dialysate is introduced into the peritoneal cavity following the insertion of a special catheter. An explanation of the purpose and the procedure is made to the patient and family and written consent for the dialysis is obtained.

The patient is weighed before and upon completion of the treatment. Serum electrolyte, creatinine, and blood urea levels are noted before commencing and may be checked during and upon completion. The vital signs are checked and serve as a baseline during and following the dialysis. The patient empties his bladder just before the start of the treatment to prevent possible trauma from insertion of the catheter. He is then placed in the dorsal-recumbent position.

Following local anesthesia of the subumbilical site to be used, the physician makes a small skin incision and passes a trocar and cannula through the abdominal wall into the peritoneal cavity. The cannula is then replaced by a catheter which has several openings, and is secured to the abdominal wall by tape or a purse-string suture. A sterile dressing is fitted snugly around the tube to protect the incision. Two liters[7] of sterile dialysate are warmed to body temperature and the flasks suspended on an infusion pole. Their tubes are connected by a Y tube which in turn connects to a tube leading to the catheter (Fig. 19–7). The solution is allowed to flow fairly rapidly into the peritoneal cavity; this generally takes 10 to 15 minutes. When the bottles with the specified volume are almost empty, the tubing is clamped; this leaves fluid in the system to initiate siphonage drainage later. The dialysate remains in the abdomen for a prescribed 15 to 30 minutes (dwell time). The dwell time is varied according to the patient's symptoms. For example, if overhydration and edema are a problem, the dwell time is short. The bottles are then lowered to the floor and the clamp released or a separate

---

[7]If the patient is a child, the amount is reduced to 1000 to 1500 ml.

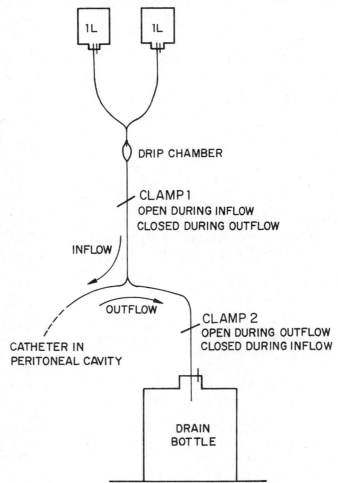

IRRIGATION SOLUTION

DRIP CHAMBER

CLAMP 1
OPEN DURING INFLOW
CLOSED DURING OUTFLOW

INFLOW

OUTFLOW

CLAMP 2
OPEN DURING OUTFLOW
CLOSED DURING INFLOW

CATHETER IN
PERITONEAL CAVITY

DRAIN
BOTTLE

FIGURE 19–7 Schematic drawing of peritoneal dialysis. (After Harrington, J., and E. R. Brener, Patient Care in Renal Failure, Philadelphia, W. B. Saunders Co., 1973.)

drainage bottle to receive the outflow may be used. It takes approximately 15 to 20 minutes for the solution to return. The outflow is measured and recorded.

The recent introduction of a peritoneal dialysis cycling machine has greatly facilitated this procedure. The automatic cycling machine provides a closed system and is set to introduce a prescribed volume of warm dialysate over a specified time, and to allow a preset dwell time and drainage period. The newer machines are set up so that measured amounts of the solid constituents of the dialysate are mixed with an appropriate volume of sterile warmed water and then pumped into the dialyzer. Most dialyzers also have an alarm system which is sensitive to malfunctioning.

The alternating infusion of fresh sterile dialysate and drainage is repeated for the period of time specified by the physician; this may vary from 10 to 36 hours. The duration is determined by the blood chemistry levels and the patient's reactions.

If the drainage becomes very slow or stops, the openings into the catheter are probably blocked by omentum or viscera. *Gentle* pressure with the flat of the hand on the lower abdomen, having the patient turn from side to side, or lowering or elevating the head of the bed may free the catheter and reestablish drainage. If these measures are not successful, the physician is notified. The first return may be expected to be slightly tinged with blood from the parietal tissues. If this persists in subsequent exchanges, the physician is consulted.

The blood pressure and pulse are recorded every 15 minutes during the first exchange, and then every 30 to 60 minutes if they are stable. Any untoward signs or symptoms such as abdominal pain, vomiting, sharp rise or fall in blood pressure, rapid weak pulse, pallor, severe headache or reduced level of consciousness are reported promptly. The patient's behavior and responses are also noted; extreme apprehension, restlessness, sleeplessness, headache and disorientation develop rarely, and are referred to as the *disequilibrium syndrome*. The patient is usually nauseated and vomits. This is attributed to urea being removed from the brain more slowly than from the blood. Osmosis results in the movement of water into the brain, causing cerebral edema. If the patient experiences the problem of disequilibrium, the dialysis may be performed more frequently but for shorter periods and the osmolality of the dialysate may be increased. If the latter measure is used the patient is observed very closely for possible hypotension. If the dialysate is hypertonic (has a high glucose content), the blood pressure and pulse are recorded every 15 minutes throughout the entire procedure so that too great a loss of intravascular fluid will be recognized quickly, before severe hypotension and shock develop. If the return fluid should be 500 ml. more than the volume of dialysate used, the physician is consulted before any further exchange is undertaken. This indicates the necessity for an accurate record of the volume of dialysate infused and the amount returned with each exchange. Blood chemistry studies (BUN, electrolytes) are made at intervals during the dialysis and upon completion. The serum protein levels are monitored, since protein may be lost in the dialysate. If there is a decrease, diet protein may be increased.

Since the patient remains on his back during dialysis, frequent turning of the pillows, massage of pressure areas and limbs, the placing of sheepskin under the patient, and a brief change of position between exchanges are used to relieve the discomfort of the long periods of immobilization. The patient may be more comfortable with the head of the bed elevated; this position reduces the pressure of the dialysate on the diaphragm, which may cause some distress. The patient is encouraged to take several deep breaths hourly and to cough if secretions are noted on chest auscultation.

When the treatment is completed, the catheter is removed, and sterile gauze and dressing pads are applied. The site is observed at frequent intervals for drainage; moist dressings are changed for sterile dry ones. The temperature and pulse are recorded every 3 or 4 hours. Fever, rapid pulse, complaints of abdominal pain and any abdominal rigidity are reported promptly to the physician since they may indicate complicating peritonitis. A culture of the return dialysate is made routinely with each dialysis so that an antibotic administration may be commenced promptly if organisms are present.

Peritoneal dialysis is generally reserved for short-term therapy only; the risk of peritonitis is too great. However, there are a few patients who for some reason are placed on a chronic peritoneal dialysis program. A sterile catheter may be introduced each time the dialysis is performed or a permanent peritoneal catheter may be inserted. The catheter has two cuffs to anchor it within the abdomen; the end of the external portion is closed off by a rubber cap between dialyses. The cuffs also tend to seal off the pathway into the peritoneal cavity.

HEMODIALYSIS. In hemodialysis, an extracorporeal flow of the patient's blood is separated from a specially prepared dialysate by a semipermeable membrane. Water and some solutes may move to or from the blood. The direction of movement is always toward reducing concentration gradients; water will move toward the solution of greater osmolality. Solid particles will shift by diffusion from the area of greater to lesser concentration in an effort to equilibrate the concentration on both sides of the membrane.

Hemodialysis is the more efficient method of dialysis but is a more complex procedure than peritoneal dialysis and requires more sophisticated equipment. As cited earlier, the principles in both methods of dialyses are the same but the procedure and equipment vary greatly. In hemodialysis, the blood from an artery is directed extracorporeally through an exchange unit and is returned to a vein. The components of the exchange unit include porous tubes through which the blood flows and a compartment containing the dialysate. A second essential unit is the dialysate supply system which mixes and delivers the solution to the exchange unit (Fig. 19–8). The membrane-like tube which transports the blood requires priming with blood or a prescribed intravenous solution to exclude all air before being connected to the patient's artery and vein.

Various models of hemodialyzers are avail-

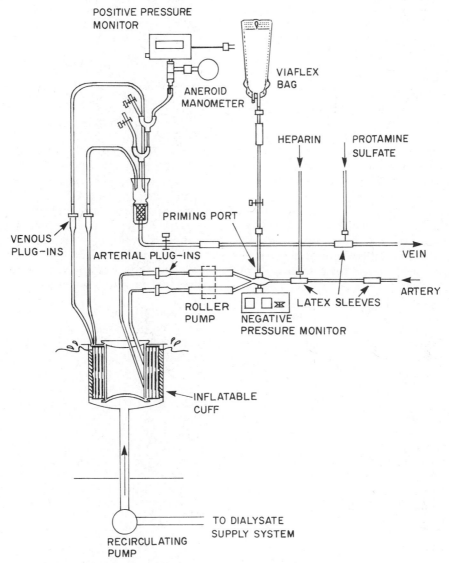

FIGURE 19–8 Schematic drawing of hemodialysis. (After Harrington, J., and E. R. Brener, *Patient Care in Renal Failure*, Philadelphia, W. B. Saunders Co., 1973.)

able; each type has individual features. They may vary in composition, structure and size of the dialyzing unit, priming volume, ease of assembly, dialysate delivery system and whether or not the blood has to be pumped through the system. The types commonly used have a coil dialyzer, flat parallel plate dialyzer or a hollow fiber or capillary dialyzer. Each functions on the same basic principles.

The pressure of the blood in the dialyzing tube is monitored and can be raised by applying a special clamp on the venous end of the tube. The latter procedure is used to establish a pressure gradient between the blood and dialysate to increase the filtration of water and salts from the blood. This process is referred to as *ultrafiltration*. In some instances, the dialysate may be made hypertonic to create an osmotic pressure that will remove excess water from the blood.

Blood is delivered to the dialyzer via an established subcutaneous arteriovenous fistula or arteriovenous shunt. The *arteriovenous (A-V) fistula* is surgically constructed by the side-to-side or end-to-side anastomosis of an artery and a vein (Fig. 19–9). The anastomosis may be between the cephalic vein and radial artery, or between the cephalic vein and brachial artery. A lower limb artery and vein may be the site of choice. A bruit can be detected over the fistula site, which indicates its patency. The fistula is not used for dialysis for several days after its establishment to insure firm healing. The vein and its branches enlarge with the rerouting of the arterial blood.

Hemodialysis with an A-V fistula involves the insertion of two needles into the *vein*. A local anesthetic may be used to reduce the discomfort associated with the introduction of the needles for each dialysis. One needle is inserted at least 2 cm. above the fistula and is connected to the outflow or arterial line of the dialyzer. The second needle is inserted 1½ to 2 inches above the outflow needle and is connected to the tube that returns the blood from the dialyzer. Blood flows out from the distal needle through the dialyzer and back into the patient via the proximal needle (Fig. 19–10). A tourniquet may be placed loosely around the limb between the needles if necessary to insure blood flow to the dialyzer as well as to prevent the return flow from reentering the dialysis line. *The limb in which an arteriovenous fistula is developed should not be used in taking blood pressure.*

The arteriovenous fistula access route in hemodialysis has several distinct advantages. It is completely subcutaneous, thus lessening the possibility of infection. Since it does not require a cannula and a bulky dressing, the patient's activity is less restricted and it also reduces the risk of hemorrhage and thrombosis.

An *arteriovenous shunt* is established by exposing an artery and an adjacent vein and implanting a cannula in each (Fig. 19–11). The ends of the cannula tubes are brought through the skin and are joined by a short connecting tube. The cannula and tubing are of inert synthetic materials (Teflon and Silastic) so reaction is avoided. The incisions are sutured around the tubes and a sterile dressing and bandage are applied. Two small clamps are attached to the bandage at all times so that they are readily available should the tubes become disconnected and bleeding occur. The distal portion of the loop of the external U-shaped tube is left exposed so that the patency of the shunt can be checked frequently.

To start dialysis, the connecting tube on the A-V shunt is removed; the arterial cannula is connected to the inflow (arterial) line of the dialyzer and the venous cannula is attached to the outflow dialyzer tube (that is, to the tube which returns the blood to the patient). The advantage of the A-V shunt is its ready and painless accessibility for commencing dialysis. During the interval between dialyses, however, it requires frequent checking, protection and surgical care. Since available sites for establishing an A-V shunt are limited, precautions and care are necessary to prevent complications and maintain the patency of the

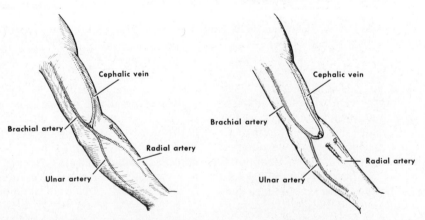

FIGURE 19–9 Construction of an arteriovenous fistula at the antecubital fossa: *left,* between the cephalic vein and brachial artery (end to side), and, *right,* between the cephalic vein and the radial artery (end to end). (From Kuruvila, K. C., and Beven, E. G.: Arteriovenous shunts and fistulas for hemodialysis. *Surg. Clin. N. Amer.,* 51:5, 1229, 1971.)

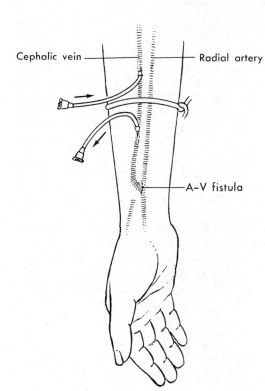

Cephalic vein ─── Radial artery

─── A–V fistula

FIGURE 19–10 The position of the needles when an arteriovenous fistula is established for hemodialysis.

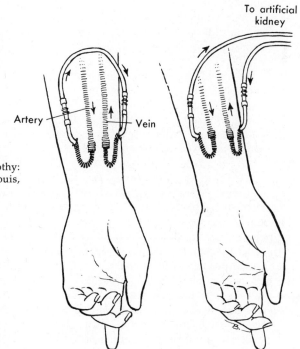

To artificial kidney

Artery ─── Vein

FIGURE 19–11 A-V shunt. (From Brundage, Dorothy: Nursing Management of Renal Problems. St. Louis, C. V. Mosby, 1976, p. 95.)

bypass. The average period of time that an A-V shunt remains patent is about 6 months.

The loop of the tube is checked at least every 2 hours for blood flow. Clotting in the shunt system and obstruction of the flow may occur with kinking or malalignment of the tubes or pressure being exerted on them. The blood becomes dark blue, and the bruit that is normally heard with a stethoscope over the venous side is absent. *The tube must not be pinched to check cannula patency.* If clotting is suspected, no attempt is made to clear the tube by "milking." The problem is reported immediately to the physician or dialysis unit. Efforts will be made to remove the clots by aspiration and the use of heparinized saline.

The site is also checked for bleeding. If the tubes become disconnected, free bleeding is quickly recognized and the clamps previously mentioned are applied promptly to the tubes. If the clamps do not control the bleeding, a tourniquet may be applied to the limb, releasing it every 5 minutes for 5 seconds. Subcutaneous bleeding may result from the displacement of a cannula or erosion of the artery or vein. This is reported promptly; pressure is applied over the site and a tourniquet used.

The limb in which there is an A-V shunt must not be used to determine blood pressure or administer intravenous infusions. Following the establishment of an A-V bypass in a leg, the patient is usually confined to bed, and all weight-bearing is avoided for about a week.

Specific directions are received from the physician as to the care of the cannula site. Some suggest daily cleansing of the skin around the exit areas of the tubes with an antiseptic solution. Others prefer that the site be cleansed and redressed only at dialysis, unless there is infection or oozing of blood. If infection occurs, the skin of the area and the bypass tubing are cleansed daily with the prescribed antiseptic solution. Aseptic dressing technique is used, and a mask is worn by the person carrying out the procedure.

In order to prevent clotting of the blood in the extracorporeal circuit, heparin is added to the patient's inflow blood at intervals during the dialysis. The clotting time is checked at intervals during the treatment. The heparin may be introduced into the tube with a syringe and needle or, on some dialyzers, is automatically infused with a pump. The dose prescribed by the physician is based on the person's weight in kilograms and their clotting and prothrombin times. At the end of the return line, protamine sulfate may be added to the blood to neutralize the heparin just before it reenters the patient.

When *nursing the hemodialysis patient,* there are a number of factors to be considered.

EMOTIONAL AND SOCIOECONOMIC CONCERNS. When the patient's chronic renal failure necessitates hemodialysis, it is natural that the patient and family will be concerned and react. It is likely to have many implications; knowing that the disease has progressed to this stage and that his life becomes dependent upon the procedure is extremely threatening. Severe anxiety may be manifested due to concern for the future and life expectancy. Acceptance may be very difficult for some patients and they may manifest resentment and anger at first, followed by a period of depression. A regular schedule of dialysis two or three times weekly imposes modifications on the patient's and family's life pattern. The therapeutic regimen may curtail his role in business; it may mean changing his occupation or giving up employment or, at best, working only part-time unless home dialysis can be provided. The adjustments that have to be made may cause both social and economic changes for family members, especially if the patient has been the main source of income or is the mother. Special diet requirements and transportation to and from the dialysis unit may incur worrisome additional expense. A referral to a social service agency may be helpful.

It is important for the nurse to be a willing listener and encourage the patient and family to reveal their concerns and problems; these vary from patient to patient and family to family. An understanding of their situation and recognition of their reactions are essential to providing the appropriate support and planning care, and in assisting them to accept the necessary modifications. A positive attitude on the part of the health personnel promotes realistic patient and family acceptance and adaptation. Many patients obtain support and pleasure through socialization and the establishment of close relationships with other dialysis patients.

Gradually, as the uremic toxicity is reduced, the patient experiences physical and emotional improvement and, by degrees, becomes more active and interested in living and may lead a relatively normal productive life.

PREDIALYSIS RESPONSIBILITIES. The patient and family receive a simple explanation of the purpose of dialysis and what it involves. Many units have prepared a brochure that is given to the patient to provide information and reinforce verbal explanations and instruction. Prior to the initial treatment, if the patient's condition permits, he visits the dialysis unit, meets the dialysis staff and may have the opportunity to chat with a patient on a regular dialysis program. Such preparation is helpful in reducing the patient's fears. A consent form is signed by the patient or next of kin and an A-V fistula or shunt is established.

For dialysis, the patient is positioned comfortably on his back in bed with the limb with the A-V fistula or shunt exposed and supported. His temperature, pulse, respirations, blood pressure and weight are recorded before the dialysis is commenced. Blood specimens are obtained when the needles are introduced (or cannulae are opened) for laboratory determination of the hematocrit, electrolyte (K^+, Na^+), blood urea, and creatinine levels and clotting time. Rarely, a sedative is prescribed if the patient is restless or extremely apprehensive.

CARE DURING DIALYSIS. Periodically, during dialysis, the head of the bed may be raised or lowered if the blood pressure is satisfactory, the pillows turned, gentle massage given to pressure areas and slight adjustments made to reduce the discomfort incurred by the hours of immobilization. Some patients like some form of diversion such as reading, radio, or crafts, while others prefer to rest and sleep.

The sphygmomanometer remains on the patient's arm throughout dialysis, as frequent recordings of the blood pressure are necessary since the flow rate through the dialyzer is regulated accordingly. A sharp fall in the blood pressure occurs if the blood flows out of the patient more rapidly than it is being returned or if there is an excessive loss of water into the dialysate, reducing the patient's total intravascular volume.

The pulse is checked at least every 15 minutes at first, gradually lengthening the interval to ½ hour if it is satisfactory. Continuous cardiac monitoring by oscillograph tracing may be required with some patients so that there will be prompt recognition of a cardiac arrhythmia should it develop. The rate of respirations is noted and any difficulty in breathing, coughing, moist sounds or complaint of chest pain are reported promptly.

Blood analysis for potassium, sodium and urea levels may be repeated at intervals during dialysis. Adjustments may be necessary in the dialysate in accordance with the electrolyte values.

The clotting time is usually checked hourly. Repeated checks are made for any indication of bleeding. The mouth, cannula sites, and all excreta are examined for any sign of blood. The dialyzing fluid is inspected frequently for any discoloration that would occur with the leaking of blood from the circuit.

Headache, vomiting and twitching may develop, and should be brought to the physician's attention. Rarely, a patient becomes disoriented or has a convulsion. These disturbances are attributed to cerebral edema associated with the disequilibrium syndrome (see p. 634). If blood is used to prime the dialyzing tubes, the patient is observed for possible transfusion reaction (urticaria, shortness of breath or dyspnea, tightness in the chest, hypotension or rapid pulse).

Fluids are given, if tolerated, within the daily allowance. The patient is fed his regular meal and, in some instances, the dietary restriction on protein may be relaxed to some extent for that one meal. He is usually asked if there is something he would especially like to have.

If the patient is on regular medication, the administration of these during dialysis is approved by the physician. Antihypertensive preparations are not usually given, since they may cause hypotension.

The temperature of the dialysate is monitored and automatically controlled on the newer machines. If the dialysate is too cool, the patient will complain of being cold. If the dialysate temperature is too high, hemolysis may occur.

The dialyzer has an alarm to alert attending staff of malfunction; the fistula or shunt area is checked first to determine if a blood line has become detached. Fast action is necessary to prevent a serious blood loss. A clamp may be placed on the line until it is reconnected; the alarm is then reset. If the malfunction is in the dialyzer unit or elsewhere in the machine, the dialysis may have to be discontinued or the patient may have to be transferred to another dialyzing machine.

If the bedpan is needed during dialysis, sufficient assistance is provided to prevent possible disturbance of the needles or cannulae and tubes. The fluid intake and output are measured and recorded.

The length of time the patient is kept on the dialyzer varies with the patient's condition and type of machine used. The average range is 4 to 8 hours for patients on a regular dialysis program, but may be longer for a patient with an acute renal shutdown. The frequency also varies with patients. In acute renal failure, daily dialysis may be necessary until renal function is reestablished. Patients with chronic renal insufficiency are dialyzed two or three times weekly and may lead a relatively normal productive life the remainder of the week. The chronic dialysis program may be long-term, extending over years, or may be a temporary measure for the patient who is awaiting a kidney transplant.

POSTDIALYSIS CARE. Upon completion of the dialysis the arterial line is clamped and as much blood as possible in the dialyzing tubes is returned to the patient. Blood samples are again obtained for determination of urea, creatinine and potassium levels; these are recorded. The needles are removed or, in the case of a shunt, the dialyzing lines disconnected and the cannulae reconnected. Dressings are applied and the area observed until there is no evidence of bleeding; it may be necessary to apply some pressure for a brief period. The patient's weight, blood pressure, pulse and temperature are recorded.

INSTRUCTION. When a regular dialysis program is recommended, the patient and a family member receive detailed instruction concerning diet and fluid intake, care of the fistula site or cannulae, activity, and recognition of disturbances that should prompt immediate notification of the physician or dialysis clinic. The brochure given out by the dialysis unit that explains dialysis also discusses these factors.

The diet prescribed varies from patient to patient and with physicians. The food intake must be balanced with the renal capacity to eliminate protein waste and prevent excesses of electrolytes (K^+, Na^+) and water. The protein content may be 60 to 80 Gm. per day, allowing 0.75 to 1 Gm. per kg. of body weight.

Potassium-containing foods may have to be restricted and low sodium is usually necessary because of the associated hypertension. Food values and meal planning are discussed. The suggested fluid intake is usually 500 ml. plus the amount excreted the previous day.

The patient and family need help in interpreting the patient's limitations and activities. His occupation and usual activity are determined and suggestions made as to advisable modifications, if necessary. The patient is encouraged to lead as normal a life as possible. Contact sports such as hockey and football should be avoided because of the fistula or shunt.

Care and maintenance of the A-V fistula or shunt are taught, and the patient takes over the necessary observations and care before his discharge from the hospital. In addition to the care procedure, the importance of observing the shunt every 1 to 2 hours, the recognition of complications (bleeding, clotting and infection) and the appropriate action should complications occur are discussed. Advice is given as to how the patient may protect the A-V bypass and also have maximum freedom.

The patient is given written instructions which outline the prescribed diet, fluid intake, activities and required rest, necessary observations, and the maintenance and care of the A-V shunt. In some instances, it is necessary to teach the patient and a family member how to take temperature and blood pressure.

After discharge from the hospital, the dialysis unit may request the patient to record exactly the food and fluid taken between dialyses. This helps to determine if the restrictions are being understood and followed. The success of a dialysis program is largely dependent upon the ability of the patient to protect and maintain his A-V fistula or shunt, and upon his adherence to the dietary, fluid and activity regulations. This is conveyed to the patient and family tactfully throughout the teaching and discussions.

The patient is advised that if he experiences persisting headache, nausea and vomiting, itching, numbness and tingling in his feet or hands or retention of fluid he should get in touch promptly with his physician or go to the dialysis unit or clinic.

Kidney Transplantation

The development of donor selection by tissue typing, and the steady progress that has been made in managing the rejection process, have resulted in an increase in the number of kidney transplants. The candidates are carefully selected by a team of physicians, surgeons and a psychiatrist. Prospective recipients are those whose life expectancy is limited to a few months at most due to severe renal insufficiency, those with renal failure whose responsibilities are not compatible with a dialysis program, or those who have had a bilateral nephrectomy because of serious hypertension attributed to the release of excessive renin by the kidneys. The patient must be free of chronic infection in other systems, and the lower urinary tract must be structurally normal and free of disease.

An advantage of a kidney transplant for the person who has severe renal failure is the discontinuance of the demanding dialysis schedule; considerable time is saved, and the individual's occupation is uninterrupted and more productive. Dietary restrictions are lifted and constraint of activity is slight.

REJECTION PROCESS. The greatest hazard associated with any organ or tissue transplant from another person is the incompatibility of the recipient's tissue with that of the donor, and the ensuing rejection process. Secondary to this are the effects of the immunosuppressive drugs used to depress the rejection process; the most formidable is the recipient's increased susceptibility to infection.

The rejection process is an antigen-antibody reaction or immune response; the recipient's immune system recognizes the graft as a foreign substance, and specific antibodies and sensitized lymphocytes attack the foreign tissue. In the case of a renal homograft, the kidney becomes swollen, edematous and congested. Thrombosis occurs in the blood vessels, and tissue necrosis due to ischemia follows. Rejection is manifested by fever, tenderness and swelling in the kidney region, general malaise, headache, anorexia, an elevation in the leukocyte count, decreased urinary output, edema, hypertension and elevated blood levels of urea, creatinine, sodium and potassium. The patient becomes anxious at first, and then appears gradually apathetic and lethargic.

The intensity of the rejection process and the rapidity with which it develops correspond to the degree of difference in the cellular antigens between the recipient and donor; the greater the difference, the more severe and rapid is the rejection. *Hyperacute rejec-tion* occurs within minutes or hours of the transplant, due to preformed antibodies attacking the homograft. This severe type of reaction may be attributed to presensitization to donor antigens as a result of previous transfusions or several pregnancies. Widespread intravascular coagulation occurs in the transplanted kidney, and failure develops.

Acute or early rejection may develop in the postoperative or convalescent period or it may occur 1 to 4 months following the transplantation. Oliguria and increasing blood urea and creatinine levels are manifested. Rejection can usually be reversed by high doses of immunosuppressive drugs (e.g., corticosteroids).

Chronic or late rejection develops insidiously after 3 or 4 months, or it may occur several years after the homograft was received. This type of rejection is characterized by arterial impairment due to intimal hyperplasia. It is attributed to chronic reaction between circulating antibodies and the antigens of the vascular endothelial cells.

The antigenicity and compatibility of the donor and recipient in tissue and organ transplants are determined by heredity. The antigens of concern, being determined by genes, are specific for each individual and are located on the surfaces of nucleated cells and red blood cells. Erythrocyte antigens compose the ABO antigen system used in blood typing and matching in blood transfusions, and may be present in vascular endothelium of the graft. Blood types are not crossed in organ transplant.

The donor-recipient relationship is an important factor in influencing acceptance or rejection of a graft. The closer the relationship, the greater is the possibility of compatibility. Because cellular proteins and antigens are specific for each individual, donor tissue is rejected by the recipient's body unless it is taken from an identical twin. In this case, the transplant is compatible because the antigens of both the host and donor are identical, having been determined by the same genetic blueprint of a single fertilized ovum. Such a graft (with identical cellular proteins and antigens) is referred to as an *isograft*. A graft between two genetically dissimilar persons is known as an *allograft* or *homograft*.

The antigens located on the nucleated cells belong to the system designated HL-A (human leukocyte antigen). Most of the antigens are represented on the leukocytes and blood platelets, which are readily accessible for tissue typing and clinical tissue tests for histocompatibility of potential donor tissue. Histocompatibility is defined as "the quality of a cellular or tissue graft enabling it to be accepted and functional when transplanted to another organism."[8]

Currently, 11 antigens are recognized in testing. These are numbered and divided into two series; those in one series are controlled by a gene in a different locus from that of the one responsible for those in the other series. One series contains HL-A 1, 2, 3, 9, 10 and 11; the other has HL-A 5, 7, 8, 12 and 13. Currently, it is recognized that each individual has a total of four HL-A antigens; two from series 1 and two from series 2.[9, 10]

HISTOCOMPATIBILITY DETERMINATION. The principal methods used to determine the recipient's immunologic response to potential donor tissue are the lymphocyte cytotoxicity test and mixed lymphocytes culture (MLC).

The *lymphocyte cytotoxicity test* (Terasaki test) is the typing of lymphocytes from the recipient and each potential donor for HL-A antigens by use of a series of standard sera which contain HL-A antibodies. The reaction of the donor's and patient's cells to each serum is observed; the more similar the nature and intensity of the reaction, the closer is the histocompatibility between the donor and patient.

The *mixed lymphocytes culture* involves making a culture of a mixture of the recipient's and potential donor's lymphocytes. The response of the recipient's lymphocytes to donor antigens is observed; reaction is demonstrated by the degree of change in the recipient lymphocytes in response to the other lymphocytes' antigens. The donor cells are treated before culturing to inhibit their response to the recipient's antigens.

Currently, histocompatibility tests may be reported as A, B, C, D, E, or F. According to Falk and Falk, A represents the match characteristic of identical twins. B indicates that the HL-A antigens of donor cells are present in the recipient, but the recipient has

antigens not present in the donor. The C match has one HL-A antigen not in the recipient; D has two that are not present in the recipient. In an E match, the donor has three antigens not represented in the recipient and an F match indicates that the recipient has antibodies active against the donor's HL-A antigens.[11]

A second system of recording the degree of histocompatibility is the net histocompatibility ratio (NHR). A report of 1.0 represents a matching of the four HL-A antigens identified for both donor and recipient. If all four are mismatched the NHR is 0. Intermediate grades of similarity are given in fractions and the greater the number (e.g., 0.5 as opposed to 0.05), the closer the match.[12]

IMMUNOSUPPRESSIVE DRUGS. Unless the organ is taken from an identical twin, some degree of rejection will occur. Fortunately, the process can be modified by therapeutic agents which depress the tissues responsible for the production of lymphocytes, plasma cells and antibodies that attack donor tissue. The immunosuppressive drugs used include azathioprine (Imuran), corticosteroids (prednisone), dactinomycin (actinomycin D), cyclophosphamide and antilymphocytic globulin (ALG) (see Table 19–2). ALG is produced by the injection of washed lymphocytes into a horse, whose system reacts by forming antibodies against the antigens. Blood is then withdrawn from the horse and the globulin fraction extracted from the serum. Suppression of the patient's immune reaction makes him extremely vulnerable to any infection.

DONOR. In early transplants, the kidney was always obtained from a live blood relative. Now, cadavers serve as the principal donor source. The cadaver is frequently an accident victim or someone who has had a sudden death and who is known to have been in good health.

If a living donor is used, he is usually related to the patient. As cited earlier, the donation is more likely to be successful if the relative is close (e.g., sibling, parent) than if the donor is a genetically nonrelated person (e.g., cousin, uncle by marriage).

[8]Benjamin F. Miller and Claire B. Keane: Encyclopedia and Dictionary of Medicine, Nursing and Allied Health, 2nd ed. Philadelphia, W. B. Saunders, 1978, p. 472.

[9]Dorothy J. Brundage: Nursing Management of Renal Problems. St. Louis, C. V. Mosby, 1976, pp. 154–155.

[10]Joan DeLong Harrington and Etta Rae Brener: Patient Care in Renal Failure. Philadelphia, W. B. Saunders, 1973, p. 174.

[11]J. A. Falk and R. E. Falk: "HL-A antigens in Clinical Transplantation." Med. Clin. North Am., Vol. 56, No. 2 (March 1972), pp. 403–417.

[12]David C. Sabiston, Jr. (Ed.): Textbook of Surgery, 11th ed. Philadelphia, W. B. Saunders, 1977, pp. 464–474.

TABLE 19–2 IMMUNOSUPPRESSIVE DRUGS

Drug	Dosage	Action	Side Effects
Azathioprine (Imuran)	1–5 mg./kg. body weight, oral. Regulated by leukocyte count.	Inhibits the synthesis of nucleic acids in cell production. Depresses the production of leukocytes (especially lymphocytes) and antibodies.	Bone marrow depression, mouth ulcers and, rarely, hepatitis.
Adrenocorticosteroid (e.g., prednisone, oral; Solu-Cortef, intravenous)	20–200 mg./day orally. Up to 2 Gm./day may be given intravenously during a rejection crisis.	Suppresses the inflammatory response; suppresses lymphocyte and antibody formation.	Lowered resistance to infection, gastrointestinal ulceration and bleeding, edema due to sodium retention, mood swings, weight gain, moon facies and cataracts.
Dactinomycin (actinomycin D)	200 micrograms intravenously during a rejection crisis.	Inhibits RNA synthesis, suppressing cell division and reproduction.	Bone marrow depression, irritation and ulceration of mucous membrane, nausea and vomiting and alopecia.
Antilymphocyte globulin (ALG)	Daily intramuscular injection(s) for a period of 2 weeks following the transplantation. (Dosage may be in units or mg.)	Suppresses lymphocyte action.	Anaphylaxis. Patient requires very close observation; the reaction may be manifested by urticaria, chills and fever, joint pains, or the patient may complain of dyspnea and develop shock.
Cyclophosphamide (Cytoxan)	1–5 mg./kg. body weight, oral.	Suppresses cell reproduction.	Bone marrow depression, alopecia and cystitis.

Obviously, the living donor must be in good health. He undergoes a thorough investigation which includes an intravenous urogram and a renal angiogram to insure normal kidneys with a normal vascular supply. He must have volunteered willingly and made the decision without pressure from others. The decision is a major one; it requires a mature, stable person. The immunologic and other investigations preceding the operation to remove the kidney, the nature of the surgery, the inherent risk in being left with one kidney and the possibility of rejection of the graft by the recipient are explained and discussed freely with the prospective donor. He is informed of the time it will take, since it may necessitate a period of absence from his job. A consent is signed for the removal of the kidney following the investigation period.

Immediate preoperative preparation and postoperative care of the donor is similar to that cited in the section on nursing in renal surgery (see p. 654). The function of the remaining kidney is monitored closely.

Blood urea and serum creatinine levels are followed for 2 to 3 weeks to assess compensatory efficiency. The patient's reactions are observed, since he may suddenly be alarmed by the risk he has taken and need support.

When a cadaver is sought as a donor, the next of kin is approached when it is known that the patient cannot recover. Consent is obtained prior to actual decease, so that the organ can be removed promptly when death occurs to avoid damage from ischemia. Rarely have relatives been known to refuse. Permission from the coroner is also necessary in case of accidental and sudden death. Several persons are usually awaiting a kidney transplant. When a donor becomes imminent a selection of two recipients is made on the basis of tissue matching, since both kidneys of the cadaver are used.

When death occurs, the kidneys are removed with their arteries, veins and ureters. The blood vessels are flushed out with cold saline and the kidneys perfused with cold saline (4° C.) or lactated Ringer's solution containing heparin and procaine. The procaine promotes dilatation of the vessels. The organs are kept cool in a refrigerator until implantation. They may be stored in this way for a period of up to about 16 hours. Precautions are taken to avoid freezing which incurs permanent tissue damage. Storage up to 2 to 3 days requires pump oxygenator perfusion, and some surgeons indicate that there is a greater risk of damage to the kidneys by this method of preservation. When a cadaver kidney is used in a transplant, the source remains anonymous to the recipient and his family.

The donor kidney is placed in the recipient's iliac fossa on the side opposite to that from which it was taken — that is, a left donor kidney is placed in the recipient's right iliac fossa. Its renal artery is anastomosed to the host's hypogastric artery, and the renal vein of the graft is anastomosed to the common or external iliac vein. The ureter is implanted in the recipient's bladder via a submucosal tunnel; the latter prevents urinary reflux. His kidneys are removed because they are a potential source of infection. In some instances, the patient may have had a previous bilateral nephrectomy and have been maintained entirely on hemodialysis.

In the case of a living donor, the removal of the kidney and the surgical implantation in the recipient are synchronized in adjacent operating rooms; this greatly reduces the period of ischemia and the risk of tissue damage.

PREOPERATIVE PREPARATION OF THE RECIPIENT. When a person is selected as a candidate for a renal transplant, the physician discusses in detail all that is involved with him and his family. They are advised that his disease is irreversible and is likely to prove fatal before long. They are informed of what is entailed in the surgery — that the kidney graft may be rejected, necessitating the resumption of a chronic hemodialysis program; that continuous drug therapy and close supervision will be needed; and that precautions against infections will be necessary. A special consent is signed, indicating that the extent of the disease, the prognosis and what a transplant involves have been fully explained.

If the patient has not been having hemodialysis, treatments are instituted twice weekly in an effort to bring him into an optimal condition for the transplant. Cultures are taken from the skin and all body orifices to check for infection. If any are found to be present, he receives appropriate antibiotic therapy. All personnel in contact with the patient should be free of colds and other infection, and strict medical asepsis is observed between patients.

A psychological assessment is made by a psychiatrist, since any psychosis that the patient might have is likely to be exaggerated by the corticoid medication he will receive following the transplant, as well as by the constant fear of rejection that he is likely to have.

If the patient's anemia is severe, he receives washed or packed cells; whole blood provides exposure to the donor's leukocyte antigens. Generally, transfusions are avoided if possible because of the increased risk of sensitization and provocation of an immunologic reaction. This predisposes the patient to more severe and rapid rejection of the donor kidney.

The blood pressure, which is likely to be elevated, is followed closely. If an antihypertensive drug is being administered, the nurse is alert for side effects and sharp pressure swings up or down. An accurate record is made of the fluid intake and output; the intake is regulated daily according to the output of the previous day to avoid overloading the cardiovascular system and promoting electrolyte imbalances.

Efforts are made to improve the patient's nutritional status and to meet his caloric requirements. His diet is catered to fit the protein and sodium restrictions prescribed.

When the death of a suitable donor becomes imminent, the patient is started on immunosuppressive drugs. If the period is likely to be short, Imuran and Solu-Cortef may be given intravenously. If the drugs are given orally over several days, the dosage may be adjusted according to the daily leukocyte count.

The patient's hair is washed, and a bath with a prescribed antiseptic solution may be ordered to minimize bacterial flora on the skin. Preoperative skin cleansing and shaving extend from the axillae to midthighs and include the perineum. A nasogastric tube may be passed to control postoperative vomiting and distention, and an intravenous infusion is started as part of the immediate postoperative preparation. A central venous pressure line may also be established so the intravascular fluid volume can be monitored. A retention

(Foley) catheter is introduced into the bladder in the operating room under strict aseptic conditions.

POSTOPERATIVE CARE. The nursing care of the patient who has received a kidney transplant is similar to that cited on page 655, and includes measures to prevent infection and graft rejection. The immediate care is the same as that for any patient recovering from anesthetic.

PREVENTION OF INFECTION. The patient is nursed in a single room using reverse isolation technique for a period of 7 to 10 days. The staff is screened for infection, and the same personnel care for the patient on each shift from day to day when possible.

Visitors are limited to close family members who are screened for infection and are required to wear sterile gowns, caps and masks during the visit. Direct contact with the patient is not permitted. Originally, efforts were made to maintain an almost aseptic environment for transplant patients during their hospitalization. Some details have been relaxed since it was found that most complicating infections are endogenous.

Frequent cleansing of the mouth is important, especially during the initial postoperative period when oral fluids are not given. It is cleansed with a mild antiseptic every 2 hours, and then four times daily (p.c. and h.s.) when the patient is allowed regular meals. A soft toothbrush is recommended to avoid trauma to the gums and oral mucosa, and the mouth is inspected daily for any infection. Deep breathing, coughing and turning are carried out every 2 hours until the patient is ambulatory to prevent the accumulation of mucus in the respiratory tract.

The female patient's perineum is cleansed thoroughly three times a day and after every bowel movement. In the case of the male patient, the area around the urinary meatus is cleansed two or three times daily to reduce the possibility of infection entering the urethra.

If infection develops, an antibiotic is prescribed and the dosage of immunosuppressive drugs may be decreased, or prednisone may be discontinued for a brief period.

OBSERVATIONS. Vital signs, urinary output, fluid intake and electrolyte concentrations are monitored, and frequent observations are made for bleeding from the wound and early signs of infection and rejection. The nurse must be constantly aware of the patient's lowered body resistance to infection due to depression of his most important defense mechanisms (lymphocytes and antibodies). The recognition of early signs of infection is necessary so that prompt antibiotic therapy may be instituted. Any oral or skin lesion, cough, nasal discharge, gastrointestinal disturbance, elevation of temperature or complaint of general malaise, pain or discomfort is promptly brought to the physician's attention. The leukocyte count is recorded daily and compared with the preoperative count. Any elevation is brought to the physician's attention; if it falls below 4000 per cu. mm. it is also reported. Immunosuppressive drug dosage is adjusted according to the leukocyte count.

The retention catheter is connected to a sterile closed-drainage system; the urinary output is recorded half-hourly for several hours and then hourly. Frequent urinalyses and cultures are made. Blood-colored urine may be expected at first but should progressively clear over 3 to 4 hours.

The transplanted kidney usually begins to excrete urine soon after the surgery. The volume may increase rapidly, resulting in profuse diuresis. Unless there is adequate replacement during this diuretic phase, dehydration, shock and electrolyte imbalance may develop. The patient may experience bladder spasm and pain with the large urine volume, because the bladder has not been used to receiving urine for some time preoperatively. If the transplant fails to excrete sufficient urine for several days, hemodialysis may be used until kidney function improves. Twenty-four hour collections of urine are continued for at least 10 to 14 days. Once the kidney function appears to be stabilized and the hourly measurement can be discontinued, the catheter is removed. The patient is encouraged to void frequently to avoid overdistention of the bladder and pressure on the ureteral implantation area, and an aliquot of each voiding is analyzed.

The nasogastric tube is attached to low suction and the drainage measured accurately. The drainage and all excreta are observed for blood. Gastrointestinal bleeding may occur as a result of peptic ulcer incurred by the steroid (prednisone) medication.

The patient is placed on a weighing bed (if available) on return from the operating room to facilitate the daily recording of his weight.

The central venous pressure is recorded every 1 to 2 hours; the physician is consulted if it is below 8 cm. or above 18 cm. The former indicates the need for more fluid; the latter signifies retention of fluid and overloading of the intravascular system. The increased intravascular volume places an increased demand on the heart and predisposes to pulmonary edema.

The fluid balance is determined every 6 to 8 hours by comparing the total intake with the total fluid loss (urine and gastric drainage). Any deficit or excess determines the intake volume. The electrolyte composition of the intravenous fluids is based upon the laboratory reports.

The nurse must be constantly alert for early manifestations of the rejection process, which may occur as early as the second or third day. There may be swelling and increasing tenderness over the kidney, fever, general malaise, headache, an elevation in the leukocyte count, anorexia, decreased urinary output, edema and elevated levels of serum creatinine, sodium and potassium and blood urea.

PREVENTION OF REJECTION. The administration of immunosuppressive drugs is resumed in the immediate postoperative period and continued. These drugs depress the body's responses to the donor kidney's antigens. The drugs used most commonly are azathioprine (Imuran) and a corticosteroid preparation (prednisone). Antilymphocytic globulin (ALG) may be given intramuscularly at regular intervals in the initial postoperative period, then gradually decreased and eventually discontinued.

As cited earlier, the dosage of azathioprine and prednisone are adjusted according to the leukocyte count and the patient's reactions to these drugs. It is necessary for the nurse to be familiar with their side effects. Imuran may depress the bone marrow production of leukocytes and produce leukopenia. Reactions to prolonged administration of prednisone may include the retention of sodium and water, an elevation of blood pressure, hirsutism, development of a round puffy face ("moon face"), euphoria, gastrointestinal ulceration, impaired liver and pancreatic function, and arrested growth in a child. Since ALG is a serum, one must be alert for an anaphylactic reaction; an intracutaneous sensitivity test is done before the initial dose.

The signs and symptoms of rejection are cited above under observations. When rejection is manifested the patient is given higher doses of prednisone; it may be given intravenously as well as orally. Dactinomycin may also be administered. The patient may receive local irridation of the kidney daily for 3 days. If the reaction is severe and there is marked fluid retention and elevation of serum potassium and creatinine and blood urea, dialysis may have to be resumed. Fluid intake and dietary restrictions may also be necessary.

If the rejection process is irreversible, the immunosuppressive drugs are discontinued and the graft is removed. The patient becomes discouraged and the nurse should be prepared to offer support and reassure the patient that he may be considered for a second graft.

OTHER MEDICATIONS. Since most medications are eliminated through the kidneys, as few drugs as possible are given following a renal transplantation. Small doses of an analgesic may be prescribed, if necessary, for the relief of pain and discomfort when nursing measures do not provide adequate palliation.

WOUND CARE. A gown and mask and sterile gloves are worn when changing the dressing on the wound. A tube may have been placed in the retroperitoneal cavity at operation, or a hemovac may have been applied to drain the area of any fluid. Observations are made for any sign of infection, swelling or leakage of urine.

DIET. The nasogastric tube is usually removed within the 48 hours after surgery, and the patient receives clear fluids by mouth. If tolerated, the diet then progresses through fluids to soft foods and then to a light diet. Roughage and highly seasoned foods are avoided because of the predisposition to gastrointestinal ulceration created by the corticosteroid medication. During a rejection crisis, renal function is impaired. The fluid intake and diet are adjusted to the reduced urinary output and the changes in blood chemistry which occur. That is, the fluid intake will be approximately 400 ml. in excess of the volume of urine for the preceding day, and protein and sodium are restricted in the diet according to blood urea and serum electrolyte levels.

POSITIONING AND AMBULATION. The patient may lie on his back or operative side and the bed may be elevated to a 30° or 45° angle when his blood pressure is stable. He is advised not to lie on the unoperative side to avoid displacement of the graft. The sitting position is also avoided as much as possible to reduce the possibility of increasing the tension on the anastomoses of vessels and ureter, and kinking of the ureter.

The patient is ambulatory after 48 hours and may walk or stand, but periods of sitting are discouraged.

PREPARATION FOR DISCHARGE. The patient may become apprehensive about leaving the hospital and becoming independent. He is likely to become fearful as he learns he must follow a prescribed pattern of living indefinitely and be constantly alert for early signs of rejection and complications. He and a member of his family receive a planned series of instruction which provides them with the opportunity to become informed about all aspects of his care. The hospital usually provides an outline of the information the patient requires in booklet or brochure form.

A social service worker is usually available in a center where organ transplants are done, and can be of considerable assistance to the patient and family in planning for the future. The patient may not be able to resume his former occupation even if it is still available to him, since strenuous physical activity is not advisable. The social worker may provide assistance in finding suitable employment or, if work is not possible, may help in obtaining welfare assistance to provide for the patient and family. For instance, the provision of medications will be costly and may cause financial embarrassment for them. Suitable forms of recreation and sports in which he is interested are discussed. Body contact sports should be avoided, and it is usually recommended that seatbelts should not be worn across the lower abdomen.

The drugs which he must continue to take are discussed fully. It is helpful if a sample of each is attached to a card on which the name of the drug, its strength, and directions for taking are clearly printed. The nurse stresses the importance of these drugs, and that if they cannot be taken or retained because of illness, the patient must contact the physician or clinic promptly. The cards are taken to the clinic or the physician when visits are made so that if the dosage is changed the directions on the cards may be changed.

The patient is instructed to keep a daily record of his weight and fluid output. Verbal and written explanations are made of the content and preparation of his bland diet. Foods that are restricted are listed. Since the prednisone may increase his appetite, the patient is advised to guard against exceeding his normal weight.

Suggestions are made as to how he may protect himself as much as possible from infection. Close contact with persons with a cold or other types of infections should be avoided. Good hygienic practices in food handling and the frequent washing of the hands are stressed. A daily bath is recommended to minimize skin bacteria, and good oral hygiene is reviewed.

The early signs of rejection are reviewed with the patient and family. By this time the patient is usually quite familiar with them and realizes that prompt action is necessary. The patient and family are cautioned to report immediately a cold, sore throat, fever, dysuria, frequency or other disturbances which may indicate infection. The patient is also urged to contact promptly his physician or the clinic if there is a sudden gain in weight (for example, 2 or more pounds in a day), swelling of the ankles or puffiness of the face, pain, tenderness and/or swelling in the area of the graft, decrease in urinary output, headache, unaccounted for fatigue, or elevation in temperature.

The patient is usually in the hospital for about 6 weeks. Following discharge he is followed closely by weekly visits to the clinic, since constant surveillance plays an important role in his progress and the development of acceptance of the situation with less fear. If his progress is satisfactory, and he indicates understanding and efficient management of his care, the intervals between visits are gradually lengthened. A referral may be made to a visiting nurse association. Prior to visiting the patient at home, the visiting nurse is informed of his history and the details of his care.

Fellowship develops between transplant patients while they are in the hospital. They share common problems which include restrictions, fears and an uncertainty of life. Continued communication between these persons is encouraged; they can offer considerable support to one another.

COMPLICATIONS. In addition to infection and the rejection process, complications which may develop in the recipient after a kidney transplantation include the following:

Tubular Necrosis. This is attributed to the ischemia of the kidney during the period between its removal and grafting. It is manifested by oliguria and the effects of the retained metabolic wastes and excess fluid.

Gastrointestinal Ulceration and Bleeding. These may be caused by the corticosteroid preparation which the patient receives to suppress the immunologic response to the graft. Any vomitus or feces containing blood is reported to the physician.

Cataracts. These are also a side effect of the prednisone. Patients are advised to have their eyes examined annually.

Urinary Fistula. This may be due to failure of healing of the ureter at the site of anastomosis with the bladder.

Lack of Wound Healing. This may be caused by the steroid medication or urine leakage.

Bone Marrow Depression. This is due to the immunosuppressive drugs. Leukopenia develops, which predisposes the individual to serious infections; erythrocyte production is depressed, and the signs and symptoms of anemia develop; normal coagulation may be impaired when the thrombocytes are decreased, and bleeding from mucous membranes, petechiae and ecchymoses may become evident.

OTHER DISORDERS INVOLVING RENAL DYSFUNCTION

Glomerulonephritis

At the onset, this disease is characterized by a diffuse, noninfectious inflammation of the glomeruli of both kidneys. Since the blood supply that supports the tubules normally passes through glomerular capillaries before reaching them, fibrous scarring and obliteration of some glomeruli lead to secondary degenerative changes in the associated tubules. It is more common in children and young adults and has a higher incidence in males. It may be acute or chronic.

ETIOLOGY. The inflammation is attributed to an antigen-antibody reaction. Wrong suggests that two types of immune reactions cause glomerulonephritis.[13] In one, antigen-antibody complexes formed extrarenally are trapped in glomeruli and initiate the inflammatory process; this is the more common reaction responsible for glomerulonephritis. The second immune reaction involves antibodies that are formed against an antigen in or produced by the glomerular basement membrane, initiating glomerular inflammation.

The most common cause of glomerulonephritis is the beta-hemolytic streptococcus (group A). The patient's history usually reveals that the renal disturbance follows an infection, such as a sore throat or respiratory infection of some form, by a latent period of 2 to 4 weeks. In some instances, the infection may have been so mild that little or no attention was given to it at the time.

Glomerulonephritis may also be associated with other infections or autoimmune diseases such as systemic lupus erythematosus, polyarteritis nodosa and scleroderma.

SIGNS AND SYMPTOMS. The onset is generally abrupt but in some instances may be insidious. The affected glomeruli are partially or completely obstructed, resulting in reduced filtration. Some glomeruli rupture, permitting the escape of blood into the tubules. The permeability of the glomeruli that remain patent is increased. The scant output of urine is cloudy and contains albumin, blood cells and casts.

Edema develops and is usually seen first in the periorbital areas and ankles. The patient complains of pain and tenderness in the back, headache, and weakness. Visual disturbances may also be manifested. The blood pressure is elevated, and decreased filtration results in a gradual accumulation of nitrogenous wastes in the blood; the blood urea and serum creatinine levels may be elevated.

Nasal and throat cultures may be done to determine if streptococci are still present. Examination of the blood may reveal an elevation in antistreptolysin O titer (ASO titer).

Neurological signs and symptoms corresponding to the degree of hypertension and cerebral edema may be present (see p. 617).

---

[13] Paul B. Beeson and Walsh McDermott (Eds.): Textbook of Medicine, 14th ed. Philadelphia, W. B. Saunders, 1975, p. 1128.

Unless the renal insufficiency is reversed, uremia, pulmonary edema and cardiac failure may ensue.

MANAGEMENT. The treatment of patients with acute glomerulonephritis consists mainly of rest, fluid and diet regulation, and chemotherapy to eliminate possible residual streptococcal infection. The patient is confined to bed with restricted activity to minimize the production of metabolic wastes. The daily fluid intake is restricted to 400 to 500 ml. in excess of the urinary output of the previous 24 hours. The blood chemistry is followed closely and the sodium, potassium, and chloride intake regulated according to the findings. The patient is sustained chiefly on carbohydrate; a minimum of 100 Gm. is given daily to reduce the breakdown of tissue protein. Protein in the diet is regulated according to the BUN level and the amount of urea excreted in the urine. Similarly, salt restriction in the diet is regulated according to the degree of edema and hypertension.

If the low output of urine is prolonged and the blood potassium and nitrogenous waste levels are progressively increasing, either peritoneal dialysis or hemodialysis may be instituted (see p. 631).

Precautions are necessary to protect the patient from chilling and exposure to infection. A superimposed infection could aggravate the disease or produce pneumonia that could prove fatal.

The frequent association of glomerulonephritis with respiratory infections emphasizes their potential danger and the importance of prevention and prompt, adequate treatment of such infections. Too often they are ignored, considered as unavoidably seasonal and treated very lightly. Women who have a history of acute glomerulonephritis are advised to consult a doctor before planning a pregnancy, since they are more likely to develop toxemia and eclampsia.

According to the literature, the majority of patients with acute glomerulonephritis associated with infection (e.g., streptococcal) recover with no residual kidney damage. These patients generally show an increase in the volume of urine and a decrease in the blood pressure and BUN within 1 week. The albuminuria and microscopic hematuria may persist for much longer. A few patients progress through a subacute phase to chronic glomerulonephritis. Others may be asymptomatic for a period of months or years and then experience an insidious development of the chronic disease which may progress to chronic renal failure.

Pyelonephritis

This is an inflammation of the pelvis and parenchymal tissue of the kidney due to infection. The predominant causative organisms are the gram-negative enteric bacilli which have invaded the lower urinary tract and ascended to the kidney via the ureters. In rare instances, the pathogen, such as the staphylococcus or streptococcus, may be bloodborne.

Significant predisposing factors are defective urinary drainage and reflux of urine from the bladder into the ureters. Obstructions to the flow of urine from the kidney may be the result of a renal calculus, new-growth, stricture of a ureter due to pressure, scarring or congenital anomaly. Stasis of urine in the lower urinary tract due to bladder or urethral dysfunction may increase the intravesical pressure sufficiently to produce a reflux into the ureters.

Pyelonephritis is more common in females than males. The incidence is relatively high in female infants and children, due perhaps to fecal soiling and *Escherichia coli* contamination of the urethral meatus. Its frequent occurrence in pregnant women is attributed to stasis of urine incurred by pressure from the enlarging uterus and atonia of the ureters due to the effect of progesterone. Pyelonephritis in males in the later years of life is generally associated with defective urinary drainage as a result of an enlarged prostate.

MANIFESTATIONS. The onset is usually sudden. In children it may be accompanied by a convulsion. Manifestations include chills, fever, headache, nausea and vomiting, pain and tenderness in the loins, leukocytosis, and frequent and painful micturition (dysuria). The urine is cloudy and contains bacteria, pus, blood, and epithelial cells.

TREATMENT. The patient is confined to bed and is encouraged to take liberal amounts of fluid unless there is complete obstruction of urinary drainage. An accurate record of the fluid intake and output is necessary. An antibiotic or sulfonamide preparation is prescribed. A culture may be made of the urine and the causative organism antibiotic sensitivity determined. A urinary antiseptic such as methenamine mandelate (Mandelamine) or nitrofurantoin (Furadantin) may also be ordered. If nitrofurantoin or a sulfonamide preparation such as Gantrisin is used, the patient is observed for possible reactions which usually appear in the form of nausea and vomiting and a skin rash.

Unless there is complete eradication of the infection, pyelonephritis may become chronic with insidious destruction of nephrons, leading to chronic renal failure and uremia. Following the initial episode of acute pyelonephritis, the patient generally undergoes a thorough investigation for a predisposing obstructive lesion. Antimicrobial therapy and a high fluid intake are prolonged beyond the disappearance of acute signs and symptoms. Specimens of urine are examined and cultured at regular intervals after the antimicrobial drug is discontinued.

Tuberculosis of the Kidney

Tubercular infection in the kidney is usually secondary to tuberculosis elsewhere in the body; most often the primary site is a lung or lymph node. The tubercle bacilli are carried by the blood to the kidneys. Scattered characteristic granulomatous lesions (tubercles) develop, eroding renal tissue and leaving cavitations. The infection may involve pyramids and calyces, interfering with tubular drainage and leading to hydronephrosis. The infection may spread to involve the bladder.

The systemic symptoms characteristic of any tubercular infection are usually present — namely, low-grade fever, night sweats, loss of weight, fatigue and a positive tuberculin skin test. The urine contains pus and blood; smears and a culture reveal the presence of tubercle bacilli. The patient complains of back pain, which may become quite severe in advanced disease. An intravenous pyelogram is done to determine whether the disease is unilateral or bilateral.

The patient receives a prolonged, intensive course of antituberculous drugs (see p. 456). He is observed for possible reactions to the drugs which may take the form of dermatitis, fever, dizziness and impaired hearing. The patient may not be required to remain in bed but is placed on a regimen that will provide extra rest and prevent excessive exertion. A nutritious full diet is encouraged without restrictions if there is adequate renal function to prevent edema, hypertension and the accumulation of wastes in the blood. Frequent urine smears and cultures are made to determine the progress of the patient's disease. The patient is advised against sexual intercourse because the disease can be spread by genital contact. Treatment is continued for a period of at least 18 months even if the cultures become negative for tubercle bacilli.

The Nephrotic Syndrome (Nephrosis)

The characteristic symptoms of the nephrotic syndrome are proteinuria, hypoproteinemia, generalized edema and usually hyperlipemia. It may develop in a patient with primary renal disease, or it may be associated with other conditions in which kidney involvement is secondary (e.g., disseminated lupus erythematosus). In many instances, the syndrome occurs without any known preceding primary or secondary renal impairment and is then referred to as idiopathic nephrosis or idiopathic nephrotic syndrome.

The idiopathic form has a much higher incidence in children, and males are more often affected than females. It is suggested that it may be the result of an immunologic process (antigen-antibody reaction).

The proteinuria, which is chiefly albumin, is the result of some change in the glomeruli that causes an increase in their permeability to the plasma proteins. Obviously, the loss of the proteins reduces the colloidal osmotic pressure of the blood, contributing to increased movement of fluid into the interstitial spaces as well as to its decreased reabsorption into the capillaries (see p. 75). The resulting decrease in intravascular volume leads to retention of sodium and water by the kidneys. The excessive concentration of serum fatty components, which is determined by estimation of the cholesterol level, is not understood.

The urine is reduced in volume and usually contains casts as well as large amounts of albumin. In contrast with other forms of impaired renal function, the blood pressure and nitrogenous waste levels of patients with idiopathic nephrosis usually remain within a normal range in the absence of advanced damage to glomeruli.

The severity of the nephrotic syndrome is variable. In some, the edema may cause only slight puffiness in the periorbital areas and ankles, yet in others it may be so extreme that ascites (accumulation of fluid in the peritoneal cavity) and pleural effusion develop. The edematous areas are generally soft and readily pit on pressure. The patient is usually pale, complains of fatigue and may experience anorexia, which further complicates the problem of hypoproteinemia. The onset may be insidious or abrupt.

TREATMENT. When the nephrotic syndrome is secondary, the treatment is directed toward the initial cause. The treatment of the idiopathic nephrotic syndrome is directed toward inducing diuresis, reducing edema, producing and maintaining a normal serum albumin level and reducing the lipid level in the blood.

The patient receives a low-sodium, high-protein full diet. The recommended daily protein intake is usually 1 Gm. per kg. of body weight plus an amount equivalent to the daily loss in urine. This implies that 24-hour collections of urine are made for estimation of the amount of protein excreted. Because of the anorexia, it may be necessary to use low-sodium milk powder and protein concentrate in order to have the patient receive an adequate amount of protein. Intravenous infusions of plasma or albumin may be given.

The patient is particularly susceptible to infection because of the lowered resistance of edematous tissues and reduced plasma gamma globulin which is essential in the formation of antibodies. Precautions are necessary to avoid exposure to infection.

A diuretic may be used in some instances if there is not a satisfactory response to the corticoid preparation and a reduction of the edema. Spironolactone (Aldactone A), which counteracts the effect of aldosterone on the renal tubules, may be the drug of choice, or a thiazide preparation such as chlorothiazide (e.g., Diuril) may be indicated. An adrenocorticosteroid preparation such as prednisone may be prescribed. It is usually given for a period of 3 to 4 weeks, with the dosage gradually being reduced until the minimum maintenance level is reached. It is then continued in that dosage.

The patient is not usually hospitalized after a satisfactory therapeutic regimen is established, nor is he confined to bed. Activity within his tolerance is encouraged. Treatment is generally required over a long period, and frequent medical checkups are necessary. A referral to a visiting nurse agency may be made to insure regular supervision and guidance in dietary preparation, the taking of the prescribed drugs and the prevention of infection.

Nephrolithiasis (Renal Calculi)

Stones or small concretions may develop in the collecting tubules, calyces or the pelvis of a kidney. They are formed by the precipitation of various substances in the urine; if retained, the initial precipitation forms a nucleus or matrix which promotes further precipitation and calculus enlargement. The substances commonly involved in calculus formation are calcium, oxalate, phosphate, uric acid, cystine, xanthine and ammonia, but most often the stones are of mixed composition (e.g., mixed phosphates and oxalates). They vary in size from tiny particles to large smooth or irregular masses. The irregular stone that forms in the pelvis and has projections into the calyces is referred to as a *staghorn calculus*.

ETIOLOGY. The constituents of renal calculi are present in normal urine; any condition which increases their concentration, reduces their solubility or promotes retention of the urinary salts favors their precipitation and calculus formation and possible obstruction to urinary flow. Conditions favorable to their formation include hypercalcemia, as occurs with hyperparathyroidism, excessive vitamin D, an excessive ingestion of milk or an alkali or prolonged immobilization, hyperuricemia associated with gout (an error in uric acid metabolism), cystinuria, a genetic metabolic disorder in which cystine and other amino acids are excreted in excess by the kidneys, dehydration, and a highly acid urine.

SYMPTOMS. The manifestations of renal calculus depend upon the size of the stone and whether it remains stationary. It may remain latent over a long period, producing no symptoms. Small, gravel-like stones may be passed without any disturbance.

The majority cause some pain, hematuria, infection and, if large, kidney damage and renal insufficiency. Renal calculi may obstruct renal drainage by impaction of the tubules, by completely filling calyces and the pelvis, or by lodging in a ureter. The urine accumulates in the pelvis and tubules, dilating them and creating a back pressure; this condition is known as *hydronephrosis*. Compression of the blood vessels and nephrons by the mass of fluid leads to their destruction and obliteration and to renal insufficiency.

The patient may complain of pain in the back which may be caused by irritation of tissues by movement of the stone or the back pressure and accumulation of fluid if the stone is obstructing renal or ureteral outflow. A small stone may enter the ureter and initiate *ureteral colic*. The patient complains of excruciating pain radiating from the back to the front along the groin into the genitalia. He becomes pale, perspires, is extremely restless and may vomit. Frequently he thrashes about, assuming unusual positions in an attempt to obtain some relief.

Hematuria results from injury to the membranous lining of the pelvis or ureter. Infection is frequently associated with a calculus and, if present, chills, fever, leukocytosis and pyuria are likely to be manifested.

Complete obstruction of the kidney outflow is eventually reflected in renal insufficiency and a palpable mass in the renal area as a result of the hydronephrosis. The total volume of urine is less than normal, and blood investigations indicate reduced elimination of waste products.

Investigation of the patient for nephrolithiasis includes a simple roentgenogram of the kidneys, ureters and bladder. Preparation for this x-ray usually involves a cathartic the night before the x-ray followed by a cleansing enema in the morning. This is to prevent shadows on the film caused by feces and gas in the intestine. Calculi will show up as dense areas. More detailed information is then obtained from intravenous pyelography (see p. 620). Serum calcium and uric acid levels are determined and renal function tests may be done (for the latter, see p. 619). Investigation includes examination of the urine for crystals, 24- or 48-hour serial pH analysis in which the pH of each voiding is recorded, and 24-hour quantitative calcium and magnesium determination.

TREATMENT AND NURSING CARE. If the pyelogram indicates that the calculus is small and may be passed by the patient, he is allowed up and encouraged to be active. Liberal amounts of fluids are given. All urine is strained through several layers of gauze and observation made for concretions. All concretions or solid particles passed are saved and submitted for identification of their composition.

During an attack of ureteral colic, the patient usually receives an analgesic such as meperidine hydrochloride (Demerol) to relieve the pain and an antispasmodic drug such as propantheline bromide (Pro-Banthine) to promote relaxation of the ureter. When the pain subsides, he is allowed to rest in bed and is given fluids.

If the stone is not passed and is lodged in the ureter, the physician may pass a ureteral catheter through a cystoscope past the calculus. It is usually left in place for 24 hours. This promotes drainage of urine from the renal pelvis and dilates the ureter. Instructions are usually left by the doctor about irrigating the catheter in the event that it becomes blocked by pus and blood in the urine. The patient remains in bed and precautions are taken to avoid dislodging the catheter. If patency of the catheter cannot be reestablished by irrigation or the patient experiences pain, the physician is notified at once. When the catheter is removed, the calculus may pass spontaneously. If the calculus is in the lower third of the ureter, a special ureteral catheter with a looped or corkscrew tip may be passed and an attempt made to withdraw the stone. This procedure is referred to as "*removal by instrumentation.*"

When a stone in the kidney or ureter is too large to be passed, open surgery may be undertaken. Removal of a stone through the renal parenchyma is called a *nephrolithotomy*. Removal of a stone directly from the renal pelvis is known as a *pyelolithotomy*. The operation for extracting a stone from the ureter is a *ureterolithotomy*. If the calculus is in the lower part of the ureter, it is approached through an abdominal incision. When it is lodged in the upper part of the ureter, the approach is through an incision in the flank. For the nursing care of a patient undergoing renal surgery, see page 654.

Calculi are prone to recur in patients with a history of previous episodes. In an effort to prevent the formation of new stones or the enlargement of existing stones, the pH of the urine is controlled according to the type of stone involved by a special diet and medication, and measures are used to eliminate any known or suspected infection. For the latter, an antibiotic or sulfonamide preparation such as Gantrisin is prescribed.

The patient is advised that a high fluid intake of at least 3000 ml. daily is essential to maintain a dilute urine. A portion of this should be taken at bedtime and during the night to prevent the concentration of urine that normally occurs at night. If the climate or patient's occupation are such that there is an excessive loss of fluid in perspiration, the intake should be increased by 1000 ml.

If the principal calculus component is calcium (and about 90 per cent of the stones are calcium[14]) the prescribed diet is low in calcium and vitamin D. If the stone is of calcium phosphate, acidification of the urine with three to four glasses of cranberry juice daily is recommended. If uric acid is involved, alkalinization of the urine is important. Solubility is promoted by the administration of sodium bicarbonate or a citrate mixture. The pH of the urine is monitored and an effort made to maintain it at a level above 6.5. Allopurinol is prescribed to lower the serum uric acid level.

The formation of cystine stones is usually seen in children. Alkalinization of the urine and a diet low in methionine are recommended. For details as to the foods which are high and low in the different substances involved in calculus formation, the reader is referred to a diet therapy or urology text. A problem in relation to dietary restrictions is that most stones are of mixed composition.

If the patient should become ill, prolonged immobility should be avoided. The patient is seen at frequent intervals by his physician, and roentgenograms at regular periods may be considered advisable.

Neoplasms in the Kidneys

Newgrowths in the adult kidney are of lower incidence than those in many other areas of the body. When they occur, they are usually malignant and are seen more often in males than in females. The most common form in adults is adenocarcinoma, which usually originates in the tubules. It readily invades the blood vessels, causing early metastasis to bones, lungs or liver, which may be the lesion that brings the person to the physician. Wilms' tumor is a highly malignant adenosarcoma which occurs in young children and may grow very large before being discovered.

MANIFESTATIONS. In the adult, the first symptom is usually hematuria. As the neoplasm enlarges, the kidney becomes a palpable mass and the patient experiences pain, abdominal discomfort from pressure, anorexia and loss of weight. Ureteral colic may occur as a result of a blood clot entering the ureter. Polycythemia develops in some patients due to an overproduction of erythropoietin by the affected kidney. Others may have marked anemia. In children, the newgrowth is frequently noted first as an abdominal mass or swelling by the mother.

A cystoscopy with ureteral catheterization is done to determine if the source of the bleeding is unilateral or bilateral. Roentgenographic studies are made, using an intravenous or retrograde pyelogram to determine filling defects and the location of the neoplasm. A renal angiogram may also be done to assess the extent of blood vessel involvement.

TREATMENT. If the disease is localized to one kidney, a nephrectomy is performed, followed by radiation or chemotherapy or both. If the renal pelvis is involved, the ureter is removed along with the kidney (*nephroureterectomy*). For nursing care required following renal surgery, see page 654. When both kidneys are affected or the patient's condition is considered inoperable, radiation and chemotherapy may be used. For the care of the patient receiving radiation and anticancer drug therapy, see Chapter 8.

Polycystic Disease of the Kidneys

This disorder is characterized by the widespread distribution of cysts of varying sizes throughout both kidneys. The disease is congenital and familial and affects both sexes. It is predominant in infants and adults over 40 years of age. In infants and young children, other abnormalities may be present. The disease is often found in more than one member of the family and in successive generations. Because of the distinct difference in the age of the groups in which the disease is manifested, it is suggested that there are two different genetic types. When it occurs in infants and young children, it is considered to be autosomal recessive, but the polycystic disease which becomes manifest in adults is autosomal dominant.

The adult form is more common and progresses slowly; the patient remains asymp-

---

[14]Felix O. Kolb: "Medical Management of the Patient with Renal Stones." Primary Care, Vol. 2, No. 2 (June 1975), p. 318.

tomatic during the first three to four decades of life. As the cysts enlarge, functional tissue and blood vessels are compressed and, eventually, serious renal insufficiency develops. Pressure on abdominal viscera may interfere with normal functioning and cause discomfort. The symptoms are intermittent gross hematuria from the rupture of blood vessels, pain in the back and abdomen and a palpable mass. The patient may experience episodes of ureteral colic due to blood clots entering the ureters. The degree of compression and damage of parenchymal tissue by the cysts determines the length of survival of the patient. With progression of the disease, he gradually manifests signs of increasing renal failure. The blood pressure and blood nitrogenous waste levels rise, electrolyte and fluid imbalances and anemia develop, and the patient eventually enters the terminal uremic phase.

Conservative treatment of the patient is similar to that for chronic renal failure. The patient may be maintained and kept active by regular hemodialysis and is considered a candidate for renal transplantation.

Since polycystic disease of the kidneys is an inherited disorder, when a patient is discovered to be affected, other members of his family are examined and followed by routine checkups.

Trauma of the Kidneys

Accidental blows and injury to a kidney are not uncommon and may cause contusion or laceration or rupture of the capsule. In laceration and rupture, hemorrhage and the escape or urine into the surrounding tissues are serious problems. Gross or microscopic hematuria occurs and there is pain and tenderness in the kidney region. If the injury is severe and massive hemorrhage occurs, shock develops rapidly. Blood transfusions are given, and surgical intervention is used promptly to bring the bleeding under control. The kidney may be repaired, or a partial or complete nephrectomy may be necessary, depending on the damage revealed.

Contusion of the kidney will usually heal spontaneously. The patient is kept at rest, the fluid intake and output are recorded, and a frequent check is made of the urine for blood. If the damage is extensive, nephrons may be replaced by fibrous scar tissue, resulting in residual impaired function.

NURSING IN RENAL SURGERY

The more common surgical procedures used in the treatment of kidney disease include the following: *nephrectomy* (the removal of a kidney—may be partial or complete), *nephrolithotomy* (the removal of a calculus from the parenchymal portion of the kidney), *pyelolithotomy* (the removal of a calculus through an incision into the renal pelvis), *nephrostomy* (an incision into the kidney and the insertion of a tube for drainage), and *nephroureterectomy* (the removal of a kidney and its ureter).

Preoperative Preparation

Surgery on a kidney is preceded by a period of investigation of kidney function and the patient's general condition. If a nephrectomy is anticipated, the ability of the opposite kidney to compensate and assume the full responsiblity for renal function must be determined. The patient and his family are generally very apprehensive of this major surgery. Aware of this, the nurse observes their behavior to determine their level of anxiety, concerns, and the reassurance needed. By showing an interest in them, providing opportunities for them to express their feelings, answering their questions and explaining what may be expected, the nurse helps to reduce the patient's and family's anxiety and promotes their confidence in those responsible for his care. They are advised by the physician that the removal of the kidney is necessary but need reassurance that normal function can be maintained by one kidney.

The physical preparation is similar to that cited in Chapter 10. Unless contraindicated by a condition such as hydronephrosis, the fluid intake is increased to promote the maximum excretion of metabolic wastes before surgery as well as optimal hydration. Since the incision is usually made in the flank of the affected side, the area of skin to be shaved and cleansed extends from the anterior midline to beyond the spine and from the nipple line to the symphysis pubis (see Fig. 10-1). The surgeon may request that an indwelling catheter and a nasogastric tube be passed the morning of operation. The latter is used because renal surgical patients are prone to develop a reduction or cessation of peristalsis and severe abdominal distention. The catheter is introduced so that a frequent check may be made of the urinary output.

Postoperative Care

The general nursing care presented in Chapter 10 is applicable to the patient who has had renal surgery.

The nurse must be familiar with what was done at operation in order to understand the purposes and care of drainage tubes and make pertinent observations. The operative site is checked at frequent intervals for bleeding. If the kidney was removed, the wound may be sealed with only a tissue drain inserted. If the kidney remains, a tube may have been inserted, necessitating frequent observation for patency and characteristics of the drainage. The tube may become obstructed by a clot, which will cause back pressure unless promptly cleared. Irrigation with a small amount (approximately 10 ml.) of sterile normal saline may be ordered to remove clots. If the tube is connected to a drainage receptable, the amount is measured and recorded every 6 to 8 hours. The volume of the urinary drainage from the indwelling catheter is noted, and less than 25 to 30 ml. per hour is reported. The urine is also checked for any sign of bleeding. An accurate record of the daily intake and output is kept and the balance estimated.

A regular schedule of deep breathing, coughing and turning is established. A directive is received from the surgeon as to positioning. Some patients are not permitted to lie on the operative side for 36 to 48 hours; in other instances, the patient may be encouraged to lie on that side to promote drainage. With each change of position, caution must be used to avoid displacing the tube or leaving it compressed, kinked or with traction on it. Because of the location of the incision, deep breathing is likely to be painful, predisposing to shallow respirations and pulmonary complications. The nurse assists the patient and supports the operative area while prompting the patient to take 8 to 10 deep respirations and cough every 1 to 2 hours.

If the dressings become moist, they are reinforced and the surgeon consulted. He may not want them disturbed for the first day or two. If there is urine drainage, the dressings are changed frequently to prevent maceration of the skin and an offensive odor.

The patient is sustained on intravenous infusions for 36 to 48 hours. Serum electrolyte determinations and the fluid balance serve as a guide to the volume and composition of the fluids used. Clear fluids may then be given orally in small amounts and increased gradually as tolerated. Solid food is introduced as soon as intestinal peristalsis is reestablished; this is evidenced by bowel sounds, the passage of flatus and absence of abdominal distention. If distention develops, the nasogastric tube is left in place, and a rectal tube is inserted. A heat application (e.g., electric heating pad) to the abdomen may be ordered. An intramuscular injection of neostigmine (Prostigmin) may be prescribed to stimulate peristalsis, and an enema is given.

Considerable pain is usually experienced in the first 2 to 3 days. Some aches and discomfort may be the result of the hyperextended lateral position used during operation. Support, change of position and analgesics are necessary. A small pillow placed between the lower costal margin and the iliac crest when the patient is on his side may reduce the discomfort by relieving strain on the incision.

Hospitalization for a minimum period of 12 to 14 days is usually considered necessary following renal surgery, since secondary hemorrhage may develop due to delayed healing and the sloughing of renal tissue. Necessary limitations of activity, any dietary restriction, and the optimal fluid intake are discussed in detail with the patient and a family member before hospital discharge. If the wound still requires a dressing, they are taught how to care for it, or a referral is made to a visiting nurse agency. The expense of the necessary dressing supplies may pose a problem for the patient. An application may be made to an appropriate source of assistance, such as a service club or a community welfare organization.

DISORDERS OF THE BLADDER

Manifestations of Bladder Dysfunction

RETENTION OF URINE. The inability of a patient to void is a relatively common problem. It may be due to obstructive disease of the bladder or urethra but occurs frequently after surgery, in acute illness and neurogenic disease, and as a postpartum complication. The resulting distention of the bladder and stasis of urine predispose to the development of ureteral back pressure, reflux of urine into the ureters, and infection of the bladder and kidneys. The reaction of the bladder to progressive obstruction of the outflow is hypertrophy of the detrusor muscle. Diverticula may develop; these are saccular protrusions of the mucosa between the muscle fibers. The sacs fill with urine which becomes stagnant and is readily infected. Calculi may also form within the diverticula.

The retention of urine is suspected if the patient has had a normal fluid intake and has not voided within a period of 8 to 10 hours or if there is distention of the lower part of the abdomen. A distended bladder may also be manifested by frequent voiding of small amounts (30 to 50 ml.), which is termed *retention with overflow*. The patient may experience a constant desire to void but efforts to do so are ineffective.

Nursing measures used to induce voiding include increasing the fluid intake, providing adequate privacy, the pouring of warm water over the perineum, the application of heat (such as a hot water bottle or electric pad) over the bladder region (*if permitted*), having the patient hear running water and, unless contraindicated, assisting the patient to assume the normal position for voiding. The female patient may be supported in the sitting position in bed or may be allowed to use a commode at the bedside. The male patient may be allowed to stand beside the bed. A warm tub bath may prove effective with some patients.

When urethral catheterization is necessary, extreme precautions are used to avoid the introduction of organisms and trauma of the mucosa; sterile gloves are worn, and strict aseptic technique is observed throughout the procedure as well as gentle handling of the catheter to minimize trauma. If the retention has been acute and severe, at first not more than 1000 to 1200 ml. of urine are removed. The sudden, complete emptying of an overdistended bladder favors atony of the bladder wall and capillary bleeding. The sudden release of pressure on the blood vessels in the bladder region causes a sudden inflow of blood; rarely, the patient may experience faintness. The catheter is clamped after 1000 to 1500 ml. are removed and is then opened hourly to drain off 100 ml. until the bladder is empty. The catheter rarely may be attached to decompression drainage. The latter method requires a Y tube positioned at a prescribed height (e.g., 5 to 6 inches) above bladder level; the catheter is attached to one arm of the Y tube. The tubing to the drainage receptacle is attached to the lower arm, while the third is left open to the air. Sufficient urine must collect in the bladder to raise the urine in the tube to the height of the Y tube before there is drainage. The access of air prevents a suction-siphonage action and complete emptying.

FREQUENCY, URGENCY AND DYSURIA. Irritation of the bladder or urethral mucosa may give rise to an abnormally frequent desire to void, urgency and painful micturition. The irritation is most frequently associated with infection in the lower urinary tract and less often with bladder calculi or chemicals excreted in the urine. The frequency of voiding may also be increased by nervous apprehension or the taking of a diuretic or increased fluids but is not considered abnormal. Frequency due to a urological disturbance is generally accompanied by an urgency which implies that there is an intense desire to void immediately. The normal voluntary control to retain the urine cannot be maintained, and some urine may escape before the patient can reach the toilet or be placed on a bedpan.

When voiding is accompanied by pain or a burning, smarting sensation, the exact location and the time at which the discomfort occurs in relation to the flow of urine should be determined; that is, the patient must determine whether it is before, during or after the passage of urine that the pain occurs. This information may be helpful to the physician in locating the problem. *Strangury* is a term used occasionally when the dysuria is unusually severe and there is increasing frequency of decreasing amounts of urine.

RESIDUAL URINE. Micturition may not completely empty the bladder, leaving a residue of urine. It is recognized and the amount determined by catheterizing the patient immediately after he has voided. Residual urine is usually the result of an obstruction to the bladder outlet and causes a stagnation that predisposes to bladder and kidney infection and calculus formation.

ALTERATIONS IN THE URINARY STREAM. The patient may have difficulty in initiating the urinary flow. This symptom of hesitancy is usually due to some obstruction in the bladder-urethral orifice or the urethra. Pressure within the bladder must be increased beyond the normal to force the urine past the obstructing lesion. This is most often seen in males as a result of prostatic hyperplasia but may also occur with newgrowths or constrictions resulting from scarring and fibrosis. The inability to maintain a continuous stream and dribbling may develop as the lesion encroaches further upon the outflow passage.

Intermittent abrupt cessation of the urinary stream during voiding may occur if the bladder-urethral orifice is suddenly occluded by a calculus or a portion of a papillary tumor near the orifice. This may also occur as a result of fatigue of the detrusor muscle. Because of resistance to the urinary outflow, the muscle tires before the bladder is empty; after a few moments, it contracts again and voiding is resumed.

INCONTINENCE. As a symptom of dysfunction of the lower urinary system, the involuntary passage of urine is most often due to infection or irritation of the bladder or urethra. It may also be the result of some congenital anomaly (e.g., hypospadias) or incompetency of the bladder and urethral sphincters due to degenerative tissue changes (as seen in the elderly) or relaxation of the pelvic floor muscles. Incontinence is frequently associated with neurological disease or injury which results in loss of bladder sensation and voluntary control of micturition (e.g., spinal cord injury or cerebral damage). Reflex incontinence develops in which filling of the bladder initiates reflex emptying as occurs in infancy. Incontinence may also develop in any acute illness because of a loss of cerebral awareness and voluntary control of the sphincter.

ABNORMAL CONSTITUENTS IN URINE. Blood, pus, bacteria and mucus may be present in the urine as a result of infection, inflammation, tissue necrosis or a newgrowth in the lower urinary tract. The urine may be cloudy or blood-colored and have an unpleasant or ammoniacal odor.

Cystitis

This is an acute or chronic inflammation of the urinary bladder characterized by frequency, urgency, dysuria and abnormal urinary constituents. It is most often due to infection caused by the ascent of organisms by way of the urethra, but it may also be associated with the administration of certain drugs (e.g., cyclophosphamide) and radiation therapy of the lower abdomen. Predisposing factors in infective cystitis are trauma of the tissues, stagnation of the urine, and distortion or compression of the bladder by an enlarged neighboring organ. The latter condition is a factor in the cystitis that not infrequently develops in the pregnant woman, especially in the last trimester; the enlarging uterus compresses the bladder. Cystitis has a higher incidence in females; this is attributed to the shorter urethra of a relatively wide caliber. Organisms from rectal and vaginal discharge can enter readily. In the male, it is usually secondary to prostatic hyperplasia or infection or to congenital malformation (e.g., hypospadias).

The inflammation is generally confined to the mucosa and submucosa which are hyperemic and edematous. Scattered hemorrhagic areas are present, and small ulcerative lesions may develop as a result of sloughing of the lining tissue. The urine contains blood cells, pus, bacteria and mucus. If cystitis becomes chronic, the inflammation may extend into the detrusor muscle. Fibrosing of the tissues occurs with persisting inflammation, which reduces the bladder capacity and increases the problem of frequency.

TREATMENT. In some instances, cystitis is of brief duration, being resolved spontaneously. There is always the danger that the infection may ascend via the ureters and cause pyelonephritis. The infection is treated by the administration of an antibiotic or urinary antiseptic such as sulfonamide (Gantrisin), nitrofurantoin (Furadantin) and pyridium. A urine specimen obtained before any antimicrobial drug is given may be cultured to determine the infective organism and its drug sensitivity. A specific antibiotic may then be ordered. Sodium bicarbonate or sodium citrate may also be prescribed for the purpose of alkalinizing the urine to decrease the bladder irritation and dysuria. Warm sitz baths may reduce bladder spasm and provide considerable relief. The patient is encouraged to drink copious amounts of fluids which should include citrus fruit juices. He usually remains ambulatory unless there is fever.

If the condition persists, the cystitis is suspected of being secondary. The patient is then investigated for a primary condition which might be pyelonephritis, a bladder calculus, urethral stricture or, in the case of the male, an enlarged prostate.

Since cystitis is frequently the result of an ascending infection and occurs readily in females, good personal hygiene and efficient cleansing of the perineum, especially after defecation, are extremely important and require emphasis in health teaching. Adequate cleansing is often very difficult for the ill person who is weak or handicapped and confined to bed. It becomes the nurse's responsibility to see that the patient is thoroughly cleansed.

Bladder Calculi

Stones in the urinary bladder nearly always form as a result of urinary stasis as occurs in prostatic hypertrophy, neurological disease or injury that has resulted in the loss of voluntary bladder control or interruption of the sacral reflex arc, bladder diverticula, urethral stricture or prolonged immobility.

The patient may complain of sudden cessation of the urinary flow before the bladder is emptied which is due to occlusion of the bladder-uretheral orifice by the calculus. He may find that he is able to void only in certain positions, which are those that keep the stone away from the outlet. Irritation of the mucosa by the stone may result in hematuria, and infection is usually present. Small concretions may pass into the urethra and become lodged there, causing urinary obstruction and severe pain. A bladder calculus may be recognized on an x-ray film of the bladder or visualized by cystoscopy (see p. 621). The stone(s) may be removed through a suprapubic cystotomy (incision into the bladder) or by litholapaxy, depending on the size of the stone(s). For nursing care following a cystotomy, see page 662. *Litholapaxy* involves the passage of special crushing forceps (lithotrite) through a cystoscope into the bladder. The stone is grasped by the forceps and crushed. The bladder is then irrigated to wash out the concretions; the returned fluid is strained through gauze and the residue checked for amount and composition of the stone particles. The patient is given large amounts of fluids to help wash out the bladder.

Prior to the litholapaxy, the bladder is irrigated frequently with an acid solution (Suby's or G. solution)[15] which may soften the stones (depending on their composition), making them easier to crush. If the patient complains of irritation when the solution is instilled, it is reported to the physician and the composition of the solution may be adjusted to reduce the acidity.

The condition causing the stasis of urine which promotes calculi formation receives attention to avoid recurrence. If the patient has an obstructing prostate, it may be removed at the same time that the stone is removed. Patients who are immobilized must be turned and moved about frequently; a bed that can be tilted at different angles may be used. The patient who spends most of his day immobile in a wheelchair is equally as susceptible as the bed patient and should receive attention.

Bladder Injury

Accidental injury of the urinary bladder, causing perforation and ensuing extravasation of urine (escape of urine from the bladder), is not uncommon. It may occur when the pelvis is fractured or as a result of direct blows to the lower abdomen. If the bladder is full and distended at the time of accident, it is more vulnerable.

If the laceration occurs in the upper portion, the rupture is intraperitoneal. Urine escapes into the peritoneal cavity and produces peritonitis. The patient exhibits shock (see p. 372) and experiences abdominal pain and tenderness. The abdomen becomes rigid and distended, and a paralytic ileus is likely to develop (see p. 545).

Rupture of the lower part of the bladder is usually extraperitoneal; urine escapes into the surrounding tissues, and infection, cellulitis and necrosis of tissue may ensue. Occasionally an abdominal or perineal fistula develops.

When there is a history of an injury or blow to the lower abdomen followed by pain and tenderness, injury to the bladder is suspected. A urine specimen is obtained promptly, either by having the patient void or passing a catheter, to determine if there is hematuria. If blood is present in the urine, a cystogram may be done to confirm the diag-

---

[15]Suby's or G. solution has a pH of 4 and contains citric acid (monohydrated), magnesium oxide (anhydrous) and sodium carbonate (anhydrous).

nosis and locate the laceration. A cystogram is an x-ray of the bladder following the instillation of a radiopaque dye through a urethral catheter.

TREATMENT. The injury is a serious threat to life and requires prompt treatment. The shock and hemorrhage are treated with a blood transfusion and intravenous infusions. An indwelling catheter is placed in the bladder, and the patient is prepared for abdominal surgery. The site of injury is repaired and a temporary cystostomy (incision of the bladder and introduction of a drainage tube) done to establish urinary drainage and prevent the possibility of pressure on the repair suture line. If the rupture was intraperitoneal, the extravasated fluid is aspirated before closure.

Following the surgery, the patient is observed closely for signs of infection. The patient may be placed on an antibiotic immediately. An accurate record of the fluid intake and all drainage is very important. (See section on nursing care of the patient having had a cystostomy, p. 663. For the care of the patient with peritonitis and paralytic ileus, see p. 563.)

Exstrophy of the Bladder

This is a developmental defect in which the anterior wall of the bladder has failed to fuse. The degree of failure of fusion varies. The opening may be small, forming a fistula that opens and drains urine onto the external surface of the abdomen, or the entire anterior bladder wall may be absent, accompanied by a wide defect in the abdominal wall, resulting in full exposure of the bladder interior. Urine spurts onto the abdominal wall from the ureters. The more extensive defects are nearly always associated with other anomalies in the genitourinary system. The pelvic bones may fail to meet to form the symphysis pubis. Epispadias (absence of the anterior wall of the male urethra) is a frequent counterpart. In the female, the urethra may be lacking. Exstrophy of the bladder is more common in males than females.

Infection of the bladder usually supervenes and may extend to the kidneys, seriously impairing their function. The corrective procedures used depends on the extent of the malformation and concomitant defects. If the exstrophy is not extensive, the bladder opening and the abdominal fistula are closed. If the defect is extensive, permanent urinary diversion may be undertaken (see p. 665). The defective bladder is removed and the abdominal wall repaired. The surgery is usually undertaken early in the child's life in order to prevent kidney infection and chronic renal failure.

Bladder Neoplasms

Newgrowths in the bladder may develop at any age but occur more frequently after the age of 50 and have a high incidence in males. The majority arise from the epithelial lining as papillomas and may be benign or malignant. Those that are benign and recur tend to become malignant eventually. Others appear as ulcers which are usually malignant and are more invasive of deeper tissue layers. Prolonged exposure to aniline dyes is recognized as a predisposing factor. It is recommended that the period of working with these chemicals should be limited to 3 years and that during this period such persons should have routine Papanicolaou smears (Pap tests) made of the urine. Workers are also advised of the importance of prompt reporting of any blood in the urine or slight bladder irritation. Smoking has also been cited as a predisposing cause of bladder cancer.

The first symptom is usually intermittent painless hematuria, or cystitis may be the initial factor that brings the patient to a physician. The lesion may encroach on the urethral orifice, giving rise to hesitancy and a decreased force and caliber of the urinary stream. Suprapubic pain and a palpable mass generally indicate that the condition is in an advanced stage. The patient may experience pain in the flank region if the growth obstructs a ureteral orifice which causes hydronephrosis. The lesion ulcerates, which accounts for the hematuria, and readily becomes infected. If the infection is severe and anemia has developed, the patient manifests weakness and loss of weight.

Diagnostic procedures include a cystoscopy and biopsy. In some instances, the patient may be given several does of tetracycline before a cystoscopic examination. The tetracycline produces fluorescence of the neoplastic tissue under the ultraviolet ray used in a special cystoscope. Cytologic studies may also be made of a urine specimen.

TREATMENT. The treatment used depends upon whether the neoplasm is benign or malignant and, in the case of malignancy, upon the stage and the depth of the tissue involved. Surgery, radiation, chemotherapy, or a combination of these may be used. Small papillomatous new growths may be treated by transurethral resection followed by fulguration (electrocoagulation) of the base tissue. An indwelling catheter is placed in the bladder on completion of the operation, and the urinary drainage is observed frequently for possible bleeding. Bladder spasm and irritability may cause considerable discomfort which may be reduced by the application of heat to the lower abdomen or by a warm sitz bath. The patient is encouraged to take a minimum of 2000 ml. of fluids daily.

Since papillomas, benign as well as malignant, tend to recur, these patients are followed closely for 5 to 6 years. They are advised to report any bleeding or bladder irritability promptly. A cystoscopic examination is usually done every 3 months during the first year following the resection, every 6 months during the second year, and then annually for 3 or 4 years.

If the neoplasm is malignant, a segmental resection of the bladder or total cystectomy (removal of the bladder) may be done.

SEGMENTAL RESECTION. A partial cystectomy is only used if the cancer is in the upper part of the bladder well above the urethral orifices. At operation, a tube or catheter is placed in the bladder and brought out through the incision, and an indwelling catheter is also introduced through the urethra. Removal of a part of the bladder obviously reduces its capacity. Adequate drainage in the postoperative period is necessary to prevent distention and possible disruption of the suture line. The tube in the incision may be connected to gentle intermittent suction. The length of time it remains in the bladder will depend on the rate of healing.

The urethral catheter usually remains in place for approximately 2 to 4 weeks. On its removal, frequency becomes a problem for the patient because of the reduced bladder capacity. He is likely to become discouraged and depressed at this time, and understanding support from the nurse is essential. He may attempt to reduce the frequency by cutting down his fluid intake, which must be guarded against. The importance of a minimum fluid intake of 2000 ml. and the spacing of the fluids so the intervals between voiding may be increased during certain periods (e.g., at night) are discussed with him. The traumatized bladder gradually becomes less irritable and increases its capacity.

CYSTECTOMY. A total cystectomy with ureteral transplantation for permanent urinary diversion is used when the cancer is situated in the lower part of the bladder or is quite extensive. Permanent urinary diversion may be achieved by cutaneous ureterostomy, ureterointestinal anastomosis, or the formation of an ileal conduit (Fig. 19–12).

In *cutaneous ureterostomy*, the detached ends of the ureters are brought through the abdominal wall and secured at skin level. This is rarely the procedure of choice. Maintaining the patency of the ureters is difficult because of strictures that tend to develop. If catheters are placed in the ureters to maintain drainage, they readily block and are difficult to keep in place. Chronic kidney infection is a frequent complication with subsequent renal failure.

URETEROENTEROSTOMY (*ureterosigmoidostomy*) provides a completely internal diversion. The ureters are implanted into the sigmoid colon and the urine and feces leave the body via a common channel—the rectum and anus. The urine draining from the ureters is retained in the lower bowel until approximately 200 ml. accumulate. The "defecation" impulse is initiated and the urine is expelled by voluntary relaxation of the anal sphincters. This is a more acceptable procedure to the patient; it provides continence and eliminates an abdominal orifice, skin problems and the constant use of special drainage appliances. Unfortunately, the direct connection with the bowel predisposes the patient to ascending infection of the kidneys and subsequent renal insufficiency and to disturbances in blood chemistry. The latter are attributed to the absorption of substances from the accumulating urine in the intestine. Acidosis is a frequent problem, resulting from the reabsorption of chlorides.

In still another procedure that involves the lower bowel, the ureters are transplanted into the rectum which is severed from the

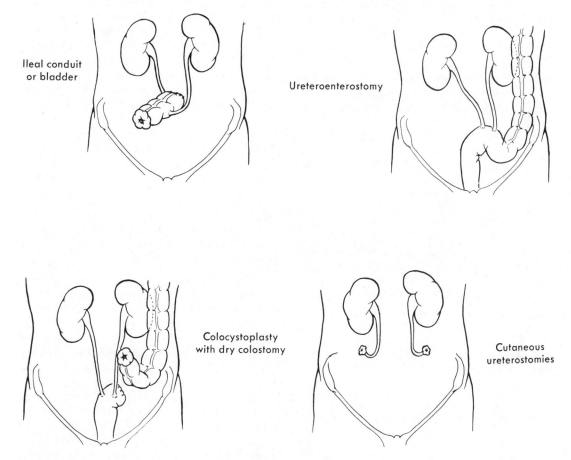

FIGURE 19–12 Types of urinary diversion. (From Bouchard, R., and Owens, N.: Nursing Care of the Cancer Patient, 3rd ed. St. Louis, C. V. Mosby, 1976, p. 257.)

sigmoid, forming what is sometimes referred to as an *anal bladder*. The free end of the colon is brought out to the skin surface, forming a colostomy. The urine and feces are kept separate by this method.

The *ileal conduit (ureteroileostomy)* currently appears to be the procedure most favored. A segment of the ileum with its mesentery and blood supply is removed. The open ends of the ileum left by the resection are anastomosed to reestablish intestinal continuity. One end of the resected ileal section is closed. The open end is brought through the abdominal wall to the skin surface and secured. The detached ends of the ureters and implanted in the ileal segment near its closed end.

For the nursing care of a patient with urinary diversion, see page 666.

RADIATION. Internal or external radiation may be used in treating cancer of the bladder. It may be used alone, as an adjunct to surgery, or with chemotherapy. Intracavitary radiation may be achieved by the enclosure of a radioisotope (e.g., Co^{60}, Au^{198}) in a catheter balloon which is placed within the bladder. The catheter is connected to a drainage receptacle, and all urine is saved and sent to the radioisotope department. In some instances, radon seeds or radiotantalum (Ta[182]) needles may be implanted around the lesion. Certain precautions are necessary in the handling of these radioactive materials and are cited on page 142. Internal radiation causes cystitis, and the patient usually experiences considerable bladder spasm and discomfort. Fluids are given freely and analgesics may be necessary. The application of heat over the bladder region may provide some relief.

External radiation therapy is usually reserved for those patients whose cancer is deeply invasive and highly malignant. When it is used, the patient is likely to experience some gastrointestinal disturbances (nausea, vomiting and diarrhea) as well as cystitis, since the intestine proximal to the bladder will be exposed to the rays. For care of the patient receiving external radiation therapy, the reader is referred to page 140.

In advanced carcinoma of the bladder and when metastases are suspected, chemotherapy may be used as well as surgery and irradiation (see p. 143).

NURSING IN DISORDERS OF THE BLADDER

The Bladder Surgery Patient

Operative procedures used in the treatment of bladder disease may be transurethral or by open surgery. Open surgery involves an incision through the abdominal wall. Transurethral operative procedures may be performed to obtain a biopsy, remove a neoplasm or calculus, or resect the prostate gland. The resectoscope, which is used to resect tissue, is similar to a cycstoscope but has insulated walls and is equipped with a wire loop which is activated by a high frequency current to cut tissue and control hemorrhage by electrocoagulation. The procedure is referred to as a transurethral resection (TUR). For resection of the prostate, see page 723. A lithotrite, which is a special crushing instrument, is used to remove a stone, and the procedure is called litholapaxy.

Open surgery on the bladder may be undertaken for repair of a perforation or laceration, the removal of a neoplasm, calculus, or the prostate gland, or a segmental resection or removal of the bladder. The open operative procedures include *cystotomy* (an incision into the bladder and closure without a drainage tube), *cystostomy* (an incision into the bladder and the insertion of a drainage tube which is brought out on to the abdominal surface), *segmental resection* (the removal of a section of the bladder) and *total cystectomy* (the removal of the bladder, involving ureteral transplantation and urinary diversion). A suprapubic approach is most commonly used in open bladder surgery, with the bladder being opened below the peritoneum.

The Patient Having a Cystotomy, Cystostomy or Segmental Bladder Resection

PREOPERATIVE PREPARATION. Unless the bladder is injured or there is acute retention that cannot be relieved by urethral catheterization, the patient who is to have bladder surgery usually undergoes several days of investigation and preparation. Kidney function is assessed and certain blood chemistry levels are determined (e.g., urea, creatinine, potassium, sodium, chloride, calcium). The urine is examined microscopically and, if infection is present, a urinary antiseptic such as a sulfonamide preparation (e.g., Gantrisin) or an antibiotic is prescribed. The patient is encouraged to take 2500 to 3000 ml. of fluid daily unless a large amount of fluid is contraindicated by cardiac or renal insufficiency. The fluid intake and output are recorded and the balance noted. The patient's nutritional status frequently requires attention. Many of these patients are elderly and the existing condition may have contributed to their lack of interest in food, resulting in deficiencies. In encouraging the patient to take nourishment, its importance in his recovery is explained. Dietary adjustments and supplements may be necessary to meet his nutritional needs.

During the preparatory period, an indwelling catheter may be used to provide adequate drainage and reduce the residual urine. The patient is usually allowed to remain ambulatory. If there is an indwelling catheter, he is given a plastic drainage receptacle that may be attached to his thigh or gown while he is up. He should understand that it must be kept low enough to accommodate gravity drainage of the urine.

When the patient has been advised of the necessity for surgery, the nurse is alert to his need for psychological support. Opportunities are provided for him to express his feelings and concerns and to ask questions. He and his family are advised as to what may be expected following the operation. If the patient is to have a partial cystectomy, this explanation will include a discussion of the frequency of voiding that will be experienced when the tubes are removed because of the reduced capacity of the bladder. Reassurance is given that this gradually becomes less troublesome. If the period of waiting for the surgery is prolonged, some form of diversion in which the patient is interested may be provided, and his family is encouraged to visit regularly. If the patient's anxiety is interfering with his rest and he is unable to sleep, the physician is consulted and a sedative may be ordered.

The immediate preparation for open bladder surgery is similar to that for any patient having abdominal surgery (see p. 164). The skin cleansing and shaving extend from the lower costal margin to midthighs and include the perineal area. If the operation is scheduled for late in the morning or for the afternoon, an intravenous infusion may be given earlier in the day to prevent preoperative dehydration.

POSTOPERATIVE NURSING CARE.   Preparation to receive the patient after operation includes the assembling of sterile tubing and drainage receptacles ready for prompt connection to an indwelling urethral catheter and a cystostomy tube. A suction machine and bottles for setting up a closed drainage system may be necessary for the cystostomy. A tray of sterile equipment and solution (sterile water or normal saline) for irrigating the catheters in the event of obstruction by clots should be readily available.

DRAINAGE.   The patient is returned from the operating room with an indwelling urethral catheter which is secured to the upper thigh to prevent traction. It is connected to sterile tubing leading to a closed sterile drainage receptacle. The length of the tube should allow for turning and moving the patient without tension being exerted on the catheter. The excess tubing lies free on the bed and is secured so there is no loop between the bed and drainage receptacle; that is, the tube must hang straight from the edge of the bed for gravity drainage.

If there is a cystostomy as well, a tube is anchored in the bladder by a suture at the time of operation. This tube may be a special right-angled tube with a mushroom, winged or straight tip, or it may be a straight tube which requires a right-angled glass connecting tube. The cystostomy tube is attached to a sterile tube and receptacle, and the same precautions are necessary as those cited in the previous paragraph. Rarely, the cystostomy tube is connected to a suction machine which can be regulated to provide a *very low* constant or intermittent negative pressure. It must be carefully controlled to avoid trauma by suction of the bladder mucosa against the tube.

Both drainage systems are checked frequently (at least hourly for the first 36 to 48 hours) for patency. The characteristics (color, consistency, and content or sediment) of the drainage are noted at the same time. The urine will be blood-colored for the first 2 to 3 hours, gradually becoming lighter. The drainage is best examined at the glass or plastic connecting tubes before it becomes mixed with what is already in the receptacles.

The cystostomy tube, urethral catheter or tubing may become obstructed by a blood clot. A sterile towel or pad is placed under the connecting tube and the catheter or cystostomy tube is disconnected and held over a sterile basin to see if it is draining. If blockage of the tubing is indicated, it may be "milked" or flushed with sterile water. The water is either collected in a separate container, or the exact amount used is noted if it is allowed to flow into the regular drainage receptacle. If the obstruction is within the catheter tube in the bladder, an order may be given to irrigate with sterile normal saline or sterile water. Fifty to 75 ml. of the fluid are introduced; if the initial fluid does not return, no more fluid is instilled and the physician is consulted. Adequate postoperative drainage is very important to prevent bladder distention and pressure on the suture line.

The drainage from each system is measured and recorded every 6 to 8 hours. A fresh sterile receptacle replaces the one being emptied. Care of the tubing varies in different institutions; it may be replaced daily with a fresh sterile set or is changed every second day or twice weeky.

The cystostomy tube usually remains in place from 4 to 7 days, depending on the patient's healing. The urethral catheter is generally left for a few days longer or until the incisional opening in the bladder heals. When the cystostomy tube is removed, some urine will escape onto the dressing for a few days until the fistula heals over.

Following the removal of the urethral catheter, a close check is made of the patient's frequency of voiding and the volume of the daily output for several days. If the patient is ambulatory, he is asked to record the necessary information. When a urethral catheter that has been in place for several days is removed, dribbling is a usual problem because the bladder-urethral sphincters have been continuously dilated for a period of time. Frequent perineal exercises, which consist of contracting the abdominal, gluteal and perineal muscles while continuing to breathe normally, may help the sphincters recover their tone and control. Occasionally, a patient may not be able to void and the catheter may have to be replaced if he has not voided within 8 hours.

A permanent cystostomy is sometimes done as a palliative measure with a patient who has an inoperable obstruction of the urethra (e.g., advanced carcinoma of the urethra, bladder neck or prostate). A urethral catheter is not inserted in this patient; bladder drainage is entrirely dependent upon the cystostomy tube.

OBSERVATIONS. As well as frequent checking of the drainage system(s), the patient's blood pressure, pulse, color and level of consciousness are noted and recorded at frequent intervals, which are gradually lengthened if the vital signs are satisfactory. Hemorrhage and shock are common complications following either transurethral resection or open bladder surgery. Bleeding may be evident in the drainage, but the dressing, surrounding skin areas and groins are also examined.

The daily fluid intake and output are recorded for a longer period than with most surgical patients. The ratio of the intake to the output is examined by the nurse so that she is alert to possible renal insufficiency or retention of urine. The characteristics of the urine are noted for a period of 10 to 14 days. The appearance of sediment, blood, shreds of mucus-like material, cloudiness or the presence of an unusual odor is reported. Sloughing and ensuing bleeding may occur 8 to 10 days following the removal of a lesion.

EXERCISE AND POSITIONING. The patient is urged to take five to ten deep breaths and cough every 1 to 2 hours to prevent pulmonary complications until he becomes ambulatory and active. If approved by the surgeon, active flexion and extension of the feet and lower limbs are encouraged three or four times daily to prevent venous stasis. If these cannot be carried out actively, passive movement of the limbs through the normal range of motion is done by the nurse.

A regimen of turning every 1 to 2 hours is established; some patients may be able to assume responsibility for this soon after operation but others, particularly elderly persons, may require assistance. Following each change of position the full length of each tube is checked to make sure it is not kinked, that it is not under the patient and being compressed, and that there is no loop between the bed and drainage receptacle. The patient is taught to make these checks when he changes his position.

The patient is allowed out of bed as soon as his condition permits, and ambulation is encouraged to promote normal physiological processes and prevent complications. When the patient is up, the drainage tubes may be connected to smaller plastic receptacles which may be attached to the patient's thigh or gown. When the patient becomes more independent in his activity, he must be advised that when he returns to bed, the drainage receptacle is transferred to the side of the bed in order to maintain gravity drainage.

DRESSINGS AND SKIN CARE. Compared with other abdominal surgery, the dressing is changed earlier and more frequently for patients who have had open bladder surgery. There is almost certain to be some leakage of urine through the incision and around the tube. The skin is cleansed of urine frequently and is kept as dry as possible to prevent excoriation and infection. Following each cleansing, an application of a protective preparation such as petroleum jelly, zinc oxide ointment or karaya gum powder is made to the skin. The lower back, buttocks, groin, inner thighs and perineum are examined each time the dressing is changed. If any areas are moist with urine drainage, they are washed and thoroughly dried to prevent excoriation. The bedding is changed as often as is necessary to ensure dryness and comfort.

PAIN. Bladder trauma and irritation cause bladder spasms which are very painful, and the patient may also experience the desire to void frequently, even though the bladder is emptied by tube drainage. In the case of the sensation of frequency, it may be necessary to explain to the patient that the bladder is empty and that trying to void only increases bladder spasms and pain. An analgesic such as morphine or meperidine hydrochloride (Demerol) is usually necessary at intervals during the first 48 hours. If the pain and discomfort persist, the surgeon is consulted. Either the catheter or cystostomy tube may require adjusting to relieve the contact and pressure of its tip on the bladder wall.

FLUIDS AND NUTRITION. A daily fluid intake of at least 2500 to 3000 ml. (unless contraindicated by other coexisting disease) is necessary to insure adequate irrigation of the bladder as well as to maintain satisfactory hydration. Most of it usually has to be administered by intravenous infusion the first day or two. A soft diet is given and is progressively increased to a regular diet as tolerated.

BOWEL ELIMINATION. The patient may be given a mild laxative after 2 days, or a cleansing enema may be given. Constipation and straining at stool are prevented, since they tend to increase the patient's pain.

PREPARATION FOR DISCHARGE. Most patients who have had a cystotomy or cystostomy remain in the hospital until the wound is healed and normal micturition is reestablished. The nurse discusses the resumption of their previous activities with them and explains any restrictions indicated by the physician. They are advised to continue taking a minimum of 2000 to 2500 ml. of fluid daily. Some may require reassurance that no special care of the wound is necessary and that they may resume tub baths.

If the cystostomy is permanent or a urethral catheter is to remain in place, the patient and a family member are given detailed instruction about the necessary care. This instruction is given over several days and should be completed soon enough for the patient to carry out the care himself before going home. This gives him confidence and provides the opportunity to clarify certain points. Verbal and written instructions will include an explanation of the necessary equipment, its use and maintenance, how it may be acquired, and any precautions to be observed in its use. An inconspicuous, oval-shaped, plastic or rubber urinal (drainage receptable) that may be strapped to the thigh is available. The inlet tube which is attached to the upper end of the bag is connected to the catheter or cystostomy tube by means of a plastic connecting tube. The other end of the urinal has a screw stopper or clamp which permits emptying of the bag into a toilet at necessary intervals. The importance of thorough washing of the hands with soap and running water before connecting or disconnecting the equipment is stressed to reduce the possibility of ascending infection. The patient and a family member are also taught how to anchor the tube that is in the patient to the abdomen or thigh to prevent traction on it.

The bag and tubing are cleansed daily with a detergent and warm water, flushed with vinegar, thoroughly rinsed with water, and aired. They are advised to have two sets, if possible, so that one set may be well aired after the cleansing. This helps to prevent odor which could cause considerable embarrassment and discouragement for the patient. The patient is reminded of the need to continue taking at least 2000 to 2500 ml. of fluid daily to provide adequate bladder irrigation. Odor is likely to be less of a problem with less concentrated urine, and there is less danger of infection with constant washing out of the bladder.

A referral may be made to a visiting nurse agency for assistance and supervision when the patient goes home. This is likely to be needed when the patient is elderly and finds it difficult to cope with the necessary care. The patient and family are advised as to how often the bladder tube or catheter is to be changed at the clinic or by the physician and of the need to promptly contact the physician or clinic if the tube slips out of the bladder.

The Cystectomy and Ureteral Transplantation Patient

Complete removal of the bladder necessitates establishing a new urinary outlet; this may be achieved by cutaneous ureterostomy, ureteroenterostomy (ureterosigmoidostomy) or ileal conduit (ureteroileostomy). For a description of these procedures, see page 660.

Following operation, the patient who undergoes a cystectomy and ureteral transplant is seriously ill. The amount of surgery usually involved predisposes the patient to severe shock. Frequently, considerable surrounding tissue is resected with the bladder (e.g., lymphatics, prostate gland), and if the ileal conduit procedure is used, an intestinal resection and anastomosis are done. The patient will have a large vertical or transverse incision through which the bladder is removed, the ureters are freed for transplant, and the intestine is resected. The stoma through which the urine will drain is made separately in the right abdominal wall. Care of the patient requires consideration of the needs incurred by the cystectomy, the intestinal surgery, the ureteral transplantation and urinary diversion as well as the individual patient's psychological and physiological responses to such radical surgery.

PREOPERATIVE PREPARATION. The operative procedure and the permanent change in urinary drainage that will ensue are explained to the patient and his family by the physician. This is likely to produce considerable anxiety and despair and will prompt many questions. The nurse observes the patient closely for his reactions and conveys her acceptance and appreciation of his concerns. Opportunities are provided for him and his family to express their feelings and ask questions and, when they are ready, the necessary adjustments and care associated with urinary diversion are outlined in simple terms. They are told that a relatively normal, active life is possible. This may be reinforced by having a person who has had a permanent urinary diversion and has made a successful adjustment talk with them. If such a person is not available, someone with an ileostomy may prove helpful. The nurse who is willing to take time to talk freely with the patient, help him to make plans for his future, and is patient in repeating answers and reinforcing what has probably already been said can provide immeasurable support. A rapport is developed that contributes to acceptance of the situation and the development of positive attitudes on the part of the patient and family.

There will be several days of investigation and preparation. Kidney function is assessed and the blood levels of nitrogenous wastes, potassium, sodium and chloride are determined. The patient usually receives a blood transfusion during and probably following the surgery, so typing and cross matching are necessary. At least 2500 ml. of fluid daily are given unless contraindicated by cardiac insufficiency or urinary obstruction.

If the intestine is to be entered, the patient receives a low-residue diet for 3 or 4 days, then clear fluids only for 2 days before operation to reduce the fecal content. The reasons for these restrictions are explained in order to gain the patient's cooperation and acceptance. Laxatives and enemas are also used for cleansing purposes, and a course of an antimicrobial drug that is poorly absorbed from the gastrointestinal tract is given orally to destroy intestinal organisms (e.g., Sulfasuxidine, neomycin). The skin preparation includes the abdomen, upper thighs and perineum. A nasogastric tube is passed the morning of operation to provide drainage of secretions and prevent intestinal distention after the surgery. The remainder of the preparation is similar to that for any major abdominal surgery (see p. 164).

The operation is a lengthy procedure; if the members of the family decide to go home, they are assured that they will be called as soon as the operation is over and advised of the patient's condition. If they choose to remain in the hospital, they are directed to a room where they may wait. A brief visit with them at intervals by the nurse and suggestions made as to where they may have a cup of coffee or lunch are appreciated and indicate a sympathetic understanding of their anxiety and concern.

THE PATIENT WITH A URETEROILEAL CONDUIT. Preparation to receive the patient after operation includes the assembling of a sterile urinary drainage receptacle with tubing, gastrointestinal suction machine, intravenous infusion standard, sterile irrigation tray and sterile normal saline.

A large part of the required care is essentially the same as that for any patient having an intestinal resection, cited on page 548.

DRAINAGE. On completion of the operation, a catheter may be inserted into the ileal segment and anchored by a skin suture. The catheter is connected directly to sterile tubing leading to a drainage receptacle. The tubing should be long enough to permit turning the patient without traction being exerted on the catheter. Since the drainage is by gravity, the tube is positioned to hang straight from the bed to the drainage receptacle. The system is checked at least hourly, and the volume of urine is recorded; less than 15 ml. per hour is reported. The catheter may become obstructed by mucus secreted by the isolated ileal segment and may require periodic irrigation. If the nurse is responsible for the irrigations, a specified directive is received as to the quantity of sterile normal saline to be introduced at one time. The return is carefully measured. Distention of the ileal segment must be avoided; it causes pressure on the suture lines, urinary reflux and back pressure in the ureters. If the solution introduced is not returned, no more is added and the physician is consulted. The catheter is usually left in place 4 to 7 days, and then a disposable ileostomy bag is applied.

If a catheter is not inserted into the ileal conduit at operation, a disposable plastic ileostomy bag is secured to the skin around the stoma by means of an adhesive disk. The lower end of the bag is then connected to the tubing and drainage receptacle. With this arrangement, the ileostomy bag is examined when checking the drainage. The bag may require moving to empty any accumulation of urine into the lower bag. A cessation of drainage may indicate occlusion of the stoma by mucus or by swelling and edema of the tissues, and the physician is notified immediately. The stoma may be dilated manually, and the bag changed daily by the surgeon for a few days, after which the procedure may be repeated daily or every 2 days by the nurse. A sterile rubber glove or finger cot is worn, and the finger used is lubricated with a water-soluble jelly and introduced gently. The interval between stomal dilations is gradually lengthened and once weekly is usually sufficient as the tissues and the stoma heal and shrink. Eventually, this becomes a part of the care procedure taught to the patient and a family member. The stoma must be kept well dilated to promote free drainage and prevent an accumulation of urine in the ileal conduit. The physician may insert a sterile catheter periodically to determine if there is residual urine. The temporary ileostomy bag is changed when dilatation of the stoma is done and, when this becomes less frequent, it is changed every 2 or 3 days. When the bag is removed, the stoma is covered with sterile wipes while the skin is gently washed and thoroughly dried. The skin is likely to show some irritation, particularly during the first few weeks. A protective coating of tincture of benzoin, karaya gum powder or Neo-Karaya (a combination of aluminum hydroxide gel and karaya) may be applied after each cleansing and before a new bag is applied. If excoriation of the skin persists or is severe,

the physician may decide to insert a catheter to prevent the escape of urine onto the skin, giving it a chance to heal.

When the stoma has shrunk to a permanent size and drainage is satisfactory, the patient is fitted for a permanent ileostomy bag (see p. 553).

Abdominal pain, distention or rigidity, nausea, vomiting or fever is reported promptly. Any of these symptoms may indicate peritonitis, resulting from the escape of intestinal content from the site of the intestinal anastomosis or from a leakage of urine from the ileal conduit or ureters into the peritoneal cavity. The nurse is also constantly alert for a positive fluid balance, fever and any complaint of back pain, which might indicate renal infection or insufficiency.

POSITIONING AND AMBULATION. The patient is turned every 1 to 2 hours. Since the ileal conduit opens onto the right side of the abdomen, more complete drainage occurs when he is on his right side or back with the trunk elevated. The physician may suggest that the patient be turned on the left side for only very brief periods and that as soon as the blood pressure and pulse have stabilized, the head of the bed should be gradually elevated. With each change of position, the bag and tubing are checked for any kinks or compression.

Early ambulation is encouraged to foster adequate drainage as well as to promote normal physiological processes and prevent complications. If his condition is satisfactory, the patient will probably be allowed up 36 to 48 hours after operation. The plastic drainage receptacle may be carried by the nurse or may be attached to the patient's gown. If an ileostomy bag is applied to the stoma, the drainage tube may be detached while the patient is out of bed.

FLUIDS AND NUTRITION. Gastrointestinal decompression suction is used to prevent vomiting and distention so that there is a minimum of pressure on the intestinal anastomosis. The nasogastric tube remains in place for 3 to 4 days and the patient is given intravenous fluids. The suction is discontinued, and the patient is observed for any signs of distention. Small amounts of water are given and the tube is clamped. If the water is tolerated and bowel sounds indicate the reestablishment of peristalsis, and there is no distention, the nasogastric tube is removed.

The intake of clear fluids is gradually increased and the diet progresses through soft foods to a light solid diet. Gas-forming foods are avoided for 4 to 6 weeks and then added gradually as tolerated.

PREPARATION FOR SELF-CARE. The patient and a family member are taught the care of the stoma, skin and appliance following the same plan as that outlined under instruction of the ileostomy patient on page 560. Emphasis is placed on the precautionary measures necessary to prevent infection. The patient should have his permanent appliance and the opportunity to develop complete familiarity with the necessary care, including dilation of the stoma, before being discharged from the hospital. During this period, he is advised of the importance of continuing a daily intake of 2500 to 3000 ml. to keep the ureters and ileal conduit well irrigated. The patient and family are cautioned that the physician is to be consulted immediately if there is a decrease in urinary drainage, abnormal constituents such as blood in urine, fever, pain in the back or abdomen, severe skin excoriation or general malaise. The patient is followed closely after hospital discharge. A referral may be made to a visiting nurse association, and the patient is seen at regular intervals at the clinic or by his physician. These visits may be frequent at first, and the intervals are gradually increased to 3 to 6 months if the patient's progress is satisfactory.

THE PATIENT WITH A URETEROSIGMOI-DOSTOMY. The patient who has the ureters transplanted into the sigmoid has the advantage of not having continuous external urinary drainage. No special appliance is necessary. The problem of skin irritation is eliminated. The colon retains the urine drainage from the ureters, and the anal sphincters control the expelling of urine just as they do feces. Approximately 200 ml of urine collect between anal voidings. The patient's stool becomes softer or liquid as the feces become mixed with urine.

A rectal tube with several openings is inserted when the operation is completed and remains in place for several days. It may be anchored by a suture or by securing the ends of a tape which circles the tube to the thighs. The tube is connected to a sterile tube leading to a drainage receptacle. Irrigations of sterile normal saline or water may be ordered to keep the tube clear of mucus and feces. Not more than 30 ml. are introduced at one time. Distention of the intestine is avoided to prevent pressure on the suture lines at the sites of the ureteral implants as well as reflux from the bowel into the ureters. The drainage is checked hourly the first 2 or 3 days and is measured and recorded. If at any time there is no drainage for 1 hour, the physician is notified.

When the tube is removed, the patient is instructed to establish a voiding schedule. The urine should be expelled at least every 4 hours to minimize the reabsorption of urinary waste products (e.g., chlorides and urea). The amount is measured and recorded each time. The patient may be wakened at regular intervals at night, or the physician may order a rectal tube inserted each night at bedtime to prevent an overaccumulation of urine in the colon. The tube is connected to a receptacle at the bedside. The patient is taught to insert and care for the tube, since the procedure may be continued when he goes home.

After the operation, the patient receives only clear fluids for 2 to 3 days, then a low-residue diet for 4 to 6 days to minimize the fecal content of the large intestine. The antimicrobial drug given preoperatively may be continued postoperatively for several days. A daily intake of 2500 to 3000 ml. fluid is necessary, and the patient is told of the importance of continuing this after his discharge from the hospital. The fluid intake and output are measured and the balance noted.

A family member and the patient are also instructed to report promptly any pain, fever, nausea, vomiting or generalized weakness. These symptoms may indicate kidney infection or electrolyte imbalance. The latter may occur as a result of reabsorption of urinary constituents from the bowel. Laxatives should not be taken without a physician's order; if one is necessary, a small dose of milk of magnesia may be prescribed. An adequate balanced diet and the suggested fluid intake generally are sufficient to promote normal bowel elimination.

If a surgical procedure which establishes an "anal bladder" and a permanent colostomy is used, the care relating to the urinary excretion is similar to that cited following a ureterosigmoidostomy. The patient will also require the nursing considerations as outlined on page 553 because of the colostomy.

THE PATIENT WITH CUTANEOUS URE-TEROSTOMY. This method of urinary diversion is used less often than the others because it is difficult to maintain adequate drainage. Stenosis of the ureters is prone to develop. The detached end of each ureter is brought out to the skin surface and everted to form a slightly protruding ureteral bud. The patient comes from the operating room with a catheter secured in each ureter. There are labeled right and left corresponding to the ureters, and are connected to separate drainage receptacles which are also labeled, respectively, right and left. The drainage is checked frequently and, if either catheter stops draining, the physician is notified and sterile equipment is prepared for irrigation. The catheters are left in place 7 to 12 days to minimize the urinary flow over the stomata while healing of the ureters to the abdominal wall takes place. The surgeon may order the application of normal saline compresses to the stomata around the catheters to prevent drying of the mucous membrane of the ureteral buds.

When the catheters are removed, an ileostomy bag may be applied over the stomata. The free end of the bag has an opening by which the urine drains into a connecting tubing and larger drainage receptacle. When the patient is ambulatory, the tubing may be connected to a plastic urinal strapped to the patient's thigh. There is also a special ureterostomy cup available, which is placed over the ureteral buds and may be held in place by a strap around the patient or by adhesive disks similar to those used with ileostomy bags. The cup is connected to a plastic urinary bag that can be attached to the patient's thigh. The urinal bag is replaced at night by a drainage receptable at the side of the bed. The bag or cup is changed every 2 or 3 days, and the connecting tubing and bags are changed daily. If an adhesive disk is used to hold the appliance in place, it is removed with a special commercial solvent available from the companies supplying the equipment. The skin around the ureteral buds requires frequent examination and attention. It is washed and thoroughly dried with each change of the appliance, and requires the application of a protective preparation such as tincture of benzoin, karaya gum powder or zinc oxide ointment. If the skin becomes excoriated, the physician is consulted. Exposure of 15 to 20 minutes to a radiant heat lamp may be ordered. Precautions must be taken to cover the stomata with sterile gauze during the treatment and, to prevent burning, the lamp should not be closer than 24 inches to the site.

The patient and a family member are given detailed instruction in the care of the stomata, skin and appliance. Two sets of equipment are desirable to allow efficient cleansing and airing. Opportunities are provided for the patient to become competent in the necessary care before he is discharged from the hospital. As with other methods of urinary diversion, the importance of a daily fluid intake of 2500 to 3000 ml. is stressed. There is always the danger that a patient may restrict his fluids so he will have less drainage to cope with, not realizing the need for continuous internal irrigation of the ureters. The patient and his family are cautioned to get in touch with the physician at once if drainage from either stoma stops, fever develops, or pain in the back or abdomen is experienced. Continuous drainage of urine from both ureters is necessary to prevent back pressure and ensuing hydronephrosis as well as ascending infection of the kidneys. The patient is followed closely; the stomata may require periodic dilatation. A referral to a visiting nurse agency for frequent supervision is recommended and the patient is seen regularly in the clinic, or by the physician.

SUMMARY CONCERNING URINARY DIVERSION. Factors to be considered in caring for a patient who undergoes permanent urinary diversion, regardless of the method used, include the following:

The patient's psychological reaction to a change in body image and normal pattern of function requires thoughtful understanding on the part of the nurse, with sincere efforts to reduce the patient's despair and promote acceptance and motivation.

Preoperative cleansing and "sterilization" of the bowel are necessary if the operative procedure involves resection of or entry into the intestine.

Maintenance of continuous, adequate urinary drainage from the ureters postoperatively is essential to prevent renal complications.

Drainage of urine through an opening onto the skin necessitates special skin care to prevent excoriation and maceration.

Drainage of urine into the sigmoid or rectum and its accumulation there necessitates scheduled anal voiding at least every 4 hours to minimize the reabsorption of urinary waste products which may incur electrolyte imbalance, acidosis and an elevation of blood urea.

A daily fluid intake of 2500 to 3000 ml. of fluid is important to provide good internal irrigation of the renal pelvis and ureters.

A planned program of instruction in the care of the stomata, skin and appliance is given to the patient and a family member. It should be given over a period of time that will allow them to acquire a satisfactory understanding and competence by the time the patient leaves the hospital. The instruction includes an explanation of the need for ample fluids and prompt reporting of decreased urinary drainage and significant symptoms.

Information about the patient's previous employment is obtained, and consideration is given as to whether it is suitable for him to resume his position or whether a referral to a social service worker would be of assistance in finding another occupation.

The patient requires a close follow-up. Frequent home visits by a visiting nurse, especially during the first few weeks after leaving the hospital, can provide assistance and considerable support to the patient and his family. Regular visits to a clinic or the physician are necessary.

DISORDERS OF THE URETHRA

Urethritis

Inflammation of the urethra is most often due to infection but may also follow trauma. The patient complains of dysuria and frequency. The causative organism may be identified by cultures and smears of the urine or discharge from the urinary meatus. A urinary antiseptic or an antibiotic (depending on the causative organism) is prescribed, and the patient is encouraged to force fluids.

Urethral Stricture

Stricture of the urethra may be congenital or acquired. A congenital stricture may go unrecognized for a period of time and only be discovered when it causes retention and stasis of urine that lead to urethritis or cystitis. An acquired stricture is usually the result of infection or trauma which has caused inflammation and ensuing fibrous scarring. The patient with a stricture may experience hesitancy in initiating voiding and a small, slow urinary stream.

Treatment consists of gradual dilatation by the introduction of bougies or catheters weekly or every 2 weeks over several months. In some instances, a catheter may be left in place to maintain dilatation or to provide adequate urinary drainage. Rarely, a temporary cystostomy is necessary because of severe retention.

Urethral Caruncle

A caruncle is a small, vascular, benign tumor that develops on the urethral wall near the urinary meatus. It occurs in females, usually appearing after the menopause. It bleeds easily and may be very sensitive. The patient may complain of pain on voiding and while sitting.

The caruncle is removed by cautery or excision. An indwelling catheter may be inserted and left in place for 24 to 48 hours because edema of the urethral tissues may interfere with voiding. The patient may find the pressure of the catheter on the site very uncomfortable. For this reason, some physicians avoid the use of a catheter unless acute retention develops. A dressing of petroleum jelly is applied to the site to avoid irritation and friction until the area heals.

References

Books

Beeson, Paul B., McDermott, Walsh, and Wyngaarden, James W. (Eds.): Textbook of Medicine, 15th ed. Philadelphia, W. B. Saunders, 1979, Part XV.

Brundage, Dorothy J.: Nursing Management of Renal Problems. St. Louis, C. V. Mosby, 1976.

Chapman, Warren H., et al.: The Urinary System: An Integrated Approach. Philadelphia, W.B. Saunders, 1973.

Ganong, William F.: Review of Medical Physiology, 7th ed. Los Altos, Cal., Lange, 1975. Chapters 38, and 39.
Guyton, Arthur C.: Textbook of Medical Physiology, 5th ed. Philadelphia, W. B. Saunders, 1976. Part VI.
Harrington, Joan DeLong, and Brener, Etta Rae: Patient Care in Renal Failure. Philadelphia, W.B. Saunders, 1973.
Krupp, Marcus A., and Chatton, Milton J.: Current Medical Diagnosis and Treatment. Los Altos, Cal., Lange, 1975. Chapter 15.
Macleod, John (Ed.): Davidson's Principles and Practice of Medicine, 11th ed. Edinburgh, Churchill Livingstone, 1974, pp. 579–620.
Sabiston, David C. (Ed.): Textbook of Surgery, 11th ed. Philadelphia, W. B. Saunders, 1977, Chapter 48.
Thorn, G. W., et al. (Eds.): Harrison's Principles of Internal Medicine, 8th ed. New York, McGraw-Hill, 1977.

Periodicals

Altshuler, Annie, et al.: "Even Children Can Learn Clean Self-Catheterization." Am. J. Nurs., Vol. 77, No. 1 (Jan. 1977), pp. 97–101.
Anger, Diane, and Anger, Daniel: "Dialysis Ambivalence: A Matter of Life and Death." Am. J. Nurs., Vol. 76, No. 2 (Feb. 1976), pp. 276–277.
Beaumont, Estelle: "Urinary Drainage Systems." Nurs. '74, Vol. 4, No. 1 (Jan. 1974), pp. 52–55.
Cross, Pamela S.: "Ureteral Reimplantation: Nursing Care of the Child." Am. J. Nurs., Vol. 76, No. 11 (Nov. 1976), pp. 1800–1803.
D'Afflitti, Judith Gregorie, and Swanson, Donna: "Group Treatment for the Wives of Home-Dialysis Patients." Am. J. Nurs. Vol. 75, No. 4 (April 1975), pp. 633–635.
Danielson, B. D., and Shapiro, F. L.: "Early Management of Renal Insufficiency." Mod. Med., Vol. 4, No. 26 (Dec. 24, 1973). pp. 21–28.
DeGroot, Jane: "Catheter-Induced Urinary Tract Infections: Can We Prevent Them?" Nurs. '76, Vol. 6, No. 8 (Aug. 1976), p. 34–37.
Dolan, Patrician O'Connor, and Greene, Harry L.: "Renal Failure and Peritoneal Dialysis." Nurs. '75, Vol. 5, No. 7 (July 1975), pp. 41–45.
Federspiel, Billie: "Renin and Blood Pressure." Am. J. Nurs. Vol. 75, No. 9 (Sept. 1975), pp. 1462–1464.
Flegle, Janice M.: "Teaching Self-Dialysis to Adults in a Hospital." Am. J. Nurs., Vol. 77, No. 2 (Feb. 1977), pp. 270–272.
Fry, J. E., and Majumdar, B.: "Basic Physical Assessment." Can. Nurse, Vol. 70, No. 5 (May 1974), pp. 17–22.
Fulton, Barbara (Ed.): "Symposium on Patient Care in Kidney and Urinary Tract Disease." Nurse. Clin. North Am. Vol. 4, No. 3 (Sept. 1969), pp. 393–482.
Garner, Julia S.: "Better Urinary Catheter Care." Nurs. '74, Vol. 4, No. 2 (Feb. 1974), pp. 54–56.
Gault, Patricia: "Six Patients with Bladder Cancer — and How They Fared After Surgery." Nurs. '77, Vol. 7, No. 11 (Nov. 1977), pp. 48–55.
Geis, W. Peter, and Iwatsuki, S.: "Acute and Chronic Renal Failure." Surg. Clin. North Am., Vol. 57, No. 6 (Dec. 1977), pp. 1263–1280.
Gittes, Rita, R. S.: "Retrograde Renal and Ureteral Brush Biopsy." Am. J. Nurs., Vol. 78, No. 3 (March 1978), pp. 410–412.
Henneman, Philip H.: "Management of Renal Stones by Internist-Urologist Collaboration." Mod. Med., Vol. 46, No. 1, (Jan. 15, 1978), pp. 34–39.
Irwin, M. A., et al.: "Plan of Care: The Young Child on Dialysis." Can. Nurse, Vol. 72, No. 10 (Oct. 1976), pp. 41–43.
Jensen, Vicki: "Better Techniques for Bagging Stomas: Part 1: Urinary Ostomies." Nurs. '74, Vol. 4, No. 7 (July 1974) pp. 60–64.
Juliani, Louise: "Kidney Transplant: Your Role in Aftercare." Nurs. '77, Vol. 7, No. 10 (Oct. 1977), pp. 46–53.
_____: "Assessing Renal Function." Nurs, '78, Vol. 8, No. 1 (Jan. 1978), pp. 34–35.
Kobrzycki, Paula: "Renal Transplant Complications." Am. J. Nurs., Vol. 77, No. 4 (April 1977), pp. 641–643.
Kolb, Felix O.: "Medical Management of the Patient with Renal Stones." Primary Care, Vol. 2, No. 2 (June 1975), pp. 317–341.
Kronfield, S. Jack: "Chronic Renal Failure: Diagnosis and Management." Primary Care, Vol. 1, No. 4 (Dec. 1974), pp. 583–601
Kurtzman, N. A. (Ed.): "Symposium on Renal Pathophysiology." Arch. Int. Med., Vol. 131, No. 6 (June, 1973). Symposium.
Lang, Gordon R., and Levin, Stuart: "Diagnosis and Treatment of Urinary Tract Infections." Med. Clin. North Am., Vol. 55, No. 6 (Nov. 1971), pp. 1439–1452.
Langford, Teddy Lynn: "Nursing Problem: Bacteriuria and the Indwelling Catheter." Am. J. Nurs., Vol. 72, No. 1 (Jan. 1972), pp. 113–115.

672

Linton, A. L.: "Acute Renal Failure." Can. Med. Assoc. J., Vol. 110, No. 8 (April 20, 1974), pp. 949–957.

Mott, M. G.: "Nephroblastoma — Wilm's Tumor." Brit. J. Hosp. Med., Vol. 13, No. 2 (Feb. 1975), pp. 161–180.

Muehrcke, Robert C., et al.: "Home Hemodialysis." Med. Clin. North Am., Vol. 55, No. 6 (Nov. 1971), pp. 1473–1491.

O'Neill, Mary: "Symposium on Care of the Patient with Renal Disease." Nurs. Clin. North Am., Vol. 10, No. 3 (Sept. 1975), pp. 411–615.

Peart, W. S.: "Renin-Angiotensin System." N. Engl. J. Med., Vol. 292, No. 6 (Feb. 6, 1975), pp. 302–306.

Pollack, Victor E., and Mendoza, Nina: "Rapidly Progressive Glomerulonephritis." Med. Clin. North Am., Vol. 55, No. 6 (Nov. 1971), pp. 1397–1414.

Prout, George R.: "Bladder Cancer." N. Engl. J. Med., Vol. 287, No. 2 (July 13, 1972), pp. 86–89.

Read, Martha, and Mallison, Mary: "External Arteriovenous Shunts." Am. J. Nurs., Vol. 72, No. 1 (Jan. 1972), pp. 81–85.

Sapperstein, Michael: "Dialysis." Am. J. Nurs., Vol. 72, No. 1 (Jan. 1972), p. 85.

Schumann, Delores: "The Renal Donor." Am. J. Nurs., Vol. 74, No. 1 (Jan. 1974), pp. 105–110.

Shapbell, N. June, and Sweigart, James E.: "A Urinary Device for Patients with Problem Stomas." Nurs. Clin. North Am., Vol. 9, No. 2 (June 1974), pp. 381–386

Schaffer, E.: "Do-It-Yourself Dialysis." Can. Nurse. Vol. 69, No. 7 (July 1973), pp. 29–32.

Willey, Maxine: "Care of the Patient with a Kidney Transplant." Nurs. Clin. North Am., Vol. 8, No. 1 (March 1973), pp. 127–135.

Wolf, Zane R.: "What Patients Awaiting Kidney Transplant Want To Know." Am. J. Nurs., Vol. 76, No. 1 (Jan. 1976), pp. 92–94.

Woodrow, Mary: "Suprapubic Catheters: Part 1, A Direct Line to Better Drainage." Nurs. '76, Vol. 6, No. 10 (Oct. 1976), pp. 40–45.

_____: "Suprapubic Catheters: Part 2, A Direct Line to Better Drainage." Nurs. '76, Vol. 6, No. 11 (Nov. 1976), pp. 40–42.

20

Nursing in Disorders of the Reproductive System

by DONNA SHIELDS, B.Sc.N., C.N.M., M.S.N.

EMBRYOLOGY

The reproductive system is unique in mammals in that it differs markedly between sexes. Sex is determined at the time of fertilization by the inclusion of the XX chromosomal pair of the female or the XY genotype of the male. In this early period of human development, sex differentiation can be determined microscopically by the presence or absence of Barr bodies in a cell nucleus which has been taken from the embryo. These Barr bodies, which are always one less than the number of X chromosomes, indicate the genotype of the embryo.

As the embryo grows, a genital ridge develops but remains undifferentiated in either sex until the seventh week of intrauterine life. At this time sex differentiation can be made morphologically because the genital ridges of the embryo, accompanied by the primordial germ cells, have grown and differentiated into a rudimentary testis or ovary, depending on the sex of the cell.

An elaborate bilateral duct system also develops. In the male much of this duct system degenerates, and the remaining portion forms the epididymis and ductus deferens, which then join the male urethra. In the female the duct systems develop bilaterally and, as growth continues, the two ducts meet and fuse in the midline. The portion which fuses becomes the uterus, cervix and vagina.

This process of fusion takes some weeks to complete and, indeed, may never occur, giving rise to paired uteri and vaginas. Fusion may be incomplete, causing some abnormalities of the uterus (Fig. 20–1).

While internal development proceeds the external genitalia are also becoming differentiated. In the "neuter" phase of development three small protuberances appear caudally on the external surface of the embryo. These protuberances consist of the "genital tubercle" and, on either side of this tubercle, the genital swellings. In the male the tubercle becomes elongated and develops into the male phallus while the genital swellings become the scrotal tissue. These two swellings must develop, descend and fuse, closing the urethra in the male penis and forming the pendulant scrotum. Should fusion not be complete on the dorsal surface, a condition known as hypospadias occurs (Fig. 20–2). Epispadias, a rarer malformation, may also occur. Here the failure of the urethra to fuse completely occurs on the ventral side of the penis. From these swellings, the prepuce, or foreskin, of the penis also arises. The foreskin is attached to the penile shaft at the base of the glans. The foreskin then drops down like a hood over the glans and remains partially fixed until sometime between birth and 3 years of age. During this time the congenital adhesions break down and the prepuce is then easily retractable over the glans penis.

673

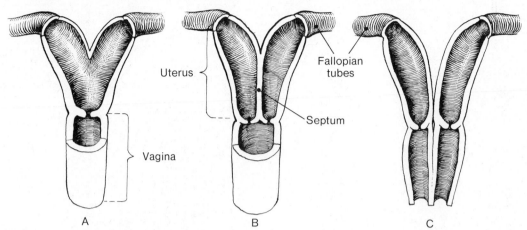

FIGURE 20–1 Some abnormalities of the uterus resulting from incomplete fusion of the ducts. *A,* Bicornate uterus. *B,* Uterus septus and a double cervix. *C,* Double uterus, cervix and vagina.

The female genitalia arise from the same three ridges. The tubercle becomes the clitoris, and the genital swellings develop into the labia majora and minora. As the labia meet anteriorly, they form a loose-fitting, hood-like fold over the clitoris. This fold is similar to the prepuce of the male penis. Posteriorly, the labial folds fuse just before the anus. Thus, male and female reproductive systems have homologous counterparts.

By the sixteenth week of embryologic life the sex of the infant can be determined externally. At this time the testes of the male, which normally reside in the scrotum, are not there. In early development the testis and ovary are abdominal organs. As further growth takes place, they descend over the pelvic brim in the case of the ovaries or into the scrotum in the case of the testes. The descent of the testes appears to be in response to hormonal and mechanical control. As the fetal testes begin to produce testosterone, in about the seventh month of fetal life, descent occurs, and they pass through the inguinal canal and the external inguinal ring to enter the scrotum by the ninth month. During descent the testis is surrounded by a tube of peritoneum known as the processus vaginalis. After descent has occurred, this tissue generally becomes obliterated, leaving the testis covered by the tunica vaginalis. Following descent, the testis shows a decline in its production of testosterone until puberty. As in all processes, descent may not

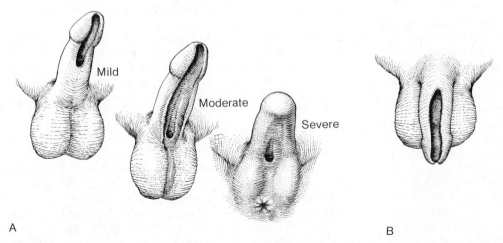

FIGURE 20–2 *A,* Hypospadias—mild, moderate and severe. In severe hypospadias note the similarity to the female. *B,* Epispadias.

occur or may occur imperfectly. This may result in maldescent of the testes.

PHYSIOLOGY

THE MALE REPRODUCTIVE SYSTEM

The system consists of the paired testes, epididymis, vas deferens, common ejaculatory ducts, urethra, penis and the scrotum. The accessory organs are the seminal vesicles, prostate gland and the bulbourethral glands (Fig. 20–3). A cross section of the testis (Fig. 20–4) demonstrates the relationships between the seminiferous tubule, rete testis, efferent ductules, epididymis and vas deferens.

The Testes

Each lobe of the testis contains a seminiferous tubule surrounded by tissue. In this tissue are interstitial, or Leydig, cells, which are endocrine in action, producing the male hormones of which testosterone is the most prominent. These cells become activated to produce some androgens in the fetal period but remain nearly dormant until puberty. At puberty, under the complex control of the hypothalamus and pituitary glands, the

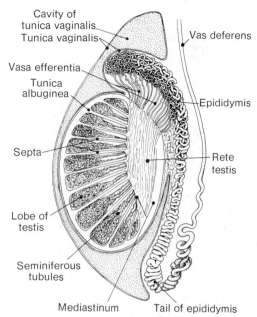

FIGURE 20–4 Section of the testis.

testes are stimulated to produce male hormones. Under the influence of these androgens, the body begins the process of puberty. The external organs of reproduction grow and develop. The distribution of body hair changes to that of the adult male. The larynx and musculoskeletal systems develop and change. Concurrently, the testes begin to produce sperm. Puberty ends with the sexual and reproductive maturity of the individual.

SPERMATOGENESIS. Spermatogenesis begins in the seminiferous tubule (Fig. 20–5). Here a basilar membrane around the lumen of the tubule is lined with two major cell types which project into the lumen of the tube. The first of these, the germ cells, are called spermatogonia. These cells undergo growth and multiplication to become primary and secondary spermatocytes and then spermatids. Until this phase is complete the cell appears to have sufficient nutrients in itself. Now, however, the second type of cell, the Sertoli or sustentacular cell, is apparently necessary to provide nutrition for the spermatid. The spermatid is engulfed by the sustentacular cell and begins a metamorphosis which produces viable spermatozoa.

When growth is complete, the sperm is released into the lumen of the seminiferous tubule and is rapidly transported to the epididymis and thence through the duct system.

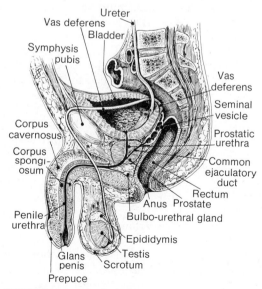

FIGURE 20–3 Sagittal view of the male reproductive system and pelvis.

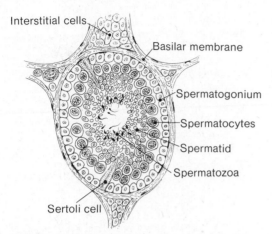

Interstitial cells

Basilar membrane

Spermatogonium

Spermatocytes

Spermatid

Spermatozoa

Sertoli cell

FIGURE 20–5 Transverse section of a seminiferous tubule in the interstitial tissue of the testis.

Although sperm may appear to be mature at the time of release into the tubule, they do undergo further maturation, increasing in fertility and vigor as they progress through the ducts. Sperm removed from the tail of the epididymis rather than the head are more fertile. If sperm are not ejaculated, they degenerate rapidly and are absorbed. Spermatogenesis is continuous and new sperm are constantly being produced. The exact time of spermatogenesis is unknown but the whole process probably takes some days. This is in contrast to the female, who does not produce ova throughout her lifetime but merely matures ova present from her own primordial germ cells.

Spermatogenesis is also sensitive to heat, and occurs at a temperature a few degrees lower than body temperature. It is for this apparent reason that the testes are suspended in the scrotum, allowing the temperature of the testes to be regulated by the body. The dartos muscle within the scrotum contracts or relaxes in response to varying temperatures. Coldness causes it to contract, bringing the testes closer to the body for extra warmth. The reverse is true in heat. It is also known that men with uncorrected cryptorchism remain sterile, possibly because the body temperature intra-abdominally is incompatible with successful spermatogenesis.

Duct System and Accessory Glands

The viable sperm must be transported from the testis to the penis and thence to the female reproductive tract so that fertilization may take place. Here the duct system and the accessory glands play a major role. As the vas deferens ascends into the pelvic cavity, it widens into a broad ampulla. The duct of each seminal vesicle and the ampulla of the adjacent vas deferens meet to form the common ejaculatory duct. As a secretory organ, the seminal vesicle does not store sperm but rather produces a fluid which is rich in nutrients. These nutrients provide for the sperm until fertilization. At ejaculation, the seminal vesicles contract and seminal fluid is forced into the common ejaculatory ducts and into the prostatic urethra where the prostate gland also discharges its fluid.

The prostate gland, which is fused to the neck of the bladder, is divided into three lobes which surround the urethra. The prostate develops in puberty and is easily palpable on rectal examination. During the years of sexual maturity the prostate secretes a thin, milky-looking solution. This solution is alkaline and is believed to reduce the acidity of seminal fluid and vaginal secretions. This is an important reproductive function, as the motility and viability of sperm are greatly reduced in an acid solution. Sperm are more motile in a neutral or slightly alkaline solution. At ejaculation the muscle layers of the prostate gland contract rhythmically, forcing prostatic fluid into that portion of the urethra near the prostate. Simultaneously with these contractions of prostatic muscle, the fibers at the neck of the bladder continuous with muscle fibers in the prostate gland also contract, closing the internal urethral orifice.

Further fluid is added to the semen by the bulbourethral glands. These paired glands lie posterior to the urethra and discharge their fluid into it when they contract at ejaculation. This fluid seems to function merely as a lubricant and fluid medium for the sperm.

When all fluids are pooled in the prostatic portion of the urethra the first phase of ejaculation has been completed. The next phase is accomplished by powerful rhythmic contractions. The result is that the semen is forced along the length of the urethra in the erect penis and expelled from the urinary meatus under pressure.

Deposition of the semen in the vagina of the female is one function of the penis. The penis also serves as an excretory organ. In order to obtain intromission, the penis must move from its normally flaccid state to one of erection. Such a change is due to engorgement with blood of the corpora cavernosa and the corpus spongiosum.

Semen is a milky, viscous fluid varying at one ejaculation from 2 to 7 ml. in quantity and containing about 60,000,000 to 100,000,000 sperm per ml. The alkaline fluid is rich in nutrients and minerals to support the sperm. It coagulates a few minutes after ejaculation and then reliquefies later. The sperm, which are actively motile by lashing their tails, move rapidly up through the uterus into the outer third of the uterine (fallopian) tube where fertilization usually takes place. It is believed that the acrosome or projection on the head of the sperm releases hyaluronidase, an enzyme which dissolves the outer wall of the ovum. This allows a sperm to enter the ovum and fertilization to take place.

THE FEMALE REPRODUCTIVE SYSTEM

The female reproductive tract consists of paired ovaries, uterine tubes, a uterus and vagina (Fig. 20–6). Externally, the labia, clitoris, and Skene's and Bartholin's glands are part of the reproductive system (Fig. 20–7).

The external area may be collectively referred to as the vulva, perineum or pudenda. Generally, perineum refers to the area stretching from the symphysis pubis laterally to the thighs and posteriorly to the tip of the coccyx. This is arbitrarily divided into the anterior and posterior perineum by an imaginary line drawn between the ischial tuberosities. Anteriorly, this contains the urogenital triangle and posterially the rectal triangle, including the perineal body. The area between the labia majora is referred to as the pudendal cleft. That area which lies between the labia minora and extends from the clitoris to the fourchette is referred to as the vestibule. Bartholin's glands, whose ducts open into the vestibule, may be referred to as the greater vestibular glands, Skene's being the lesser.

The female reproductive system functions to produce the female hormones (estrogen and progesterone), to ripen ova for fertilization, and for intercourse which permits fertilization of ova and the release of sexual tension. In addition, the organs of reproduction incubate the human conceptus, providing it with safety and nourishment until the fetus is expelled from the uterus to continue its growth and development externally.

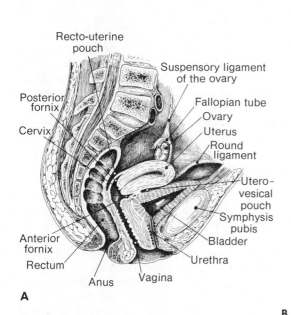

A

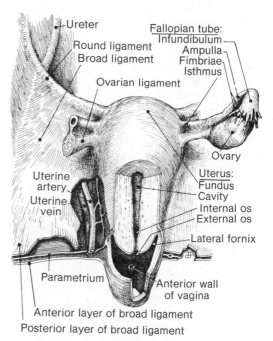

B

FIGURE 20–6 *A,* Median sagittal section of the female pelvis. *B,* Uterus and adnexa, posterior view (uterus, cervix and vagina wedge sectioned).

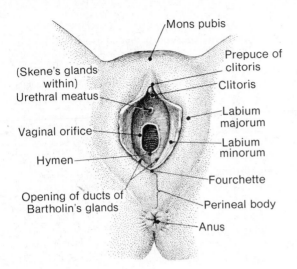

Mons pubis

Prepuce of clitoris

(Skene's glands within)

Urethral meatus

Clitoris

Vaginal orifice

Labium majorum

Hymen

Labium minorum

Opening of ducts of Bartholin's glands

Fourchette

Perineal body

Anus

FIGURE 20–7   Female external genitalia.

The Ovary

The ovary is a small, almond-shaped organ lying posterior to the broad ligament of the uterus and attached to it by the mesovarium. Cross sections of the ovary show a cortex and a medulla. The cortex, or outer layer, is composed of connective tissue and cells, among which are scattered the ova and developing follicles. Over this outer layer of the cortex is a thin layer of germinal epithelium. The medulla is composed of connective tissue containing blood vessels and smooth muscle fibers.

The fetal ovary is recognizable very early. By the fourth month of intrauterine life some cells in the ovary have differentiated enough to be recognizable as primary oocytes. Such oocytes, numbering only 300 to 400 in each woman, are determined at fertilization. Throughout childhood certain of these oocytes develop but never reach maturity and ovulate. Then, under the influence of the maturing hypothalamus, which stimulates the anterior lobe of the pituitary to produce hormones, puberty begins.

The secondary sex characteristics begin to develop. First there is growth and development of the breast tissue. Pubic hair appears and the internal and external organs of reproduction become fully developed and functional. The vagina, under the influence of estrogens, thickens and develops several layers of squamous epithelium. This makes it more resistant to infection. Previously, the vaginal pH had been neutral or alkaline; now

it becomes acidic. This is largely due to Döderlein's bacillus which oxidizes the glycogen which has been deposited in the vagina to form lactic acid. Concurrently, the ovaries are developing and menarche, or the beginning of menstruation, occurs.

THE OVARIAN CYCLE. Under the influence of the follicle-stimulating hormone (FSH) released by the pituitary gland, the primary follicle begins to mature. The primary follicle is composed of an oocyte and follicular cells. Growth is eccentric and the oocyte or ovum gradually comes to lie at one side of the group of follicular cells. Fluid collects between these cells and the ovum. A clear membrane, the zona pellucida, develops and surrounds the ovum. As the follicle grows, the cells surrounding it begin to form and are termed thecal cells. Now the interstitial cell-stimulating hormone (ICSH, luteinizing hormone) works with the FSH to allow the thecal cells to function. These cells, which are similar to the Leydig cells of the male, produce estrogens which are released into the blood. Eventually, the high level of circulating estrogen triggers the hypothalamus to stop releasing the FSH-releasing factor. As the level of FSH-releasing factor declines, the anterior pituitary gland responds by reducing the amount of FSH released. ICSH continues to be produced. Many follicles may start to ripen, but usually only one continues on to ovulation. The others undergo degeneration in the ovary. The thecal cells surrounding these degenerated (atretic) follicles also produce estrogens. The mature

follicle may now be termed a graafian follicle, after de Graaf who first described it in
1672 (Fig. 20–8).

As the graafian follicle approaches ovulation, it comes to lie close to the surface of the
ovary. The tissue over it becomes thin and
taut. Soon the follicle wall ruptures and the
ovum, surrounded by the zona pellucida and
some attached granulosa cells, is expelled
into the abdominal cavity. The time of rupture is designated as ovulation. Although it is
felt that a buildup of pressure within the follicle is not the principal cause of rupture, the
precise mechanism is still not perfectly understood. However it is accomplished, ovulation marks the end of the preovulatory, or
follicular, phase.

The ovary now embarks on the luteal
phase of its cycle. Immediately following
ovulation, the wall of the follicle collapses
inward and some hemorrhage may occur into
this cavity. In a few hours the remaining
granulosa cells hypertrophy and begin to
show the characteristic yellow of the corpus
luteum. These yellowed granulosa cells are
now called luteal cells. The luteal cells are
stimulated by ICSH to become the corpus
luteum and to begin producing progesterone.
Estrogen continues to be produced as well.
The corpus luteum reaches full maturity by
about the ninth day following ovulation. At
this time it is easily recognizable on the surface of the ovary as a raised yellowed area
and may constitute nearly half the volume of
the ovary. Near this time the corpus luteum

may receive a message that the ovum has
been fertilized. If it does so, the corpus luteum is maintained and becomes known as
the corpus luteum of pregnancy. If fertilization does not occur, the luteal site begins to
degenerate, and progesterone production
drops. As the site degenerates, so do the
thecal cells. Estrogen production from this
source declines. The luteal site shrinks to
form a small mass of whitish scar tissue on
the surface of the ovary which is known as
the corpus albicans.

In response to the falling estrogen and progesterone levels, the hypothalamus signals
the pituitary gland to release FSH and ICSH
and the cycle repeats itself. This cycle recurs
roughly every 28 to 32 days in the vast majority of adult women from menarche to menopause, unless it is interrupted by periods of
pregnancy. However, in response to this
cycle, the endometrium of the uterus also
undergoes cyclic phenomena. These phenomena are known as the uterine cycle. The
two cycles, uterine and ovarian, are intimately related and occur simultaneously.

The Uterus

The uterus is a thick-walled, muscular,
pear-shaped organ about 3 inches in length in
the adult virgin. It is held in position by its
ligaments and by the pelvic floor. The uterus
is composed of three layers: (1) an inner
mucous layer, or endometrium; (2) a middle
muscular layer, or myometrium; and (3) an
outer serous layer which covers the entire
body of the uterus except where it is reflected up and over the bladder. The uterus is
divided into two distinct parts, the body and
the cervix.

The cervix projects into the vagina. It appears to be mainly connective tissue, and
only 10 per cent is muscle. The endometrial
lining of the body of the uterus extends
downward, undergoing certain modifications
in the cervical canal and terminating just
above the external os of the cervix where it
meets the stratified squamous epithelium of
the vaginal wall.

THE UTERINE CYCLE. In the uterine
cycle the endometrium plays a major role.
The endometrium is a thin, pink membrane
which is attached directly to the underlying
muscle layer. It is composed of surface epithelium, uterine glands and connective tissue, and is richly supplied with blood vessels

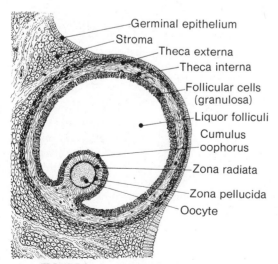

Germinal epithelium
Stroma
Theca externa
Theca interna
Follicular cells
(granulosa)
Liquor folliculi
Cumulus
oophorus
Zona radiata
Zona pellucida
Oocyte

FIGURE 20–8 Mature graafian follicle.

and tissue spaces. The thickness of the endometrium varies with the cycle. At the beginning of a new cycle it is probably about 0.5 mm. thick. In response to the estrogens of the preovulatory phase of the ovary it begins to proliferate and continues to do so throughout the cycle until it reaches a peak of proliferation and secretion several days following ovulation. In addition to the effect of estrogen, the progesterone released in the luteal phase of the ovary further promotes the secretory activity of the endometrium. In this secretory stage the endometrium is edematous, the glands are large and sacculated, the arteries have developed their typical coiled, tortuous pattern and some connective tissue has undergone hypertrophic stages. The rich, succulent endometrium now contains much glycogen. At this time the endometrium may be 5 to 6 mm. in depth. In short, all is ready for the implantation of the fertilized ovum, should it appear. In perfect timing the endometrium reaches its peak development approximately 7 to 8 days following ovulation, or just when the fertilized ovum should appear in the uterine cavity ready for implantation.

If the ovum has been fertilized and the corpus luteum is continuing to secrete progesterone, the endometrium is maintained and implantation may occur successfully. However, should the corpus luteum not receive this message, it begins to degenerate. Estrogen and progesterone production decline. This decline in progesterone causes the endometrium to retract and degenerate. Vasoconstriction of blood vessels occurs and the uterus becomes ischemic. Shortly thereafter the endometrium begins to slough away and menstruation begins. The process of sloughing takes from 3 to 7 days, with each woman usually establishing her own pattern. Menstrual flow is composed of endometrial tissue, mucus and some blood. As the tiny arterioles constrict and relax, bleeding occurs. Usually not more than 50 to 60 ml. of blood per menstrual period is lost. This blood does not clot because of the action of fibrinolytic enzymes released into the uterine cavity during menstruation. Occasionally, a heavy menstrual loss neutralizes the available fibrinolysins and clots occur. At the completion of menstruation the endometrium has returned to its unproliferative state. It is now ready to respond again to the rising estrogen levels.

Ovulation

THE MENSTRUAL CYCLE. The uterine and ovarian cycles are often referred to as the menstrual cycle. This cycle begins on day one, which is the day menstruation begins, and continues until the day before menstruation begins again. Ovulation occurs on or around the fourteenth day of a 28-day cycle. However, this is subject to many factors, and the timing of ovulation in any one woman is often a matter of considerable variation.

The hypothalamus is subject to a measure of control from the cerebral cortex. Events associated with excitement, stress, a change of environment or anxiety can delay the ripening of a follicle and, consequently, ovulation. All follicles do not appear to mature at the same rate each month. This produces a month-to-month variation in the timing of the ovulation in any one woman. The variation in timing is perceived by most women as a change in the onset of menstruation. However, the onset of menstrual flow appears to be controlled by the corpus luteum of the ovary. Once ovulation occurs, menstruation follows 14 days (±1 day) after. Hence, ovulation occurs 14 days before menstruation, and this relationship appears to be constant. Fluctuations in the length of the cycle arise in the preovulatory phase.

ANOVULATION. Not all cycles are ovulatory, and it is known that women can have an anovulatory cycle and still menstruate. The precise mechanisms for these phenomena are not clearly understood. Some believe that in such cases a follicle develops, becomes cystic and degenerates. Certainly, some such mechanism appears possible, particularly in adolescent girls, in whom the first menstrual periods may be anovulatory, and at the menopause.

Cervical, Vaginal and Tubal Cycles

Changes also occur in the cervix, vagina, and uterine tubes in response to stimuli from the ovary. Estrogen prompts the endocervical glands to respond by increasing their secretions and becoming longer and more tortuous. This is accompanied by increased vascularity and tumescence of the cervix. From about the seventh day of the menstrual cycle to about the twenty-first the cervical mucus gradually increases in amount. The mucus contains an increasing concentration of sodium chloride, which causes it to show a typical ferning pattern when allowed to dry on a slide. During the other periods of the cycle and during pregnancy the dried cervical mucus shows a beaded pattern. The mucus reaches its peak of production at ovulation. The consistency changes at ovulation and becomes thinner and can be drawn out into long, thin threads; this is called spinnbarkeit. These changes demonstrate the timing of the body as the mucus will permit easy entry of the sperm at ovulation, the most logical time. Indeed, it appears that the cervical mucus permits passage of sperm through the cervix only at this particular time.

Changes in the vagina and uterine tube are minimal compared to the changes in the ovary, uterus and cervix. The vaginal epithelium proliferates and reaches a peak at ovulation time. The uterine tube becomes swollen. Its secretory cells enlarge and project beyond the ciliated cells. Maximum development is timed to occur simultaneously with ovulation and the passage of the ovum through the tube. The ovum is also assisted in its passage by the wave-like contractions of the uterine tube and the beating of the tubal cilia toward the uterus. These contractions appear to be under the influence of estrogens. The uterine tube secretes fluids, which provide nutrients first for the ovum and then for the conceptus until implantation occurs.

The Vagina

The vagina, a fibromuscular tube from 3 to 4 inches long, is the female organ of intercourse. Here sperm are deposited. It also serves as a passage for the fetus from intrauterine to extrauterine life. The vagina is protected by the labia, which usually remain in close approximation over the introitus. During sexual excitement the labia become engorged and swollen and gape, thus exposing the vestibule.

Under neural stimulus, Bartholin's glands secrete a fluid which serves to lubricate the vaginal introitus. However, the mucus these vulvovaginal glands secrete is minimal and not of sufficient quantity to lubricate the entire vagina. Hence, most vaginal lubrication arises from the vaginal walls themselves. Very quickly following sexual stimulation the vaginal walls exhibit a "sweating"-like appearance as beads of mucoid material appear throughout the rugal folds. Soon the droplets run together and form a complete coat of lubrication over the inner surface of the vagina. Since there are no glandular elements in the vaginal wall, it is hypothesized that the exudation is a result of marked dilatation of the venous system which surrounds the vagina. The cervix, once thought to be the source of much of the lubrication of the vagina, also appears to play a relatively minor role. This seems to be confirmed by the fact that little or no secretory activity of the cervix has been observed during sexual activity. Also, women who have undergone total hysterectomy and bilateral salpingo-oophorectomy produce reasonable vaginal lubrication in response to sexual stimulation. Indeed, the same response will develop in artificially constructed vaginas, and the source of the lubricating material is presumed to be the same.

The vagina also responds to sexual stimuli by enlarging. The inner two-thirds of the vagina expand and lengthen, forming a basin for the seminal pool which will form in the posterior fornix of the vagina just below the cervical os. The outer third of the vagina becomes engorged and constricted, serving to assist the vagina to form a reservoir for the semen. Engorgement of pelvic organs also results in a slight elevation of the uterus and cervix.

An orgasm may occur as a generalized systemic feeling, with sensation localized in the clitoris, and rhythmic muscular contractions of the outer third of the vagina and the uterus. With orgasm, pelvic engorgement of blood vessels is rapidly resolved. This causes the uterus to return to its normal position, placing the cervix very near to or in the seminal pool, thus facilitating movement of sperm through the cervix.

The clitoris seems to be a unique organ in human anatomy. As the primary focus of sensual response, it appears to serve no other function. Made of fibrous tissue with two corpora cavernosa and richly innervated, it undergoes engorgement and enlargement when the female is sexually stimulated either physically or mentally. It also appears to be the translator of sexual stimuli to other organs of the reproductive tract. There is no apparent observable response in the clitoris at orgasm.

Menopause

. The reproductive functions of the male and female continue throughout adult life. Given health and opportunity, the male's sexual and reproductive capabilities are lifelong; the only major change is a slowing of sexual response and a gradual reduction in libido (sexual drive).

Women, however, present a different picture. Reproductive function, usually demonstrated by menses, continues until middle age. Then, at the average age of 50, women cease menstruating. The climacteric or cessation of menstruation is perhaps the most obvious sign of menopause, or "change of life." Actually menopause, in onset and duration, resembles puberty, which was a gradual awakening of reproductive function over a period of 6 months to 2 years. Menopause also may take a few months to several years and is the result of altered ovarian function. Ovarian follicles cease to ripen. The endometrium does not respond as richly, and menstruation becomes scantier and shorter in duration. The woman may have several anovulatory cycles, just as she may have had in puberty. Eventually the menses may become irregular and finally cease. Menopause is said to be complete when the woman has had no menses for 1 year. As the perimenopausal woman may ovulate erratically, family planning advice is important to her. She cannot assume she will not become pregnant until menopause is complete, after which the risks of pregnancy occurring are very slight.

Decreasing estrogen levels stimulate gonadotropic hormones (FSH, ICSH) which show a proportionate rise, but the ovary does not respond fully. The vascular system, once functioning smoothly under hormonal control, begins to respond to these imbalances and the woman may experience "hot flashes," feelings of tingling and faintness. She may have periods of sweating, especially at night. Hypertension may develop, for estrogen appears to have inhibiting effects on the development of atherosclerosis. Osteoporosis has also been linked to declining estrogen levels. She may feel depressed and experience swings in mood for no apparent reason. Much of this may be unsettling to the woman, especially when accompanied by cessation of reproductive function and fears of advancing age and of loss of usefulness, sexual function and love of her husband.

Most women accept the changes with some minor disturbances. It would seem that an understanding of menopause and some reassurance of her usefulness and worth will help most women. Only about 25 per cent of women require hormone replacement treatment. This is in the form of short-term therapy with oral estrogens. The dosage is individualized to relieve the symptoms and is continued for 2 to 3 months, at which time a reassessment is made to decide whether to continue or stop treatment. Because the prolonged use of estrogens in the perimenopausal woman is associated with an increased risk of cancer of the endometrium, women should be alerted to the risks of long-term estrogen therapy.

It should be understood that all estrogen production does not cease at menopause. The ovaries do not appear to be inert postmenopausally, and it is thought that they continue to excrete small amounts of hormones. This is in addition to estrogens from the adrenal gland. Over the years estrogen production declines further and the development of other organ changes occurs. The vulva becomes atrophic and thin from a resorption of fatty tissue. The uterus decreases in size; the endometrium becomes thin and atrophic. The vaginal epithelium thins out and is more susceptible to injury and infection. Lubrication of the vagina may require supplementation so that dyspareunia (painful sexual intercourse) need not occur.

Sexual function can continue with little change in the vast majority of postmenopausal women. The most important factors in the continuance of sexual function appear to be the opportunity for and the frequency of intercourse, so that the changes of menopause themselves do not mean this phase of a woman's life must cease. Indeed, relief from fear of pregnancy may make the experience a more enjoyable one.

DISORDERS OF THE REPRODUCTIVE SYSTEM

GENERAL NURSING CONSIDERATIONS

The patient with a disorder of the reproductive system presents some special concerns for the nurse. In many ways a human being is defined by his sex. Knowing he or she is a man or a woman gives the person a set of behaviors, culturally and physiologically determined, which help to guide his or her actions. The normal functioning of the reproductive system gives constant reassurance of a person's essential maleness or femaleness. The distortion or interruption of these processes may prove very disturbing to the individual and family.

The person may fear loss of reproductive function. The ability to reproduce is seen by many as a criterion of usefulness and sexuality. The loss of function may be followed by feelings of uselessness or of being only half a person. These feelings can be particularly distressing to the woman who has defined herself in terms of her reproductive and sexual function. To her the removal of her uterus or ovaries may be tantamount to removing her femaleness. Because she may feel less a woman, she fears her husband will see her as less a woman. Indeed, in some unfortunate situations, he may. Thus, to the fear of loss of reproductive function may be added the fear of loss of a loved one. For some the fear of loss of libido as well as sexual function may be very frightening and can cause the patient much anguish.

Also, most patients have been culturally conditioned to the idea that these areas of the body should not be discussed, much less exposed, in examination or discussion. Thus, it should not be difficult for a nurse to understand why a patient may be nervous, anxious, embarrassed and perhaps uncooperative, demanding or irritable.

The nursing approach to all patients requires a double focus. With one inner eye the nurse must see the disease and understand the nature of its cause, transmission, course and resolution. Accompanying this must be a knowledge of the nursing care as well as some understanding of the medical treatment and prevention for the disease. With the other inner eye the nurse must focus on the patient. It is the ability to apply this double focus which seems to allow the nurse to remain sensitive to the patient as an individual — to see, always, a person with a disease, a person sick, a person in the hospital.

As each human being is a unique individual, so shall each person's response to a life situation be a unique one. Illness is another life experience to which a person responds. This response is governed by many factors. The person's age, past experiences, cultural group and social class are but a few. Some reactions are personality characteristics, either inborn or learned. Others are responses to transient stresses and pressures on the patient which appear prominent at that time and place. These stresses may be so important to the patient that they appear to dominate his thoughts, preventing him from concentrating on other situations. The patient's response to illness and hospitalization, and the resulting effect of this response on the course of the disease and the effectiveness of medical treatment, has long been hotly debated and ill defined. Research does indicate that very anxious preoperative patients do not tolerate surgical procedures and anesthesia as well as calm, confident patients. Unfortunately, too little study has been done to show the relationship between the response to illness or medical therapeutics and the course of the patient's illness.

The nurse is frequently left with a frightened, lonely patient who, too often, is confounded by the strange processes which, unasked for, have gripped his or her body, and by the hospital and its therapeutics which hope to restore the patient to health. A nurse who approaches the patient warmly and with a general air of confidence usually communicates these feelings to the patient. With the patient who talks freely and verbalizes well, she usually has an easier time and can offer her explanations and interpretations of the illness and treatments in response to the patient's particular need and at a time which appears appropriate. With other patients who are more reserved, verbalize less easily or are more timid, she may have to work harder. Here a nonverbal approach such as touching the hand, providing physical care and answering the call bell readily and willingly will communicate much to the patient. As a result, the patient becomes more relaxed and secure in the environment. Anticipating the need for explanations and interpretations may have to be done, for the patient may not realize that an explanation would help to ease his tensions and feelings of insecurity or helplessness. Generally, relatives need as much consideration and nursing as the patient. Since the lives of family members are so intimately interwoven, a crisis for one is a crisis for all.

By reassuring the relatives, you may be reassuring the patient, as often the anxiety and tension of one family member are easily communicated to the others. Allowing the family to work together to cope with a situation with some assistance from the medical team may also be a wise adjunct to therapy. Many families have faced other crises together and have developed methods of handling crises which were compatible with their way of life.

As in all things, knowledge will help the patient. Such knowledge should ideally begin at an early age. The nurse has a role to play in the teaching of the normal anatomy and physiology of reproduction to all age groups in whatever professional capacity she occupies at the time — that is, public health nurse, occupational health nurse, etc. In addition, she must deliberately provide opportunities for patients in the hospital to ask her questions and to help provide solutions and interpretations. This will require skill in interviewing in order to determine what the patient really wants to know and skill in phrasing answers, since the nurse must communicate with the patient. The nurse must also cope with her own feelings and culturally determined responses. Her sense of modesty may be offended. She may have difficulty accepting attitudes which differ radically from her own. This conflict may be particularly acute when she is nursing patients who have obtained abortions or contracted venereal disease or pelvic inflammatory disease. A nonjudgmental acceptance of the patient is required of the nurse. However, the nurse may find this difficult until she has reconciled her own feelings with the requirements of a professional in the situation.

CONGENITAL ANOMALIES OF THE REPRODUCTIVE SYSTEM

Hereditary Disorders in the Male

Maldescent of Testes

Approximately 4 per cent of newborn males will exhibit some form of maldescent of the testes. Unilateral maldescent of testis is about four times as prevalent as bilateral maldescent. The cause of this condition is not known but may be related to defects in the surrounding structures of the fetal testes, defects in the testes themselves or hormonal deficiencies. The majority of testes descend during the first 3 months of extrauterine life. Many more descend at puberty under the influence of rising testosterone levels. Probably less than 1 per cent of men remain with undescended testes following puberty. The principal sign is an inability to palpate one or both testes in the scrotal sac.

It is important to distinguish between three possible types of maldescent. Retractile testes are those which, under the influence of a strong muscular reflex, are drawn up to the external inguinal ring. This gives a false impression on palpation that the testes are not in the scrotum. No treatment is required. Ectopic testes are those which have descended to an abnormal site. Commonly this is the superficial inguinal pouch but may be almost anywhere near the normal path of descent. Cryptorchidism is a condition in which the descent of the testis is interrupted anywhere along the normal path of descent.

Because histologic changes can be observed in undescended testes as early as 6 years of age, treatment is usually initiated earlier than puberty to insure maximum functioning of the testes. Orchiopexy (surgical placement and fixation of the testes in the scrotal sac) is the primary method of treatment and should be completed by the age of 1 year. Hernioplasty may also be done to repair the inguinal hernia which is often present in these cases. The patient will be on complete bed rest or bed rest with restricted activity for several days. Thereafter, excessive physical activity should be avoided for about 6 weeks. Hormone therapy in the form of chorionic gonadotropins or methyltestosterone may be given in rare cases of bilateral undescended testes where a hormone deficiency exists. Successful descent usually indicates that these testes would probably have descended spontaneously at puberty. Hormone therapy is less successful with unilateral conditions.

Should the condition not be diagnosed until after puberty, most authorities agree that orchiopexy is indicated even though the man may be sterile. First, the Leydig cells of the testes continue to produce male hormones which will sustain the secondary sex characteristics. Secondly, such testes have a higher incidence of malignancy than do normally positioned testes and can be more easily examined yearly for malignancy in the scrotum than in the abdomen. In unilateral conditions, the extrascrotal testis will be removed to reduce the possibility of malignancy further. This leaves the man with one functioning testis as a source of sperm and male hormones.

Absence or Duplication of Organs

Congenital absence of the penis, scrotum and vas deferens is very rare. However, in certain genetically determined syndromes, the testicular tissue may be absent or nonfunctioning. One such example is Klinefelter's syndrome. The person with this syndrome has an XXY genotype; this produces atrophic testes and sterility. The person may also have eunuchoid development, and mental retardation may or may not be present. Androgens are administered to prevent feminization. Other examples are hermaphrodites, or persons who have some characteristics of both sexes. This could be genetically determined as true hermaphroditism or could be due to a feminizing lesion, producing pseudohermaphroditism.

Hypospadias

Hypospadias arises from a failure of the folds to fuse (Fig. 20–2). Chordee, a curvature of the penis, usually accompanies hypospadias and epispadias. Since the sex of the child may be doubtful, chromosome studies will be carried out and treatment based on the results of these findings. In mild cases of hypospadias, no treatment is necessary, as function is usually not impaired. In more severe cases, surgical repair will be necessary. This repair will straighten the penile shaft so that normal intercourse is possible. In addition a urethra will be formed which extends as near as possible to the tip of the glans so that semen is deposited deep in the vagina. Surgery is usually not immediately indicated and may be done in a series of operations beginning at about the age of 2 in a child in whom the condition has been detected early. In a few unfortunate cases the child is assumed to be female from birth, and these extreme cases may not be discovered until puberty and the development of secondary sex characteristics. For this reason, it is important that the nurse carefully examine the external genitalia of the newborn and report to its physician any baby which she feels does not appear normal.

Epispadias

Epispadias is much rarer than hypospadias and is often associated with exstrophy of the bladder (Fig. 20–2B). Because of the possible bladder involvement, the patient may be incontinent as a result of imperfect or absent urethral sphincters. Surgical repair provides the child with a functioning penis and urethra.

Preoperatively, a cystostomy may be done. The patient may also return from the operating room with a splinting catheter in the urethra until healing takes place. If the patient is discharged home with a cystostomy, the parents will need instruction in the care of the child.

Hereditary Disorders in the Female

Absence or Duplication of Organs

The uterus, cervix and vagina can undergo duplication or incomplete fusion (Fig. 20–1). The exact incidence of such anomalies is unknown, since they are largely asymptomatic. Some may cause sterility in women or an increased risk of abortion. Rarely an organ is completely absent. Also, as in the male, some absence (agenesis) or maldevelopment of tissue (dysgenesis) is genetically determined. Ovarian agenesis may be the result of an XO genotype (Turner's syndrome). The patient with this genotype may present a characteristic appearance from birth with a webbed neck, multiple anomalies, small birth weight or irregularities of the hairline. However, in others, the patient may present in adolescence because of the failure of the menarche to appear. Treatment is usually estrogen replacement therapy, with 1 mg. being given every day for 3 weeks followed by withdrawal. Withdrawal of estrogen permits the endometrium to slough away, thus simulating a menstrual period. Because the ovaries do not exist, the patient remains sterile.

Imperforate Hymen

Normally the hymen is patent. Rarely, it may not be. Usually the condition is not discovered until adolescence when the girl may present herself because of absence of menstrual flow. Menstruation occurs but the menstrual blood is retained behind the closed hymen. The patient may complain of crampy, lower abdominal pain occurring monthly. She may also notice dysuria, frequency, and urinary retention as the growing mass of retained menstrual blood accumulates in the vagina, putting increasing pressure on the bladder and urethra. Treatment consists of a cross-shaped incision of the hymen which allows drainage of the debris. This debris is often a thick, chocolate-like material. Because of this old blood, the risk of postoperative infection is greatly increased. Antibiotics are usually ordered. The nurse must pay careful attention to good aseptic technique postoperatively to reduce the risk of infection further. She must see that adequate drainage is maintained, frequent cleansing of the perineum occurs, and perineal dressings are changed frequently.

The hymen may also be rigid. This is usually discovered when the patient presents with a complaint of dyspareunia. In mild cases the patient will be instructed to dilate the hymen digitally, usually while sitting in a tub of warm water. If this does not succeed, vaginal dilators may be inserted by the physician or nurse and later by the patient. In difficult cases, hymenotomy is performed. This is one rationale for a premarital examination. The discovery of a rigid hymen and its treatment premaritally may be of great importance to a newly married couple.

FERTILITY AND INFERTILITY

Control of Fertility

Perhaps one of the greatest problems facing the world today is the control of fertility. One is constantly bombarded with news of the population explosion and its disastrous implications for the future of the world. These implications have usually been stated in terms of the developing nations, but more recently they have taken on a global context. In addition, there is a feeling that contraception be considered a matter of personal decision — that it can exercise an important liberalizing potential for the family or the single person. In the light of these discussions it would seem that the health professional has a responsibility to extend the knowledge and availability of contraception to anyone who requests it. With more family practice units and conception control clinics in the outpatient department or the public health department, the nurse has an expanding role in the control of fertility.

Nursing Responsibilities

Generally, the nursing responsibilities include referral of the patient to the appropriate clinic or physician and education and interpretation. Depending on the nurse's situation and knowledge, these may be taken care of in an initial interview (or group discussion) with a patient (or a group of patients) seeking birth control advice. The nurse can assist the patient or couple in making a decision by presenting concise, factual information about the methods available. The couple should choose a method which will be most compatible with their personal circumstances. Most certainly this should be the one they will use and feel comfortable in using. No method of birth control is effective unless it is used constantly. This final decision is usually made with medical counsel. As the physician reviews the patient's history, he may make other recommendations which will affect the person's or couple's choice. The patient or couple will need counsel in the proper use of the method they have chosen and what to expect in the period of initial adjustment. The nurse should validate the patient's real understanding of the method chosen and provide explanations and interpretations if necessary. In a simple fashion the knowledge of an alternate emergency method should be provided as well, for it is this which may prevent a pregnancy. Emergencies do occur. The patient forgets to take her pills with her on vacation, or she discovers the intrauterine device is missing at 1:30 A.M., and is too embarrassed to call the physician at that hour. Be sure the patient leaves the clinic or office with knowledge of an alternate method. Usually, the use of spermicidal foam or the use of a condom by the husband will overcome these situations. The nurse is responsible for gaining sufficient knowledge of the complex subject of contraception to be able to present factual knowledge to couples and to discuss the pros and cons of each method. In addition, the nurse will need to understand much of the emotional, social and religious aspects of contraception. A detailed presentation of family planning is beyond the scope of this work, but a brief outline of methods follows.

Methods of Contraception

COITUS INTERRUPTUS. This method consists of the male withdrawing his penis from the vagina before ejaculation occurs and ejaculating outside the vagina. Coitus interruptus, or withdrawal, is better than no attempt at birth control but is still very unreliable. Care must be taken not to ejaculate on or near the vulva, as the sperm may make their way into the vagina and pregnancy can result. The method requires the man to have advance awareness of ejaculation. This control and knowledge may be difficult to establish and may require more sexual experience than the man or couple possesses. Also, some sperm may escape before ejaculation occurs. The method has also come under considerable criticism for its psychological effects. These have been associated principally with frustration as a result of unresolved sexual tensions on the part of one or both partners. However, if the method is accepted by the couple and orgasm and ejaculation do occur, the resulting psychological stresses are probably minimal.

CONDOM. The condom is a thin rubber sheath which is placed over the penis before intromission. It prevents pregnancy by acting as a mechanical barrier to the sperm. Proper use includes application before intromission to avoid the possibility of a pre-ejaculatory emission of semen into the vagina and careful withdrawal of the penis and condom following intercourse to be sure that some semen is not lost into the vagina or over the vulva. Some physicians advise the use of a spermicidal jelly as a lubricating agent over the condom. This is a method of additional safety, particularly if the condom should be defective. However, newer methods of manufacture have greatly reduced this hazard. The condom is reasonably priced and is available without prescription. This greatly increases its availability and hence makes it one of the most widely used methods in the world.

Some couples find it objectionable as a method of birth control because it may interrupt sexual foreplay, it can lessen sensation, and its effective use relies heavily on the motivation of the male. These objections can be overcome if it is used by a highly motivated man who is taking mature responsibility for his behavior. Fortunately, many such men exist and the condom is classified as a highly effective form of birth control.

DIAPHRAGM. The diaphragm is a thin rubber cup which is inserted into the vagina by the woman and placed over the cervical os. The cap provides a mechanical barrier to the sperm. In addition a spermicidal jelly is placed in the dome of the cap. When the diaphragm is in place the spermicidal jelly will be in touch with the cervix.

The diaphragm is not dispensed without a prescription and requires individual fittings by a physician initially, after a few months of use and following pregnancy or miscarriage. The woman also requires careful teaching in the proper insertion and care of the diaphragm. The diaphragm is inserted manually or with an inserter which is provided. The position of the diaphragm should be checked following each insertion. The woman stands with one foot elevated or squats. The diaphragm is squeezed between two fingers, thus narrowing it, and the drop of jelly is kept facing up as the woman slips the diaphragm into her vagina. In its proper position, the diaphragm cups the cervix with its anterior side behind the pubic bone and its posterior side in the posterior fornix of the vagina. Following insertion the woman must be taught to check the position of the diaphragm to see that it is properly situated. Properly positioned, it is not felt by either partner. It can be left in place for 24 hours but should then be removed and cleansed with soap and water. Removal should not take place until at least 6 hours postcoitus to insure death of all sperm present in the vagina.

Used by intelligent, well instructed, highly motivated women it is a highly effective method of birth control. However, some women find it distasteful to insert the diaphragm and to check its position. For these women it is probably a very poor method of birth control.

SPERMICIDAL PREPARATIONS. In more recent years chemicals with a spermicidal action have been placed in gels, creams, aerosol foams, suppositories and foam tablets. These are inserted into the vagina about ½ hour before intercourse. The foam or jelly coats the cervix and inner vaginal walls. It should remain in the vagina for at least 6 hours to be sure that all sperm are dead. Used consistently, the method is very effective. Objections to the method revolve around the messiness which can result after coitus and a distaste in some people for the idea of killing a living sperm. Some men may complain of a slight urethral irritation when some foaming types of preparations are used.

DOUCHE. The vaginal douche or irrigation may be used for cleanliness following coitus or may be considered to be a method of birth control by those who are under the impression that it "washes the sperm away." In fact, it may force the sperm into the uterine cavity and merely speed them on their way. It is not a reliable method of contraception.

BREAST-FEEDING. Under the stimulus of breast-feeding many women remain anovulatory for several months. Others quickly regain their fertility. Hence, breast-feeding should not be considered a method of birth control.

THE RHYTHM METHOD. This method requires temporary abstinence from coitus during the possible ovulation time of the woman. It is the only method of birth control officially sanctioned by all religions. The rationale for the method is based on several assumptions. First, a woman is only fertile at the time of ovulation, which occurs once monthly at a predictable time, and the ovum lives for approximately 24 hours. Secondly, sperm will survive in the genital tract for only 3 days. Placing these facts together, and allowing 3 days before and after ovulation for the life span of the sperm, we arrive at 6 days. Since we know that the time of ovulation varies in any one woman we must allow 1 or 2 days for extra safety on either side. This now gives us a fertile period of approximately 8 days' duration, falling near the middle of the menstrual cycle.

The crux of the problem is the timing of ovulation. Since no anticipatory method of timing ovulation has been discovered, we must rely on a retrospective view of the time of ovulation in any one woman. Under the influence of the rising progesterone levels following ovulation, the basal body temperature in women shows a rise. This rise should be noticeable within the first 24 hours following ovulation. The temperature remains slightly elevated for the remainder of the cycle (Fig. 20–9). Also, at the time of ovulation, the cervical mucus changes. There is an increase in amount and a reduction in viscosity. Women can be taught to recognize and record these changes. Most physicians will attempt to predict the time of ovulation for any one woman after she has carefully recorded the dates of her menstrual periods, the mucus changes, and her temperatures taken

daily at a uniform time. Depending on the woman, physician or clinic, this may be done for 3 to 6 months. An average is then calculated from these dates and her individual period of likely fertility is plotted. In the graph (Fig. 20–9) the fertile period can be seen for a regular 28-day cycle. The calculated fertile period should be reviewed at specified intervals. At periods of her life when ovulation is being established or reestablished — that is during postpartum and lactation or menopause — the method is highly unreliable. In women of very regular periods and with high motivation the method has had success. However, until a foolproof method of anticipating ovulation is achieved, this method will have to be regarded merely as reliable even in highly motivated couples. One major objection by some couples is that the period of abstinence is long and occurs at a time when the libido in the woman may be very high.

THE INTRAUTERINE DEVICE. An intrauterine device is an object placed inside the uterus which remains in the uterus and prevents pregnancy. The action is not completely understood. Some physicians believe that the intrauterine device (IUD) creates a hostile intrauterine environment either for sperm or for the fertilized ovum. The addition of copper to the IUD is thought to intensify those changes, thus producing a more effective IUD. Others feel that it is implantation which is prevented.

Most intrauterine devices used today are made of a flexible plastic and are in several shapes. The device must be inserted by a physician, or other suitably trained personnel. It is a sterile procedure.

First, the physician will sound the uterus, confirming its depth and position. Then, having threaded the IUD into the inserter, he will insert this through the cervix, push down the plunger and retract the inserter. The use of the uterine sound and the skill of the inserter greatly reduce the risk of perforating the uterus. However, uterine perforation remains a rare complication of the IUD. Removal of the device is by a small hook. Many devices are equipped with strings which hang into the vagina just below the cervix. The device can usually be removed by gentle traction on the strings. The woman is also taught to check for the presence of these strings weekly; during her menstrual period she checks them daily. If she checks her pad or tampon, she usually satisfies this safety precaution. IUD's can be

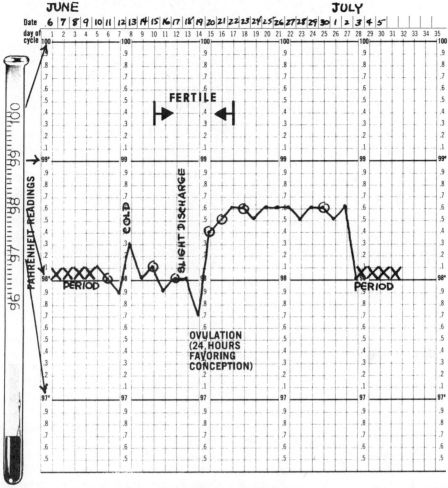

FIGURE 20–9 Basal body temperature chart showing fertile period. (Modified from Bleier, I.: Maternity Nursing, 3rd ed. Philadelphia, W. B. Saunders Co., 1971, p. 188.)

expelled from the uterus, and this is most likely to occur during the menstrual period. Women who have never been pregnant have an increased tendency to expel the device, as do women who have previously expelled it. Also, because of the tightness of the cervical os in the nullipara, insertion and removal of the IUD may be more difficult. If the woman notices that the IUD appears to have been expelled, she should report this to the physician so that he may confirm this. In some women the IUD causes cramping and spotting. Also, the first menstrual periods following insertion may be considerably heavier. The patient should report these to her physician. In earlier years infection associated with IUD's discouraged their use. This has not proven to be a problem in recent years.

Pregnancies do occur in about 2 to 3 per cent of women using an intrauterine device. The device is left in place and is removed following the birth of the placenta. No damage to the fetus has been reported.

However, the IUD does rank as a very effective method of birth control in about 80 per cent of the women who try it. The 20 per cent failure rate arises from pregnancies, expulsions and removals because of cramping or bleeding.

ORAL CONTRACEPTIVES. Birth control pills are synthetic chemical hormones which resemble the female hormones of the ovary. In suppressing ovulation they mimic the action of pregnancy. The high hormone levels depress the hypothalamus, which in turn inhibits the release of pituitary gonadotropins which stimulate ovulation. Thus, the woman is anovulatory. Protection is established as soon as the woman begins taking the pills.

The pills are divided into two types, the combined form and sequential form. The combined pill contains synthetic estrogen and progesterone hormones in each pill. This pill is more effective in preventing pregnancy apparently because it induces changes in the cervix, making the mucus thicker and more impenetrable by sperm. Also, changes occur in the endometrium which would discourage implantation should fertilization occur.

The sequential pills are given in sequence. The first 14 pills contain estrogen only, and the last 7 pills contain a combination of estrogen and progesterone. The sequential pills appear to be slightly less effective than the combined ones. Pregnancies have occurred with women following the sequential regimen. However, the risk of pregnancy in both types is minimal if used as prescribed. If taken correctly, the pills are the most effective method of contraception today.

Both types of pills are dispensed in the same way. The oldest method is a pill a day for 21 days (sometimes 20) and no pill for the next 7 days, regardless of the woman's period. Confusion frequently arises over when to start the pill. Initially, the first pill is taken on the last day of the woman's menstrual period unless she has an unusually long one. Then the fifth day of the menstrual cycle is used as a beginning day for the pill. Now the pill will regulate her menstrual cycle and she takes them as prescribed. It is wise for her to cross them off on a calendar or devise a method of knowing when to start again because each succeeding 21-day series of pills is begun on the basis of when she took the last pill, not on her subsequent menstrual period. She begins again regardless of the state of her menstrual period.

To make this regimen easier another regimen is the "pill-a-day" packet. This contains 28 pills. The final 7 pills are placebos and simply correspond to the 7 pill-free days of the other method. This does make it easier for women to follow, for no timing, counting or remembering other than to take the pill is required. Also, to maintain consistently high hormonal levels in the body, the pill should be taken at approximately the same time each day.

Withdrawal bleeding is regulated by the pill and occurs regularly at some time during the 7 pill-free days. This withdrawal bleeding stimulates true menstruation. With the withdrawal of the high hormone levels, the endometrium sloughs away. However, menstruation is usually scantier and shorter, since the endometrium is thinner and scantier. A woman may miss one period but, should she miss two, this should be reported to the physician immediately.

Much discussion has occurred over the possible side effects or complications attendant on the use of oral contraceptives. For many women, adjustment to oral contraceptives may take some months. During that time she may experience nausea, fullness and tingling in her breasts, headache, some spotting between menstrual periods, weight gain, chloasma or masking of pregnancy, acne, loss of libido or changes in vaginal discharge. On the other hand she may feel better, have relief from menstrual cramps and have an increased libido. Sometimes changes in dosages or in the timing of taking the pill helps. If she takes the pill with supper or lunch, she may feel less nauseated later.

The missed pill is cause for concern in many women. The woman should take the pill when she remembers it and take the next pill as she is accustomed to do. This may mean taking two pills in one day. On the sequentials, the omission is more serious. The couple should plan to use an additional method of birth control for the remainder of that cycle. Should more than one pill be missed in either the combined or sequential pills, then the couple should use an alternate form of birth control for the remainder of that cycle. If several pills are missed, the physician should be consulted, as the cycles may be sufficiently interrupted as to require some further regulating under medical supervision.

The major complications of the pill are rare but not inconsiderable. For some women the hazards of the pill are still less than the hazards of a pregnancy or an abortion. Major concern revolves around the increased incidence of diseases of the circulatory system in women using the pill. Research in Britain indicates that a woman classified as an ever-user of oral contraceptives has a five (4.7) fold increase in her chances of death from circulatory disease over a woman who has never used the pill. The major circulatory diseases include thromboembolic disease, coronary artery disease, cerebrovascular accidents and hypertension. The risks rise with age, cigarette smoking, and duration (over five years) of pill use.

Mortality rates for continuous users of the pill for over five years were ten times in excess of those for non-users. Age and smoking considerably modify the risks. For example, mortality rates were 1 per 10,000 in non-smoking users of the pill versus 3.3 per 10,000 in smoking users of the pill. Thus the smoking woman who has been using oral contraceptives for five years or more and is over 35 is placing herself at considerable risk if she continues use of the pill. Such women should be counseled to give up smoking and if unable to do so, to consider another method of birth control.

These studies have brought prolonged use of oral contraceptives into question. However, medical opinion still supports widespread use of the pill for carefully chosen women. The role of the family planning counselor is of great importance. Simply handing out a pill does not meet the requirements. The factors of past health, age, and smoking history are important, as is the duration of use. Safe birth control, compatible with the woman's life style, will demand the use of several different methods of birth control throughout her life. The pill is best during periods of high risk for pregnancy and a strong desire to avoid pregnancy; the I.U.D., diaphragm, or condom for periods of higher risk but less desire to avoid pregnancy or to space children; finally, sterilization for those who wish no more worries in this direction. Oral contraceptives continue to be contraindicated for patients with conditions aggravated by higher levels of estrogens.

STERILIZATION. Sterilization means the termination of reproductive capacity and is the most extreme case of fertility control. However, it may be chosen as a method of birth control. In other cases, when the hazards of pregnancy are life-threatening, it may be strongly indicated. In others, it is a sad sequel to necessary treatment to save or prolong the life of the patient.

Removal of any or all of the major organs of reproduction in either male or female results in sterility. Generally that is considered too extreme. A simple method of mechanically barring sperm and egg from meeting is required which will neither reduce natural hormone levels nor affect sexual capacity.

VASECTOMY. In men vasectomy will accomplish this purpose. This simple operation can be done in the physician's office. On the surface of the scrotum the ascending spermatic cord is palpated and identified. Under local anesthetic a small incision is made slightly to one side of each cord. The vas deferens is dissected and ligated in two places. It may or may not be severed after ligation. Thus, new sperm are barred from reaching the vagina. Other sperm are still present in the tract above the ligation. For this reason a man is not considered sterile until he has had two negative sperm counts postoperatively. There have been no significant reports of side effects, either physical or emotional, following this procedure. The majority of men tolerate it very well; sexual function, libido and self-concept remain unaltered. Some cases are recorded of reconstructing the vas deferens. However, the rate of successful reconstruction is low. Thus, the patient should regard a vasectomy as irreversible. A vasectomy may also be done abdominally.

TUBAL LIGATION. Tubal ligation is the comparable operation in women. It can be done vaginally but is usually done abdominally. Under a general anesthetic two small incisions are made in the abdomen. The uterine tube is dissected, a loop of tube is lifted up, ligated, and above the ligation is either crushed with a clamp or severed. In some operations the uterine end of the tube may be turned back and embedded in the posterior wall of the uterus. Various names for these techniques include Madlener, Pomeroy and Irving, respectively. Tubal coagulations, in conjunction with a laparoscopy, may also be done. The physician identifies the tubes through the laparoscope and then applies the heat source which coagulates the tube. In the hands of a skilled operator the procedure is safe and associated with few side effects. In an attempt to make sterilization temporary some physicians use clips on the tubes. These can be released at a later date should the patient desire another pregnancy. Experience with this method is limited, but the clips should not damage the tubes so that later function will be impaired, yet they should occlude them sufficiently to be effective. As in the male the tubes can be reconstructed, but the incidence is not high. Thus, the patient should see the operation as irreversible. The operation is not entirely harmless. Rare major complications postoperatively can be pulmonary embolism and later tubal pregnancy. These make the operation a more hazardous procedure than a vasectomy.

Nursing responsibilities in both operations include regular pre- and postoperative care. However, in addition to the consent for operation, there is a separate consent for sterilization which must be signed before the operation.

Infertility

Infertility is defined as the failure to conceive after 12 months of adequate exposure without the use of contraceptives. Primary infertility refers to a couple who has never conceived. Secondary infertility refers to a couple who has had a previous pregnancy but now cannot conceive. Approximately 12 per cent of couples prove infertile. Of this 12 per cent about 40 per cent of the problem rests with the man, 40 per cent with the woman and from 5 to 10 per cent with the couple as a unit.

Causes of Infertility

The possible causes of infertility are too numerous to list. However, the major causes can be grouped under several headings. Any impairment of ovarian function which interrupts ovulation creates infertility. This may be caused by hormonal imbalances or may be due to some intrinsic defect in the ovaries themselves. The same is true of the testes. The conducting system may not be patent. Infections leading to adhesions are a major cause in both men and women. Malformations or displacements of the organs of the reproductive tract may contribute to infertility. The problem may arise because of unique factors particular to the union. Vaginal secretions may not be compatible with the seminal fluid, causing the sperm to die.

Nursing Responsibilities

The patient will usually go through a series of investigative tests. During these tests the nurse's supportive presence is of great value. The nurse should understand the technique and procedure well enough to prepare the patient for the test or to teach the patient how to perform some tests. Some women may feel more at ease discussing such problems with the nurse. Use should be made of this opportunity to listen to and reassure the patient. This may happen when the nurse is told several facts which the patient "forgot" to tell the physician. Also, the nurse may be asked questions which the patient hesitated to ask the physician. Any pertinent information should be relayed to the appropriate medical advisor as well as those questions the nurse did not feel capable of answering.

Diagnosis and Assessment

The investigation usually begins when the woman presents herself to the gynecologist with a complaint of failure to conceive. By this time the problem may have become a nagging fear for both her and her husband. Often reassurance and ventilation of the anxiety seem to help the patient, for many patients are reported as returning shortly thereafter as pregnant. A persistent infertility case will require thorough investigation. Many gynecologists prefer to see the couple together so that both partners may receive an outline and discussion of the approach which will be used. The physician's assessment of the possible cause of the infertility will guide the direction of the investigation. Some techniques which are used in investigating infertility are described.

MEDICAL HISTORY AND PHYSICAL EXAMINATION. A detailed medical history and physical examination are done for both partners. Particular attention will be paid to the development of the secondary sex characteristics and any evidence of virilizing or feminizing effects. Any history of infections and injuries involving the genitourinary tract will be carefully noted. In addition the physician will take a marital history to gain an adequate picture of the couple's sexual pattern. The woman will be asked to give a detailed menstrual history. At this point some education in human reproduction may help the couple.

Before other tests are begun, infections, particularly cervicitis and prostatitis, are likely to be treated, as they may contribute to infertility. Anemia, poor health, exhaustion, overwork, stress and other psychosocial situations all may be causative factors, and the physician often tries to relieve these first if they seem of sufficient magnitude to be affecting the sexual adjustment of the couple.

OVULATION. Whether or not ovulation

occurs monthly may have to be established. The patient is asked to keep a basal body temperature chart. This also helps the physician to estimate hormonal levels. The woman is asked to come to the office or clinic near ovulation time. Cervical smears will be taken and tested for spinnbarkeit and ferning. Respectively, these tests help to time ovulation and indicate how receptive the cervical mucus is to sperm. If ferning appears to be unsatisfactory, the patient may be given small oral doses of stilbestrol daily for several cycles. The patient may be requested to return for serial vaginal smears, which give indications of ovulation.

URINALYSIS. Urine tests may be done to determine whether adequate levels of pituitary gonadotropins are present and, if the physician feels it is warranted, the presence and amount of 17-ketosteroids are established. This may be done for both partners.

ENDOMETRIAL BIOPSY. This is done to indicate whether or not a healthy endometrium is present. If it is not, then the problem may be one of failure of the fertilized ovum to achieve successful implantation. Occasionally tuberculosis, hitherto unsuspected, is discovered, and may be the cause of the infertility.

PATENCY OF THE TUBES. The Rubin test is performed by insufflating the uterine tubes with carbon dioxide under pressure. Auscultating the sounds of gas bubbling through the tubes, complaints of referred shoulder pain by the patient or x-ray evidence of air beneath the diaphragm give evidence of at least one patent tube. The shoulder pain is the result of the gas escaping from the ends of the patent tube, collecting beneath the diaphragm, and exerting pressure on the phrenic nerve which is felt as referred pain to the shoulder. This test is being replaced by the hysterosalpingogram.

HYSTEROSALPINGOGRAM. A hysterosalpingogram is the injection of a radiopaque dye into the genital tract. It serves to outline the uterine cavity and uterine tubes. The patient may not be anesthesized. The test is done in the x-ray department under sterile technique. The patient is usually asked to move from side to side after the injection in order to promote spilling of the dye into the abdominal cavity. This test provides information about the exact location of any abnormality.

POSSIBLE COMPLICATIONS OF TUBAL PA-TENCY TESTS. Pain, collapse and vomiting may be experienced shortly after the test is done, especially in women who were not anesthetized. The patient should be observed for these signs for approximately 3 hours following a test. Helping the patient to assume a knee-chest position for a few minutes before standing up may prevent further discomfort. Cramps and vomiting may be more prevalent following cervical dilatation.

Other complications may include exacerbation of pelvic infections, air embolism or sensitivity reactions to the dye and inadvertent abortion.

On the other hand, either of the tests may be therapeutic because they may have opened the tract. This is supported by many patients who conceive with no further treatment.

SIMS-HUHNER POSTCOITAL TEST. Postcoitally, a specimen of seminal fluid from the posterior fornix of the vagina and the cervical canal is aspirated. The specimen is examined for motility of the sperm and their ability to survive in the cervix or vagina. This test is best performed at the time of ovulation. The patient will be instructed not to douche or use lubricants for 2 days before the test. Following intercourse she will remain supine, hips elevated on a pillow for 30 minutes. Within the next 2 to 4 hours she will come to the physician's office or the fertility clinic, at which time the specimen will be taken. A reading will assess how many live, motile sperm are in the specimen. Should the sperm not be present, the investigation may be directed toward the male. Does he have sperm? If he does, why is he not capable of depositing them near the cervix? If they are dead or nonmotile, the vaginal environment may be hostile to them. One such reaction is due to the stimulus a foreign protein (sperm) evokes in the woman's body. Consequently, antibodies develop. The antibodies in the female inactivate the sperm before fertilization can take place. Following a 3- to 6-month period of abstinence or the use of a condom by the male, circulating antibodies may be sufficiently reduced to permit sperm to live in order to fertilize.

SEMEN ANALYSIS. A specimen of seminal fluid will be examined for volume and the number, morphology and mobility of sperm. Ideally, 2 to 5 ml. of fluid should be present. The fluid should gel and then reliquefy after 15 to 20 minutes. The sperm should number above 60 million per ml. of ejaculate, and 60 per cent should still show vigorous activity when examined at room temperature 2 hours after ejaculation. Not more than 20 per cent of the sperm should show abnormal forms.

The specimen is collected after a 3-day period of abstinence from coitus. It is collected in a dry, sterile jar by masturbation or coitus interruptus and is brought to the clinic for examination within 2 hours of collection.

If no sperm are present in the ejaculate, the patency of the duct system may be assessed. Testicular biopsy may be indicated. If the biopsy shows living sperm, then the failure of the sperm to arrive in the seminal fluid may be due to a blockage in the tube.

Treatment

SURGERY. In both male and female, surgery is aimed at restoring function. Adhesions may be released; the ducts are reconstructed. In certain cases polyethylene tubes are inserted into the uterine tubes to help maintain patency. Cysts and tumors are removed as indicated. The nursing care would be the same as that for any pelvic operative procedure.

ALPHA AMYLASE. Should the seminal fluid not reliquefy, a suspension of alpha amylase introduced into the vagina postcoitally has attained some success. The woman must be instructed to insert 1 ml. of the suspension into her vagina and to remain supine with hips elevated for 30 minutes following insertion. The solution should be kept refrigerated.

HORMONE THERAPY

CLOMIPHENE. Hormones may be administered to induce ovulation. Clomiphene (Clomid) is an antiestrogenic substance which stimulates the hypothalamus to stimulate the pituitary to increase the output of FSH and LH (ICSH). By displacing the circulating estrogens, the hypothalamus is released from the inhibiting effects of high levels of estrogen. In addition, clomiphene may increase ovarian sensitivity to FSH and LH.

Treatment consists of administering 50- to 100-mg. pills daily for 5 days. These tablets may be started on the fifth day of the cycle or at any time if no cycles are occurring. Ovulation is expected 7 to 12 days following treatment. The patient must be instructed to monitor her basal body temperature carefully, as a rise in temperature is expected with ovulation. Coitus should occur close to ovulation. Treatment may be repeated several times until pregnancy occurs or the treatment is judged ineffective. Good rates of success are recorded. Clomiphene is more successful when used in situations of altered function, such as amenorrhea following the oral contraceptives or anovulation in Stein-Leventhal syndrome.

The drug does stimulate the growth of benign ovarian cysts which usually disappear after its use. The incidence of multiple births is increased in couples using this medication. There do not appear to be any long-term effects.

GONADOTROPINS. The gonadotropins may be supplied artificially. Hypothalamic-releasing factors may be given to stimulate the pituitary. Human pituitary gonadotropins made from freeze-dried human pituitaries may be administered. These are, in effect, the FSH and LH hormones. The patient receives injections of FSH to ripen a follicle and then LH to stimulate ovulation. The process is complex, necessitating close monitoring of the patient for ovulation and for overstimulation of the ovaries. Ovarian cysts follow its use, as do multiple pregnancies. Like clomiphene, good pregnancy rates have been achieved. Because of abortions and high fetal wastage associated with prematurity and multiple births, the overall success rate in terms of live children is lower.

Hormone therapy may also be instituted in the man. Gonadotropins may be prescribed and have achieved some success in raising the sperm counts of men with low counts. Sometimes vitamin B will be prescribed to insure the normal inactivation of estrogens by the liver. Varying doses of testosterone may be tried with varying rates of success.

DISORDERS OF THE MENSTRUAL CYCLE AND MENSTRUATION

Mittelschmerz

Mittelschmerz is a feeling of lower abdominal pain on one side on or near ovulation day. It is thought to be caused by fluid or blood escaping from the ruptured follicle site and causing peritoneal irritation. It occurs in about 25 per cent of women. Occasionally, when the right side is involved, fear of appendicitis may bring the woman to the physician.

Premenstrual Tension

This syndrome is probably experienced by most women in mild forms. However, extreme cases are seen. The symptomatology includes a feeling of fullness or heaviness in the lower abdomen, backache, painful breasts, irritability, headache, weight gain premenstrually, nervousness, depression and insomnia.

The favored etiology relates the symptoms to an imbalance in the estrogen-progesterone ratio. The high levels of estrogen result in sodium retention, which is characterized by increased intercellular fluid and edema. This edema gives the bloated feeling, headaches, irritability and breast tenderness. Secondary to these hormonal imbalances, the patient may become hypoglycemic. This accounts for feelings of faintness and weakness. Other theories of the possible etiology are concerned with overproduction of the antidiuretic hormones and adrenocortical hyperactivity.

Treatment consists in taking a sympathetic and understanding approach, as the patient may be very upset by the changes of mood and behavior which she experiences. The patient will be instructed to restrict sodium intake in the latter half of the cycle. She may also be given oral diuretics for some days immediately before menstruation. In most cases the nurse is responsible for giving the patient whatever guidance in food selection and preparation that the patient requires to assist her to follow this regimen. While she is on diuretics, it is also wise to instruct the patient to take her pill with orange juice. This guards against possible excessive loss of potassium from the use of diuretics. In conjunction with this treatment, the physician may prescribe a mild tranquilizer to ease her nervousness.

Dysmenorrhea

Dysmenorrhea is defined as pain with menstruation. Two types, true and congestive dysmenorrhea, are commonly distinguished.

TRUE DYSMENORRHEA. True dysmenorrhea is a spasmodic type of pain, occurring at the onset of the menstrual period and lasting from 1 to 24 hours. It is most common among young girls, rarely beginning with the menarche and fading away spontaneously around 24 years of age or following the delivery of a full-term infant. No pathology in pelvic structures is associated with this type of dysmenorrhea. In addition to the cramps, there may be shivering, a feeling of tension, nausea, vomiting and pallor. Some girls faint easily at this time.

The etiology remains unclear. It appears to be connected to ovulation, as anovulatory cycles are rarely accompanied by dysmenorrhea. This probably explains why the first few cycles are pain-free and dysmenorrhea in some girls is synchronous with ovulation. Also, the daughters of women who suffer or have suffered from dysmenorrhea are more frequently dysmenorrheic. Whether this is learned or inherited is still disputed. In any case the psyche can play a role in aggravating the symptoms but is very rarely the sole explanation. A woman's personal tolerance for discomfort undoubtedly affects her response to any pain, dysmenorrhea being no exception.

Physiological explanations implicate an imbalance in neural-hormonal control of uterine muscle. Progesterone, following ovulation, causes increased tone in the isthmus and upper cervix. An overactive sympathetic nervous system causes hypertonus of the muscles of the isthmus and internal os. As the uterus contracts to empty the fundus of menstrual flow and clots, resistance is met in the lower half of the uterus. This sets up a pattern of incoordinate uterine action which is felt as a cramp by the patient.

Treatment consists of a kind and sympathetic approach by all members of the health team. Mild analgesics may be prescribed. Often, the physician may prescribe a course of oral contraceptives. This induces anovulatory periods and may be followed by very good results. It may also be diagnostic. Should dysmenorrhea continue, the physician may look for other causes. In more extreme cases, surgery may be chosen. The cervix is dilated with varying success. A presacral sympathectomy or, in desperation, a hysterectomy may be done.

NURSING RESPONSIBILITIES. The school

and occupational health nurses commonly deal with the girl or young woman suffering from dysmenorrhea. She may present herself in their office, or the nurse may be asked to interview the girl or woman who frequently misses school or work because of dysmenorrhea. Frequent, severe dysmenorrhea should always be investigated by the physician, and it is the nurse's responsibility to suggest this to the patient and assist her in obtaining this care.

In regard to general care, the patient may need instruction in the normal anatomy and physiology of menstruation. This serves to eradicate misconceptions and lessen the fear and anxiety which may be associated with her periods. She may need some instruction in menstrual hygiene so that her period does not seem distasteful and restricting. This may simply mean a switch from sanitary pads to tampons, frequent bathing or the use of a deodorizer. The patient may need to be encouraged to get more exercise and be sure that she is not constipated before her period.

Immediate care involves providing a sympathetic, understanding approach, a place to lie down, a warm blanket, if necessary, and usually a mild analgesic. When the symptoms are relieved, the girl often continues with her work. However, before returning to work or home, she might appreciate a cup of tea or coffee. If the patient has been given a prescription for medication, she should be instructed to take the tablet before dysmenorrhea becomes acute. This will prevent the symptoms and has the double advantage of breaking a cycle. The girl can feel some control over the events which are happening to her rather than being totally subject to them.

CONGESTIVE DYSMENORRHEA. Congestive dysmenorrhea is a constant type of pain which often starts 2 to 3 days before the period and persists well past the first day. It may continue for a day or two following the period. Pain may radiate through the abdomen into the back and down the thighs. It occurs after several years of normal painless menses and is frequently associated with pelvic pathology. The most frequent causes are tumors, inflammatory diseases, endometriosis and fixed malpositions of the uterus. It is essentially a symptom of disease. Should the nurse be consulted by a woman describing these symptoms, the woman should be referred to a physician immediately.

Amenorrhea

Amenorrhea, or absence of menstruation, may be primary or secondary. Secondary amenorrhea is that which occurs after several months or years of normal menses.

Menorrhagia

Menorrhagia is excessive bleeding at the time of normal menses.

Polymenorrhea

Polymenorrhea refers to cyclic bleeding which is normal in amount but occurs too frequently.

Epimenorrhagia

Epimenorrhagia is cyclic bleeding which is both excessive and too frequent.

Metrorrhagia

Metrorrhagia refers to any bleeding which occurs between menstrual periods. Any bleeding per vaginam at any time other than abnormal menses is included, even if it amounts only to slight staining.

Dysfunctional Uterine Bleeding

True dysfunctional uterine bleeding refers to that which occurs in the presence of endocrine dysfunction rather than organic disease. It can present a very real challenge to the physician, as the cause of the bleeding is often difficult to discern. It may be seen as chronic epimenorrhagia or as an episode of acute bleeding. Some episodes of hemorrhage are caused by unexplained high levels of estrogen in the proliferative phase of the cycle. These high levels depress the hypothalamus-pituitary complex and no ovulation occurs. Because there is no ovulation, no progesterone is produced and the endometrium remains proliferative and becomes cystic. As estrogen levels fall, usually after a 6- to 8-week period of amenorrhea, bleeding occurs.

Treatment consists of administering progesterone for some days to convert the endometrium to the secretory phase. The progesterone is then withdrawn and the patient sheds the endometrium and is placed on oral contraceptives so that progesterone is assured. The cycle usually stabilizes in 2 to 3 months. Mild cases may be placed on the pill initially. The condition occurs more commonly during puberty and menopause or in nulliparous women over 35. In most cases of bleeding investigation begins with dilatation and curettage, then proceeds to hormone therapy or further surgery such as a hysterectomy.

Endometriosis

Endometriosis is the location of endometrial-like tissue outside the uterine cavity. Although the location may be varied, the most frequent locations are in or near the ovaries, the uterosacral ligaments and the uterovesical peritoneum. Extrapelvic sites may be as varied as the umbilicus, an old laparotomy scar, vulva or even lungs. The tissue responds to the hormones of the ovarian cycle and undergoes a small menstruation just like the uterine endometrium. Statistics vary, but perhaps 5 per cent of all patients seen by the gynecologist suffer from endometriosis.

ETIOLOGY. Causes may be varied. Two major theories are prevalent. One concludes that small bits of endometrial tissue are forced or regurgitated back up the uterine tube and escape into the abdomen during menstruation. The other theory points out that the peritoneum and reproductive tract derive from the same early embryologic tissues. Some of the tissues may be misplanted from that early time. Under sufficient stimulation, these cells respond and differentiate into a functioning endometrial tag. Rare cases seem to be caused by small pieces of endometrium being transported to other parts of the body through the lymphatics or by the blood. This seems to be true of endometrial tissue in the limbs or in lung tissue. As the ectopic endometrium menstruates, the blood collects in little cyst-like nodules which have a characteristic bluish-black look. Usually they are pea-sized but may be much larger. Those in the ovary and uterosacral area often attain a size of 3 to 6 cm. These ovarian cysts are sometimes termed "chocolate cysts" because of the thick, chocolate-colored material which they contain. The cysts become surrounded by fibrous tissue which makes them easy to palpate, as they feel firm and well defined. Frequently the cyst perforates and spills its sticky contents into the abdomen. The resulting irritation promotes the formation of adhesions which readily fix the ovary or the affected area to the broad ligament or other pelvic structures.

The disease is seen most frequently in the white, nulliparous woman, aged 30 to 40. It occurs more commonly in the upper economic and social groups, presumably because of less frequent and later childbearing.

SIGNS AND SYMPTOMS. The patient may have no symptomatology, and the disease may only be discovered incidental to abdominal surgery. More commonly, the patient complains of pain. Congestive dysmenorrhea may appear with pain becoming severe 1 to 2 days before menstruation. The pain gradually becomes worse and may be described as "boring." This is due to the distention and pain of the swollen, shedding areas contained within the fibrous capsule of the cysts. The patient may also complain of backache, dyspareunia of a deep nature localized in the posterior fornix of the vagina or persistent lower abdominal pain occurring throughout the cycle. Pain may be of an acute nature, localized in the abdomen when a cyst ruptures. The physician may suspect endometriosis when a patient is infertile, since this is a common symptom of this group. Sometimes the adhesions become severe enough to cause a bowel obstruction or painful micturition.

Diagnosis is frequently confirmed on bimanual examination when firm nodular lumps are felt in the adnexa. Visualizing the typical bluish nodules may be done by culdoscopy, laparoscopy or during a laparotomy.

TREATMENT. This is based on the age of the patient, her desire for more children and the severity of the disease. Pregnancy relieves the symptoms and may be advised if the couple wants more children. Pseudopregnancy may be achieved by the administration of progesterone for varying periods of time.

Treatment may be surgical and is directed at preserving reproductive function. Affected areas are removed, and fixed organs released. Infertility often ceases following surgery. In severe cases a hysterectomy may be done.

Depending on the extent of the cystic involvement, oophorectomy may also be performed. The symptoms usually disappear at menopause as ovarian atrophy begins and hormonal stimulation declines.

Adenomyosis Uteri

This condition is similar to endometriosis in that it is characterized by ectopic endometrium within the muscular wall of the uterus or the uterine tube. While it is often classified as "intrauterine endometriosis," Novak suggests that the disease processes are quite different.[1] Adenomyoma is also a poor way of referring to the process, for it is not a true tumor. The cause is unknown.In any case, the uterine endometrium appears to grow downward between the muscle bundles of the myometrium. This produces a uniform, moderate enlargement of the uterus. The patient may complain of menorrhagia and congestive dysmenorrhea. Often pelvic endometriosis is also present. Then the uterus may be fixed (frozen) in the pelvis, and pelvic nodules may be palpated. The patient may complain of pain in the sacral or coccygeal area as well.

INTERRUPTIONS OF PREGNANCY

Abortion

An abortion is the termination of a pregnancy before the fetus is viable. Some confusion exists over when a fetus becomes viable. Arbitrarily, viability has been set as above 20 weeks of gestation, 500 Gm. of weight or a crown-rump length of 18 cm. The definition is not universal and varies from country to country. "Miscarriage" also refers to abortion but is the lay term for designating lack of criminal involvement.

The incidence of abortion is difficult to state accurately. Estimates place it at between 10 and 20 per cent of all conceptions. See Table 20–1 for classification of abortions.

CAUSES.   Most known causes can be separated into three major groups: fetal, maternal and faulty environment. Fetal causes are often associated with chromosomal or other abnormalities which are incompatible with life. This has been considered to be as high as 40 per cent of all causes of abortion. Maternal and faulty environment causes are more varied. Endotoxins, as a result of severe infections in the mother, may invade the fetus, usually causing its death and later expulsion. Drugs ingested by the mother may damage the fetus directly or may damage the placenta and hence the nutrition of the fetus. Hormonal imbalances may be the cause of some abortions, especially in cases in which the thyroid gland is involved. Lack of progesterone may result in a poorly developed endometrium. As a result, nidation does not occur or does so ineffectively. Anatomic uterine defects or uterine pathology causes some abortions. Nutritional factors are linked to abortion and premature labor, for adequate nutrition of the woman bears an important part in her reproductive capacity. The emotional state of the woman is also considered a possible contributing factor. This often centers on fear, grief or emotional trauma in susceptible women. Physical trauma can also induce an abortion. This may be true of surgery performed during pregnancy.

A threatened abortion is one in which the threat to the pregnancy is slight. With care, the woman may carry the pregnancy to term. Since any bleeding, however minor, per vaginam is abnormal in the pregnant woman, any evidence of such bleeding is taken as a sign of threatened abortion until proven otherwise. In addition, some backache or mild intermittent lower abdominal pain may be present. If the abortion is not to be immediate, cramping and bleeding may stop. Should the cramping and bleeding increase in spite of treatment, the abortion may now be called imminent. It becomes inevitable when bleeding continues, cramps become stronger and regular, the cervix dilates and the membranes rupture. The inevitable abortion becomes the complete abortion when all products of conception are expelled. This usually occurs before the twelfth week of gestation. The abortion is incomplete when some of the products of conception are retained. This is usually the placenta and membranes and is more frequent following the twelfth week, when the placenta is more firmly embedded.

[1]Edmund R. Novak and J. Donald Woodruff: Novak's Gynecologic and Obstetric Pathology: With Clinical and Endocrine Relations, 7th ed. Philadelphia, W. B. Saunders, 1974.

The umbilical cord breaks, leaving the placenta and membranes in utero. A missed abortion is one in which the fetus dies; symptoms of abortion cease and the products of conception are retained in the uterus for 2 or more months. Following this, the uterus is not observed to increase in size. Indeed, it begins to regress slightly as the amniotic fluid is absorbed. No fetal heart is heard. The patient remains amenorrheic, and the breasts regress. The abortus is usually expelled spontaneously but may be retained for many months or years. In such cases it becomes a shriveled sac with areas of dense calcification.

A woman is considered to be an habitual aborter when she aborts three or more consecutive pregnancies. The causes can be any of the causes of a single abortion but persist through several pregnancies. In addition, an incompetent cervix is frequently sited as a cause of habitual abortion. Possibly because of inherent problems in the cervix or trauma to the cervix during surgery, the cervix dilates easily and will not retain the pregnancy. Loss of the pregnancy usually occurs later at about 16 to 20 weeks. Dilation of the cervix is rapid, with little pain and bleeding. Rupture of the membranes occurs, followed by the expulsion of the fetus.

Treatment and nursing care

THREATENED ABORTION. The treatment of threatened abortion is aimed at preserving the pregnancy. Every pregnant patient should be told the danger signs of pregnancy. Often this instruction is the responsibility of the nurse in either the clinic or the office. Thus, the woman should recognize bleeding as abnormal and be aware that she should notify her physician immediately. She should then go to bed and rest unless otherwise instructed by her physician. Because of the association of malformed fetuses with spontaneous abortions, a conservative approach toward saving the pregnancy may be taken. If the bleeding is slight, the patient is managed at home and advised to get extra rest for a few days. For some patients this may be impossible, and admission to hospital is necessary. In other situations a more aggressive approach is taken toward conserving the pregnancy.

On admission to the hospital, the patient is placed on bed rest. Temperature, pulse and blood pressure are noted as frequently as the patient's condition warrants. All the pads, linens and clothing stained with blood are kept for inspection by the physician. This helps in the estimation of blood loss. The possibility of losing the pregnancy may be very distressing to most women. The patient should be given sympathy, reassurance and support. This assists in keeping the patient quiet and calm and allows her to get the physical and mental rest which is considered advisable. Sedatives may be ordered. In addition, the patient is observed for any increased bleeding or cramping which would indicate a change in status. A diet low in roughage is usually ordered with supplementary iron and vitamin C. Purgatives and enemas are not given in order to avoid stimulation of the uterus. Rectal and vaginal examinations are contraindicated. Bleeding usually ceases within 24 to 48 hours if the pregnancy is going to continue. At this time the physician will probably perform a careful speculum and bimanual examination, since other possible causes of bleeding must be ruled out. These causes could be carcinoma or other complications of pregnancy.

On discharge home the patient is instructed to get extra rest and to avoid strenuous exercise, heavy lifting, excitement or fatigue. Coitus may be restricted for a period of 2 weeks or longer. Should bleeding recur, the patient is advised to notify her physician and remain in bed.

MISSED ABORTION. The patient will be followed by her physician to see that the pregnancy progresses normally. If it does not and a persistent brownish discharge recurs, missed abortion may be suspected. The diagnosis may be difficult for the physician to make until it is quite clear that the uterus has ceased to enlarge and that the fetus is dead. A positive pregnancy test may only indicate that placental tissue still remains living. The physician is faced with the choice of interfering to evacuate the uterus or waiting until it is done spontaneously. Physically, there is usually no pressing need. Emotionally, however, it is very distressing to the woman and her family to know that she is carrying a dead fetus. The danger from afibrinogenemia as a complicating factor to intervention by the physician increases as the dead fetus is retained. Presumably this occurs as some of the degenerating products of the fetus enter the maternal blood stream. This danger appears to be most serious about 4 to 6 weeks after fetal death. Therefore, fibrinogen studies may be done before intervention is attempted.

For these reasons the physician usually intervenes approximately 2 weeks after death of the fetus. The dead fetus may be aborted by means of an intravenous oxytocic administered in high concentrations. The patient may be started on 20 I.U. of Pitocin in 1000 ml. of 5 per cent dextrose in water. Each hour the dose may be increased until effective contractions occur. The therapy will continue until abortion ensues or for 8 to 10 hours. Then the drip may be discontinued and resumed at the original beginning levels of Pitocin the next day. The procedure is emotionally and physically exhausting for the patient. She requires much supportive nursing care. Also, the contractions are painful, and some analgesic should be administered. Since no danger can result to the fetus, the mother need not suffer unduly. Close observation of the patient's condition for overhydration is necessary because of the danger of overhydrating her with large amounts of fluid containing Pitocin, which has an antidiuretic action. An intake and output record should be kept.

INEVITABLE ABORTION. The treatment of an inevitable abortion is similar to that of a threatened abortion. The patient is placed on bed rest. Blood will be taken for hemoglobin, typing and cross matching. The amount and character of the bleeding is observed carefully. Blood pressure and pulse may need to be taken every 10 minutes if bleeding is profuse, and the patient must be observed for other signs of shock. Any tissue or suspicious clots are saved to be examined for traces of fetus and placenta. Good perineal care is maintained by frequent cleansing of the vulva to reduce the risk of infection and to promote the patient's comfort. Procedures for perineal care will vary. Generally, soap and water are sufficient. The perineum is swabbed from the pubes to the perineal body (front to back) and from the vulva out to the thigh. The rectal area is washed last. This is to prevent the spread of bacteria from the rectum upward into the vagina and thence to the endometrium. A perineal shave may be ordered. Support and encouragement are provided by the nursing and medical staff, as the patient may be very distraught at the impending loss of her infant. If the abortion seems to be approaching a conclusion, it is not assisted. However, with the membranes ruptured, the cervix dilated and contractions tapering off, the process may be hastened by the administration of intravenous Pitocin.

If the abortion has been complete and the physician is satisfied of this, the woman is treated similarly to a postpartum patient. If the patient is Rh negative blood group, she receives RhoGAM (anti-D immunoglobulin) to prevent complications in further pregnancies. A slight lochial discharge is expected and the woman must be taught perineal care. She will be discharged home in 3 to 4 days, depending on the state of her health. To reduce the risk of infection, coitus is contraindicated until lochial discharge has ceased. This usually occurs within 2 weeks.

When the products of conception are retained, the uterus must be emptied. Two of the major causes of bleeding associated with pregnancy result from the partially separated placenta and retained fragments of conception. The uterus cannot contract effectively; the torn blood vessels remain open and bleed. Also, the risk of infection is much increased by the debris lying in the uterus. If the bleeding is acute, the patient is usually taken to the operating room and an emergency dilation and curettage (D and C) is done. Under a general anesthesia, the cervix is gently dilated until the passage of a curette is possible. Dilation is accomplished by using the dilators or by the use of a special vibrating dilator. The curette is used to scrape the tissue from the walls of the uterus.

Following this operation the patient receives perineal care and is observed for signs of hemorrhage and infection. She may receive an intravenous oxytocic solution to help involution of the uterus. Because of the danger of accidental perforation of the uterus with the instruments, the patient is observed postoperatively for signs of peritoneal irritation or abdominal (concealed) hemorrhage. Packing may or may not have been inserted in the vagina to help control or prevent hemorrhage. This should be carefully noted on the chart. If packing was inserted, the nurse must watch the patient even more carefully for signs of shock, since any bleeding may be concealed by the packing. If there is packing, it will have to be removed within several hours to allow free drainage of lochia and thus help prevent infection. By altering urethrovesical relationships, vaginal packing increases a woman's inability to void postoperatively. Inability to void with subsequent bladder distention should be avoided, either by removing the packing or inserting a catheter.

The nurse should anticipate some postoperative vomiting, since these women appear to have an increased incidence of vomiting. Good preoperative care may do a great deal to present us with a more relaxed, confident patient. This may lessen vomiting to some extent. However, often the patient goes to the operating room on an emergency basis, either to control hemorrhage or to prevent its occurrence. To prepare this patient adequately for the operating room requires a smooth blending of supportive nursing care and the accomplishment of all the necessary tasks as quickly as possible. The easiest and least skilled method is to do the technical tasks efficiently. The most accomplished method, and therefore the most difficult, is to do the necessary preparation efficiently and at the same time reassure the patient and explain the procedure to her while going about these tasks in a calm, quiet manner. This invites the respect and confidence of the patient and her family.

INCOMPETENT CERVICAL OS. The patient who has had several abortions will probably receive a thorough assessment between pregnancies in an attempt to ascertain her problem. Should the cause be considered an incompetent cervical os, the physician may attempt to tighten the cervix with a suture. This is usually done during the twelfth to sixteenth week of pregnancy. The Shirodkar technique consists of running a nondissolving suture around the cervix like a drawstring or purse string. The Lash operation involves removing a small piece of tissue from the cervix and closing the gap with sutures. The Lash operation particularly may be done between pregnancies.

On return from the operating room, the pregnant patient is observed for signs of labor and imminent abortion. Should the abortion appear inevitable, the suture must be removed or serious tearing of the cervix might occur. At term, the suture is removed and vaginal delivery follows, or the suture is retained and delivery is by cesarean section.

The patient who has aborted will often be distraught at losing another pregnancy. She may experience the loss of the desired child acutely, and in the immediate period following the abortion she may derive little consolation from being told that she can have other children or that she has children at home. It is the loss of this child which she feels. Sympathy, understanding and someone to talk to are greatly appreciated by these women. The nurse who deals with these patients should further acquaint herself with the patterns of normal grieving so that she may understand these patients more fully.

BAPTISM OF FETUS. If the patient who aborts is Roman Catholic, the fetus must be baptized. In addition, some Protestants may feel strongly that the fetus should be baptized. The nurse may ascertain this by tactfully inquiring what the patient's wishes are. Baptism may be performed by any person, regardless of his religious beliefs. If a clergyman is immediately available, he should be asked to perform this rite. In his absence, the nurse may have to baptize the fetus. Clear water must be poured over the head of the fetus while the nurse pronounces the words, "I baptize you in the name of the Father and of the Son and of the Holy Spirit." The water must come into direct contact with the fetus. Therefore, if the fetus is still in the amniotic sac, the sac must be broken before baptism is performed. The procedure is similar for all religions. If the fetus is very small; it may have to be immersed in water to insure that water reaches the head. Sometimes a conditional baptism is given with the words, "If thou art living, I baptize thee...." This is done in cases in which the fetus may have died before delivery, but the exact state is unknown.

THERAPEUTIC ABORTION. The past few years have seen an explosive increase in the number of therapeutic or induced abortions performed throughout the world, in response to the liberalization of abortion laws. It is estimated that legal abortion for social and medical reasons is now available to over half the world's population, making the therapeutic abortion one of the most common medical procedures performed.

Because an abortion concerns the life and death of at least two people, it is governed by religious and legal codes. Complex issues surround the topic of induced abortions and a discussion of all of them is beyond the scope of this work. Only a brief discussion of the law and medical and nursing management is presented here.

The laws governing abortions vary from country to country and from state to state. In all nations legal codes exist defining the conditions under which an abortion may be done. They outline who may do an abortion, where it may be done (in or outside the hospital), and when it may be done in relationship to the length of gestation. The law also defines the social and medical conditions which constitute cause for an abortion. All abortions performed outside the limits of the legal condition are illegal. In many countries assisting a patient to procure an abortion outside the law is also punishable by law. For these reasons the nurse should be acquainted with the law pertaining to the area in which she practices.

Abortions can be divided into two groups on the basis of risk to the woman and her future childbearing potential. Low-risk or early abortions are those done before 12 weeks of gestation. Late or high-risk abortions are done from the thirteenth week of gestation onward. As the upper limits of abortion are defined by the law they will vary from 20 to 28 weeks of gestation, depending upon the jurisdiction. An abortion may carry greater risk if the patient has a serious accompanying medical condition.

EARLY ABORTIONS. Most abortions performed before 12 to 14 weeks of gestation are done by suction D and C. If done before 8 weeks of gestation the cervix usually does not require dilation. The procedure may be done in the hospital or on an outpatient basis. A general anesthetic may be given, but many abortions, particularly those not requiring cervical dilation, may be done without anesthesia or with a local anesthetic such as a paracervical block. Some physicians administer intravenous Syntocinon before suctioning to insure a strong firm contraction of the uterus; others do not feel this is necessary.

Following these initial steps the doctor determines the size, shape and position of the uterus by bimanual examination. The cervix is then visualized and immobilized by forceps and the cervical canal sounded for direction and the uterus for depth. Should the cervix require dilating it will now be done to the size of the cannula required to perform the D and C. The size of the cannula is deter-

mined by the length of gestation. A suction tip, which may be nonflexible or flexible (not requiring cervical dilation), is then slipped through the cervix. It is attached to a vacuum source which sucks out the uterine contents. The pressure of the pump is carefully regulated to achieve evacuation while avoiding damage to the walls of the uterine cavity. The physician judges when the uterus is empty by the grating feel of the denuded uterine walls, the contractions of the uterus and the content and character of the aspirated fluid. The aspirated tissue is caught in a gauze trap to facilitate recovery for immediate inspection and for examination by the pathologist. Immediate identification of fetal tissue is important to confirm the diagnosis of an intrauterine pregnancy which has been completely evacuated. As the operator becomes more experienced, the need for postsuction curettage of the uterus declines but may still be performed in cases of doubtful complete emptying of the uterus. It is necessary to confirm the intrauterine pregnancy to avoid an ectopic pregnancy continuing unnoticed. Immediate inspection and, later, pathology reports may confirm a molar pregnancy which, if left undetected, would deprive the patient of important follow-up care.

Following the procedure the patient recovers as determined by the anesthetic she received. Many patients experience some cramping postabortion, which is normal. The cramps are frequently gone by the time the effects of the anesthetic, either general or paracervical, are over, but may persist for longer. A mild analgesic may be required. The patient is then observed for a few hours more or allowed to go home with instructions, depending upon her condition.

Laminaria stents are used to reduce the risks of traumatizing the cervix and uterus during dilation. They are small cylinders of the seaweed *laminaria digitata*, dried and compressed into a stick shape. The weed is extremely hygroscopic and, in a moist environment such as the cervix, gradually swells to several times its size. The cervix is slowly dilated over 6 to 12 hours. The size of the stent chosen is one which the cervical canal will readily admit. Smaller ones are used for nulliparous patients. Because of the time involved the patient is admitted to the hospital the day before and the laminaria stent inserted the evening before the abortion. The insertion is a sterile procedure, and vagina and cervix are painted with an antiseptic solution before insertion.

Complications of the stents are few. Many women experience cramping and occasional fainting on insertion and intermittent cramps thereafter. The patient may require a mild analgesic for these cramps. Occasionally, a patient will expel the stent. Further dilation has been required for some patients when the stent was used for abortions beyond the twelfth week of pregnancy. Because the use of the stent is associated with a small risk of infection, the patient is monitored for signs of infection during the process and postabortion.

Very early aspiration of the contents of the uterus with a flexible plastic cannula and a specially designed hand pump or 50-ml. syringe is referred to as menstrual regulation. It is done within 14 days of a missed menstrual period before pregnancy can be confirmed by a urine test. The cervix does not require dilating and the procedure is done without anesthesia on an outpatient or office basis. Some physicians administer a paracervical block, especially to a nullipara. The procedure is most effective between the seventh and fourteenth days following a missed menstrual period. Incomplete evacuation of the uterus is more common if menstrual regulation is done before the seventh day or after the fourteenth day (35 to 42 days of amenorrhea). Unnecessary surgery is also avoided, as the incidence of pregnancy rises as amenorrhea continues. After the procedure the patient rests and is observed for any untoward effects for 10 to 30 minutes and is then discharged home.

The procedure is not without controversy. Is it an abortion or not? Is it done too frequently on nonpregnant women, thereby exposing them to unnecessary surgery and wasting medical resources? Does it promote a laissez-faire attitude toward the use of birth control? Or is it merely a simple, effective way of reducing troublesome anxiety in a woman and/or performing an abortion with reduced risk and less use of medical resources? For many women it undoubtedly avoids the much greater anxiety, stress and risk of a later abortion. The method is also proving useful in obtaining endometrium for biopsy.

LATE ABORTIONS. When the pregnancy is above 12 to 14 weeks a D and C becomes more difficult. Other methods must be selected by the physician. He may decide to induce labor by the use of an intra-amniotic injection. The technique and preparation are similar to a paracentesis, but an amniocentesis is done. With strict sterile technique the patient's abdomen is prepared and draped. A skin wheal is made with a local anesthetic agent. Then a needle is inserted through the abdomen, and into the amniotic cavity. Some amniotic fluid is withdrawn and replaced by an equal amount of 20 per cent saline solution. The fetus dies, and the uterus is apparently irritated and begins to contract within 36 to 48 hours. The contractions may need to be assisted with an oxytocic medication given intravenously.

Later pregnancies of 16 to 20 weeks' gestation may be terminated by the performance of a hysterotomy. This means that an incision is made into the uterus and the contents removed. It is a miniature cesarean section. The pre- and postoperative care is similar to abdominal surgery. However, perineal and abdominal shave preparations may be ordered. Postoperatively, the fundus must be checked for firmness and position. Lochia is observed for color, amount and odor, since hemorrhage or infection may occur postoperatively. Perineal care is done.

PROSTAGLANDINS. Prostaglandins are naturally occurring fatty acids which were first isolated in semen and thought to arise in the prostate gland. Since then they have been found in many body solutions, and are involved in many important physiological functions. One of their actions is the ability to make smooth muscle contract. This ability is pronounced in relation to uterine muscle. Two forms of prostaglandins, E_2 and $F_{2\alpha}$, are used therapeutically. E_2 is several times stronger than $F_{2\alpha}$. The most common side effects described are nausea, diarrhea, pyrexia and local tissue reactions at the site of injection. Synthetic analogues of both F and E groups are now made. They produce fewer side effects and still stimulate uterine contractions. One of their major uses is to induce abortion and to stimulate labor in full-term pregnancies.

Prostaglandins may be given in an intravenous drip which is carefully regulated by an infusion pump. The dosage is started at very low levels; the responses of the patient, fetus and uterus are carefully monitored. The dose is gradually increased until the uterus is con-

TABLE 20–1 CLASSIFICATION OF ABORTIONS

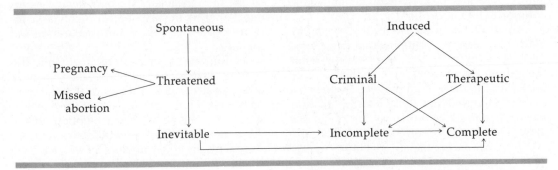

tracting satisfactorily. Labor and delivery or abortion will follow for most patients in 12 to 24 hours. If the stimulation is not sufficient, additional stimulation with Pitocin may be given. This is associated with an increased risk of rupture of the cervix and uterus, so the response of the contracting uterus must be carefully monitored. The patient's complaints of discomfort or pain should be carefully heeded.

Intra-amniotic injections of prostaglandins may also be given. The procedure is similar to the injection of saline but may be given in divided doses. Therefore, a tiny polyethylene tube is left in the uterus to avoid multiple injections. Prostaglandin is added at hourly intervals for a total of three doses. Some give an initial dose slowly over 5 minutes, observe how this is tolerated and, after a few minutes more, inject the total dose. The prostaglandins are absorbed and the uterus begins to contract. Delivery usually occurs about 20 hours after the injection. If the attempt fails, the dose may be repeated the next day. Occasionally additional stimulation with a Syntocinon drip is required. Side effects include, rarely, sudden abdominal pain due to hypertonus of the uterus, transient hypotension, vasovagal collapse, increased intraocular pressure, difficulty in breathing and the more common vomiting, diarrhea and pyrexia.

Extra-amniotic injection is a more common method of inducing abortion with prostaglandins. The systemic effects are fewer, although vomiting remains a problem. Vomiting and diarrhea may be lessened by the administration of antiemetics and drugs which reduce gastric motility. A polyethylene tubing or a Foley catheter is passed under aseptic conditions through the cervix, and is directed between the uterine wall and the membranes. The bag of the Foley catheter is inflated to help retain the catheter in the uterus. The tube is attached to further tubing attached to a syringe containing the solution. The rate of infusion is controlled by an infusion pump. Small amounts are injected and the uterine response observed. The dose is gradually increased. Abortion occurs in anywhere from 12 to 24 hours.

NURSING RESPONSIBILITIES. The therapeutic abortion is not a totally benign procedure. Physical and mental complications can arise. Thus, the decision to perform an abortion is a weighty one for the physician as well as for the woman. She and her family will need support and acceptance. Some patients will benefit from counselling beforehand, especially those for whom the abortion involves conflict. All patients require an explanation of the procedure. Unfortunately, many patients are so driven by the overriding need to have the pregnancy terminated that detailed explanations or teaching is not absorbed. Most patients appear less tense, more relaxed and less hostile once they know that the pregnancy is terminated. They are then more receptive to teaching and explanations about follow-up. Anxiety, loneliness and fear are the problems expressed by patients waiting for their contractions to start. Some have told no one, and have no friends or family to support them through the procedure. The nurse can be an important factor in their experience of the event.

Postoperatively the patient is nursed similarly to the patient who has had a spontaneous abortion and a D and C to complete the process. In late abortions the patient requires more intensive nursing care. While the intra-amniotic injections are being given the patient must be observed for reactions to the drug injected. Hypertonic saline may be absorbed into the circulatory system. To avoid this a small amount is injected, the patient's response assessed, and then the remainder injected. If saline is being absorbed intravascularly she may complain of confusion, heat sensations, headache, tinnitus, a dry mouth and tachycardia. In this event the saline is stopped and the injection site altered. When the injection is completed, the patient then awaits the beginning of contractions. To reduce the risk of infection, oxytocin is usually begun within 12 hours if uterine contractions are not adequate. The patient may express some thirst during this period of waiting. All patients who have been given saline absorb a portion of it, thus producing some electroyte imbalance. Fluid is required and she should be allowed to drink. The patient experiences labor and requires the support and nursing care which is given to a laboring patient. The contractions are distressing, especially since they appear to be for a negative purpose. Analgesia is required by some patients and should not be withheld. Bed rest is usually maintained after active labor begins or after administration of a sedative. In extra-amniotic injection of prostaglandins the catheter may be expelled as the uterus contracts and the cervix dilates. To maintain labor Pitocin stimulation may be required.

As progress is difficult to assess, the patient frequently aborts in bed alone or with the nurse in attendance. If previously warned she may call the nurse when she feels pressure. However, the patient herself frequently receives little warning.

All products of conception are retained for examination by the physician and the pathologist. Often the placenta is retained and only the fetus expelled. The nurse should clamp and cut the cord and remove the fetus. Now the patient enters one of the hazardous periods during an abortion, and requires close observation by the nursing staff. Severe hemorrhage may result from the partially separated placenta or the retained products of conception. Hemorrhage may take several forms: the sudden gush, a steady trickle, or smaller gushes interspersed with periods of minor loss. In all cases the nurse must assess the cumulative loss as well as the immediate one. Individual episodes of bleeding might not alert the nurse to hemorrhage but she must assess the loss over the period of time from the beginning of bleeding to the present. In this way morbidity is reduced, since evacuation of the uterus is begun before the patient has suffered severe loss. If the placenta is not expelled spontaneously within 2 hours and bleeding does not indicate immediate removal, the patient will be scheduled for a D and C for a convenient time within a few hours. Meanwhile, frequent observations of the lochia must be maintained, as the patient's status may change at any time. Following the D and C she is nursed as other patients post-abortion D and C.

Infection may develop, and the patient is monitored for signs of pelvic infection every 4 hours during the hours when she is aborting. Regular daily checks of temperature, general well-being and the character of the lochia follow.

Most abortion patients are discharged within hours of being aborted or within 1 or 2 days. They need clear discharge instructions so that they may take care of themselves in the days that follow. Each patient should be told:

1. To resume normal activities, except for hysterotomy patients who as postoperative patients may do so more gradually.
2. To expect intermittent menstrual-like discharge for the next week or two, but no heavy, bright-red bleeding.
3. Some cramping may occur but should not persist or be severe.
4. To report any fever or unusual discomfort.
5. To expect her menstrual period within 4 to 5 weeks after the procedure. If it does not occur, it may indicate a continuing intra- or extrauterine pregnancy or a new pregnancy. Ovulation occurs as early as 18 days following an abortion and pregnancy is possible immediately. Birth control advice and teaching should be given to the patient as necessary.
6. It is wise to limit coitus while the menstrual-like flow continues to reduce the risk of infection.
7. To contact her physician or clinic immediately if any of the unusual signs should occur.

8. When, or if, she is to return for a follow-up visit.

While the therapeutic abortion is now associated with low maternal morbidity and mortality statistics (lower than pregnancy in many countries), it does carry some serious risks which need to be considered. Psychiatric sequelae are rare but do occur. The main concern appears to be an increased incidence of spontaneous abortion and premature labor in those women who have had a prior abortion. The risk is greatest with the older methods of dilation and curettage, and is greater still when damage to the cervix has been documented. It is hoped that earlier abortions involving less traumatic methods of dilating the cervix will refute these findings. In the meantime it appears important to educate women to seek abortion as early as possible so that the need for dilating the cervix, particularly by older methods, will be reduced. Prevention is better than cure, and birth control should be seen as the first line of defense. Nursing has an important role to play by providing knowledge of and access to birth control to those who need it.

CRIMINAL ABORTION. The criminal abortion is a dangerous procedure. Often women attempt to abort themselves by the use of strong douches or instruments which they insert into the uterus. Frequently, the instrument used punctures the posterior fornix of the vagina, the cervix or perforates the uterus. The bowel may be involved should the instrument be inserted far enough. Conditions are furtive, untrained people frequently officiate, and sterility is not maintained. These patients frequently contract an infection and may present a grave situation. The situation is known as a septic abortion. Infection is essentially an endometritis, which may spread to peritonitis or to septicemia.

Ectopic Pregnancy

Implantation of the fertilized ovum anywhere outside the uterine cavity is considered an ectopic pregnancy. Most frequently this occurs in the ampullary portion of the uterine tube, but it may be ovarian, abdominal or cervical. Ectopic pregnancies are estimated as occurring once in every 250 pregnancies. Women with a history of one ectopic pregnancy have an increased risk of having a second one.

An ectopic pregnancy results when the passage of the zygote to the uterine cavity is impeded or slowed. Any blocking of the tube or reduction in tubal peristalsis will achieve this. Former salpingitis, tumors and hormonal imbalances may all play a part.

As implantation occurs, the chorionic villi burrow into the thin tubal wall. Eventually, they burrow into a blood vessel, and bleeding occurs. If the bleeding is sufficient, the fetus dies. This is the fate of most. The abortus may be retained in the tube as a tubal mole or may be extruded through the end of the uterine tube as a tubal abortion. Occasionally, the trophoblast burrows through the wall of the tube and out into the peritoneal cavity. This is known as a ruptured tubal pregnancy and often occurs as the result of a pregnancy in the narrow isthmus of the tube. A secondary abdominal pregnancy may follow if the chorionic villi settle elsewhere in the abdominal cavity and begin to grow. This is rare.

SIGNS AND SYMPTOMS. The accurate diagnosis of an existing ectopic pregnancy or a recently aborted ectopic pregnancy may require much skill, since the picture may be confusing. Fortunately, many are diagnosed by bimanual examination of the early pregnant woman. Others abort before the patient sees a physician. These women may first be seen in the emergency department or in the clinic with a variety of symptoms.

The woman has a history of the early signs of pregnancy, including amenorrhea usually of 6 to 10 weeks' duration. Soon after her first missed period she may have complaints of a localized pain on one side, due probably to the distention of the tube. Following this she may have sharper intermittent pain in the same area. This may be due to strong peristaltic waves of the tube attempting to pass the embryo or abortus along the tube. At some point the patient may experience a sharp, severe pain. This is probably synchronous with separation of the embryo and some hemorrhage. The sharp pain may be followed by generalized abdominal discomfort as blood spills into the abdomen. Referred shoulder pain may occur. Four or 5 days following this episode there is bleeding per vaginam due to falling hormone levels, which occur following the death of the fetus and cause the endometrium to regress and menstruation to occur.

ACUTE RUPTURED TUBAL PREGNANCY. Sometimes the patient reports no early symptoms but experiences one episode of acute abdominal pain shortly after her missed period. This acute pain is often accompanied by vomiting and fainting. Some vaginal bleeding may be present but appears too minimal to warrant the reaction of the patient. The patient may rapidly go into shock with a drop in blood pressure, rapid weak pulse, pallor, sweating, low temperature and cold extremities. The abdomen is distended with blood and may be tight and tender to the touch. A pelvic examination of the patient may be difficult because of the exquisite tenderness. The patient presents as an emergency situation.

NURSING RESPONSIBILITIES. Nursing care includes notifying the physician immediately and treating the patient for shock by elevating the foot of the bed and checking vital signs every 10 minutes. The nurse will be responsible for having equipment on hand for the doctor to start an intravenous infusion and to take blood for hemoglobin, typing and cross matching. Catheterization is usually ordered. The nurse should be ready to prepare this patient for surgery, which is frequently a laparotomy.

LAPAROSCOPY. In other situations the patient presents with atypical signs and symptoms. The physician may feel that direct visualization of the pelvic organs is necessary. Examination under anesthesia involving colpotomy, culdoscopy and culdocentesis may be used. However, these procedures are being largely replaced by laparoscopy as the method of choice. It provides better lighted, direct visualization of the anterior aspect of the tubes and ovaries, unlike the posterior and frequently less satisfactory view seen by culdoscopy. The knee-chest position is avoided, and frequently the necessity for a laparotomy. The procedure is done under a general anesthetic and aseptic conditions.

To avoid damage and to obtain better visualization of abdominal and pelvic contents, the cavity is distended with carbon dioxide. Now the abdominal wall is lifted by the gas above the underlying organs. The patient is tilted head downwards to about a 45° angle, shifting the abdominal contents up and away from the site of insertion of the laparoscope and from the pelvis. Through a small incision in the lower rim of the umbilicus a trocar and sleeve are inserted on an angle; the trocar is then withdrawn and the endoscope inserted. It enters the peritoneal cavity approximately halfway between the umbilicus and symphysis pubis. The contents of the abdomen and pelvis are observed, and the uterus may be manipulated from below by a clamp in the cervix. This changes angles and brings the organs into better view. At the close the endoscope is withdrawn, the gas is expressed from the abdomen through the cannula, and the incision closed with a clip or stitch which is removed in 24 to 48 hours.

There are few complications, but cardiac arrhythmias, collapse and death have been recorded. These are very rare. The patient may complain of some mild abdominal or shoulder pain following the procedure. This is usually abdominal gas which collects beneath the diaphragm and is not intestinal colic. The gas is absorbed gradually over a few days, but a change of position such as the knee-chest may help. Severe pain or signs of abdominal tenderness or tightness should be reported.

The patient receives pre- and postoperative care as usual, but does not require a shave "prep." She is ambulatory on return from the recovery room and generally returns to a full diet immediately.

When the diagnosis of a tubal pregnancy is confirmed, a salpingectomy (removal of the uterine tube) with the removal of the fetus is performed. This is usually done within 24 to 48 hours of diagnosis unless the situation is acute, in which case it is done immediately. Sometimes the ovary on the same side as the salpingectomy is also removed. This is thought to reduce the risk of another ectopic pregnancy occurring and to increase fertility. The remaining ovary then ovulates each month rather than alternate ones, on the same side as the remaining functioning uterine tube.

Ectopic pregnancies in other locations will be investigated in a similar fashion. Treatment is usually surgical removal of the fetus. However, abdominal pregnancies have carried to term and been delivered by laparotomies.

Tumors of the Trophoblast

Trophoblastic tumors are a group of neoplasms which arise in the chorionic villi of the fertilized ovum during the trophoblast stage. The condition is rare in Europe and North America, occurring about once in every 2500 pregnancies. However, it is more prevalent in

TABLE 20–2 TROPHOBLASTIC TUMORS

Benign ⇐⇒	Intermediate ⟶	Malignant
1. Hydatidiform mole	1. Metastasizing mole	1. Choriocarcinoma (chorionepithelioma malignum)
	2. Chorioadenoma destruens	

the Far East. The reason for this is not known. The tumors range from benign to malignant (Table 20–2). Not all benign tumors become malignant, nor are all malignant tumors preceded by a benign stage.

HYDATIDIFORM MOLE. Hydatidiform mole is an abnormal development of the chorionic villi of the conceptus. It begins to form about the fifth week of embyronic life. The mole appears to occur when the fetal cardiovascular structure fails to develop, but an intact trophoblast and a functioning maternal structure remain. As the fluid accumulates, the chorionic villi distend into small clear vesicles, clinging to thin threads of connective tissue in a grape-like pattern. Few blood vessels are present in the mass. Characteristically, there is no fetus. Rarely, some mole-like degeneration may be present on one part of an otherwise normal placenta.

The condition is the most common of all the tumors. Thus, the majority of women who have a molar pregnancy do not need to fear malignancy. Only 3 to 7 per cent of benign moles will proceed to malignancy.

The intermediate stages are characterized by an increased ability to invade uterine musculature and to send bloodborne deposits of trophoblast cells throughout the body. However, in some cases, the host, or pregnant woman, seems able to contain the spread of the tumor and it disappears. The intermediate stage is frequently not identified clinically, but is obvious only on pathologic examinations of specimens of tissue. This means that all moles must be treated as potentially malignant until demonstrated otherwise.

SIGNS AND SYMPTOMS. The patient exhibits the signs and symptoms of early pregnancy. Vomiting may be more frequent. The uterus is often much larger than expected for the weeks of gestation. About the twelfth week, some vaginal bleeding may occur, and this is often the first sign of some abnormality. No fetal movements are reported by the mother, and no fetal parts can be palpated. On palpation the uterus may have an elastic consistency. There is an increased incidence of preeclampsia. Urine tests for the quantity of chorionic gonadotropins excreted show very high titers which persist and do not fall as is usual in a normal pregnancy. These high levels also stimulate the formation of theca lutein cysts in the ovary. The cysts regress following the abortion of the mole.

TREATMENT AND NURSING RESPONSIBILITIES. The patient is usually admitted to the hospital and nursed as a threatened abortion until proven otherwise. All perineal pads are carefully inspected for pieces of the mole, as this would be diagnostic. Thyroid function tests may be ordered, for, in rare cases, trophoblastic tumors secrete thyroid-stimulating hormone.

An ultrasonic scan of the abdomen will most likely be done. The scan plots a "snowflake" pattern, which is typical of a mole and is considered diagnostic. In preparation for an ultrasound scan the patient is instructed to drink 6 to 8 large glasses of water in quick succession. The bladder fills within 15 to 20 minutes, after which the scan is done. The full bladder pushes the bowel away from the uterus and tubes, permitting better penetration of sound waves. At the same time the uterus is pushed up and away from the symphysis pubis, allowing better visualization. The full bladder provides a water path or window through which to look, a landmark in the abdomen, for it is clearly outlined, and an internal reference standard for density comparisons.

In scanning soft tissue two types of scans are done; one outlines tissue and the other estimates density of the mass or tissue outlined. The operations are separate and require different manipulations of the ultrasound equipment. The snowflake pattern of a mole reflects an irregular shaped mass with areas of alternating density. Because sound waves can be dispersed or lost, a contact gel is used between the transducer and the skin of the patient. This keeps the sound waves on track as it were. The area is carefully mapped out as the transducer is moved in lines 1 cm. apart up and down and across the area. The findings are displayed on a monitor screen. Printouts can be obtained for permanent record.

Ultrasound is being used increasingly in gynecology for the localization of foreign objects in the uterus, the diagnosis of tumors of the uterus, ovary and tubes, ectopic pregnancy, and as a device to outline precise areas for irradiation. The patient suffers no discomfort save that of a full bladder during the procedure.

Often the mole is partially aborted spontaneously. Hemorrhage may be acute. Oxytocics will be given to control the bleeding, and a careful and complete evacuation of the uterus will be done. Because of the danger of perforating the uterus in areas weakened by the erosion of the mole, a curette is usually not used. Instead, a suction D and C is done. Postoperatively the patient must be observed for signs of hemorrhage.

Because of the possibility of a malignancy occurring, the patient receives close follow-up care during the next 12 to 18 months. The first signs of the recurrence of the mole or the development of a malignancy is a rising chorionic gonadotropin level. Therefore, the urinary levels of gonadotropin will be monitored at regular intervals. Amenorrhea, metrorrhagia or persistent cystic ovaries may alert the physician to look for rising hormone levels. The patient is advised against pregnancy during this period, as early pregnancy also produces high chorionic gonadotropin levels which could mask the signs. Cytotoxic drugs (such as methotrexate) are given in all intermediate cases, and may be given as prophylaxis to all women who have had a molar pregnancy.

CHORIONEPITHELIOMA MALIGNUM. Chorionepithelioma is a malignant tumor of the embryonic chorion and is marked by invasion of the uterine musculature by malignant trophoblastic cells which have lost their original villous pattern. Destruction of uterine tissues with accompanying necrosis and hemorrhage is the result. The growth quickly metastasizes, and the most frequent site is the lung. The condition is extremely rare but because of its rapid advancement is considered to be one of the most malignant of all pelvic neoplasms. Death usually occurs within 12 months unless the patient receives early treatment. Fifty per cent of all cases of chorionepithelioma are preceded by a mole. The others are preceded by a normal pregnancy or abortion. Because of careful follow-up of patients who have had a molar pregnancy, the number of deaths from this disease have been reduced.

The chemotherapeutic agent methotrexate is the treatment of choice but may be combined with surgery. The drug is a folic acid antagonist and may be administered orally or parenterally for 5 consecutive days and then withdrawn for a week. The course may need to be repeated several times if chorionic gonadotropin titers do not regress. Actinomycin D may also be used alone or in combination with methotrexate.

INFECTIONS OF THE REPRODUCTIVE TRACT

Infections in the Male

Balanitis

Balanitis[2] is an infection of the glans penis. Many different organisms may be causative. It is generally associated with poor personal hygiene in the uncircumcised male, but it may be due to venereal diseases. Symptoms include redness, swelling, pain and a purulent discharge. The disease may be chronic and may cause the formation of adhesions and scarring.

TREATMENT. The infection is treated with the appropriate antibiotic following culture and sensitivity tests. Once the inflammatory process is controlled, circumcision, the excision of the prepuce, is advised.

On return from the operating room, the patient has a small petroleum jelly gauze dressing which is changed following each voiding. The patient may be taught to do this and how to care for the dressing at home.

Should bleeding occur, a pressure dressing is applied. The dressing may make voiding impossible or difficult. Usually the dressing can be removed within a short period of time.

PHIMOSIS. Phimosis is a condition in which the preputial orifice is too small to permit retraction over the glans. It may be congenital but is most frequently a sequel to infection or trauma. Circumcision is advised.

---

[2]*Balanos* is the Greek word meaning acorn; in reference to the glans, it is a combining form indicating relationship to the glans penis.

PARAPHIMOSIS. Paraphimosis occurs when a narrowed prepuce is either forced back over the glans or is gradually retracted over it. It then forms a tight, constricting band around the glans; venous return is impaired, and swelling and pain follow. Usually pain is too severe to permit manipulation, so a general anesthetic is given, and the foreskin is pulled forward. Occasionally the foreskin may have to be incised, and a slit is made up the dorsal surface. This is usually followed by circumcision after the treatment of any infection which may have been present.

Prostatitis

Prostatitis is usually an ascending infection of the genitourinary tract, but it may also be the result of the hematogenous spread of the organism. It is often secondary to urethritis or instrumentation of the urethra, as occurs in the use of an indwelling catheter.

In the acute stage, fever and chills are accompanied by hematuria, frequency and dysuria. A urethral discharge may be noted. Rectal examination usually reveals an enlarged, tender, "hot" prostate. Since infection of the seminal vesicles almost invariably accompanies prostatitis, the seminal vesicles can be palpated as well. Prostatic massage and instrumentation of the urethra are avoided to prevent possible spread of the infection to the epididymis, bladder and kidney. Exceptions are made only to relieve acute urinary retention, which may be a sequel to the enlarged prostate. A small urethral catheter will be used. In severe cases, drainage may be by suprapubic cystostomy rather than by catheterization. Prostatic abscesses may develop and usually drain through the urethra. Occasionally, excision and drainage are required.

The patient is placed on bed rest. Appropriate antibiotic therapy is ordered, and the tetracyclines are frequently chosen first. The patient is in considerable pain. The nurse often sees a tense, anxious and frightened patient who needs reassurance and support. Explanations to clarify that the infection is not venereal may be necessary. Analgesics, warm sitz baths and rectal irrigations help to relieve the pain and bladder spasms. The irritable bladder may require special attention, and antispasmodics and bladder sedatives are frequently ordered. Fruit juices and bicarbonate of soda help to alkalinize the urine.

In cases in which treatment is early, excellent results usually follow. However, the acute picture may become chronic. The symptoms are mild and include a low-grade fever and some bacteria and pus in the urine. Fertility and potency are not affected unless complications ensue. The chronic infection may stubbornly resist treatment. Antibiotics and chemotherapy are given. Prostatic massage four to five times every 7 to 14 days is done by the physician and helps by draining the bacteria away. Sexual intercourse accomplishes the same purpose. Daily sitz baths also help resolve the infection, and the patient will need instruction in taking a sitz bath at home.

Epididymitis

Epididymitis may be caused by any pyogenic organism. It frequently follows prostatitis and may be a complication of prostatectomy. Fever, malaise and chills accompany swelling and pain in the scrotum. The patient may be so uncomfortable that he may walk in a waddling fashion. Symptoms of cystitis may be present, and a hydrocele often develops. The swelling and irritation cause congestion of the testes which impedes the circulation of blood. Sterility follows from necrosis of the tubular epithelium and fibrosis which occludes the ducts.

The patient is placed on bed rest. The scrotum is elevated on towel rolls or with a Bellevue bridge during the acute stage. Local applications of heat or cold may be ordered. Sitz baths often relieve symptoms of congestion and pain. After the patient is ambulant, a roomy scrotal support is worn.

Antibiotics are given but are not usually curative. If the disease is diagnosed early, a local anesthetic agent is injected into the spermatic cord above the testes. Symptoms are usually absent in a day or two following this treatment. Chronic epididymitis may follow an acute episode. If the involvement is bilateral, sterility follows.

Orchitis

Inflammation of the testes may follow any infectious disease or may be acquired as an ascending infection from the genital tract.

Most commonly it follows mumps parotitis. The mumps virus is excreted in the urine; therefore, the spread to the testes in this case appears to be by descent. The onset is sudden, manifested by pain and swelling of the scrotum followed by fever and prostration. Urinary symptoms are usually not present. A hydrocele may develop, and the involvement may be unilateral or bilateral. Sterility probably follows death of the spermatogenic cells from ischemia. Bed rest, scrotal support and local applications of heat are necessary. A padded athletic support may be worn continuously.

Antibiotics are used in some situations but are not of value against the mumps virus. Local infiltration of the spermatic cord with a local anesthetic may relieve the symptoms. The prevention of mumps in the postpubertal male has some value. If a man who has not been immunized as a child against mumps or who has not previously had mumps has been in contact with the virus, gamma globulin is usually administered.

Infections in the Female

Bartholinitis

Bartholinitis is an infection of the greater vestibular gland and may or may not be gonorrheal in origin. The infection is an ascending one, progressing up the ducts to the gland. Symptoms are usually those of an acute infection — pain, swelling, inflammation and a purulent discharge. Cellulitis of the surrounding tissues aggravates the situation, but the infection may localize and become an abscess. This is usually excised and drained. Sometimes the infection subsides, leaving the duct scarred and occluded. This may be followed by a cyst filled with the secretions of the gland which now cannot escape. The cyst is usually a painless swelling in the lower third of the labium minus. Treatment is to excise the cyst and gland. Alternatively, a marsupialization of the cystic duct may be done. This leaves the functioning gland in place.

Hot sitz baths or saline soaks may be ordered following surgery. The patient may need instruction on how to take a sitz bath at home. Following the daily bath, a fresh tub of hot water is run. The patient sits in this for 10 to 15 minutes. The water is not above the level of the iliac crest.

Vaginitis

PHYSIOLOGICAL LEUKORRHEA. Physiological leukorrhea is a normal whitish discharge which helps to keep the vagina moist. It is composed of endocervical secretions, leukocytes, desquamated epithelial cells and other normal flora of the vaginal tract. The pH is normally 4 to 5 but varies during the life cycle of the woman. At birth, it may be as low as 5 under the hormonal stimulus of the mother. As a child it is 6 to 7. At menarche the pH becomes acidic again, and assumes the adult pH of 4 to 5. Postmenopausally, estrogen is withdrawn, and the pH rises to 6 to 7 again. The quantity of the discharge also varies among women, during stages of the menstrual cycle and during pregnancy. An increase is usually noticed at ovulation, during sexual stimulation and during pregnancy. The most characteristic symptom of a vaginitis is a change in the normal vaginal discharge.

TRICHOMONIASIS. The most common cause of vaginitis is a flagellated protozoon, known as a trichomonad, which grows and thrives in a vaginal pH of 5 to 6. Trichomonads may be found in the large bowel and occasionally in the bladder and vestibular glands. They can be transmitted to a man at intercourse and from him can be communicated to other women or serve as a source of reinfection. In men, trichomonads may be harbored in the urethra, bladder or prostate.

The woman presents with symptoms of a heavy, yellow, frothy discharge which has a slight odor. This heavy discharge may be irritating to the vulva, causing pruritus and excoriation. The vaginal mucosa is reddened and is slightly edematous. The patient may complain of dyspareunia and, if the bladder is involved, of dysuria and frequency. As the condition becomes chronic, the woman has fewer symptoms. Diagnosis is confirmed when trichomonads are seen microscopically in a vaginal smear.

Men frequently have few symptoms. There may be some urethral itching and a slight discharge. Invasion of the bladder may produce frequency and burning on micturition. Wet smears are made of the urethral discharge, and the protozoa seen microscopically confirm the diagnosis.

Treatment is usually the oral administration of metronidazole (Flagyl) 250 mg. three times a day for 10 days. Repeat smears will then be done, and a repeat course of therapy may be necessary. During the treatment, a condom should be worn until both partners are considered cured. Women may be given vaginal suppositories instead of oral therapy. A suppository is inserted morning and night daily for 4 to 8 weeks. This is continued through the menstrual period, for the menstrual flow is alkaline and provides an excellent medium for the protozoa. Insertion is like that of a vaginal tampon. The patient is instructed to remain flat for about 10 minutes following insertion.

MONILIAL VAGINITIS. Monilial vaginitis occurs when the vagina is invaded by the fungus *Candida albicans*. The vaginal pH is usually 5 to 7. Pregnant women and diabetics are predisposed because of glycosuria and the increased glycogen present in the vagina during pregnancy. Contamination may be from the rectum. A thick, white, curdy vaginal discharge is present which frequently causes pruritus and irritation of the vulva. The vaginal walls are reddened and covered with typical white patches. When the patches are swabbed off, bleeding may occur. Diagnosis is confirmed microscopically from a vaginal smear.

The patient is instructed in careful perineal care and hand washing to avoid reinfection and spread of the fungus to others, especially children. Mycostatin orally or in suppository form achieves good results. It may be given to pregnant women.

ATROPHIC VAGINITIS (SENILE). Because of hormonal changes following the menopause, the pH rises and the glycogen stores are reduced in the vagina. The vagina loses its rugae and becomes smooth and shiny. It is now more susceptible to invasion by organisms. A sticky, mucoid discharge may appear. The patient complains of a burning in the vagina, dyspareunia and pruritus of the vulva. Occasionally, the discharge is blood flecked, as areas of the vagina ulcerate and adhesions develop and tear. Infection is controlled by the use of systemic antibiotics or sulfa drugs. Estrogens are administered orally or vaginally. When the vaginitis is relieved, medication is stopped, and the patient may be advised to have cleansing vinegar douches periodically.

Cervicitis

The cervix is the main barrier against ascending infections of the genital tract. As such it is exposed to many insults. The majority of these are small lacerations which occur during childbirth or injuries associated with surgery, instrumentation or venereal disease. Bacteria invade these slits in the cervix. When the cervical epithelium is damaged, the infection easily spreads to the endocervix. Congestion and edema follow. An increase in cervical mucus results in an elevation in vaginal pH. The cells of the endocervix begin growing out around the external os. This outgrowth of cells produces a red, granular raised lesion. As the cervix is exposed to further trauma, the eroded areas become infected again and again. Chronic cervicitis results.

The symptoms vary. Usually a heavy vaginal discharge exists. The patient may notice deep dyspareunia or some bloodstained discharge following intercourse or douching.

The diagnosis depends on the characteristic appearance of the lesion. Cytologic studies are usually done to distinguish cervicitis from early carcinoma. When carcinoma is ruled out, the condition is generally treated by cautery of the endocervix. After cautery the old tissue sloughs away, followed by the regeneration of the new from the outside edges of the lesion. The patient should expect a brownish discharge for 1 to 2 weeks as the old tissue sloughs away.

Often patients with cervicitis need to be taught proper perineal care. The use of strong, irritating douches should be discouraged, and perineal hygiene is stressed.

Pelvic Inflammatory Disease (P.I.D.)

Pelvic inflammatory disease has come to mean all ascending pelvic infections once they are beyond the cervix. Many organisms may be responsible for the symptoms. However, among the most frequent are the gonococcus and *Staphylococcus aureus*. On occasion, tuberculosis and anaerobic bacteria can be causative. Symptoms may follow labor and delivery, a criminally induced abortion, surgical procedures, or a contact with gonorrhea or cervicitis. Other, rarer

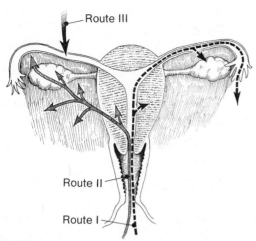

FIGURE 20–10 Common routes of the spread of pelvic inflammatory disease. Route I: commonly gonococcus and staphylococcus. Route II: frequently streptococcus. Route III: tuberculosis, usually a descending infection from another source.

causes exist as well. The condition may be acute or chronic.

SIGNS AND SYMPTOMS. The typical picture is one of a systemic infection with fever, chills, malaise, anorexia, nausea and vomiting. This is usually accompanied by lower abdominal pain which is either unilateral or bilateral. In more chronic cases, this pain is increased before and during menstruation. Pain is experienced on movement of the cervix. Leukorrhea is present. With gonorrheal or staphylococcal infections the discharge is usually heavy and purulent; streptococcal infections cause a thinner, more mucoid discharge.

Spread of the infection occurs by two typical routes, which are demonstrated in Figure 20–10. Symptoms depend on which route the infection follows. In Route I the bacteria spread along the surface of the endometrium to the tubes and into the peritoneum. The consequences of this route may be adhesions or cysts of the tube, with consequent infertility. In more advanced cases abscesses develop about the ovary or in the cul-de-sac. Infection following Route II is spread mainly through the lymphatics and produces a pelvic cellulitis in contrast to the more localized endometritis or salpingitis (infection of the uterine tube) of Route I. Thrombophlebitis may follow this cellulitis. Advanced and virulent infections admitted by either route may become systemic and may show all the signs of septicemia.

TREATMENT AND NURSING CARE. The patient with an acute episode is usually admitted to the hospital. She may or may not be isolated, depending on the cause of her infection. The patient is placed on bed rest in semi-Fowler's position to promote drainage of pus into the vagina and the cul-de-sac. Perineal care should be done as needed to keep the patient clean and comfortable. Douching is usually avoided, since it may only advance the infection further. Heat to the lower back and abdomen may be soothing. Analgesics and sedation may be ordered. The patient will receive antibiotics following culture and sensitivity studies. In some cases blood cultures may be obtained. Surgical treatment is deferred, if possible, until the infection is controlled. A culdocentesis or colpotomy may be done to drain a pelvic abscess. Tubo-ovarian abscesses may require an abdominal approach. In cases of prolonged, debilitating infections which are resistant to conservative treatment, salpingectomy or hysterectomy may be done.

VENEREAL DISEASE

The most common venereal diseases are gonorrhea and syphillis. Nonspecific urethritis is becoming of greater importance. A brief review of these follows.

Gonorrhea

The specific organism causing gonorrhea is *Neisseria gonorrhoeae*, and it is transmitted almost exclusively by sexual intercourse. The organism dies quickly when not harbored in the human body.

SIGNS AND SYMPTOMS. Symptoms appear 2 to 10 days after the initial contact. In the male urethritis occurs, heralded by a purulent urethral discharge. Some itching and burning about the meatus are also present. The urethral meatus is red and edematous. The infection may remain localized. However, an ascending infection involving the prostate, seminal vesicles, bladder and epididymus may result. If adhesions develop, they may damage the urethra and duct system with consequent urethral stricture and infertility.

Diagnosis is confirmed when the gonococcus is seen microscopically in smears or cultures taken from the urethra. If discharge is slight, the first urethral washings may be used. These are obtained by collecting the first portion of a voided urine specimen. The penis is not swabbed off before collecting the specimen.

In the adult female the vagina with its layers of squamous epithelium is resistant to the gonococcus. Therefore, the vulnerable areas are the vestibular glands, the urethra and the endocervix. The glands become red, swollen and sore. A purulent discharge may drain from the urethra and the ducts of the glands. Leukorrhea is present in cases in which cervicitis accompanies the picture. Dysuria and frequency often occur. Sometimes the symptoms may be mild and vague in the female. The infection may ascend above the cervix and may form the characteristic picture described in pelvic inflammatory disease.

Diagnosis is made on the basis of organisms seen in smears or cultures. To obtain these specimens the patient is instructed not to void or douche for approximately 2 hours before the cultures are taken. The vulva are not cleansed first. With the patient in a lithotomy position, smears are taken from the urethra, cervix and the ducts of the vestibular glands.

TREATMENT. Treatment with antibiotics, notably penicillin, is highly successful and has succeeded in reducing the incidence of complications. However, there is evidence of strains of gonococcus showing an increasing resistance to penicillin. Other antibiotics can be employed if penicillin does not eradicate the infection. Treatment is successful in cases in which repeated cultures are judged to be negative.

Nonspecific Urethritis

Nonspecific urethritis is an infection of the male urethra. The man complains of mild gonorrhea-like symptoms which may become severe. It is important to rule out gonorrhea as a cause. The onset of the symptoms is frequently related to coitus, often during menstruation when vaginal bacteria are increased, but in other cases no obvious link exists. In most cases no causative organism can be identified. Because no bacteria exist sensitivity tests are of little value. Treatment is frequently a combination of sulfonamides and tetracyclines. It may be resistant to therapy. Nonspecific urethritis appears to be less common among women.

Syphilis

Syphilis is a more serious disease and, fortunately, is less common than gonorrhea. The causative organism is the spirochete *Treponema pallidum*.

SIGNS AND SYMPTOMS. Incubation varies between 10 and 90 days. In most cases the disease is spread by sexual intercourse. As with the gonococcus, the spirochete does not survive outside the host. In the untreated condition, three stages are distinguished. The stages may overlap or be widely separated. The primary lesion is a small, painless chancre or ulcer. It is deep and has indurated edges. Usually this chancre heals spontaneously, giving the false impression that the disease is cured. This primary lesion appears most commonly on the penis of the male. In the female, it may appear on the labia, vagina or cervix. The secondary stage is usually characterized by a rash appearing over the body. This rash may be accompanied by condylomata lata on the female vulva. This is a cauliflower-appearing collection of flat, gray vulvar warts. As are all lesions of syphilis, these are teeming with spirochetes and are highly infectious. The rash is usually accompanied by malaise and fever. In a short period the rash regresses and the patient enters the latent stage. Latency refers to the absence of symptoms in the infected individual. Pregnant women can still infect their fetus in utero, thus demonstrating the infectiousness of the blood. However, progress of the disease in the individual seems arrested and only rarely can others be infected in this stage. Three outcomes are now possible: (1) the patient proceeds immediately or after a delay of 10 to 30 years to the third stage; (2) the disease remains latent for the rest of the person's life; or (3) a spontaneous cure occurs. In the tertiary stage the bones, heart, and central nervous system, including the brain, can be affected. Personality disorders arise and the typical ataxic gait of the tertiary syphilitic appears. A large, ulcerating necrotic lesion known as a gumma now occurs. Rarely is it seen in the genital tract, but it may occur on the vulva or in the testes. At this stage the disease may be arrested but not reversed.

Diagnosis is made by a careful history, clinical findings, and cultures or biopsies from the lesions. Blood serology is also assessed. Since blood serology is not positive for about 4 weeks after the onset of the disease, the early diagnosis is made from scrapings of the lesions. They can be seen on dark-field examination. These scrapings are made before antibiotic therapy is initiated so that the diagnosis can be confirmed. Blood serology tests such as the Kahn, Wassermann and VDRL are all reliable.

TREATMENT AND NURSING CARE. Treatment is by antibiotic, and penicillin is the drug of choice. Usually a series of injections is necessary.

Most cases of venereal disease are treated on an outpatient basis, and the patient must be taught how to protect himself and others. First, the nature and transmission of the disease should be understood. No immunity develops and reinfection can occur easily. Strict personal and perineal hygiene should be observed. Hand washing following any handling of the genitalia is imperative, as the gonococcus can be readily carried to the eye, which quickly becomes infected. Blindness may ensue if treatment is not received. Women who are handling small children need to be especially careful. Also, the vagina of a prepubertal girl is extremely sensitive to the gonococcus because it lacks the protective layers of squamous epithelium. A particularly distressing form of vulvovaginitis may occur as a result of contamination from a family member. Sexual intercourse is to be avoided until the physician notifies the patient he or she is cured. The nurse must practice all she teaches by following strict medical asepsis while caring for patients who are in the infectious stages of the disease. All equipment must be sterilized following use, and dressings or swabs are disposed of in a safe way. The disease may be transmitted by direct contamination with living spirochetes of a laceration. For this reason, the nurse who has a break in her skin must be very careful when dealing with the lesions of syphilis. Gloves may be indicated. Once therapy has been initiated, the patient is usually noninfectious within 48 hours.

The disease may be very distressing to the patient. The patient may experience guilt feelings, and marital difficulties may arise when one partner infects the other. The disease carries a social stigma. For these reasons, confidentiality must be maintained by the nurse at all times. Indeed, the issue is protected by law. However, the disease is reportable. Contacts must be identified and discreetly followed by the public health nurse. The nurse, by explaining the nature of the disease, usually obtains the patient's cooperation in identifying contacts. In addition, the nurse should include venereal disease in any lectures she prepares on general health education in the schools so that the population may become more aware of the signs and symptoms as well as the modes of transmission of these diseases.

DISPLACEMENTS AND RELAXATIONS OF THE FEMALE GENITAL ORGANS

Retroversion and Retroflexion of the Uterus

The normal position of the uterus is one of some anteversion and anteflexion (Fig. 20–11). It is not a fixed organ. The filling of the bladder or bowel may cause a change in uterine position. On occasion, the uterus assumes a retroverted or retroflexed position. When retroverted, the fundus points toward the sacrum and the cervix toward the anterior vaginal wall. Retroflexion refers to the position of the fundus of the uterus in rela-

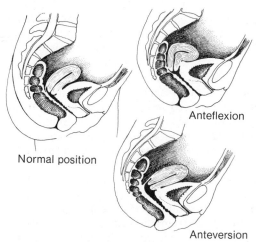

Anteflexion

Normal position

Anteversion

FIGURE 20–11 Normal position of the uterus, anteflexion, and anteversion.

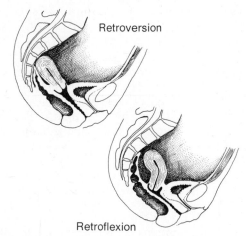

Retroversion

Retroflexion

FIGURE 20–12 Retroversion and retroflexion of the uterus.

tion to the cervix. In retroflexion the fundus bends back over the cervix (Fig. 20–12). Degrees of retroversion and retroflexion are possible so that the case may be mild or extreme.

The etiology appears to lie in a weakness of the supporting structures which may be either congenital or acquired. The acquired weakness is frequently due to injuries during the maternity cycle. Adhesions and tumors may pull or push the uterus into this position.

The patient may complain of backache, infertility, dyspareunia or dysmenorrhea, but she is frequently symptomless unless the situation is extreme. Backache and dysmenorrhea are probably associated with pelvic congestion. Infertility may arise because the cervix does not reach the seminal pool. Frequently, the ovaries prolapse into the cul-de-sac and become congested and enlarged. Because of this, intercourse may be painful.

TREATMENT AND NURSING RESPONSIBILITIES. Usually the uterus is manually replaced, and a vaginal pessary is inserted to hold the uterus in place. The most common pessaries used are the Smith-Hodge type. The pessary functions by holding the cervix in a posterior position. This in turn rotates the uterus forward. When the pessary is properly in position, the patient is unaware of its presence and no difficulty is experienced on voiding or during intercourse. The patient will return in about 4 to 6 weeks to have the pessary checked and removed for cleaning. The physician may then give the patient a 6-week trial period without the pessary to see if she remains free of symptoms. If not, a further trial with the pessary may be given.

The nurse frequently has to instruct the patient in proper personal hygiene after the insertion of the pessary. All pessaries are irritating, especially those which are rubber and have some degree of movement. An offensive-smelling leukorrhea usually develops, and chronic ulceration may occur. The patient will need to return for checkups as advised. Also, she will be instructed to douche every 2 to 3 days. This is best done when lying flat in the bathtub. The douche is held about 2 feet above the vagina and the inflow is by gravity. Occasionally, if warm water seems inadequate, a weak (0.5 per cent) solution of lactic acid may be used.

In other cases the uterus will be surgically suspended by shortening the round ligaments. This is done when the pessary does not correct the situation.

Prolapse, Cystocele and Rectocele

Uterine prolapse refers to the downward displacement of the entire organ. Prolapse (Fig. 20–13) may occur in varying degrees. First-degree prolapse describes the condition existing when the uterus descends within the vagina. Second-degree prolapse occurs when the cervix protrudes through the introitus. Procidentia, or third-degree prolapse, refers to the entire uterus protruding through the introitus with total inversion of the vagina.

Cystocele, urethrocele, rectocele and enterocele refer to herniations or relaxations of the bladder, urethra, rectum and small bowel into the vagina (Fig. 20–14). They may occur singly or in combinations with some degree of uterine prolapse.

The single most important etiologic factor in the development of these conditions is thought to be injury at childbirth. The pelvic floor and supporting structures may be stretched and torn during the process of delivery and are thereby weakened. Further relaxation results after menopause as the tissues atrophy following estrogen withdrawal. Large intra-abdominal tumors may also place an added strain on already weakened tissue. In some rare cases, the structures seem to be congenitally weak.

The patient with a prolapse often complains of a feeling of "something coming

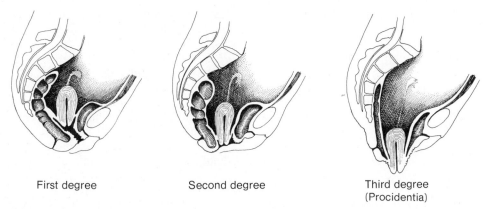

First degree

Second degree

Third degree
(Procidentia)

FIGURE 20–13 Uterine prolapse, showing first-, second- and third-degree (procidentia) prolapse.

down.'' She may have a dragging or heavy feeling in the pelvis, accompanied by backache. She may have bladder symptoms of either retaining or losing urine. She may have recurrent cystitis. When the cervix protrudes through the introitus, it may become ulcerated from constant friction. This may produce pain and bleeding. The patient with a cystocele frequently has symptoms of stress incontinence.

Diagnosis is usually confirmed by bimanual and rectal examinations. The patient will be asked to bear down, cough or strain while the doctor estimates the degree of prolapse or herniation.

TREATMENT AND NURSING RESPONSIBILITIES. The best treatment is prevention. Better care during the maternity cycle has helped to reduce the incidence of these complications. Exercises should be taught by the nurse to all patients in the postpartum period and the same exercises may be taught to help relieve mild prolapse. These consist of alternately tightening and relaxing the gluteal and perineal floor muscles. Practicing starting and stopping the stream of urine also helps the patient regain good perineal muscle tone. She should continue to practice these exercises several times a day for several weeks.

In situations in which surgery is contraindicated, the use of pessaries may be employed. A variety are available for different degrees of prolapse.

Surgical intervention is frequently necessary to correct the situation. An anterior and posterior colporrhaphy and perineorrhaphy repair a cystocele and rectocele, respectively.

If some prolapse of the uterus is present and future childbearing is not an issue, a Manchester repair may be done. This combines the amputation of an elongated cervix and shortening of the cardinal ligaments with an anterior and posterior repair. Although childbearing is not precluded by an anterior and posterior repair, delivery by cesarean section is usually recommended in order to retain this repair. Vaginal hysterectomy with an anterior and posterior repair is usually performed for more severe uterine prolapse. The uterine tubes and the uterus with all or part of the cervix will be removed. The ligaments and blood vessels are ligated, and a cuff is made in the upper portion of the vagina.

The nursing care of these patients is similar to that given to any patient undergoing surgery. However, the patient will receive a perineal shave preparation. Orders may be

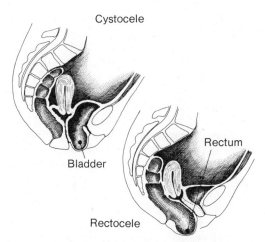

Cystocele

Bladder

Rectum

Rectocele

FIGURE 20–14 Cystocele and rectocele.

given outlining special perineal or vaginal preparations. The nurse should assist the patient in understanding the limitations, if any, surgery will impose on sexual and reproductive capacity, since many misunderstandings frequently occur.

During surgery the patient may receive intravenous vasoconstrictors to reduce the danger of hemorrhage. Blood loss during vaginal surgery tends to be heavy and is heavier still in premenopausal women.

The patient's legs are carefully lifted together to be placed into and removed from the stirrups. No one should lean or apply pressure on the anesthetized leg. These measures will reduce postoperative discomfort, avoiding strain on the repaired perineal muscles and help reduce the incidence of postoperative emboli. These same measures should be used whenever a patient's legs are placed in stirrups.

Following vaginal surgery, the nurse observes the patient for signs and symptoms of hemorrhage, urinary tract infection, thromboemboli and infections at the surgical site. Hemorrhage may be frank, oozing or in the form of a large hematoma. The oozing of blood may not be readily noticed by the patient or the staff; therefore, the nurse must be careful to observe the estimated blood loss over a period of time, not just each time she checks the patient. A hematoma is a form of concealed hemorrhage; the blood vessels bleed into the tissue of the vagina or perineum. The patient complains of discomfort or pain over the site. The tissue bulges and may be so taut as to glisten. The nurse should notify the physician immediately and be prepared to assist with treatment and the possible return of the patient to the operating room. Blood transfusions may be required. The clot may be evacuated, the bleeding vessels ligated or the site firmly packed. Antibiotics may be ordered to lessen the chance of infection.

Postoperatively the patient returns with a cystostomy tube. This is a small polyethylene tube which has been threaded through a needle into the bladder. The abdomen is surgically prepared, the bladder filled with sterile water, and the needle inserted. The tube is taped or caught with a stitch to the skin to avoid accidental removal and attached to a sterile drainage system. It drains freely for 3 to 4 days and the patient voids as she can. Seventy per cent of women void spontaneously for periods of time, before the tube is clamped, starting on the fourth day. If the tube leaks, tape may be placed around the base. The tube can be used to obtain residuals, but occasionally a catheter may have to be used. Cystostomy tubes have reduced the incidence of postoperative urinary tract infections by reducing the need for catheterizations. They also reduce the emotional tension surrounding first voiding.

In some cases the patient may have catheter drainage. She is catheterized preoperatively, and the catheter remains in place for 7 to 9 days until the edema has been resolved. The catheter is clamped and released for periods of time, finally removed, and then the patient attempts voiding. She is usually catheterized twice daily for residual urine during the first 24 to 36 hours without the catheter. If the amount of urine remaining in the bladder is above 75 to 100 ml., a Foley catheter may be reinserted or the cystostomy tube opened.

Voiding in sufficient quantities should occur at least every 6 hours. To induce the patient who is unable to void to do so requires all the nurse's skill in an attempt to avoid catheterization. Patients are usually ambulated early and getting up to void helps. If sitz baths or perineal irrigations are allowed, having the patient take one immediately before attempting to void usually helps. When catheterization is necessary, the strictest aseptic technique should be followed.

Perineal care is important to the prevention of infection. Depending on the extent of the surgery, sterile technique may be required. It should be as frequent as necessary to keep the perineal area clean and dry. General principles of working from front to back are followed. In addition, sterile pads are applied. Sitz baths may be ordered. The patient sits in a tub of water up to the level of the iliac crest. An irrigation may be ordered with sterile or plain water or some solutions. The nurse or patient runs the solution from a bag and tubing over the perineum into a basin. If the patient is well enough, she is frequently taught how to do these procedures.

Straining at stool is avoided by a low residue diet and the avoidance of constipation.

On discharge the patient may receive further instructions; some physicians definitely restrict heavy lifting and prolonged standing, walking and sitting. Intercourse is contraindicated for approximately 6 weeks.

Stress Incontinence

Stress incontinence is the involuntary loss of small amounts of urine when a woman coughs, sneezes or otherwise suddenly increases the intra-abdominal pressure and, therefore, the intravesical pressure. It should be distinguished from urge incontinence and frequency.

Continence is thought to be maintained at the junction of the urethra and bladder by continuous spiral muscles from the base of the bladder to the upper urethra. Assistance is also received from the muscles surrounding the urethra, as well as a tight supporting perineal floor. In the continent woman these relationships can be demonstrated radiologically by observing that the angle between the urethra and posterior wall of the bladder is approximately 90° (Fig. 20–15). Normally, this angle is only obliterated at micturition (Fig. 20–16) when an increased intra-abdominal pressure combines with a relaxed urethrovesical muscle and perineal floor to lower the base of the bladder. However, in stress incontinence, the slight effort of straining, coughing or sneezing is sufficient to reduce this angle, and an involuntary loss of urine occurs. This explanation is thought to describe about 90 per cent of cases of stress incontinence. A woman may have a cystocele (Fig. 20–15) and still be continent if the relationships demonstrated by the angle are maintained. However, many women with a cystocele also have accompanying stress incontinence.

Occasionally, stress incontinence follows a cystocele repair. This is probably due to elevation of the bladder to a position which obliterates the angle. For this reason many surgeons check the angle following repair to be sure it will be adequate.

The symptoms may become distressing to the woman. Frequent small dribbles of urine cause wetness, irritation and an offensive odor. The woman may have to wear a perineal pad or plastic pants continuously. Gradually she may become shy of social contacts and may confine herself to home.

Diagnosis is made on examination by the physician. Cystourethrograms may also be indicated. In this procedure a dye outlines the urethra and bladder, demonstrating the state of the angle at rest, during straining and, if possible, on micturition. A small chain may also be inserted to further outline the urethra on x-ray.

TREATMENT AND NURSING RESPONSIBILITIES. Treatment consists of prevention of injury by good maternity care and the practice of postpartum exercises in the immediate postpartum period. In some mild cases exercises may be prescribed and will help if practiced. In the older woman, the symptoms seem to be aggravated by a weakening of structures secondary to reduced estrogen stimulation.

Surgery may be necessary in order to sup-

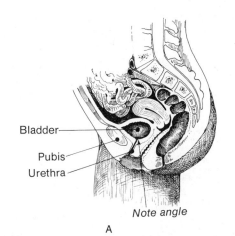

Bladder
Pubis
Urethra

Note angle

A

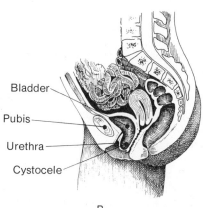

Bladder
Pubis
Urethra
Cystocele

B

FIGURE 20–15 *A,* The bladder at ease—no stress incontinence. *B,* Cystocele without stress incontinence.

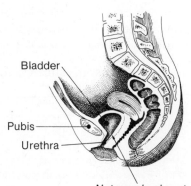

Note angle absent

FIGURE 20–16 The bladder during micturition.

port the urethra and restore the proper urethrovesical relationship. Two types of operations are commonly used.

In the Aldridge sling operation the surgeon makes a sling of fascia. This sling is then attached to the anterior abdominal wall. This serves to support the urethra, which can be demonstrated by observing the restoration of the angle. The approach may be abdominal, vaginal or both. Occasionally, the sling is too tight and the patient has difficulty micturating and emptying the bladder properly. Cystitis and other complications may occur. Teaching the patient to bend her body forward when attempting to void postoperatively helps. This relaxes the muscles of the abdomen, thereby loosening the sling and lowering the base of the bladder.

The Marshall-Marchetti-Krantz operation supports the urethra by suturing the anterior vaginal wall on each side to the periosteum of the pubic bone and the anterior wall of the bladder to the pubic bone.

Fistulae

Fistulae may occur between the vagina or uterus and the bladder, urethra or rectum (Fig. 20–17). They can occur as a sequel to injury during labor and delivery, surgery, and disease processes, such as carcinoma, and radiation therapy.

When urinary fistulae develop, some urine leaks into the vagina or uterus. Rectal fistulae cause the escape of flatus and feces into the vagina. In both instances, irritation to the tissues occurs. An offensive odor develops and causes much embarrassment for the patient. Since many fistulae spontaneously heal within a matter of several weeks, treatment may be postponed. During that period nursing care is very important to the patient. Frequent perineal care is required to keep the patient clean. Cleansing and deodorizing douches may be ordered. High enemas may be given to reduce the constant flow of feces. Care should be taken to go above the fistula with the rectal tube. If the fistula does not heal spontaneously, surgery may be indicated. Following surgery involving the bladder, the patient may return from the operating room with a urethral as well as a suprapubic catheter. Drainage must be maintained so that pressure on the repaired area is kept at a minimum. Repair may also include implantation of the ureters elsewhere. Rectal fistulae may be repaired and a temporary colostomy established in order to provide time to heal. Ambulation may be postponed for a few days. The woman may be discharged home on restricted activity until the physician advises that the repair is complete.

BENIGN AND MALIGNANT DISORDERS OF THE REPRODUCTIVE TRACT

In the Male

Spermatocele

A spermatocele is a cyst of the spermatic cord which contains sperm in a thin white fluid. It lies above the testis and is separate

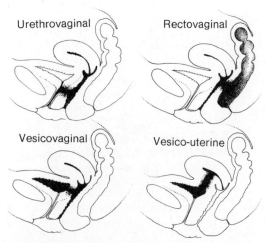

FIGURE 20–17 Fistulae: urethrovaginal; rectovaginal; vesicovaginal; and vesicouterine.

from it. The mass will transilluminate. Usually a spermatocele requires no treatment. Sometimes it may become large enough to be confused with hydrocele and to be aggravating to the patient. Then it may be excised. The etiology is unclear.

Varicocele

Varicocele is the dilatation of the venous plexus about the testis. It occurs most frequently on the left side. Its appearance on the right side may indicate that a tumor is occluding the vein above the level of the scrotum. Some testicular atrophy may occur if the circulation is impeded for long periods of time. This may result in subfertility. On palpation behind and above the testis the physician feels a mass of tortuous veins which empties when the patient lies down.

Treatment may consist of a scrotal support which relieves the dragging sensation. If fertility is an issue or the condition is severe, the internal spermatic vein may be ligated. The results are usually excellent. A scrotal support may be worn for 4 to 5 days following surgery, since scrotal edema may be present.

Hydrocele

A hydrocele is a collection of fluid in the tunica vaginalis. It may occur following local injury, infection or a neoplasm and may be unilateral or bilateral. More often it is chronic, and the cause is unknown. In newborn babies, the cause is usually a late closure of the processus vaginalis. This frequently closes spontaneously. In some young men a chronic type exists because the processus vaginalis never closes completely, and a connection remains between the peritoneal cavity and the tunica vaginalis.

Treatment is not required unless the testis cannot be palpated to rule out abnormality, circulation to the testis is impaired or the hydrocele becomes large, unsightly and uncomfortable. Then the hydrocele is aspirated, and a sclerosing drug may be injected. In chronic cases the tunica vaginalis is excised (hydrocelectomy). Postoperatively the scrotum is elevated on a pillow or bridge dressing, and a pressure dressing is applied. Depending on the operation, there may or may not be a drain present in the incision. The patient must be observed for hemorrhage which may be concealed in the hydrocele sac. When ambulatory the patient usually requires a fresh scrotal support daily. Immediately after the operation he may need a larger support than usual.

Torsion of the Testis

Torsion of the testis occurs when the testis rotates within the tunica vaginalis. Often this is due to spasm of the cremaster muscle which rotates the testis in what is usually an abnormally large vaginalis. The young man experiences a sudden severe pain in the area of the testis which is unrelieved by rest or support. Because the torsion reduces the blood supply to the testis, testicular atrophy follows rapidly. Sometimes under local anesthesia the physician will attempt to reduce torsion. If this is unsuccessful, surgical reduction follows.

Benign Hyperplasia of the Prostate

The reason benign enlargement of the prostate gland occurs is unknown. However, it is estimated that over 50 per cent of men over 60 show some signs of prostatic enlargement. Of these, about 25 per cent will require treatment.

In the young adult male the prostate gland is encased in a thin capsular membrane which is closely adherent to the underlying tissue. Gradually tissue begins to enlarge by new growth (hyperplasia) and the capsule of the prostate becomes thick and is loosely attached to the underlying tissue. This inner tissue can now be easily stripped away, leaving the thickened capsule intact.

However, there is much debate about what actually happens in a prostate gland undergoing hyperplasia. One theory states that the hyperplasia occurs in the periurethral glands (Fig. 20–18), which then press the true prostatic tissue outwards to form the thick capsule. In this case a procedure which leaves the capsule intact is not a prostatectomy. Others reason that the growth is primarily prostatic tissue, with periurethral glands included. Here prostatectomy is indeed performed, but only partially, as the posterior prostatic lobe which forms part of the capsule is not removed (Fig. 20–19). In any case the enlarging prostate en-

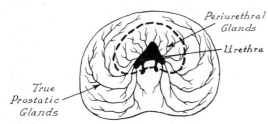

FIGURE 20–18 Transverse section of the adult prostate.

croaches on the urethra and the base of the bladder, producing certain symptoms.

SIGNS AND SYMPTOMS. Gradually, the man may experience hesitancy in beginning the flow of urine. The stream of urine is reduced in force and size. Incomplete emptying of the bladder produces residual urine which reduces bladder capacity so that urgency and frequency result. Nocturia occurring three or more times in one night is a good indication of frequency. Often, cystitis occurs as well. In severe cases, the bladder becomes overdistended, and hypertrophy and small diverticula follow as weakened areas of bladder mucosa bulge out between the bands of muscle fibers. The back-up of urine causes hydroureter or even hydronephrosis. Over long periods of time renal function may be impaired.

Frequently, the patient does not seek medical attention until acute retention of urine occurs. Overdistension of the bladder is usually the precipitating factor. The patient is catheterized and decompressed. Decompression allows for the slow release of urine from the bladder. This prevents a sudden

release of pressure in the abdomen which could cause shock and hemorrhage. Shock follows the rush of blood from vital centers to fill the newly released blood vessels. This sudden filling may cause small blood vessels in the bladder mucosa to rupture. The catheter remains in place for 2 to 3 days, after which normal voiding patterns usually return. The patient is then encouraged to maintain regular ejaculation to relieve prostatic congestion. He is cautioned to avoid an excessive intake of fluid in a short period of time, as this rapidly distends the bladder, precipitating retention. He should void frequently when he has the urge to do so in order to avoid overdistension of the bladder. If followed, these instructions should help the individual to avoid acute retention. However, one should remain alert for the patient with retention with overflow who voids frequent small amounts of urine. This may be seen in the chronic case with progressive upper urinary tract involvement.

Backache and sciatica may also bring the patient to the physician, since the enlarged prostate exerts pressure on nerves.

DIAGNOSIS AND TREATMENT. Treatment is indicated to relieve the symptoms and to prevent infections of the urinary tract and renal damage. If the amount of residual urine in the bladder is above 75 to 100 ml., the physician may feel treatment is necessary even though the symptoms are not severe. Residual urine is estimated in several ways. Immediately after voiding, a catheter may be passed and any remaining urine is drawn off and measured. A radiopaque dye can be injected into the bladder. The man is then asked to void and postvoiding films are made. Direct visualization of the bladder may be done by cystoscope, and any bladder changes will be noted. Intravenous pyelograms will indicate the extent of ureter and kidney involvement. Renal function tests may be ordered as well.

Treatment is usually surgical removal of the enlarged structures. A period of preoperative preparation may be necessary. Residual urine and hydroureter are treated by catheterization for a period of 1 to 2 weeks. The patient is prepared for surgery by explaining what may follow the operation so that the postoperative period is not so traumatic. Because of the incidence of postprostatectomy epididymitis, the vas deferens may be ligated to prevent this complication.

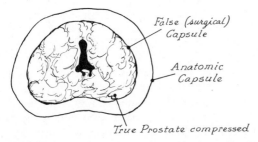

FIGURE 20–19 Transverse section of a hyperplastic prostate.

The operation may be done concurrently or preoperatively. A signed consent is required.

Several operations are commonly used to treat this condition. The choice of operation seems to depend on the size of the prostate, the condition of the patient and the preference of the surgeon. A prostate in excess of 50 Gm. is considered by most surgeons to be too difficult to remove transurethrally. Therefore, an open route is chosen.

TRANSURETHRAL PROSTATECTOMY. This procedure is the most frequently performed operation and is the closed method. Postoperative recovery is usually rapid; sexual potency is maintained, and urinary results are good. The operation is performed with a resectoscope, an instrument similar to a cystoscope but equipped with cutting and cauterizing attachments. This slender instrument is inserted up the urethra to the prostatic urethra, and the enlarged prostate is chipped away. The capsule remains intact. During the operation, the bladder and urethra are continuously irrigated with a sterile, isotonic, nonconductive clear fluid. In this manner, debris and blood are washed away. Following removal of the intracapsular tissue, a Foley catheter with a 30-ml. bag is passed. The catheter bag is pulled down into the prostatic fossa where it exerts pressure on blood vessels and helps to prevent hemorrhage. The catheter is usually attached to straight drainage, but it may be attached to medium or high decompression drainage. If hemorrhage has been a problem, the patient may have a cystostomy tube attached to continuous irrigation. This acts as a safety valve should clots plug the catheter.

The decompression drainage aids hemostasis by keeping constant pressure on the prostatic fossa. Also, the partially full bladder may help reduce bladder spasm. However, care should be taken to check that the catheter is draining and that the bladder is not full. A full bladder may cause hemorrhage by "milking" the blood vessels in the fossa.

Immediately after the operation the catheter drainage is bloody. The nurse must be alert for signs of hemorrhage by paying close attention to the blood pressure and pulse of the patient and the amount of drainage. Frequent irrigations of the catheter are usually ordered. If the catheter becomes plugged, the physician is notified.

The fluid used to irrigate the bladder during the operation may be absorbed, causing hemodilution. The signs and symptoms of this may be those of sodium deficiency or excessive blood volume. Complaints of headache, nausea, vomiting or muscle weakness should not be ignored by the nurse but must be reported. Hypertension, restlessness, apprehension, shortness of breath or blurred vision likewise should be reported. If the physician expects that the operation may be more than 2 hours long, fluid intake may be restricted for 12 hours before the operation. Following the operation, 200 to 300 ml. of normal saline may be given intravenously over 2 hours. The nurse must observe the patient for signs of pulmonary edema.

Frequently, the irritation of the catheter gives the patient the urge to void. With a properly draining catheter this usually passes. However, if the patient attempts to void around the catheter, the bladder muscles contract and make the patient more uncomfortable. Careful preoperative preparation of the patient so that he understands the phenomenon and therefore does not try to void postoperatively usually is the greatest help to the patient. In severe cases, the patient will need sedation or an analgesic to obtain relief. If the catheter causes the patient great discomfort postoperatively, the nurse should check for other causes. Frequently, this increased discomfort is due to an overdistended bladder produced from a catheter which is not draining properly or from hemorrhage into the bladder. Occasionally, the bladder has been perforated during the operation and the hemorrhage is perfusing into the abdominal cavity. All of these require immediate attention — complaints of pain by the patient should never be ignored or go uninvestigated by the nurse.

Because hemorrhage remains a threat, even in the later postoperative period, care is taken to prevent its occurrence. The patient is cautioned against straining to pass stool, and a light diet is usually ordered. Enemas, rectal tubes and rectal thermometers are frequently contraindicated during the first postoperative week.

Because of the danger of a urinary tract infection, prophylactic antibiotics are frequently given for approximately 2 weeks postoperatively. The catheter is removed 3 to 7 days postoperatively and, for a short period following this, the patient is usually instructed to record and measure each voiding. If difficulty in voiding is still present, the catheter may be reinserted. The nurse should watch for signs of incontinence which may follow or signs of urinary retention which may indicate a urethral stricture. Before being discharged the patient should be told that an episode of bleeding may occur about the second to fourth week postoperatively. In that event, he should contact his physician and come to the emergency department of the hospital. Also he is warned to avoid any straining, heavy lifting or vigorous exercise for about 1 month postoperatively.

SUPRAPUBIC PROSTATECTOMY. This operation may be chosen when the prostate is large and when some bladder surgery is indicated as well. Sexual potency is maintained following the operation.

A small abdominal incision is made above the pubis and directly over the bladder. The bladder is opened and, through another incision into the urethral mucosa, the prostate is excised. The prostatic capsule remains intact. Various methods of draining the bladder and applying pressure to the operative site may be used postoperatively. A Foley catheter with a large bag and a cystostomy tube may be used. Sometimes a cystostomy tube with packing or a hemostatic bag in the prostatic fossa is used. Traction to maintain pressure on the hemostatic bag is achieved by attaching it to a birdcage apparatus which is placed between the patient's thighs. The packing and the hemostatic bag may have to be removed in the operating room at a later date. Sometimes only a Penrose drain in the abdominal incision is all that is judged necessary. It is usually removed after 36 hours. Special urethrostomy cups may have to be used in these cases to keep the patient dry and to collect urine for measurement. If a cystostomy tube is present, it is removed 3 to 4 days postoperatively. The indwelling catheter usually stays until the abdominal incision is nearly healed. The suprapubic incision may take time to heal. The nurse will need to have skill in keeping the patient dry and odorless. Bladder spasm is a frequent difficulty to these patients. Usually the muscles become fatigued in 24 to 48 hours and the bladder spasms become fewer. Recovery may be prolonged, since ambulation is slower.

RETROPUBIC PROSTATECTOMY. This method is preferred by many surgeons. Urinary results are excellent and potency is maintained. An abdominal incision is made above the bladder. The bladder is not incised, but the surgeon dissects down between the pubis and the bladder to reach the prostate. The capsule is opened and the tissue is removed. A large Foley catheter is inserted postoperatively. Since the bladder has not been opened, discharge on the abdominal dressing should not contain urine. If it does, the surgeon should be notified. The postoperative care is the same as for any prostatectomy patient. These patients seem to have fewer bladder spasms and less difficulty voiding.

PERINEAL PROSTATECTOMY. In a perineal prostatectomy the surgeon excises the prostate through a semicircular incision in the perineal body. The prostatic capsule is opened and the gland is removed. The pre- and postoperative care resembles that of other prostatectomies. A perineal shave preparation will be necessary. Because of the risk of rectourethral fistula, the large bowel may be surgically prepared preoperatively. Unfortunately, after this operation is performed the patient may be impotent, and some difficulty may be experienced in establishing urinary continence following surgery.

CRYOSURGERY. For patients unable to tolerate regular surgery, cryosurgery is being performed. The patient is prepared as though he were going for a cystoscopic examination. A local anesthetic with sedation is used. To protect the bladder walls the bladder is distended with sterile water or air. Then the probe with the freezing agent, either liquid nitrogen or nitrous oxide, is inserted into the prostatic urethra and the tissue destroyed. The patient returns to the ward with a self-retaining catheter attached to straight drainage until he can void on his own. This usually occurs within 10 to 21 days. The advantages of the method include little hemorrhage and early ambulation. However, there is some danger of retaining the sloughed tissue and damage to the surrounding tissues.

Carcinoma of the Prostate

Carcinoma of the prostate gland is one of the most common tumors seen in men. Perhaps 16 per cent of all malignancies in the adult male are due to prostatic lesions. The tumor most often arises in the posterior prostatic lobe and is hormone-related, depending upon androgens to retain its integrity. The tumor also causes an increase in the secretion of acid phosphatase which is normally high in prostatic secretions. This increased production is reflected in blood serum levels and may indicate a prostatic tumor. Cancer of the prostate is frequently seen in association with benign hyperplasia but does not result from it. In addition, surgery for benign hyperplasia is not prophylactic against cancer as the posterior prostatic lobe is retained.

Because of its frequency and the fact that early diagnosis can be made in most cases by a rectal examination, all men should be advised to have an annual checkup after the age of 40. Nurses are advised to include this advice whenever it is related in their health teaching to the community.

SIGNS AND SYMPTOMS. The symptoms are essentially those of benign enlargement of the prostate. On rectal examination, the surgeon palpates a hard nodule. Since the nodule may resemble other conditions, a biopsy is often done. Two types are commonly used. A *needle biopsy* is safely done on an outpatient basis. The perineum is cleansed and draped. The surgeon palpates the nodule with one finger in the rectum, and simultaneously guides a needle, passed through the perineum, to the site. Several samples are usually collected. On discharge, the patient is instructed to watch the injection site for signs of redness, pain and swelling and to report their occurrence to his physician. This technique is not judged to be as complete as *direct biopsy*. Under anesthesia, the perineum is cleansed, and a small incision is made. Direct biopsy of the prostate is made and sent to the laboratory. If immediate results are positive, a prostatectomy may be done before the patient leaves the operating room. If negative, the incision is closed, and the surgeon awaits the more extensive laboratory report. Because of the possibility of an immediate prostatectomy, the patient is prepared for the operating room as if he were undergoing major surgery.

CLASSIFICATION. Carcinoma of the prostate is classified into four stages. These stages are based on the results of rectal examinations, serum acid phosphatase levels, x-rays of the skeleton and metastases. Stage I, or carcinoma in situ, is often called latent, or focal. Usually there are no symptoms. In Stage II the nodule may be palpated on rectal examination, and serum acid phosphatase levels will be elevated in approximately 50 per cent of men. When Stage III is reached, the growth has spread to the seminal vesicles, the base of the bladder and outside the prostatic capsule, but no distant metastases are present. Seventy-five per cent of men will show elevated serum acid phosphatase levels. With Stage IV carcinoma excessive levels of serum acid phosphatase circulate in the blood stream. Previously, the thick prostatic capsule has kept the lesion localized and prevented spread into the abdominal cavity. Now the blood and lymphatics have carried the disease to distant sites. The bones of the pelvis are most frequently affected, and elevated serum alkaline phosphatase levels reflect this spread. Also, because of bone and liver involvement, severe anemia may occur, accompanied by the other symptoms of a terminal disease.

TREATMENT AND NURSING CARE. Stages I and II are treatable. Stages III and IV usually receive palliative therapy. Treatment is by radical prostatectomy by the retropubic or perineal routes. The entire gland and seminal vesicles are removed. The bladder neck is sutured to the urethral stump. A large Foley catheter is inserted which serves as a splint for the urethra as well as a drain for the bladder. Drains may be placed in the incision lines as well. Pre- and postoperative care are similar to that of any prostatectomy.

Incontinence may follow temporarily or on a longer basis. Immediately after the operation the man may be incontinent of feces as well. The patient is usually greatly relieved to be assured that this is usually temporary and that control can be regained by practicing perineal floor tightening and relaxing a few times periodically throughout the day. This also aids in the reestablishment of urinary continence. Some surgeons ban the use of incontinence clamps or bags, feeling that the patient comes to rely on them and will never regain function. In particularly resistant cases, a prosthesis with an inflatable bulb may be inserted below the urethra in an attempt to restore normal anatomy. Hopefully, this will restore continence.

If the perineal route was used, care must be taken to avoid infection. The incision must be kept clean by cleansing frequently and following bowel movements. A heat lamp and sitz baths may be ordered for several days postoperatively. The scrotum may be elevated on an adhesive bridge in order to acquire adequate exposure of the incision. In the presence of hemorrhoids, a heat lamp is usually contraindicated.

In Stages III and IV palliative therapy includes the administration of estrogens in high doses. This suppresses the production of androgens upon which the tumor is dependent. The patient experiences relief, and life is prolonged. However, the side effects may be severe, so that estrogen is usually reserved for patients with metastases. Some physicians may give lower doses of estrogens in the earlier stages to shrink the tumor before surgery. The side effects include edema of the ankles, tender gynecomastia, some nausea and vomiting, impotence with loss of libido, and a significant increase in the incidence of death from thromboembolic disease. The patient on estrogens is observed for these side effects. Sodium intake is reduced in order to reduce edema, and prior radiation of breast tissue will make the breast unresponsive. Eventually the effect of the estrogens is reduced, and an orchiectomy (removal of testes) may be done to reduce the amount of androgens in the body.

This combination of estrogens and orchiectomy may produce good results for about 18 months. Then the adrenals seem to recover from the estrogen-induced hormonal imbalance and begin producing androgens again. Cortisone may be given now in an attempt to depress this source of androgens. In extreme situations an adrenalectomy may be performed. Deep x-ray therapy reduces discomfort from bone metastases. Radioactive phosphate given orally or intravenously also lodges in the bone, bringing relief from pain. In the case of a bladder obstruction, a transurethral prostatectomy is done. Since the operation is merely palliative, no attempt is made to remove all of the growth.

The patient will require nursing care related to the special needs of the cancer patient (Chap. 10) and to the aforementioned prostatectomy therapies.

Carcinoma of the Testes and Penis

Most tumors of the testes are malignant. However, only about 0.5 per cent of all malignancies occur in this area. Frequently, the man is in the prime of his reproductive years. Treatment is bilateral orchiectomy followed by radiation therapy to the lumbar lymph nodes.

Malignancies of the penis are essentially malignancies of the skin. The glans and prepuce are nearly always affected. The disease is less frequent among circumcised men. Treatment is by excision of the affected areas or by partial or total amputation of the penis.

In the Female

Polyps

Polyps are common benign growths occurring mainly in the endometrium and cervix. The polyp has a characteristic smooth, shiny surface and is pink to deep red in color. They are small in size, seldom exceeding more than 3 cm. in length. The cause is unknown. No symptoms are usually present, but occasionally postcoital bleeding occurs. Treatment is by surgical excision of cervical polyps and may be followed by dilation and curettage to remove endometrial polyps. The patient receives nursing care as for minor vaginal surgery.

Myomas of the Uterus

A myoma (fibromyoma, leiomyoma) is a benign tumor of the uterus composed of myometrium and fibrous tissue. Colloquially, myomas are known as "fibroids." At least 25 per cent of women over 35 years of age show some evidence of myomas. The cause is unknown.

Myomas occur mainly in the uterine body. According to their position they are classified as subserous, submucous and intramural (Fig. 20–20), and may become pedunculated. A pedunculated fibroid in the uterine cavity may be referred to as a fibroid polyp. This may be extruded through the cervix and may come to lie in the vagina. Myomas in the broad ligament or cervix are recorded, but these locations are rare. Several fibroids of varying sizes may be present in any one uterus. As the fibroids become larger, their blood supply may be reduced, causing some degeneration. The most common is a hyaline degeneration in the middle of the myoma. This causes a loss of cellular structure and, in extreme cases, a collection of gelatinous fluid lies at the center. Sometimes the tumor

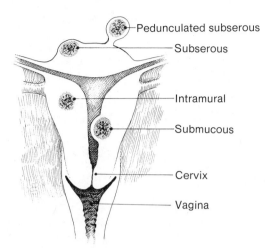

- Pedunculated subserous
- Subserous
- Intramural
- Submucous
- Cervix
- Vagina

FIGURE 20–20 Uterine fibroids.

shows signs of fatty changes and may even become calcified (womb-stone). A so-called red degneration may occur, usually in association with pregnancy. The tumor looks like raw beef on the inside. The patient shows signs of malaise with fever, rapid pulse and pain over the fibroid. Following menopause all myomas atrophy and show slight shrinkage.

SIGNS AND SYMPTOMS. Symptoms vary with the size and location of the tumor. Frequently, with small tumors, there are no symptoms. Occasionally hypermenorrhea occurs. Pain is rarely a symptom but most frequently is associated with torsion of a pedunculated myoma. Sometimes the myoma passing through the cervix causes cramps. Dysmenorrhea may occur as a result of mechanical interference. Large myomas can cause frequency or retention of urine. Pressure on veins, lymphatics, and nerves of the pelvis may cause varicosities, unilateral or bilateral edema of the lower extremities, or a radiating pain through the thighs. Occasionally, these tumors may be the cause of abortions or infertility. Some tumors become infected.

TREATMENT. Treatment depends on the age of the woman, her desire for more children and the size of the myoma. In the young woman who wishes children, a myomectomy is usually done. This is the enucleation of the myoma, but the uterus is retained. Blood loss during the operation may be extensive as the surgeon excises multiple myomas from a large uterus which may not contract efficiently. Persistent oozing of blood may

occur postoperatively for the same reasons. The nurse should be alert to this possibility. In cases of very large myomas the treatment is hysterectomy.

In the young woman, myomas are not a contraindication to pregnancy and usually cause no difficulty. Rarely, they may obstruct labor or cause a postpartum hemorrhage.

TUMORS OF THE OVARY. Tumors of the ovary are many and varied. The etiology of most is unknown. For purposes of clarity they are roughly divided into non-neoplasms and neoplasms. Only a few are described in each group.

NON-NEOPLASMS. Non-neoplasms are usually simple cysts or collections of fluid surrounded by a thin capsule. They do not grow but expand only as more fluid accumulates. These physiological cysts are seen mainly during the reproductive years. The follicular cyst is the most common of this group. Corpus luteum cysts may occur as well. Theca lutein cysts develop under the stimulation of high levels of chorionic gonadotrophins.

Occasionally, the Stein-Leventhal syndrome or polycystic disease of the ovary is distinguished. The syndrome appears in the late teens and early twenties with variable symptoms. These may include a history of sterility, secondary amenorrhea, hirsuitism and bilateral cysts in the ovary. The ovary shows some enlargement and presents a glistening white appearance. Microscopically, many atretic follicular cysts are present. The syndrome is thought to follow an endocrine imbalance, probably arising in the ovary but affecting the hypothalamus. Treatment is usually surgical, and a wedge resection of the ovary is performed. Ovulation, menstruation and pregnancy may follow a wedge resection in a sizable proportion of cases. The nursing of the patient is the same as that for any patient undergoing abdominal surgery. Clomiphene has also attained some success.

NEOPLASMS. Pseudomucinous cystadenomas are the single most common neoplasms, occurring in about 40 per cent of patients with a neoplastic ovarian growth. Also, they may attain the largest size of any ovarian tumor. The tumor is characterized by multiple pockets filled with a thick fluid called pseudomucin. They may be bilateral and may become malignant.

Serous cystadenoma is the second most

common of this group and appears to arise from germinal epithelium. The cyst contains a serous fluid. These cysts are frequently bilateral and often become malignant.

The dermoid cyst or teratoma may be cystic or solid. When it is soft, the cyst is filled with sebaceous material, hair and ordinary skin. The solid cyst frequently contains cartilage, bone, teeth, thyroid, and similar material. Rarely is the cyst malignant. It occurs most frequently in young women and may be bilateral.

Neoplasms of the ovary may also be divided into those which have some hormonal effect and those which do not. One tumor with no hormonal effect is a *dysgerminoma*. It arises from the primitive germ cells and is usually malignant. A *fibroma* is a benign solid neoplasm occurring most frequently in the postmenopausal patient. The fibroma arises from connective tissue in the ovary and may be associated with Meigs' syndrome, which is characterized by ascites and pleural effusion.

Those tumors which have hormonal effects may be further subdivided into feminizing and virilizing lesions. The most common of the rare feminizing tumors is the *granulosa cell tumor*. The tumor produces estrogen and may induce precocious puberty or cause hypermenorrhea or postmenopausal bleeding. It may be malignant or may be associated with carcinoma of the endometrium. The most common of the even rarer masculinizing tumors is *arrhenoblastoma*. By the production of androgens, presumably from the primitive male cell elements in the ovary, the woman is masculinized. In about 15 to 25 per cent of cases it proves to be malignant.

Carcinoma of the Ovary

Primary carcinoma of the ovary is usually the common adenocarcinoma. However, a review of ovarian growths is indicated, as almost any one of them has the potential to become malignant. The most common malignancy arises from the serous cystadenoma. Only one ovary may be affected but the other quickly follows, apparently because of the close lymphatic connections. About 5 per cent of all cancers in the female arise in the ovary.

Secondary tumors represent metastases from almost any other cancer. However, the Krukenberg tumor deserves mention. In this case bilateral, equal involvement is usually secondary to tumors in the stomach or gallbladder. Back-up of the lymphatic drainage appears responsible for this particular tumor, especially since other metastases usually occur later.

SIGNS AND SYMPTOMS. The ovarian tumor in its early stages is often symptomless. At regular yearly checkups, palpation of the adnexa will reveal a mass. Often this may be the first discovery of the tumor. The symptoms commonly result from the size of the tumor or its position. An increase in girth may be noticed but ignored. Pressure on the bladder causes frequency or a feeling of fullness. Constipation, edema of the legs, anorexia and a full feeling in the abdomen may be present. Pain may be associated with stretching of the tissues as the tumor enlarges. Ascites may be present, accompanied by difficulty in breathing.

TREATMENT. Because of the danger of malignant growth, any ovarian mass is observed suspiciously. A rule of thumb says that any soft mass below 5 cm. may be watched closely for 2 to 3 months. If no further growth occurs, then conservative treatment may be considered. Other tumors demand biopsy, and a laparotomy is indicated. Following diagnosis, the surgeon strives to preserve as much ovarian function as is possible. In premenopausal women benign growths, if size permits, will be enucleated and ovarian function retained. Malignant growths are treated with total hysterectomy and bilateral salpingo-oophorectomy (removal of the tubes and ovaries). Surgery is followed by irradiation. Unfortunately, many malignancies have metastasized before discovery of the tumor. Prognosis is poor and surgery may be only palliative. Further treatment is directed toward relieving the symptoms of the terminally ill patient. Recurrent ascites may be a problem, and frequent paracentesis may be indicated. Occasionally intraperitoneal colloidal gold or chemotherapy will be used.

COMPLICATIONS OF OVARIAN TUMORS. Torsion or twisting of the growth on its stalk frequently occurs. Circulation is impeded, and necrosis may follow. The patient usually feels a sudden severe pain in the lower abdomen. Treatment is by excision of the tumor at an immediate laparotomy.

The cyst may rupture. Often the "chocolate cyst" of endometriosis ruptures and drains fluid into the abdomen. Again the patient may present with an "acute abdomen."

Hemorrhage and infection occur in tumors as well. Usually, they are more common in the malignant tumor.

Postsurgical menopause is the result of a bilateral oophorectomy. The symptoms are similar to those of the regular menopause, but may be more severe because of the sudden withdrawal of hormones. Replacement therapy with estrogens may begin before the patient leaves the hospital if it is not contraindicated by malignancies which are aggravated by estrogens.

Carcinoma of the Cervix

Carcinoma of the cervix is the second most frequent malignancy in women. The woman who has borne children, married young, or had an early active sex life with several partners is more apt to develop the disease. She is more likely to be above the age of 35.

Cancer of the cervix is a complex disease which is preceded by several earlier cervical changes (Table 20–3).

These changes usually occur at the squamocolumnar junction of the cervix (Fig. 20–21), and initially are evident only on histologic examination. They reflect a varied pattern of development. Some cases arise with no known precursor stage, while others appear to have gone through all the changes or any combination of them. The earlier changes may be reversible, and so do not always herald cancer. How many of these will reverse is unknown, but about 50 per cent of women with carcinoma in situ are thought to develop invasive cancer; this development may take an average of 10 years. The Pap smear is the best method of early detection of these changes. Combined with treatment of these changes it is largely re-

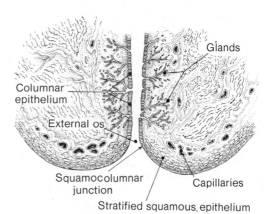

FIGURE 20–21 Squamocolumnar junction of the cervix.

sponsible for the declining mortality rates associated with cervical cancer.

Because 5-year survival rates are excellent in those cases which are discovered early, all women who are sexually active or over 25 should have yearly medical examinations and Pap smears. The nurse has a responsibility to disseminate this knowledge. The nurse should dwell on the hopeful aspects of cure following cases of early recognition. This may encourage more women to seek medical attention by reducing their anxiety. Fear of what she may discover often seems to prevent the patient from consulting her physician. The nurse should do her utmost to persuade the woman confiding irregular bleeding to her to seek medical attention immediately.

SIGNS AND SYMPTOMS. A small lesion develops which, in the early stages, can be confused with other cervical conditions. The early stages may be asymptomatic, but eventually some bleeding from the vagina occurs. An unusual vaginal discharge may be present. This may become foul-smelling, suggesting an infection. Pain is a late symptom and is followed by weight loss, anorexia and cachexia.

Carcinoma of the cervix is divided into stages. Stage 0 is carcinoma in situ, or focal carcinoma. There is an intact basement membrane containing the malignant cells. To some, Stage 0 is not considered in a staging of cancer as it is thought to be a separate condition. Stage I is invasive cancer, which means that the basement membrane has been breeched and the cells are invading the surrounding tissue. Stages IA and IB refer to

TABLE 20–3   PATTERNS OF DEVELOPMENT OF CANCER OF THE CERVIX

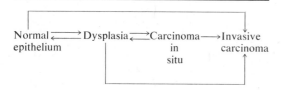

degrees of this invasion which is still within the confines of the cervix. Unfortunately, about 20 per cent of Stage I will already have spread to the lymphatics. A small lesion similar to an erosion may be present on the cervix. In Stage II the carcinoma has spread to close adjacent structures, and the upper third of the vagina may be involved. By Stage III invasion has reached the pelvic walls and lower vagina. Stage IV is marked by extensive pelvic involvement, including the bladder or bowel, and distant metastases may be present.

TREATMENT AND NURSING CARE. Treatment is usually guided by the stage assigned to the situation by the physician. Since the main method of diagnosing Stage 0 carcinoma is the Pap smear, the results of this test help to guide treatment. The Pap smear results are organized into five classes. In Classes I and II the cells are nonmalignant, and no treatment is necessary. Class III is suspicious and arouses concern. The patient is asked to have repeat smears done in 3 months or is biopsied. Classes IV and V are positive, indicating that definite changes are present which require biopsy.

BIOPSY. A *punch biopsy* may be done with special punch biopsy forceps. Because of the paucity of nerve endings in the cervix, the biopsy may be done with relative comfort for the patient. She may feel something like a pinch when the biopsy is taken. A Schiller test can be done. Normally the cervix contains glycogen. This is depleted in areas of abnormal cell change. When Lugol's solution (iodine in potassium iodide) is swabbed on the cervix, the normal epithelium stains a dark brown. Glycogen-deficient areas are a pale color by contrast, and these are the areas biopsied.

Further treatment may be a *cone biopsy*. It is an operative procedure in which a cone-shaped segment of the central cervix is removed. The internal os remains intact (Fig. 20–22). On examination the section may contain all of the malignant area. In these cases the biopsy may be considered sufficient treatment. Pre- and postoperative care for the biopsy is similar to any minor vaginal surgery. The major difference is that these patients face the threat of a malignant disease and may be extremely anxious. Considerable skill in providing supportive nursing will be demanded of the nurse. Hemorrhage is a threat, and the patient should be warned of this.

The biopsy results may indicate normal cells, dysplasia, carcinoma in situ or invasive carcinoma. Many situations contribute to dysplasia, and the patient is usually treated for these and followed closely with repeat Pap smears. Some of these will revert back to normal epithelium. If they do not, a cone biopsy may be performed or, in the older woman, a hysterectomy. Carcinoma in situ may be treated with close follow-up or coning if the woman wishes more children or by total hysterectomy. All carcinoma in situ must be treated to insure prevention of most invasive carcinoma. Invasive carcinoma of the cervix will be treated according to the stage in which it is classified.

SURGERY AND RADIATION THERAPY. Stages 1A and 1B and some early Stage II's are treated by radical surgery (modified Wertheim's hysterectomy), which attempts to eliminate the cancer, and radiation therapy. There is much debate over the optimum approach. Some prefer radiation alone; others prefer surgery with or without radiation. In major medical centers, with highly

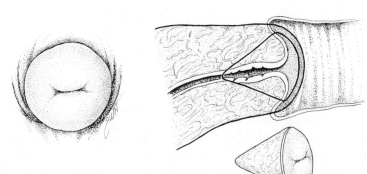

FIGURE 20–22 Cone biopsy of the cervix.

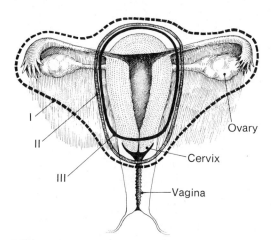

FIGURE 20–23 Types of hysterectomy. I: total hysterectomy with bilateral salpingo-oophorectomy (panhysterectomy). II: total hysterectomy. III: subtotal hysterectomy.

qualified surgeons and sophisticated radiation equipment and radiologists, higher cure rates have been recorded with a combination of surgery and radiation. In smaller centers lacking highly experienced surgeons some quote higher cure rates for radiation alone. Most seem to agree that Stages III and IV are best treated by radiation and some palliative surgery. In cases where the surgeon feels that the tumor is surgically excisable a pelvic exenteration is done. Surgery is, of course, used in cases of a radioresistant tumor.

The patient who is having a total hysterectomy (Fig. 20–23) for carcinoma in situ will have the uterus, cervix and upper third of the vagina removed. The ovaries are conserved in most cases of the premenopausal woman but may be removed in the older woman. The patient is prepared as for abdominal surgery. A perineal shave preparation may be ordered as well, and the mons pubis, vulva, perineal body, and the upper third of the thighs are shaved. Postoperatively, any vaginal discharge must be observed. Some staining may occur from the vaginal cuff. A Foley catheter may be inserted and may remain in place for 1 or 2 days postoperatively. The nurse should be alert to possible signs of hormonal imbalance following removal of the ovaries as well as signs of a urinary tract infection and thromboemboli.

In a Wertheim's hysterectomy the uterus, ovaries, broad ligaments, surrounding tissue, upper half of the vagina and pelvic lymph nodes are removed. Sometimes the ovaries will be retained, especially in a younger woman. In a more extensive Wertheim's operation, the pelvic fascia and further lymph tissue will be removed. Preoperatively the patient has a cystostomy examination and her ureters are catheterized. This allows them to be easily identified during the extensive pelvic dissection. The patient's vagina and cervix are painted with an iodine solution to identify any glycogen-deficient areas which would indicate further vaginal resection.

When the patient returns to the ward she will require general postoperative care, as with any other surgical patients. However, she may have several drains. Two red rubber drains may have been inserted, one in either lower quadrant, and attached to drainage bottles or low Gomco suction. These are advanced about the fourth postoperative day and removed when there is no drainage. Drainage is usually more extensive if no radiation has been given before surgery, and less if radiation has been given. Two Penrose drains, one on either side, may be draining into the vagina. They are advanced about the third postoperative day and removed about the fifth day if drainage has ceased. If oozing of blood was a problem during surgery, the pelvis may have been packed with a gauze pack, the tail of which is brought out through the vaginal cuff into the vagina. This is usually advanced in 48 hours and removed in 72 hours. The ureters and bladder have been handled during surgery and may be atonic. Care must be taken to see that the catheter is draining properly and that bladder distention does not occur. The catheter should drain clear urine. Special attention should be directed toward observing for signs of thromboemboli postoperatively. Femoral areas as well as the calves should be observed. Early ambulation is encouraged, but does not merely mean sitting in a chair by the bedside for extended periods of time. Better venous return is achieved by having a patient lie in bed with her legs elevated to about 15° than by sitting for long periods of time in a chair at the bedside. Ambulation refers to movement — getting up to sit in a chair for 10 to 15 minutes, back to bed with feet slightly elevated, getting up to walk to the bathroom, getting up to eat lunch and back to bed to rest. Leg exercises, coughing and deep breathing exercises are important in promoting good circulation.

Fistula formation is a hazard and the risk is greater if radiation therapy has been given prior to surgery. Because these fistulae are a result of poor blood supply and the sloughing of tissue they are a later development, usually appearing in the second postoperative week. The most common are vesicovaginal and ureterovaginal. Thus, any unusual drainage of urine must be noted. In addition, any unexplained fever or lower quadrant or flank pain should alert the nurse. The fistula is usually not repaired immediately, but postponed until a more favorable time.

A pelvic exenteration includes all of the Wertheim's hysterectomy plus a total vaginectomy and removal of portions of the bladder or bowel, depending upon the spread of the disease. The patient may return postoperatively with an ileostomy, a colostomy or an ileal conduit. Nursing care for such conditions is elaborated elsewhere. In these operations preoperative bowel preparations are done. Postoperatively, drains may be left in areas of node dissection to prevent the pooling of blood and serum which may easily lead to infection. The drains may be draining freely or may be attached to suction. Usually they are advanced daily and removed by the fifth postoperative day.

The postoperative adjustment to life may be difficult. Preoperative discussions with the physician and nurse should help to prepare the patient. In pelvic exenteration sexual function of the vagina is lost; in a Wertheim's operation it may have to be modified. Menopause may occur as estrogen therapy is frequently contraindicated. The care of the colostomy or ileostomy must be learned and accepted. The patient will require much understanding and support from the nursing staff while the nurses gently encourage her to retain as much independence as is compatible with her situation.

Frequently external and internal radiation therapy is used in conjunction with, or instead of, surgery for these patients. Because a high oxygen concentration in the tissues and blood increases the radiosensitivity of the tumor, anemia and low circulating blood volumes are corrected before radiation therapy by medication or blood transfusions. Radium in special containers is inserted into the cervical canal and into the lateral fornices of the vagina. The insertion of the radium is an operative procedure. The patient receives a cleansing enema the day before and a perineal shave preparation. During the procedure a urinary catheter with a small bag is passed. This prevents a distended bladder from coming into contact with the radium, which would greatly increse the chance of a vesicovaginal fistula. After the radium is inserted, packing is placed in the vagina and may be sutured in place to maintain the position of the radium. Because the tight packing prevents voiding, the catheter drains the bladder. The patient's temperature is monitored, as radiation may stimulate a latent infection. The patient remains on bed rest with head and shoulders nearly flat. A slipper bedpan is used, and straining at stool is discouraged. The catheter is checked to see that it is draining. These measures help to insure that the radium remains where it has been placed. Complaints of pain and any bloody discharge should be reported to the physician. The time for removal should be carefully observed. Removal may be uncomfortable for the patient because of the tight packing, and the patient may need an analgesic for this. Care must be taken to dispose of the radium in a safe manner. The nurse must also protect herself while taking care of the patient and must teach visitors to protect themselves as well. The patient and her family will need explanations of the procedures and understanding from the nurse. In later observations the nurse watches for signs of radiation sickness. Also, any leaking of urine may indicate a fistula is forming and should be reported to the physician.

Carcinoma of the Endometrium

This is a frequently occurring malignancy which appears to be increasing in incidence. Since it is a disease largely of older women, this may be due to a lengthened life span. The postmenopausal woman is at greater risk, as is the black American woman, who has a higher incidence than her white sister. The reason for this is unknown. Estrogens aggravate the tumor and prolonged estrogen therapy, especially in the premenopausal or postmenopausal woman, has been implicated as a contributing cause of endometrial cancer.

The first symptom is a painless, bloody vaginal discharge. Thirty to 40 per cent of women with postmenopausal bleeding have cancer of the endometrium. Bleeding postmenopausally should therefore never be ignored but investigated immediately. A careful endometrial biopsy is usually done. The growth is usually in the fundus of the uterus, but may arise in or spread to the isthmus. The thick body of the uterus contains the growth and it metastasizes late in its growth.

Treatment is by intracavitary radiation followed by a careful total hysterectomy and bilateral salpingo-oophorectomy. Care is taken to pack the vagina or suture the cervix, and tie the tubes to prevent spread by seeding from the uterus. Surgery is often followed by radiation of the vagina as well in order to reduce the risk from stray malignant cells spread during surgery. Some physicians may do the hysterectomy first and follow with radiation. More advanced cases are treated with combinations of external and internal radiation with surgery to relieve symptoms. Where radium is inserted, several containers attached to strings may be placed in the body of the uterus to irradiate the endometrium. Cure rates are excellent when the tumor has been discovered early. This is, of course, the case with all cancers of the genital tract.

Carcinoma of the Vagina and Uterine Tubes

Both of these conditions are rare. Treatment is by surgical excision.

Carcinoma of the Vulva

Carcinoma of the vulva is a less frequent malignancy, occurring mainly among women in their fifth and sixth decades of life. It is frequently preceded by vulvar changes.

DYSTROPHY OF THE VULVA. Dystrophy of the vulva refers to changes in vulvar epithelium which are most often associated with aging but may occur in the younger woman. Most are benign but some are premalignant. Because premalignancy must be assessed at the cellular level, all lesions are biopsied.

The patient complains of a shrinking of vulvar structures which progressively narrows the introitus. Dyspareunia, pruritus and soreness are frequent complaints. Smooth red or white patches of thick or thin epithelium may be evident. They may be only in the vestibule or scattered over the vulva and perineum. These patches crack easily, and fissures and excoriated areas develop. Pruritus is common and secondary infection of the scratched lesions occurs. Ulceration may develop.

Mild symptoms usually respond to improved perineal hygiene, control of pruritus and infection and topical application of estrogen. Patients with more severe symptoms are admitted to the hospital. Nursing care will then involve keeping the vulva dry, cool and clean by daily baths and sitz baths. No pants or pajamas are allowed. The patient is nursed as much as possible with her legs apart and a bed cradle over the perineum to keep it dry and cool. A hair dryer may be used at intervals to blow cool dry air over the perineum. This helps relieve pruritus and promotes healing. It is wise to avoid powders and creams. Medication to reduce the pruritus may be needed as well. If the condition resists treatment or recurs a simple vulvectomy may be done. Those patients who show signs of cellular changes consistent with an increased risk of developing cancer will have periodic examinations and biopsies done or a simple vulvectomy.

In addition the nurse must observe the vulva and perineum of any patient for whom she cares in order to identify changes which would require further investigation. She should encourage patients who confide symptoms in her to seek medical attention.

TREATMENT. Carcinoma of the vulva is treated by radical vulvectomy. Here the dissection is extensive for the clitoris, labia and all the perineal subcutaneous tissue; all the perineal glands and the femoral and inguinal lymphatics are removed.

Preoperative preparation includes all the measures common for perineal and abdominal surgery. The patient and nursing staff may react with repugnance at the thought of this surgery. It is frequently seen as mutilating. However, the results of the operation are quire favorable. Sexual function is retained, as the vagina is not removed. Young women have conceived following simple vulvectomy and have been delivered by cesarean section.

Postoperatively, the patient returns to the ward with an indwelling catheter. Much edema is present and great care must be taken not to dislodge the catheter. It may be very difficult to replace. The operation may be done in two stages or all at once. In the former, the patient returns with an open area, requiring future skin grafting. Barrier isolation may be required for this patient both before and after skin grafting. A bed cradle over the pubic area will keep bed linen away. When the procedure is completed in one operation the patient may return with a bulky pressure dressing held in place by a T binding. In other cases there are bilateral stab wounds near the iliac fossa containing drains which are attached to a suction machine; this arrangement may replace the pressure bandage. Thus, the fluid is drained away and the skin flap is kept in close approximation to the underlying tissue so that it becomes firmly attached to the tissue. Some necrosis along the incision lines may be expected, and occasionally skin grafting may be necessary to replace a necrotic area. The stitches are usually not removed for 2 to 3 weeks. Close observation must be maintained for thromboemboli. Once ambulation is begun, the patient may need elastic stockings to avoid swelling of her legs. Standing for long periods of time should be avoided.

References

Books

Behrman, S. J., and Gosling, J. R.: Fundamentals of Gynecology, 2nd ed. New York, Oxford University Press, 1966.

Dumas, R. C., et al.: "The Importance of the Expressive Function in Preoperative Preparation." In

Ellis, H., and Calne, R. Y.: Lecture Notes on General Surgery, 4th ed. Oxford, Blackwell Scientific Publications, 1972.

Garland, G. W., Quixley, J., and Cameron, M.: Obstetrics and Gynecology for Nurses, 3rd ed. London, English Universities Press, 1971.

Guyton, Arthur C.: Textbook of Medical Physiology, 5th ed. Philadelphia, W. B. Saunders, 1976.

Hamilton, W. J., and Mossman, H. W.: Hamilton, Boyd and Mossman's Human Embryology, 4th ed. Cambridge, W. Heffer and Sons, 1972.

Jacob, Stanley W., Francone, Clarice Ashworth, and Lossow, Walter J.: Structure and Function in Man, 4th ed. Philadelphia, W. B. Saunders, 1978.

Jeffcoate, Norman: Principles of Gynecology, 4th ed. London, Butterworths, 1975.

Kleinman, R. L. ed.: Family Planning Handbook for Doctors. London, International Planned Parenthood Federation, 1974.

Lockhart, R. D., Hamilton, G. F., and Fyfe, F. W.: Anatomy of the Human Body. London, Faber and Faber, 1959.

Masters, William H., and Johnson, V. E.: Human Sexual Response. Boston, Little, Brown, 1966.

Novak, Edmund R., and Woodruff, J. Donald: Novak's Gynecologic and Obstetric Pathology: With Clinical and Endocrine Relations, 7th ed. Philadelphia, W. B. Saunders, 1974.

Smith, D. R.: General Urology, 7th ed. Los Altos, Cal., Lange, 1972.

Stallworthy, John and Bourne, Gordon, editors, Twelve Recent Advances in Obstetrics and Gynecology, Edinburgh, Churchill, Livingstone, 1977.

Te Linde, R. W., and Mattingly, R. F.: Operative Gynecology, 4th ed. Philadelphia, J. B. Lippincott, 1970.

Winter, C., and Roehm, M.: Sawyer's Nursing Care of Patients with Urologic Diseases, 2nd ed. St. Louis, C. V. Mosby, 1968.

: A Cancer Source Book for Nurses. New York, American Cancer Society, 1975.

: Syphilis and Gonorrhea, A Manual for Physicians. Ottawa, Department of National Health and Welfare, 1968. Revised Treatment Schedule, 1975.

Periodicals

Alford, D. M.: "Nursing Care of the Patient with Endometriosis." Nurs. Clin. North Am., Vol. 3 (June 1968), pp. 217–227.

Ballinger, C. B.: "Mental Health Aspects of the Menopause." R. Soc. Health J., Vol. 96 (April, 1976), pp. 78–80.

Barglow, P., et al.: "Hysterectomy and Tubal Ligation: A Psychiatric Comparison." Obstet. Gynecol., Vol. 25 (April 1965), pp. 520–527.

Bennett, E. A.: "Abortion." Nurs. Clin. North Am., Vol. 3 (June 1968), pp. 243–251.

Cavanagh, D.: "The Vaginal Examination." Hosp. Med., Vol. 5 (Jan. 1969), pp. 35–51.

Clark, M. M., and Storrs, J. A.: "The Prevention of Postoperative Vomiting After Abortion: Metoclopramide." Br. J. Anaesthiol., Vol. 41 (Oct. 1969), pp. 890–893.

Cranston, J.: "Benign Enlargement of the Prostate Gland." Nursing Times, May 11, 1978, pp. 789–794.

Durbin, Sister M. S.: "Geriatric Gynecology." Nurs. Clin. North Am., Vol. 3 (June 1968), pp. 253–261.

Goldsmith, S., and Margolis, A. J.: "Aspiration Abortion without Cervical Dilation." Am. J. Obstet. Gynecol., Vol. 110 (June 15, 1971), pp. 580–582.

Gottesfeld, K. R.: "The Use of Ultrasound in Gynecological Diagnosis." Applied Radiology, Vol. 7 (July/August 1978), pp. 132–140.

Harper, M., et al.: "Abortion." Nurs. Res. Vol. 21 (July-Aug. 1972), pp. 327–331.

Horenstein, D., and Houston, B. K.: "The Effects of Vasectomy on Post-operative Psychological Adjustment and Self-concept." J. Psychol., Vol. 89 (March 1975), pp. 167–173.

Kendall, P., et al.: "A Retrospective Study of 191 Cases of Pelvic Inflammatory Disease." Canadian J. Public Health, Vol. 68 (July/August 1977), pp. 318–322.

Kohli, K. L.: "Motivational Factors and Socio-Economic Characteristics of Vasectomized Males." J. Biosoc. Sci., Vol. 5 (1973), pp. 169–177.

Langley, F. A.: "Premalignancy in Gynecology." Nurs. Mirror, Vol. 42 (Jan. 29, 1976), pp. 57–58.

Maudsley, R. F., and Robertson, M. B.: "Common Complications of Hysterectomy." Can. Med. Assoc. J., Vol. 92 (April 24, 1965), pp. 908–911.

McQueen, A.: "Termination of Pregnancy using Extra-Amniotic Prostaglandin." Nurs. Mirror, Vol. 142 (June 17, 1976), pp. 45–47.

Main, J. M.: "Prostatitis." Nurs. Times (May 11, 1978), pp. 787–788.

———: "Mortality among Oral-contraceptive Users. Royal College of General Practitioners' Oral Contraceptive Study." Lancet (8 Oct. 1977), pp. 727–731.

Newton, J., et al.: "Nurse Specialists in Family Planning" Br. Med. J., (April 17, 1976), pp. 950–952.

Richardson, J., and Dixon, G.: "Effects of Legal Termination on Subsequent Pregnancy." Br. Med. J. (May 29, 1976), pp. 1303–1304.

Scott, J. S., Lynck, E. M., and Anderson, J. A.: "Surgical Treatment of Female Infertility." Br. Med. J. (March 13, 1976), pp. 631–634.

Skegg, D. C. G., et al.: "Hormonal Assessment Before and After Vasectomy." Br. Med. J. (March 13, 1976), pp. 621–622.

Talbot, H., and Leeton, J.: "The Role of Laparoscopy in 1,400 Patients." Med. J. Austr. (Jan. 12, 1974), pp. 36–38.

Tomkinson, J. S.: "Carcinoma of the Vulva." Nurs. Times, Vol. 72 (June 3, 1976), pp. 854–855.

Underhill, R.: "Gynecological Problems in Children." Nurs. Times, Vol. 72 (May 27, 1976), pp. 812–815.

Williams, T. J.: "Preoperative and Postoperative Care in Radical Pelvic Surgery." Clin. Obstet Gynecol., Vol. 8 (Sept. 1965), p. 629.

Williamson, J.: "Carcinoma of the Body of the Uterus." Nurs. Times, Vol. 72 (May 27, 1976), pp. 822–823.

Wright, B. M.: "Uterine Aspiration Techniques." Population Rep., Washington, D.C., The George Washington University Medical Center, Series F, No. 3 (June 1973).

———: "Menstrual Regulation Update." Population Rep., Washington, D.C., The George Washington University Medical Center, Series F, No. 4, (May 1974).

21

Nursing in Disorders of the Breast

THE NORMAL BREAST

The breasts, or mammary glands, lie on the anterior chest wall. The base of each rests on the fascia of the pectoralis major muscle, and supporting ligaments extend from the skin through the breast to the fascia. The breasts are undeveloped in both sexes until puberty. At this time, the female breasts enlarge and develop secreting cells and ducts in response to increased concentrations of ovarian and certain adenohypophyseal (anterior pituitary) hormones. Estrogen is responsible for the growth of the duct system, and the luteotropic hormone and progesterone are considered the chief stimulants for the development of the secreting cells. The cylindrical projection on the skin surface forms the *nipple,* which is perforated by duct orifices. The pinkish area of skin around it is referred to as the *areola;* it becomes markedly pigmented during pregnancy and retains the darker color following delivery. The male breasts remain rudimentary throughout life.

Following growth and maturation, the female breast is composed of 15 to 20 lobes, each with a duct that opens onto the surface of the nipple. Each lobe consists of clusters of secreting cells which form lobules (Fig. 21–1). The main ducts (lactiferous ducts) are formed by the union of smaller ducts which drain the lobules. They are dilated just before entering the base of the nipple to form reservoirs, or ampullae, for the milk during active secretion. The lobes and ducts are separated and support-ed by areolar, fibrous and fatty tissues. The size of the breasts is mainly determined by the amount of fatty tissue rather than by glandular tissue.

The blood supply to the breasts is abundant and is derived from the internal mammary arteries and branches of the thoracic and intercostal arteries. A large proportion of the lymph in the breasts is channeled through the axillary lymph nodes; the remainder drains through mediastinal nodes.

The breasts are subject to menstrual, cyclic changes associated with alterations in the concentrations of various hormones. Varying degrees of enlargement, tenderness and discomfort develop during the few days preceding menstruation and disappear in a day or two.

During pregnancy, the lobes and ducts enlarge in preparation for the secretion of milk. Lactation is the function of the breasts and occurs only after the birth of a child, continuing as long as the milk is withdrawn. After menopause, the lobes and ducts undergo some atrophy and replacement with fibrous tissue.

DISORDERS OF THE BREASTS

The most common disorders of the breasts are fibrocystic disease, fibroadenoma, carcinoma and infection. The symptoms which most commonly lead to investigation include a lump or mass in the breast, nipple bleeding or discharge, nipple

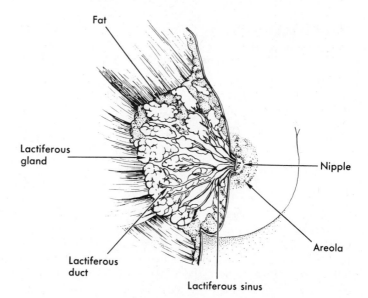

FIGURE 21–1 The female breast. (From Bouchard, R., and Owens, N.: Nursing Care of the Cancer Patient, 3rd ed. St. Louis, C. V. Mosby, 1976, p. 160.)

retraction, a lump (lymphadenopathy) in the axilla or supraclavicular region, change in breast contour due to dimpling or retraction of an area, pain and tenderness, an inflamed area and an ulcerated area.

Diagnostic Procedures

Investigation of the patient for breast disease includes the following procedures.

SELF-EXAMINATION OF THE BREAST. Early recognition and prompt treatment of cancer offer the patient the most promise for control of the disease. Women are urged to examine their breasts monthly and to see a physician promptly if any changes are observed. They are also advised of the necessity of an annual examination by a physician.

Every nurse has the responsibility, as well as frequent opportunity, to teach patients and friends the importance and procedure of regular self-examination of the breasts. A pamphlet outlining the process is published by the American Cancer Society and is available for distribution, free of charge, from local branches. A film demonstrating the procedure is also available from the same source.

The examination should be made regularly each month, a few days after menstruation, and should be continued after menopause. It involves inspection before a mirror and palpation while bathing and then in the supine position. See Figure 21–2 for a description and diagrams of the techniques of breast self-examination.

MEDICAL INVESTIGATION. Prompt, thorough medical investigation is indicated when any changes or symptoms are observed. The following procedures may be used in the examination.

HISTORY. A detailed history is taken of the individual's: (1) age; (2) health history, family history of illness; (3) parity and nursing of infant(s); (4) menstrual history (age of onset, regularity, menopause); (5) date of discovery of lesion; and (6) detailed description of symptoms that prompted her visit to the physician.

INSPECTION AND PALPATION. The breasts are examined for: (1) nipple inversion, retraction and discharge; (2) retraction or dimpling of an area; and (3) redness, excoriation, discoloration, edema, and changes in contour and symmetry.

The patient assumes the supine position while the physician palpates the breasts and examines the infraclavicular, cervical and axillary areas for enlarged lymph nodes.

MAMMOGRAM. This is a roentgenographic procedure used in breast examination without the injection of a contrast medium. A series of x-rays of the breasts is made from two planes, from above and lateral. The films are examined for any areas of increased density and, if present, their

How to examine your breasts

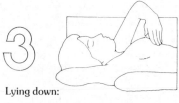

In the shower:

Examine your breasts during bath or shower; hands glide easier over wet skin. Fingers flat, move gently over every part of each breast. Use right hand to examine left breast, left hand for right breast. Check for any lump, hard knot or thickening.

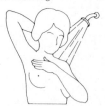

Before a mirror:

Inspect your breasts with arms at your sides. Next, raise your arms high overhead. Look for any changes in contour of each breast, a swelling, dimpling of skin or changes in the nipple.

Then, rest palms on hips and press down firmly to flex your chest muscles. Left and right breast will not exactly match—few women's breasts do.

Regular inspection shows what is normal for you and will give you confidence in your examination.

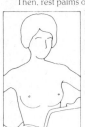

Lying down:

To examine your right breast, put a pillow or folded towel under your right shoulder. Place right hand behind your head—this distributes breast tissue more evenly on the chest. With left hand, fingers flat, press gently in small circular motions around an imaginary clock face. Begin at outermost top of your right breast for 12 o'clock, then move to 1 o'clock, and so on around the circle back to 12. A ridge of firm tissue in the lower curve of each breast is normal. Then move in an inch, toward the nipple, keep circling to examine *every part of your breast*, including nipple. This requires at least three more circles. Now slowly repeat procedure on your left breast with a pillow under your left shoulder and left hand behind head. Notice how your breast structure feels.

Finally, squeeze the nipple of each breast gently between thumb and index finger. Any discharge, clear or bloody, should be reported to your doctor immediately.

FIGURE 21–2 Self-examination of the breast. (Courtesy of the American Cancer Society.)

characteristics (location, size, shape, regularity of borders). A lesion may be detected in a mammogram that is not palpable.

XEROGRAPH. Xerography involves the use of an aluminum plate with an electrically charged coat of selenium. On x-ray exposure, an electrostatic image is transferred to paper by a special process. The xerogram provides more accurate, detailed information about the soft tissues of the breast than the mammogram.

THERMOGRAM. The skin over some tumors of the breast is warmer than that over normal areas. A thermogram may be made of the breast with an infrared camera to detect these areas of higher temperature. The thermography is carried out in a room in which the temperature is controlled at 21° C. or 70 ° F.; the patient is brought to the room 30 minutes before the thermogram is made.

BIOPSY. Biopsy provides a specimen of tissue for cytologic examination; the specimen may be obtained by aspiration, resection or excision. In the case of breast tumors, most physicians prefer an excision biopsy, since it permits an examination of the complete tumor.

FIBROCYSTIC DISEASE (MAMMARY DYSPLASIA)

This is a relatively common disorder of the female breast and is characterized predominantly by fibroplasia, epithelial hyperplasia and the formation of cysts. It is attributed to a hormonal imbalance, is usually bilateral and occurs most often in women 30 to 50 years of age, with a higher incidence in those approaching menopause. A painless mass is usually the first and only manifestation; occasionally there may be some tenderness. The patient may experience more severe soreness and pain of the breasts than is usual in the premenstrual period.

The cysts may be aspirated under local anesthesia. If a solid mass is encountered or the aspirated fluid contains blood, an incisional biopsy may be done to rule out carcinoma. Following the initial aspiration, the patient is reexamined periodically and aspiration of recurrent or newly formed cysts may be necessary. The disease regresses with the onset of menopause.

FIBROADENOMA

Fibroadenoma is a benign tumor which develops most frequently in young women. It generally occurs singly, but rarely there may be more than one. Although it is not usually encapsulated, it remains localized and is freely movable. Medical authors indicate no increased tendency to subsequent carcinoma in patients who have had a fibroadenoma.

The treatment consists of local excision of the tumor, which is submitted for cytologic examination for confirmation of the diagnosis of nonmalignancy.

CARCINOMA

The breast is the most common site of cancer in the female. The incidence is high, and it accounts for a large number of deaths annually. It rarely occurs under the age of 25, and the incidence progressively increases with age. The greatest number of patients develop their disease between the ages of 40 and 50.

Most breast cancers originate in the epithelial tissue of the ducts; the remainder arise from the secreting cells of the lobules. Forty-five per cent of breast carcinomas develop in the upper outer quadrant, 10 per cent in the lower outer quadrant, 15 per cent in the upper inner quadrant, 5 per cent in the lower inner quadrant and 25 per cent are diffuse.[1]

The cause is unknown. As with cancer of other areas, heredity may be a factor, since there is significant evidence of familial incidence — that is, a person is more likely to develop cancer of the breast if there is a history of the disease in the mother, aunt or sisters.

Many malignant tumors of the breast appear to be influenced by ovarian hormones, especially estrogen. It has been demonstrated that some patients with cancer of the breast have a remission of their disease when the estrogen concentration is reduced by oophorectomy, adrenalectomy, hypophysectomy or by the administration of antiestrogenic agents.

Manifestations

The earliest symptom is generally a single, painless, nontender mass which is poorly circumscribed and may have a nodular surface. It is usually discovered by the patient when bathing or during a routine self-examination of the breasts. Other symptoms which may develop include a change in the size or contour of the affected breast, retraction of the nipple or an area of the skin over the breast, bleeding or discharge from the nipple, a scaly rash around the nipple, enlargement of axillary or infra- or supraclavicular lymph nodes or a bleeding, ulcerated area on the breast surface.

As the cancer grows, it spreads to adjacent tissues, such as the skin and underlying fascia and muscle. Retraction is due to involvement of the supporting fibrous tissue; there is a proliferation of fibroblasts and ensuing scar tissue within the breast and fascia of the chest muscles. The breast becomes firmer and cannot be moved as freely. Ulceration is associated with advanced disease which has spread to involve the skin.

Metastases

Cancer of the breast may spread directly into adjacent structures or may metastasize to distant structures by emboli of tumor cells being transported through the lymphatics or the blood vessels. The axillary, supraclavicular or mediastinal lymph nodes are usually the first site of secondary involvement. Other structures which frequently become the site of metastases are the lungs, liver, spine, pelvic bones and femora.

Records show that progress relative to

[1]Marcus A. Krupp and Milton J. Chatton: Current Medical Diagnosis and Treatment. Los Altos, Cal., Lange, 1975, p. 398.

cure and survival of persons with cancer of the breast has been disappointing. It is suggested that a majority of the women have metastasis at the time of diagnosis and primary treatment.[2]

Types of Breast Cancer

Cancers of the breast may be classified according to the primary breast tissue involvement or according to certain tissue changes. The most common type is *scirrhous carcinoma* characterized by marked fibrosing and hardness. The *medullary breast cancer* grows rapidly, forming a larger mass which is softer in consistency than the scirrhous type. There is less fixation of the breast. A third type which occurs rarely is the *inflammatory carcinoma*, which involves the skin and more superficial tissues as well as the lymphatics. *Lobular cancer* involves primarily glandular tissue and is less invasive than other types. *Intraductal carcinoma*, which has a high incidence, originates in the epithelial tissue of one or more mammary ducts. *Papillary carcinoma* is characterized by small papillary growths within the duct system and usually causes bleeding from the nipple. *Paget's disease* is also an intraductal cancer that extends to involve the nipple and areola; a scaly rash and erosion of the nipple accompany this type.

The patient's disease may be classified in stages (clinical staging) according to the characteristics of the primary breast *tumor*, regional lymph *node involvement* and *distant metastasis*. This classification is referred to as the TNM System:[3]

T_1 Tumor of 2 cm. or less. No skin involvement.
T_2 Tumor over 2 cm. Skin attachment or nipple involvement. No pectoral muscle or chest wall attachment.
T_3 Tumor of any size with skin infiltration, ulceration, peau d'orange, skin edema, or pectoral muscle or chest wall attachment.

N_0 No palpable axillary lymph node(s).
N_1 palpable axillary lymph node(s) that are not fixed. Metastasis suspected.

N_2 Palpable homolateral axillary or infraclavicular lymph nodes that are fixed to one another or to other structures. Metastasis suspected.

M_0 No distant metastasis.
M_1 Clinical and radiographic evidence of metastasis except those to homolateral or infraclavicular lymph nodes.

A second classification that may be adopted to indicate the stage of the individual's disease uses the following categories:[4]

Stage I   Tumor confined to the breast. No regional lymph node involvement or evidence of distant metastasis. Some early signs of skin involvement or nipple retraction may be present.
Stage II   Palpable, movable axillary lymph node(s). Primary tumor as in Stage I. No evidence of distant metastasis.
Stage III   Involvement of the skin or chest wall. Palpable fixed axillary nodes. No evidence of distant metastasis.
Stage IV   Evidence of distant metastases.

Treatment

The forms of treatment used in carcinoma of the breast are surgery, radiation, alteration of hormonal concentrations (either by administering certain hormones or by removing certain hormone-producing structures), chemotherapy and combinations of these. There is no unanimous opinion as to the best method of treatment; the search continues for treatment that will provide more encouraging statistics than those currently recorded.

Currently, the choice of treatment is influenced by the stage of the disease, the age and general condition of the patient, and the physician's personal philosophy as to the best therapy. In relation to the latter, radical mastectomy may be advocated, or a modified radical or simple mastectomy may be the procedure selected, combined with radiation or chemotherapy.

SURGICAL TREATMENT. *Radical mastectomy* is the operation adopted by many surgeons and involves removal of the complete breast, the underlying pectoralis (major and minor) muscles and the axillary lymphatics and lymph nodes. A large area

[2]Bernard Fisher: "Adjuvant Chemotherapy in the Primary Management of Breast Cancer." Med. Clin. North Am., Vol. 61, No. 5 (Sept. 1977), pp. 953–961.

[3]David C. Sabiston (Ed.): Textbook of Surgery, 11th ed. Philadelphia, W. B. Saunders, 1977, p. 644.

[4]Krupp and Chatton, op. cit., p. 401.

of the overlying skin is removed and, if the remaining skin flaps cannot be approximated without a good deal of tension, a skin graft is done. The anterior surface of the thigh is the usual donor site.

A *modified radical mastectomy* is a more conservative procedure which removes the breast, axillary lymphatics and lymph nodes and leaves the pectoral muscles. This is frequently the operation performed when the patient's disease is found to be in Stage I or II. Removal of the breast leaving the axillary lymphatics, lymph nodes and pectoral muscles intact comprises a *simple mastectomy*.

RADIATION THERAPY. External radiation therapy may be used as an adjunct to surgery or alone in cases in which the disease is advanced and inoperable, or in which there is a local recurrence after surgery. For the care of the patient receiving radiation therapy, see p. 140.

CHEMOTHERAPY. There is an increasing use of chemotherapeutic agents as an adjunct to mastectomy in the treatment of breast cancer. A single anticancer drug may be used, or a combination of several. Examples of drugs used singly are fluorouracil, L-phenylalanine mustard (Alkeran, L-PAM) and cyclophosphamide (Cytoxan). An example of a combination used in therapy is CMF, which is cyclophosphamide (C), methotrexate (M) and fluorouracil (F). The schedule for administration may vary with patients; if a single drug is used it is usually given intravenously daily for five consecutive days every month. In the case of CMF, Cytoxan may be taken orally for 2 weeks and the other two drugs (methotrexate and fluorouracil) are given intravenously on certain days.

Adjuvant chemotherapy is prescribed over a long term — one or more years. The drugs are circulated in the blood throughout the body, reaching areas of metastatic disease. They are toxic to many normal cells in addition to cancerous cells, and have severe side effects. It is important that the nurses caring for patients receiving these drugs be familiar with the action and side effects, and be prepared to provide the patients with the necessary support and guidance. Adequate instruction may mean the difference between the patient coping with the chemotherapy with minimal interference to her accustomed way of life and

being a chronic invalid. See Chapter 8 for side effects of these chemotherapeutic agents and their nursing responsibilities.

HORMONE DEPRIVATION. As cited earlier, some patients with carcinoma of the breast experience a remission of their disease when the concentration of certain hormones (mainly estrogen) is reduced. Their cancer is said to be hormone-dependent. It is suggested that there are cells in some breast cancers that have a high affinity for estrogen; these cells are referred to as estrogen-receptor cells. Haskell indicates that they have been found in 45 per cent of breast cancer.[5] Those patients whose breast cancer tissue has a high estrogen-receptor content are considered candidates for hormone deprivation by endocrine ablative surgery or antiestrogenic chemotherapy.

The patient may have an oophorectomy (removal of the ovaries), especially if she is premenopausal. This reduces the production of both estrogen and progesterone. An adrenalectomy or hypophysectomy may also be done to decrease the production of estrogen if the patient has shown a favorable response to an oophorectomy. The patient who has an adrenalectomy will require cortisone replacement therapy (see p. 779 for care following adrenalectomy). If a complete hypophysectomy is done, the administration of cortisone and thyroid extract will be necessary because of the removal of the respective tropic hormones (ACTH and TSH), as well as a Pitressin preparation to replace the antidiuretic hormone (ADH).

The administration of an androgen (male hormone) such as calusterone (Methosarb) may be prescribed alone or in conjunction with one of the above surgical procedures. Androgen therapy is likely to cause masculinization; there is a deepening of the voice, growth of hair on the face and the development of other secondary male characteristics. Cortisone may be ordered even though no adrenalectomy is done; it suppresses adrenocortical activity, thus reducing the secretion of sex hormones by the adrenal glands.

Breast Cancer in the Male

Carcinoma of the breast is relatively rare in the male, usually occurring in the fifth or sixth

---

[5]Charles M. Haskell: "Management of Metastatic Breast Cancer." Med. Clin. North Am., Vol. 61, No. 5 (Sept. 1977), p. 968.

decade. The course of the disease is similar to that in the female; it readily metastasizes to regional lymph nodes and other structures. It is often unrecognized and neglected in the early stage because of the low incidence in men; as a result, metastases have frequently developed when the patient is first seen. Treatment involves radical mastectomy and radiation therapy or chemotherapy. A bilateral orchidectomy (removal of the testes) and hormonal therapy may also be used.

Nursing Care in Breast Surgery

PREOPERATIVE PREPARATION. If there has not been a previous biopsy to determine if the mass is benign or malignant, the patient is prepared as for a radical mastectomy. The tumor is excised and the surgical team waits while a quick frozen section is examined by the pathologist. If the mass indicates malignancy, a radical mastectomy is then performed. Before operation, the surgeon explains to the patient and the family the procedure that will be followed and the operative consent indicates "biopsy and possible radical mastectomy."

PSYCHOLOGICAL PREPARATION. The general public has become more aware of cancer but, unfortunately, many persons do not realize that a large number of cancer patients who receive early treatment are cured. To many, the word cancer only implies suffering, mutilation and death. In many instances fear of learning the truth leads to delay in seeking medical advice.

The impact of being advised of the need for a biopsy and possible radical mastectomy if the mass is cancerous understandably evokes fears and emotional reactions in the patient. Her anxiety may be focussed upon suffering, disfigurement, loss of femininity, or death. How she will react is unpredictable; responses and behavior are individualized, depending on background and previous experiences. One patient may appear quite unconcerned but actually is in turmoil underneath her composure. Some may be withdrawn and unresponsive, others are angry and resentful that this should happen to them, and a few may be actually disorganized. The patient may have feelings of helplessness, loneliness and abandonment. Each patient requires the support of a nurse who understands and appreciates what the implications of the situation may be for the woman and her family.

The nurse needs to know what the physician has told the patient and should observe her closely for her reactions. The patient is encouraged and is given opportunities to talk about the situation and ask questions. In this way, the nurse learns of the patient's particular concerns and can discuss them, appropriately clarifying misconceptions and informing the patient that she will be able to resume former activities, that excellent prostheses are available, and that, hopefully, her tumor is one in which good results may be expected. Being able to express her fears openly and being aware of the nurse's understanding and available support generally help to reduce the patient's level of anxiety and promote acceptance of the situation.

PHYSICAL PREPARATION. Usually, there is a minimal period of preparation; the surgery is considered urgent in order to prevent spread of the disease, if possible. Investigation to detect metastases may include a chest x-ray, liver and bone scanning and determination of the alkaline phosphatase concentration in the blood. The patient's blood is typed and cross matched, and blood is made available for transfusion. Her general condition is assessed, and erythrocyte and hemoglobin estimations are made. If anemia is present, a transfusion may be ordered preoperatively. The fluid intake is increased to insure optimum hydration.

An explanation is made to the patient of what she may expect following operation. This will include the deep breathing, coughing and arm exercises that she will be required to do, and a description of the drainage system that may be used.

The local skin preparation (shaving and cleansing) extends from above the clavicle to the umbilical level, and from the nipple line on the unaffected side to the back on the affected side, and includes the axilla and the arm to the elbow. If the surgeon anticipates the need for skin grafting, preparation of an indicated donor site will be necessary. A sedative is generally given the night before operation to insure adequate rest. The remainder of the preparation conforms to general preoperative preparation (see Chapter 10).

POSTOPERATIVE CARE. If the patient's surgery involves only resection of a tumor and not mastectomy, no special care is required. A nurse remains with the patient until she recovers from the anesthetic; she is then made comfortable and is left to rest. The physician visits to advise her of the pathologic findings. She may be permitted to be up later that day or the next morning and, if no further surgery is required, she is usually discharged from the hospital on the second or third postoperative day. The sutures are removed in 5 to 7 days in the physician's office or surgical clinic.

If a mastectomy was done, care includes the following considerations.

ASSESSMENT. The breast has an abundant blood supply, which increases the blood loss during surgery and the risk of postoperative hemorrhage. Close observation of the patient is maintained during the first 36 to 48 hours to detect early signs of shock or hemorrhage. The dressings are inspected for blood, and the bedding under the affected side is also checked since blood may not be visible on the dressing because of its flow over the patient's side or from the axillary area. The space between the chest wall and the skin may be drained by a tube brought out through a stab wound and attached to a wound suction receptacle (Hemovac). The amount and color of the drainage are noted at frequent intervals, and any indication of bleeding is reported at once. The removal of the serosanguineous fluid promotes healing as the underlying space is reduced and the skin flaps are brought into apposition with the chest wall.

The patient's blood pressure, pulse, color and responses are recorded at frequent intervals. Her reaction to the mastectomy is also noted, since emotional disturbance may contribute to shock. Throughout the patient's hospitalization, the affected arm is checked frequently for edema and, after 48 hours, the range of motion.

POSITIONING. When the patient is responding fully, the head of the bed is gradually elevated to promote wound drainage. The patient is turned on the unaffected side every 2 hours. The affected arm is immobilized for 36 to 48 hours to prevent hemorrhage and wound strain. The immobilization is usually achieved by enclosing the arm within the strapping or binder that is used to hold the dressings in place. If it is not incorporated with the dressing, the arm is supported and elevated on a pillow above the level of the right atrium to promote lymphatic and venous drainage. The hand is raised so that it is higher

than the elbow. When moving or turning the patient, the arm is *gently* lifted, and any abduction and extension that might increase wound tension are avoided. After 2 or 3 days, the physician usually permits some movement. The patient tends to hold the arm close to the trunk, predisposing to contracture and limited range of shoulder movement. To prevent this a firm pillow is placed between the trunk and the arm to maintain abduction.

RELIEF OF PAIN. An analgesic such as morphine or meperidine (Demerol) is prescribed for the relief of pain during the first 48 hours. A milder analgesic such as codeine or propoxyphene (Darvon) is then used if necessary. Turning the patient, slight change of position and alternate flexion and extension of the fingers and hand and forearm of the affected arm to promote relaxation or adjustment of supporting pillows may also contribute to the relief of discomfort.

DEEP BREATHING AND COUGHING. The respirations are likely to be shallow because of the chest wound. To prevent pulmonary complications, the patient is encouraged to take several deep breaths and cough at frequent intervals during the period she is confined to bed. Gentle support to the affected side while deep breathing and coughing may lessen the discomfort and be reassuring to the patient.

FLUIDS AND NUTRITION. There is a considerable loss of blood and fluid during a radical mastectomy. A blood transfusion is frequently given during the surgery or immediately after. Fluids are given intravenously the day of operation to replace the loss and may be continued until sufficient quantities are taken orally. The patient is given fluids by mouth as soon as she can tolerate them and is progressed to a regular diet accordingly.

WOUND CARE. The dressing is quite bulky and, unless there is bleeding, is usually left undisturbed for several days. The drainage tube may be removed the second or third day, depending on the amount of drainage. Sutures are removed in 7 to 9 days; the surgeon may remove every other one, leaving the remainder for a few days longer, depending on the healing that has taken place and the degree of tension on the incision. If a skin graft has been done, the donor site dressing may be removed in 3 to 4 days, leaving the area exposed. It may be quite sensitive and require protection from the bedding.

The patient is encouraged to view the

wound while it is being dressed so that she gradually becomes accustomed to the permanent change in her appearance prior to discharge from hospital.

EMOTIONAL SUPPORT. The patient who has had a mastectomy requires a great deal of support and needs to know that someone understands her problems. The psychological impact of having cancer and experiencing the loss of a breast is great and, even though the patient was well prepared before operation, shock and depression follow, especially when the dressing is removed and the operative area is seen. The nurse indicates a willingness to listen to the patient, acknowledging and accepting her reactions. If she is withdrawn, efforts are made to have her talk and express her despair.

It is helpful to talk with the family, especially the husband, to alert them to the patient's depression and fear of rejection and seek their cooperation. The family should tactfully show that their relationships have not changed and that the patient is still acceptable to them. The husband is advised of the marked change in his wife's physical appearance and told that this can be corrected by prosthesis.

AMBULATION AND EXERCISES. The patient is usually assisted out of bed the day after the operation if her vital signs are stable. If the arm is not incorporated in the dressing, it is supported in a sling the first few times she is up if the surgical procedure was radical. A nurse remains with her to determine her reaction and provides support when she is walking or going to the toilet because her balance and accustomed pattern of movement are interfered with by the immobilization of the arm.

Exercise of the affected arm is necessary soon after the operation to promote circulation and lymph drainage, prevent contracture and limited range of movement and restore normal function. The surgeon indicates when exercises may commence. This may vary from a few days to a week or two, depending on the condition of the wound.

During the first few days, the patient is encouraged to alternately flex and extend the fingers, hand and forearm several times, three or four times a day. Squeezing a soft rubber ball is also a very useful exercise. Then gradual abduction of the arm and raising it over the head are introduced when indicated. The purpose of the exercises is explained, and the

patient is advised that to regain the full use of her arm she must begin to use it now. The initial exercises are begun slowly; the frequency, vigor and range of movement are progressively increased from day to day according to the patient's tolerance. Using the affected arm in the performance of self-care activities such as washing the face, bathing, cleansing the teeth and brushing and combing the hair is encouraged by the nurse. See Figure 21–3.

A more formalized program of exercises is planned and started with the consent of the surgeon. These generally include pulley motion, rope-turning, pendulum-swinging, climbing the wall with the hands, and rod raising. Additional exercises may be included later.

Pulley motion is achieved by throwing a rope over a shower curtain rod or overhead bed bar. The patient takes an end of the rope in each hand, stands straight with arms abducted and extended and pulls the rope up and down in seesaw fashion. When one arm is pulling the rope down, the other arm is raised.

The rope-turning exercise involves circumduction of the arm. A 7- or 8-foot rope is tied to a door knob or a firm, stationary object. The loose end of the rope is held in the hand of the affected arm, which is kept straight. The rope is then swung around in circles as one turns a skipping rope. The range may be limited at first, but the patient is encouraged to progressively make larger circles.

In pendulum-swinging, the patient bends forward from the waist, allowing her arms to fall forward in front of her. They are then swung from side to side in a pendulum motion.

Climbing the walls with the hands requires the patient to stand close to and face a wall and place the palms of her hands against it at shoulder level. Using the fingers in a crawling motion, the hands are moved up the wall as far as she can reach and then down again to shoulder level. The objective is to reach full extension of the arm.

In the rod-raising exercise, a rod (similar to a broom handle) approximately 4 feet long is grasped with the hands as far apart as possible. It is raised over the head, lowered behind the head, raised again and returned to the original position. An exercise which may be substituted for this one entails raising the arms out from the sides to shoulder level,

FULL RANGE OF MOTION

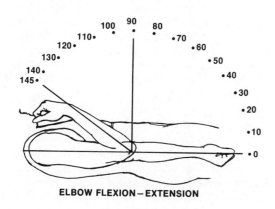

ELBOW FLEXION – EXTENSION

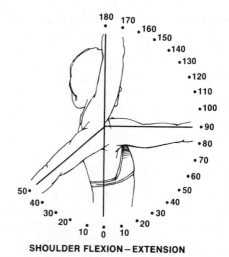

SHOULDER FLEXION – EXTENSION

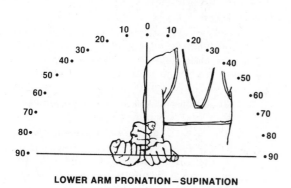

LOWER ARM PRONATION – SUPINATION

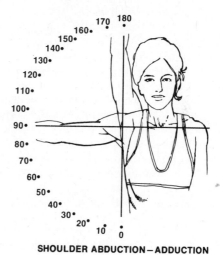

SHOULDER ABDUCTION – ADDUCTION

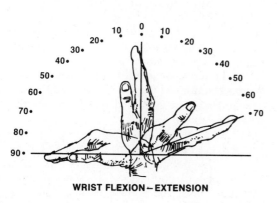

WRIST FLEXION – EXTENSION

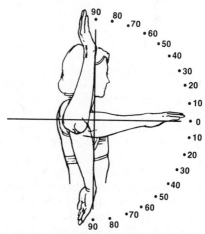

INTERNAL – EXTERNAL ROTATION OF SHOULDER

FIGURE 21–3 Range of motion exercises for the postmastectomy patient. (From Foss: Nursing '74, 4:23, June, 1974.)

placing the hands behind the neck, extending the arms again, and then lowering them to place the hands behind the lumbar region of the back.

All exercises are done only twice the first day; then, gradually, they are increased from day to day until each is repeated ten times two or three times daily. When the patient is discharged a written outline of the exercises which she is expected to continue is prepared for her and reviewed by the nurse. Local branches of the American Cancer Society have a booklet entitled "Help Yourself to Recovery." This illustrates and gives directions for postmastectomy exercises and activities as well as useful information on prostheses. A supply of these booklets should be kept available on the surgical ward for use by the nurse in teaching the patient exercises. A copy is also given to the patient if her physician approves.

EDEMA OF THE ARM. The removal of axillary lymphatics and lymph nodes in radical mastectomy predisposes to edema and swelling of the arm after operation. If it develops, an elastic or crepe bandage is applied, extending from the wrist to the shoulder. The arm is elevated on pillows during the night. During the day, it is recommended that the patient rest the arm several times on the back of a sofa or a table or something comparable for a brief period.

PROSTHESIS AND CARE OF THE WOUND AREA. Before the patient is discharged from the hospital, she is advised as to how to care for the wound area. The area may be bathed as usual but should be gently patted dry. Vigorous rubbing is discouraged in case of wound separation. Gentle massage of the area with petroleum jelly or lanolin may be suggested to increase the elasticity of the skin, which is generally drawn very tightly over the chest wall. The patient is cautioned that if any irritation, redness, open sore or swelling occurs she should see her physician. She is also advised that if swelling (edema) of the arm occurs, it should be reported.

The patient is encouraged to be fitted for a brassiere with a prosthesis. The improvement it makes to her general appearance will raise her morale. The various types of prostheses (e.g., sponge rubber, silicone, or padding) may be described and a list of reliable supply firms with experienced fitters is given to the patient. Prosthesis manufacturers have brochures that should be kept available for exploration by the patient. The nurse shows the patient how to pad the brassieres she has with absorbent cotton covered with soft cotton so they can be used until a properly fitted prosthesis can be worn. The surgeon will indicate when the wound is sufficiently healed that she may wear a prosthesis. The nurse avails herself of the opportunity to describe the wound to the patient's husband or a close relative and emphasizes that the patient may be sensitive about this alteration in her appearance.

If the wound is not completely healed and requires cleansing and dressing, the patient or a member of her family is taught the necessary procedure, or a referral may be made to the visiting nurse agency. A visiting nurse may also be helpful in supervising the patient's exercise program and care during radiation therapy if it is given.

The patient is advised that extra precautions should be taken to protect the arm on the operative side. This is necessary because of the loss of the defense mechanisms (lymph nodes, and the lowered resistance associated with the disease), irradiation and chemotherapy. Cuts, scratches, hangnails, burns and constrictions (e.g., blood pressure cuff) should be avoided. The arm is protected by carrying the purse and heavy articles on the other arm. The arm should not be used for the withdrawal of blood specimens or receiving injections. Jewelry (watch, bracelet, rings) should not be worn in case the arm or hand becomes edematous, resulting in constriction and difficulty in removing rings or a bracelet. The identification card carried by the individual should indicate that needle injections and constriction should not be used on the affected arm, and why (mastectomy lymphedema). A Medic Alert pendant or bracelet may be obtained that indicates the need for caution.

If a series of radiation treatments or chemotherapy is to be given, the surgeon discusses this with the patient and advises her when the treatment will commence. It is not usually instituted until the wound is healed, and it may be given on an outpatient basis. The physician also informs the patient as to when she may resume her household activities or return to her former occupation. The resumption of former activities is encouraged just as soon as the patient is well enough. It relieves her depression and leaves her less time to concentrate on her disease.

A close follow-up is done on the patient;

she is required to make frequent visits to her physician or the cancer clinic during the first year or two. Then, if there has been no evidence of recurrence of her disease, the interval between examinations is lengthened to 6 months or 1 year.

BREAST RECONSTRUCTION (MAMMO-PLASTY). Following a mastectomy the patient may be a candidate for reconstructive surgery. A team of physicians usually assesses the patient and decides whether the procedure should be undertaken. Contraindications are the suspicion of recurrence of the disease locally or regionally, or the presence of systemic metastases. The risk of poor healing of the area is frequently a concern that negates the plastic surgery.

The mammoplasty usually consists of the insertion of a Silastic implant under the subcutaneous tissue. A dermal-fat tissue graft (from the lower abdomen or buttocks) may also be used to provide soft tissue over the mound. More extensive surgery may involve the formation of an areola and nipple with tissue from other areas (e.g., labia minora). Postoperatively, the area is observed closely for drainage. The dressing is removed by the surgeon and is then replaced by a comfortable brassiere which provides the same support as that given to the contralateral breast. The brassiere is worn day and night for at least a month. The patient will require at least two similar brassieres so a change may be made when necessary.

Physical activity which involves the arm is restricted for at least 6 weeks but *gentle* exercise of the arm is necessary to preserve the normal range of motion and functions.

INFECTION OF THE BREAST

Infection of the breast causes acute mastitis and most commonly occurs during lactation. The causative organism enters through a fissure or abrasion of the nipple which might have been prevented by careful cleansing and protection. The patient's temperature is elevated, and the breast becomes firm, red, painful and very tender. The patient is given an antibiotic and kept at rest. The baby is taken off the breast temporarily, and hot or cold applications may be ordered. Unless the infection is checked in the early stage, suppuration may develop, necessitating surgical drainage.

References

Books

Bouchard, Rosemary, and Owens, Norma F.: Nursing Care of the Cancer Patient, 2nd ed. St. Louis, C. V. Mosby, 1972. Chapter 13.

Del Regato, Juan A., and Spjot, Harlan J.: Cancer: Diagnosis, Treatment and Prognosis. St. Louis, C. V. Mosby, 1977.

Hardy, James D. (Ed.): Rhoad's Textbook of Surgery, 5th ed. Philadelphia, J. B. Lippincott, 1977. Chapter 29.

Horton, John, and Hill, George J., II (Eds.): Clinical Oncology. Philadelphia, W. B. Saunders, 1977. Chapter 12.

Krupp, Marcus, and Chatton, Milton J.: Current Medical Diagnosis and Treatment. Los Altos, Cal., Lange, 1975. Chapter 11.

Sabiston, David C. (Ed.): Textbook of Surgery, 11th ed. Philadelphia, W. B. Saunders, 1977. Chapter 24.

Schwartz, Seymour I., et al. (Eds.): Principles of Surgery, 2nd ed. New York, McGraw-Hill, 1974. Chapter 15.

Periodicals

Bacon, Monica: "Mammatherm." Can. Nurse, Vol. 72, No. 6 (June 1976), pp. 23–25.

Butler, Ada: "Breast Cancer." Can. Nurse, Vol. 72, No. 6 (June 1976), pp. 17–22.

Carter, Stephen K.: "What You Can Do for Your Patients With Breast Cancer." Med. Times, Vol. 106, No. 3 (March 1978), pp. 50–63.

Coburn, Dorothy: "Anticipating Breast Surgery." Am. J. Nurs., Vol. 75, No. 9 (Sept. 1975), pp. 1483–85.

Fisher, Bernard: "Adjuvant Chemotherapy in the Primary Management of Breast Cancer." Med. Clin. North Am., Vol. 61, No. 5 (Sept. 1977), pp. 953–965.

Folk, Frank A., "Breast Surgery." Surg. Clin. North Am. Vol. 57, No. 6 (Dec. 1977), pp. 1173–1183.

Foss, Georgia: "Postmastectomy Exercises: How To Make Them Painless, More Effective." Nurs. '74, Vol. 4, No. 6 (June 1974), pp. 23–27.

Haskell, Charles M.: "Management of Metastatic Breast Cancer." Med. Clin. North Am., Vol. 61, No. 5 (Sept. 1977), pp. 967–978.

Kemmerer, William T.: "The Mastectomy Controversy." Nurs. '72, Vol. 2, No. 6 (June 1972), pp. 12–13.

Kennerly, Sadie: "What I've Learned About Mastectomy." Am. J. Nurs., Vol. 77, No. 9 (Sept. 1977), pp. 1431–32.

Leven, Martin B.: "A New Role for Radiation Therapy." Am. J. Nurs., Vol. 77, No. 9 (Sept. 1977), pp. 1443–44.

Mahoney, Leo J.: "Early Diagnosis of Breast Cancer: The Breast Self-Examination Problem." Can. Family Physician, Vol. 23, No. 4 (April 1977), pp. 91–93.

_____: "Clinical Examination of the Breast." Can. Family Physician, Vol. 24, No. 4 (April 1978), P. 368.

Mamaril, Aurora P.: "Preventing Complications After Radical Mastectomy." Am. J. Nurs., Vol. 74, No. 11 (Nov. 1974), pp. 2000–2003.

McCorkle, Margaret Ruth: "Coping With Physical Symptoms in Metastatic Breast Cancer." Am. J. Nurs., Vol. 73, No. 6 (June 1973), pp. 2034–38.

Miller, Beverly A., et al.: "Mastectomy's Challenge." Nurs. '72, Vol. 2, No. 6 (June 1972), pp. 7–11.

Owen, Margaret L.: "Special Care for the Patient Who Has a Breast Biopsy or Mastectomy." Nurs. Clin. North Am., Vol. 7, No. 2 (June 1972), pp. 373–382.

Puhaty, Henrietta Doltz: "Two Rehabilitative Approaches." Am. J. Nurs., Vol. 77, No. 9 (Sept. 1977), p. 1437.

Robbins, Guy F.: "The Rationale for the Treatment of Women with Potentially Curable Breast Carcinoma." Surg. Clin. North Am., Vol. 54, No. 4 (Aug. 1974), pp. 793–800.

_____, et al.: "Inflammatory Carcinoma of the Breast." Surg. Clin. North Am., Vol. 54, No. 4 (Aug. 1974), pp. 800–810.

Schwartz, Morton K.: "Hormone Receptor Assay." Am. J. Nurs., Vol. 77, No. 9 (Sept. 1977), pp. 1445–46.

Thomas, Sally Galbraith, and Yates, Marilyn Mann: "Breast Reconstruction After Mastectomy." Am. J. Nurs., Vol. 77, No. 9 (Sept. 1977), pp. 1443–44.

Todd, Ann: "Prophylactic Mastectomy." Am. J. Nurs., Vol. 77, No. 9 (Sept. 1977), pp. 1447–49.

Tully, Joanne, and Wagner, Beatrice: "Breast Cancer: Helping the Mastectomy Patient Live Life Fully." Nurs. '78, Vol. 8, No. 1 (Jan. 1978), pp. 18–25.

Turnbull, Ellie: "Breast Examination Practices." Am. J. Nurs., Vol. 77, No. 9 (Sept. 1977), pp. 1450–51.

Winkler, Win Ann: "Choosing the Prosthesis and Clothing." Am. J. Nurs., Vol. 77, No. 9 (Sept. 1977), pp. 1433–36.

Wynder, E. L., et al.: "The Epidemiology of Breast Cancer in 785 United States Caucasian Women." Cancer, Vol. 41, No. 6 (June 1978), pp. 2341–2353.

22

Nursing in Disorders of the Endocrine System

THE ENDOCRINE SYSTEM

Introduction

A gland is an organ which extracts substances from the blood and produces one or more new chemical substances, referred to as secretions. Glands may be classified as exocrine or endocrine. The secretion of an *exocrine gland* is carried along a duct into a body cavity or to the external surface of the body. Examples of such glands are the salivary, gastric, mammary and sweat glands. *Endocrine glands* do not have ducts; their secretions, which are called *hormones,* pass directly into the blood and act on remote tissues.

The glands usually cited as composing the *endocrine system* are the hypophysis (pituitary gland), thyroid gland, four parathyroid glands, two adrenal (suprarenal) glands, islets of Langerhans and two gonads (ovaries or testes) (see Fig. 22–1). Unlike other body systems in which the component organs are located close together and are connected, the glands are situated in various parts of the body. There are other organs which are known to demonstrate endocrine action through their liberation of chemical agents into the blood. They are not considered to be part of the endocrine system since they are a more in-

tegral part of other major systems. These include the gastrointestinal glands, which secrete gastrin, secretin and cholecysto-kinin-pancreozymin (see p. 482), and the kidneys, which secrete renin and the renal

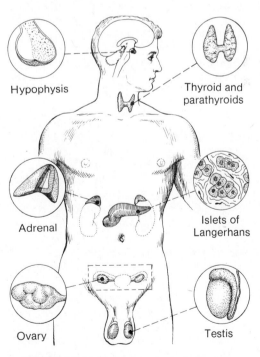

Hypophysis

Thyroid and parathyroids

Adrenal

Islets of Langerhans

Ovary

Testis

FIGURE 22–1 Endocrine glands in the body.

erythropoietic factor into the blood (see p. 614). The placenta, formed in pregnancy, also serves as an endocrine gland because of its production of progesterone, estrogen and chorionic gonadotropin.

Coordination and integration of the development and functions of the body are dependent upon the nervous system and the endocrine system. The endocrine system is concerned mainly with growth, maturation, metabolic processes and reproduction. The action of each hormone is specific. One hormone may modify the activity of all body cells (e.g., thyroxine); others affect the activity of only one particular organ (e.g., adrenocorticotropin). The site of action of any hormone is referred to as the *target organ or tissue*. Some hormones are necessary for survival (e.g., adrenocorticoid); others are not essential to life (e.g., gonadal secretions).

REGULATION OF SECRETION. The production of endocrine secretions is generally controlled according to the need for their action; that is, production and release into the blood stream are stimulated when their action is needed and are inhibited when the effect is achieved. The control mechanism may be mediated by the blood concentration of the secretion of the target organ, or by physicochemical processes. For example, regulation of secretion by the thyroid, adrenal cortices and the gonads is maintained by hormones which are produced by the adenohypophysis (anterior pituitary gland) and are liberated in response to the blood concentration of the hormones of those glands. To illustrate, the adenohypophysis secretes a thyroid-stimulating hormone (thyrotropin), and, the output of thyrotropin is controlled by the level of thyroid hormones in the blood. This reciprocal arrangement is referred to as a *feedback mechanism*. A hormone which stimulates the secretion of another hormone is referred to as a *tropic hormone*. An example of control by a *physicochemical process* is the influence of the osmotic pressure of the blood on the output of the antidiuretic hormone (see p. 753).

DYSFUNCTION. Disorders of an endocrine gland may incur an excess or deficiency of its hormone(s). Signs and symptoms of the disorder are predominantly manifestations of dysfunction in the target organ or tissues. Enlargement or outgrowths of a gland may also impose on neighboring structures, interfering with their function(s).

HYPOPHYSIS (PITUITARY GLAND)

The hypophysis is a very small gland located at the base of the brain in the sella turcica, a depression in the sphenoid bone. It lies just below the anterior part of the third ventricle and adjacent to the optic chiasm.[1] It is attached to the brain by a stalk, the *infundibulum*, which contains nerve fibers and blood vessels. The gland has two distinct parts: the anterior lobe, or adenohypophysis, and the posterior or neural lobe, or neurohypophysis. The adenohypophysis is an embryologic outgrowth of the roof of the mouth and is completely separated from its origin. The neurohypophysis develops from the base of the brain, remaining connected to the hypothalamus by many nerve fibers (see Fig. 22–2).

The cells of the adenohypophysis are truly glandular in that they extract substances from the blood and secrete new chemicals (hormones). The neurohypophysis consists mainly of many terminal nerve fibers which originate with nerve cells (neurons) in the hypothalamus. The fibers are supported by nonsecreting cells called *pituicytes*. The hormones released by the neurohypophysis are secreted by the neurons of the hypothalamus.

Adenohypophysis (Anterior Pituitary Lobe)

The cells of the adenohypophysis comprise "several largely independent functional units, each composed of a specific cell type, synthesizing and releasing one of the pituitary hormones."[2] On this basis, cells may be classified as follows:[3, 4]

---

[1]For a description of the *optic chiasm,* see p. 981.
[2]Robert H. Williams (Ed.): Textbook of Endocrinology, 5th ed. Philadelphia, W. B. Saunders, 1974, p. 33.
[3]Loc. cit.
[4]Richard S. Dillon: Handbook of Endocrinology. Philadelphia, Lea and Febiger, 1973, p. 166.

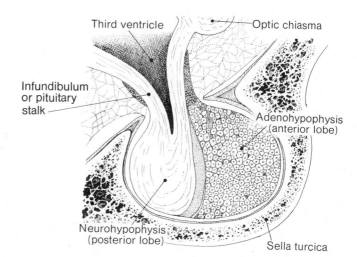

FIGURE 22–2   The hypophysis.

Somatotropic cells secrete somatotropin (STH) and are located in the lateral areas of the adenohypophysis.

Thyrotropic cells secrete thyrotropin (TSH) and are located centrally in the adenohypophysis.

Gonadotropic cells secrete the gonadotropin hormones (follicular-stimulating hormone (FSH) and luteotropic hormone (LH) and are widely distributed in the adenohypophysis.

Corticotropic cells secrete corticotropin (adrenocorticotropic hormone, ACTH) and are mainly located in the adenohypophysis. Some are also found in the area of the neurohypophysis that approximates the adenohypophysis.

Lactotropic cells, which increase during pregnancy and secrete prolactin (LTH), are located in the adenohypophysis.

Melanotropic cells secrete melanocyte-stimulating hormone (MSH). It is suggested that MSH and ACTH may be produced by the same cells as ACTH. The secretion of the two hormones by the same cells is not established, but a relationship is supported by the fact that in adrenocortical insufficiency increased pigmentation is a common symptom.

Nonsecretory cells are also found. Many pituitary cells have been recognized as having no identifiable secretory function, but are suspected of having some contributory overall function.

The older classification of the cells of the anterior pituitary lobe distinguishes three major types according to their ability to be stained by certain dyes: *acidophils* or *alpha cells*, *basophils* or *beta cells*, and *chromophobes*.[5] The cells are arranged in columns or groups surrounding blood sinuses.

The hormones TSH, ACTH, FSH, LTH and LH stimulate other glands; STH acts directly on almost all tissues of the body.

A branch of the internal carotid artery supplies the adenohypophysis, but the blood is circulated through the lower hypothalamic tissue before entering the gland. It is carried from the hypothalamus in hypothalamic-hypophyseal portal vessels in the infundibulum (pituitary stalk) to the sinusoids of the adenohypophysis. Control of the various adenohypophyseal secretions is mediated by neurosecretory substances or releasing factors which are liberated by special hypothalamic neurons into the hypothalamic-hypophyseal portal system. On reaching the sinusoids, these substances influence the secretory activity of the respective glandular cells.

FUNCTIONS OF THE ADENOHYPOPHYSEAL HORMONES. *Somatotropin* is concerned with the growth of the body and plays an important role in determining a person's size. It is most freely secreted from infancy until late adolescence. The most striking effect of the hormone is evidenced in the skeleton. Bones increase in

---

[5]Pituitary neoplasms are frequently indicated as being *eosinophilic*, *basophilic* or *chromophobic*.

length and thickness, the muscles enlarge and there is a corresponding growth of the viscera. Many metabolic processes are influenced by STH, and a positive nitrogen balance develops because of the increased use of proteins in tissue synthesis. Growth is also dependent upon the secretion of normal amounts of other hormones. The thyroid hormones are necessary to maintain an adequate metabolic rate, and insulin must be available to promote glucose metabolism for the provision of energy. The growth hormone is diabetogenic; it increases the breakdown of glycogen in the liver, promotes the release of glucose into the blood and also produces an anti-insulin effect in muscle.[6]

The secretion of somatotropin is controlled by a feedback mechanism. The hypothalamus is sensitive to the blood level of the hormone and, when it falls below normal, the hypothalamus produces a somatotropin-releasing factor (SRF) which is transmitted to the appropriate cells in the adenohypophysis.

Thyrotropin (thyroid-stimulating hormone) promotes the growth and secretory activity of the thyroid gland, the function of which is the production of hormones which regulate the metabolic rate of all tissues. The production of thyrotropin is regulated by a feedback mechanism. A decrease in the blood concentration of thyroid hormones increases the secretory output of thyrotropin; conversely, when the thyroid hormones reach a normal or above normal level, there is a reciprocal decrease in the release of thyrotropin.

Corticotropin (ACTH) has as its target organ the adrenal cortices, influencing their secretory output of several cortical secretions. ACTH secretion is regulated by a corticotropin-releasing factor produced in the hypothalamus in response to a decreased blood level of cortisone, or to nerve impulses initiated by biological stress (e.g., trauma, pain).

The *follicle-stimulating hormone (FSH)* causes the development of the ovarian follicle and the secretion of estrogen. The secretion of FSH is reciprocally related to the blood level of estrogen; FSH production is increased as the estrogen level declines (See p. 678 for details of its role in the female menstrual cycle). In the male, FSH promotes the production of spermatozoa in conjunction with the male hormone testosterone.

The *luteotropic* (luteinizing) hormone (LH) promotes ovulation and is necessary for the formation of the corpus luteum in the ruptured follicle. When the corpus luteum develops and secretes progesterone, the production of LH is suppressed. In the male, this hormone may be called the interstitial cell–stimulating hormone (ICSH) because it stimulates the production of the male hormone testosterone by the interstitial cells of the testes.

Lactotropic (LTH) *hormone* (prolactin) stimulates the corpus luteum to secrete progesterone and initiates and stimulates the secretion of the mammary glands which have undergone preparatory changes in response to the estrogen and progesterone blood levels. It is similar to luteotropin. Its action in the male, if any, is undetermined.

A seventh adenohypophyseal hormone which is normally secreted in very small amounts in man is the *melanocyte-stimulating hormone (MSH),* which increases skin pigmentation. Its chemical structure is similar to that of ACTH, and pigmentation of the skin may occur in the human with a high blood concentration of ACTH. Pigmented areas of the skin are frequently seen in persons with a deficiency of adrenocortical secretion which results in an increased, compensatory output of ACTH.

Functions of the Neurohypophyseal Hormones

Two hormones, the antidiuretic hormone (ADH) and oxytocin, are released by the neurohypophysis. The *antidiuretic hormone,* also called vasopressin, increases the permeability of the distal and collecting tubules of the kidneys, resulting in increased reabsorption of water. Release of ADH by the posterior pituitary lobe is regulated by osmoreceptors in the hypothalamus. When the osmotic pressure of the blood is elevated (for example, because of dehydration or increased salt ingestion) the neurons sensitive to changes in the osmotic pressure of the blood transmit

---

[6]William F. Ganong: Review of Medical Physiology, 7th ed. Los Altos, Cal., Lange, 1975, p. 304.

impulses to the neurohypophysis to release ADH into the circulating blood. Conversely, if the solute concentration of the blood is below normal, nerve impulses are not produced and release of ADH is inhibited. The reduction in the blood concentration of ADH decreases the permeability of the renal tubules to water. A decrease in effective intravascular volume, regardless of osmolality, also results in a decrease in the secretion of vasopressin. This hormone plays an important role in maintaining normal fluid balance. When it is present in large amounts, ADH stimulates a relatively transient, generalized vasoconstriction — hence the term vasopressin. It is not considered to have any significant role in regulating blood pressure. ADH released into the general circulation is destroyed rapidly by enzymatic action, mainly in the liver and kidneys.

Oxytocin excites contractions of the pregnant uterus, especially during the latter part of gestation. It also stimulates other smooth muscle in the body to a lesser extent, which accounts for its use occasionally to stimulate peristalsis in abdominal distention. The mechanism that prompts the release of oxytocin to initiate labor contractions is not known. Sensitivity of the uterine muscle to the hormone is thought to gradually increase throughout pregnancy, reaching a maximum at term. This hormone plays an important role in lactation; suckling initiates afferent nerve impulses which on reaching the hypothalamus bring about the liberation of oxytocin from the neurohypophysis. The hormone is carried by the blood to the mammary glands, stimulating the release and flow of milk.

Disorders of the Hypophysis (Pituitary Gland)

Manifestations of disorders of the hypophysis vary greatly, depending on which lobe is involved, the nature of the disease (hyperplasia, neoplasm or destruction of tissue), and the particular type of cell of the adenohypophysis that is involved. Dysfunction may be manifested in one or more of the gland's target organs, reflecting either an excessive or deficient output of one or more hypophyseal hormones. Secondary neurological disturbances may also occur as a result of pressure on neighboring brain tissue by a pituitary neoplasm. For example, early symptoms may be persisting headache or visual disturbances. The visual disturbances frequently occur because of the proximity of the visual tract. Conversely, primary pathologic lesions in the brain, especially in the hypothalamic region, may cause secondary involvement of the hypophysis.

The more commonly recognized disease entities associated with the adenohypophysis include: gigantism, the result of an excessive secretion of somatotropin in childhood; acromegaly, due to an excessive secretion of somatotropin commencing in adulthood; dwarfism, resulting from a deficiency of somatotropin in childhood; Cushing's disease, the result of a hypersecretion of adrenocorticotropin; and Simmonds' disease (panhypopituitarism), which occurs with a deficiency of all the adenohypophyseal hormones. Hyperthyroidism (Graves' disease) may also be secondary to an excessive production of thyrotropin or an abnormal form of the hormone and is discussed in the section on disorders of the thyroid, page 762.

The most common disorder associated with the neurohypophysis is diabetes insipidus, which is a result of a deficiency of the antidiuretic hormone.

Gigantism and Acromegaly

An overproduction of somatotropin before closure of the epiphyses causes a rapid overgrowth of the bones, producing the condition known as *gigantism*. It may commence in early childhood or not until adolescence. A person with this disturbance may attain a height of 7 to 8 feet. Most cases are attributed to an adenoma of the somatotropic or acidophilic cells (alpha cells). When the person passes adolescence, acromegaly is superimposed on the gigantism.

If the adenoma develops after the epiphyses have closed, longitudinal growth cannot occur, but marked thickening of the bones occurs and *acromegaly* develops. Enlargement of the head, jaws, hands and feet becomes apparent. Increased growth of cartilage produces an increase in the size of the nose, ears, costal cartilages and larynx. Hypertrophy of the larynx may be accompanied by a deepening of the voice, and the change in the costal cartilages results in an increase in the thoracic circumference. The skin, subcutaneous tissues and lips thicken, the chin lengthens and the lower teeth separate because of the overgrowth of the mandible. Viscera enlarge and may become overactive, leading to disturbances.

As well as the evident skeletal changes and alteration in appearance, the patient experiences lethargy, weakness, increased metabolic rate and excessive sweating due to hypertrophy of the thyroid. Common complaints are joint pains, stiffness in the limbs, and tingling or numbness in the hands. Impaired carbohydrate metabolism and hyperglycemia develop owing to the diabetogenic effect of STH. Pressure from the causative expanding neoplasm may cause headache, insomnia and loss of visual acuity. Increased gonadal function may be associated with the early stage of acromegaly but, later, loss of libido and amenorrhea are common. Osteoporosis, rarefaction of bones due to loss of calcium, may develop, especially in the vertebrae, and kyphosis (forward curvature of the spine) may be seen in the advanced stage. Hypertension is a common complication. The course of the disease varies considerably from one patient to another; it may develop slowly over many years in some, but in others it may prove fatal in 3 or 4 years. Destruction of hypophyseal tissue by progressive growth and spread of the tumor may cause a general hypopituitarism.

Diagnostic investigation involves x-rays of the skull in which the sella turcica is checked for widening. A small dose of insulin is administered intravenously, after a period of fasting; blood specimens are obtained every half hour for 2 hours for blood sugar, somatotropin and corticoid determinations. Normally, hypoglycemia is induced — the blood sugar may fall to 50 mg. per cent. Glucose is kept available for rapid administration to prevent a dangerously low level. An excessive secretion of STH causes hyperglycemia and insulin resistance.

TREATMENT. Gigantism and acromegaly may be treated by external or internal irradiation of the hypophysis or by a hypophysectomy (see p. 000). Internal radiation may be achieved by the implantation of radioactive gold (Au^{198}) or yttrium (Y^{90}) seeds in the hypophysis. The gland is approached through the nasal cavity and sphenoid bone. The disease is likely to cause emotional reactions and depression in the patient and his family. Support and understanding from the nurse may help them to accept and adjust to the situation. A high-calorie, well-balanced diet is necessary to meet the increased metabolic rate. With some, it may have to be modified because of the decreased carbohydrate metabolism. Substitution hormonal preparations are prescribed if a hypophysectomy is done or if the patient manifests insulin, thyroid, adrenal or gonadal insufficiency in the advanced stage of the disease. Treatment arrests further changes but the changes in bony structures are irreversible.

Cushing's Disease

A basophilic tumor of corticotropic cells or disturbance in the hypothalamus may give rise to an excessive production of ACTH and, in turn, hyperactivity of the adrenal cortices. The adrenal cortices respond by hyperplasia and an excessive secretion of glucocorticoids, producing the characteristic features of Cushing's disease. The syndrome is more often a consequence of a primary disorder of the adrenal gland (see p. 776).

Pituitary Dwarfism

A deficiency of somatotropin in childhood produces dwarfism. The deficiency most often becomes apparent when the child is 2 to 4 years of age. He may be normally formed, but his proportions are not characteristic of the age at which growth ceases and the head is relatively larger than the rest of the body. In some instances, the head and trunk develop normally, but growth of the legs and arms is stunted. Dwarfism due to a somatotropic deficiency is differentiated from that due to a deficiency of the thyroid hormone (cretinism) in that the mental development is normal in the former. The deficiency in some patients may be limited to somatotropin or it may involve other hormones. Sexual development and maturity may or may not be normal.

A second type of dwarfism which is rarely seen is referred to as Fröhlich's syndrome, in which there is obesity and failure of sexual development; mental retardation may be present in some. An adult form of Fröhlich's syndrome occurs in which obesity, atrophy of the genitals and loss of reproductive ability occur. The obesity in Fröhlich's disease is attributed to hypothalamic involvement.

Simmonds' Disease (Panhypopituitarism)

This disease denotes a deficiency of all the adenohypophyseal hormones. The condition may be the result of a primary lesion, such as a tumor or cyst, within the anterior lobe itself, or it may be secondary to a space-occupying lesion in neighboring structures or to inferference with the blood supply to the gland. The latter may occur with thrombosis of the hypophyseal vessels rarely associated with postpartum shock (Sheehan's syndrome). Frequently the causative lesion is a craniopharyngioma which is derived from vestigial cells of Rathke's pouch.[7] This tumor occurs most often in children but may not give rise to symptoms until adulthood because it grows slowly. A second neoplasm that may be responsible for panhypopituitarism is an adenoma of the chromophobe cells. The cells of both these tumors are nonsecreting and, as they enlarge, they compress and destroy the secreting cells. Surgical excision or irradiation of the gland for the purpose of suppressing the secretion of certain hormones in the treatment of carcinoma of the breast (see p. 741) or acromegaly may incur hyposecretion of all the adenohypophyseal hormones.

MANIFESTATIONS. The multiple hormone deficiency results in a lack of stimulation to the thyroid, adrenal cortices and gonads. Secondary atrophy and a hyposecretion of their hormones ensue. If the condition occurs in childhood, failure of the secretion of somatotropin along with the others produces dwarfism. Growth and development are arrested, the skin becomes wrinkled and the child develops an appearance characteristic of a "wizened old person."

In the adult, there is also a general wasting of all body tissues and the person exhibits emaciation and severe weight loss. The skin is dry and wrinkled and may assume a yellowish cast. The body hair becomes sparse. Decreased thyroid activity causes a reduction in the metabolic rate, leading to a subnormal temperature and extreme weakness. Arrested function of the gonads results in failure of ovulation and amenorrhea in the female and an absence of spermatogenesis and impotence in the male. Concomitant hypoglycemia and hypotension are seen and may lead to shock and coma. The low blood sugar is attributed to the decreased somatotropin and adrenocorticoid secretions. If the panhypopituitarism is due to an expanding neoplasm, the neurohypophysis and the infundibulum (neural stalk) may become involved, manifested by polyuria and extreme thirst, which is characteristic of a deficiency of the antidiuretic hormone. An expanding lesion may impose itself on the optic tract, impairing vision. The hypothalamus may also be affected and varied neurological disturbances become evident; for example, the patient may experience severe anorexia.

TREATMENT AND NURSING CARE. Treatment includes the administration of substitution hormones of the target glands. The patient receives cortisone and desiccated thyroid in dosages adjusted to his individual needs. Gonadal hormones may be prescribed, depending on the patient's age. Testosterone (male hormone) may be administered to both sexes for its anabolic effect. Estrogen may be used with the female to preserve female secondary sex characteristics.

If the cause is a tumor, it is removed by surgery and/or treated by irradiation.

The nurse plays an important role in encouraging these patients to take a high-calorie, high-vitamin diet. Since anorexia is a frequent problem, resourcefulness is necessary to gain the patient's cooperation and to tempt him to take adequate nourishment. Various methods and approaches must be

---

[7]*Rathke's pouch* is the embryologic structure which arises from the roof of the mouth to form the adenohypophysis.

tried. It is usually helpful to provide small servings of high-calorie foods at frequent intervals rather than the usual three or four regular meals. Varying the foods, adding concentrates to fluids, determining the patient's preferences, having favorite "dishes" prepared at home and brought to him, eating with others and a change of environment are just a few suggestions that may prove beneficial. If the patient is emaciated and inactive or confined to bed, bony prominences and pressure areas require frequent and special care to prevent pressure sores. The lethargy and apathy generally associated with Simmonds' disease predisposes to the patient's immobility. Prompting the patient to change his position and exercise within his tolerance is necessary to stimulate circulation and prevent complications.

Diabetes Insipidus

The etiologic factor in this disorder may be a deficiency of the antidiuretic hormone (ADH or vasopressin) or failure of the renal tubules to respond to ADH. In the latter, the disorder may be referred to as nephrogenic diabetes insipidus and is a rare sex-linked, recessive hereditary condition present at birth. A deficiency of ADH is most commonly due to hypoactivity or destruction of a part of the hypothalamic-neurohypophyseal system resulting from primary or metastatic neoplasms or infection, such as encephalitis or meningitis. In some instances, no apparent cause can be identified.

MANIFESTATIONS. Diabetes insipidus is characterized by a very large urinary output (polyuria) and extreme thirst (polydipsia). The daily output may range from 5 to 20 liters and the patient may experience anorexia, headache, muscular pains, loss of weight and strength, and electrolyte imbalance. The urine has an abnormally low specific gravity and does not contain any abnormal constituents. If fluid is withheld or does not keep pace with the output, an excessive loss of urine continues, leading to severe dehydration and shock. The persisting symptoms of polyuria and polydipsia day and night interfere with rest and normal activities.

DIAGNOSIS. Investigation of the dis-

order usually involves the withholding of fluids for 8 hours; the urinary output is measured, and the specific gravity of the urine of each voiding is determined. Plasma osmolality determinations are made during the test and the patient's weight loss over the period of water deprivation is recorded. Failure to increase the specific gravity of the urine and an elevation of plasma osmolality are characteristic of diabetes insipidus. If these studies are positive for diabetes insipidus, a trial dose of vasopressin (Pitressin) is given; if the polyuria and thirst are not relieved, nephrogenic diabetes insipidus is suspected and kidney function studies may be done.

Investigative procedures may also include neurological examination, x-rays of the skull, visual field tests and an encephalogram for detection of a possible brain tumor.

TREATMENT. The patient is treated by replacement therapy; a preparation of posterior pituitary extract or vasopressin is prescribed. The preparations used include an aqueous solution of vasopressin (Pitressin), given daily by subcutaneous or intramuscular injection, and vasopressin tannate (Pitressin Tannate) in oil, given intramuscularly every 2 or 3 days. The latter preparation is absorbed more slowly; less frequent administration is necessary since one dose can be large enough to provide the relief of symptoms over a longer period. If the patient is allergic to the above animal vasopressin preparations, a synthetic substitute is available in the form of a nasal spray, lypressin (Diapid). One spray (or two may be necessary) is generally used in each nostril four times daily. The use of the nasal spray is more convenient but irritation of the nasopharyngeal mucosa may develop.

The patient is usually hospitalized during diagnostic investigation and regulation of the optimal dosage of the substitutional hormone. It is difficult for the patient to accept the fact that he will most likely be dependent upon the drug for the remainder of his life. The nurse can help the patient to plan for necessary readjustments and should reassure him that he can resume a normal pattern of life.

The patient and a family member are taught the details of how to administer the drug, including care of the equipment. The instructions are also given in writing. They may require further explanation of the disorder to appreciate the importance of regular administration of the drug, and should be advised that it is ineffective if taken orally because it is inactivated by the digestive enzymes. The patient is advised to record his weight every 2 or 3 days and note the urinary volume. Water retention indicated by weight increase and scanty urine may necessitate a decrease in vasopressin dosage.

Hypophyseal Ablation

The hypophysis (pituitary gland) may be removed or destroyed because of hyperfunction or a neoplasm of the gland. Hypophysectomy is also employed in the treatment of diabetic retinopathy and cancer of the breast and prostate. Malignant disease of the latter organs in many instances is supported by the sex hormones estrogens and androgens, respectively. Removal of the source of gonadotropic hormones reduces support for the primary neoplasm and its metastasis. Withdrawal of the hormones does not cure the disease, but usually produces a remission for a period of several months.

Pituitary ablation may be carried out by radiation therapy, surgical excision or destruction by stereotactic cryosurgery (freezing). Irradiation may be from an external source or radioactive yttrium-90 may be implanted. Access to the gland may be by a craniotomy or by a transfrontal or nasaltranssphenoidal approach. The first two approaches are used to provide a greater view of the operative field. Transsphenoidal surgery involves the use of televised radiofluoroscopy and a binocular microscope. Hypophysectomy results in the withdrawal of the adrenocorticotropic hormone (ACTH), the thyroid-stimulating hormone (TSH), and probably the antidiuretic hormone (ADH) as well as the gonadotropins. In some instances, the neural stalk, which transmits the nerve fibers from the hypothalamus to the neurohypophysis, may be preserved at operation, thus preventing diabetes insipidus. The patient requires cortisone, thyroxine and possibly ADH replacement for the remainder of his life. Gonadal function ceases, and the patient becomes infertile. If the surgery was done because of disease of the hypophysis, the male patient may be given testosterone to prevent impotence.

PREOPERATIVE PREPARATION. Because of the location and the infrequency of this particular operation, the patient and family are very apprehensive. The nurse, cognizant of their anxiety, encourages them to verbalize their fears and ask questions and provides necessary emotional support. The permanent results of the surgery will have been explained by the physician but the nurse, knowing what the patient has been told, is prepared to answer their questions and explain the hormonal replacement.

Specific directions are received from the surgeon for the skin preparation. For transfrontal surgery, usually an area of approximately 2 inches from the hairline across the front of the head is shaved and cleansed. The patient is advised that there will be frequent recording of his blood pressure, temperature, pulse and respirations following the operation and that he may not receive anything by mouth for a day or two but that his fluid and nutritional needs will be met by continuous intravenous infusion. A corticosteroid preparation is usually given the day before operation and again before going to the operating room. An indwelling catheter may be passed before the surgery so that a frequent, accurate check may be made of the urinary output to determine if there is a need for ADH replacement. A venous cannula is inserted, and continuous intravenous infusion is started to establish a route for the quick administration of drugs and fluids as needed.

POSTOPERATIVE CARE. The care following a hypophysectomy is similar to that of any patient who has had intracranial surgery (see p. 864). Close observation is made for early signs of acute adrenal insufficiency (see p. 775) or fluid imbalance. An adrenocorticoid steroid is given intravenously until the patient can tolerate it orally. The dose is gradually decreased until the maintenance dose is established. Vasopressin (Pitressin) may be necessary to control the fluid loss; the dosage is adjusted to the urinary volume. Thyroid extract is generally started orally on the second or third postoperative day.

The patient is allowed out of bed with assistance on the second or third postoperative day. The period of hospitalization is relatively short (approximately 10 days); instruction about the taking of the necessary hormones (cortisone, vasopressin and thyroxine) is begun as soon as the patient is well enough.

THYROID GLAND

The thyroid is situated in the neck and consists of two lateral lobes, one on each side of the trachea immediately below the larynx. These lobes are connected by a band of tissue, the thyroid isthmus, lying across the anterior surface of the trachea (Fig. 22–3). The lobes contain numerous vesicles or follicles, and the walls of the follicles are composed of a layer of secreting cells. The follicles contain a clear, colloidal protein-iodine compound called thyroglobulin. The gland has an abundant blood supply; paired superior and inferior thyroid arteries arise from the external carotid and subclavian arteries.

Two hormones are produced and released into the blood; these are *triiodothyronine* (T_3) and *tetraiodothyronine* (*thyroxine*, T_4). The latter (T_4) occurs in greater amounts than the former (T_3). The thyroid hormones are formed by the combination of the amino acid tyrosine and iodine. The tyrosine molecule first combines with one or two iodine atoms to form monoiodotyrosine (MIT) or diiodotyrosine (DIT), respectively. Oxidative reactions, promoted by enzymes, combine these compounds to form *triiodothyronine* (T_3) and *thyroxine* (T_4) (MIT + DIT $\rightarrow$ T_3; DIT + DIT $\rightarrow$ T_4). T_3 and T_4 are stored in the thyroglobulin in the follicles. They are freed from the thyroglobulin and released into the blood as needed. In the blood most of the thyroid hormone combines loosely with a globulin fraction of the blood proteins from which it readily separates at cellular level.

The thyroid hormones (T_3 and T_4) increase the metabolic rate in most of the cells by stimulating oxidative processes. There is a notable increase in cellular activity, oxygen consumption and heat production. The hormones are essential for normal physical growth, maturation and mental development. The production and release of the thyroid hormones are controlled by thyrotropin (TSH) secreted by the adenohypophysis. It may also be influenced indirectly by the nervous system through the hypothalamus, which is closely linked with the adenohypophysis. TSH promotes the uptake of available tyrosine and iodine as well as the release of the hormones from the thyroglobulin into the blood. A reciprocal or feedback relationship exists between thyrotropin and the thyroid hormones. When the blood concentration of the thyroid hormones decreases, the hypothalamus produces a releasing factor (TRH) which alerts the adenohypophysis to release thyrotropin. Conversely, with an increase in the thyroidal hormone concentration of the blood, a corresponding decrease of the thyrotropin output occurs.

The thyroid gland is also considered to be a source of a third hormone called *thyrocalcitonin* or *calcitonin*. It is secreted in response to an above-normal elevation in the blood calcium or an excess of glucagon in the blood. It lowers the serum calcium and phosphate levels by promoting their excretion in urine and movement into the bones.[8]

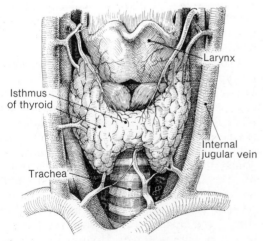

Larynx

Isthmus
of thyroid

Internal
jugular vein

Trachea

FIGURE 22–3 The thyroid gland.

[8]Dillon, op. cit., p. 282.

Disorders of the Thyroid

Disease of the thyroid may cause a hypo-secretion or hypersecretion of the thyroid hormones and a change in the size and contour of the gland. A deficiency in the secretion is called *hypothyroidism*; an excessive secretion is referred to as *hyperthyroidism*. The normally functioning gland is designated as *euthyroid*.

Tests Used in Assessing Thyroid Function

SERUM PROTEIN-BOUND IODINE (PBI) TEST. Since most of the thyroid hormone in circulation is bound to plasma protein, a measurement of the iodine precipitated with plasma protein provides information about the amount being produced. False results are presented if the patient has received iodine in the form of a medication or radiopaque contrast dye within the preceding month or two. The PBI level is also higher in the second and the third trimesters of pregnancy.

Normal value: 4.0 to 8.0 micrograms per cent.

SERUM THYROXINE (T_4), TOTAL AND FREE. The total amount of the thyroid hormone in the blood and the concentration of free thyroxine are determined.

Normal: Total, 4.4 to 9.9 micrograms (μg.)/100 ml. Free, 1.0 to 2.1 nanograms (ng.)/100 ml.

THYROTROPIN RADIOIMMUNOASSAY. The serum level of the thyroid-stimulating hormone is determined to detect if the problem is at pituitary or thyroid level. This is a particularly valuable test if there is a deficiency of thyroid hormones.

Normal: 0 to 7 microunits/ml. (μu./ml.).

THYROTROPIN-RELEASING HORMONE TEST. A dose of the synthetic preparation of the thyrotropin-releasing hormone is administered intravenously. Laboratory examination for the thyrotropin level follows, usually 30 minutes and 60 minutes after the administration. Normal thyrotropic cells of the adenohypophysis are stimulated by the injection to release increased amounts of thyrotropin.

BASAL METABOLIC RATE. Measurement of the patient's oxygen consumption over a given period of time when he is at rest provides an indirect estimate of cellular activity. Since the rate of cellular metabolism is influenced by the thyroid hormones, the amount of oxygen used reflects the amount of these hormones in circulation. This test is less reliable than several others since an increase in the metabolic rate is associated with a number of disorders (e.g., fever, neoplastic disease). The person's temperature must be normal, and an undisturbed rest period of at least 1 hour and a fasting period of 14 hours precede the test. A record is made of the height, weight and age. An explanation of what the test involves is made to the patient to reduce apprehension, which could influence the results obtained. The test is done in the morning in a comfortably warm room, and the patient remains lying down at complete rest. A clamp is placed on the nostrils and he is asked to breathe through his mouth from a tube supplying oxygen, usually for 6 minutes. A table of the mean oxygen consumption according to sex, weight and height has been compiled with which those of the patient are compared. The difference in oxygen consumption (which represents heat production and metabolic cellular activity) with the comparable mean is expressed as a percentage above or below the normal. Because of the influence of subjective factors, the test is not considered particularly reliable unless repeated several times. Usually, those subsequent to the first test provide lower results because the patient is less apprehensive of the procedure.

Normal value: 10 to 15 per cent above or below the normal for the patient's sex, height and weight.

RADIOACTIVE IODINE THYROID UPTAKE (RAIU). This test determines the rate at which the thyroid is removing iodine from the blood and utilizing it. The patient receives a small (tracer) oral dose of radioiodine (I^{131}) in water. The amount concentrated in the thyroid in 6 hours and in 24 hours is estimated by placing a Geiger counter over the neck. A hyperactive thyroid will have a high uptake, and an underactive gland will show a lower concentration than normal. The distribution of radioactivity may also indicate a difference in the degree of activity in different areas of the gland. The uptake of the radioiodine may also be determined by measuring the amount excreted in the urine in 24 or 48 hours. The patient voids when the iodine is administered and that urine is discarded. All urine is then saved for the prescribed 24 or 48 hours and submitted to the isotope laboratory. The fraction of the dose of I^{131} not excreted is assumed to have been localized within the thyroid.

Normal value: 5 to 35 per cent of that administered is taken up within 24 hours.

RADIOIODIDE SUPPRESSION TEST. This test of thyroid function is based on the homeostatic balance between the production and release of thyroid hormones and their blood concentration which is regulated by the hypothalamic-adenohypophyseal system. When a preparation of thyroid hormone is administered, raising the blood concentration of the hormone, the activity of a normal thyroid is suppressed; the output of hormones is decreased in order to establish the normal blood level. If the thyroid is hyperactive, the administration of thyroid hormone will not suppress its activity.

The suppression test involves a 24-hour radioiodide uptake test which is followed by the daily administration of thyroid hormone for 7 days. The RAIU test is then repeated. The uptake of the normal thyroid will be considerably less in the second test. Failure of the increased blood concentration of the hormone to decrease thyroid activity and the iodine uptake indicates hyperthyroidism.

T_3 TAGGED WITH I^{131} UPTAKE. In this test, triiodothyronine tagged with radioiodine is added to a specimen of the patient's blood. The normal T_3-binding proteins are saturated and then the amount of binding of the remainder of T_3 by the erythrocytes is noted. In hyperthyroidism, the binding is high; conversely, it is low in hypothyroidism.

THYROID SCAN. The uptake or lack of uptake of radioiodide by a limited area of the thyroid can be determined by a scan or scintigram. Following the administration of a tracer dose of I^{131} a scanner is passed over the thyroid and automatically makes a graphic record of the radiation emitted, showing the distribution of the isotope in the gland. Areas of greater concentration show greater density on the record. This procedure is helpful in determining the presence of a localized hyperactive lesion such as an adenoma.

ACHILLES TENDON REFLEX TIME. The extent of the response of the foot to a tap on the Achilles tendon and the time involved in the rise and fall of the foot are measured and recorded by a special machine. The patient with an overactive thyroid records a more rapid and greater response; a lesser response over a longer period is characteristic of hypothyroidism.

THYROID STIMULATION TEST. This test is used to determine if the cause of hypothyroidism is within the thyroid or is secondary to a deficiency of thyrotropin. The response of the thyroid to an injection of thyrotropin (TSH) is measured by a radioiodine uptake or by a serum protein-bound iodine estimation. Obviously, if the uptake of I^{131} or the PBI remains abnormally low, the problem is primarily in the thyroid. If the radioiodine uptake and PBI are normal following the thyrotropin injection, the problem may be attributed to a deficient secretion of thyrotropin by the adenohypophysis.

Hypothyroidism

The effects and manifestations of a deficiency of thyroid hormone differ with the age at which it develops as well as with the degree and duration. The deficiency of thyroid hormones may be primary, due to a disorder in the thyroid itself, or may be secondary as a result of a pituitary or hypothalamic disturbance. If the dysfunction is congenital or develops in infancy or early childhood, it gives rise to cretinism. In the adult it produces myxedema.

CRETINISM. A deficiency of thyroid hormone in infancy or early childhood is characterized by the failure to achieve normal physical growth and mental development. The child may become a mentally deficient dwarf. The symptoms of cretinism are rarely present in the newborn but more often appear gradually in infancy or early childhood. Suggestive signs include limpness and inactivity, feeding problems, pale, dry, cool skin, thick tongue, coarse features, coarse hair, and a puffy appearance. The circulation is sluggish, the temperature is usually subnormal and the pulse slow. Constipation is a common problem. The child's growth is stunted, and there is a distinct lag in the development of normal behavioral responses. If the deficiency is recognized in the early stages and a thyroid preparation administered, normal growth and development may occur. If the deficiency is allowed to persist, irreversible damage results, and both physical growth and mental development are retarded.

The fact that cretinism may be corrected if recognized and treated early emphasizes the nurse's role in promoting adequate infant and child supervision. Mothers should be taught the characteristics of normal growth and development. Simple, authentic information is available to parents in pamphlets and booklets published by provincial and state health departments. The mother is encouraged to take the child to well-baby or pediatric clinics for regular examinations.

MYXEDEMA. Adult hypothyroidism is known as myxedema. The *symptoms* and the rate at which they develop correspond to the degree of thyroid inactivity. An abnormal decrease in thyroid hormone causes a general reduction in cellular metabolism, producing mental and physical sluggishness. The person gradually exhibits apathy and slowness in responses. An abnormal deposition of a mucopolysaccharide, which tends to hold water, occurs in the subcutaneous tissues, giving the person an edematous appearance. The skin becomes dry and thick, the face (particularly the eyelids) appears puffy and the lips and tongue enlarge. The person experiences weakness, fatigue and an increased sensitivity to cold. His appetite is poor although he may show a gain in weight. The temperature, pulse and blood pressure are abnormally low. Mental processes are retarded, and the patient sleeps a great deal. Impaired function of the reproductive system is manifested by menstrual disorders, such as metrorrhagia and amenorrhea, and loss of sexual drive. Hoarseness and slow, monotonous speech may be noted. Because of his complacency and dull mental processes, the condition is of much less concern to the patient than to his family or friends witnessing the changes. Allowed to progress, the disorder may lead to arteriosclerotic changes, cardiac insufficiency or coma.

Causes of myxedema include destruction of the gland by a disease such as thyroiditis and Hashimoto's disease (autoimmune thyroiditis), irradiation, prolonged iodine deficiency, a disorder of the hypothalamic-adenohypophyseal system which results in a deficiency of thyrotropin, and complete thyroidectomy.

TREATMENT AND NURSING CARE. Hypothyroidism is treated favorably by the administration of thyroid extract or thyroxine. Preparations used are desiccated thyroid (thyroid), thyroglobulin (Proloid), sodium levothyroxine (Synthroid sodium), liotrix (Euthroid) and sodium liothyronine (Cytomel). Sodium liothyronine is a preparation of triiodothyronine (T_3) and acts very rapidly, but the effect is sustained for a shorter period than the others, which are not fully effective before 7 to 10 days. The dosage is usually small to start with and is gradually increased to guard against a too sudden and excessive demand on the heart by rapid acceleration of metabolism. The pulse is checked and recorded frequently until the maintenance dose is established. Reactions to overdosage include rapid pulse rate, palpitation, restlessness or hyperactivity, nervousness and insomnia. The maintenance dose is individualized on the basis of the responses observed and recorded.

It may be necessary for the nurse to explain the condition to the patient and his family and emphasize that replacement therapy must be continued indefinitely. The patient may neglect taking the medication when he feels better. During the myxedematous state, it is important that the family appreciate that the patient's lethargy and dullness are a part of his disease. They may be prone to criticize and drive the patient. The nurse and his family must be patient and tolerant of his slowness. He should be encouraged and given time to complete responses and activities. Early indications of improvement and response to the drug therapy may be pointed out to them for reassurance that the condition is reversible.

Much of the nursing care is symptomatic. For example, extra warmth is provided because of the patient's lower heat production and consequent decreased tolerance to cold. Without extra clothing and bedding, he may be uncomfortable in an environmental temperature that is comfortable to others. A minimum of soap is used on the patient's skin, and oily lotions or creams are applied to relieve the dryness. A low-calorie, high-protein diet is served with added roughage to combat the problem of constipation. Laxatives or enemas may be necessary to avoid impaction. The hypothyroid patient is seen at the clinic or by his physician at regular intervals; adjustment of the drug dosage may be necessary from time to time.

Severe hypothyroidism may be complicated by coma which may be precipitated by exposure to cold, infection, trauma or the taking of medications which depress the central nervous system. Older persons with hypothyroidism are more predisposed to develop coma. Their temperature falls to hypothermic levels and respiratory insufficiency may develop. An endotracheal tube may be inserted or a tracheostomy may have to be done and mechanical respiratory assistance provided. Thyroxine and hydrocortisone are given intravenously along with glucose. Gradual rewarming by additional covers is used rather than the application of heat.

Goiter

The term goiter simply indicates enlargement of the thyroid gland. It may be a compensatory hypertrophy as occurs in iodine deficiency or in cases in which there is an increased demand for the thyroid hormone, as in pregnancy and puberty. Enlargement may be the result of a neoplasm, thyroiditis or hyperplasia associated with pathologic hyperactivity, as in Graves' disease (exophthalmic goiter). Rarely, it is due to a congenital defect in which a specific enzyme which is necessary in the process of forming the hormones is missing or defective. A goiter may be classified as: diffuse or nodular; endemic or sporadic, depending on the frequency with which it occurs in a given geographical area; and toxic, nontoxic or simple, depending on whether the enlargement is accompanied by hyperthyroidism.

Goiter most commonly refers to an enlargement that is endemic and due to a deficiency in the natural supply of iodine in the water and soil. It is seen most often in mountainous areas and inland areas distant from the sea (e.g., Great Lakes districts, the Rocky Mountains and the Alps). Terms used to describe it include simple endemic goiter, iron-deficient goiter, and simple colloid or nontoxic goiter. In most areas where the natural source is inadequate, the simple, inexpensive prophylactic measure of adding iodine to salt used in food has been adopted. Residents of such districts should be informed of the significance of using iodized salt.

The enlargement of the thyroid in iodine deficiency occurs because of stimulation by an increased release of thyrotropin by the adenohypophysis in response to the low thyroxine concentration of the blood. The follicles increase in number and size and the thyroid becomes more vascular. If the iodine deficiency and excessive thyrotropin stimulation are prolonged, the gland tends to develop nodules which contain greatly distended follicles that may eventually undergo degeneration.

The enlarged gland may cause disfigurement which creates embarrassment for the person. More serious symptoms are pressure on the larynx and trachea, manifested by a chronic cough and respiratory difficulty, interference with swallowing, and compression of nerves in the area.

The simple nontoxic goiter is treated with an iodide preparation (e.g., potassium iodide) or, if there is evidence of hypothyroidism, the patient receives a thyroid preparation. In the early stages, with an adequate supply of iodine, the goiter gradually becomes smaller. If the gland has been enlarged over a period of years and has become nodular, drug therapy is likely to be less effective. The gland remains large and surgical removal of a large portion may be indicated to relieve pressure on the trachea, larynx, esophagus or nerves and to improve the patient's appearance.

Hyperthyroidism

Hyperthyroidism implies an excessive secretion of the thyroid hormones and may be called *thyrotoxicosis, toxic goiter, exophthalmic goiter, Graves' disease* or *Basedow's disease*. The terms exophthalmic goiter, Graves' disease or Basedow's disease are reserved for hyperthyroidism that is accompanied by exophthalmos and extreme nervousness.

The exact cause of hyperactivity of the thyroid in most patients is not clear. It is suggested that it may be due to a primary disorder within the gland, rarely to an excessive secretion of thyrotropin (TSH), or to the production of a long-acting thyroid stimulator (LATS). The latter is a protein that has been found exclusively in the serum of approximately 60 per cent of patients with thyrotoxicosis. It is thought that it stimulates thyroid activity and hyperplasia of the gland,

and that it is an immunoglobulin G which "can be synthesized by the lymphocytes of patients with Graves' disease." This suggests that LATS is an antibody, but the antigen which initiated its development is not known.[9] Hyperthyroidism affects females more often than males, and is rare in childhood. Frequently, the onset is closely related to an emotional crisis in the person's life.

MANIFESTATIONS. Some enlargement of the gland may be evident owing to a diffuse hyperplasia of the gland or the development of one or more adenomas. It may be readily seen to move upward with the larynx in swallowing.

The increased blood level of thyroid hormones accelerates the metabolic rate. The patient's appetite increases and, unless the food intake keeps pace with the rapid metabolic rate, there is a marked loss of weight. Lowered heat tolerance and excessive sweating are manifested. The hyperthyroid patient is uncomfortably warm in an environmental temperature quite acceptable to others.

Nervousness, apprehension, emotional instability and restlessness are evident, and the hands are warm and moist in contrast to the cold, moist extremities associated with anxiety. Although the patient is eating more, he complains of weakness and quick fatigue. The pulse is rapid and exhibits a sharp rise on exertion. The increased pulse rate is due to the increased metabolic demands and the effect of thyroxine on the sympathetic nervous system. Shortness of breath on exertion and palpitation are experienced as a result of the increased metabolic rate. The diastolic blood pressure is usually lower than normal because of widespread vasodilation. A fine, rapid tremor develops in the hands and is accentuated when they are outstretched. Diarrhea, resulting from increased gastrointestinal activity, may be troublesome. Menstrual disorders, such as oligomenorrhea (scant flow) or amenorrhea, are common.

Eye changes may appear in hyperthyroidism (Graves' disease or exophthalmic goiter) which are unexplained. It has been suggested that the hypophysis may produce a substance that causes these changes.[10] Exophthalmos, a protrusion of the eyeballs, occurs as a result of an increase in the retrobulbar tissue within the orbit which pushes the eye forward. The upper eyelids are retracted, showing the upper sclerae. The lids fail to follow the movement of the eyes when the person looks down (von Graefe's sign).

TREATMENT. Hyperthyroidism may be treated by antithyroid drugs, radioactive iodine (I^{131}) or surgery.

DRUG THERAPY. The drugs most commonly used interfere with the formation of the thyroid hormones. They include propylthiouracil (Propyl-Thyracil) and methimazole (Tapazole). The drug is generally taken over a prolonged period of 1 to 2 years if the patient remains free of side effects. These antithyroid drugs are potentially toxic. Side effects which may develop are dermatitis, agranulocytosis and fever. Rarely, hepatitis, joint and muscle pain and neuritis have been reported. The patient is advised to report promptly a sore throat, swollen tender "neck glands," fever, rash or jaundice. It is important that he understand the necessity for taking the drugs regularly and at the hours suggested in order to obtain the desired effect and prevent a remission. Some compensatory enlargement of the gland may occur and the patient is reassured that this is not serious.

The patient is followed closely; weekly visits to the physician or clinic are usually required for 4 to 6 weeks and the interval is gradually lengthened. A blood specimen is taken for determination of protein-bound iodine (PBI), and a leukocyte count is made on each visit. The reports may indicate a need for an adjustment in the dosage of the antithyroid drug.

Drug therapy usually includes a sedative to reduce the hyperthyroid patient's nervousness and agitation; for example, a small dose of sodium amytal or phenobarbital may be given four times a day.

RADIATION TREATMENT. If the patient is unable to tolerate the antithyroid drugs, radioactive iodine (I^{131}) may be administered. Treatment by radioiodine (I^{131}) is very sim-

[9]Maxwell M. Wintrobe, et al. (Eds.): Principles of Internal Medicine, 7th ed. New York, McGraw-Hill, 1974, p. 475.

[10]John Macleod (Ed.): Davidson's Principles and Practice of Medicine, 11th ed. Edinburgh, Churchill and Livingstone, 1974, p. 641.

ple. It is given orally and the radioiodine is trapped in the thyroid, where its radiations destroy tissue, reducing the functioning mass. Improvement is usually evident in 3 weeks and the metabolic rate is expected to reach a normal level in 2 to 3 months. Radioiodine is not generally given for therapeutic purposes to persons under 20 years of age, and is never given during pregnancy. The therapeutic dose is not considered large enough to constitute a radiation hazard to those in the person's environment.

The patient is observed closely for signs of aggravation of his disease and thyroiditis, manifested by tenderness and soreness in the area of the gland. Rarely, a thyroid storm (thyrotoxic crisis) may develop (see p. 768). After receiving the I^{131}, regular visits to the clinic or the physician are necessary. The patient is examined for remission of his disease and for possible hypothyroidism. The protein-bound iodine blood level is determined and the basal metabolic rate may be checked. If hypothyroidism is indicated, a replacement preparation (e.g., a thyroxine preparation) is prescribed.

SURGICAL THERAPY. A partial thyroidectomy may be done if antithyroid drug sensitivity precludes its prolonged administration, if radioactive iodine is contraindicated or if the gland is very large, causing disfigurement or pressure on the respiratory tract or on the esophagus. In hyperthyroidism, approximately three-quarters of the gland is removed; in the case of cancer of the thyroid, a complete thyroidectomy is done which necessitates continuous replacement drug therapy during the remainder of the patient's life.

NURSING THE PATIENT WITH HYPERTHYROIDISM. The care of a hyperthyroid patient, whether in the hospital or at home, requires the following considerations.

ENVIRONMENT. Because of the patient's nervousness and hyperexcitability, quietness and serenity in his environment are very important. An established routine, so that he knows what to expect and what is expected of him at given times, may prevent unnecessary disturbance which only aggravates his condition. If the patient is being cared for at home, the family must be made fully aware of these needs. They are advised that his irritability, restlessness, and emotional lability are characteristic of his illness and that to argue with him or criticize him will worsen it.

In the hospital, the patient is placed in a single room; if this is not possible, careful consideration is given to his placement on the ward. Exposure to very ill, talkative or otherwise disturbing patients is avoided. Since the patient is producing more than the normal amount of body heat, he is only comfortable in an environment of lower temperature than normal persons tolerate. Scant, lightweight bedding is used, and the room is kept well ventilated.

OBSERVATIONS. An accurate record of the patient's temperature, pulse and respirations is made at least every 4 hours, and the patient's responses and degree of restlessness and agitation are noted frequently. This is necessary so that any early indication of increasing thyrotoxicosis and cardiac insufficiency may be recognized and receive prompt attention. The patient is told that his vital signs will be checked at regular intervals so he will not be unduly apprehensive about his condition because of the frequent checking. The physician may request the recording of a sleeping pulse; in hyperthyroidism, the elevated rate persists during sleep. The patient is weighed daily or every second day to determine if his caloric intake is keeping pace with his metabolic rate. Reactions to visitors are noted; an elevation in pulse rate and increased agitation and excitement may indicate the need for additional limitations on visitors.

REST AND ACTIVITY. Activity is restricted because it increases the metabolic rate, but the patient's nervous excitability makes it difficult for him to rest. Efforts are made to provide some interest or occupational therapy that expends little energy. Depending on the severity of the patient's condition and his pulse rate, he may be allowed up, since enforced confinement to bed may cause greater irritation and restlessness. He is discouraged from wandering about the ward aimlessly. Regular doses of a sedative, such as phenobarbital (Luminal) or amobarbital sodium (Amytal Sodium), may be ordered at regular intervals. A stronger preparation may be necessary at bedtime to insure adequate sleep.

Keeping the patient as comfortable as possible by frequent turning of the pillows, changing of the bed linen and patient's gown when they become moist because of the excessive perspiration, and gentle, soothing back rubs help to promote rest. Situations which tend to annoy or frustrate the patient are avoided. Needs should be anticipated, and things that prove awkward for him because of tremor are unobtrusively done for him. Whenever possible, the same nurse cares for the patient, since adjusting to strange personnel may be stressful.

DIET. The patient requires a high-protein, high-carbohydrate, high-calorie diet (4000 to 5000 calories) to prevent tissue breakdown by the high metabolic demand and to satisfy the patient's increased appetite. A snack between meals and at bedtime is provided. Tea and coffee are usually restricted to eliminate caffeine stimulation. Decaffeinated coffee may be used as a substitute.

FLUIDS. The patient's excessive heat production and resulting perspiration increases his fluid loss, necessitating extra fluids. Also, there is an increased production of metabolic wastes, requiring dilution for elimination by the kidneys. A minimum intake of 3000 to 4000 ml. daily is recommended, unless contraindicated by cardiac or renal dysfunction. An explanation of the importance of this amount of fluid is made to the patient to gain his cooperation, and a variety of fluids are provided.

SKIN CARE. A daily bath is necessary because of the profuse perspiration. If the patient is extremely restless and is confined to bed, special attention is given to the pressure areas. Soft linen is selected and talcum applied to the skin to prevent friction irritation.

EYE CARE. If the patient has exophthalmos, the eyes should be protected from irritation by sunglasses. Methylcellulose (a conjunctival lubricant) drops (0.5 to 1 per cent) may be recommended to prevent drying of the conjunctiva and cornea. Sleeping with the head of the bed elevated has also been suggested to promote drainage of fluid from the orbital region. The patient's vision is tested frequently, especially if the exophthalmos is progressive; compression of the optic nerve and artery may occur, with ensuing visual impairment.

VISITORS. Visitors are restricted to those persons who do not excite the patient and who use judgment in their conversation with him. Obviously, those who focus on the patient's condition, transmit disturbing information, or are themselves excitable could aggravate the patient's symptoms.

NURSING THE PATIENT WHO HAS THYROID SURGERY. In caring for the patient who has had a thyroidectomy, pertinent factors to be kept in mind are the *location of the gland in relation to the trachea and larynx;* its *proximity to the recurrent laryngeal nerve,* which controls the vocal cords; its *abundant blood supply;* and that the *parathyroid glands,* which influence neuromuscular irritability through their control of the blood calcium level, lie on the posterior surface of the thyroid. The nurse must be constantly alert for manifestations of disturbances due to these factors.

PREOPERATIVE PREPARATION. The hyperthyroid patient who is to have surgery is given an antithyroid drug for several weeks prior to operation to reduce the metabolic rate, and return the gland to as near the euthyroid state as possible. During this period, whether at home or in the hospital, the care cited in the preceding section is applicable. The antithyroid drugs produce some compensatory enlargement of the gland and an increased blood supply. When the metabolic rate has been reduced to a satisfactory level, the drug is discontinued. Then, in a few days, a course of Lugol's solution (a strong iodine preparation) is commenced and continued for approximately 10 days. This reduces the size and vascularity of the gland, facilitating surgery and lessening the problem of bleeding. Since Lugol's solution has a disagreeable taste and may also irritate the mucous membrane, it is well diluted in fruit juice (e.g., grape juice) or milk.

Preparation includes an electrocardiogram to obtain further information about the patient's cardiac status and blood typing and cross matching for transfusion. The female patient may have some concern for the cosmetic effect of the operation. She is assured that consideration is given to this and that the scar becomes barely perceptible in a few months. During the interval, it may be concealed by a scarf or necklace. Remembering that the hyperthyroid patient is hyperexcitable and apprehensive, judicious explanations are made of what may be expected after the operation. If the patient still responds by extreme nervous reactions and tachycardia to stressful situations, he may be heavily sedated before being transferred to the operating room. Specific orders are received about the local skin preparation. For the female patient, the surgeon may require only thorough cleansing of the entire neck, upper shoulder aspect and upper chest. In the case of the male patient, shaving as well as cleansing is necessary.

PREPARATION TO RECEIVE THE PATIENT AFTER OPERATION. Special equipment to be assembled and ready for use when preparing to receive a patient following a thyroidectomy includes: (1) sandbags or small firm pillows to immobilize the head; (2) suction machine and catheters for clearing mucus from the throat; (3) a humidifier to relieve tracheal and laryngeal irritation and facilitate the removal of mucus; (4) intravenous infusion equipment; (5) a sterile emergency intubation and tracheostomy tray in the event of respiratory obstruction; (6) equipment for obtaining a blood specimen quickly for blood calcium determination; and (7) ampules of calcium chloride or calcium gluconate, with the necessary equipment for intravenous administration in the event of the complication tetany (hypocalcemia).

POSTOPERATIVE CARE. A nurse remains in close attendance on the thyroidectomy patient, especially during the first postoperative 48 hours. He is usually very apprehensive, and serious complications may *develop rapidly.*

Observations. The blood pressure, pulse and respirations are recorded every 15 minutes; the frequency is gradually reduced if they remain stable. The rectal temperature is recorded every 4 hours; after the second day the temperature may be taken orally. The degree of restlessness and apprehension is noted and, if not relieved by the prescribed sedation, is brought to the surgeon's attention. Particular attention is paid to the patient's respirations; any complaint or sign of respiratory distress and cyanosis is reported promptly, since it may indicate laryngeal paralysis or compression of the trachea by accumulating blood. Some hoarseness is common and is due to irritation of the larynx by the surgery and the endotracheal tube used in administering the anesthetic. The physician is advised if the hoarseness and weakness of the voice persist beyond 3 or 4 days.

The fluid intake and output are measured, and the balance is noted.

Positioning and Activity. When the patient has recovered from the anesthetic, he is placed on his back and the head of the bed is moderately elevated. The head and neck are supported by a pillow and are positioned in good alignment, preventing flexion and hyperextension. A sandbag or firm pillow may be necessary at each side of the head for immobilization. The patient is advised not to move his head but to relax, since it is adequately supported; he tends to develop tension in an effort to keep it still. Gentle massage of the back of the neck may promote relaxation and reduce his discomfort. When the patient's position is changed, the nurse lifts and supports the head, preserving good alignment. After the first or second postoperative day, if his progress is satisfactory, the patient is taught to lift and support his head by placing his hands at the back of his head when he wishes to move.

While the patient is confined to bed, foot and leg exercises are encouraged, as with other surgical patients. If the vital signs are stabilized and normal, the patient is assisted out of bed on the first or second postoperative day.

Following removal of the sutures or skin clips and firm healing of the incision, head exercises which include flexion (forward and lateral), hyperextension and turning are gradually introduced with the surgeon's approval. To prevent contraction, the patient may be taught to massage the neck gently twice daily, using lanolin, cold cream or an oily lotion.

Respiratory Secretions. During the early postoperative period there is likely to be increased mucus secretion in the respiratory tract which proves troublesome and difficult to raise. The patient is helped by suctioning and by being assisted to a sitting position, with support given to his head and neck, while he coughs and clears away secretions.

The throat may be sore, and tracheal irritation may also be a source of discomfort. Analgesic throat lozenges and humidification of the room air may be used to provide some relief. The moisture may also help to make the secretions less tenacious and easier to raise.

Fluids and Food. Some difficulty in

swallowing is usually experienced for a day or two, but fluids by mouth are encouraged as soon as tolerated. Intravenous fluids are given until an adequate amount can be taken orally. The patient progresses through a soft diet to a full diet in 2 to 3 days.

Medication. Meperidine hydrochloride (Demerol) or morphine may be ordered to keep the patient comfortable and less apprehensive during the first 48 hours. Judicious use must be made of the narcotic; the drug is not repeated without consulting the physician if there is evident depression of the respirations to 12 or less per minute or if there is increased difficulty in raising mucus secretions. On the other hand, unnecessary withholding of sedation increases the patient's metabolism and restlessness and may precipitate tachycardia.

Complications. The nurse must be aware that hemorrhage, respiratory difficulty, loss of voice and tetany are serious complications which may occur following thyroid surgery. The first three may develop with startling rapidity and are usually seen within 48 hours of operation.

Hemorrhage may be manifested by a rapid thin pulse, fall in blood pressure and evident bleeding. The bleeding may only be discovered by frequent checking of the dressing and by sliding the hands under the shoulders and behind the neck. Blood may collect quickly within the tissues and cause pressure on the trachea. The patient may complain of a choking sensation and shortness of breath; cyanosis and dyspnea develop and, unless the pressure is relieved quickly, asphyxia may occur. The surgeon is notified immediately at the earliest sign or change. The dressing is loosened to promote freer, outward drainage. Instruments for removing the sutures or skin clips are brought to the bedside and the emergency tracheostomy tray is made ready, since the surgeon may consider an immediate tracheostomy necessary. On reporting the situation, the nurse may be instructed to remove the skin clips to allow the escape of blood. A thick sterile dressing is then applied until the surgeon arrives. The patient will probably be returned to the operating room to bring the bleeding under control. Blood replacement may be necessary.

Occasionally, *injury to one or both recurrent laryngeal nerves* may occur during thyroid surgery. These nerves control laryngeal muscles, the opening of the glottis and voice production. Injury to one nerve produces hoarseness and weakness of the voice but no serious respiratory disturbance. Bilateral nerve injury causes paralysis of muscles on both sides of the larynx, resulting in closure of the glottis and respiratory obstruction. The patient is unable to speak, the respirations suddenly become stridulous (i.e., have a shrill, crowing sound), cyanosis develops and loss of consciousness ensues unless respirations are quickly reestablished. Prompt endotracheal intubation or emergency tracheostomy is done, and oxygen is administered via either tube. The injury and paralysis are rarely permanent; function is usually gradually restored, and the tracheostomy tube is removed.

During surgery, interference with the blood supply to the parathyroid glands or injury or removal of parathyroid tissue may occur which depresses secretion by the glands. Decreased parathyroid hormone concentration leads to *hypocalcemia*, resulting in increased neuromuscular irritability and the condition known as *tetany*. Early signs of this complication include complaints of numbness and tingling in the hands or feet, muscle twitching and spasms, and gastrointestinal cramps. A change may be evident in the voice; it may become high-pitched and shrill because of spasm of the vocal cords. To confirm increased neuromuscular irritability due to hypocalcemia, the patient is examined for a positive Chvostek's or Trousseau's sign. Chvostek's sign is demonstrated by twitching of the upper lip and contraction of the facial muscles in response to tapping of the facial nerve in front of the ear. Trousseau's sign is elicited by the inflation of a blood pressure cuff around an arm; if the blood calcium level is low, spasmodic contraction of the forearm muscles occurs, producing a claw-like flexure of the hand and fingers. A blood specimen is obtained for serum calcium determination with the appearance of early symptoms. Calcium gluconate 10 per cent may be slowly administered intravenously by the physician; then, an oral preparation is given until normal parathyroid function resumes. The patient is encouraged to take milk and calcium-containing foods.

Thyrotoxicosis or thyroid storm rarely

complicates the postoperative period following a thyroidectomy (see further on).

CARE AFTER DISCHARGE FROM HOSPITAL. The patient's hospitalization is usually brief if no complications develop. Information as to the amount of activity he may resume is obtained from the physician and discussed with the patient. Extra rest will still be necessary, and the patient is advised to continue neck exercises until there is freedom of movement without any feeling of pulling. He is usually followed at the clinic or by the physician for about a year, being examined for any residual laryngeal damage and hypoparathyroidism, recurring hyperthyroidism, or developing hypothyroidism. If no problems develop during that year, an annual checkup is then recommended.

Thyroid Storm (Thyrotoxic Crisis)

This is a serious complication of hyperthyroidism that usually proves fatal but, fortunately, it is rarely seen since the advent of antithyroid drugs and radioiodine. The crisis may be precipitated in a hyperthyroid person by a severe infection, such as pneumonia, or by an emotional crisis. It must also be kept in mind as a possible, but rare, complication of a subtotal thyroidectomy or radioiodine treatment. It is attributed to the sudden release of large amounts of the thyroid hormones into the circulation.

MANIFESTATIONS. The metabolic rate rises rapidly and the patient manifests hyperpyrexia, an extremely rapid pulse, inordinate restlessness, disorientation, diarrhea and vomiting, and eventually shock and coma due to heart failure and circulatory collapse.

TREATMENT. The patient receives a continuous intravenous infusion of glucose and electrolyte solutions. A corticosteroid preparation is given intravenously, and an antithyroid drug may be administered via a nasogastric tube. A sedative or tranquilizer is also given intravenously to reduce restlessness. Oxygen is administered, and a hypothermic blanket is used to reduce the patient's body temperature. The patient requires constant observation and attention; a nurse remains in constant attendance.

Thyroiditis

Inflammation of the thyroid occurs rarely and may be acute or chronic. Acute thyroid-itis may be the result of viral or bacterial infection or may follow irradiation therapy of the gland. The thyroid area of the neck is tender, warm and reddened; the patient's temperature is elevated and signs of hyperthyroidism may develop. The patient may be treated by bed rest, an antimicrobial preparation if the condition is of infectious origin, and local cold applications.

Chronic thyroiditis occurs in a form which may be referred to as *Hashimoto's disease*. This disease is an autoimmune reaction; that is, the patient develops antibodies in response to antigens originating in his own thyroid. It is suggested that substances which normally remain within the thyroglobin escape into the general circulation. The production of lymphocytes and plasma cells with antibodies is stimulated, and these cells infiltrate and attack the thyroid, resulting in destruction of the functioning tissue. The gland becomes swollen and congested, and eventually hypothyroidism develops. The condition may be treated with cortisone or, because of the increased incidence of cancer in Hashimoto's disease, a complete thyroidectomy may be done. Replacement therapy is used for the associated thyroxine deficiency.

A type of chronic thyroiditis, which is extremely rare, is known as *Riedel's thyroiditis*. The etiology is unknown. The condition is characterized by the slowly progressive involvement of the thyroid and adjacent tissues by dense, fibrous connective tissue. The affected areas become very hard and may cause pressure on the trachea and esophagus. Surgical resection may be undertaken to relieve pressure, and various drugs used may include thyroxine, and corticosteroid and immunosuppressive drugs.[11]

Carcinoma of the Thyroid

The most common malignancy of the thyroid is adenocarcinoma. Signs and symptoms include rapid and progressive enlargement of the gland without an appreciable increase or decrease in thyroid hormone secretion, hardness and fixation of the gland, lymph node enlargement in the neck and supraclavicular areas, hoarseness due to involvement of the recurrent laryngeal nerve, and respiratory distress because of pressure on the trachea.

---

[11]Dillon, op. cit., p. 261.

The condition may be treated with internal radiation by the administration of radioiodine (I^{131}), relatively large doses of desiccated thyroid to suppress the gland's activity, or total thyroidectomy followed by radiation therapy and hormonal replacement. Thyroidectomy may include neck dissection to remove involved lymph nodes.

PARATHYROID GLANDS

The parathyroid glands are small oval bodies attached to the posterior surface of the lateral lobes of the thyroid (Fig. 22–4). The number may vary but is usually four. The principal secretion of the parathyroid glands is *parathormone* (PTH), which regulates the concentration of calcium and inorganic phosphorus in the blood through its action on the intestine, bone tissue and kidneys. It promotes absorption of calcium in the intestine and demineralization of bone and the movement of the calcium into the extracellular fluid. In the kidneys, the hormone increases the excretion of phosphorus by decreasing its reabsorption from the glomerular filtrate and conversely, the reabsorption of calcium is increased, decreasing its excretion in urine.

Parathormone, through its regulation of blood calcium and phosphorus levels, plays an important role in normal physiology. A normal concentration of calcium is essential for the normal structure of bones and teeth,

coagulation of blood, maintenance of normal cardiac rhythmicity, normal neuromuscular excitability and cellular membrane permeability. The greater part of the absorbed calcium is deposited in bones. The optimal blood calcium level for meeting these functions is 9 to 11 mg. per cent (5 mEq/liter). Phosphorus functions in cellular metabolism, bone structure and the maintenance of a normal pH of body fluids. The normal blood concentration of inorganic phosphorus is 3 to 4 mg. per cent (2 mEq./liter).

The rate of secretion of the parathyroid hormone is controlled by the concentration of calcium in the blood. When the calcium level rises above normal, the glands are inhibited and less hormone is produced. A fall in the blood calcium level stimulates the glands, resulting in an increased output of parathormone.

Some *calcitonin* (thyrocalcitonin) is also secreted by the parathyroid glands. Its output is stimulated by an elevation in the calcium of the blood or an excess of glucagon. It is an antagonist to parathormone; as cited previously (p. 758) it inhibits bone resorption and promotes the excretion of calcium and phosphorus in urine and the movement of calcium into the bones.

In summary, a feedback system exists between the parathyroid glands and the circulating blood calcium level. Following a decrease in calcium concentration there is an increased secretion of parathormone. The hormone thus acts to: (1) raise the serum calcium level; (2) lower the serum phosphorus level; (3) decrease the urinary output of calcium; (4) increase the renal excretion of phosphate; and (5) promote the movement of calcium from the bones and the absorption of calcium from the intestine. A feedback mechanism also operates to regulate the secretion of calcitonin; hypercalcemia stimulates its production.

Parathyroid Disorders

Primary disease of the parathyroid glands is rare; the disturbances seen are most often secondary to thyroid disease.

Hypoparathyroidism

Parathyroid insufficiency may be the result of idiopathic atrophy of the glands or surgery

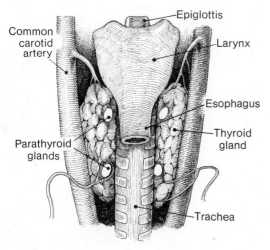

FIGURE 22–4 Posterior surface of the thyroid gland, showing the parathyroid glands.

on the thyroid. In the case of surgery, there may have been interference with the blood supply to the glands, injury which inhibits secretion or, rarely, inadvertent removal of them.

EFFECTS. The deficiency of parathormone causes hypocalcemia, and symptoms of increased neuromuscular excitability and tetany are usually the first manifestations (muscle cramps, carpopedal spasms, laryngeal spasm affecting the voice, dysphagia, convulsions). Wheezy respirations may be heard due to bronchospasm. Less calcium than normal is excreted in the urine because of the low blood calcium level, and the bones tend to become more dense. Renal excretion of phosphorus is reduced and the serum phosphate level is elevated, which predisposes the patient to acidosis. If the hormone deficiency is prolonged, calcium deposition may develop in the lens and conjunctiva of the eyes, the brain, lungs or gastric mucosa. The hair becomes thin and gray; areas of alopecia and loss of eyebrows are common. The skin becomes coarse and scaly and the nails are brittle and have horizontal ridges.

TREATMENT. The hypocalcemia is corrected initially by the intravenous administration of calcium gluconate 10 per cent. The patient is then given regular oral doses of a calcium salt, such as gluconate or lactate, along with a preparation of vitamin D to promote the absorption of the calcium. The patient is followed closely; frequent determinations of blood phosphorus and calcium levels are made. Phosphorus-containing foods may have to be limited to avoid complications; these are principally dairy products. An alternative may be the prescription of aluminum hydroxide gel which binds the phosphorus in the intestine, preventing its absorption. The patient is encouraged to take extra fluids to promote renal excretion of phosphorus.

Hyperparathyroidism

The cause of an excessive secretion of parathormone is usually an adenoma but may rarely be hyperplasia or carcinoma of the glands.

MANIFESTATIONS. The high parathormone concentration in the blood causes decalcification of the bones, and hypercalcemia occurs. The blood level of inorganic phosphorus falls as its renal excretion increases, and the concentration of calcium in the glomerular filtrate is higher than normal, predisposing to the formation of renal calculi. Neuromuscular excitability is depressed and loss of muscle tone is evident. Demineralization of the bones may be so marked that fibrous cystic areas develop which frequently lead to deformities and pathologic fractures. In some instances bone tumors consisting of an overgrowth of osteoclasts develop. When bone changes occur, the disorder may be referred to as *von Recklinghausen's disease* or *osteitis fibrosa cystica,* and the patient may experience tenderness and pain in the bones, especially with weight-bearing.

The patient with hyperparathyroidism may, over a period of time, develop a resistance to insulin. He may complain of muscular weakness, loss of appetite, nausea, vomiting and constipation. The urinary volume is usually increased because of the excessive amounts of calcium and phosphorus to be excreted. Renal function may become impaired; the tubular epithelium may be damaged by the excessive excretion of calcium or the formation of renal calculi. Frequently, the disease is only recognized when some deformity develops or a pathologic fracture occurs.

TREATMENT. The patient with hyperparathyroidism should receive 3000 to 4000 ml. of fluid daily. If anorexia, nausea and vomiting are problems, intravenous infusions may be necessary to insure an adequate intake. Foods containing calcium are restricted in the diet.

Hyperparathyroidism is treated by surgical excision of the gland with the adenoma or, in the case of hyperplasia, removal of all the glands but one. Following surgery, the patient is observed closely for the early signs of possible hypocalcemia (tetany; see p. 767). Frequent serum calcium and phosphorus determinations are made. A diet high in calcium and phosphorus may be necessary to restore normal bone structure.

ADRENAL GLANDS

The two adrenal or suprarenal glands are situated immediately above the kidneys. Each one is enclosed within a capsule and consists of two distinct parts, the cortex and medulla, which are functionally unrelated and are of different embryologic origin. The cortex develops from germinal mesodermal cells. The medulla is derived from the ectoderm in close association with the sympathetic division of the autonomic nervous system with which it is functionally related. The adrenal glands have an abundant blood supply through branches of the aorta and the inferior phrenic and renal arteries.

The Adrenal Cortex

The cortex forms the outer part as well as the greater portion of the gland and produces hormones essential to life. These are steroids and collectively are called the *adrenocorticoids,* corticosteroids or corticoids. Cells of the cortex have a high cholesterol and vitamin C content which is used in the production of many steroid substances. Those secreted in physiologically significant amounts fall into three classes: mineralocorticoids, glucocorticoids and sex hormones. The steroids in each of these classes have some predominant characteristics or actions, but may overlap into another class. There are three zones or groups of cells: the outer one (zona glomerulosa) secretes the mineralocorticoids; the middle, thicker area of cells (zona fasciculata) secretes the glucocorticoids; and the inner layer of cells (zona reticularis) adjacent to the medulla secretes the adrenal sex hormones (androgens and estrogen).

MINERALOCORTICOIDS. The most significant mineralocorticoid is *aldosterone,* which influences electrolyte concentrations and fluid volume. It stimulates the renal tubules to reabsorb sodium and excrete potassium, and it decreases the sodium concentration while increasing the potassium content of saliva, gastric secretion and sweat. An increase in the level of circulating aldosterone causes an increase in the serum sodium level, and that in interstitial fluid. The consequent elevation in their osmotic pressure causes an increased release of the antidiuretic hormone and a resultant retention of water. Conversely, a decreased output of aldosterone reverses these reactions.

The secretion of aldosterone is regulated in the interest of maintaining a normal sodium concentration and normal fluid volume. Factors which influence the amount of aldosterone released are the blood sodium and potassium levels and the blood volume. A decrease in the sodium concentration stimulates an increased output of aldosterone and, conversely, a rise in sodium to above the normal level decreases the output of the hormone. The effect of potassium is the reverse of that of sodium; that is, the adrenal cortices respond to an elevated potassium concentration by an increased secretion of aldosterone and vice versa. Decreases in renal arterial blood pressure such as occur in shock, physical trauma and hemorrhage increase renin secretion by the kidneys. The production of angiotensin II that results from the release of renin (see p. 613) stimulates the adrenal cortex to secrete aldosterone. The adrenocorticotropic hormone (ACTH) also stimulates the secretion of aldosterone as well as glucocorticoids, but more is required than that necessary to initiate an output of glucocorticoids.

GLUCOCORTICOIDS. Several glucocorticoids have been recognized, but *cortisol* (hydrocortisone) is considered to be the most important, since it is more potent and is produced in much greater amounts than the other cortical hormones. Cortisol influences the metabolism of glucose, protein and fat, and is involved in the body's responses to physical and mental stress. Its actions are complex and not clearly understood; for example, it enables a person to deal more effectively with stress, but how this is achieved is not known. Cortisol elevates the blood sugar level and the liver glycogen stores are increased. Tissue protein is broken down and the amino acids are converted to glycogen or glucose in the liver (gluconeogenesis). Fat is also mobilized, some of which is also converted to glucose.

Glucocorticoids are secreted in response to circulating adrenocorticotropic hormone (ACTH). In turn, the production and release of ACTH by the adenohypophysis depends upon the release of corticotropin-releasing factor (CRF) which is secreted by the hypothalamus and delivered to the corticotropic cells of the adenohypophysis. The production of CRF is influenced by a feedback mechanism; that is, a low concentration of adrenocorticoid secretions in the blood initiates the hypothalamic responses. With an elevation of blood glucocorticoids the output of ACTH is depressed. Physical and psychological stress and hypoglycemia also stimulate the release of CRF through impulses delivered from the cerebral cortex or midbrain to the hypothalamus. ACTH is secreted in diurnal rhythm; the secretory output is highest in the morning and lowest in the evening.

A concentration of cortisol in excess of the normal is of clinical significance because it suppresses local inflammatory responses to irritating substances (antiinflammatory effect), delays healing through depressed fibroplasia and reduces tissue sensitivity reactions to antigens (antiallergic reaction). Glucocorticoids have a tissue-wasting effect; they promote the breakdown of body proteins and tend to inhibit amino acid uptake and tissue synthesis. Other effects also associated with an excess of cortisol are atrophy of the lymphoid tissues, a decreased production of lymphocytes and eosinophils, an increased secretion of gastric hydrochloric acid and pepsinogen which predisposes to the development of ulcers, and increased cerebral excitability manifested by restlessness and euphoria. The glucocorticoids, as well as the mineralocorticoids, may also cause some sodium retention, resulting in a positive fluid balance.

ADRENAL SEX HORMONES. The adrenal cortices of both sexes secrete both male and female hormones — namely, *androgens, estrogen* and *progesterone*. Estrogen and progesterone are produced in lesser amounts than the androgens but, normally, the quantity of any of these hormones is considered to be physiologically insignificant compared with the amounts produced by the gonads. Occasionally, tumors of the adrenal cortex may result in an excessive production of the sex hormones, leading to precocious sexual development in childhood, masculinizing changes in the female adult or feminization in the case of an adult male.

Adrenal Medulla

The medulla forms the central portion of each adrenal gland and is composed of specialized neurons (nerve cells) which secrete two hormones, *epinephrine* (adrenalin) and *norepinephrine* (noradrenalin). Because of their chemical composition, they are frequently referred to as catecholamines. During any stress or threat to the organism, the hormones are released and serve with the autonomic nervous system to produce defensive reactions throughout the body. Their production is controlled by nerve impulses transmitted to the medullae by sympathetic nerve fibers, and their effects are similar to those produced by sympathetic innervation. Approximately 80 per cent of the secretion is epinephrine, and the remainder is norepinephrine.

Epinephrine causes constriction of the peripheral and renal blood vessels and dilatation of the coronary and skeletal muscle vessels. The rate and force of contraction of the heart and skeletal muscle is increased. The smooth muscle of the bronchioles, gastrointestinal tract and urinary bladder relaxes. The dilator muscle fibers of the irises contract, resulting in dilatation of the pupils. The blood sugar is elevated by increased glycogenolysis (conversion of glycogen to glucose) in both the liver and skeletal muscles. The metabolic rate is accelerated, and there is an increased alertness and awareness due to stimulation of the brain. Epinephrine also promotes the release of adrenocorticotropin, which in turn increases the secretion of glucocorticoids.

Norepinephrine causes a more generalized vasoconstriction and does not cause dilatation of any vessels. Because of this action, it is more effective in raising the blood pressure; both systolic and diastolic blood pressures rise.

Disorders of the Adrenal Cortices

As with other endocrine glands, dysfunction of the adrenal cortices may involve hyposecretion or hypersecretion of their hormones. Adrenocortical hypofunction produces Addison's disease. Hyperfunction may cause Cushing's syndrome or primary aldosteronism.

Assessment of Adrenocortical Function

Investigation of adrenocortical activity includes the following tests:

PLASMA CORTISOL CONCENTRATION. A venous blood specimen is collected for estimation of the concentration of this principal glucocorticoid.

Normal: 4 to 30 micrograms (μg.)/100 ml.

The initial evaluation may be followed by an injection of ACTH and a second plasma cortisol determination. Normally the level rises; if there is no increase, adrenocortical insufficiency is suspected.

PLASMA CORTISOL DIURNAL RHYTHM. Normally, plasma cortisol concentration is greatest approximately 1 to 2 hours after awakening and is lowest 2 to 3 hours after going to sleep at night. Determinations are made of the concentration at various times over a 24-hour period. The 8 A.M. plasma cortisol level is usually in the range of 15 to 30 μg./100 ml. At 8 P.M., the concentration is normally only 50 per cent of the 8 A.M. level.

An abnormal rhythm of cortisol secretion usually indicates some dysfunction in the adrenal cortices.

METYRAPONE TEST. This drug blocks the formation of cortisol at the stage of 11-desoxycortisol; the latter is released and may be measured in the serum and urine. Normally, a low plasma level of cortisol stimulates the hypothalamus to deliver corticotropin-releasing factor to the adenohypophysis to increase the output of ACTH. An accumulation of the precursor to cortisol (11-desoxycortisol) in the serum indicates that ACTH is being released and that the adrenal cortices are responding. The test procedure involves the oral administration of metyrapone; it is usually given every 4 hours for 6 hours. Twenty-four-hour urine specimens are collected the day prior to the test, the day the metyrapone is given and the day following. The urine is examined for 17-hydroxycorticosteroid content. Blood specimens may be taken at intervals after the drug has been administered to determine the plasma ACTH or 11-desoxycortisol level.

The test evaluates both pituitary and adrenal function; if 11-desoxycortisol is not produced and the plasma ACTH level is elevated, there is adrenal dysfunction. If the 11-desoxycortisol production is below normal and the ACTH level is low, the problem may lie in the hypothalamic-adenohypophyseal system.

URINARY EXCRETION OF 17-KETOSTEROIDS. An estimation of the concentration of 17-ketosteroids in a 24-hour urine collection provides some indication of the secretory activity of the adrenal cortices. These ketosteroids are metabolic products of androgens and glucocorticoids. If the concentration is less than normal, an intravenous infusion of ACTH in normal saline is given *slowly* over 8 hours, and the urine is collected for a second 24-hour specimen. If the low level of 17-ketosteroids still persists, it suggests dysfunction of the adrenal cortices. An elevation in the urinary steroids following the administration of the ACTH indicates a deficiency in the secretion of ACTH by the adenohypophysis.

Normal 24-hour urinary steroids: adult male, 8 to 20 mg. per 24 hours; adult female, 6 to 15 mg. per 24 hours.

EOSINOPHIL COUNT. Normally, an elevated concentration of glucocorticoids reduces the number of circulating eosinophils. Using this as a means of testing adrenocortical function, the eosinophil count is taken in the morning before breakfast. Then the patient receives an intramuscular injection of ACTH. The response of normal adrenal cortices is an increased output of glucocorticoids and a corresponding fall in eosinophils. If there is no appreciable decrease in the circulating eosinophils, it suggests adrenocortical hypofunction.

Normal eosinophil count: 200 per cu. mm. or 1 to 3 per cent of leukocytes.

Normal following ACTH injection: approximately 20 to 30 per cent decrease of the initial count.

WATER EXCRETION TEST. Adrenocorticoid insufficiency reduces the renal ability to excrete water rapidly. The patient is given 1500 ml. of water in the fasting state. Normally, the urine output will be 1000 ml. or more within 5 hours. A decrease to 50 per cent or less of the volume of water given is common in adrenocortical hypofunction.

BLOOD CHEMISTRY. Blood electrolyte concentrations are determined, and the ratio of sodium to potassium is noted. In adrenocortical insufficiency, the sodium level is below normal and that of potassium is elevated, decreasing the ratio of sodium to potassium.

Normal sodium: 132 to 142 mEq./liter.

Normal potassium: 3.5 to 5.0 mEq./liter.

Normal ratio Na to K: Approximately 1:30.

The fasting blood sugar concentration is determined and is found to be below normal with decreased adrenocorticoid secretion and above normal with hypersecretion.

Normal blood sugar: 70 to 100 mg. per cent.

Addison's Disease (Primary Adrenal Insufficiency)

Primary failure of the adrenal cortices to produce corticoids is most often the result of atrophy of the glands but may also be caused by tubercular infection or a neoplasm. Atrophy of the glands is attributed to an autoimmune reaction; antigens escape from the adrenals, resulting in infiltration and ultimate destruction of the glands by lymphocytes, plasma cells and antibodies.[12] Secondary hypofunction of the adrenal cortices occurs with hypopituitarism and the concomitant deficiency of adrenocorticotropin. The patient undergoes various diagnostic procedures to distinguish between primary and secondary adrenocortical insufficiency. This is important since, in secondary insufficiency, the secretion of aldosterone usually remains normal and mineralocorticoids should not be administered.

MANIFESTATIONS. In Addison's disease there is a deficiency of cortisol which interferes with the maintenance of a normal blood sugar level; the body cannot compensate by gluconeogenesis, liver glyocgen is depleted and hypoglycemia develops, especially between meals. There is a general depression of metabolic activity and energy production. The ability to cope with even mild stress is greatly diminished and minor infections, slight injuries, exposure to extremes of temperature, or emotional problems that are relatively insignificant to the normal person may prove very serious to these individuals.

The patient complains of weakness and constant fatigue which becomes progressively more severe and incapacitating unless treatment is instituted. Listlessness, irritability and impaired mental ability may be manifested. Anorexia, nausea, abdominal pain and constipation alternating with diarrhea are common complaints. The patient loses weight. The skin takes on a dusky, bronze hue and brown pigmented areas appear, especially in sites normally exposed to light pressure or friction such as the backs of the hands (particularly over the knuckles), face,

---

[12]Williams, op. cit., p. 272.

neck, axillae and "belt" areas. Patchy areas of pigmentation may also be observed in the oral mucosa and conjunctivae.

The adrenocortical insufficiency causes an outpouring of the adrenocorticotropic hormone (ACTH). As noted earlier in this chapter, ACTH is similar in chemical structure to the melanocyte-stimulating hormone (MSH) and, in high concentration, may produce similar effects. As a result, pigmented areas of the skin are common to the patient with Addison's disease.

The aldosterone deficiency incurs decreased reabsorption of sodium by the renal tubules with a consequent excessive loss of water as well as sodium in the urine. Severe dehydration may develop, leading to a depletion of the intravascular volume and ensuing reduced cardiac output, hypotension and shock. There is not the normal exchange of hydrogen ions for reabsorbed sodium ions in the kidneys, and acidosis may develop. Increased reabsorption of potassium by the tubules produces an elevated blood level, and hyperkalemia may develop (see p. 89) and cause cardiac arrhythmias.

TREATMENT AND NURSING CARE. Addison's disease is treated by maintenance doses of corticoid preparations. The glucocorticoids are replaced by the oral administration of a cortisol preparation two or three times daily. The deficiency of mineralocorticoid (aldosterone) associated with primary adrenocortical insufficiency is met by giving desoxycorticosterone intramuscularly or fludrocortisone (synthetic aldosterone) orally once daily. If desoxycorticosterone is used, after the maintenance dose is determined, a preparation in which the drug is carried in an oil solution (desoxycorticosterone trimethylacetate) may be given intramuscularly at intervals of 3 or 4 weeks instead of the daily dose. The patient with secondary adrenocortical insufficiency does not require the aldosterone replacement.

The nurse caring for a patient receiving corticoid preparations must be familiar with the potential adverse effects of these drugs. If the patient receives corticoids in doses even slightly in excess of the amounts normally secreted, certain changes are likely to occur, especially with prolonged administration. Constant observation is necessary for early signs of side effects. Restlessness, insomnia, euphoria and swings in mood may be manifested. The patient's susceptibility to infection may be markedly increased by the drug's suppression of lymphocyte and antibody production and local inflammatory responses. Muscle wasting and weakness may occur as a result of an excessive protein breakdown and increased loss of potassium in the urine. Sodium and water retention may be evidenced by edema. Increased fat deposition on the trunk and face may develop, changing the patient's general appearance. Increased fullness and rounding of the face produces the characteristic change referred to as the "moon facies." Females may develop secondary male characteristics accompanied by growth of hair on the face, and growth of the breasts in males is occasionally seen. Prolonged administration of corticoids in excess of normal secretion may produce hyperglycemia and glycosuria. The patient also becomes predisposed to the development of gastrointestinal lesions, such as peptic ulcers.

The patient with Addison's disease is encouraged to take a high-carbohydrate, high-protein diet. The danger of hypoglycemia which may occur with glucocorticoid deficiency may be offset by the patient taking nourishment between meals and at bedtime. In primary adrenal insufficiency the patient may require additional sodium chloride. A directive as to the amount of salt to be included in the diet should be received from the physician; the average amount served with meals may be sufficient. The patient with secondary adrenocortical insufficiency will not require additional salt.

Acute corticoid insufficiency, which is also referred to as *Addisonian crisis,* may develop when corticoid replacement is inadequate or omitted, or it may be what brings the patient for medical attention before the disease is diagnosed. Frequently a crisis is precipitated by some physical or psychological stress such as infection, exposure to extremes of temperature, gastrointestinal upset (e.g., vomiting and diarrhea), fever, profuse perspiration, strenuous activity, anxiety or grief. Acute insufficiency is serious and, unless treated promptly, can rapidly lead to death. Early symptoms are nausea, vomiting, diarrhea, abdominal pain, fever and extreme weakness. Severe hypoglycemia and dehydration develop rapidly; the blood pressure falls, and shock and coma may follow.

Blood glucose, sodium and cortisol levels are low and the potassium and urea concentrations are markedly elevated.

Addisonian crisis is treated by continuous intravenous infusion of dextrose in normal saline to which hydrocortisone (cortisol) is added for at least the first 24 hours. Hydrocortisone is also given orally or intramuscularly. The large doses of hydrocortisone which the patient receives usually exert a sufficient sodium-retaining effect, eliminating the need for supplementary administration of a mineralocorticoid preparation. A vasopressor such as levarterenol (Levophed) or metaraminol (Aramine) may be ordered intravenously to raise the blood pressure. This will be given in a separate intravenous solution, since the rate of flow is slow and must be carefully controlled according to the blood pressure.

Frequent recordings of the blood pressure, temperature, pulse, respirations and level of response are made. The patient is kept at absolute rest to avoid expenditure of energy and is turned, bathed and fed by the nurse. He is kept flat and any change of position is made slowly because of the hypotension. Frequent, high-carbohydrate feedings are given as soon as they can be tolerated. When the patient's blood pressure and other vital signs have returned to normal and are sustained, and the condition which precipitated the crisis has been controlled, the corticoid dosage is gradually reduced to maintenance level.

PATIENT INSTRUCTION. An important nursing function in caring for the patient with Addison's disease is teaching him and his family about his disease and the necessary care. A simple explanation is given of the nature of the condition, and he is told that, although hormone replacement will be necessary during the remainder of his life, if the prescribed therapeutic regimen is followed, he can live a relatively normal life.

The importance of regular and adequate hours of rest, stopping activities short of fatigue and avoiding exposure to cold are stressed, indicating the effect of exposure and overexertion on cellular activity and the blood sugar level. No medications, including laxatives, except those ordered by the physician should be taken. Explicit instructions are given regarding the taking of the prescribed corticoid preparations; directions are written clearly, and the importance of taking the exact amounts at the prescribed times is emphasized. If the patient is to have desoxy-corticosterone acetate in oil intramuscularly every 3 or 4 weeks instead of fludrocortisone by mouth, a referral is made to a clinic or to a visiting nurse agency for the administration. The high-carbohydrate, high-protein diet with the amount of sodium recommended by the physician is discussed in detail, explaining the need for nourishment between meals and at bedtime to maintain a normal blood sugar level.

The patient and family are advised of the need for avoiding contact with those with an infection as much as possible, and suggestions are made as to how this may be achieved. They should understand that a stressful situation or illness demands more corticoids. To prevent a serious crisis or acute corticoid insufficiency, prompt medical attention is necessary with any disorder such as a respiratory infection, vomiting, diarrhea, fainting or sudden weakness. The role of worry and emotional situations in precipitating a crisis is emphasized. The patient with Addison's disease should always carry an identification card or wear a Medic Alert bracelet or pendant which clearly indicates that he has a corticoid insufficiency and what should be done in the event of injury or sudden collapse.

In teaching, the nurse does not attempt to provide all the necessary information at one time. The instruction is planned to cover several sessions; salient points are clarified and reinforced by repetition, and opportunities are provided for the patient and family members to ask questions.

Cushing's Syndrome (Adrenocortical Hyperfunction)

This is a rare disorder which is more common to females and results from an excessive secretion of adrenal corticoids. It may be due to primary hyperfunction of one or both of the adrenal cortices or may be secondary to a pathologic hypersecretion of adrenocorticotropin (ACTH) by the adenohypophysis. Primary hyperactivity of the adrenal cortex is usually caused by a neoplasm, most frequently an adenoma, but may also occur as a result of unexplained hyperplasia.

MANIFESTATIONS. These will vary in individual patients according to age and the amount of corticoid being produced in excess of the normal. The increased output of cortisol causes excessive protein catabolism, gluconeogenesis, an abnormal distribution of fat and atrophy of lymphoid tissue. The patient manifests a decreased glucose tolerance, hyperglycemia, and muscle wasting and weakness. The appearance changes because of the increased deposition of fat on the trunk, thin wasted limbs, and a round, bloated-looking face ("moon" face). Purple striae may appear, notably on the abdomen, buttocks and thighs, and are due to increased fragility of the blood vessels and atrophy of the skin. Ecchymoses are common. The production of lymphocytes is suppressed, increasing the patient's susceptibility to infection. Osteoporosis may occur, usually in the vertebrae, because of calcium mobilization; the patient frequently complains of backache.

The excessive secretion of mineralocorticoids results in electrolyte, fluid and acid-base imbalances. Hypernatremia, water retention and hyopkalemia develop. The increased reabsorption by the renal tubules of sodium ions in exchange for hydrogen ions (see p. 97) depletes the acid ions, producing alkalosis. The low blood level of potassium may cause extreme weakness and cardiac dysfunction. Hypertension due to the sodium and water retention is common.

As a consequence of the increased production of androgens, the female patient develops secondary male characteristics. There is a marked growth of hair on the face, the voice deepens, breasts atrophy, amenorrhea occurs and the clitoris may enlarge. If the disease occurs in childhood, precocious sexual development is evident in the male. The female child manifests masculinization with marked enlargement of the clitoris.

If the disease is secondary to a hypersecretion of ACTH, the disturbances are associated principally with an excessive production of the glucocorticoids only.

TREATMENT AND NURSING CARE. The treatment of Cushing's syndrome depends upon whether the hypersecretion of corticoids is due to primary dysfunction of the adrenal cortices or is the result of a hypersecretion of ACTH. In the case of an adrenocortical neoplasm, the affected gland is removed. If the cause is hyperplasia, a bilateral adrenalectomy is usually done. The patient then receives hormonal replacement therapy as outlined under Addison's disease (p. 774). If the condition is secondary to a pituitary tumor, the tumor is usually treated by irradiation or surgical removal.

Nursing care of the patient with Cushing's syndrome is mainly symptomatic. If he is ambulatory, precautions are necessary to prevent accidental falls which may occur because of his weakness. The fluid intake and output are recorded to determine the amount of water retention, and the sodium intake is restricted. The blood pressure and pulse are taken at regular intervals so that early changes may be detected. Changes in mood and behavior are common and should be reported. Exposure to persons with infection is avoided because of the patient's lowered resistance.

Primary Aldosteronism

An excessive production of aldosterone occurs rarely and is usually caused by an adenoma or hyperplasia of the particular adrenocortical cells which secrete the hormone. The most striking features of the disease are the excessive renal loss of potassium, retention of sodium and hypertension. The patient experiences severe generalized muscular weakness due to the hypokalemia. Depletion of the body potassium reduces the kidneys' ability to concentrate the urine, and polyuria occurs. Despite an increased retention of salt, there is no corresponding retention of water or edema. This is attributed to an increased glomerular filtration rate and the polyuria. As a result of the hypernatremia and polyuria, the patient usually experiences severe thirst. An elevation of arterial blood pressure is characteristic. In addition to hypernatremia and hypokalemia, laboratory investigation reveals elevated urinary and plasma aldosterone levels and normal renin concentration. Treatment consists of surgical removal of the adenoma or affected gland preceded by administration of potassium salts.

Secondary hyperaldosteronism due to an excessive secretion of renin by the kidneys may occur. It may be treated with spironolactone, an aldosterone antagonist, or renal surgery.

Dysfunction of the Adrenal Medullae

Pheochromocytoma

Disease of the adrenal medullae is rare and most commonly occurs in the form of a neoplasm known as a pheochromocytoma, which produces an excessive amount of epinephrine and norepinephrine. The tumor is usually unilateral and benign and causes hypertension, hyperglycemia and hypermetabolism. The increased liberation of large amounts of the hormones is usually paroxysmal at first, lasting from a few minutes to hours, but is likely to eventually become persistent. The patient frequently complains of a pounding headache, nausea, vomiting, palpitation, air hunger, nervousness, tremor and weakness. Sweating, pallor, dilatation of the pupils, tachycardia and a sharp rise in the blood pressure are also manifested. The increased glucogenolysis and subsequent elevated blood sugar may result in glucosuria.

Tests used to establish the diagnosis of pheochromocytoma include the phentolamine (Regitine) test and estimation of the blood and urinary content of the hormones or their major metabolite. Phentolamine is given intravenously and neutralizes circulating epinephrine. If the hypertension is due to a pheochromocytoma, there is a rapid, brief decline in the blood pressure. The pressure usually returns to its previous level in 10 to 15 minutes. The patient lies flat in bed during the test, and vasopressor drugs (e.g., Levophed) should be available for prompt administration in the event of a vasomotor collapse and hypotension.

Determination of the catecholamines in the urine is usually done on a 24-hour specimen. The normal varies from 8 to 165 micrograms per 24 hours; this may range from 300 to 4000 micrograms in the case of pheochromocytoma. The normal blood content is 0.2 to 7.0 micrograms per liter.

The principal metabolite of the hormones is vanillylmandelic acid (VMA) and is excreted in the urine. An estimation of the amount of VMA in a 24-hour specimen may be done. Normally 2 to 9 mg. are excreted in 24 hours; this is markedly increased in patients with pheochromocytoma.

The patient with pheochromocytoma is treated by surgical removal of the tumor of the affected gland.

Nursing in Adrenal Surgery

Surgery of the adrenal glands may be done on patients with hypersecretions of hormones due to hyperplasia or tumors of one or both glands. The procedure may involve the removal of both adrenal glands (bilateral or total adrenalectomy), the removal of one gland (unilateral adrenalectomy) or resection of a part of a gland (subtotal adrenalectomy). Bilateral adrenalectomy is occasionally undertaken in patients with cancer of the breast and occasionally in those with cancer of the prostate. Malignant disease of these organs is dependent to some extent on sex hormones, and, since the adrenal cortices produce both estrogens and androgens, their removal eliminates a source of the supporting hormones. In the case of cancer of the breast, adrenalectomy is preceded by oophorectomy (removal of the ovaries). The patient with cancer of the prostate undergoes orchidectomy (removal of the testicles) before adrenalectomy is considered.

PREOPERATIVE PREPARATION. Preparation of the patient for adrenal surgery includes the general preparation cited in Chapter 10. Blood studies are done to determine electrolyte concentrations, and corrections are made as indicated. Because of an excessive potassium excretion, a solution of potassium chloride may be ordered to restore the normal level of potassium in the blood. The blood sugar level and glucose tolerance are investigated. The patient is given a high-protein diet because of the protein depletion due to excessive glucocorticoid secretion. The fluid intake and output are measured, and the balance is noted. The blood pressure is recorded at least once daily to serve as a postoperative comparative baseline. The patient with hyperfunction of the adrenal cortices frequently has experienced hypertension for some time. Phentolamine (Regitine) and/or phenoxybenzamine hydrochloride (Dibenzyline) may be prescribed preoperatively to reduce vasomotor tone and hypertension because the anesthetic and actual surgery may precipitate severe hypertension.[13]

If both adrenal glands are to be removed, the patient and his family must understand that constant hormone replacement will be necessary for the remainder of the patient's life. They may indicate some concern about meeting the expense of the drugs; the nurse may suggest sources of assistance or refer the problem to the social service department.

After operation, the patient's respirations tend to be shallow because the incision is close to the diaphragm. In discussions with the patient as to what he may expect postoperatively, emphasis is placed on the need for frequent deep breathing, coughing and early ambulation to prevent complications. He is taught how to cough and is assured of support.

The surgeon's approach to the adrenal gland is usually through a high flank incision or occasionally through the abdomen. When a bilateral adrenalectomy is done, two incisions are made unless the transabdominal approach is used. The entire trunk from the nipple line down to and including the pubis is shaved and cleansed. A nasogastric tube is passed before the sedative is given on the morning of operation. This prevents postoperative vomiting and abdominal distention.

Cortisol may be administered before and during as well as following the operation to prevent adrenal insufficiency in the immediate postoperative period. An intravenous solution is run slowly and continuously. This is in preparation for prompt administration of corticosteroids or a vasopressor as indicated.

POSTOPERATIVE CARE. During the first few postoperative days, and until the maintenance dosages of cortisol and desoxycorticosterone or fludrocortisone are established in the case of adrenalectomy, special attention is paid to the patient's blood pressure, fluid balance and blood chemistry. Constant nursing care is necessary until the vital signs and the corticoid, sodium and potassium concentrations are stabilized. The blood pressure, respirations and pulse are recorded every 15 minutes for several hours and the interval gradually lengthened if they remain satisfactory. Any rapid or significant fall in the blood pressure, dyspnea, or tachycardia is reported promptly. The fluid intake and output are accurately measured, and any imbalance is brought to the physician's attention. Frequent checks are made of the blood sodium, potassium and glucose levels which influence the amount of corticoids given. Vomiting after the nasogastric tube is removed, increased weakness, dehydration,

---

[13]David C. Sabiston, Jr. (Ed.): Davis-Christopher: Textbook of Surgery, 11th ed. Philadelphia, W. B. Saunders, 1977.

hypotension and an elevated temperature may indicate acute corticoid insufficiency.

As indicated previously, deep breathing and coughing are very important while the patient is confined to bed and are encouraged at least every 2 hours. The patient's position is also changed every 1 to 2 hours. Any complaint of chest pain is reported at once.

Intravenous corticoids are given continuously for a day or two with the dosage and rate of flow adjusted to the patient's clinical manifestations and the electrolyte and fluid balances. Oral doses of cortisol are started as soon as tolerated by the patient; a daily intramuscular injection of desoxycorticosterone is also given and is usually replaced by oral fludrocortisone in a few days. The dosage of both corticoid preparations is gradually tapered off until maintenance amounts are established. When the intravenous corticoids are withdrawn, an intravenous infusion of glucose in water or normal saline is continued slowly even though the patient may be tolerating fluids by mouth. The purpose of this is to keep the route available for quick administration of corticoids or a vasopressor (e.g., Levophed, Aramine) if needed. The patient's condition tends to be labile and may change quickly. The nurse must be constantly alert for signs of corticoid insufficiency or indications of excessive corticoid administration. When the nasogastric tube is removed, the patient is started on fluids containing glucose and progresses to a regular diet as tolerated.

When surgery is performed to remove a pheochromocytoma, monitoring of the blood pressure is necessary every ½ to 1 hour for at least 36 to 48 hours; severe fluctuations may occur. A marked rise may occur during or immediately following surgery because of an excessive liberation of epinephrine and norepinephrine from the tumor during removal. An adrenergic blocking agent such as phentolamine (Regitine) is kept available for quick intravenous administration to neutralize the medullary hormones.

More often the problem following surgery is severe hypotension and concomitant shock. The blood pressure is maintained by giving a vasopressor such as levarterenol (Levophed) or metaraminol (Aramine) in an intravenous solution. The rate of flow must be carefully controlled and adjusted according to frequent blood pressure recordings and the physician's directives. The patient is kept flat, and any change in position achieved slowly.

When unilateral adrenalectomy or a subtotal resection of one or both glands is done, the patient may receive some cortisol following operation. Less will be required than in total adrenalectomy and it is gradually withdrawn.

Following adrenal surgery, the patient usually remains in bed for 2 or 3 days or until the blood pressure remains at a satisfactory level. Before commencing ambulation, the head of the bed is elevated and the blood pressure checked. When the patient is permitted to get out of bed a nurse remains with him, and the blood pressure is checked every 15 minutes the first time he is up. If a significant decrease in blood pressure occurs, the patient is returned to bed and kept flat. The application of elastic or crepe bandages to the lower extremities may be made before getting the patient up in order to maintain a greater blood volume in vital areas.

In preparation for discharge, the patient who has had a bilateral adrenalectomy receives the same instruction as the patient with Addison's disease (see p. 775). If he has had one gland removed or a subtotal resection done, he is cautioned to avoid overfatigue, exposure to extremes of temperature (especially cold), infections, and emotional disturbances as much as possible. It is possible that stress may precipitate an acute adrenal insufficiency or crisis because the remaining adrenal tissue cannot meet the increased hormonal demand. He is advised to contact his physician immediately if he experiences weakness, fainting, fever, or nausea and vomiting, as he may require a corticoid supplement.

Following any adrenal surgery, the patient should resume activity very gradually and is followed closely at the clinic or by his physician. Usually several months are required to adjust the hormonal replacement satisfactorily. The patient who has had hypertension due to pheochromocytoma may not regain a stable blood pressure level for 3 to 4 months.

ISLETS OF LANGERHANS

The pancreas is both an exocrine and endocrine gland. Its exocrine secretions are carried by a system of ducts to the duoden-

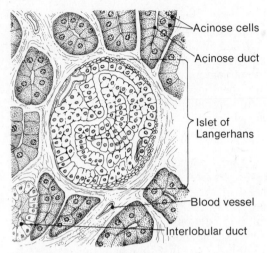

FIGURE 22–5 Location of cells of islets of Langerhans between lobules of pancreas.

um and contain enzymes which play an important role in digestion (see p. 482). The islets of Langerhans form the endocrine component of the pancreas and consist of irregularly scattered groups of cells which are totally independent of the pancreatic system of ducts (see Fig. 22–5). The islets are highly vascularized and consist mainly of two types of cells — alpha cells, which secrete the hormone glucagon, and beta cells, which produce insulin. Both of these hormones are protein and are rendered inactive in the gastrointestinal tract by the proteolytic enzymes; therefore when necessary, they must be administered parenterally.

Secretions and Functions

INSULIN. This hormone plays a dominant role in carbohydrate, fat and protein metabolism, especially in the liver and muscular and adipose tissues. Knowledge of the ways in which insulin promotes specific metabolic cellular activities is incomplete, but it has been established that it stimulates: (1) the transfer of glucose into most cells and its metabolism by those cells;[14] (2) the formation of glycogen by the liver and muscle cells; (3) formation of triglycerides and the synthesis of fat from glucose in adipose tissue; (4) the uptake and incorporation of

amino acids into cell proteins; and (5) an increased uptake of potassium by cells. These activities result in a lower concentration of glucose in the blood.

The chemical structure and composition of the insulin that is initially secreted by the beta cells differs from that normally released and has been named *proinsulin*; it may be referred to as the precursor of insulin. Proinsulin undergoes chemical changes which are activated by proteolytic enzymes within the cells to form insulin.

The secretion of insulin is regulated by the concentration of the blood glucose. An elevation increases the production of insulin and, conversely, a decrease below the normal blood level of glucose suppresses its secretion. Thus, a feedback mechanism is established which controls the output of insulin in order to maintain the blood sugar level within a normal range. The release of insulin is also stimulated by an excess of growth hormone and glucocorticoids. The amount of insulin circulated in the blood increases when carbohydrate foods are ingested; this is attributed to the effect of the gastrointestinal hormones (e.g., gastrin, secretin, cholecystokinin-pancreozymin) on the beta cells. Glucose given intravenously does not produce the same effect as when it is taken orally. It is suggested that there also may be a specific unidentified factor secreted by the gastrointestinal mucosa that stimulates the secretion of insulin.[15]

Calcium ions are necessary for the release of insulin by the beta cells. Other factors that result in an increased insulin level include plasma amino and fatty acid concentrations, right vagal nerve stimulation, acetylcholine and sulfonylurea drugs.[16]

GLUCAGON. This hormone may also be referred to as the hyperglycemic factor, since its primary effect is stimulation of glycogenolysis (the conversion of glycogen to glucose) and its release into the blood by the liver to increase the blood glucose concentration. It also promotes gluconeogenesis and lipolysis. Its secretion by the alpha cells is stimulated by a low blood sugar level. An oral intake of proteins initiates an increased secretion of glucagon, greater than that seen in response to intravenous adminis-

---

[14]Not all cells are insulin-dependent for the transfer of glucose; notable in this respect are the brain cells and erythrocytes.

[15]Ganong, op. cit., p. 260.
[16]Williams, op. cit., p. 517.

tration of amino acids. This suggests a gastrointestinal hormone that stimulates the secretion of glucagon. Sympathetic nervous stimulation of the pancreas also increases the glucagon output.[17]

BLOOD SUGAR LEVEL. The normal blood sugar (glucose) level 3 to 4 hours after a meal varies from approximately 70 to 110 mg. per cent. Fluctuations occur as a result of energy expenditure and the ingestion of foods. The types of food taken also influence the degree of change; obviously, a meal high in carbohydrate produces a greater concentration of glucose for a period of time than a meal with a low carbohydrate content. An elevation of the blood sugar level above the normal is known as *hyperglycemia*. A level below normal is referred to as *hypoglycemia*.

As cited previously, the blood sugar level is regulated by the hormones of the islets of Langerhans. It may, however, be influenced by several other endocrine secretions. An excess of the somatotropic hormone (growth hormone) produces a tendency toward hyperglycemia by decreasing the utilization of glucose and stimulating the production of glucagon. The release of glucocorticoids (cortisol) by the adrenal cortices promotes gluconeogenesis (formation of glucose from amino acids and the glycerol portion of fat), resulting in an elevation of the blood sugar. Epinephrine and norepinephrine stimulate liver glycogenolysis and the metabolism of muscle glycogen to lactic acid, which is then converted to glucose by the liver. The thyroid hormones also increase the blood sugar level by an acceleration of gluconeogenesis.

Disorders of the Islets of Langerhans

Diabetes Mellitus

Diabetes mellitus is a chronic disorder of carbohydrate, fat and protein metabolism characterized by hyperglycemia, degenerative vascular changes and neuropathy. It tends to accelerate degenerative changes throughout the body by widespread vascular changes.

MANIFESTATIONS. As a result of an absolute or relative deficiency of insulin, there

---

[17]Ganong, op. cit., p. 262.

is an inadequate transfer of glucose into the cells; the utilization of glucose for energy and cellular products and its conversion to glycogen or fat and storage as such are depressed. Glucose accumulates in the blood, causing hyperglycemia.

Fat may be mobilized from adipose tissue and broken down to provide a source of energy. The mobilized fat is withdrawn from the blood by the liver and broken down to glycerol and fatty acids. The fatty acids are oxidized by the hepatic cells to ketone bodies (acetoacetic acid, β-hydroxybutyric acid and acetone), which are then circulated and may be metabolized by cells to produce energy, carbon dioxide and water. Only a limited amount of ketone acids can be utilized by the cells. If ketogenesis proceeds rapidly, exceeding the rate at which they can be metabolized, the ketone acids accumulate in the blood, causing ketosis or ketone acidosis.

Tissue protein may also be broken down to amino acids which are used in gluconeogenesis, contributing to the hyperglycemia. Both the uptake of amino acids by the cells and body protein synthesis are decreased.

Diabetes mellitus in young persons usually has a sudden onset in a severe, acute form. In older persons, the onset is most frequently insidious, going undetected and untreated for a considerable period of time. Their diabetes may be recognized in a routine examination in which glucosuria is discovered, or eventually a distressing symptom presents which prompts them to consult a physician.

The most striking symptoms are the result of abnormal carbohydrate metabolism and the resultant hyperglycemia, but the disorder is also marked by disturbances in protein and fat metabolism and degenerative changes, especially in the vascular system. The patient excretes an excessive volume of urine (polyuria) as a result of the increased concentration of glucose in the glomerular filtrate. The glucose increases the osmotic pressure of the filtrate, preventing the reabsorption of water. As a result of the excessive water loss, the patient experiences a persisting thirst (polydipsia), and dehydration and electrolyte imbalance may develop. The blood sugar concentration exceeds the capacity of the renal tubules to reabsorb it from the glomerular filtrate, and sugar is excreted in the urine (glucosuria). The maximum capacity of the renal tubules to reab-

TABLE 22–1 ENDOCRINE GLANDS, THEIR HORMONES AND ASSOCIATED DISORDERS

Gland	Hormones	Functions	Disorders
Hypophysis			
A. Adenohypophysis (anterior lobe)	Somatotropin (growth hormone, STH, GH)	Growth. Aids in determining size; accelerates metabolism, diabetogenic action	Simmonds' disease— decrease of *all* adenohypophyseal hormones Gigantism—increase of STH in childhood Acromegaly—increase of STH in adulthood Dwarfism—decrease of STH in childhood
	Thyrotropin (TSH)	Promotes growth and secretory activity of the thyroid	Hyperthyroidism (Graves' disease)—secondary to increase of TSH
	Corticotropin (adreno-corticotropic hormone, ACTH)	Stimulates secretion of adrenal cortices	Cushing's syndrome—increase of ACTH
	Gonadotropins 1. Follicle-stimulating hormone (FSH)	Causes development of ovarian follicle and secretion of estrogen	Tumors
	2. Luteotropin (LTH)	Promotes ovulation; required for formation of corpus luteum	
	3. Luteinizing hormone (LH) (lactogenic hormone, prolactin)	Stimulates secretion of progesterone; initiates secretion of mammary glands	
	Melanocyte-stimulating hormone (MSH)	Regulates production of pigment of cells in skin	Increase—pigmented areas
B. Neurohypophysis (posterior lobe)	Antidiuretic hormone (vasopressin, ADH)	Increases permeability of distal and collecting tubules of kidneys; therefore, increases reabsorption of water	Diabetes insipidus—decrease of ADH Tumor
	Oxytocin	Excites contraction of pregnant uterus; some effect on smooth muscle; stimulates release and flow of milk	

Thyroid	Triiodothyronine (T$_3$)
	Tetraiodothyronine (T$_4$)
		Increases metabolic rate by stimulating oxidative processes; promotes normal physical growth, maturation, mental development	Hypothyroidism
			  Cretinism in child
			  Myxedema in adult
			Goiter
			Hyperthyroidism
			Thyroid storm
			Thyroiditis
			Carcinoma

	Calcitonin	Promotes excretion of serum calcium and phosphate and movement into bones	
Parathyroid	Parathormone (PTH)	Controls concentration of calcium and inorganic phosphorus in blood	Hypoparathyroidism (tetany) Hyperparathyroidism
	(Calcitonin)		
Adrenal glands A. Adrenal cortex	Adrenocorticoids (corticosteroids, corticoids)		Addison's disease (hypofunction of cortices) Cushing's syndrome (hyperfunction of cortices)
	1. Mineralocorticoids, aldosterone	Influences electrolyte concentration, fluid volume, blood pressure	Primary aldosteronism (increase of aldosterone)
	2. Glucocorticoids, cortisol (hydrocortisone)	Influences metabolism of glucose, protein and fat; concerned with body's responses to physical and mental stress	
	3. Sex hormones (androgens, estrogen and progesterone)		

TABLE 22–1 ENDOCRINE GLANDS, THEIR HORMONES AND ASSOCIATED DISORDERS (Continued)

Gland	Hormones	Functions	Disorders
B. Adrenal medulla	Epinephrine (adrenalin)	Constricts peripheral and renal blood vessels; dilates coronary and skeletal muscle vessels; relaxes smooth muscle of bronchioles, gastrointestinal tract, urinary bladder; dilates pupils; elevates blood sugar; promotes release of adrenocorticotropin; accelerates metabolic rate	Pheochromocytoma (increase of production of both hormones)
	Norepinephrine (noradrenalin)	Generalized vasoconstriction	
Islets of Langerhans	Insulin	Active in carbohydrate metabolism	Diabetes mellitus Hyperinsulinism

sorb glucose represents what is referred to as the glucose renal threshold. The normal is 165 to 180 mg. per cent.

Weakness and fatigue are common complaints because the glucose cannot be utilized to produce energy. There is a loss of weight which is attributed to the mobilization of fat from adipose tissue and the breakdown of protein. Some patients also experience an increased appetite (polyphagia).

Older female patients may develop pruritus of the vulva, usually due to infection by fungi which thrive on the glucose deposit from the urine. The vulva becomes swollen and inflamed. In some instances it is this distressing condition that brings the patient to the physician and leads to the diagnosis of her diabetes. Rarely, male patients develop pruritus and inflammation of the prepuce and glans penis.

Other manifestations generally associated with long-term disease are impaired vision due to retinal changes and opacity of the lens (cataract) and pain, numbness and tingling in the extremities due to peripheral neuritis.

INCIDENCE. Diabetes mellitus is one of the most common chronic disorders and is seen more often in middle-aged and older persons, but it cannot be considered rare in children and young adults. The incidence is higher in women than men, in persons who are obese or have a history of obesity, and among relatives of diabetics. The incidence is also higher in urban populations and among those in sedentary occupations.

It has been estimated that there are 200 million diabetics in the world.[18] Many thousands are known diabetics, and it is believed that those diagnosed represent only a relatively small fraction of those undetected. In many countries the increase corresponds with increased food consumption, reduced physical exercise and obesity. The increased number of diabetics may also be attributed to: (1) increased longevity — more persons survive to the high-incidence age; (2) a lower mortality rate among young diabetics because of improved treatment and control of their disease; (3) extended education of the public about the disease; and (4) the increased number of detection facilities.

ETIOLOGY. The exact cause of diabetes mellitus is not known, but the following factors are considered significant in the development of the metabolic derangement.

INSULIN DEFICIENCY. A common factor in all cases of diabetes mellitus is a lack of sufficient metabolically effective insulin to promote normal carbohydrate metabolism and maintain a normal blood sugar level. The deficiency may be absolute or relative. The former is due to failure of the pancreatic beta cells to produce and/or release sufficient insulin. With a relative deficiency, the insulin production and release are normal but the hormone is ineffective. A greater concentration may be necessary for normal metabolic processes, or cells may have developed an insulin resistance, or the problem may be an

---

[18]Wintrobe, op. cit., p. 532.

unidentified circulating antagonist to the insulin.

HEREDITY. It is now generally accepted that persons who develop primary diabetes mellitus have an inherited. predisposition to the disease. It is transmitted as a recessive genetic trait, which implies that those likely to develop diabetes must have received a defective gene from each parent. The penetrance of the defective genes appears to vary; some homozygotes (persons who have inherited a gene for the predisposition from each parent) do not develop the disease even in their advanced years.

The expected incidence according to the Mendelian law of heredity is as follows. If both parents are diabetic, all their children will most likely become diabetic if they live long enough. When a diabetic marries a carrier,[19] there is a 50 per cent chance that each child will develop diabetes. If the child does not receive a defective gene from each parent, he will receive one from the diabetic parent and will be a carrier. If both parents are carriers, the child has a 25 per cent chance of being a diabetic, a 50 per cent chance of being a carrier and a 25 per cent chance of receiving normal genes. In the case of a marriage of a diabetic to a noncarrier, none of their children will become diabetic, but they will all be carriers (see Table 22-2).

OBESITY. The majority of diabetics who develop their disease after the age of 40 are obese or have a history of obesity. The relationship is not understood. It is thought that persons with a predisposition to the disease who take an excess of food probably create increased demands for insulin which results in eventual exhaustion of the beta cells of the islets. The association of diabetes with obesity is a very significant factor in considering prevention.

DIAGNOSTIC PROCEDURES. The diagnostic procedures used in the investigation for diabetes mellitus are simple in comparison with those used for many other conditions. They include the following urine and blood tests.

URINALYSIS. A urine specimen is examined for the presence of glucose and ketone bodies (acetone, acetoacetic and β-

---

[19]A *carrier* is a person who is free of the disease but has one gene bearing the predisposition to diabetes.

TABLE 22–2 GENETIC COMPOSITION OF OFFSPRING WHEN PARENTS ARE: (A) A DIABETIC AND A CARRIER, (B) TWO CARRIERS, (C) PROBABLE DIABETIC AND A NONCARRIER

	D*	d			D	d
d	dD	dd		D	DD	Dd
d	dD	dd		d	dD	dd

A   B

	D	D
d	dD	dD
d	dD	dD

C

*D = dominant normal gene; d = recessive gene for predisposition to diabetes
DD = Noncarrier
Dd = Carrier
dd = Person likely to develop diabetes

hydroxybutyric acid). Normally, glucose is almost completely reabsorbed from the glomerular filtrate by the renal tubules, and what remains in the urine is insignificant and not detected by the usual tests. If sugar is present (glucosuria), the amount is noted on the basis of the intensity of the reaction and is indicated as a trace, one plus, two plus, and so on. Simple, quick methods of testing the urine for sugar have been devised in the form of a tablet, powder or strip of paper impregnated with the necessary reagent. Directions for their use and a color comparison chart accompany each product. The color chart indicates the characteristic color change associated with certain glucose concentrations. The presence of glucose in the urine may only be suggestive of diabetes mellitus; for instance, the person may have a low glucose renal threshold. If glucose is found, blood sugar determinations are then made for more conclusive evidence.

A 24-hour urine specimen may be ordered to determine the amount of sugar the patient excretes in that period. The collection usually begins in the morning. The patient voids and that urine is discarded. The time is noted and all urine that is voided until that time the next morning is saved. The patient is asked to empty his bladder at the time the test is completed, and that urine is included in the specimen.

Ketone bodies may be present in the urine of a diabetic because of the mobilization and breakdown of fat. Ketonuria occurring with glucosuria generally indicates the presence of diabetes mellitus. Materials similar to those cited in testing for sugar are available for simple quick testing for ketonuria.

BLOOD SUGAR. A blood sugar determination is made from a specimen of venous blood following a period of *4 to 8 hours of fasting*. The normal range is 70 to 110 mg. per cent. In mass surveys for diabetes mellitus and in detection clinics, the blood specimen does not provide a fasting blood sugar level, but the patient is questioned as to when he last ate; a note is made of this and the information is taken into consideration when assessing the report. Persons with abnormally high or borderline levels are followed for further investigation.

GLUCOSE TOLERANCE TEST. This test determines the patient's ability to clear the blood of excess glucose following the ingestion of sugar and to return the blood sugar to a normal level. Preferably, the patient should receive approximately 250 or 300 Gm. of carbohydrate in his diet for 2 or 3 days preceding the test. Food is then withheld overnight, and in the morning a urine specimen and venous blood sample are collected for glucose determinations. Instead of high-carbohydrate meals, the patient may be given 100 Gm of glucose dissolved in 300 to 500 ml. of water orally; it may be flavored with lemon juice. Urine and blood specimens are collected ½, 1, 2 and 3 hours after the ingestion of the glucose. These are examined for the glucose concentration. Normally, the blood sugar level rises to approximately 140 to 160 mg. per cent but returns to normal within 2 hours. In the diabetic, the elevation in the blood sugar will be much higher and several hours (3 to 5) may be required for the original level to be attained.

Rarely, glucose may be given intravenously rather than orally, and urine and blood specimens are collected 30, 60, 90 and 150 minutes following the administration. The amount of glucose used is based on the patient's weight (0.5 Gm. per kg.) and is given in sterile distilled water (20 Gm. of glucose to 100 ml. of water) over a period of 30 minutes. The blood sugar should reach a normal level in 90 minutes.

Normally, with either method, no sugar appears in the urine. In the diabetic the elevation in the blood sugar exceeds the glucose renal threshold and glucosuria occurs. With any glucose tolerance test all medication that may affect the blood sugar level should be withheld (e.g., thiazides, prednisone and estrogen).

TOLBUTAMIDE TEST. This test determines the patient's response to an intravenous injection of sodium tolbutamide which normally results in an increased secretion of insulin. After an overnight fast, blood is taken for blood sugar determination, and the patient is then given 1 Gm. of sodium tolbutamide dissolved in 10 or 11 ml. of sterile distilled water over a period of 2 minutes. The blood sugar level is determined 20, 30, 40 and 60 minutes following the tolbutamide administration. The blood sugar level falls rapidly in normal persons. In diabetes, even in those with a very mild form of the disease, the decrease in blood sugar is less and the decline takes longer.

GLUCOCORTICOID TEST. The administration of glucocorticoid normally increases the output of insulin.

INSULIN ASSAY. Recently techniques for determining the plasma insulin level have been used. Following the administration of glucose to a nondiabetic, the plasma insulin level immediately rises and then quickly falls. Diabetics manifest a low plasma insulin level and there is a limited or sluggish increase in response to the glucose administration.

CLASSIFICATION OF DIABETES. The disorder may be classified in a variety of ways. It may be categorized as *primary diabetes* or idiopathic, although several factors are considered to contribute to the onset of the disorder. In a small number of diabetics the disorder is *secondary* to primary pancreatic or endocrine disease. Pancreatic diabetes occurs as a result of the destruction or removal of islet tissue. Endocrine diabetes is associated with an excess of a hormone that opposes the action of insulin (e.g., corticosteroid, epinephrine, somatotropin). Diabetes may be referred to as *juvenile* or *adult-onset,* depending upon the period in life when the disorder was manifested.

Karam uses a classification based upon the

circulating insulin level.[20] The diabetes may be insulinopenic or insulin-plethoric. *Insulinopenic* (Type 1) diabetes is divided into two types, 1A and 1B. *Insulinopenic 1A* diabetes is a serious form of the disorder seen most often in children and nonobese individuals. Pancreatic beta cell function is impaired, and there is an absence or marked deficiency of insulin. *Insulinopenic 1B* diabetes is less severe; those with it are not usually obese and their circulating insulin level is less than normal, but is certainly higher than is found in the 1A type. The disorder can usually be controlled by diet alone, or by diet and an oral hypoglycemic agent.

Insulin-plethoric (Type II) diabetes is a milder form of the disorder and occurs most commonly in obese adults. It is attributed to end organ unresponsiveness to insulin action; the insulin level is relatively normal and the treatment consists of controlled diet.

Other terms applied to indicate types of diabetes are *genetic* or hereditary, which are synonymous with primary and idiopathic, and *iatrogenic,* which is secondary and due to the treatment used for a primary condition (e.g., corticosteroid administration).

Heredity is considered to play an essential role in primary diabetes, and the individual is considered to have the disorder although he may be asymptomatic for many years. Based on this, the disorder is "staged" according to the presence or absence of hyperglycemia and degree of glucose tolerance. The stage of *prediabetes* or *potential diabetes* is suspected because of family history and is characterized by a normal fasting blood sugar level and glucose tolerance test. Some slight delay may be evident in the insulin response to glucose. *Subclinical (stress) diabetes* is reflected in a normal fasting blood sugar level, but during stress or pregnancy, there is an abnormal glucose tolerance, abnormal cortisone-glucose tolerance and a decreased insulin response to glucose. *Latent (chemical or asymptomatic) diabetes* shows a normal fasting blood sugar level but an abnormal glucose tolerance and a decreased insulin response to glucose. *Overt or frank diabetes* manifests an elevated fasting blood sugar level and a marked decrease in insulin response to glucose.[21, 22]

PREVENTION AND CASE-FINDING. With the knowledge now available, preventive measures in diabetes mellitus are limited chiefly to the prevention and correction of obesity. This is especially important for those with a family history of diabetes or a suggestive obstetrical history. As indicated previously, the majority of diabetics are either obese at the time their disease is manifested or have a history of obesity. The incidence of diabetes among women who have previously given birth to an infant of 4.5 kg. (10 lb.) or more is sufficiently significant to recommend that they maintain their ideal weight and be checked annually for diabetes mellitus. The hospital and visiting nurse have a responsibility to advise persons who are overweight of the many adverse effects of obesity and that they are possible candidates for diabetes mellitus. Occasionally, the nurse is questioned by a diabetic about whether he should marry and whether his children will be diabetic. The hereditary predisposition and the possible chances of transmission may be explained; with that information, the persons concerned must decide for themselves. They are also urged to discuss the problem with a physician or may be referred to a genetic counseling clinic.

Programs for case-finding and education of the general public about diabetes mellitus are organized by national diabetic associations and their local branches. The nurse should be familiar with these associations so that patients and their families may be advised to avail themselves of the services. Detection clinics may be set up, or industrial or community surveys may be made by mobile laboratory units. A blood sugar determination is done on each registrant, and those with a definite or borderline elevation are followed. Obese persons, those in the most susceptible age group (over 40 years of age), those with a family history of diabetes, and women with a history of having had a large baby are urged especially to visit the clinic or participate in the survey.

Informing the public as to the characteristics of diabetes mellitus, susceptibility factors (obesity and family history), possible

[20]John H. Karam: *In* Marcus A. Krupp and Milton J. Chatton (Eds.): Current Medical Diagnosis and Treatment, Los Altos, Cal., Lange, 1975, pp. 719–720.

[21]Ibid., p. 533.
[22]Williams, op. cit., pp. 556–557.

consequences of undetected and uncontrolled diabetes and available sources of screening is being promoted by the distribution of brochures by diabetic associations and life insurance companies and through the use of mass media.

TREATMENT AND NURSING CARE. Treatment is directed toward correcting the hyperglycemia and glucosuria, maintaining the patient's normal weight and strength (and in the case of a child, normal growth and development), encouraging appropriate activity and the prevention of complications commonly associated with diabetes. The treatment of all patients includes a carefully regulated diet, moderate exercise and education about the disease and necessary care; for some it may include the administration of insulin or an oral hypoglycemic drug. The plan of treatment for each patient is *determined on an individual basis;* the therapeutic requirements for control in the case of one diabetic may be quite different from those of another. Some diabetics are satisfactorily treated by diet alone; others require an oral hypoglycemic drug or parenteral insulin in varying dosages.

PSYCHOLOGICAL CONSIDERATIONS. The impact of being advised of a chronic condition such as diabetes causes psychosocial stresses for the patient and family. The limitations imposed by a therapeutic diet, fear of continuous medication if insulin or a hypoglycemic preparation is needed, fear of complications (blindness, insulin shock, stroke) of which they have heard and the measures suggested to prevent these initiate varying reactions. Some immediately see themselves as a chronic invalid. Some patients may express despair by saying, "What is the use? Life is not worth living." Others may be depressed and withdraw or show anger that this should happen to them. The patient and family are encouraged to discuss how they feel about the situation and to indicate their concern. The nurse listens willingly and, when the patient and family have overcome their initial shock and reaction, begins to help them understand the disorder and necessary treatment. They must be reassured that, although the person's disease cannot be cured, it can be controlled so that he can live a reasonably normal life. Many centers have facilities for group discussions among diabetics which prove helpful. Some express many of their concerns more freely with fellow diabetics than with professionals.

DIET. Diabetes does not preclude the need for all the essential food principles, but it does necessitate careful selection and control of the amounts of the major food elements to provide a balance between the caloric intake and energy expenditure. The caloric intake should equal the energy output to avoid a positive balance, with a resultant hyperglycemia and weight increase, or a negative balance that may lead to an excessive fat breakdown with the risk of ketoacidosis. The diet can be quite similar to that of the normal person and provide sufficient variety to make it appetizing and palatable.

The *dietary prescription* indicates the number of calories required each day and the proportions of these calories to be allocated to carbohydrate, protein and fat. The number of calories is determined by the patient's ideal and present weight, age and activity. Initially, if the patient is overweight, the number of calories may be lower than the figure indicated as needed for his ideal weight. The objective is to bring about a gradual and steady loss of weight until the normal or slightly subnormal weight is achieved. Appropriate increases in calories are usually made as the weight approaches normal. Principles and methods used in the calculation of the diabetic diet vary among physicians.

The diabetic child's caloric intake must provide for growth and considerable activity and may be based on the rule of 1000 calories for the child at the age of 1 year plus 100 calories for each additional year; that is, the 2-year-old would receive 1100 calories, the 3-year-old 1200 calories, and so on. The child's caloric requirement may be calculated on the basis of weight by some physicians: 100 calories per kg. of weight at the age of 1 year, 75 calories per kg. at 5 years, 50 calories per kg. at 10 years, and 40 calories per kg. at 15 years.

Apportionment of the calories into carbohydrate, protein and fat differs from the normal diet in that the carbohydrate is usually lower. The protein allowance is usually the same as that recommended for the normal diet: 1.0 to 1.5 Gm. per kg. of body weight for adults and 2.0 to 3.0 Gm. per kg. for children. Generally, 40 to 45 per cent of the adult diabetic's caloric intake is provided as carbohydrate; this is about 10 per cent less than in the normal diet. Approximately 20 per cent of the total calories are in protein, 40 to 45 per cent in carbohydrate, and 35 to 40 per cent in fat. For children, the amount of carbohydrate prescribed may be within normal limits (i.e., 50 per cent of the caloric requirement) because of their activity and growth.

In providing the necessary carbohydrates, concentrated forms such as sugar, candy, jam, jelly, preserves, honey, ice cream, sherbets, pastries, cake, and sweetened beverages are avoided. The carbohydrates most commonly used are bread, cereals, milk, fruits and vegetables. In the selection of fat, the substitution of unsaturated for saturated fats is recommended because of the diabetic's predisposition to the development of atherosclerosis and vascular lesions.

As a guide for selecting the kinds and amounts of food in the diabetic diet in keeping with the physician's dietary prescription, foods have been divided into six basic classes — milk, vegetables, fruits, breads, meats and fats. The vegetables are subdivided into classes A and B according to their nutrient and carbohydrate value. Foods are listed in each class, indicating the amount in household measurements of each which comprises one serving and the value of one serving in terms of Gm. of carbohydrate, protein and fat. These lists are referred to as *exchange lists,* and one serving is called an exchange. All exchanges in a list are equal in value in the suggested amount for a serving; thus, one may be substituted for another *in the amount indicated.* The exchange system permits the diet to be varied and planned according to the availability of foods as well as to the patient's preferences. To illustrate, if the patient's meal allows one fruit exchange, he may select ½ cup of unsweetened applesauce, one medium orange, ½ cup of raspberries (raw), *or* one-half of a 6″ banana from the multiple exchange list of fruits; each has the same value of 10 Gm. of carbohydrate and provides 40 calories.[23]

The patient's daily food allowance is outlined as to the amount of food or number of exchanges he may have from each exchange list. This must then be allocated to his meals and snacks. The *division of the day's allowance* depends upon the associated treatment.

If diet is used without insulin or a hypoglycemic drug, it is simply divided into three equal parts and intermediate snacks. If an oral hypoglycemic drug is used, the carbohydrate is evenly distributed throughout the day. When insulin is used, the division of the carbohydrate and the number of feedings are specified by the physician. The distribution of the carbohydrate depends on the type of insulin used; it must provide an adequate concentration at the time of peak action of the insulin administered to prevent hypoglycemia and insulin shock. The exchange lists and sample menus for various daily caloric requirements (1000 to 3000 calories) are available from the diet counseling service of national and local diabetic associations,[24] hospital dietary departments and diabetic clinics, and diet therapy textbooks.

It must be impressed upon the patient that all of his daily food allowance should be eaten, especially if he receives insulin or a hypoglycemic drug, and that nothing else of caloric value is taken. When the patient is unable to take a portion of his diet, the caloric requirement is made up in some way (e.g., orange juice, milk), especially if he is receiving insulin. Meals should be taken regularly; the delay or missing of a meal may upset the blood sugar level and promote the breakdown of fat. The carbohydrate is distributed over the day to avoid abnormal fluctuation in the blood sugar concentration. Foods of no significant nutrient value which the patient may have as desired include clear broths and consommé, clear tea and coffee, Jello made with sugarless jelly powder, tomato juice, and artificially sweetened carbonated beverage. Commercially prepared dietetic foods are available. An artificial sweetener is used in these, and they tend to be expensive. However, they may help to vary the patient's diet occasionally. If the patient becomes ill and cannot tolerate solid foods, he may be given fruit juices (unless diarrhea is a problem), ginger ale, gruel and milk.[25] If these are not

---

[23]Canadian Diabetic Association; Meal Planning for Diabetics in Canada, 5th ed. Toronto: Burns and McEachern, 1975.

[24]American Diabetes Association, New York, N. Y., U.S.A. The Canadian Diabetic Association, 123 Edward St., Suite 601, Toronto, Ontario M5G1E2.

[25]One-half cup of orange juice is equivalent to 10 Gm. of carbohydrate and provides 40 calories; 6 oz. of ginger ale is equivalent to one slice of bread and has 15 Gm. of carbohydrate (60 calories); ½ cup of gruel is equivalent to 15 Gm. of carbohydrate and 2 Gm. of protein (70 calories); 1 cup of skim milk is equivalent to 12 Gm. of carbohydrate and 8 Gm. of protein (80 calories).

tolerated, intravenous infusions of glucose may have to be administered.

The diabetic diet is very much an individual factor. Following the initial dietary prescription, the patient is followed closely to determine if it is satisfactory; the urine is checked daily for sugar, frequent blood sugar determinations are made, his weight is recorded daily, and his general reactions (physical and psychological) are noted. Adjustments of the total caloric intake and in the amount of carbohydrate and fat may be necessary. Consideration is given to adapting the prescribed diet to the patient's food habits, which are influenced by his cultural and economic background, family, and individual preferences.

INSULIN. If the diabetic on a regulated diet does not have sufficient effective insulin in his body to use and store his carbohydrate requirement and prevent fat and protein catabolism, insulin may be prescribed. The majority of diabetics requiring insulin therapy tend to be children and adults who have developed their disease before the age of 40. The person whose diabetes is normally controlled by diet regulation may require insulin during periods of increased body demands and stress (e.g., infection, surgery, pregnancy, emotional crisis).

Insulin is a protein which is still being prepared from a natural source — the pancreas of cattle, hogs and sheep. The preparation of a synthetic form has been reported, but the product has not been perfected for therapeutic use. Because it is a protein, insulin is destroyed in the gastrointestinal tract by proteinases; therefore, it must be given parenterally. Several types are available and may be classified as rapid-acting with shorter period of action, intermediate-acting with longer period of action, and slow-acting with prolonged period of action. The rapid-acting preparations include regular (unmodified; Toronto; crystalline) and semilente insulins. The *intermediate-acting* insulins include neutral protamine Hagedorn (NPH; isophane) and lente. Those which are *absorbed more slowly* and have a prolonged effect on lowering blood sugar are protamine zinc insulin and ultralente insulin. See Table 22–3 for the onset and duration of action of each type of insulin.[26] These figures are approximate, since individual differences in responses do occur.

It is important that the nurse caring for or counseling diabetics be familiar with the action characteristics of the various types of insulin so that complaints and disturbances can be considered in relation to the onset, peak and duration of the type being received. A summary of these, kept readily accessible for reference on the hospital ward, in the clinic or in the visiting nurse's bag, can prove very helpful.

Insulin is measured in units. Dosage is determined individually on the basis of the

---

[26]Connaught Laboratories: Insulin and Insulin Preparations, 13th ed. Toronto, Connaught Laboratories, 1975, p. 11.

TABLE 22–3   ONSET, PEAK AND DURATION OF ACTION OF VARIOUS INSULINS

Type	Onset of Action (hours after injection)	Peak of Action (hours after injection)	Duration of Action (hours after injection)
Rapid, short action			
Regular (Toronto, unmodified, crystalline)	½–1	2–3	5–7
Semilente	½–1	5–8	12–16
Intermediate action			
NPH (neutral protamine Hagedorn)	1–3	10–18	18–28
Lente	1–3	10–18	18–28
Long action			
Protamine zinc	3–7	15–22	24–36 or more
Ultralente	5–8	16–24	28–36 or more

amount of glucose in the diet which the person is unable to metabolize as manifested by the blood sugar level and glucosuria. Insulin is supplied in 10-ml. vials in 100-unit (U.-100) strength; that is, each ml. contains 100 units of insulin. Until recently, insulin of 40- and 80-unit strengths were used, but these have been replaced by the U.-100 insulin. The use of one strength of insulin only (100 units per ml.) reduces error in dosage. Insulin syringes are calibrated for measuring U.-100 insulin.

Fast-acting insulin is given 20 to 30 minutes before breakfast and may be repeated before lunch and supper if the urine still shows sugar. Following the administration of rapid-acting insulin, food must be given within 1 hour to prevent hypoglycemia. The slower-acting insulins are generally given only once daily, usually in the morning at breakfast time. *If the patient is ill and cannot take his meal or for some reason the meal is delayed, the insulin is omitted.* If it is given and the patient does not eat or he vomits, the incident is reported promptly and the patient is given glucose in some form to prevent hypoglycemia.

Insulin is given by hypodermic below the subcutaneous fat to prevent lipodystrophy. The arms, thighs and abdomen are the areas used, and the site is rotated (Fig. 22–6). Too

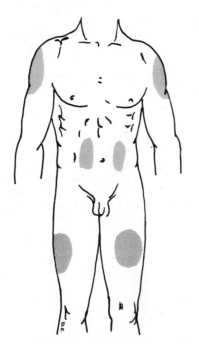

FIGURE 22–6 Suitable locations for insulin injections.

frequent use of one site causes fibrosing and scarring which delay absorption as well as make the injection more difficult.

All insulin other than the regular must be thoroughly mixed before use to insure uniform suspension and concentration throughout. This is done by rotating the bottle and inverting it slowly from end to end; vigorous shaking is avoided to prevent the formation of froth.

Some patients require a combination of fast-acting and slower-acting insulins. Before mixing two types for one administration, the nurse checks with the physician; some prefer to have them given separately. Generally, regular insulin may be mixed with protamine zinc, NPH or lente insulin. To avoid contamination of the regular insulin in the vial, it is drawn into the syringe first and separate needles are used. When both types are loaded, the syringe is then slowly tipped up and down until the two preparations are well mixed.

Each bottle of insulin bears an expiration date beyond which the content should not be used. Insulin should be kept in a cool place, preferably a refrigerator; freezing is avoided. Extremes of temperature and exposure to sunlight are likely to cause deterioration.

Reactions. Various local and general reactions to insulin may occur. The *local reactions* are minor in nature and include local sensitivity, lipodystrophy and fibrosis. Frequently, when insulin therapy is first started, sensitivity may be manifested at the site of injection because the insulin is a foreign protein and antigenic. The area becomes red, swollen and itchy but the response is generally temporary and disappears as the patient becomes desensitized by the repeated doses of insulin.

The local action of insulin on the adipose tissue cells may incur a swelling of the fatty tissue followed by atrophy which leaves a hollow space in the area. These atrophic areas are not serious but present an undesirable cosmetic effect. They may be prevented by making sure that the insulin is introduced below the subcutaneous tissue. Frequent and repeated injections into one area of tissue may result in fibrosing of the tissue and induration of the site. Fibrous tissue has poor vascularization which decreases the rate of absorption of the insulin. This complication may be prevented by systematic rotation of the injection sites and avoiding the use of any one spot oftener than once every 2 to 3 weeks.

General insulin reactions include insulin resistance and hypoglycemia. *Insulin resistance* is said to be present when diabetes cannot be controlled with less than 200 units of insulin per day.[27] It may occur secondary to some other diseases, such as severe adrenocortical hyperfunction, acromegaly and thyrotoxicosis. As a primary condition, it is attributed to an antigen-antibody reaction. Antibodies are developed in response to the foreign protein (insulin). It is more likely to occur with insulin extracted from cattle than with that prepared from the pancreas of hogs. Insulin resistance usually develops insidiously several months after insulin treatment has begun. Treatment includes the use of pork insulin and cortisone to reduce the patient's antibody production.

Hypoglycemia is discussed on page 799.

ORAL HYPOGLYCEMIC DRUGS.   There are two groups of drugs which lower blood sugar — sulfonylurea compounds and biguanides (Table 22–4). The fact that they may be taken orally provides a distinct advantage. Their use is limited mainly to diabetics whose disease is mild and stable and generally has developed after the age of 40.

The *sulfonylurea compounds* lower the blood sugar by stimulating the secretion of insulin and are usually used for non-obese patients. These preparations include tolbutamide (Orinase), chlorpropamide (Diabinese), acetohexamide (Dymelor) and tolazamide (Tolinase). The principal difference between these preparations is in the duration of their action; tolbutamide has some effect in lowering the blood sugar for 6 to 12 hours, chlorpropamide is effective up to 60 hours, acetohexamide acts for 12 to 24 hours, and tolazamide acts for 12 to 24 hours. The *biguanide* preparations are phenformin (DBI, Meltrol), which is effective for 4 to 6 hours, and long-acting phenformin (DBI-TD), which is effective in lowering the blood sugar over a period of 12 to 14 hours. The action of the biguanide preparation is not clearly understood, but it is thought to enhance the effectiveness of insulin, increasing the cellular uptake of glucose.[28]

It must be remembered that it is still important for the patient receiving oral hypoglycemic agents to respect his prescribed diet, exercise and supervision. Although the risk of hypoglycemia is less than with insulin therapy, it may occur, and the patient must be made aware of the early manifestations. Hypoglycemia is more likely to occur in elderly persons and patients with renal or liver dysfunction, and with the concurrent taking of certain drugs. Examples of the latter are barbiturates, alcohol, aspirin, phenylbutazone, sulfonamide and methyldopa (Aldomet). Occasionally, oral hypoglycemic agents produce some side effects, such as gastrointestinal disturbances (heartburn, nausea, vomiting, diarrhea), headache, skin rash and itching.

There has been some concern expressed in

[27]Wintrobe, op. cit., p. 546.

[28]Gail B. Askew and Kenneth I. Letcher: "Oral Hypoglycemic Agents." Nurs. '75, Vol. 5, No. 8 (Aug. 1975), pp. 45–50.

TABLE 22–4   ORAL HYPOGLYCEMIC DRUGS

Group	Duration (hours)	Action
Sulfonylurea compounds		Stimulate the secretion of insulin
Tolbutamide (Orinase)	6–12	
Chlorpropamide (Diabinese)	up to 60	
Acetohexamide (Dymelor)	12–24	
Tolazamide (Tolinase)	12–24	
Biguanide preparations		Thought to enhance effectiveness of insulin, increasing cellular uptake of glucose
Phenformin (DBI, Meltrol)	4–6	
Long-acting phenformin (DBI-TD) (time-released)	12–24	

recent years about the use of tolbutamide and phenformin. In reference to a controlled study that was done, Fletcher indicates that the findings suggested an increased cardiovascular mortality in those patients who received tolbutamide and phenformin. As a result, recommendations have been made that the use of oral hypoglycemic agents should be reserved for those rare patients who cannot be controlled by diet and cannot be treated with insulin.[29, 30]

GENERAL HYGIENIC MEASURES. Particular attention is paid to the patient's skin and feet, especially if he spends the greater part of the day in bed. The diabetic's skin is less resistant to pressure and irritation and, when broken, it readily becomes infected and is difficult to heal. This is attributed to the vascular changes. The skin is kept clean and dry; a mild soap is used for bathing, and a light application of lanolin or oil may be made to prevent cracking if the skin is dry. Foot soaks in *warm* water followed by oiling may be necessary to remove thick dry skin, calluses and corns. The toenails are cut straight across to avoid ingrown toenails and possible infection. For the bed patient, a footboard is used to relieve the weight of bedding on the feet, and a routine of frequent regular foot and leg exercises is established, especially with older persons. Vulnerable pressure areas are gently massaged every 3 or 4 hours and are protected by frequent turning and the placing of a square of synthetic sheepskin under the patient. When ambulatory, the patient is discouraged from sitting and standing for prolonged periods; brief periods of walking about, changing position and flexing and extending the limbs assist in improving circulation.

Exposure to infection is avoided since any infection tends to increase the demand for insulin and may interfere with the diabetic's normal food intake, predisposing him to ketosis. Any indication of a respiratory infection, gastrointestinal disturbance or skin lesion is promptly brought to the physician's attention, since such conditions require more prompt and careful attention than in the nondiabetic.

EXERCISE. A moderate amount of exercise is an important part of diabetic treatment. It promotes the use of glucose and may diminish the amount of insulin or oral hypoglycemic needed to control the blood sugar level. It also stimulates and improves the circulation, helps to maintain muscle tone, prevents obesity and promotes a sense of well-being. Some diabetics have sufficient exercise in their occupation, but those in sedentary jobs or who are retired should have a planned program which is introduced gradually. Since the prescription for diet and a hypoglycemic is based on the patient's physical activity, the regimen should be approximately the same each day to minimize fluctuations in the blood sugar concentration. When variations in daily energy expenditure are necessary, adjustments in the diet may be needed. Extra carbohydrate in the form of fruit, milk or bread may be added if activity is increased. When the usual amount of activity is decreased for some reason (other than illness or infection), some decrease in the caloric intake is usually indicated.

Active exercise at regular intervals is encouraged during hospitalization unless contraindicated for other physical reasons. With an anticipated increase of activity on discharge from the hospital, the insulin dosage may be decreased and the carbohydrate and fat or protein intake may be increased. For the older diabetic a daily routine of walking and light home chores (house and garden) is recommended.

The aim is to maintain a balance between energy expenditure and the prescribed treatment (diet and insulin or oral hypoglycemic). More than the usual amount of exercise lowers the blood sugar; less than the usual amount will raise it.

The diabetic participating in strenuous activity, particularly if he is on insulin therapy, should advise a coworker or, in the case of sports, a friend or sports supervisor that he is a diabetic in case of a hypoglycemic reaction. The physician will probably advise him to increase his carbohydrate intake and/or decrease his insulin dose before he undertakes the increased energy expenditure. He should also carry sugar cubes or candy which he can take at the first sign of weakness and hypoglycemic reaction. When making a

[29]H. Patrick Fletcher: "The Oral Antidiabetic Drugs: Pro and Con." Am. J. Nurs., Vol. 76, No. 4 (April 1976), pp. 596–599.

[30]Edgar C. Boedeker and James H. Dauber (Eds.): Manual of Medical Therapeutics, 21st ed. Boston, Little, Brown, 1974, p. 346.

change in occupation that involves either a decrease or increase in activity, the diabetic should have his plan of therapy reviewed by his physician or at the clinic.

EDUCATION. Diabetes mellitus is a disease with which the patient will have to live the rest of his life. To maintain successful control of his disease which will permit him to live an independent satisfying life, the diabetic must have an understanding of his disorder, the treatment and care prescribed for him and the possible complications. Patient and family education is a responsibility of the nurse caring for the diabetic, and plays as important a role in successful treatment as diet and insulin.

Before launching a program of instruction, it is necessary to assess the patient's attitude toward his disease and to determine his readiness to accept the teaching. The patient may become quite emotional when told he has diabetes and its implications. His behavior may manifest depression, fear, withdrawal or resentment that this has happened to him. The nurse, recognizing the patient's reaction, conveys to him a willingness to listen and to talk about his future when he is ready. Most patients work through their immediate reactions and reach a phase in which they verbalize their feelings and are prepared to listen and accept the reassurance that their disease can be controlled and that the necessary treatment and care will become a routine part of their life without seriously altering it.

In planning the instruction, it is necessary to know the patient's background so that care can be adapted as much as possible to his accustomed way of life. The physician and dietitian may participate in the program, but the nurse should be familiar with their advice so that she can answer the patient's and his family's questions and reinforce certain areas when necessary. The amount of information given at one time depends on the patient's ability and willingness to receive it. Generally, brief periods of discussion are more effective than the presentation of a large amount of information at one time. Group instruction may be used in the hospital or clinic for some topics, but it must be remembered that each diabetic's treatment is individualized. A large part of the discussion must be on an individual basis.

Teaching is begun as soon as possible to avoid giving too much at one time, leading to confusion and discouragement, and to allow time for the patient to practice self-care, read and ask questions.

Explanations are made in simple lay terms; and demonstrations are broken into steps, made slowly, repeated as often as necessary, and sufficient opportunity is provided for the patient to practice. Illustrations, films and written explanations and directions are used for clarification. Reading material (books, pamphlets) written for diabetics should be made available; several publications are available from diabetic associations.

The instruction program covers the following: (1) an explanation of diabetes; (2) diet; (3) insulin therapy or oral hypoglycemic agents, if appropriate; (4) urine testing; (5) hypoglycemia; (6) uncontrolled diabetes; (7) identification card; (8) special personal care; (9) regular supervision; and (10) sources of information and assistance.

Explanation of Disorder. A simple basic explanation is made of the nature of diabetes, relating it to the symptoms experienced by the patient. To illustrate, the patient may be told that sugar and starches (such as bread and cereal) are converted by digestion to a simple form of sugar called glucose, which is the body's chief source of energy. In order for the cells to extract it from the blood and use it, the chemical insulin is necessary. In diabetes, there is not sufficient insulin being produced to use the amount of sugar and starches being taken, so glucose accumulates in the blood in excess of the normal. The kidneys remove some of the excess, which is why the diabetic voids a lot and the urine contains sugar. The loss of large amounts of urine results in thirst. Weakness, fatigue and hunger occur because the sugar is not being "burned" to produce energy. The body, in an effort to provide energy, may break down body tissue, causing a loss of weight. Some diabetics produce enough insulin to handle the amount of sugar they actually need to still maintain their normal weight. Others may require more glucose because of their activities but are not producing sufficient insulin to use that amount, so they require a drug which may be taken by mouth or insulin which must be taken by an injection.

Diet. The prescribed diet must be clearly and carefully interpreted to the patient. The initial instruction is usually given by a dietitian, but considerable clarification and reinforcement by the nurse, who is with the patient more often and for longer periods, is usually necessary. The prescription, sample meal plan and exchange lists are explained. The foods allowed each day, their division into meals and snacks, and the selection from exchange lists are reviewed several times. It is helpful to have the patient plan meals for several days. The purchase and preparation of food and how it may be worked in with the family meals are discussed. The following general principles which apply to the diabetic diet are cited. Only standard measuring cups and spoons are used; amounts used should be accurate and correspond with that indicated on the exchange lists; concentrated sweets such as sugar, candy, jams, jelly, preserves, honey, cake and pastries should be avoided; labels are carefully read when purchasing canned and prepared foods, and only those indicating that no sugar has been added are used; to satisfy hunger, foods of no caloric value may be taken which include clear tea and coffee, sugarless jelly powder, consommé, clear broth, bouillon and artificially sweetened beverages; the daily food allowance should all be eaten; and meals should be taken at regular hours. The patient is advised that he should check his weight at least weekly and should be informed that obesity is a distinct hazard. A frequent question raised by patients is whether liquor, beer and wine are allowed. The question is referred to the attending physician; if an alcoholic beverage is permitted, it should be counted in the total caloric intake, since it is fairly high in calories.[31] The patient is encouraged to read and obtain for his personal use books and pamphlets which contain considerable detail on diabetic diets. The national diabetic associations have a diet counseling department which is prepared to provide assistance in meal planning.

Insulin Therapy. If the patient is on insulin therapy, he is advised of the necessary equipment and where it may be obtained. An explanation is made of what insulin is and of and several types and unit strengths, indicating the name and nature of that prescribed for him, and how it is identified. Unit dosage is explained and measurement by units is

demonstrated. The patient is encouraged to practice handling the syringe and needle and the measurement of his prescribed dose. Instruction and demonstrations are then given to familiarize him with the sterilization of the equipment, aseptic handling, rotating of the vial to equalize the suspension of insulin, withdrawal of the required amount of insulin, the necessary rotation and cleansing of sites for injection, the actual injection and the aftercare of the equipment. Storage and maintenance of an adequate supply of insulin are discussed. Free insulin is available to many patients but can usually only be obtained by a special requisition form signed by the patient's physician. Automatic injectors are available which may be of assistance to those patients who find the injection of the needle difficult. The injector has a mechanically controlled spring which, when released, pushes the needle quickly through the skin. If it is used, a metal-tipped syringe is usually necessary. The need to plan and break down all this information into small logical teaching units or blocks is again emphasized. If discouragement and frustration are evident, further instruction is delayed and another approach considered.

Oral Hypoglycemic Drugs. If an oral hypoglycemic agent is prescribed, the importance of taking the drug in the exact dosage at the times ordered is stressed. Written directions are given, and the patient is advised that if headache, nausea, vomiting or other disturbances are experienced, he should contact the physician. The patient is reminded that he must not experiment with the dosage of the drug on his own and that adherence to the diet prescribed for him is most important even though he is receiving medication.

Urine Testing. The diabetic may be required to test his urine regularly for sugar and ketone bodies using one of the commercial preparations (e.g., Clinitest, Clinistix or Tes-Tape), and the procedure and interpretation of the result are demonstrated. The time(s) at which he should make the test will depend upon whether his therapy is diet alone, diet with insulin or diet with an oral hypoglycemic drug. Those receiving insulin are more likely to be required to test daily or more often. Occasionally, the patient may have to be taught to adjust his insulin dosage according to the results of the urine tests. The patient should know that if sugar or acetone appears

---

[31]Caloric value of 240 ml. (8 oz.) of beer is 114 calories; 45 ml. (1½ oz.) of whiskey is 120 calories; and 120 ml. (4 oz.) of wine is 114 calories.

in the urine it is likely that his blood sugar level is elevated. He is advised to review his diet and insulin or medication as taken to find the cause. If the disturbance persists and cannot be explained he should report to the clinic or physician. A written record of the urine tests is recommended; this is reviewed by the physician on each visit.

Hypoglycemia. The diabetic who is receiving insulin or an oral hypoglycemic should know that under certain circumstances the blood sugar level may fall below normal, resulting in what is called an insulin or hypoglycemic reaction. The patient and family should be familiar with the symptoms (see p. 799) and know what to do. The possible causes of hypoglycemia are cited (see p. 799), and the patient is advised that on experiencing early symptoms he should immediately take a concentrated form of sugar that is available quickly. Two or three cubes of sugar, tea or coffee with 2 or 3 teaspoonfuls of sugar, two or three small candies, orange juice or grape juice (4 oz.), or 1 teaspoonful of honey, corn syrup or jelly may be used. If the symptoms do not disappear in 10 minutes, the administration is repeated. The patient on insulin is advised to always carry lump sugar or hard candies with him.

Following a reaction, he should rest for 2 or 3 hours to reduce the demand on his blood sugar and should take more "sugar" and some form of protein (cheese, milk or peanut butter). The latter will slowly provide some glucose and contribute to the maintenance of a more constant blood sugar level. The family should know that if the diabetic cannot swallow or retain sugar, a physician is summoned at once, or he is taken as quickly as possible to a hospital emergency department. Friends and associates as well as the family should know that the diabetic receives insulin and may experience a reaction. The patient is advised that insulin reactions should be reported to the physician; his insulin dosage or diet may require adjustment.

Hyperglycemia. The patient should also be able to recognize early symptoms of uncontrolled diabetes, which causes hyperglycemia. If it is not corrected in the early stage it may lead to the serious complications of diabetic acidosis and coma. Hyperglycemia and ketosis develop more slowly than hypoglycemia, usually over several days. The disturb-

ance is usually manifested by loss of appetite, nausea, vomiting, thirst, weakness, drowsiness and general malaise. Sugar will be present in the urine. It is frequently associated with infection or stress or may be due to dietary indiscretion or omission of insulin or oral hypoglycemic. The patient is advised that his physician should be contacted as soon as symptoms are experienced. Until medical attention is obtained he should remain in bed, keep warm, drink hot clear fluids *without sugar* freely and repeat them even if he vomits; if possible, someone should remain with him.

Identification Card. Every diabetic should carry a diabetic identification card at all times so that his condition will be made known quickly in the event of a reaction, illness or accident. Cards which carry appropriate information are available from physicians, the diabetic clinic and the National Diabetic Association or its local branches; a written one may be carried temporarily. The diabetic may also acquire a membership in the Medic Alert Foundation, which provides a Medic Alert emblem in the form of a bracelet or medallion to be worn at all times. The emblem indicates the medical problem and the number of the diabetic's file from which information can be obtained at any time.

Skin and Foot Care. The patient is advised that, because of his diabetes, he may be more susceptible to infections and will tend to heal more slowly when breaks occur in the skin. Any infection predisposes to uncontrolled diabetes, and persons whose disease is uncontrolled appear to develop infection more readily. The diabetic avoids contact with persons who have an infection as much as possible. The skin should be kept clean, warm and free of irritation and pressure as much as possible. Precautions are taken to prevent cracks and breaks in the skin. Scratches, cuts, abrasions and hangnails are cleansed with alcohol or an antiseptic and are protected by a dressing. The use of strong antiseptics (such as iodine) and adhesive is avoided. Prolonged exposure to sunlight and the use of local heat applications (electric heating pad, hot water bottle) are discouraged. If heat applications are necessary, extra precautions are necessary because of some loss of sensation; a lower degree of heat and extra covers are used.

The adult diabetic's feet require constant

special attention because of the increased susceptibility to circulatory disorders as well as infection. The patient is directed to bathe his feet daily with warm (not hot) water, using a mild antibacterial soap, and to dry them thoroughly, especially the areas between the toes, using gentle pressure rather than vigorous rubbing. Talcum powder may be used sparingly if the feet tend to be moist and perspire; if they are dry and scaly, a light application of lanolin or prescribed lotion is rubbed into the skin. The toenails are cut straight across with scissors. If calluses and corns cannot be controlled by rubbing them lightly with a pumice stone, they should be treated by a podiatrist who is advised of the person's diabetes. The patient is cautioned against attempting to remove them by cutting or applying commercial preparations. Stockings or socks should fit well to avoid any constriction or wrinkles that might cause irritation or pressure and are changed daily. To prevent possible interference with the circulation, round garters are not worn. Shoes should be well-fitting so there is no irritation or pressure on any part of the foot, and new shoes are worn only for brief periods until "broken in." The foot and leg exercises introduced during hospitalization should be continued, particularly if the patient is likely to be inactive. Walking barefoot and the application of heating appliances are discouraged. Numbness, persisting coldness, discoloration, a burning feeling, pain or any unusual condition of the lower limbs is reported to the physician.

Eye Examination. It is advisable for the diabetic to have an annual eye examination because of the predisposition to visual change which can only be detected by an ophthalmologist.

Medical Supervision. The newly diagnosed diabetic will be required to make more frequent visits to his physician or the clinic. These will become fewer as his disease and treatment are stabilized. The patient is instructed to take a urine specimen with him on each visit. The nurse in either situation checks with him as to how he is managing and gives him the opportunity to ask questions. Some phase of his care may require repetition and reinforcement. Before leaving the hospital, the importance of keeping the scheduled appointments is stressed. In the case of older persons, assistance may be necessary in making some arrangements for transportation to the clinic.

Sources of Assistance. The patient and family are made aware of the available sources of help and information. These include the national and local diabetic associations, visiting nurse agency and public health nursing department. The services provided by the various organizations and recommended publications are cited. Patients are encouraged to join a diabetic association; membership may be obtained through a local chapter or directly from the national association. This entitles them to the regular periodical and additional literature published by the association.

The Child Diabetic. The care of the child or adolescent diabetic requires the understanding and cooperation of the entire family. Because of their growth and the vigorous activity characteristic of these young persons, closer medical supervision is necessary. They tend to be less stable, and more frequent adjustments in their insulin dosage and diet are necessary. The child is taught self-care and self-administration of his insulin as soon as possible. He must be able to recognize early symptoms of hypoglycemia and know when to take the sugar cubes or a concentrated form of glucose that he always carries with him. It must be emphasized in discussions with the parents that the child be encouraged to assume responsibility for his own care and that he be permitted to live as much like a normal child as possible so that he and his associates will not think of him as being "different."

Throughout all patient and family education, emphasis is placed on the positive — that is, control can be maintained, permitting the diabetic to carry on an active satisfying life. Certainly they must be made familiar with signs of certain complications and know what action to take to avoid serious consequences, but one must guard against creating unnecessary anxiety and discouragement.

COMPLICATIONS OF DIABETES MELLITUS. The most common complications of diabetes are diabetic acidosis, degenerative changes and hypoglycemia. Hypoglycemia occurs in those receiving insulin or oral hypoglycemic therapy.

DIABETIC KETOACIDOSIS. Diabetic ketoacidosis is a serious complication which develops in uncontrolled diabetes. The glucose in the blood cannot be utilized by the cells, and fat is broken down to provide energy. Fat is mobilized and broken down rapidly, producing ketone bodies (acetoacetic acid, β-hydroxybutyric acid and acetone) in excess of the tissue cells' ability to metabolize them. The acids and acetone accumulate in the blood. At first the normal pH is maintained by the buffer systems,[32] but eventually the alkali reserve becomes depleted and the pH of the body fluids falls, resulting in acidosis. At the same time, the increased concentration of glucose causes an increased output of urine (osmotic diuresis), and dehydration develops. The increased osmotic pressures of the extracellular fluid result in the movement of fluid out of the cells accompanied by electrolytes. Serious sodium, potassium and phosphate deficiencies develop.

Symptoms. Ketoacidosis has an insidious onset over several days, being preceded by symptoms characteristic of uncontrolled diabetes (polyuria, thirst, glucosuria, weakness). The symptoms related to the accumulation of ketones and reduced alkalinity of body fluids include anorexia, nausea, vomiting, deep and rapid respirations (Kussmaul's breathing), drowsiness, weakness which progresses to prostration, and abdominal pain or muscular cramps. The skin and mouth are dry, and the eyeballs are soft because of dehydration. The patient may appear flushed in the early stages but later becomes pale owing to hypotension. The pulse is rapid and may be weak because of severe dehydration and the reduced intravascular volume. Unless the condition is recognized and treated promptly, the blood pressure falls, the patient becomes comatose, and his condition is critical.

The patient's urine shows a high concentration of sugar and ketones. The blood sugar is elevated and the sodium and chloride blood levels are lower. The potassium level may be low at first owing to polyuria and vomiting; then it may become normal or elevated as the electrolyte moves out of the cells. The blood

urea level is usually higher, and the leukocyte count is generally elevated. The carbon dioxide concentration and combining power are lowered as well as the pH.

Causes. The most common causes of diabetic ketoacidosis are acute infection and gastrointestinal disorders. These conditions not only incur metabolic changes and demands but may lead to neglect of diet and insulin therapy. Other causes include dietary indiscretion, omission of insulin doses and undiagnosed diabetes mellitus.

Treatment and Nursing Care. The patient with diabetic ketoacidosis requires immediate treatment which is directed toward stimulating the utilization of glucose by the cells and decreasing the production of ketone bodies by the administration of insulin, and correction of dehydration and the electrolyte imbalance. Any causative disorder is also treated.

The nurse who is notified that a patient with ketoacidosis is to be admitted may assemble the following equipment to prevent delay in treatment: (1) regular insulin; (2) vasopressor drugs; (3) intravenous infusion equipment; (4) sterile syringes and needles for subcutaneous and intravenous injections; (5) necessary equipment for taking blood samples; (6) catheterization tray with an indwelling catheter and urine drainage receptacle; (7) sphygmomanometer and stethoscope; and (8) mouth care tray.

Immediate blood determinations are made of the glucose, carbon dioxide, potassium, sodium, chloride, phosphate, and urea concentrations. The hematocrit is also checked to determine hemoconcentration. An indwelling catheter is passed so that the hourly urinary output may be noted and the urine examined frequently for glucose and ketones. The patient receives repeated doses of regular (rapid-acting) insulin intravenously and a continuous intravenous infusion. The solution for the infusion and the dosage of insulin are based on the laboratory blood and urine findings. An electrocardiogram is done to detect changes in heart action characteristic of an abnormal potassium blood level. The initial solution used is usually normal saline; sodium lactate or sodium bicarbonate and potassium chloride or potassium phosphate may be added later. As cited previously, potassium moves out of the cells and at first the serum concentration may be normal or

---

[32] Example of the type of reaction that occurs:
$NaHCO_3$ (sodium bicarbonate) + acetoacetic acid $\rightarrow$ sodium acetoacetate + H_2CO_3 (carbonic acid)
The sodium acetoacetate is excreted in the urine, causing a loss of the base sodium. The weaker carbonic acid dissociates to H_2O and CO_2 and the CO_2 is eliminated through ventilation.

even elevated. With the administration of the intravenous insulin and solutions, plasma potassium moves into the cells and hypokalemia may develop which may then necessitate the administration of a potassium solution. Repeated blood electrolyte and sugar determinations and urinalyses are done. When the blood sugar level approaches normal, the frequency of administration and the dosage of insulin are decreased, and an intravenous glucose solution (5 per cent in water or saline) may be ordered. If the patient's blood pressure is low and shock is present, a blood transfusion may be given, or a vasopressor such as levarterenol (Levophed) or metaraminol (Aramine) may be administered intravenously. This administration will necessitate frequent checking of the blood pressure, since the rate of flow of the solution containing the vasopressor is regulated according to the blood pressure response.

If the patient is comatose, the positioning, precautions to maintain respiration and prevent aspiration, safety measures (side rails), frequent change of position and constant nursing attention which are appropriate for any unconscious patient must be applied (see p. 159). The blood pressure, pulse and respirations are recorded every 30 to 60 minutes, the temperature is recorded every 2 to 3 hours, an hourly check is made of the urinary output, and the patient's level of consciousness is noted. A gastric intubation and lavage with sodium bicarbonate solution may be done by the physician. The tube may be left in to reduce the risk of aspiration if the patient is vomiting frequently.

The patient should be kept warm with extra blankets. Frequent mouth cleansing and the application of an oil or cream to the lips are necessary. As soon as the patient regains consciousness and oral fluids can be tolerated, water, salty broth, orange juice, ginger ale, sweetened tea, milk, *or* gruel is given freely. The fluid intake and output are recorded, and the balance is noted. As soon as possible, the patient receives a prescribed soft diet, and if tolerated, it is increased to a prescribed light diet. When the patient is taking sufficient nourishment by mouth and a satisfactory blood sugar level is maintained, intravenous infusions are discontinued and regular subcutaneous doses of insulin reestablished.

Unless the cause of the ketoacidosis was evident at the onset, efforts are made to determine why it occurred. Further patient and family education may be indicated.

DEGENERATIVE CHANGES. The blood vessels of practically all diabetics undergo degenerative changes to some extent. Atherosclerosis (deposits of the fatty substance cholesterol) develops in the arteries, narrowing their lumen, and the endothelial walls of the capillaries thicken. These changes may eventually interfere with the normal cellular nutrition and oxygen supply, contributing to tissue change and impaired function. The structures which most frequently manifest lesions and reduced efficiency are the eyes, coronary arteries, kidneys, lower limbs and nerves.

The higher incidence of these vascular changes in diabetics is not understood, nor is there agreement as to whether the severity and rate of progression may be correlated with the control of the diabetes.

Diabetic retinopathy occurs in the form of minute aneurysms in the retinal vessels. These dilatations are prone to rupture and cause a hemorrhage into the eye. The condition is only revealed by ophthalmoscopic examination. Depending on the location of the lesions, the diabetic's vision may or may not be affected.

Atherosclerosis of the coronary arteries of the diabetic frequently leads to angina pectoris and myocardial infarction, especially in older persons.

Renal function may be slowly impaired by changes in the glomerular capillaries (intercapillary glomerulosclerosis or Kimmelstiel-Wilson syndrome) and by sclerotic changes in the larger renal vessels. The patient may manifest albuminuria and some degree of hypertension.

Defective circulation, due to vascular changes in the lower limbs, frequently leads to gangrene. A small superficial injury may be a precipitating factor. The gangrene may necessitate the amputation of a toe, foot or leg. Restricted circulation may be manifested by abnormal coldness of the extremities, numbness, discoloration, muscular cramps, weakness, burning pain or a small ulcer that does not heal. When impaired circulation is manifested, Buerger's exercises may be recommended. While the patient lies on his back, he raises one or both legs, allowing them to rest on a support until they blanch (approximately 1 to 3 minutes). A straight-backed chair, which is padded, may be used as a support; the top of the back and the front of the seat rest on the bed. A regular Buerger board may be available and can be adjusted to different heights (45° to 60° angle). Following the elevation and blanching of the limbs, the patient sits up, allowing the legs to hang over the side of the bed until they become red (5 to 10 minutes). The physician may suggest that repeated flexion, extension, and inward and outward rotation of the feet be carried out while in this position. When color is restored to the legs and feet, the patient lies in the horizontal position for a few minutes (5 to 7 minutes) before repeating the exercise. The physician indicates the number of times the exercise is to be done and may state a specific number of minutes for each stage.

Peripheral neuritis is a painful complication of diabetes. The patient may experience muscular cramps, tingling, numbness or burning pain in the extremities; this is usually most troublesome at night. The condition frequently responds to vitamin supplements, especially the vitamin B complex, increased protein in the diet, and better control of the diabetes.

HYPOGLYCEMIA. Hypoglycemia implies an abnormally low blood sugar concentration. Signs and symptoms usually begin to appear when the blood sugar level falls below 60 mg. per cent. The onset of symptoms varies with individuals; some may develop symptoms at a higher level of blood sugar, while others may not manifest the disturbance until a lower level is reached. Adults tend to have symptoms earlier than child diabetics.

Causes. The causes of hypoglycemia in the diabetic may be the delay or omission of a meal after having taken insulin or an oral hypoglycemic agent; an undue amount of energy expenditure; an overdosage of insulin; a gastrointestinal disorder which produces anorexia, vomiting or diarrhea; or improvement in the diabetic's ability to utilize glucose.

Manifestations. A hypoglycemic reaction in a patient receiving regular insulin usually occurs approximately 2 to 6 hours after the injection. In the patient receiving an intermediate-acting insulin given in the morning, it happens more commonly in the afternoon or evening. Hypoglycemic reaction to a slow-acting insulin generally occurs during the night or early in the morning of the following day.

It should be kept in mind that it is possible also for the patient receiving an oral hypoglycemic to develop hypoglycemia. It develops insidiously and may occasionally go unrecognized.

The signs and symptoms manifested by an abnormally low blood sugar are a reflection of its effect on the central nervous system. The brain is very dependent on a constant, adequate supply of glucose. Any deprivation, even for a relatively brief period, may seriously impair cerebral activity and result in permanent damage. Similarly, repeated occurrences of hypoglycemia, even of short duration, especially in children, may incur some permanent cerebral impairment. The manifestations of hypoglycemia vary from one patient to another but tend to be the same with each reaction for the same person, which makes it more easily recognizable by him. The earlier signs and symptoms include sweating, tremor, apprehension, hunger, weakness, tachycardia and palpitation. Symptoms usually do not appear until the blood sugar level is about 50 to 60 mg. per 100 ml. More advanced symptoms are faintness or dizziness, blurring of vision or diplopia, headache, slow reactions, uncoordinated movement which occasionally leads to mistaking the patient's condition for alcohol intoxication, muscular twitching that may progress to convulsions especially in children, disorientation and confusion, stupor and eventual loss of consciousness. The urine is negative for sugar. All diabetics, their immediate family and close associates should be familiar with the early signs and symptoms of hypoglycemia and should know what to do.

Treatment. If the patient can still swallow, he is immediately given some form of rapidly absorbable concentrated sugar. Ten to 15 Gm. of carbohydrate are usually sufficient to restore the blood sugar level. Orange juice (120 ml.) or other sweetened fruit juice or 2 teaspoonfuls of corn syrup, honey or sugar with a glass of water may be used. If there is no improvement in 5 to 10 minutes, the administration is repeated. If the patient is unconscious or uncooperative, a physician is summoned and 30 to 50 ml. of 50 per cent glucose are given intravenously. Glucagon (1 to 2 mg.) or epinephrine 1:1000 (0.5 ml.) sub-cutaneously may be ordered to promote gly-cogenolysis and subsequent increase in blood glucose. A venous blood specimen is collect-ed as soon as possible and is repeated at frequent intervals for blood sugar determina-tions until the patient is stabilized.

Following a reaction, the patient is en-couraged to rest for several hours in order to decrease the utilization of his blood glucose. Carbohydrate administration may be repeat-ed and some form of protein (cheese or milk) should be given the patient to provide addi-tional glucose which is produced gradually as a result of protein metabolism. The nurse always checks with the physician be-fore giving the next scheduled dose of insulin. Adjustments are usually made in the carbohy-drate content of the diet and in the insulin dosage. The patient may learn from the expe-rience if encouraged to examine the reaction in retrospect. A discussion of the possible cause and the early symptoms may be helpful in preventing further reactions and in having the patient recognize hypoglycemia at the onset.

SURGERY AND DIABETES MELLI-TUS. The emotional stress, physical trauma and physiological responses associated with surgery present a greater problem for the diabetic than for the normal person. A de-crease in the utilization of glucose and an increased demand for insulin are likely to occur, predisposing the diabetic to acidosis. The diabetic who is to have elective surgery is usually hospitalized several days before the operation. During this period, his diabetes is thoroughly checked and brought under op-timum control. The blood sugar level is brought within normal range, and the urine must be free of sugar and ketones. The patient undergoes a thorough investigation for com-plications of his disease (degenerative changes), and his fluid and electrolyte bal-ances and nutritional status are assessed. The total caloric intake and the carbohydrate and protein portions of the diet may be increased; this may necessitate additional insulin to in-sure metabolism. The increase in carbohy-drate is to provide an adequate reserve of liver and muscle glycogen.

The morning of operation, intravenous glu-cose 5 per cent in normal saline and a dose of regular insulin may be ordered. If a long oper-ative period is anticipated, an indwelling cath-eter may be passed so that a urine specimen may be analyzed during surgery and addition-al intravenous solutions and insulin given if indicated.

Postoperatively, constant nursing attention is necessary; responses and reactions vary greatly with individuals. The insulin require-ment may increase sharply with some pa-tients and not with others. The pulse, respira-tions and blood pressure are usually recorded frequently and for a longer period than usual, and a frequent check is made of the patient's level of consciousness. If the patient does not recover consciousness following the opera-tion in a reasonable period of time, it is brought to the physician's attention. An in-dwelling catheter is passed if drainage was not established before operation. Blood and urine specimens are obtained immediately after operation and are repeated every 2 to 4 hours; glucose and electrolyte levels are determined. Intravenous solutions and regular insulin are usually given; the type of solution and insulin dosage are based on the urine and blood find-ings. The nurse must be constantly alert for signs of hypoglycemia and acidosis.

Oral feedings are started just as soon as they can be tolerated, and specific orders are given as to what liquids may be given and how much the patient is to receive. The sooner he is returned to his usual diet, the better. Fre-quent foot and leg exercises are especially important because of the diabetic's predispo-sition to vascular changes and circulatory problems. Precautions are taken to provide the maximum protection against infection; any slight indication of possible infection such as an elevation of temperature, cough or sore throat is reported immediately. Early ambulation is encouraged to promote greater utilization of glucose as well as to stimulate the patient's circulation.

Hypoglycemic State

An abnormally low blood sugar may be due to a variety of factors. It may be fasting or postprandial.

An excessive secretion of insulin by the islets of Langerhans occurs rarely. It may be due to a functioning-cell neoplasm in the pan-creas, involving the islet cells, or to an un-explained hyperactivity of the islets. The overproduction of insulin produces periodic hypoglycemic episodes which are usually precipitated by fasting or exercise. The patient manifests the signs and symptoms cited on page 799. Because of the repeated attacks, changes in personality and reduced intellectual ability may be evident as a result of permanent brain damage. The patient is treated by surgical excision of the newgrowth or a subtotal pancreatectomy.

It may occur after a meal following a gastrectomy, or it may be functional and postprandial which is attributed to increased parasympathetic innervation to the beta cells of the islets of Langerhans by the vagus nerve resulting in an excessive secretion of insulin.

It may be associated with a marked deficiency of cortisol or the growth hormone. In some instances, especially in children, it is idiopathic.

In postprandial hypoglycemia, the protein and fat content of the patient's diet is increased to insure a more "continuous" production of glucose (gluconeogenesis), since carbohydrate is used quickly from the blood. Glucagon may be prescribed for the patient; regular doses may be given subcutaneously. The patient is advised to take four or five regular meals and to carry candy or sugar or a ready source of simple sugar.

References

Books

Canadian Diabetic Association: Cookbook for Diabetics and All the Family. Toronto, Burns and MacEachern, 1975.

Connaught Laboratories: Insulin and Insulin Preparations, 13th ed. Toronto, Connaught Laboratories, 1975.

Dillon, Richard S.: Handbook of Endocrinology. Philadelphia, Lea and Febiger, 1973.

Ellenberg, Max, and Rifkin, Harold (Eds.): Diabetes: Theory and Practice. New York, McGraw-Hill, 1970.

Ezrin, Calvin, et al. (Eds.): Systematic Endocrinology. New York, Harper and Row, 1973.

Ganong, William F.: Review of Medical Physiology, 7th ed. Los Altos, Cal., Lange, 1975. Chapters 18–22.

Gormican, Annette: Controlling Diabetes with Diet. Springfield, Ill., Charles C Thomas, 1971.

Harper, Harold A.: Review of Physiological Chemistry, 15th ed. Los Altos, Cal., Lange, 1975. Chapter 20.

Kaplan, Dorothy: Comprehensive Diabetic Cookbook. New York, Frederick Fell, 1977.

Krupp, Marcus A., and Chatton, Milton J.: Current Medical Diagnosis and Treatment. Los Altos, Cal., Lange, 1975. Chapters 18 and 19.

Minneapolis Diabetes Education Center (Conference: An Interdisciplinary Approach to the Education and Management of the Patient with Diabetes Mellitus): Education and Management of the Patient with Diabetes Mellitus. Elkhart, Ames, 1973.

Sabiston, David C., Jr. (Ed.): Davis-Christopher: Textbook of Surgery 11th ed. Philadelphia, W. B. Saunders, 1977. Chapters 25–27.

Schwartz, Seymour I., et al. (Eds.): Principles of Surgery, 2nd ed. New York, McGraw-Hill, 1974. Chapters 37 and 38.

Spencer, Roberta T.: Patient Care in Endocrine Problems. Philadelphia, W. B. Saunders, 1973.

Williams, Robert H. (Ed.): Textbook of Endocrinology, 5th ed. Philadelphia, W. B. Saunders, 1974.

Wintrobe, Maxwell, M., et al. (Eds.): Principles of Internal Medicine, 7th ed. New York, McGraw-Hill, 1974. Chapters 82–90.

Periodicals

Bell, Mercedes: "Pre-operative Teaching and Post-operative Care of the Hypophysectomy Patient," J. Neurosurg. Nurs., Vol. 4, No. 2 (Dec. 1972), pp. 165–171.

Burrow, Gerard N. (Ed.): "Symposium on Current Concepts of Thyroid Disease." Med. Clin. North Am., Vol. 59, No. 5 (Sept. 1975).

Edis, Anothony J.: "Surgical Treatment for Thyroid Cancer." Surg. Clin. North Am., Vol. 57, No. 3 (June 1977), pp. 533–542.

Esmeraldo, R., et al.: "Thyroidectomy, Parathyroidectomy and Modified Neck Dissection." Surg. Clin. North Am., Vol. 57, No. 6 (Dec. 1977), pp. 1365–1377.

Gann, Donald S. (Ed.): "Symposium on Endocrine Surgery." Surg. Clin. North Am., Vol. 54, No. 2 (April 1974).

Gillies, Dee Ann, and Alyn, Irene Barrett: "Caring For Patients With Thyroid Disorders: How Good Are Your Skills?" Nurs. '77, Vol. 7, No. 10 (Oct. 1977), pp. 71–80.

Hallal, Janice C.: "Thyroid Disorders." Am. J. Nurs., Vol. 77, No. 3 (March 1977), pp. 417–432.

Hurley, James R.: "Thyroiditis," D. M., Vol. 24, No. 3 (Dec. 1977).

Jackson, Charles E., and Frame, Bay; "Diagnosis and Management of Parathyroid Disorders." Ortho. Clin. North Am., Vol. 3, No. 3 (Nov. 1972), pp. 699–712.

Jarman, Wayne T., et al.: "Cancer of the Parathyroids." Arch. Surg., Vol. 13, No. 2 (Feb. 1978), pp. 123–125.

Manns, L., and Boechler, N. E.: "Two Disorders of the Thyroid Gland." Can. Nurse, Vol. 68, No. 9 (Sept. 1972), pp. 42–45.

McConahey, William M.: "Diagnosing and Treating Myxedema and Myxedema Coma." Geriatrics, Vol. 33, No. 3 (March 1978), pp. 61–66.

Morrow, Lewis B.: "How Thyroid Disease Presents in the Elderly." Geriatrics, Vol. 33, No. 4 (April 1978), pp. 42–45.

Neelon, Francis A., and Sydnor, Charles F.: "The Assessment of Pituitary Function." D. M., Vol. 24, No. 4 (Jan. 1978).

Purnell, Don C., et al.: "Diagnosis of Primary Hyperparathyroidism." Surg. Clin. North Am., Vol. 57, No. 3 (June 1977), pp. 533–542.

ReMine, William H., and McConahey, William M.: "Management of Thyroid Nodules." Surg. Clin. North Am., Vol. 57, No. 3 (June 1977), pp. 523–531.

Schultz, Alvin L.: "Diagnosing and Managing Hyperthyroidism." Geriatrics, Vol. 33, No. 2 (Feb. 1978), pp. 77–81.

Tripp, Alice: "Hyper and Hypocalcemia," Am. J. Nurs., Vol. 76, No. 7 (July 1976), pp. 1142–45.

Walton, Joseph, and Ney, Robert L.: "Current Concepts of Corticosteroids – Uses and Abuses." D. M., June 1975.

Diabetes

Askew, Gail B., and Letcher, Kenneth I.: "Oral Hypoglycemic Agents: A Little Teaching Makes Therapy Go a Long Way." Nurs. '75, Vol. 5, No. 8 (Aug. 1975), pp. 45–50.

Cranley, Mecca S., and Frazier, Sue A.: "Preventive Intensive Care of the Diabetic Mother and Her Fetus." Nurs. Clin. North Am., Vol. 8, No. 3 (Sept. 1973), pp. 489–499.

Crosby, Elizabeth F.: "Childhood Diabetes." Can. Nurse, Vol. 73, No. 9 (Sept. 1977), pp. 20–23.

Davies, Derek: "Advances Toward Understanding Diabetes Mellitus." Geriatrics, Vol. 3, No. 11 (Nov. 1975), p. 79.

Duncan, Theodore G. (Ed.): "Symposium — Diabetes: Diagnosis and Management in the Older Patient." Geriatrics, Vol. 31, No. 10 (Oct. 1976).

Dwyer, Lois, and Fralin, Florence.: "Simplified Meal Planning for Hard-to-teach Patients." Am. J. Nurs., Vol. 74, No. 4 (April 1974), pp. 664–655.

Ehrlich, Robert M.: "Diabetes Mellitus in Childhood." Primary Care, Vol. 1, No. 4 (Dec. 1974), pp. 613–624.

———: "Is Diabetes Mellitus Preventable?" Can. Family Physician, Vol. 24, No. 7 (July 1978), pp. 680–682.

Engle, Veronica: "Diabetic Teaching — How To Win Your Patient's Cooperation in His Care." Nurs. '75, Vol. 5, No. 12 (Dec. 1975), pp. 17–24.

Fletcher, H. Patrick: "The Oral Antidiabetic Drugs: Pro and Con." Am. J. Nurs., Vol. 76, No. 4 (April 1976), pp. 594–599.

Fulton, Mary, et al.: "Helping Diabetics Adapt to Failing Vision." Am. J. Nurs., Vol. 74, No. 1 (Jan. 1974), pp. 54–57.

Guthrie, Diana W.: "Coping with Diabetic Ketoacidosis." Nurs. '73, Vol. 3, No. 11 (Nov. 1973), pp. 14–23.

———: "Diabetes in Adolescence." Am. J. Nurs., Vol. 75, No. 10 (Oct. 1975), pp. 1740–1744.

———: "Exercise, Diets and Insulin for Children with Diabetes." Nurs. '77, Vol. 7, No.2 (Feb. 1977), pp. 48–54.

——— and Guthrie, Richard A.: "DKA: Breaking the Vicious Cycle." Nurs. '78, Vol. 8, No. 6 (June 1978), pp. 54–61.

Hayter, Jean: "Fine Points in Diabetic Care." Am. J. Nurs., Vol. 76, No. 4 (April 1976), pp. 594–599.

Hornback, May: "Diabetes Mellitus — The Nurse's Role." Nurs. Clin. North Am., Vol. 5, No. 1 (March 1970, pp. 3–12.

Laugharne, E., and Duncan, F.: "Gestational Diabetes — When Teaching is Important." Can. Nurse, Vol. 69, No. 3 (March 1973). pp. 34–36.

Laugharne, E., and Steiner, G.: "Tri-Hospital Diabetes Education Centre." Can. Nurse, Vol. 73, No. 9 (Sept. 1977), pp. 14–19.

Leahey, M. D., Logan, S. A., and McArthur, R. G.: "Pediatric Diabetes: A New Teaching Approach." Can. Nurse, Vol. 71, No. 10 (Oct. 1975), pp. 18–20.

Levine, Myra (Ed.):"Insulin Reactions in a Brittle Diabetic." Nurs. '72, Vol. 2, No. 5 (May 1972), pp. 6–11.

McConnell, Edwina A.: "Meeting the Special Needs of the Diabetic Facing Surgery." Nurs. '76, Vol. 6, No. 6 (June 1976), pp. 30–37.

Mirsky, Stanley: "Adult-Onset Diabetes." Primary Care., Vol. 1, No. 1 (March 1974), pp. 53–62.

Palumbo, P. J.: "How To Treat Maturity-Onset Diabetes Mellitus." Geriatrics, Vol. 32, No. 12 (Dec. 1977), pp. 57–63.

Petrokas, Judith C.: "Commonsense Guidelines for Controlling Diabetes During Illness." Nurs. '77, Vol. 7, No. 12 (Dec. 1977), pp. 36–37.

Polowich, Carol, and Elliott, M. Ruth: "The Juvenile Diabetic." Can. Nurse, Vol. 73, No. 9 (Sept. 1977), pp. 24–27.

Porter, Anne Lynn (Ed.): "Symposium on Diabetes: Patient Education and Care." Nurs. Clin. North Am., Vol. 12, No. 3 (Sept. 1977), pp. 361–445.

Reynolds, Clayton, and Garg, Arun K.: "Who is a Diabetic?" Can. Family Physician, Vol. 24, No. 7 (July 1978), pp. 687–690.

Schaffrin, M.: "The Adolescent Diabetic." Can. Family Physician, Vol. 24, No. 7 (July 1978), pp. 682–686.

Schumann, Delores: "Coping with the Complex, Dangerous, Elusive Problems of Those Insulin-Induced Hypoglycemia Reactions." Nurs. '74, Vol. 4, No. 4 (April 1974), pp. 56–60.

————: "Assessing the Diabetic." Nurs. '76, Vol. 6, No. 3 (March 1976), pp. 62–67.

Skelton, J. M.: "A Diabetic Teaching Tool." Can. Nurse, Vol. 69, No. 12 (Dec. 1973), pp. 35–38.

Wiley, Loy (Ed.): "Diabetic Out of Control." Nurs. '73, Vol. 3, No. 5 (May 1973), pp. 10–15.

Wolfe, Lawrence: "Insulin: Paving the Way to a New Life." Nurs. '77, Vol. 7, No. 11 (Nov. 1977), pp. 38–44.

Yue, Dennis K., and Turtle, John R.: "New Forms of Insulin and Their Use in the Treatment of Diabetes." Diabetes, Vol. 26, No. 4 (April 1977), pp. 341–345.

Associations

American Diabetes Association Inc., 18 East 48th St., New York, N.Y., U.S.A. 10017.
Canadian Diabetic Association, 123 Edward St, Suite 601, Toronto, Ontario, Canada M5G1E2.

23

Nursing in Disorders of the Nervous System

MARYLEA KENLY, R.N.

JEANNETTE E. WATSON, R.N., M.Sc.N.

INTRODUCTION

The nervous system is the dominant system of the body. It provides an elaborate communication system and directs and integrates (along with the endocrine system) body activities.

The manifestations of dysfunction within the nervous system depend on the location of the lesion. This necessitates some understanding of the areas of the nervous system involved in various activities. Space does not permit an extensive review of the anatomy and physiology of this system, but some basic information of selected areas especially pertinent to nursing is presented.

All body movements, including much of the visceral activity, are brought about by contraction of muscle tissue which, in practically all instances,[1] is initiated and coordinated by the nervous system. Relatively few primary disorders of muscle activity occur, but loss of movement (paralysis) and abnormal movement (e.g., spasticity) resulting from nervous dysfunction are common. For this reason, this section includes a brief consideration of muscle tissue.

---

[1]Exceptions: Inherent capacity of cardiac and intestinal muscle.

THE NERVOUS SYSTEM

The component structural parts of the nervous system are the brain, spinal cord, nerves, ganglia, receptors and effectors. The brain and spinal cord comprise the *central nervous system;* the other parts form the *peripheral nervous system.* There are two main functional divisions: the cerebrospinal or *somatic nervous system,* which is concerned mainly with activities at conscious level (perception and willed responses), and the *autonomic or involuntary nervous system,* which innervates visceral muscle and glands. These divisions are useful for descriptive purposes; the activities of the total system are interrelated.

Neuron

The microscopic structural unit of the nervous system is the neuron (nerve cell), which consists of a cell body and cytoplasmic processes (Fig. 23–1). Each neuron has a single process called an *axon,* which conducts impulses away from the cell body, and one or more processes known as *dendrites* that carry impulses toward the cell body. Dendrites have many branches, increasing the surface area over which impulses may be picked up. Axons frequently extend over great distances and give off branches nearer to their terminations. The processes (axons and dendrites) may be referred to as nerve fibers if they are outside the central nervous system, or as tracts if within the brain or spinal cord.

Unlike most body cells, neurons are incapable of reproduction by mitosis; when they are destroyed they are not replaced. A neuronal process may be replaced under favorable conditions (see p. 814).

Nerve cells may be classified as motor (efferent), sensory (afferent) or connecting (internuncial). The axon of a motor neuron transmits impulses which leave the central nervous system to stimulate muscle or glandular tissue. The sensory neuron's axon transmits impulses to areas of the brain or spinal cord. One or more of its dendrites end in a receptor of some type in the periphery. Connecting neurons occur only in the gray matter of the brain and spinal cord. Nerve

impulses must pass from the sensory neuron through one or more connecting neurons before being dispatched to a muscle or gland by a motor neuron. The connecting neurons play an important role, especially within the cerebral cortex, since they comprise the association areas which are discussed with the cerebral cortex. They "decide" the responses to the incoming (sensory) impulses and prompt the initiation of the appropriate motor neuron response.

Nerve Impulse

The functions of the nerve cells are to receive, initiate and conduct "messages" known as nerve impulses. An impulse is a physicochemical process initiated at the point of stimulation. It occurs as the result of a mechanical, chemical or electrical change at some point in the immediate environment of the neuron. This change temporarily alters the permeability of the cell membrane at that point and is referred to as the stimulus. The

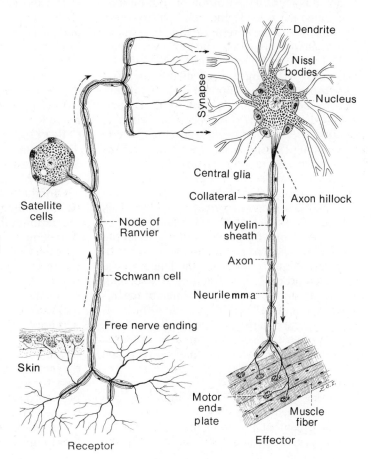

FIGURE 23–1 Diagram of 2 neurons. (From King, B. G., and Showers, M. J.: Human Anatomy and Physiology, 6th ed. Philadelphia, W. B. Saunders Co., 1969, p. 59.)

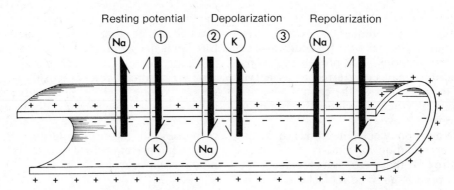

FIGURE 23–2 Resting state, depolarization and repolarization.

series of events that result from the change in the membrane permeability produces an electrical current (Fig. 23–2).

When a normal neuron is in a resting state, the outer surface of its membrane is electropositive, but the inner surface is electronegative. As a result, it is said to be polarized. This electrical polarity is attributed to the selective action of the cell membrane by which a higher concentration of sodium ions is maintained outside the cell. The positive sodium ions, which are normally attracted to the negative ions within the cell, are not allowed to cross the membrane; if they do so, they are ejected by the cell membrane. The electronegativity within the cell is mainly due to the nondiffusible protein anions and retained chlorine anions. When the stimulus occurs, the membrane becomes permeable to sodium. The influx of cations depolarizes the membrane; a reversal of the electrical potential develops as the outer surface of the membrane becomes electronegative and the inner surface becomes electropositive. This change alters the electrical relationship of the excited area to the adjacent portions; the shift of ions acts as a stimulus, and a wave of depolarization passes along the length of the neuronal process. In a fraction of a second, following depolarization, the membrane recovers its normal permeability and the resting electrical polarity is restored. The electrical currents that are generated as impulses sweep over the fibers and may be recorded and used in assessing function (e.g., electroencephalogram).

During the conduction of impulses, the neurons consume oxygen and glucose and produce heat and carbon dioxide. Impulse velocity is determined by the size of the neuronal process (nerve fiber) and whether or not it has a myelin sheath. The smaller unmyelinated fibers conduct more slowly than the larger, myelinated ones.

SYNAPSE. Neurons occur in a chain-like arrangement to provide a pathway for impulses. The axon of one neuron passes the impulse to a dendrite or the cell body of the successive neuron in the pathway. The point of transmission is referred to as a synapse. A slight gap exists between the end of the axon and the receptive neuron. The transmission is brought about by the release of a chemical from the terminal portion of the axon which acts as a stimulus to initiate the impulse in the succeeding neuron. The chemical transmitter is then rapidly destroyed or removed.

REFLEX ARC, RECEPTOR, EFFECTOR. The functional unit of the nervous system is called a reflex arc; structurally, it consists of the pathway over which impulses are conducted from a receptor to an effector. At the ending of afferent (sensory) fibers in the peripheral nervous system are receptors. A receptor, in a few instances, consists of bare nerve fibers; in others the afferent fibers end in specialized structures which are sensitive to specific stimuli. When the receptor is stimulated by a change in its environment (pressure, temperature, chemical, stretching) it evokes an impulse in the nerve fibers. The impulse is carried through the cell body of the sensory neuron and via its axon into the central nervous system. Here, it may pass through one, several or many connecting neurons before it excites a motor neuron whose axon (efferent or motor fiber) carries the impulse out of the central nervous system to muscular or glandular tissue. The ter-

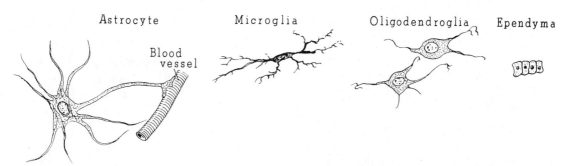

FIGURE 23–3 Neuroglial cells of the central nervous system. (From Jacob, Stanley W., Francone, Clarice Ashworth, and Lossow, Walter J.: Structure and Function in Man, 4th ed. Philadelphia, W. B. Saunders Co., 1978, p. 226.)

minal portion of the efferent fiber releases a chemical at its junction with the effector, initiating its response. This response is contraction in the case of muscle and is secretion if it is a gland that is innervated.

Neuroglia

Lying among the neurons of the central nervous system are supporting cells referred to collectively as neuroglia. There are three types of glial cells, which vary in size, shape and function, but all have many processes which interlace with the neuronal processes and frequently attach to cerebral blood vessels (Fig. 23–3). The *astrocytes* are star-shaped, and some of their processes attach to adjacent small blood vessels. *Oligodendroglia* have fewer and shorter processes, and the third type, which are smaller, are called *microglia*.

Knowledge of the function of the glial cells is limited. The astrocytes increase during infection and probably play a role in transporting fluid and nutrients from the blood into the neurons. The microglia are capable of enlarging and becoming phagocytic to remove exudate and degenerative tissue following injury. It has been suggested that the oligodendrocytes are active in the formation and maintenance of the myelin around the neuron processes. It is also thought that the glial cells contribute to the blood-brain barrier by which certain substances in the blood are prevented from entering the brain neurons. In contradistinction to the neurons, glial cells can divide and multiply; the majority of brain tumors arise from the uncontrolled growth of neuroglia.

THE CENTRAL NERVOUS SYSTEM

Brain

The brain is protected by the skull and for purposes of description may be divided into the cerebrum, basal ganglia, thalami, hypothalamus, midbrain, pons varoli, medulla oblongata and cerebellum (Fig. 23–4).

CEREBRUM. The cerebrum is divided by a longitudinal fissure into two hemispheres which are joined at their bases by bands of nerve fibers, collectively forming the corpus callosum. Each hemisphere is subdivided into four main lobes: frontal, parietal, temporal and occipital, corresponding approximately in location with the overlying skull bones. The lobes are separated by fissures: the central fissure (fissure of Rolando) lies between the frontal and parietal lobes; the

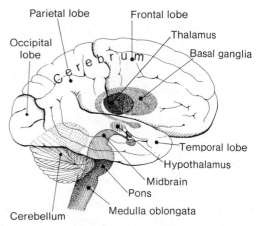

FIGURE 23–4 Diagram of the brain and its major parts.

lateral cerebral fissure (fissure of Sylvius) separates the temporal from the parietal and frontal lobes; and the parieto-occipital fissure separates the occipital from the perietal and temporal lobes. Lying deep within the lateral cerebral fissure is a small lobe referred to as the insula.

The brain contains areas of gray and white matter. The gray matter is an aggregation of neuronal bodies and unmyelinated processes; the white matter consists primarily of myelinated fibers. The surface of the cerebrum (cerebral cortex) consists of gray matter which is arranged in a series of coil-like elevations called gyri. The shallow crevices between the gyri are sulci (Fig. 23–5).

The *cerebral cortex* is a highly specialized area involved in all conscious processes. It is responsible for the intellectual processes such as learning, thought, memory, reasoning, verbalization and willed (voluntary) body movement, all of which are dependent on the information received through the afferent pathways.

Some parts of the cortex are receptive areas for incoming impulses and are called *sensory areas or centers*; others are concerned with dispatching outgoing impulses to prompt action responses in peripheral structures and are referred to as *motor areas or centers* (Fig. 23–6). Around the sensory and motor areas lie the *association areas,* which occupy the greater portion of the cortex. A maze of connections exists between the association areas themselves as well as between them and sensory and motor centers. The association areas "analyze" the data received by the sensory areas, giving them meaning and making decisions as to appropriate responses which are then initiated. In some instances, the response may be to store the perception in memory; in others, it may involve stimulation of motor centers to bring about body movement or speech.

Certain areas of the cerebral cortex have been recognized as being primarily responsible for particular functions. The motor area that initiates all voluntary movements of the body occupies the strip of the frontal lobe immediately in front of the central fissure (Fig. 23–7). The area in one hemisphere controls the movements on the opposite side of the body. The muscles are represented from the lower lateral surface of the lobe medially in the following order: head, throat, hand, arm, trunk, thigh, leg and foot.

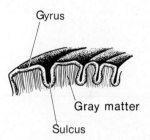

FIGURE 23–5   The surface of the cerebrum.

The medial end of the motor strip terminates on the surface of the lobe in the longitudinal fissure. The size of the cortical area representing the muscular control in the various parts of the body is quite irregular and is proportional to their functional importance. The muscles of the fingers and hands have a large representation because of the frequent activity and precision movements. Similarly, the areas innervating the muscles involved in the highly developed function of speech (larynx, tongue, lips) are large. The area in front of the primary motor area is known as the *premotor or secondary motor area*. It is thought to be involved in patterns of movement requiring the coordinated contraction of groups of muscles. It has connecting pathways with the primary motor area and lower levels of the brain.

The sensory impulses that enter the cortex are conducted to various areas, depending on their origin. The impulses concerned with touch, pressure, temperature, pain and the sense of position of the body and its parts (collectively referred to as the *somesthetic senses*) are received in the area of the parie-

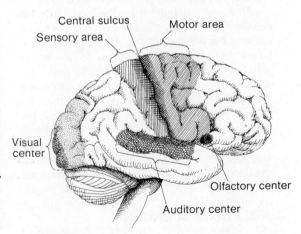

FIGURE 23–6   Major centers of the cerebrum.

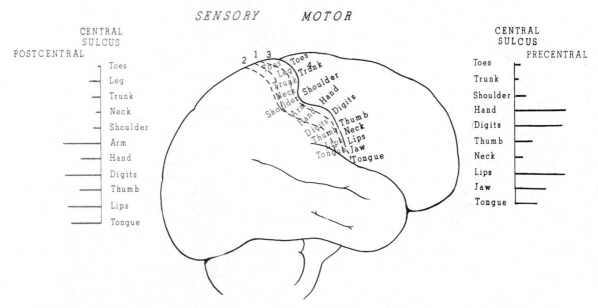

FIGURE 23–7 Lateral view of the brain showing somesthetic and primary motor areas. The amount of brain surface related to a specific part of the body is not proportionate to the size of the part but to the extent of its use, as illustrated diagrammatically. (From Jacob, Stanley W., Francone, Clarice Ashworth, and Lossow, Walter J.: Structure and Function in Man, 4th ed. Philadelphia, W. B. Saunders Co., 1978, p. 240.)

tal lobe just behind the central fissure. As with the motor areas, sensations from the lower part of the body are received at the medial portion lying within the longitudinal fissure. Those from the head are received at the lower lateral part of the strip. Sensations from the right side of the body are transmitted to the left hemisphere and vice versa.

Impulses originating in the retinae of the eyes are transmitted to the posterior part of the occipital lobe, resulting in vision. The *visual center* in the right occipital lobe receives impulses from the right half of the retina of each eye and, conversely, the left cerebral visual center receives those from the left half of each eye.

The *centers for hearing* (auditory centers) lie in the superior parts of the temporal lobes. Impulses from both ears are received in both the right and left auditory centers. The sense of smell (*olfactory sense*) is also represented in the temporal lobe. The frontal lobes anterior to the motor areas are concerned with the personality, emotional reactions, initiative and sense of responsibility for socially acceptable standards. Persons who undergo prefrontal lobotomy, in which the severing of fibers interrupts many association pathways, frequently exhibit a complete change of personality, loss of judgment and inhibitions, and reduced efficiency.

The abstract mental activities such as thought, learning, reasoning, memory and emotions involve widespread cortical activity rather than a definitive local area. Associative memory is constantly used; it provides the knowledge that a person has. For example, vision stored as memory, auditory sensation stored as memory and other sensory experiences in memory may all be recalled and associated to give incoming impulses meaning and provide an appropriate response. To illustrate, if one has been introduced to a person and gains information about him at some time, he recognizes that person when he meets him again and recalls what he knows about him. One hemisphere tends to be dominant; in right-handed persons, the left hemisphere is dominant and vice versa.

The interior of the cerebrum consists mainly of white matter. Myelinated neuronal processes are arranged in functionally related bundles called tracts. These are classified as commissural, association and projection tracts. The *commissural tracts* transmit impulses between the two hemispheres. The *association tracts* carry impulses from one area of the cerebral cortex to another in the same hemisphere. *Projection tracts* are ascending and descending pathways from one level of the central nervous system to another. One of the most important of these is the *internal capsule*.

BASAL GANGLIA (NUCLEI). Embedded deeply within the cerebral white matter of each hemisphere are four irregular masses of gray matter, collectively referred to as the basal ganglia, or nuclei. Singly, they are the *lentiform nucleus, caudate nucleus, amygdaloid body* and the *claustrum*. The lentiform nucleus is subdivided into the putamen and globus pallidus. The lentiform and caudate nuclei and the segment of the internal capsule which separates them constitute what may be called the *corpus striatum,* an important part of the extrapyramidal system. It sends impulses to the globus pallidus and is influenced by impulses delivered to it from the frontal lobe, thalamus and hypothalamus.

The functions of the basal nuclei are not clearly understood. They are concerned with skeletal muscle tone and inhibitions essential to orderly, smooth patterns of movement. Normal functioning in relation to this is influenced by dopamine, a neurotransmitter substance produced at the ends of the neuronal fibers that derive from cells in the substantia nigra, a small layer of pigmented gray matter within the midbrain. It receives fibers from the corpus striatum and frontal lobe motor areas, and fibers of nigral cells pass to the corpus striatum. Degenerative changes in the substantia nigra decrease the amount of dopamine released to the basal nuclei, resulting in increased muscle tone, rigidity and tremor (Parkinson's disease). The amygdaloid and claustrum are thought to be concerned with emotion and autonomic nervous system function.

THALAMI. A large oval mass of gray matter lies at the base of each hemisphere and forms the lateral walls of the third ventricle. Each is referred to as a thalamus and serves as an important relay center for all afferent impulses. The impulses are "sorted" and forwarded to appropriate cerebral cortical areas. Each thalamus is capable of producing a crude uncritical awareness of pain, temperature and pressure; refinement of the sensation as to precise location, quality and intensity is made at cerebral cortical level.

HYPOTHALAMUS. Lying below the thalami and forming the floor of the third ventricle is an important gray mass called the hypothalamus. It has extensive connections with higher and lower levels of the central nervous system and with the posterior lobe of the pituitary gland (neurohypophysis).

The hypothalamus integrates and coordinates the responses of the autonomic nervous system, regulating visceral activities; for example, it exerts a control on vasomotor tone, gastrointestinal motility and heart rate. It contains groups of neurons responsible for temperature regulation. Through connections with the thalami and cerebral cortex, the hypothalamus' regulation of visceral activities may be influenced by emotional impulses.

Neurons in the hypothalamus also serve as osmoreceptors (cells sensitive to changes in the osmotic pressure of body fluid) and regulate the production and release of the antidiuretic hormone, which plays an important role in maintaining fluid balance. The production and release of oxytocin (see p. 753) is also influenced by the hypothalamus. This area of the brain also has control centers concerned with appetite and sleeping and waking mechanisms.

MIDBRAIN. This portion of the brain is a short segment below the thalami and is comprised of a number of ascending and descending pathways. A narrow canal, the cerebral aqueduct, passes through the center, connecting the third and fourth ventricles. Groups of neurons form the corpora quadrigemina, which is comprised of two superior colliculi and two inferior colliculi. The superior colliculi correlate eye movements with movements of the head and trunk and initiate the protective reflexes, blinking and closure of eyelids. The inferior colliculi are groups of neurons concerned with auditory reflexes such as the startle reflex on hearing a sudden sound and the turning of the head to improve the hearing of a sound. Centers (groups of neurons) for postural and righting reflexes also occur in the midbrain.

BRAIN STEM. The midbrain continues downward into the pons varoli, which consists of many tracts linking the various parts of the brain and serving as a conduction pathway. The pons also contains portions of the reticular formation and groups of neurons (nuclei) which give rise to some cranial nerves (V, VI, VII and VIII).

Below the pons lies the medulla oblongata, which continues down to connect with the spinal cord. It is comprised of ascending and descending conduction pathways and several important regulating centers. Groups of neurons form the vital cardiac, respiratory and vasomotor regulation centers. It also contains reflex centers for salivation, sneezing, vomiting, coughing and swallowing as well as the nuclei for a number of cranial nerves (IX, X, XI and XII).

CEREBELLUM. This portion of the brain lies under the posterior portion of the cerebrum posterior to the pons and medulla. It is separated from the cerebrum by a fold of meningeal membrane (dura mater) called the tentorium cerebelli. A fissure divides the cerebellum into hemispheres which are connected at their base. The outer surface consists of smooth layers of gray matter, and the interior consists mainly of white matter with scattered nuclei. The cerebellum has wide connections with other parts of the brain and with the spinal cord through tracts running through the pons. It is linked with the motor centers of the cerebral cortex and basal ganglia. It functions in the coordination of muscular activity and orienting the individual in space. Afferent impulses are received from the proprioceptors in the skeletal muscles which result in impulses being delivered to the cerebral motor centers to provide synergic control in movements in which several muscles are involved. For example, antagonist muscles are inhibited and relax to allow contraction of the prime movers; the cerebellum is largely responsible for this type of integration to provide smooth, effective patterns of movement. Afferent impulses are also delivered to the cerebellum from the labyrinth of each internal ear. These impulses prompt appropriate reflex muscle responses to maintain balance of position or postural equilibrium.

RETICULAR FORMATION (RETICULAR ACTIVATING SYSTEM). A core of small neurons in complex intertwining networks extending from the spinal cord through the medulla, pons, midbrain and into the hypothalamus comprises the reticular formation. It has widespread afferent connections, receiving sensory impulses from all over the body. It initiates impulses which are transmitted via subcortical relay areas to most of the cortex, alerting it to deal with ensuing impulses (Fig. 23–8). In this way, it is said to produce an awareness or state of wakefulness that makes perception possible. The neurons of this area learn to be selective, making judgment as to whether the cortex should be alerted or not. For example, a mother may not be awakened by heavy, noisy traffic, but she is aroused by the slightest whimper from her infant. Injury to this area produces loss of consciousness. The reticular formation also contributes to smooth, orderly motor performance, both reflex and voluntary. Its activities also have a role in endocrine secretion and conditioned reflexes.

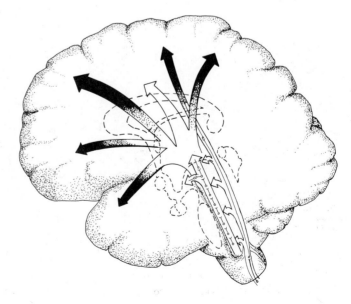

FIGURE 23–8   The reticular activating system.

BLOOD SUPPLY TO THE BRAIN. The blood supply to the brain is derived from the two internal carotid arteries and the two vertebral arteries which arise from the subclavian arteries (Fig. 23–9). At the base of the brain, the carotids give off anterior and middle cerebral arteries. The vertebrals, on reaching the brain, unite to form the basilar artery which gives rise to posterior cerebral arteries. The cerebral arteries are connected by communicating arteries, forming an arterial circle at the base of the brain called the circle of Willis which serves as a collateral channel. Branches of the cerebral arteries extend throughout the cerebrum, midbrain and brain stem; cerebellar arteries arise from the vertebral and basilar arteries and provide branches to the brain stem as well as the cerebellum. Blood from the capillaries enters veins which empty into sinuses in the dura mater (outer meningeal membrane). The sinuses are drained by the internal jugular veins.

A constant flow of blood through the brain is critical since it requires 20 per cent more oxygen than any other part as well as a continuous supply of nutrients, especially glucose. Brain cells are extremely sensitive to hypoxia, particularly those of the cerebral cortex; interruption of the blood supply to the brain produces loss of consciousness in seconds. Brain stem neurons are less sensitive to hypoxia than cortical cells; individuals experiencing prolonged hypoxia may survive because the vital centers in the medulla are more resistant and recover, but irreversible cortical damage persists, resulting in mental deficiency.

Glucose is the major energy source for the brain cells and is necessary for survival. As with oxygen, the cerebral cortex is more sensitive to hypoglycemia than neurons at brain stem level; permanent cortical damage may be incurred by a prolonged period of hypoglycemia.

Factors which affect cerebral blood flow include the pressure of the blood in the arteries and veins at brain level, conditions of the vessels (e.g., atherosclerotic), intracranial pressure, viscosity of the blood and, to a lesser extent, constriction and dilatation of cerebral vessels.

BLOOD-BRAIN BARRIER. The network of neuroglial cell processes which invest the blood vessels in the central nervous system prevents some substances from reaching the interstitial fluid (which is very limited) and entering into the neurons. This ''rejection'' of some substances develops as the brain's neuroglial cells (astrocytes) mature; the brain cells of the infant, especially if premature, are readily permeable to some substances (e.g., bilirubin, radioactive phosphorus) that are prevented from reaching the neurons when the glial cells are mature or fully developed.

VENTRICLES AND CEREBROSPINAL FLUID. Within the brain are a series of cavities called ventricles which originate with the embryonic, neural tube (Fig. 23–10). There are two *lateral ventricles,* one in each cerebral hemisphere. Each lateral ventricle communicates with the *third ventricle* by means of an interventricular foramen (foramen of Munro). The third ventricle is a small and slit-like space between the thalami, and the larger fourth ventricle lies between the pons and the cerebellum. The third and fourth ventricles are united by a narrow channel called the cerebral aqueduct (aqueduct of Sylvius). The *fourth ventricle* has openings into the subarachnoid space (see meninges) and is continuous with the narrow central canal of the medulla and the spinal cord.

Within the ventricles, complex networks

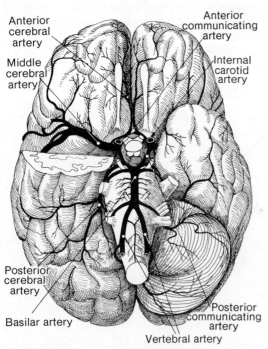

FIGURE 23–9 The blood supply to the brain.

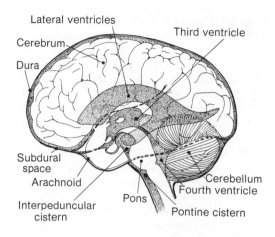

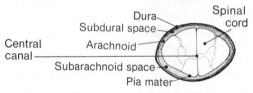

FIGURE 23–10 A diagram showing the ventricles, meninges and spaces.

of capillaries (choroid plexuses) occur from which fluid escapes into the cavities, forming what is referred to as the *cerebrospinal fluid*. The fluid flows through the communicating channels and eventually escapes from the fourth ventricle into the subarachnoid space to surround the brain and spinal cord. This distribution of the fluid provides a protective cushion for the brain and cord.

The cerebrospinal fluid is steadily and slowly absorbed from the subarachnoid space into the venous sinuses. Any interruption within the cerebrospinal fluid circuit, such as occurs with a congenital absence of openings between the fourth ventricle and subarachnoid space, results in an excessive accumulation of fluid within the ventricles. The condition is referred to as hydrocephalus. The brain tissue becomes compressed between the skull and the expanding volume of fluid.

MENINGES. The brain and spinal cord are enclosed in three layers of membranous tissue known as the meninges. The tough outermost layer is the *dura mater*. The cranial portion of the dura mater occurs in two layers; the external layer is adherent to the skull bones and does not continue into the spinal region. The two cranial layers are closely connected except where they form

sinuses to receive the venous blood from cerebral vessels.

The middle membrane is called the *arachnoid;* it is much thinner and lies free. The potential space between the dura mater and arachnoid is known as the *subdural space*.

The innermost membrane is the pia mater and is thin, reticular and elastic; it is closely applied to the surface of the brain and cord, dipping into the fissures and sulci. The space between the arachnoid and pia mater is referred to as the *subarachnoid space* and contains the cerebrospinal fluid.

Spinal Cord

The cord, continuous with the medulla oblongata, originates at the foramen magnum of the skull and extends downward in the vertebral canal to approximately the second lumbar vertebra. It tapers off into a fine cord called the *filum terminale*. A ventral and a dorsal fissure incompletely divide the cord into lateral halves. A small canal (*central canal*) extends the full length of the cord. It contains cerebrospinal fluid, and the superior end opens into the fourth ventricle at the level of the medulla oblongata.

The cord consists of gray and white matter, but in contrast with the cerebrum, the gray matter is concentrated in the interior, roughly in the form of an **H**. White matter comprised of tracts is on the outside (Fig. 23–11). Afferent impulses are received by neurons in the posterior columns or horns of

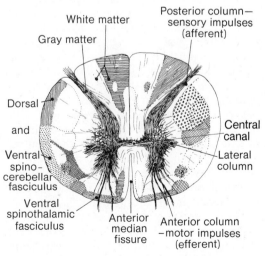

FIGURE 23–11 Cross section of the spinal cord.

gray matter. Efferent impulses are discharged by neurons in the anterior columns or horns of the gray matter. The gray matter also contains neurons which may transmit impulses from one lateral half of the cord to the other, from dorsal to ventral and to other levels of the central nervous system. The cord consists of 31 segments, each of which gives rise to a pair of spinal nerves. Two notable enlargements occur; one is in the cervical region corresponding to the origin of the upper limb nerves, and the other is in the lumbar region and gives origin to the nerves supplying the lower extremities.

The spinal cord provides conduction pathways to and from the brain and functions as a center for reflex actions which are involuntary responses following the reception of certain afferent impulses.

Nerves and Tracts

The term nerve refers to a bundle of neuronal processes which extends beyond the central nervous system. Nerves consisting only of afferent fibers which transmit impulses from the periphery to the central nervous system are called *sensory nerves*. *Motor nerves* are comprised entirely of efferent fibers, which transmit impulses from the central nervous system out into the periphery. Many of the nerves — for example, all the spinal nerves — contain both efferent and afferent fibers and are known as *mixed nerves*.

Structurally, three types of nerve fibers occur; one is enclosed in a sheath of fatty substance, *myelin,* and an outer membranous sheath called the *neurilemma* (sheath of Schwann) and is known as a *myelinated* or *medullated fiber*. The other type has no myelin sheath but does have a neurilemma and is referred to as a *nonmyelinated* or *nonmedullated fiber*. Most nonmyelinated fibers belong to the autonomic nervous system, which is concerned with visceral action. A third type of neuronal process lacks a neurilemma. All fibers within the central nervous system and the optic and auditory nerves have no neurilemma. An injured neuronal process cannot be regenerated in the absence of the neurilemmal sheath.

Nerve tracts are bundles of neuronal processes within the brain or spinal cord that transmit impulses that are usually similar in origin, termination and function. The origin and destination may be determined from the name of the tract. For example, the corticospinal tract carries impulses originating in the cerebral cortex to the spinal cord; the spinothalamic tract transmits sensory impulses from the spinal cord to a thalamus.

NERVE REGENERATION. Unlike most cells in the body, the adult nerve cells cannot reproduce by mitosis to replace any that are destroyed. Nerve fibers are outgrowths of the cell body of the neuron. If a fiber's connection with the cell body is interrupted, the distal fragment ceases to function and degenerates. The fiber may regenerate and restore function, providing it has a neurilemma. Since nerve fibers within the central nervous system have no neurilemma, they cannot regenerate to reestablish function.

When a fiber with a neurilemma is damaged, the distal fragment disintegrates and the debris is removed by phagocytic cells. The Schwann cells of the neurilemma proliferate, forming strands and a pathway along the course of the degenerated portion of the fiber. The distal tip of the viable portion of the fiber begins to extend buds or branches; one of these finds and extends into the tube-like pathway formed by the strands of Schwann cells and continues to grow until it reaches the peripheral destination. This is a slow process. Nonmyelinated fibers regenerate more rapidly than those that must form a myelin sheath. When a peripheral nerve is severed, this means that a great many fibers are separated from their cell bodies. If the two cut ends of the nerve are approximated and sutured, less scar tissue forms, favoring the regenerative process. Occasionally, because of fibrous scar tissue, a branch or bud of the viable fiber stump may not find its way into the "tube" of Schwann cells which is essential to the growing fiber. In such an instance, multiple growing tips may be produced by the fiber stump and may form a small mass referred to as a neuroma.

THE PERIPHERAL NERVOUS SYSTEM

The peripheral nervous system consists of nerves and ganglia. The nerves may be divided into two main groups — namely, the cranial and spinal nerves — according to whether they emerge from the central nervous system at the cranial or spinal level.

Cranial Nerves

Twelve pairs of cranial nerves emerge from the undersurface of the brain and are numbered according to the order in which they arise from the front to back. They are also named according to their function or distribution. Some of the cranial nerves consist mainly of efferent (motor) fibers, three are comprised of afferent (sensory) fibers only (I, II and VIII), and others are made up of both motor and sensory fibers (mixed nerves). Cell bodies of the motor fibers form nuclei within the pons or medulla. Sensory fibers originate in ganglia (groups of neurons outside the central nervous system) (see Table 23–1).

Spinal Nerves

Thirty-one pairs of nerves arise from the spinal cord and are numbered and named according to the order in which they arise and the vertebral level at which they emerge. There are *eight cervical, twelve thoracic, five lumbar* and *five sacral pairs* and *one coccygeal pair.* The cervical and thoracic nerves emerge from the vertebral column at the level they arise from the cord. The lumbar, sacral and coccygeal descend from the lower end of the cord (which terminates at first or second lumbar vertebra) and emerge from the vertebral canal at their respective vertebral levels.

All spinal nerves are mixed, and each one has two origins which are referred to as the ventral and dorsal roots (Fig. 23–12). The *ventral root* of a spinal nerve is comprised of neurons in the ventral column or horn of gray matter. The axons of the neurons emerge from the cord carrying efferent impulses and join with afferent fibers to form a spinal nerve just before emerging from the vertebral column. The *dorsal root* of a spinal nerve is formed by a ganglion (dorsal root or spinal ganglion) lying just outside the spinal cord. The dendrites of the neurons of the ganglion form the afferent (sensory) fibers of the nerve. The axons of the neurons carry the impulses into the dorsal column of gray matter of the cord (see Fig. 23–12).

After emerging from the vertebral canal each spinal nerve divides into two major branches, the *anterior and posterior rami.* The posterior rami divide into smaller branches which go directly to the muscles and skin of the posterior portions of the head, neck and trunk.

The anterior rami supply all the structures of the extremities and lateral and anterior portions of the trunk. These branches tend to form plexuses before going to the structures they innervate. A *plexus* is an intermixing of several nerves, forming a network. Several nerves emerge from the plexus; each nerve and its branches are named according to the regions they supply (e.g., femoral, ulnar, radial). Four main plexuses are formed by the anterior rami of spinal nerves — the *cervical, brachial, lumbar* and *sacral* plexuses. The cervical plexus is formed by the anterior rami of the first four cervical spinal nerves. The most important branch arising from this plexus is the phrenic nerve, which supplies the diaphragm. It contains fibers from the third, fourth and fifth cervical nerves. Injury to the spinal cord above these levels may result in respiratory paralysis.

The brachial plexus, which is located in the shoulder region, is formed by the anterior rami of the fifth, sixth, seven and eighth cervical nerves and the first thoracic. The nerves derived from the plexus supply the upper extremity (musculocutaneous, median, ulnar and radial nerves).

The lumbar plexus is formed by the intermingling of the anterior rami of the first four lumbar spinal nerves and is located in the lumbar region of the back. The nerves which emerge supply the lower abdominal wall, external genitalia, and parts of the thigh and leg (femoral, saphenous, obturator nerves).

The sacral plexus in the posterior pelvic cavity is formed by anterior rami of the fourth and fifth lumbar and first, second and third sacral spinal nerves. The nerves leaving the plexus supply the buttocks, perineum and lower extremities. The most important nerve derived from this plexus is the sciatic nerve, the longest and largest nerve of the body.

Ganglia

A ganglion consists of a group of neurons outside the central nervous system. Several different groups of ganglia occur. Those as-

TABLE 23–1 ORIGIN AND FUNCTIONS OF CRANIAL NERVES (12 PAIRS)

Number	Name	Origin of Main Nerve Fibers	Function
I	Olfactory	Sensory fibers: neurons in nasal mucosa	Olfactory sense (sense of smell)
II	Optic	Sensory fibers: neurons of retina	Vision
III	Oculomotor	Motor fibers:* nucleus in midbrain	Movements of the eyeball and upper eyelid; size of the pupil of iris (i.e., constriction and dilation of pupil to regulate amount of light admitted); control of ciliary muscle to regulate degree of refraction by the lens
IV	Trochlear	Motor fibers: nucleus in midbrain	Movement of eyeball by superior oblique muscles
V	Trigeminal Largest cranial nerve; has three sensory divisions —ophthalmic, maxillary and mandibular	Motor fibers: nucleus in pons Sensory fibers: gasserian or semilunar ganglion in temporal bone	Motor function: mastication Sensory function: sensations (pain, touch, temperature) of the face, nose, teeth and mouth
VI	Abducens	Motor fibers: nucleus in pons	Movement of the eyeball by lateral rectus muscle
VII	Facial	Motor fibers: nucleus in pons Sensory fibers: geniculate ganglion in temporal bone	Motor function: contraction of facial and scalp muscles (facial expression); secretion of saliva by submaxillary and sublingual glands Sensory function: taste (from anterior two-thirds of tongue)
VIII	Auditory (acoustic) Has two divisions: vestibular cochlear	Sensory fibers: vestibular branch: vestibular ganglion in internal ear cochlear branch: spiral ganglion in internal ear	Sensory function: vestibular branch: equilibrium (position balance) cochlear division: sense of hearing
IX	Glossopharyngeal	Motor fibers: nucleus in medulla Sensory fibers: jugular and petrous ganglia	Motor function: swallowing; reflex control of blood pressure through connection with carotid pressoreceptors; salivary secretion by parotid glands Sensory functions: taste and oral and pharyngeal sensations
X	Vagus Has very wide distribution	Motor fibers: nuclei in medulla Sensory fibers: jugular and nodosa ganglia	Motor function: muscles of pharynx, larynx, thoracic and abdominal viscera (e.g., regulates gastrointestinal motility or peristalsis; influences cardiac rate); secretion by gastric, intestinal and pancreatic glands Sensory function: sensations in pharynx, larynx, and thoracic and abdominal viscera
XI	Accessory	Motor fibers: nucleus in medulla and the spinal cord	Movement of shoulder and head by trapezius and sternocleidomastoid muscles
XII	Hypoglossal	Motor fibers: nucleus in medulla	Movements of the tongue

*Most motor nerves are considered to also contain some sensory fibers by which information as to the existing conditions in the muscles concerned (proprioceptive data) is transmitted into the central nervous system. The proprioceptive impulses result in appropriate motor responses to facilitate the required pattern of movement.

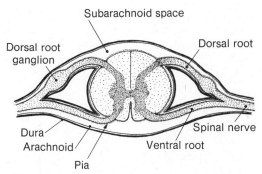

FIGURE 23–12 A spinal nerve, its dorsal root ganglion, dorsal root and ventral root.

sociated with the sensory fibers of the cranial nerves are named specifically (e.g., gasserian ganglion; dendrites of the neurons in the ganglion form the three sensory divisions of the trigeminal (V) nerve) (see Table 23–1).

The ganglia which form the dorsal or sensory root of the spinal nerves lie just outside the spinal cord and within the vertebral column. These are known as the spinal or dorsal root ganglia.

The ganglia associated with the autonomic (visceral) nervous system (Fig. 23–13) may be divided into three groups according to their location. The vertebral, sympathetic or lateral ganglia occur in two chains; one chain of 22 ganglia lies on each side of the vertebral column (three cervical, eleven thoracic, four lumbar and four sacral). A second group of autonomic ganglia is called the collateral or prevertebral ganglia. They lie in front of the vertebral column and close to large arteries for which they are named (e.g., iliac, mesenteric, splanchnic ganglia). A third group is referred to as the terminal ganglia; they lie close to or within the viscera which the nerve fibers supply.

The Autonomic Nervous System

The autonomic or visceral division of the nervous system is responsible for the regulation of smooth and cardiac muscle activity and glandular secretion. It carries only efferent impulses, and the actions are unwilled.

The anatomical arrangement differs from that of the voluntary system. Impulses are carried from the central nervous system to a ganglion from which axons pass to the viscera to be innervated. The nerve fibers which originate in the brain or spinal cord and carry the impulses to the ganglia are referred to as preganglionic fibers. Those which transmit the impulses from the ganglia to the viscera are known as the postganglionic fibers (see Fig. 23–13).

The autonomic system is divided into two parts, the parasympathetic and sympathetic systems. Most viscera have a nerve supply from each division; impulses delivered from one system excite activity, and those originating with the other division inhibit activity.

THE PARASYMPATHETIC NERVOUS SYSTEM. The preganglionic fibers of the parasympathetic autonomic division enter the periphery at the cranial and sacral levels. For this reason, the system may also be referred to as the craniosacral division. The preganglionic fibers are quite long, extending to ganglia which are located within or close to the viscera they supply. The cranial division supplies the ciliary and sphincter muscles of the eyes, salivary glands and thoracic and abdominal viscera. The sacral division innervates the muscle tissue of the colon and rectum, pelvic viscera and genitalia.

The responses to parasympathetic innervation are *localized* and specific for various parts of the body. One part alone may receive impulses. Generally, the innervation promotes a normal state; it is concerned with the restoration and conservation of body energy and elimination of body wastes. For example, parasympathetic impulses slow the heart rate and conserve cardiac energy when necessary.

THE SYMPATHETIC NERVOUS SYSTEM. The preganglionic fibers of this autonomic division are short and are derived from the thoracic and lumbar regions of the spinal cord. Because of these origins, the system is also referred to as the thoracolumbar nervous system. The associated ganglia lie in two chains of approximately 22 ganglia each, extending along either side of the vertebral column from the base of the skull to the coccygeal region (three cervical, eleven thoracic, four lumbar and four sacral). These ganglia are known as the sympathetic or vertebral ganglia. Those in each chain are connected by nerve fibers (preganglionic fibers) passing up or down to higher or lower ganglia. Most of the axons of the ganglionic neurons are distributed in the spinal nerves; a few are distributed separately and directly to the viscera concerned.

The sympathetic nervous system produces *generalized physiological responses* rather

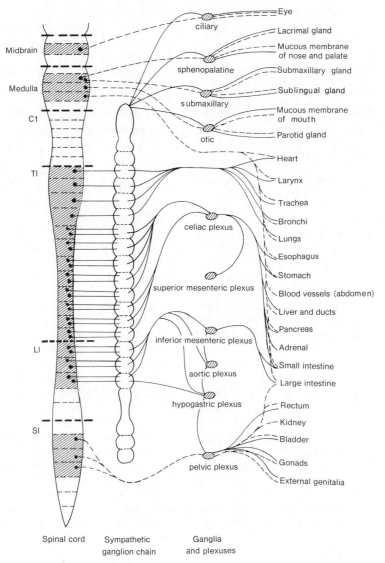

FIGURE 23–13 Ganglia associated with the sympathetic division of the autonomic nervous system.

than specific localized ones. It responds to stress, strong emotions (e.g., fear, anger), severe pain, cold, or any threat. The purpose of the responses induced is to mobilize the body's resources for defensive action ("fight or flight"). It produces vasoconstriction of superficial and abdominal blood vessels, increasing the volume to the heart, skeletal muscles and brain. Glycogenolysis is promoted, sweat gland and adrenal medullary secretions are increased, and the bronchioles and pupils of the eyes dilate. The heart rate, cardiac output and arterial blood pressure are increased.

The responses to sympathetic nervous impulses are augmented by the release of epinephrine and norepinephrine by the adrenal medullae. Stimulation of the sympathetic nervous system results in stimulation of the adrenal medullae. Their secretions are released into the blood stream, producing generalized "defensive" responses similar to those produced by sympathetic innervation.

CHEMICAL MEDIATORS. Transmission of impulses from the preganglionic fibers to the ganglia in both the sympathetic and parasympathetic nervous systems is dependent upon the release of *acetylcholine* by the terminal portion of the preganglionic axons. The postganglionic fibers of the parasympathetic system also release acetylcholine at their junction with the effector organs to facilitate the transmission of their impulses. The fibers which release the chemical mediator acetylcholine are said to be *cholinergic*. Most of the postganglionic fibers of the sympathetic system are *adrenergic*; they release *sympathin (norepinephrine)* at their junction with the effector organs or tissues.

REGULATION OF AUTONOMIC INNERVATION. Regulation and integration of autonomic activity is attributed mainly to the hypothalamus. Although the responses are unwilled, they may be influenced by cerebral cortical activity. Tracts from the cortex to the hypothalamus deliver impulses which frequently arise from emotional stress that may result in overstimulation of either the parasympathetic or sympathetic nervous system. For instance, chronic emotional stress resulting in excessive parasympathetic stimulation of gastric glands is thought to play a causative role in peptic ulcer.

MUSCLE TISSUE AND ACTIVITY

Most of man's activities, and indeed his survival, depend on functioning muscle tissue. This tissue performs vital activities such as circulation of the blood, respiration and peristaltic movement of food through the gastrointestinal tract; it also maintains posture against gravity and is responsible for movements of a part of the body as well as the mobility of the body as a whole. The capacity of the body to carry out these activities is directly dependent upon the specialized physiological properties peculiar to muscle tissue. These are: *contractility,* which is a shortening and thickening of muscle cells as a result of their ability to convert chemical energy to mechanical energy; *extensibility,* which indicates the capacity of stretching; *elasticity,* the ability to resume their original length after a stretching force is removed; *excitability or sensitivity,* which is the capability to respond by contraction to a change in the environment which may be initiated by a nerve impulse, pressure, stretching, chemical changes (e.g., calcium concentration) or temperature changes (e.g., cold stimulates contraction); and *tonus,*

which is a continuous partial contraction maintained by groups of muscle cells contracting in relays.

During muscle contraction, the chemical reactions which occur liberate both mechanical and heat energy. The heat energy contributes to the maintenance of normal body temperature. At rest, most of the body heat is produced by metabolic activities within visceral cells such as occur in the liver.

Muscle cells, because of their elongated shape, may be referred to as muscle fibers. The cell membrane is called the *sarcolemma*. Since varying degrees of muscular performance are needed throughout the body for its diversified activities, different types of muscle tissue with different types of control occur. These are *cardiac, smooth* (visceral) and *striated* (skeletal or voluntary) muscle tissues. Cardiac muscle tissue has been discussed in Chapter 13. Smooth muscle tissue is found in viscera (e.g., blood vessels, gastrointestinal tract, bladder) and is under autonomic nervous control. The muscle cells are smaller and are arranged in sheets or layers, and their sarcolemmae are not as well defined as in skeletal muscle.

Skeletal muscle tissue forms what is generally referred to as the muscle system. It comprises the muscles which are attached to the bones and are responsible for external body movements and the maintenance of position against gravity. Each muscle fiber presents the microscopic appearance of being striated. Its cytoplasm, which may be called sarcoplasm, contains many myofibrils and its sarcolemma is well defined. In contradistinction to most body cells, each striated muscle fiber has several nuclei. A skeletal muscle consists of several bundles of *muscle fibers or fasciculi*. Each bundle or fasciculus is enclosed in a sheath of connective tissue (perimysium) and the several bundles which comprise the muscle are also enclosed in strong connective tissue (epimysium) and may also have a tough fibrous coating, called the fascia (Fig. 23–14). Prolongations of the connective tissue extending beyond the actual muscle fibers form the tendinous attachments to bones. Each skeletal muscle has an *origin,* which is the fixed point of attachment, and an *insertion,* which is the attachment to the movable part. When the muscle contracts, the insertion is pulled toward the origin. The thick part of the muscle consist-

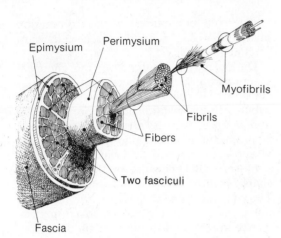

FIGURE 23–14   Cross section of a skeletal muscle.

ing of the bundles of fibers may be referred to as the *body* of the muscle.

Motor Innervation of Skeletal Muscles

Contraction of skeletal muscles normally only results from nerve impulses which are discharged by motor neurons within the central nervous system and are transmitted along peripheral nerve fibers to the muscle. Contractions are usually voluntarily produced, since the motor centers lie within the cerebral cortex. Involuntary (unwilled) contractions do occur in the form of reflex responses (see p. 823).

Each motor nerve fiber divides into many branches when it reaches the muscle, and an unmyelinated branch is distributed to each muscle fiber. The point of contact between the nerve fibril and muscle fiber is known as the myoneural or neuromuscular junction or motor end-plate (Fig. 23–15). When a nerve impulse reaches a myoneural junction, *acetylcholine* is released by the terminal portion of the nerve fiber. The sarcolemma is electrically polarized; the inside is negative to the outside. The acetylcholine initiates a wave of depolarization which sweeps over the fiber. Depolarization is followed by a series of chemical reactions within the cell which result in the release of mechanical and heat energy and the shortening and increased tension of the fiber characteristic of contraction. The acetylcholine is quickly destroyed by the enzyme *cholinesterase,* the cell membrane becomes repolarized and the fiber relaxes.

Sensory Innervation of Skeletal Muscles

Afferent nerve fibers carry sensory impulses from the skeletal muscles to the central nervous system, informing it of stretching of the muscle fibers, tension of tendons, and pain. The end organs (receptors) which are sensitive to these changes and initiate the impulses are classified as *proprioceptors. Muscle spindles,* which are excited by stretching, lie between the muscle fibers and are associated with the stretch reflex (see p. 824). *Golgi bodies* are the proprioceptors located in the tendons which are sensitive to tension; when the tension becomes excessive, impulses are initiated that result in inhibition of muscle contraction. *Free nerve endings* are also distributed within the muscle that give rise to pain impulses.

Chemical Composition and Contraction

About 20 per cent of a muscle fiber is represented by the proteins myoglobin, actin and myosin. Actin, myosin and adenosine triphosphate (ATP) are the main contractile elements of muscle fiber. Water accounts for about 75 per cent of the tissue, and the remaining 5 per cent includes carbohydrate (glycogen), phosphocreatine, creatine and inorganic salts (potassium, sodium, calcium, magnesium chloride).

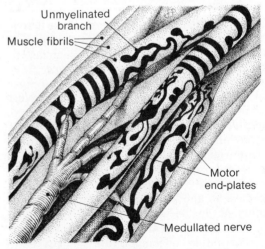

FIGURE 23–15   Innervation of a muscle.

The source of the energy for muscle contraction is a series of chemical reactions within the muscle fibers. Briefly, these include the following: the motor nerve impulse causes depolarization of the sarcolemma, leading to the sudden breakdown of adenosine triphosphate (ATP) to adenosine diphosphate (ADP) and the release of phosphate and energy; the energy promotes the interaction of actin and myosin filaments which produces the actual shortening and thickening of the muscle (contraction); phosphocreatine is hydrolyzed and gives up phosphate, which combines with ADP to quickly restore the ATP so that a constant source of energy for contraction is maintained; glycogen is then broken down, releasing phosphate and lactic acid; the phosphate molecules combine with creatine to replenish the phosphocreatine; about one-fifth of the lactic acid is oxidized to energy, carbon dioxide and water; and the remainder of the lactic acid is reconverted to glycogen. The initial reactions which provide instantaneous energy for contraction do not utilize oxygen (anaerobic). The oxidation of lactic acid requires oxygen and the energy released is utilized in the resynthesis of the basic compounds used during contraction. In hypoxemia or in strenuous exercise, the oxygen supply is generally inadequate to oxidize lactic acid and provide the required energy for resynthesis. Lactic acid accumulates and the condition is said to have incurred an oxygen debt; that is, the oxygen provided was not sufficient to keep pace with the production of lactic acid.

The *strength of the contraction* of a muscle depends on the number of fibers excited; a maximal or intense stimulus involves all fibers. When stimulated, each fiber responds on the all-or-none principle; it contracts to its fullest capacity. The force of contraction of a fiber increases proportionately with its length up to a certain point, after which it decreases. The size of the muscle also influences the force of the contraction. The larger the mass, the greater amount of energy produced. A muscle responds to repeated increased demands by hypertrophy of the individual fibers. If demands are decreased, the cells store less substance for energy and become smaller, producing muscular atrophy.

A single stimulus to a muscle produces a quick jerky contraction referred to as a *twitch*. A *tetanic contraction* is a sustained contraction with no apparent relaxation; it results from a rapid succession of stimuli being delivered to the muscle. When a muscle shortens and produces movement but the tension remains much the same, the contraction is said to be *isotonic*. An *isometric* contraction is one in which the length of the muscle does not change, but its tension is noticeably increased.

Muscles are arranged to function in pairs; the contraction of one of the pair is accompanied by relaxation of the other (reciprocal inhibition). For example, if the biceps is to contract to flex the forearm, the triceps must relax. The muscle which contracts is called the *prime mover,* and the one which relaxes at the same time is known as the *antagonist*. Other muscles may be necessary in certain patterns of movement and may be classified as *synergists or stabilizers*. They facilitate the work of the prime mover.

Voluntary Movement

Normal voluntary movements are the result of controlled contraction and relaxation of groups of muscles. All willed movements, from the simplest (which involves only a prime mover and its antagonist) to the most complex refined activity involving various groups of muscles, depend upon excitation of neurons within the cerebral cortex (upper motor neurons) and at a lower level (lower motor neurons). The neurons at a lower level may be cranial nerve nuclei in the brain stem or may be in the spinal cord. Two major pathways are involved within the central nervous system — the pyramidal and extrapyramidal tracts or systems.

PYRAMIDAL TRACT (CORTICOSPINAL TRACT). (Fig. 23–16.) Willed movement begins with the stimulation of a specific area of neurons in the motor area of the cerebral cortex (see p. 808). If the movement applies to only muscles on one side of the body, only the motor area of the cerebral hemisphere on the opposite side will be involved. The axons of the motor neurons of each hemisphere converge in the interior of the cerebrum, coming together in a compact mass referred to as the *internal capsule*. The fibers continue down through the midbrain and brain stem. In the lower part of the medulla most of them (75 to 80 per cent) cross to the oppo-

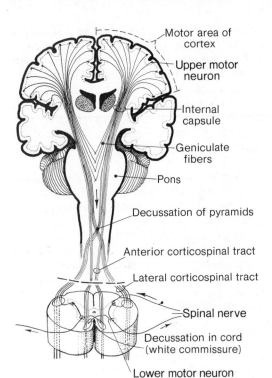

FIGURE 23–16 The pyramidal tract (corticospinal tract).

site side before descending into the spinal cord. At various levels in the cord, the fibers synapse with neurons in the anterior column or horn of gray matter. The axons of these neurons form the motor fibers of the peripheral nerves by which the impulses are delivered to the muscle fibers. Some fibers in the tract may synapse in the brain stem with nuclei of cranial nerves. The impulses are then carried out to a muscle by motor fibers of a peripheral cranial nerve.

The neurons of the cerebral cortical motor areas are referred to as the *upper motor neurons*. Those with which the axons of the upper motor neurons synapse are called the lower motor neurons. The axons of the *lower motor neurons* carry the impulses to skeletal muscles in the periphery. Interruption of the pyramidal tract at any level produces paralysis. Damage of an area above the lower motor neurons produces spastic paralysis. The muscles controlled by the affected upper motor neurons or their axons resist passive movement and exhibit increased muscle tone and exaggerated reflexes. Injury of lower motor neurons or their axons results in flaccid paralysis in the respective muscles, loss

of tone and reflexes, and wasting (atrophy) of the muscles.

EXTRAPYRAMIDAL SYSTEM. Willed movement involves much more than just activation of the pyramidal system which is mainly concerned with initiating the contraction of prime movers. Excitation of upper and lower motor neurons alone cannot achieve even the simplest movement. When a specific activity is performed, a ''pattern of movement'' occurs which requires a varying number of muscular responses. As well as reciprocal relaxation of the antagonist muscle(s), the pattern of movement may include the contraction of a group of muscles simultaneously or in coordinated, timed sequence, the stabilization of a neighboring joint, and adjustments in posture. Some movements require rapid relaxation of the antagonists; others need slow, gradual relaxation in order to provide smooth precise movement. These essential components — inhibition, facilitation and coordination — are controlled by the extrapyramidal system (Fig. 23–17), which is more complex than the pyramidal system. Extrapyramidal impulses are initiated in several different areas of the brain below conscious level. They may originate in

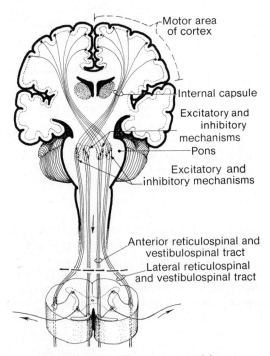

FIGURE 23–17 The extrapyramidal tract.

the basal ganglia (caudate nucleus, putamen, globus pallidus), cerebellum and reticular formation and may be influenced by impulses from the premotor areas of the frontal lobe. All of the impulses synapse in the reticular formation and are transmitted by reticulospinal tracts to lower motor neurons. The lower motor neurons provide the final common pathway for all afferent impulses (both pyramidal and extrapyramidal) to skeletal muscles.

Disturbance within the extrapyramidal system or interruption of the tract does not cause paralysis but may produce abnormal movements. There may be slowness of response, tremors, lack of coordination or excessive muscle tone.

The following activity illustrates the role of the pyramidal and extrapyramidal tracts in voluntary movement. If a person who is standing reaches out to pick up a pen from a table, he consciously concentrates on the action of his fingers and thumb necessary to grasp the object. Several muscle responses are involved as well as the flexion of fingers and thumb. The forearm is extended to reach the pen (the biceps relaxes and the triceps contracts); muscles contract to stabilize the shoulder and wrist; leaning forward to reach the pen may be necessary, so the trunk flexes and shifts the center of gravity, necessitating muscle action in the trunk and lower extremities to insure maintenance of the upright position.

The pyramidal tract transmits the impulses which were consciously initiated to produce the actual picking up of the pen by the fingers and thumb. The other essential components of the total movement (reciprocal relaxation, correlation, stabilization and adjustments in posture) are automatically contributed by the extrapyramidal system.

Reflexes

A reflex is an involuntary response which tends to be specific, or of fixed pattern for a given stimulus. Nerve impulses initiated in the periphery enter the central nervous system and automatically activate a certain response in a peripheral structure. The response may involve the contraction of muscle tissue or the secretion of a gland. The nervous pathway over which the impulses pass is called a reflex arc. The arc is comprised of receptors (e.g., proprioceptors in a muscle, cutaneous pain receptors), an afferent pathway (sensory nerve fibers), central nervous system connections (e.g., connecting or internuncial neurons of the spinal cord), motor neurons (e.g., lower motor neurons in anterior columns of spinal cord), efferent pathway (motor nerve fibers) and effector organ (muscle fibers or glandular cells).

Reflexes occur without conscious or willed initiation, but the person usually becomes conscious of the reflex activity because the impulses reach the cerebral cortex and are interpreted as sensation. For example, when a person touches a hot stove, his hand is withdrawn before he is fully aware of the burn sensation.

Reflex responses are either protective or postural. *Protective reflexes* are produced in response to irritating or painful stimuli. Examples are the closing of the eyelids when the cornea is lightly touched, excessive lacrimal secretion when the eye is irritated by a foreign particle, muscle spasm around an injured area (e.g., rigidity of abdominal wall), contraction of underlying muscles when the abdomen is stroked with a sharp object (withdrawal reflex) and rapid withdrawal of the hand from a hot stove.

Postural reflexes maintain an appropriate degree of muscle tone which is essential in supporting the body against gravity and maintaining an upright position. The body is subjected to the pull of gravity at all times. The only way the body can stay upright is by muscles exerting a continual pull on bones in the opposite direction from gravity. Two reflex mechanisms operate in regulating the muscle contraction necessary to provide the antigravity force. They are the stretch (myotatic) reflex and impulses which originate in the internal ear. When a person bends over or changes his position, movement of the fluid in the semicircular canals in the ear gives rise to sensory impulses which are transmitted by the vestibular fibers of the eighth cranial (auditory) nerve to nuclei in the brain stem. Impulses are then transmitted via vestibulospinal tracts from the nuclei to motor neurons which discharge impulses to certain muscles, resulting in an increase in their tone in support of the body's upright position.

If muscle fibers are stretched, they usually

oppose the stretching force by quickly contracting. When the muscle is stretched, proprioceptors (spindles) are stimulated and initiate impulses which are transmitted to the spinal cord. In the cord, the afferent fibers synapse with connecting neurons which in turn synapse with motor neurons whose axons conduct the impulses out of the muscle. If the reflex arc for the stretch reflex is interrupted, the muscle becomes atonic and flaccid. An extremely strong contraction exerts an excessive tension in the muscle's tendon, causing tendon proprioceptors (Golgi bodies) to initiate afferent impulses. These impulses bring about inhibition of the motor neurons concerned, reducing the strength of the contraction.

Even the simplest reflex muscle response or movement involves more than the primary contracting muscle. For instance, the antagonist must reciprocate with relaxation; this necessitates inhibition of its tone. This inhibition takes place in the central nervous system and is imposed on the lower motor neurons which innervate the muscle whose fibers are to relax. The exact inhibitory mechanism is not clear. A reflex may be complex, involving responses in several muscles, some of which may be contralateral. To illustrate, if a person steps on something sharp, the limb is quickly drawn up. The person avoids putting it down and placing his weight on the injured area again. In order to maintain his balance and upright position, the muscles in the trunk and opposite limb must adjust and compensate.

Reflex pathways or arcs are comprised of a varying number of neurons. The simplest consists of two neurons; the afferent fibers which enter the cord synapse directly with the motor neurons whose axons transmit impulses to the muscle. An example of this type of reflex arc is that associated with the patellar reflex ("knee jerk") which is elicited by tapping the tendon of the quadriceps femoris muscle. The muscle fibers are stretched, resulting in contraction of the muscle and extension of the leg. More often, a reflex arc includes one or more connecting neurons which activate the motor neurons.

Reflexes are important clinically; deviations from normal responses may provide information about the location and nature of neurological disorders. The reflexes observed clinically may be classified as superficial, deep or pathologic. *Superficial reflexes* are evoked by cutaneous stimulation. *Deep reflexes* are produced by tapping a tendon. Pathologic reflexes are responses not normally present. These reflexes are discussed on page 827.

NEUROLOGICAL DISORDERS

The cause of organic disease of the nervous system, as with other systems, may be congenital, vascular, degenerative, infectious, traumatic or neoplastic. Since it is the main control system of the body, the problems associated with a neurological disorder can be varied, multiple and complex, involving several different parts and systems. The resulting disturbances depend primarily on the area(s) of the nervous system affected, the extent of the lesion and, to a lesser degree, the nature of the pathological process. The lesion may diminish or abolish normal responses or cause defective or excessive activity.

Neurological disorders are many and complex. This section presents a discussion of only those which are most commonly encountered and their implications for nursing.

Manifestations of Neurological Disorders

The diagnosis of neurological disease frequently includes a prolonged period of observation of the patient's responses and behavior. The nurse may make an important contribution by making close, accurate observations and detailed, meaningful records. This necessitates a knowledge of what is relevant and significant and the ability in many instances to elicit responses in order to observe and assess the patient. Knowledge of the rate at which functional changes and defects develop is important. Certain conditions are known to have a sudden onset with signs and symptoms reaching maximum intensity very rapidly (e.g., traumatic and severe cerebral vascular lesions). Others have an insidious, prolonged onset with changes in actions and behavior occurring so gradually that they may be unnoticed and are recognized only in retrospect by the patient, his family and associates (see Table 23–2).

TABLE 23–2 MANIFESTATIONS OF NEUROLOGICAL DISORDERS

Motor dysfunction
Abnormal reflexes
Disturbance of sensation
Visual disturbances
Auditory disturbance
Vestibular disturbance
Speech dysfunction
Impaired intellectual ability
Emotional lability
Impaired awareness
Change in appearance
Change in food habits
Abnormal vital signs
Impaired autonomic function
Incontinence
Changes associated with pituitary dysfunction
Failure of growth and development
Disturbances in cranial nerve innervation

MOTOR DYSFUNCTION. Significant factors to be noted in relation to a patient's motor ability include the size, tone, and strength of his muscles, his performance (pattern, accuracy and success) of common purposive movements, the ease and smoothness of passive and active movements, his posture and gait, the presence and character of involuntary, purposeless movements, and any asymmetry between the two sides of the body.

Paralysis and abnormal movements are common symptoms of neurological disease.

PARALYSIS. Paralysis implies the loss of power of muscular contraction. It may be partial (exhibited by weakness) or complete and may be classified according to the extent of the involvement. *Monoplegia* indicates paralysis of one limb. *Hemiplegia* signifies the loss of muscular power in the limbs on one side of the body. It may also involve the muscles on one side of the face; if it affects the side of the face opposite to that of the paralyzed limbs, the term *alternate hemiplegia* may be used. *Paraplegia* denotes paralysis of both lower extremities, and *quadriplegia* implies paralysis of all four limbs. *Isolated paralysis* indicates the loss of the contractile ability of one muscle of a group; this symptom is usually associated with peripheral nerve injury rather than with a lesion of the central nervous system and is usually accompanied by loss of sensation in the area supplied by the affected nerve.

Paralysis may also be classified as that due to an upper or lower motor neuron lesion. Damage to the motor areas of the cerebral cortex or their projection pathways (corticospinal or pyramidal tracts) produces paralysis due to an upper motor neuron lesion or what may also be termed *spastic paralysis*. Since the lower motor neurons and reflex arc are intact, the affected muscles are still capable of reflex movements and exhibit hypertonicity (spasticity) as well as exaggerated reflexes. There is increased activity of postural (stretch) and protective reflexes (see Table 23–3). Paralysis resulting from injury of the motor neurons in the nuclei of cranial nerves or in the anterior horns or columns of gray matter in the spinal cord or damage to their axons in the periphery may be referred to as that due to a *lower motor neuron lesion* or as *flaccid paralysis*. Flaccidity occurs because the reflex arc is interrupted; there is a lack of reflex innervation and responses (see Table 23–3).

ABNORMAL MOVEMENTS. Excessive muscle tone, loss of integration and coordination, and involuntary purposeless movements are also expressions of disordered nervous function.

Hypertonicity may cause spasticity or rigidity in muscles. In spasticity, there is quick contraction of the antagonist muscle in response to sudden passive movement (resistance is offered to passive movement). After a few seconds or minutes the opposing muscle relaxes and the desired movement is achieved. Rigidity results from a steady, excessive contraction of flexor and extensor muscles; as a result, movement is inhibited.

Failure of coordination and the normal sequence of activities of a group of muscles seriously impairs movements. The disturbance may be manifested in the gait, inability to achieve the desired range in a movement (dysmetria), jerky irregular movements and a lack of steadiness and control of speed.

Spontaneous *involuntary movements* associated with impaired nervous function include a variety of tremors, athetoid and choreiform movements, spasms, tics and convulsions. *Tremors* are involuntary rhythmic movements due to alternate contractions and relaxations of prime movers and antagonists. They are seen most often in the distal portions of the extremities, but the head, jaws, lips and rarely the trunk may also be affected. The tremor is observed as to ampli-

TABLE 23–3   COMPARISON OF PARALYSIS OF UPPER AND LOWER
MOTOR NEURON ORIGIN

	Upper Motor Neuron Lesion	Lower Motor Neuron Lesion
Involvement	Muscle groups affected	Individual muscles may be involved
Tonus	Increased; muscles spastic; resist passive movement	Absent; muscles flaccid; no resistance offered
Reflexes:		
Normal	Normal tendon reflexes exaggerated (hyperactive); abdominal reflex absent or diminished on affected side	Tendon reflexes absent; abdominal reflexes diminished if lesion is at thoracic level
Pathologic	Babinski's sign present; i.e., dorsiflexion of toes, especially the great toe, in response to scratching sole of the foot Hoffmann's sign present in hand (flexion of thumb and index finger following sudden release of terminal phalanx of middle finger after it has been flexed)	Babinski's sign absent; normal response (plantar flexion of toes) present Hoffmann's sign absent
Muscle atrophy	Only slight atrophy	Marked muscle wasting
Fasciculations (involuntary contractions of small groups of muscle fibers in a muscle)	Absent	May be present

tude, frequency, distribution and its relationship to rest and voluntary movement. A fine rapid tremor, especially of the hands, is commonly associated with anxiety, fatigue and toxic conditions such as thyrotoxicosis, uremia and alcoholism. Intention or cerebellar tremor begins after a willed movement is initiated and is intensified as the action continues, especially where increasing precision is required. It may be seen when the person is reaching for a specific object or attempting to arrive at a definite goal. This tremor may be noted in the patient with multiple sclerosis. Static tremor is coarse and occurs with the part at rest. It is suppressed by willed movement but disappears also when the patient is asleep. The "shaking" is commonly seen first in the hands or the head. This tremor is usually due to degenerative changes in the substantia nigra in the midbrain and is characteristic of Parkinson's disease. An action tremor is one which develops only when the limbs assume and maintain a certain position. It has a familial tendency and may appear in early adulthood.

Athetoid movements are stereotyped, slow and writhing, following a definite pattern in the individual patient. They are continuously repeated, ceasing only during sleep, and are commonly seen in persons with cerebral palsy. Athetosis may be unilateral or bilateral.

Choreiform movements are rapid, rhythmic and forceful. They begin abruptly, are variable in pattern and distribution, and may occur when the patient is asleep. The limbs, face and tongue are most frequently involved. The forcefulness of the movements may lead to injury unless adequate protection is provided.

Spasms or cramps are produced by the involuntary contraction of a large muscle or group of muscles. Sites which are frequently affected are the leg, foot, arm and neck. The cause may be a lesion within the central nervous system (e.g., degenerative change in the extrapyramidal system), a deficient blood supply to the muscle(s), overstretching and injury of the muscle fibers, or a blood calcium or sodium deficiency.

Dystonic movements involve spasms in the proximal portions of the limbs as well as the trunk. The result is usually slow, grotesque, twisting movements and abnormal posture.

A *tic* or *habit spasm* is a stereotyped, repetitious, purposeless pattern of movement which is functional in origin. The form is variable from one person to another. The tic usually develops in childhood or adolescence and is thought to be often a symptom of underlying tension or excitement.

Apraxia is a term used to describe motor dysfunction when the person is unable to carry out a skilled or complex movement on request. Isolated movements which are a part of the more complex pattern may be achieved but the total cannot be put together. In some patients, this is attributed to an inability to grasp or retain the idea of the desired act. In others it is attributed to the memory loss of the established pattern of movement which is learned in early childhood and normally retained.

Central nervous system disturbances may be manifested by *convulsions or seizures,* which are uncoordinated, purposeless contractions of muscles. Convulsive movements may involve the entire body or only a part, and may be clonic or tonic. The term tonic is used to describe a rigid spasm resulting from prime movers and antagonists contracting simultaneously. A clonic seizure is characterized by alternate contraction and relaxation of the muscles. Generalized convulsions are accompanied by loss of consciousness.

ABNORMAL GAITS. Locomotion depends upon a normal degree of tone and close integration and coordination of the action of the involved muscles of the lower limbs and trunk. These factors are primarily dependent upon normal innervation. In neurological diseases, various abnormal gaits may be manifested.

The *ataxic gait* is associated with a loss of the proprioceptive sense in the extremities and a lack of coordination of muscle action. The person is not sure of the position of his lower limbs and is unable to judge or control placement or length of steps. As a result, he tends to watch his feet when walking. The gait is clumsy, the base too wide (the feet are placed abnormally far apart), and the feet are lifted abnormally high and slapped down hard. The steps are unsure and unevenly spaced and may deviate to one side. The ataxia is more pronounced in the dark.

The *steppage gait* (footdrop gait) is characterized by footdrop due to paralysis of the anterior tibial muscles and by the person lifting the legs abnormally high to avoid dragging and stumbling.

A *cerebellar gait* is marked by staggering, erratic steps and reeling or deviation to one side. The legs are vigorously moved forward and the feet forcefully slapped to the floor.

The gait characteristic of patients with Parkinson's disease may be referred to as a *propulsion or festination gait*. The trunk is flexed forward, the steps are short and shuffling, and the speed of walking progressively accelerates.

The *scissors gait* occurs as a result of spasticity in the lower limbs. The thighs and legs are adducted and movement is difficult, slow and irregular. When the person walks, one leg is placed directly in front of the other, and the knees rub with each step. The steps are short and jerky and may be accompanied by compensatory, forward movements of the trunk and hip.

ABNORMAL REFLEXES. Exaggerated or diminished responses of normal reflexes and the presence of pathologic reflexes are frequently among the earliest indications of neurological disturbance. Those which are most commonly checked during the examination of a patient include the following deep (tendon) and superficial reflexes. The *maxillary reflex* is elicited by tapping the middle of the chin when the upper and lower teeth are separated and the jaw relaxed; the normal response is quick closure of the jaw. The *biceps reflex* is tested by striking the biceps tendon when the forearm is extended; the normal response is flexion of the arm at the elbow. Similarly, the *triceps jerk* is examined by the tapping of the triceps tendon, with the forearm flexed; extension at the elbow may be expected. *Extension or flexion of the wrist* normally occurs when the corresponding tendon is tapped.

Stroking of the abdomen normally elicits tensing of the abdominal muscles on the side being stroked. The response may be diminished or absent in lesions of the corticospinal tracts above the lumbar level of the cord.

The *patellar reflex* (knee jerk) is tested by striking the patellar tendon; the normal response is quick contraction of the quadriceps femoris muscle, resulting in extension of the leg. *Tapping of the Achilles tendon* normally produces contraction of the calf muscles (gastrocnemius and soleus) and plantar flexion of the foot (ankle jerk).

Other reflexes commonly tested are the *corneal and pupillary reflexes*. Normally the eyelids close when the conjunctiva is irritated by gentle touch. The pupil of the eye normally constricts when light is flashed on the eye.

The more common pathologic reflexes tested in examining the patient include Hoffmann's sign, Babinski's sign, ankle clonus and Brudzinski's sign. *Hoffmann's sign* is present when the thumb and fingers flex in response to flicking of the distal phalanx of the middle finger or to its flexion and sudden release by the examiner. *Babinski's sign* is the extension of the great toe and probably fanning of the other toes in response to stroking of the sole of the foot. Normally, flexion of the toes occurs. *Ankle clonus* is characterized by repetitive, rapid flexion and extension of the foot in response to forceful, quick dorsiflexion of the foot while the leg is relaxed and extended. *Brudzinski's sign* is elicited by the forward flexion of the patient's head by the examiner; the abnormal response is flexion of the ankle, knee or thigh.

DISTURBANCE OF SENSATION. A neurological lesion may cause abnormalities of sensation characterized by a dulling, loss or intensification of one or more senses. In checking the patient's senses the physician explores the face, trunk and limbs. A sensory disturbance may be localized to one particular area of the body because of the different sensory pathways being associated with different parts. Hypo- or hypersensitivity of a particular area may provide information about the location of a lesion.

The patient's *superficial (exteroceptive) sensations* of pain, temperature and touch are noted. Impairment of the sense of position may be demonstrated by the patient's inability to recognize the position of a limb which has been moved by the examiner. A disturbance in his sense of movement may be noted by his lack of perception of passive movement of a digit or limb. A disturbance in the patient's sensory system may also be manifested by his inability to recognize a familiar object by the feel of its shape, size and texture, or by his inability to detect that a stimulus is being applied at two points simultaneously. The capacity to recognize the shape, size and texture of objects and identify them by touch is referred to as stereognosis.

During tests which are made to evaluate the patient's sensations, his eyes must be closed.

Normally, a person is aware of vibrations when a tuning fork is applied to a body prominence such as the clavicle and iliac crest. Loss of sensory acuity may be detected by the physician testing the patient's appreciation of vibration following the application of the tuning fork to several bony prominences.

VISUAL DISTURBANCES. Neurological lesions, especially within the brain, frequently cause disturbances in vision, the movements of the eye and eyelids, and the pupillary and corneal reflexes. Edema of the optic disks may also occur.

The patient may experience reduced visual acuity, diplopia (double vision), blurring of vision, or loss of vision in part or all of the visual field in one or both eyes. On examination, the pupils may be uneven in size, and one or both may remain fixed, not reacting to light. The corneal reflex may be abolished, exposing the eye to injury. Normal movements of the eyeball may not be possible because of interference with motor innervation to the extrinsic muscles. Ptosis (lid drop) due to paralysis of the muscle responsible (levator palpebrae) may be evident. Involuntary movement of the eyeballs may occur and is referred to as nystagmus. It may take the form of side-to-side, up-and-down or rotating movements. Some neurological patients manifest the inability to follow the examiner's moving finger.

Ophthalmoscopic examination of the fundus may reveal swelling, pallor and edema of the papilla or optic disk which may be associated with increased intracranial pressure.

AUDITORY DISTURBANCE. Loss of hearing may be a symptom of a disorder in the middle ear, damage to the cochlear portion of an auditory nerve, or a lesion affecting the auditory pathway within the brain. Deafness due to external or middle ear disease is classified as *conduction deafness;* that due to nerve damage or a brain lesion is known as *perception deafness*.

Any complaint of a constant or recurring

abnormal sound, which the patient may describe as roaring, ringing, buzzing or swishing, is recorded and brought to the physician's attention.

VESTIBULAR DISTURBANCE. The most common symptoms produced by a disturbance in the semicircular canals of the internal ear or of the vestibular nerve (part of auditory nerve) or pathway within the brain are dizziness and loss of position balance (equilibrium). Nystagmus, nausea and vomiting may also be present.

SPEECH DYSFUNCTION. Intracranial lesions frequently cause *aphasia*, which is the loss of the ability to understand words or use them to communicate. It occurs frequently in persons who have suffered a cerebral hemorrhage or thrombosis or who have a brain tumor. Aphasia may be classified as motor (expressive) or sensory (receptive). *Motor aphasia* implies the inability to speak; the *sensory type* is the inability to understand the written or spoken word. Mixed forms of disturbances occur, depending upon the location, size and nature of the lesions. A patient may experience both motor and sensory aphasia. Another may understand what is said and written but is unable to express his thoughts in words or writing. Another may be able to interpret the written and spoken word and communicate by writing but cannot speak. Still another patient may be able to speak but his responses are inappropriate and meaningless, or he may use one or two words repeatedly though attempting to express different ideas.

IMPAIRED INTELLECTUAL ABILITY. The patient may manifest impaired reasoning or judgment, unjustified fears, distorted ideas and loss of memory. His attention span may be abnormally short, and he may be unable to do very simple calculations or identify normally familiar objects or sounds.

EMOTIONAL LABILITY. Disordered emotional reactions may be evident in the patient's fluctuating attitudes. There may be inappropriate laughing, crying, irritability, hostility or anger. Sharp swings in mood may occur; the patient who is withdrawn and depressed or anxious may suddenly become excited or euphoric.

IMPAIRED AWARENESS. Confusion and disorientation as to time, place and person may occur with cerebral lesions. The patient's response to stimuli may vary from a coherent verbal response to no response of any sort to painful stimuli. The nurse is responsible for applying the stimuli, recording in detail the reactions and reporting to the physician any significant changes in response.

CHANGE IN APPEARANCE. Frequently, the family of a patient with a neurological disorder comments on the change in his appearance which has probably taken place over a period of time. His face may have become inexpressive (as in Parkinson's disease), his posture may have altered, or he may have become careless about his personal care and grooming.

CHANGE IN FOOD HABITS. Anorexia may be a problem, or the reverse (excessive appetite) may develop if the disorder is in the region of the hypothalamus. The patient may experience a loss of taste because of involvement of one or both of the seventh (facial) cranial nerves or their nuclei. Dysphagia (difficulty in swallowing) may occur because of interference with motor innervation to the muscle tissue of the soft palate and pharynx (glossopharyngeal nerves). Nausea and vomiting may be symptoms of increased intracranial pressure, cerebral irritation or disorders of the vestibular system. Vomiting of cerebral origin is frequently projectile and may not be preceded by nausea.

ABNORMAL VITAL SIGNS. A combination of an abnormally slow pulse and increased arterial blood pressure is usually associated with increased intracranial pressure, especially if there has been a decrease in the patient's level of consciousness. A high temperature may indicate infection or loss of control by the body temperature center in the hypothalamus.

IMPAIRED AUTONOMIC FUNCTION. Local or general flushing, a difference in the skin temperature in one area from that of others, and the absence of or excessive skin moisture (sweating) may be symptoms of disturbed autonomic nervous system function.

INCONTINENCE. Bladder and bowel incontinence are common in disease of the brain or spinal cord.

CHANGES ASSOCIATED WITH PITUITARY DYSFUNCTION. Manifestations of pituitary hormonal imbalance may be symptoms of a brain lesion in the hypothalamic and pituitary region. The pituitary disturbance is secondary to a primary neurological disorder. (See Chapter 22 for discussion of pituitary dysfunction.)

FAILURE OF GROWTH AND DEVELOPMENT. In an infant or child a neurological disorder may be manifested by either the failure of the child to grow and develop normally or the presence of a deformity such as a meningomyelocele, or by the development of a phenomenon such as an abnormally large head.

DISTURBANCES IN CRANIAL NERVE INNERVATION. Many neurological disorders can be diagnosed and localized by the signs and symptoms of a disturbance of the innervation by one or more of the cranial nerves. All initial neurological examinations include a systematic examination of the cranial nerves, as follows.

The *olfactory* nerves (number I, sensory) are tested by having the patient inhale a series of odorous substances, such as coffee, perfume and oil of cloves. Each nostril is tested separately.

The *optic* nerve (number II, sensory) is tested by examining the eyes with an ophthalmoscope and by assessing the patient's visual acuity and range of visual fields (see p. 987).

The *oculomotor* (number III), *trochlear* (number IV) and *abducens* (number VI) motor nerves are responsible for eye movement and pupillary reaction, and are tested as a group by observing eye movements and pupillary reactions to light.

The sensory function of the *trigeminal* nerves (number V, sensory and motor) is assessed by testing both sides of the face and mouth for touch, temperature and pain sensations and the cornea for the normal response of closing the eye. The motor function is assessed by having the patient make chewing and biting movements.

The sensory functions of the *facial* nerves (number VII, sensory and motor) are tested by seeing if the patient can recognize the taste of bitter, sour, sweet and salty substances, respectively, when applied to the tongue. The motor portions are tested by having the patient use his facial muscles in such expressions as smiling, frowning, closing the eyes tightly and puckering the lips.

Equilibrium functions of the *auditory* nerves (number VIII, sensory) are tested by rotating the patient and by performing the caloric test (as described on page 835). Hearing is tested by whispering in each ear, using a ticking watch and using a tuning fork (see p. 1003).

The *glossopharyngeal* (number IX) and *vagus* (number X) motor nerve functions are normally tested by observing the patient's gag reflex, swallowing ability and the strength and quality of the voice.

The *spinal accessory* nerves (number XI, motor) are assessed by checking the sternocleidomastoid and trapezius muscles for atrophy and strength. The patient is asked to shrug his shoulders against resistance and to rotate his head.

The *hypoglossal* nerves (number XII, motor) are assessed by looking at various movements of the tongue and by examining it for atrophy and circulation.

Diagnostic Procedures

Certain special investigative procedures may be used by the physician to aid in determining the location and nature of neurological lesions.

ROENTGENOGRAMS. X-rays of the skull and spine are used to detect such abnormalities as fractures, congenital deformities, unusual intracranial calcified areas, erosions and osteoporosis (demineralization of vertebra).

LUMBAR PUNCTURE. This procedure involves the introduction of a needle into the lumbar subarachnoid space below the termination of the spinal cord. It is passed through the intervertebral space between the third and fourth or fourth and fifth lumbar vertebrae. The purposes of the puncture in diagnosis are to determine the pressure of the cerebrospinal fluid and to obtain specimens of the fluid for examination.

A signed consent for the procedure may be necessary in some hospitals and the test should be carefully explained to the patient, as well as the importance of his remaining as still and relaxed as possible.

The patient is normally in a lateral horizontal position, with the back on the edge of the bed or examining table. The knees should be drawn up and the head and trunk flexed to widen the interspinous spaces. The nurse supports the patient behind the neck and knees. Strict aseptic technique is necessary to prevent the introduction of infection into the spinal canal. A local anesthetic is usually administered at the site of the needle insertion to minimize discomfort. If the needle is not introduced in the midline, it may contact one of the dorsal nerve roots and cause pain down one leg. This can be rectified immediately by moving the needle, and the patient is reassured that no damage has been done. The pressure of the fluid is measured with a manometer, and several samples of cerebrospinal fluid are collected in sterile tubes for examination.

The initial cerebrospinal fluid pressure in the recumbent position normally measures from 60 to 180 mm. of water. If the pressure is abnormally low, it may indicate a blockage in the spinal subarachnoid space above the puncture site. If the pressure is high, it could signify infection or the presence of an intracranial space-occupying lesion, such as a tumor or blood clot. Great care must be taken in this latter situation, since any removal of fluid may create sufficient vacuum to cause the brain to shift downward, causing compression of the medulla in the foramen magnum. The nurse keeps a careful watch on the patient's respirations, pulse and color, since respiratory arrest can occur if the medulla is compressed. If increased intracranial pressure is suspected, lumbar puncture is not usually done.

Cerebrospinal fluid is examined for color (normally it is clear and colorless), leukocyte count (normal: 0 to 5 leukocytes), glucose concentration (normal: 5 to 40 mg. per cent), and chloride concentration (normal: 725 to 750 mg.), and may be examined for the presence of pathologic organisms. Special tests may be done on the fluid, such as the colloidal gold reaction, if multiple sclerosis or syphilis is suspected.

The patient may complain of headache after the procedure. This is normally attributed either to the removal of cerebrospinal fluid during the test or to later leakage of the fluid into the tissues. The headache is usually relieved by having the patient remain in a horizontal position for 6 to 12 hours. An ice bag is applied to the head and a mild analgesic (e.g., acetylsalicylic acid) may be prescribed.

If signs of an increase in intracranial pressure become evident, the patient's level of consciousness, pulse, respirations, blood pressure and pupillary reactions are observed and recorded every 30 minutes for the first 2 hours and then every hour for the next 12 hours. Any adverse change is reported to the physician immediately.

CISTERNAL PUNCTURE. This procedure is similar to the lumbar puncture but carries a greater hazard and is done much less frequently. A shorter needle is introduced into the cisterna magna (the subarachnoid space between the undersurface of the cerebellum and the posterior surface of the medulla) just below the occipital bone. The procedure is explained to the patient, and the nape of the neck is shaved up to the occipital protuberance. The patient is placed on his side with his head flexed. He is observed closely for any signs of respiratory difficulty which may indicate that the needle has made contact with the medulla.

PNEUMOENCEPHALOGRAM. In this investigative procedure, air or oxygen is introduced into the subarachnoid space through a lumbar or cisternal puncture. Twenty to 30 ml. of cerebrospinal fluid are withdrawn and replaced by an equal volume of gas, which serves as a contrast medium so that the ventricles, their aqueducts and the cranial subarachnoid space may be visualized by x-rays. The patient is placed in a sitting position, so the gas rises when injected into the subarachnoid space. Abnormal shape or size or displacement of the ventricles or their failure to fill may indicate a congenital anomaly, atrophic or scarred areas of the brain or a space-occupying lesion (see Figs. 23–18 to 23–20). Similarly, distortion of the subarachnoid space or failure to fill may demonstrate a lesion.

An explanation of the procedure is made to the patient and a family member, and a written consent obtained. The patient is advised that he may have a headache after the procedure and that he will be required to remain quiet for 1 or 2 days. Vital signs are taken and recorded for comparison after the procedure. Food and fluids are withheld for 6 hours before the test. A sedative may be given prior to the procedure.

After pneumoencephalography, the patient's vital signs and level of consciousness are noted and recorded every 15 to 30 minutes for the first 2 hours and, if stable or improving, then every hour for the next 12 to 24 hours so that early signs of increased intracranial pressure may be detected. If the patient suffers headache, nausea and vomiting he should remain in bed in a quiet environment until the symptoms disappear. Side rails on the bed are advisable if the patient is restless and distraught due to headache or is

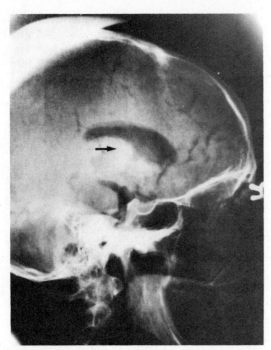

FIGURE 23-18 Pneumoencephalogram showing a normal lateral ventricle (lateral view).

confused or disoriented. An ice bag applied to his head may be helpful, and an analgesic such as acetylsalicylic acid may be ordered. He is given fluids (with the necessary assistance to avoid having to raise his head) and, if these are not tolerated, intravenous fluid may be given to prevent dehydration.

VENTRICULOGRAM. A roentgenogram of the skull is made following the direct replacement of cerebrospinal fluid in the lateral ventricles with air or another contrast medium. It involves making two burr holes (trephine openings) in the skull. A needle is then passed into each lateral ventricle and the contrast medium is introduced following the removal of the fluid. The purpose is to visualize the ventricular system; the size, shape and filling of the ventricles are noted.

The preparation of the patient is similar to that cited above for pneumoencephalogram. The posterior third of the head is shaved, and the whole head is thoroughly cleansed before the operation. The patient will have a general anesthetic for this procedure.

Following the ventriculogram, the patient may experience headache, nausea and vomiting, and the nursing measures are similar to those used for postpneumoencephalography. The same observations and recording are made. The scalp wounds are examined daily and the sutures removed in 4 to 5 days.

CEREBRAL ANGIOGRAM (ARTERIOGRAM). A radiopaque iodide preparation is injected into a carotid or vertebral artery by direct puncture. If this approach is unsatisfactory, these vessels may be entered with a catheter via the brachial, femoral or subclavian artery. As the dye is injected a series of x-ray films of the neck and head are taken rapidly to follow the flow of the contrast

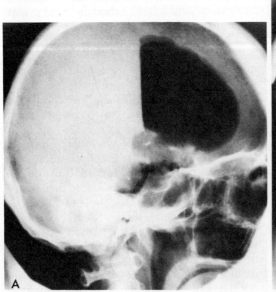
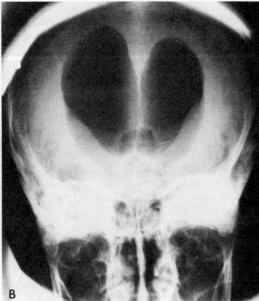

FIGURE 23-19 Pneumoencephalogram showing grossly enlarged ventricles. *A,* Lateral view; *B,* A-P view.

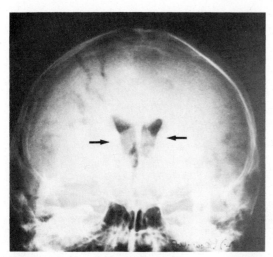

FIGURE 23–20 Pneumoencephalogram showing normal lateral ventricles (A-P view).

material. The presence of an aneurysm or an abnormal vascular mass, the occlusion of a vessel or the displacement of blood vessels by an intracranial mass may be demonstrated (see Fig. 23–21).

The procedure is explained to the patient and a family member. The patient is advised that he will probably experience a sense of warmth through his neck and face during injection of the dye. He is questioned about any allergies he may have because patients occasionally react to the contrast material; any history of sensitivities is brought to the physician's attention and clearly recorded in a conspicuous place on the patient's record. A written consent is necessary, and a sedative ordered to be given ½ hour prior to the test. A local anesthetic is used in the skin over the vessel.

If the patient is restless or confused a general anesthetic may be used, in which case food and fluids will be withheld for 6 hours prior to the test.

Before sedation is given *craniocerebral testing* is done to give the nurse a baseline with which to compare her observations after the angiography. This includes vital signs, blood pressure, level of consciousness, pupillary reaction to light and strength and mobility of limbs. Side rails are installed on the bed in case the patient is confused or restless after the test. Drugs that may be used to treat anaphylactic shock (see p. 51) and an emergency tracheostomy set should be readily available in the event of a reaction to the radiopaque dye.

Following the arteriogram, the patient lies on his back with a pillow unless he has had a general anesthetic, in which case he will be placed in a semiprone position. Craniocerebral testing, as mentioned previously, is done every 15 to 30 minutes for the first 2 hours and then every hour for the next 12 hours or until stable. Any signs of deterioration are reported immediately. Vasospasm within the cerebrovascular system may occur; it is manifested by weakness or paralysis of the face, limbs, speech or swallowing, breathing difficulty or a deterioration in the level of consciousness. Externally the puncture site is observed for bleeding. Application of an ice bag to the site is advisable to lessen edema and the development of a hematoma. If there are no complications, the patient resumes his previous routine after 24 hours.

MYELOGRAM. This procedure is a roentgenographic study of the spinal subarachnoid space, and is used to detect and localize lesions which may be compressing the spinal cord or nerves. A radiopaque liquid is injected into the subarachnoid space in the lumbar region. The flow of the contrast medium up and down the canal during tilting of the table is observed by fluoroscope. A series of x-ray films is also taken. If the canal is blocked above the lumbar region,

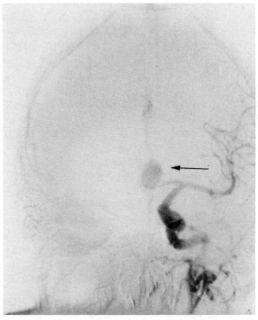

FIGURE 23–21 Arteriogram showing a large anterior communicating aneurysm.

the radiopaque liquid is injected by cisternal puncture. Upon completion of the x-rays, the radiopaque substance is aspirated to prevent meningeal irritation.

As with other diagnostic procedures, an explanation is made to the patient so that he will know what to expect. Consent to the examination is signed. Food and fluid are withheld for 4 to 6 hours preceding the test in case of nausea and vomiting.

Following the myelogram the patient remains flat in bed for several hours. He is observed for 2 or 3 days for signs of mengineal irritation. Persisting headache and pain and stiffness of the neck, especially with flexion of the head, are reported. If the contrast material is not removed, the patient's head and shoulders are elevated to prevent the fluid from rising to the cranial subarachnoid space.

COMPUTERIZED TRANSAXIAL TOMOGRAPHY (CTT). Computerized transaxial tomography is a new and revolutionary radiologic diagnostic technique. It is noninvasive and dependable; to a large extent it has replaced some invasive techniques, such as pneumoencephalography and angiography.

For this test, the patient's head is placed in a rubber cap surrounded by water in a Lucite cube. An x-ray tube is rotated around the patient's head and the rays are picked up on the opposite side by crystal detectors. Various tissues and fluids have different densities and, with the aid of a computer, information picked up via the crystals is transformed into an image whose brightness is proportionate to the tissue absorption values. The image is then photographed (see Fig. 23–22).

If the CTT scan is abnormal, an intravenous injection of a radiopaque substance may be indicated to enhance the vascular structures and make the diagnosis more exact.

An explanation is given to the patient. The test is not painful; the person is required to lie still for 20 to 40 minutes. Normal activities may be resumed immediately after the test. CTT can be done on an outpatient basis.

BRAIN SCAN (RADIOISOTOPE UPTAKE). This test is a screening procedure for the early detection of focal intracranial lesions. The patient is given an intravenous injection of a radioactive tracer, such as technetium-99m (Tc^{99m}) or mercury isotopes (Hg^{203} and Hg^{197}), which will be picked up by

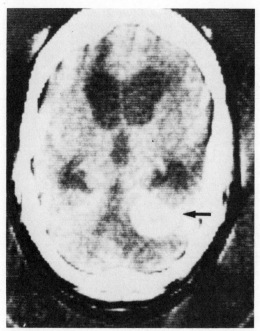

FIGURE 23–22 CTT scan showing a hemangioblastoma (round white area in the right lower quadrant).

abnormal brain cells. Normal brain cells form a blood-brain barrier which inhibits absorption of the isotopes. A scanning device is used to measure the uptake of the tracer throughout the brain. Scans are made in 15 to 30 minutes following the administration of the isotope.

No special preparation or aftercare of the patient is necessary, but the procedure and its approximate length of time are explained beforehand.

ELECTROENCEPHALOGRAM (EEG). This is a graphic record of the electrical activity of the brain. Several small needle electrodes are inserted superficially into the scalp in standard positions on the head; they are distributed over the frontal, parietal, occipital and temporal areas, and one is attached to each ear lobe. The action potentials carried by the leads from the electrodes are amplified 10,000,000 times and then recorded. Some electrical activity is recorded at all times by the brain, except during very deep anesthesia and during a severe depletion of blood to the brain.

The waves in the tracings are observed for their frequency per second, amplitude, wave forms (spike, flat, serrated), rhythm and distribution of the activity. An EEG is of value in diagnosing epilepsy, tumors and hematoma. For example, it is of assistance in localizing an area of electrically inactive tissue, such as a tumor.

The procedure is explained to the patient beforehand so that he will not be fearful of "receiving a shock." He should be relaxed; apprehension and fear will influence brain activity. If the patient has been receiving an anticonvulsant, the physician may order it to be omitted during the 24 to 36 hours preceding the EEG. The recording is made in a special insulated room. The patient is recumbent or seated comfortably with his eyes closed. Periodically, various forms of stimulation may be used to evoke or intensify responses. The stimuli may include opening of the eyes, side-to-side and up-and-down eye movements, hyperventilation, clenching of the jaw and light flashes. No special care is necessary following an EEG. This test is often done on an outpatient basis.

ECHOENCEPHALOGRAM. This diagnostic procedure involves the direction of a beam of ultrasonic waves (high frequency sound waves not perceptible to the normal human ear) horizontally through the skull and an oscilloscope recording of the echoes. The waves normally are reflected by midline structures. The time taken for the reflected waves to return can be projected and, on this basis, a shift of the midline structures can be demonstrated and may confirm the presence of a space-occupying lesion.

ELECTROMYOGRAM (EMG). This test records the electrical activity of muscle. Needle electrodes are placed in various muscle groups and electrical activity is measured when the muscles are made to contract. Normal voluntary muscle is electrically inactive when at rest. The procedure is used to help investigate peripheral nerve injuries and primary muscle disease, such as dystrophy.

CALORIC TEST. Neurological investigation may include a caloric test to assess the function of the vestibular portion of the acoustic (VIII) cranial nerve and the vestibular system. The test consists of thermal stimulation of the auditory canals and observance of the patient's reactions. Hot or cold water introduced into the external ear produces changes in the temperature of the endolymph (fluid within the semicircular canals) and sets it in motion, giving rise to certain impulses.

Before the test the patient is advised as to what will be done and that he should indicate any discomfort such as dizziness, nausea and vomiting that he experiences during it. He is tested for past pointing and Romberg's sign for comparison with the responses to the caloric test. Romberg's sign is the falling or swaying to one side when the patient stands with his feet together and his eyes closed. The past pointing test involves having the patient direct a finger to a particular mark with his eyes closed. Past pointing is manifested by deviation of the finger from the mark. Food and fluids are withheld for 4 to 6 hours before the test because of the likely responses of nausea and vomiting.

The patient may be placed in a sitting position with the head tilted backward at an angle of 60 degrees. If the recumbent position is used, the head is flexed forward at an angle of 30 degrees. The two ears are tested independently with cold water, 20° to 21° C. (68° to 70° F.), and then with hot water, 40° to 45° C. (104° to 113° F.). The solution is introduced slowly and is discontinued with the initial response. Observations are made for nystagmus; its duration is timed, and the direction of the quick phase is noted. Complaints of dizziness, nausea and vomiting are recorded. Normally, stimulation with cold water produces nystagmus with the rapid phase of the movement directed toward the side opposite to that being stimulated, past pointing deviation and postural deviation (Romberg's sign) to the side stimulated, vertigo, and probably nausea and vomiting. The characteristics of the normal responses to stimulation with hot water are nystagmus with the rapid component directed to the side of stimulation, past pointing and postural deviation to the side opposite to that stimulated, vertigo, and probably nausea and vomiting. Pathologic lesions interfering with the function of the vestibular system produce an absence of or diminishment in the responses to thermal stimulation.

Following the caloric test, the patient remains in bed with a minimum of disturbance until free of dizziness, nausea and vomiting.

CEREBROVASCULAR DISORDERS

The most common cerebrovascular disorders include cerebral atherosclerosis, cerebral aneurysm, cerebral infarction and cerebral hemorrhage. Infarction and hemorrhage cause what is commonly referred to as a cerebrovascular accident, or stroke, and are frequent sequelae to cerebral atherosclerosis or aneurysm.

Cerebral Atherosclerosis (Arteriosclerosis)

Atherosclerosis of the cerebral vessels is a chronic degenerative process characterized by the gradual development of atheroma (fatty plaques) in the intima and subsequent roughening and destruction of the endothelium, narrowing of the lumen and weakening of the vascular wall. These degenerative changes predispose to cerebral ischemia, thrombosis with regional infarction and hemorrhage. The atheromatous plaques tend to form predominantly in the carotid, vertebral and larger cerebral arteries but may be diffuse, involving both large and small cerebral vessels. The disease tends to develop more rapidly in persons with hypertension, diabetes mellitus, obesity and heart disease, and who are heavy smokers.

Generalized atherosclerosis develops slowly and insidiously, and may only be diagnosed in a routine physical examination. The physician may notice a noise or bruit over the eye or the carotid artery in the neck when a stethoscope is applied to the area.

If the patient is asymptomatic he may be placed on a low-cholesterol diet, advised to stop smoking, if relevant, and receive an antihypertensive drug. In some instances an anticoagulant is prescribed. Frequently the patient complains of brief spells of lightheadedness, dizziness, blurred vision or short periods of clumsiness. These disturbances and the intermittent presence of other phenomena, such as numbness and/or weakness of a limb, may be referred to as transient ischemic attacks (TIA); no permanent deficit is incurred. If treatment is not started at this stage, the person may go on to have a minor or even a major stroke. A stroke may leave him with a severe disability, such as hemiplegia and aphasia (the inability to speak or comprehend speech), and may render him unconscious. Diagnosis of atherosclerotic changes in the arteries is confirmed with the aid of carotid angiography.

TREATMENT. The patient with arteriosclerosis may be treated medically or may be a candidate for an endarterectomy. The latter consists of opening up the affected vessel and peeling out the fatty plaque. Conservative care involves a diet which is low in cholesterol and saturated fats. If the patient has hypertension, an antihypertensive drug is prescribed, and he is advised to avoid confusing situations, excessive physical exertion and emotional stress as much as possible. Activity within the patient's capacity is encouraged. If the patient is overweight, a diet of 1200 to 1500 calories is prescribed and the patient is urged to maintain his normal weight when attained.

The family is helped to understand the disorder and develop tolerance and patience. Increasing guidance and assistance with personal care may be required of them.

Not all patients are candidates for the surgery; those who are very elderly and have a family history of vascular disease, or who have serious cardiac or renal problems, are too great a risk. Chronological age has not proven to be a major factor.

PREOPERATIVE PREPARATION. Specific preparation of the patient for an endarterectomy includes an explanation of the procedure and what he may expect immediately after his operation. Preoperatively the patient is placed on an anticoagulant such as bishydroxycoumarin (Dicoumarol). A consent form for surgery must also be signed. The care cited in general preoperative preparation (see p. 164) is applicable, except that a specific directive is received concerning skin preparation.

POSTOPERATIVE CARE. Postoperatively, as with any patient who might develop neurological complications, the patient will be on craniocerebral testing which includes checking and recording vital signs, blood pressure, level of consciousness, size and reaction of pupils to light, and strength and movement of all limbs. After the initial postanesthetic recovery time of about 2 hours, during which the testing is done more frequently, the patient is checked every hour for the first 24 hours. Special attention is paid to the blood pressure. An elevation above normal or a hypotensive level is reported to the physician promptly. Hypotension predisposes to thrombus formation within the artery at the site of surgery, and a cerebral embolism (stroke) may ensue. Hypertension may cause increased stress on the operative site and may result in a severe hemorrhage.

The patient is kept quiet and at rest during the first 24 hours; all exertion on his part is avoided. After this period the patient is mobilized gradually, if his vital signs are satisfactory and stable; he may be out of bed on the third or fourth postoperative day. If the vessel involved in the surgery is situated outside the cranial cavity, such as the common carotid artery, the patient is observed for signs of bleeding or swelling in the neck. The nurse must check the dressing frequently for bleeding and be aware of the signs and symptoms of hypovolemic shock (weak thready pulse, poor color, low blood pressure and restlessness). The neck circumference is measured with a tape measure at regular intervals to check for increased edema. Any respiratory distress is reported promptly; swelling due to edema and clot formation may cause pressure on the trachea and interfere with respirations.

The postoperative course after the first 24 hours is generally uneventful. The patient usually receives an anticoagulant orally for about 6 months following the surgery. Regular checking of prothrombin time is necessary. The patient is advised to report any blood in the urine or stool, bleeding of gums or discolored bruised areas (ecchymoses). Former activities are resumed very gradually.

Cerebral Aneurysm

An aneurysm is the saccular dilatation of an arterial wall, thought to be caused most often by the congenital absence of the layer of muscular tissue in this area. It may also develop due to degenerative changes in the vessel. Intracranial aneurysms occur principally at the junctions of the major vessels at the base of the brain. A patient may have a single aneurysm or several. These aneurysms do not always produce symptoms and have been found incidently at autopsy. If an intracranial aneurysm develops, it may produce localizing symptoms from pressure on adjacent structures (e.g., visual impairment due to pressure on the optic nerve). More commonly the aneurysm ruptures suddenly, causing severe symptoms. These ruptures occur frequently in those in the prime of life, from the twenties to the late fifties, and those with hypertension

are more predisposed to rupture. The episode may be precipitated by mental stress or physical strain. The initial symptom is usually sudden severe headache causing nausea, vomiting and, in some cases, loss of consciousness. If the bleeding is slight, headache may be the only symptom. The more severe the hemorrhage, particularly if it is into the subarachnoid space, the more severe the symptoms.

CLASSIFICATION. Many physicians categorize the hemorrhage by the presenting manifestations.

Grade I: Patient alert, severe headache, no neurological deficit and a few red cells in the cerebrospinal fluid (CSF).

Grade II: Patient alert, severe headache, nuchal rigidity (neck stiff and painful on flexion) and cerebrospinal fluid xanthochromic (yellow-colored).

Grade III: Headache, nuchal rigidity, drowsiness, a focal deficit such as limb weakness, and confusion. Cerebrospinal fluid bloody.

Grade IV: Very evident neurological deficit; responds only to painful stimuli. Gross blood present in cerebrospinal fluid.

Grade V: Unresponsive, moribund appearance, and showing decerebrate rigidity. *Decerebrate or decorticate rigidity* results from interruption of the corticospinal tract (usually in the midbrain or pons) and is characterized by adduction of the arms and flexion of the arms, wrists and fingers, extension and internal rotation of the lower limbs and plantar flexion.

DIAGNOSTIC PROCEDURES. If subarachnoid hemorrhage (SAH) is suspected on admission, a lumbar puncture (see p. 830) is done and the presence of blood in the cerebrospinal fluid confirms the diagnosis. A cerebral arteriogram (see p. 832) is done to determine the site of the aneurysm.

TREATMENT AND NURSING CARE. Surgery is considered the treatment of choice for patients with intracranial aneurysms.

PREOPERATIVE PERIOD. The most crucial period for the patient is that between the initial rupture and surgery. Most surgeons wait 7 to 14 days before operating to allow time for the postrupture edema to decrease and for any blood clots to resolve. Nursing care during this time may well be the deciding factor in whether or not the patient survives.

If the patient is unconscious, the nursing

measures will include those which apply to any unconscious patient (see Chapter 9). Craniocerebral testing (see cerebral atherosclerosis, p. 836) is done frequently to assess his condition. It is important that the blood pressure remain in the lower range of normal to reduce the possibility of further bleeding. Antihypertensive drugs such as methyldopa (Aldomet) and hydralazine hydrochloride (Apresoline) may be prescribed. The patient is put on complete bed rest, kept very quiet and exposed to a minimum of stimuli. If he is alert, the reason for this is explained to him in a manner that will not alarm him. He may be allowed to listen to quiet music but is not usually allowed a television, telephone or reading matter. His next of kin is informed that they may sit quietly with him but are to discourage his talking. If he is very alert or is restless, a sedative such as phenobarbital or diazepam (Valium) may be prescribed.

The patient receives a soft diet and is not allowed to feed himself. Mild laxatives are administered to prevent any straining when passing stool. Enemas are contraindicated. The patient may have an indwelling catheter to prevent any exertion and to overcome the difficulty of voiding in a supine position. Fluid intake and output are monitored. If the patient is nauseated, oral fluids are withheld and an antiemetic is ordered. A mild analgesic (nothing stronger than codeine) is prescribed for relief of headache. Sedatives and analgesics are used judiciously with neurological patients since they tend to mask significant changes and symptoms.

The greatest challenge to the nurse may be the patient who is in the Grade I or II categories. He is often an intensely hard-working young businessman who is worried about his business and family while he is in the hospital. He may not feel particularly ill, and finds it difficult to understand why he must be kept totally inactive and treated as though he were "helpless." The nurse spends time talking quietly with him, reassuring him and generally trying to prevent any incidents that might increase his blood pressure.

In addition to rebleeding, other complications may occur during the preoperative phase. One is spasm of one of the cerebral vessels, the exact cause of which is still being disputed, and a second is hydrocephalus (excessive accumulation of cerebrospinal fluid).

The spasm may result in ischemia and possible infarction of the portion of the brain supplied by the vessel(s) in spasm. The hydrocephalus is due to the residue of blood in the cerebrospinal fluid blocking the arachnoid villi and preventing cerebrospinal fluid absorption. The patient in this instance will show signs of *increasing intracranial pressure;* these include an increasingly severe headache, restlessness, gradual change in level of consciousness, drowsiness, nausea and vomiting and slower pulse and respirations. If this situation does not resolve itself within a few days, a draining procedure may be undertaken to reduce the cerebrospinal fluid accumulation. This may entail either inserting a tube directly into a lateral ventricle, from which the fluid will be allowed to run out into a closed collecting system, or establishing a shunt between either a ventricle or the lumbar subarachnoid space and the peritoneal cavity where the cerebrospinal fluid can be absorbed.

A specific directive is received from the surgeon as to the immediate preoperative preparation. The surgical treatment of the aneurysm involves placing a clip around the stalk of the aneurysm or tying it off. If this is not feasible, the aneurysm may be wrapped with fascia or muscle tissue to reinforce the wall and prevent a repetition of the rupture.

POSTOPERATIVE NURSING CARE.   The care is similar to that cited for any patient who has undergone intracranial surgery (see p. 866).

If no complications arise, ambulation is started within 2 or 3 days after the operation. Progression from lying to the sitting position and then to standing is made very slowly, as the patient will have been on complete bed rest from up to or beyond 2 weeks.

Cerebrovascular Accident (Stroke)

A cerebrovascular accident, or stroke, may be defined as a sudden interruption of the blood supply to a part of the brain. It may be due to a thrombosis, hemorrhage or, rarely, an embolism. The site of the lesion may be an internal carotid or vertebral artery, the basilar artery, circle of Willis or a cerebral artery. The disorder may also be referred to as apoplexy. (See Fig. 23–9, p. 812.)

Cerebral thrombosis is most often associated with atherosclerosis; the lumen of the vessel is narrowed, impeding the flow of blood. The circulatory stasis leads to thrombus formation, occlusion of the vessel and ischemia of an area of brain tissue. Narrowing of the vessel and ensuing thrombosis may occasionally be the result of vasculitis or outside pressure by a space-occupying lesion. An inadequate delivery of blood to the brain, secondary to cardiac insufficiency, shock or reduced intravascular volume, may also cause stasis and subsequent thrombosis. The onset of a stroke due to thrombosis may be relatively gradual and usually occurs when the person is at rest. If the occlusion of the vessel persists, necrosis of the tissue follows; the infarct eventually liquefies and is absorbed. Glial and fibrous scar tissue replaces the brain tissue that was destroyed.

When a cerebral hemorrhage occurs, the artery which ruptures has usually been vulnerable because of degenerative changes (atherosclerosis) in its walls or because of the presence of an aneurysm (a weak, saccular, vascular area). The hemorrhage may have been precipitated by an elevation of blood pressure. The escaping blood forms a hematoma which presses on the surrounding tissue. The pressure, along with the deficit in the blood supply, leads to destruction of adjacent brain tissue. The onset of a stroke caused by a cerebral hemorrhage is sudden and is usually associated with physical activity or emotional stress.

Cerebral embolism is the occlusion of a cerebral vessel by a blood clot, a clump of fat or tumor cells, or bacteria which has been carried by the circulation from another area of the body. Blood clots which form emboli may originate in the heart as a result of cardiac disease or in the saphenous or femoral veins due to circulatory stasis. A fat embolism most often follows a fracture; an embolism formed of tumor cells may arise from a malignant neoplasm. An infected embolus may be associated with bacterial endocarditis. The stroke due to an embolism occurs suddenly.

INCIDENCE. Cerebrovascular accidents account for a large proportion of neurological disease and are responsible for many deaths and mental and physical disability. It is thought the majority of strokes result from cerebral thrombosis. They have their highest incidence in those over 60 years of age. The principal predisposing factors are atherosclerosis, hypertension, congenital aneurysm and conditions which provide a possible source of emboli.

EFFECTS AND MANIFESTATIONS. Obviously, the effects of a cerebrovascular accident depend upon the site of the lesion and the amount of brain tissue affected. The damage may be so severe that death ensues within a few hours or days, or the injury may be so slight that the symptoms are transient and may even go unrecognized. Between these extremes are many variants. Certain patterns of defects have been recognized as being associated with a cerebrovascular accident involving specific vessels and areas.

The following clinical features are common to the majority of patients who suffer a cerebrovascular accident.

PREMONITORY SYMPTOMS. Premonitory manifestations may be experienced which might include persistent headache, dizziness or "lightheadedness," fleeting loss of consciousness or "blackout," brief confusion, blurring of vision in one or both eyes, stumbling of speech or "thickness" of the tongue, or transient local sensory and motor deficits. Any of these symptoms are especially important and should serve as a warning, especially if the patient is known to have hypertension, arteriosclerosis or a condition which may give rise to an embolus.

LOSS OF CONSCIOUSNESS. A period of unconsciousness is common to stroke patients and may vary from hours to days. Coma lasting longer than 24 to 36 hours presents a grave prognosis. A few patients experience only a clouding of consciousness and confusion.

CONVULSIVE MOVEMENTS. The immediate onset may be accompanied by convulsive movements which may be local or general.

HEADACHE AND VOMITING. If the patient remains conscious, he may complain of severe headache as a result of increased intracranial pressure. Vomiting frequently occurs with the initial onset and may be recurring in the conscious patient.

VITAL SIGNS. The respirations are usually slow and stertorous or may be Cheyne-Stokes. The pulse is generally slow, full and bounding. The temperature may be normal during the first few hours, and then becomes elevated. Progressive hyperpyrexia is considered an unfavorable sign.

MOTOR AND SENSORY DEFICITS. Hemiplegia is one of the most common effects of a stroke. For a few days, there is a marked loss of tone in the affected structures and an absence of normal reflexes. Babinski's sign is present in the paralyzed limb. Even with the patient in coma, one may recognize a greater loss of tone in the muscles of the paralyzed limbs; when the limbs are flexed, the affected one falls more quickly in a limp, lifeless manner. Later this flaccidity in the affected limbs is replaced by spasticity and hyperactive reflexes characteristic of upper motor neuron lesions. One side of the face may be paralyzed, resulting in that side blowing out and in with each respiration. The mouth may also be drawn to one side. When conscious, the patient may experience difficulty in swallowing (dysphagia), indicating some paralysis of the swallowing muscles. There may also be loss of sensation in some parts. Motor and sensory deficits in the limbs occur on the side of the body opposite to the lesion.

SPEECH DEFECT. There may be complete or partial loss of speech. The defect may take various forms (see p. 842); he may not only be unable to communicate verbally but may manifest some impairment in comprehension of either verbal or written communication.

EYE CHANGES. The eyes as well as the head tend to turn to the side of the lesion in the early stage; later, the deviation may be reversed and the head and eyes are probably turned to the side of the paralysis. The pupils may be uneven or constricted to "pin point" size, the corneal and pupillary reflexes are most likely absent, and the physician's examination of the fundus may reveal papilledema resulting from increased intracranial pressure. The conscious patient may indicate impaired vision, and there may be a defective movement of one or both eyes.

OTHER SYMPTOMS. For the first few days the face may be flushed and, if there has been bleeding into the subarachnoid space, there may be nuchal rigidity. Incontinence is common. As the patient recovers.it may become apparent that there has been sufficient brain damage to cause some mental impairment.

TREATMENT AND NURSING CARE. At the onset, the outcome as to residual disability is unpredictable. The degree of recovery will depend on the size of the infarction or hemorrhage and to some extent on the age of the patient. When the patient regains consciousness, some functional recovery may be expected as the pressure and edema in the area of the brain lesion subside. The permanent disability is generally not confirmed for several days. If function is regained, it tends to follow a general pattern in which the facial and swallowing muscles recover first and then those of the lower limbs. Speech and arm function are regained more slowly and less completely.

During the acute phase of the illness following a cerebrovascular accident the care is principally supportive and is directed toward preventing complications and damage that may interfere later with maximum rehabilitation (e.g., subluxation and contractures). When the patient is comatose, the care will include that which is applicable to any unconscious patient (see Chapter 9). Following the acute phase, care emphasizes rehabilitation of the patient to a reasonably active, independent life compatible with his residual disabilities.

POSITIONING. While unconscious, the patient is placed in a semiprone or lateral position to facilitate breathing and prevent the aspiration of mucus and vomitus. A pharyngeal airway may be introduced to permit unobstructed breathing. Suction equipment is kept at the bedside to remove mucus and any vomitus when necessary. Good alignment of the head is maintained to avoid compression of the neck vessels; flexion may interfere with cerebral venous drainage, favoring cerebral congestion, bleeding from the lesion and increased intracranial pressure. The physician may want the patient kept turned on the side of his lesion and minimal moving of the patient for several hours to prevent the possibility of increased intracranial bleeding.

Side rails are placed on the bed in the event of recovery of consciousness accompanied by disorientation and restlessness. These remain on the bed until the patient is sufficiently rehabilitated so that he can turn and sit up in bed without danger of losing his balance.

OBSERVATIONS. In the initial acute phase, the vital signs are recorded at frequent intervals. An abnormal elevation of the blood pressure, a decrease in the pulse and slow or Cheyne-Stokes respirations may indicate increasing intracranial pressure. An abnormal fall in the blood pressure and weakening of the pulse may point to circulatory collapse. A progressively rising temperature to levels of hyperpyrexia is an unfavorable sign, generally pointing to interference with the body temperature-regulating center and loss of the controlling reflexes.

The size of both pupils and their reaction to light are observed and checked at intervals for changes, and the level of consciousness is noted by being alert to any movements made by the patient and to responses such as resistance or withdrawal offered to passive movement or other forms of care.

FLUIDS AND NUTRITION.   During the first 24 to 48 hours fluids may be administered intravenously. The rate of flow and volume are carefully controlled to avoid too rapid an increase in the intravascular volume and blood pressure. If coma is prolonged, or the patient has considerable dysphagia, nasogastric feedings may be introduced to provide sufficient nutrients (see p. 503). An accurate record of the patient's fluid intake and output in the acute phase is necessary.

When consciousness is regained, the swallowing reflex is tested before giving any fluids orally. If the patient can swallow, a soft diet is given and is progressively increased to a full, balanced diet as soon as tolerated. The patient will probably have to be fed at first, particularly if the area he is accustomed to using is paralyzed, but with the necessary assistance he is encouraged to feed himself as soon as possible to establish independence. If one side of the face is paralyzed, food is placed in the opposite side of the mouth to make swallowing easier. Mouth care is then given following the meal to remove retained food particles from the weak side to prevent aspiration and the formation of sordes.

REACTION AND BEHAVIOR.   Emotionally, a stroke is devastating to a patient and, usually, the more intellectually intact he is, the greater is the psychological impact. On regaining consciousness, he may be confused at first but, as his thoughts clear, he is shocked to find himself in a totally strange environment, unable to communicate or to move one side of his body. The depression and resentment or hostility that the patient is likely to manifest are normal responses. His immediate thought is likely to be that life is no longer worth living. The patient gradually works his way through his depression and

becomes interested and cooperative as his rehabilitative program is introduced.

He requires an explanation of what happened to him and what is going to be done for him. At this time, he is greatly in need of understanding and psychological support. A visit from a member of his family may now provide considerable reassurance. Continuing care by the same personnel, as much as possible, is helpful. If he is in a single room, he will probably be less apprehensive if transferred to a room where there is at least one other patient. Isolation tends to contribute to greater despair, but conversation with others provides verbal stimulation which plays a role in speech therapy, if necessary. Taking time to converse with the patient as a normal person may convey some assurance to him that he is still worthwhile and that people are interested in him. Such courtesy and respect are likely to promote a more positive attitude in the patient toward his recovery and usefulness.

A lack of concern for his disability on the part of the patient may reflect brain damage. Similarly, responses such as uncontrolled crying and inappropriate laughter may be manifested and are likely to be very distressing to the family. It is impressed on the family that the patient's behavior does not necessarily represent his true feelings and that such responses may disappear or become less marked. The patient may exhibit impaired intellectual ability which may affect certain areas of mental activity such as judgment, reasoning and comprehension. This intellectual loss, combined with impaired physical and possibly language abilities, may prevent the patient from resuming previous activities and responsibilities — for example, his return to gainful employment. The family is alerted to these facts so that they may avoid ensuing problems as much as possible.

Some stroke patients develop fixed ideas and rigid behavior which also relate to changes in the brain, and these persons are not apt to respond to verbal entreaties. Relatives are helped to understand and accept these as sequelae of the disease process.[2]

ORAL AND SKIN CARE.   During the acute

---

[2]Roy S. Fowler and W. E. Fordyce: Stroke: Why Do They Behave That Way? Dallas, American Heart Association, 1974. Also available from the Canadian Heart Foundation.

stage, the mouth requires frequent cleansing (every 2 to 3 hours) with a mild, antiseptic mouthwash to prevent the accumulation of secretions. Good oral hygiene plays an important role in preventing parotitis to which older patients seem to have a greater predisposition. Mineral oil or petroleum jelly is applied to the lips. Later, because of the hemiplegia, the patient may find cleaning his teeth difficult and require some assistance until he becomes more adept with the functioning arm and hand.

Because of their inability to turn and move in bed, especially in the early phases of their illness, stroke patients are particularly prone to develop pressure sores. The majority of these patients are in the older age group which increases the predisposition because their skin is less resistant and develops local anemia more readily when subjected to pressure. While confined to bed, the patient is turned every 2 hours. The vulnerable bony prominences (sacral and lateral hip areas, heels, malleoli and shoulder and scapular areas) are kept clean and dry and are massaged gently to stimulate circulation. A protective emollient or lotion may be applied if the skin is dry. An air mattress or squares of sheepskin may be used to protect pressure areas. When the patient is allowed out of bed, precautions are still necessary to prevent prolonged sitting; he must be taught to stand or shift his weight from one hip to another at intervals to relieve compression of vessels in the area.

ELIMINATION. During the acute phase, an indwelling catheter may be used to prevent skin irritation by involuntary voiding and to measure urinary output accurately. It is used for as brief a period as possible because of the chance of urethral and bladder irritation and development of infection. When the catheter is removed, the patient is placed on the bedpan or toilet at frequent, regular intervals, gradually decreasing the frequency as control is reestablished. During rehabilitation, stress incontinence is likely to occur at times when the patient becomes emotional and frustrated, further increasing the patient's discouragement. Reassurance and psychological support from the nurse are needed in these situations.

The enforced inactivity associated with hemiplegia frequently gives rise to constipation. The nurse must be alert to the possibility of impaction. An enema, laxative, or glycerin or bisacodyl (Dulcolax) suppository may be necessary at first but increased dietary roughage and fluid intake should be used to resolve the problem as soon as possible.

MEDICATIONS. On regaining consciousness, the patient may complain of severe headache. Acetylsalicylic acid or acetylsalicylic acid compounds may be prescribed, but strong analgesics are generally withheld because they tend to mask neurological symptoms. If hypertension persists following a cerebrovascular accident, a hypotensive drug such as methyldopa (Aldomet) or a diuretic (e.g., hydrochlorothiazide) may be prescribed.

APHASIA. The aphasia associated with a cerebrovascular accident is usually expressive in type (see p. 829). It occurs most frequently in those whose lesion is in the left cerebral hemisphere. Right hemispheric lesions tend to produce dysarthria in which the muscles involved in articulation (e.g., larynx, tongue) are affected.

The sudden loss of the ability to communicate creates fear and frustration in the patient, especially in the initial phase. He feels isolated, lonely and threatened. The nurse endeavors to allay some of the patient's anxiety by anticipating his needs as much as possible, acknowledging his difficulty and concern, and indicating support in working through his problem. He is likely to benefit psychologically from knowing that someone understands and is interested in helping. Most aphasic patients can recover their ability to communicate to some degree. It is not possible to predict the extent of this at the onset; speech is usually recovered very gradually and slowly and requires the assistance of those around the patient. The nurse avoids conveying what may be false optimism at first but reassures the patient and his family that special assistance will be given to help in the recovery of speech. In the early stage of recovery from the stroke, patient's gestures to indicate needs and wishes may be encouraged but should not be accepted indefinitely, since established use of them may inhibit his efforts to verbalize.

If the services of a speech therapist are available, an assessment of the patient's language capacity is made and a retraining program planned. In many situations, the nurse will be mainly responsible for helping him.

recover the ability to communicate. It is necessary, as soon as possible, to determine whether the patient can express his ideas verbally or by written word and whether he understands what is said to him and, if so, whether his comprehension is limited to short simple phrases or single words. Rarely, intellectual impairment occurs which precludes speech rehabilitation.

It is important to talk normally and with ease to the patient. Auditory stimulation and socialization play important roles and are considered as valuable as structured remedial drills. For this reason, following recovery from the acute stage of the illness, he is better off in a room with others. It must be remembered that the fact that he cannot speak is no indication that his intelligence, comprehension and hearing are impaired. The patient should not be discussed within his hearing as though he does not hear or understand. This was a very disturbing factor cited by Buck in writing of his experiences.[3] The aphasic patient should receive the courtesy and respect due every patient and be included in the conversation taking place in his presence. The nurse is cautioned against treating him as a child, since he does not necessarily think as a child. In chatting, use short simple sentences; if there is evidence of difficulty in comprehension, they should relate to the present and his immediate environment as much as possible.

When helping the patient to recover his speech, the vocabulary selected is kept to a simple, functional level. Emphasis is placed on nouns and simple responses such as "yes" and "no" first, and then progression through verbs and adjectives to short sentences is used, much the same as the process used with the young child learning to communicate. The use of several sensory avenues is usually more effective than the use of just one at a time. Hearing words in direct association with the objects they represent and the printed words contributes to recovery. As care is given, names of articles being used are enunciated slowly and clearly. The vocabulary is gradually extended to other useful words by placing actual objects or pictures of the objects and the printed name

before the patient and repeating the name several times. He is asked to say the word and is given plenty of time to respond.

The patient should be rested and relaxed and in a quiet undistracting setting during the periods of instruction, which are kept brief as he tires easily and his attention span is likely to be short. He should never be pressured to the point of frustration which leads to discouragement and withdrawal. Emphasis on exact pronunciation is avoided. Some speech therapy departments use a special language machine which may be left with the patient to use on his own. It presents a picture of an object and its name in print at the same time that the word is presented audibly. When advised as to the use of it, the patient is of course instructed to "speak" the word. The repetitive association of the object with the written and spoken word does facilitate recovery, especially in those who are highly motivated and not easily discouraged.

After the first 2 or 3 weeks, at which time the patient is returned to his home, most of the assistance in the recovery of speech must come from the family. Early in the illness, family members are helped to understand the patient's communication problem and their role in the rehabilitation program. Frequently, the patient makes more rapid progress when he goes home to the familiar relaxed environment. The importance of conversing normally with the patient, expecting a response and giving him plenty of time to respond are discussed with the family. The methods and details related to periods of instruction are explained, and it is helpful if at least one member observes a teaching session carried out in the hospital or rehabilitation center. Excellent pamphlets and booklets on aphasia are available from the local branch of the National (American or Canadian) Heart Association.[4] These may be reviewed with the family by the nurse and clarification of details made whenever necessary. Emphasis is placed on the need for patience and effort on the part of all concerned, and on the need of providing opportunities for the patient to practice and use

[3]M. Buck: "Adjustments During Recovery from Stroke." Am. J. Nurs., Vol. 64, No. 10 (Oct. 1964), pp. 92–95.

[4]American Heart Association: Aphasia and the Family. Dallas, American Heart Association, 1969. Also available from the Canadian Heart Foundation and its provincial branches.

what speech he has. The family is advised that progress is likely to be slow and may require many months. They are cautioned against placing excessive demands on the patient, which may have demoralizing effects. The patient will be slow in responding or expressing himself; but if he is cut off, he readily becomes discouraged and gives up. Progress should be acknowledged because it encourages him and prompts motivation for continued effort.

FAMILY. A stroke is usually as much of a shock and tragedy to the family as it is to the victim. Buck, a physician writing about his personal experience following a stroke, makes the following statement: "A stroke is actually a family illness and continuous counseling should be readily available for the entire household."[5] The nurse has a responsibility to talk with them, answer their questions when possible and discuss how they may help the patient and each other. If it is the wage earner who has been stricken, economic hardships may be imposed on the family. A discussion with a social service worker may be arranged or a referral to a social welfare agency made. As well as the disability, the patient may exhibit inappropriate or bizarre behavior which the family finds very distressing and hard to understand and accept. An effort is made to explain that this is due to actual tissue damage and is not controllable by the patient.

Members of the family who are informed and develop acceptance of the situation with a positive attitude play an important role in motivating and assisting the patient to regain functions and independence. To fill this role, they require the guidance and support of the health team. This is particularly important when the patient leaves the hospital. Too often the family and the patient are left to carry on entirely on their own when the patient leaves the hospital. Some follow-up should be arranged with a visiting nurse agency.

REHABILITATION. Certain aspects of the care that the stroke patient receives in the early stage of his illness play an important role in his rehabilitation. As cited previously, the muscles of the affected limbs are flaccid for a few days, then become spastic. The paralyzed arm is adducted, and flexion

occurs at the elbow, wrist, finger and thumb joints. The lower limb assumes a position of external rotation at the hip, flexion of the thigh and leg, and plantar flexion of the foot. With immobility, muscles atrophy and the collagen fibers of the connective tissue of tendons, ligaments and joint capsules tend to shorten and become dense and firm. The process may be hastened by circulatory stasis, edema and trauma. As a result, if the affected limbs are permitted to remain immobile in the positions they automatically assume, contractures and reduced range of motion may become permanent, making rehabilitation difficult and possibly creating deformities which actually increase the patient's disability. Maintenance of joint motion, support to prevent the pull of gravity on joints and subsequent subluxation, and positioning to prevent contractures and maintain good alignment are essential from the onset of the illness. In the supine position, the paralyzed arm is abducted to a 90° angle, and a pillow is placed along the side of the trunk into the axilla. Internal rotation of the shoulder is avoided. The arm and hand are supported on a pillow; a roll is placed in the hand to preserve the normal position. In some instances, marked spasticity may necessitate the use of a padded splint, especially at night, to prevent flexure contractures of the wrist and hand. If the hand is edematous, the hand and arm are elevated above the level of the heart to promote venous and lymphatic drainage and reduce stasis. A long sandbag or firm roll is placed along the outer side of the lower limb to counteract external rotation. To be effective, the sandbag must extend from above the greater trochanter to the external malleolus. The foot is kept at a near-right angle to the leg by the use of a footboard.

When the patient lies on his unaffected side, his paralyzed limbs are supported in good alignment on pillows to prevent strain on the shoulder and hip joints. Two or three times a day, the patient is placed in the prone position for 30 minutes to prevent flexion contracture of the thighs. The affected arm is adducted and extended, palm down, and the roll is kept in place. A folded bath towel or small pillow is placed under each shoulder to avoid inward rotation. A small flat pillow is placed under the ankles, and the feet are extended beyond the mattress to prevent

5Buck, op. cit., p. 93.

plantar flexion. The limbs are passively moved through a full range of motion two or three times daily. While the patient is helpless and confined to bed, his position is changed every 2 hours; he is encouraged to take eight to ten deep respirations and cough each time he changes position. Bed rest and immobility promote stasis and retention of pulmonary secretions which predispose to infection.

The stroke patient is usually assisted out of bed for progressively increasing periods as soon as his vital signs have returned to normal. This lessens muscle deterioration and the possibility of pulmonary complications, facilitates the recovery of postural reflexes, and promotes a more positive attitude on the part of the patient toward his future. When the patient is up, the affected arm is placed in a sling to prevent subluxation of the shoulder joint.

As soon as the patient is well enough, an assessment is made of his remaining abilities and disabilities to determine his rehabilitation potential. Each one must be evaluated and treated on an individual basis.

As cited previously, the location and extent of brain damage influence the nature of impaired function. Most hemiplegic patients fortunately experience extensor spasm of the affected knee and hip with weight-bearing which stabilizes the leg as the good leg is carried through a forward step. Instead of this extensor spasm, in response to the weight-bearing, some experience spasm of the flexor muscles. When the patient attempts to walk, the knee and hip flex and will not support him. This necessitates the application of a leg brace for stabilization. Others, because of interference with the blood supply to the cerebellum, suffer ataxia and marked loss of balance. This is likely to preclude ambulation, and the patient remains in a wheelchair.

Sensory function may also be impaired; as well as a reduced sensitivity to pain, pressure and temperature, there may be loss of the ability to know the location of parts of his body in space, making movement difficult. The ability to recognize objects by touch (stereognosis) may also be impaired.

A stroke may cause intellectual damage; reasoning, judgment and normal responses may be impaired and will limit the level to which the patient may be rehabilitated.

Once the assessment of the patient's abilities and disabilities is completed, a plan is made and instituted for exercises and teaching to assist the patient to function within the framework of his disability. He should be given every opportunity to recover as great a degree of independence as possible to make life more tolerable for him and his family. The program, in which the nurse has an important role, is directed toward assisting the patient to achieve self-care and mobility and regain verbal communication if speech has been impaired. A physiotherapist, in cooperation with the physician, may plan and introduce the program but frequently it is the nurse who must follow it up and give the necessary guidance and support to the patient and his family.

As soon as possible, the retraining for self-care is begun while the patient is still in bed. He learns to feed himself and to care for his person (washing himself, combing his hair, dressing and undressing). He is taught how to change his position in bed and to pull himself to a sitting position through the help of an overhead bar attached to the bed or a rope secured to the foot of the bed. Side rails on the bed also provide assistance in sitting up and insure safety against falls until he can maintain his balance. A schedule of exercises is established to strengthen the trunk and unaffected muscles so they may compensate for those paralyzed. Passive movements of the affected limbs are carried out to prevent contractures and stimulate circulation as a part of the exercise schedule. The patient is taught to do the exercises on his own, and he also learns how to do the passive movements of the affected limbs with his good limbs. Progressively, he learns to sit on the side of the bed, to stand, to transfer to a chair or commode, and eventually to walk using a walker or a regular or wide quadruple-base cane for support. When assisting the patient in walking, the nurse or family member supports him from his affected side. A leg brace may be necessary if the patient has the previously cited problem of flexor spasm in the paralyzed leg, and he will require instruction in applying it. If plantar flexion and toe-dragging interfere with walking and tend to trip the patient, a drop-foot splint may be used. The bed is lowered and made stationary when transfer techniques are being carried out.

Rehabilitation also includes retraining in simple useful functions (activities of daily living) on which every person is so dependent in normal living. These include such activities as opening doors, using the telephone, writing his name if the dominant hand has been paralyzed, handling various articles (e.g., wallet) and turning on the radio or television. The homemaker is assisted in learning to use various pieces of household equipment and is advised of simpler ways of performing some housekeeping tasks; suggestions are made for reorganizing the kitchen and other facilities so that she may be less dependent.

In relation to the aphasia which the patient may experience, the suggestions cited under speech impairment are continued. Efforts to have them regain some speech must not be abandoned too soon because of lack of early improvement.

As a guide to the exercises used for hemiplegic patients and the retraining for the activities of daily living and for suggestions for adaptations and special devices to promote independence and usefulness, the references cited below should be familiar to the nurse.[6] These booklets are readily available and may be used by the patient and family. Other useful references which are applicable to the rehabilitation of the stroke patient are also included at the end of this chapter.

The total rehabilitation program is fully discussed with a member of the family. This person should be familiar with the exercise and passive movement regimen and should understand the importance of encouraging and permitting the patient to do things for himself. The family members, as do many nurses, find it difficult to stand back, leaving the patient to persevere and struggle with activities. The brochure entitled "Strokes — A Guide for the Family," published by the American Heart Association, may be helpful to the family and should be made available.

When the rehabilitation plan is instituted,

the stroke patient is usually discharged from the hospital. Both the patient and family still require considerable support and assistance. Following discussions with the family, a referral may be made to a visiting nurse agency. It is helpful in many instances if a visit is made to the home before the patient is discharged so that the situation may be assessed and modifications of the environment suggested to facilitate the patient's care and independence. These may include the changing of rooms, handrails beside the toilet and bathtub, placement of articles for ready accessibility to the patient, making the bed stationary, arranging for a footboard, the removal of scatter rugs and wax from floors, and selection of a chair that will promote good posture and also allow the patient to rise from it with a minimum of difficulty. The visiting nurse becomes familiar with the patient's history, his potential and the rehabilitation program planned so the necessary supervision can be provided. Assistance may be given in solving the social and economic problems imposed on the family by this illness and disability. Financial supplements may be arranged, and the nurse may help the family to organize so that all share in the increased responsibility. Early signs of resentment may be recognized and, by listening to the family members' points of view and explaining the patient's condition and unusual behavior, complete rejection of him may be prevented.

The patient is encouraged to develop interests and worthwhile hobbies and to gradually assume responsibility for some household chores within his physical and intellectual capacity. The performance of some useful tasks, remunerative or otherwise, promotes the patient's morale and greater harmony within the family.

The goals of rehabilitation are not achieved in a few weeks; in most instances, attainment requires months of perseverance and patience. The patient and family naturally experience periods of depression, frustration and pessimism. The established goals should not exceed the possibility of realization. Activities are taken in steps so achievement may be experienced. Demanding too much at one time fatigues and discourages the patient, defeating progress. Complete restoration to his previous functional ability is seldom possible, but much can be done to restore the patient to

[6]Public Health Service, U.S. Department of Health, Education and Welfare: Strike Back at Stroke. Washington, D.C., U.S. Department of Health, Education, and Welfare. Distributed by the American Heart Association and Canadian Heart Foundation and its branches.

American Heart Association: Do It Yourself Again. Dallas, American Heart Association, 1969. Also available from the Canadian Heart Foundation and its provincial branches.

a degree of independence that makes life more tolerable for him and his family.

DEGENERATIVE DISEASES OF THE NERVOUS SYSTEM

Paralysis Agitans (Parkinson's Disease)

Paralysis agitans is a progressive degenerative disease within the brain that causes dysfunction of the extrapyramidal system, resulting in muscular rigidity, difficulty in initiating voluntary movements, tremor and disturbed autonomic nervous function.

ETIOLOGY AND INCIDENCE. For a long while this disease was attributed chiefly to degenerative changes in the basal ganglia. Recently, failure of the substantia nigra to produce normal amounts of the chemical dopamine is considered to play an important etiologic role. The substantia nigra (meaning black substance) is a nucleus in the midbrain and consists of neurons distinctly characterized by their high pigment (melanin) content. These cells produce dopamine and deliver it via their axons to the basal ganglia which function as part of the extrapyramidal system. The chemical appears to be essential for normal neurotransmission and functioning of the basal ganglia. It is excreted from the body in the urine. Patients with Parkinson's disease show reduced urinary levels of dopamine, and autopsies have revealed an abnormally low amount of melanin in the substantia nigra of these patients.[7]

This disease, which is relatively common, usually has its onset between the ages of 50 and 60 and has a slightly higher incidence in males.

SYMPTOMS. Tremor and muscular rigidity develop insidiously and at the onset are usually unilateral with involvement of the other side developing later. The fine tremor occurs when the part is at rest and is arrested with voluntary movement and when the person is asleep, and becomes more pronounced with emotional stress and fatigue. The tremor develops initially in the distal portions of the limbs and eventually involves the head, lips and tongue. In the upper limbs the involuntary movements are confined mainly to the wrist, fingers and thumb; in the legs, flexion and extension at the ankle occur. Tremor of the fingers and thumb produce the characteristic "pill-rolling" movement.

In the early stage of the muscular rigidity, the patient may complain of stiffness on moving but gradually, as tonic contraction of skeletal muscle increases, voluntary movements become slow and difficult. There is marked resistance of the limbs to passive movement. The patient may have difficulty in starting to walk, and his gait is characterized by short, shuffling steps. The trunk and head are flexed forward, causing a progressive acceleration of his steps (festination gait), difficulty in stopping and a predisposition to falling. The arms are adducted and semiflexed, and their normal swing during walking is absent. He may have difficulty in assuming any change in position such as sitting down, rising from the sitting position and turning in bed. Finger movements are impaired, as evidenced by the patient's small cramped writing and difficulty with tying his shoes or closing fasteners on his clothing.

Rigidity of the facial muscles produces a mask-like, inexpressive appearance. Speech becomes weak, slurred and monotonous (devoid of inflections) as the muscles concerned with articulation become involved. Late in the disease, the patient may experience difficulty in mastication and swallowing. The respiratory excursion and the ability to cough are diminished, predisposing the patient to chest complications. Pain and easy fatigue due to the continuous increased traction of muscles on their attachments are common. Dryness of the skin, coldness of the extremities and an excessive secretion of saliva may occur due to disturbances in the autonomic nervous system.

TREATMENT AND NURSING CARE. The patient with paralysis agitans is encouraged to remain active for as long as reasonably possible. Because the condition progresses slowly, generally over years, he is usually able to continue his gainful occupation. As the tremor and slower movements become more troublesome, he may have to change his occupation, depending on its nature, and may eventually be forced to give it up. It should be remembered that the patient's mask-like expression and motor impairment belie his mental capacity, which suffers no deterioration until the very late stage.

[7]A. Fangman, and W. E. O'Malley: "L-Dopa and the Patient with Parkinson's Disease." Am. J. Nurs., Vol. 69, No. 7 (July 1969), p. 1455.

Currently, treatment falls into three categories — drug therapy, physical therapy and surgery. These do not cure the disease but may be effective in reducing the distressing tremor and muscular rigidity.

DRUG THERAPY. The drugs used in treatment of Parkinson's disease include natural and synthetic anticholinergic preparations, antihistamines, and dihydroxyphenylalanine (L-dopa).

The anticholinergic preparations are thought to inhibit the transmission of the abnormal impulses responsible for the excessive muscular contraction and tremor. The earlier antiparkinsonism drugs, such as tincture and extract of belladonna, atropine, scopolamine and stramonium, are employed less often now because the synthetic preparations generally produce fewer and less severe side effects. The synthetic antispasmodic preparations most commonly used are benzhexol chloride (Artane), ethopropazine hydrochloride (Lysivane) and orphenadrine hydrochloride (Disipal). A patient receiving a natural or synthetic anticholinergic drug is observed for side effects which commonly are dryness of the mouth and skin, blurring of vision, headache, retention of urine, tachycardia and palpitation. The patient is generally started on a small dose of the prescribed preparation which is then gradually increased until side effects appear. The dosage is then slightly reduced and maintained at a level at which the patient is free of side effects. An antihistamine such as diphenhydramine hydrochloride (Benadryl) may be ordered with the drugs except with orphenadrine, to cut down on the patient's anxiety. Orphenadrine has antihistaminic as well as anticholinergic properties; side effects of diphenhydramine hydrochloride (Benadryl) may be lightheadedness and drowsiness.

L-Dopa is regarded as a very useful drug when given with an anticholinergic drug. Its initial use was based on studies which indicated that patients with paralysis agitans have less than the normal amounts of dopamine in their substantia nigra and basal ganglia. Dopamine, as such, is not given, since it does not cross the blood-brain barrier; dihydroxyphenylalanine (L-dopa) is given and is absorbed by the substantia nigra which then produces dopamine.[8] Tremor and muscular

rigidity are markedly reduced with L-dopa, facilitating normal movements and independence, and the face loses some of the inexpressiveness. At first the patient receives a small dose which is progressively increased over several days. He is hospitalized during this period, since some side effects of varying intensity may be experienced. These may be manifested in gastrointestinal or cardiovascular disturbances. He is observed for hypotension, pulse changes, anorexia, nausea, vomiting, marked weakness, restlessness, abnormal patterns of movement (e.g., athetosis), behavioral changes, confusion, and swings in mood. Frequent blood counts are made since some patients have shown a fall in granulocytes.

PHYSICAL THERAPY. Because of the difficulty in moving associated with the muscular rigidity, the patient is prone to remain immobile. As a result the normal range of joint movement may be lost and contractures develop. A program of physical therapy is instituted when the patient's disease has advanced to the stage when even slight difficulty in activity is manifested. A schedule of exercises is planned and initiated in a rehabilitation or physical therapy department. The types of exercises are prescribed according to the patient's disability and are designed to promote independence and self-care within the limits of his potential capacity. The family and visiting nurse must be familiar with the program, since the patient may reach a stage at which he is not sufficiently self-motivated to carry out the daily exercises and requires prompting and encouragement. Progression of the disease may necessitate periodic adjustments in the prescribed program.

SURGICAL TREATMENT. Certain patients may be treated by pallidotomy or thalamotomy, which may alleviate tremor and muscular rigidity; results vary and, with recent advances in medical management, surgery is attempted less often than in the past. The pallidotomy procedure produces a lesion in the globus pallidus; in the case of the thalamotomy, the lesion is produced in the ventrolateral portion of the thalamus. If surgical treatment is undertaken the thalamic procedure appears to be the surgery of choice in recent years. Either procedure is performed under local anesthesia and involves the destruction of a well-defined area of tissue by the introduction of absolute alcohol, electro-

---

[8]Ibid., p. 1457.

coagulation, freezing by means of liquid nitrogen (cryosurgery) or separation from adjacent tissue using a leukotome (fine blunt wire). The surgery is performed on the side opposite to the limbs with the greater rigidity and tremor. If this results in improvement, and there is bilateral involvement, the operation may be undertaken on the other side a few months later.

The patients for surgical therapy are carefully selected. Preferably the candidates are those who are 50 to 60 years of age who are not responding to drug therapy, are not fully incapacitated and whose disease is unilateral. In preparation for surgery, antiparkinsonism drugs are usually discontinued several days preceding the schedule date. General preoperative preparation is applicable, and a specific directive is given as to the necessary local skin preparation. The usual procedure is to shampoo the patient's hair the afternoon or evening before the scheduled operation using a germicidal soap. A small area of the scalp is then shaved in the operating room, preceding the making of a burr hole through which the surgeon works. The patient is advised that local anesthesia will be used and that he will be requested, during the procedure, to perform movements such as opening and clenching his hand or raising his arm on the side opposite to the surgery. These are made to assist in localizing the area of tissue to be treated. An explanation is also made of the frequent checking of his vital signs and responses that will be made after the operation.

Following the surgery, the head of the bed is elevated to promote venous drainage and prevent cerebral edema and increased intracranial pressure. The vital signs are recorded every half-hour for several hours; the interval is gradually increased if they remain normal. Frequent observations are made of the patient's level of consciousness, pupillary reactions, size and equality, and orientation. Tests are made for any indication of loss of motor and sensory function. Side rails are placed on the bed in the event of mental confusion or sudden seizure. A suction apparatus should be readily available in the event of excessive mucus and respiratory difficulty. The patient is usually assisted out of bed in 36 to 48 hours and is helped to walk. The limbs are passively moved through a full range of motion two or three times daily, and an active exercise program is instituted as soon as the patient's condition permits.

GENERAL NURSING CONSIDERATIONS. The majority of persons suffering from paralysis agitans are cared for at home until the advanced stage of their disease leads to marked disability and helplessness. The clinic or visiting nurse assumes the major role in providing the necessary counseling and guidance for the patient and family at the onset and through the successive months and years. It is important that the nurse understand the nature of the patient's disease and recognize the emotional, physical and socioeconomic problems incurred by it. *The fact that his intellect is unimpaired must be kept in mind as well as his tendency to become very self-conscious, depressed and withdrawn* because of his appearance and limitations. The reader will find it helpful to read Margaret Bourke-White's "My Mysterious Malady" to receive first hand the thoughts and reactions of a person with Parkinson's disease.[9]

The nurse helps the family and others around the patient to understand his problems and emphasizes his need to be treated normally, to socialize, and to do things for himself even though he may take much longer than usual. The environment should be quiet, cheerful and free of haste and confusion, since emotional stress and fatigue aggravate his tremor and rigidity. As the disease progresses, certain aspects of his care require increasing attention and modification.

The patient is encouraged to feed himself, and provision is made for the fact that he takes longer, spills food and probably has difficulty in chewing and swallowing. His nutritional status and weight are followed, since he may consume only a small part of his meals because of depression and fatigue. Inadequate food intake weakens the patient and influences his capacity to participate in an exercise program and other activities. A schedule of frequent smaller meals may be helpful, and he may find it easier to take strained or chopped foods or food prepared in a blender. The patient may be less self-conscious and take more if privacy is insured while he is eating. His clothing is protected

---

[9]Margaret Bourke-White: My Mysterious Malady. Chicago, United Parkinson's Disease Foundation. (Taken from: Portrait of Myself, New York, Simon Schuster, 1963.)

during the meal so that traces of his incapacity do not remain to increase his concern. Eventually, he may require assistance, especially with fluids.

Constipation is a frequent problem because of the reduced activity, tension, prescribed drugs and limited bulk in the diet. Impaction may develop. Additional fluids, fruits and vegetables may be included in the diet, and a bulk-producing laxative may be prescribed to establish regular bowel movements.

The patient sits for prolonged periods and may also be unable to change his position in bed because of the rigidity. Obviously, this predisposes to circulatory stasis and pressure sores. Assistance at regular intervals to prevent these prolonged periods of immobility is necessary. Assistive devices, such as a rope secured to the end of the bed or suspended from an overhead bar, may be helpful for the patient to raise himself to a sitting position from which he can shift his weight. When he is up, arms on his chair may permit him to raise himself to a standing position.

Excessive salivation and difficulty in swallowing may cause drooling, which is extremely uncomfortable and embarrassing for the patient. An adequate supply of available soft tissues, skin care with the application of a protective lotion or ointment, and frequent changes of the pillow cover are necessary.

The patient's forward flexion of the trunk, shuffling gait, and slowness of righting reflexes to maintain his balance predispose him to falls. Some simple modifications within his environment may prevent such accidents. Floors should not be waxed. Hazards such as scatter rugs, small stools and other articles which might trip him are removed. A straight chair that is not likely to tip or move as he lowers himself into it or rises from it is provided. A raised toilet seat and hand bars in appropriate places in the bathroom facilitate self-care and prevent falls. The patient's belongings and articles which he is likely to need are kept in places which are easily accessible to him.

Clothing with zippers rather than buttons and pull-on shoes instead of those with laces are suggested so that the patient can maintain his independence in dressing and undressing as long as possible. By being able to achieve these tasks, he is likely to be more interested in his personal appearance and is less likely to drift into the habit of remaining in pajamas

and a dressing gown throughout the day. The male patient usually becomes dependent on others to shave him before many other self-care activities are relinquished. A schedule is planned for a member of his family to assume this responsibility regularly so that the patient does not feel neglected or that he is a nuisance.

Participation in activities and socialization with the family and others in the home and outside are promoted. Otherwise, the Parkinson's disease patient becomes a very lonely, disillusioned person. Personality changes are fostered by isolation and frequently lead to difficult patient-family relationships. The results of group involvement in exercises and planned recreation in institutions have demonstrated the benefits derived from socialization and being one of the group.

Multiple Sclerosis (Disseminated Sclerosis)

Multiple sclerosis is a degenerative disease characterized by demyelination of nerve fibers within the spinal cord and brain. The lesions are irregular and scattered which accounts for the term disseminated. Destruction of an area of a myelin sheath occurs, followed by a proliferation of neuroglial cells, scar formation, and damage to the nerve fiber with ensuing loss of transmission of impulses.

ETIOLOGY AND INCIDENCE. The cause of multiple sclerosis is unknown despite prolonged and continuous research. At present, theories undergoing investigation are concerned with autoimmune mechanisms and viral infection as possible etiologic factors.

The disease is more prevalent in colder climates but, once established, climate does not appear to influence its progress. It has a slightly higher incidence in females and most frequently has its onset in persons between 20 and 40 years of age.

COURSE AND MANIFESTATIONS. Multiple sclerosis is characterized by remissions and relapses, and the course is extremely variable and unpredictable. Spontaneous remissions of varying length are common, especially in the early years of the disease. The manifestations may vary from one relapse to another as a result of lesions developed in tracts other than those previously involved. Gradually, the cumulative, residual effects of nerve fiber damage from recurring exacerbations lead to a chronic incapacitated state in which the patient is helpless and is confined to a wheelchair.

Early symptoms usually include transient tingling sensations, numbness and muscular weakness in one or both arms and legs and visual disturbances which may take the form of nystagmus, diplopia or blurring of vision. The patient may manifest emotional lability, evidenced by alternating periods of euphoria (false sense of well-being), depression and irritability. Later, with repeated relapses and increasing damage, the patient may develop paralysis, impaired speech, dysphagia, increasing loss of sensation, bladder and bowel incontinence, increasing visual difficulties, personality changes and intellectual impairment. Weakness of the respiratory muscles and cough reflex may also be present, predisposing him to pulmonary complications.

At present, there are no specific diagnostic tests for multiple sclerosis. The cerebrospinal fluid of many of these patients shows an elevated gamma globulin level and a positive colloidal gold precipitation test (Lange colloidal gold curve).

TREATMENT AND NURSING CARE. There is no specific treatment for multiple sclerosis, but good counseling and care may contribute to the prevention of relapses and complications as well as help to keep the patient active and independent as long as possible. Management comprises mainly general supportive measures and symptomatic care which increase in amount and complexity with the progression of the patient's disease. He is cared for at home through the early stages of his disease and as long as the family can provide adequate care. Hospitalization or care in a nursing home usually becomes necessary when complete dependence has been reached or when secondary conditions such as bladder or pulmonary infection or decubitus ulcers intervene. While being cared for at home, the patient should receive regular supervision and assistance by a visiting nurse. It may be necessary for the hospital or clinic nurse to inform the family of this available service and make the initial referral. If the illness poses socioeconomic problems for the patient and his family, a social worker may be brought in to counsel them, or they may be advised of welfare agencies from which assistance may be obtained. They are told of the Multiple Sclerosis Society[10] and of the services it provides and are urged to avail themselves of these. As well as promoting research of the disease, the association assists in securing a wheelchair and self-help devices, transports patients to clinics, contacts sources of welfare, if needed, and has voluntary workers who make home visits and plan occupational therapy and recreational programs for multiple sclerosis patients.

A plan of care for the patient with multiple sclerosis includes the following considerations.

DURING REMISSIONS. In early remissions, when the residual effects are likely to be minimal, the patient is encouraged to resume his usual pattern of life, modifying it as necessary to avoid overfatigue, emotional stress and infections, since these frequently precipitate an exacerbation. A well-balanced diet, adequate, regular rest and learning to accept what cannot be readily changed to avoid emotional upsets are stressed. In the case of a married woman, the physician usually advises her of the increased risk of a relapse incurred by pregnancy. A visit to the physician or clinic at regular intervals is recommended.

REST. During a relapse, the patient is confined to bed for a period of 2 to 3 weeks or until symptoms begin to disappear. The promotion of rest and alleviation of the patient's likely psychological concern for his condition are a challenge to the nurse. Warm baths, massage, pleasant quiet surroundings, encouraging reading and listening to the radio and the nurse's taking time to visit and chat with the patient to avoid long periods of isolation may promote relaxation and rest. The limbs are passively moved through a full range of motion twice daily but active exercises are only permitted later when indicated by the doctor.

STEROID THERAPY. An adrenocorticoid preparation such as dexamethasone (Decadron), adrenocorticotropin (ACTH) or prednisone may be used to treat acute exacerbation. The response to this therapy varies with

[10]Multiple Sclerosis Society of Canada, 130 Bloor St. West, Toronto, Canada.

The National Multiple Sclerosis Society, 257 Park Ave. South, New York, U.S.A.

Both national associations have local chapters or branches throughout the provinces and states.

patients; some manifest a remission of symptoms fairly quickly, but others may show little improvement. Generally, at first the patient receives fairly large doses, which are gradually decreased over a number of weeks. He is observed closely when receiving the drug for changes in symptoms as well as for side effects.

PSYCHOLOGICAL FACTORS. Those associated with the patient should be aware of the possible personality and behavioral changes that are likely to develop. Frequently, relationships become strained and "scenes" and situations develop because of a lack of understanding that the patient's reactions and swings in mood are an actual part of his illness. If marked depression is evident, he is not left alone, and precautions are instituted to guard against suicide. Hobbies and interests are fostered to keep the patient occupied, remembering of course that fatigue is to be avoided. A quiet, cheerful environment, free of confusion, is important; the patient is likely to become emotional when exposed to an atmosphere of pressure or haste.

MOTOR DISABILITY. The patient is kept ambulatory as long as is reasonably possible. Spasticity and muscle spasms, especially in the lower limbs, are prone to develop in the advanced stages of the disease, and walking becomes increasingly difficult. In order to prevent falls, floors are not waxed and are kept clear of scatter rugs, stools, electric light cords, and other articles over which the patient might trip. It is helpful if hand rails are installed in appropriate places to facilitate continued mobility and independence. When stairs become difficult for the patient, consideration should be given to having the patient's room on the main floor. This may necessitate additional bathroom facilities, or moving to another house or an apartment. Articles he is likely to need for self-care or for the performances of small chores are kept within easy reach.

When walking becomes impossible, a wheelchair is provided, and the patient is taught to transfer himself from the bed to chair if he has sufficient strength in his arms and trunk. He is taught to maneuver the chair from room to room and outside if possible in order to widen his horizon and prevent isolation.

In the case of the homemaker, adjustments in the kitchen may be made to permit the patient to work from her wheelchair. Rehabil-itation centers usually have personnel who will assess the situation and make work simplification suggestions.

The family members require instructions on how to transfer the patient from the bed to a chair and on guarding against injury to him in the process.

A carefully controlled program of physical therapy may be prescribed after an acute exacerbation and continued within the patient's tolerance. It is introduced very gradually, and the patient is observed for regressive symptoms. Walking between parallel bars or with the aid of a walker may be helpful in rehabilitating the patient. He and his family are instructed as to the continuance of the program at home.

When spasticity develops in the paralyzed limbs, massage, passive movements and careful positioning similar to that used with the hemiplegic patient (see p. 840) are used to prevent contractures, joint immobility and deformities.

LOSS OF SENSATION. The interruption of sensory pathways may result in the patient's loss of awareness of temperature, pressure, pain, and position of limbs. Precautions are necessary to protect the patient; local heat applications are not used, and the temperature of the bath water must be carefully controlled; prolonged pressure and malpositioning are avoided.

SKIN CARE AND MOUTH CARE. As the patient becomes increasingly inactive, the skin requires frequent care and protection from prolonged pressure to prevent decubitus ulcers. His position is changed every 2 hours, and the skin is kept clean and dry and is gently massaged to stimulate circulation. Pressure is relieved by the use of pieces of sheepskin or sponge rubber and an air mattress. A footboard or cradle is provided to keep the weight of the bedding off the feet.

Muscular weakness or paralysis of the arms may prevent the patient from cleansing his teeth himself. There may also be some difficulty in swallowing which results in the accumulation of mucus and food particles in the mouth, leading to sordes. The teeth and mouth should be cleansed after each meal, or more often if indicated.

ELIMINATION. In the early stages of multiple sclerosis, the patient may experience urgency and occasional incontinency which he finds very distressing. Atropine or propantheline bromide (Pro-Banthine) may be prescribed to relax the detrusor muscle and increase bladder capacity. Rarely, a patient develops retention of urine during an acute relapse of the disease, necessitating catheterization. In the advanced stage of the disease, sphincter control usually is lost. An indwelling catheter may be used for a period of time to protect the skin. As soon as possible it is replaced by an attachable rubber or plastic urinal, and efforts are made to establish an automatic bladder.

Constipation is a common problem as a result of inactivity and weakness of the abdominal muscles. The fluid intake and roughage in the diet are increased, and a stool softener or bulk-producing laxative may be ordered. If the patient has incontinence of feces, regular use of a glycerin or bisacodyl (Dulcolax) suppository each morning stimulates evacuation at a convenient and predictable time.

PREVENTION OF PULMONARY COMPLICATIONS. Weakness of respiratory muscles results in shallow breathing and difficulty in coughing up secretions, predisposing the patient to chest infection. He is instructed to breathe deeply and encouraged to cough several times every 2 to 3 hours. In late stages of the disease, suctioning may be helpful. The patient with multiple sclerosis is protected as much as possible from contact with persons with infection.

Myasthenia Gravis

Myasthenia gravis is a chronic disorder characterized by weakness of the voluntary muscles of the body due to a chemical defect that interferes with the transmission of impulses at the neuromuscular junction.

The cause is not known, but it has been suggested that the nerve fibers release insufficient acetylcholine (ACH) or that there is a deficiency in the number of receptors in the motor end-plate that are sensitive to acetylcholine. On the basis of the increased antibodies that react against muscle tissue elements, it is thought that the disease may be of autoimmune origin.[11] The disease is also known to be associated with disorders of the thymus gland, primarily hyperplasia of the

gland. It can affect muscles innervated by bulbar nuclei (face, eyes, lips, tongue, throat and neck) and limb musculature. Diagnosis is often difficult.

MANIFESTATIONS. Symptoms may be vague and associated with physical exertion and emotional upset. The patient may present with ptosis, diplopia, dysphagia, limb weakness and breathing difficulty. He may complain that he feels fairly strong on rising in the morning but becomes weak as the day progresses.

The disease is characterized by remissions and exacerbations. It affects women twice as often as men, with the onset usually between the ages of 15 and 30. Men develop it more often after the age of 50. It can affect the newborn babies of myasthenic mothers, causing acute symptoms in the first few days of life. Treatment of these babies is usually effective and, normally, symptoms disappear about the sixth week of life with no recurrence. Children may develop the disease up to puberty and the prognosis is usually good.

DIAGNOSTIC TESTS. There are two types of tests which may be used in diagnosing myasthenia gravis. *Confirmatory tests* are those in which anticholinesterase drugs, such as edrophonium chloride (Tensilon), which inhibit the destruction of acetylcholine are injected intravenously. After a period of 30 to 90 seconds, signs of weakness should decrease — for example, a drooping eyelid should return to normal and there should be some return to limb strength. Prostigmin in combination with atropine may be given intramuscularly instead of Tensilon. The improvement here is slower.

Provocative tests are those which involve using a depolarizing motor end-plate blocking agent, such as curare, which greatly increases any weakness. This weakness should then respond to the Tensilon test. These provocative tests are very dangerous unless used by trained staff who have equipment readily available to intubate and ventilate the patient in case of respiratory failure. Electromyographic studies (see p. 835) are also done in the process of diagnosing the disease.

TREATMENT. There is as yet no cure for myasthenia gravis, but present methods of treatment provide effective control for varying periods of time.

DRUG THERAPY. Anticholinesterase drugs such as neostigmine (Prostigmin), pyridostigmine bromide (Mestinon Bromide) and

[11]Benjamin F. Miller and Claire B. Keane: Encyclopedia and Dictionary of Medicine, Nursing and Allied Health, 2nd ed. Philadelphia, W. B. Saunders, 1978, p. 660.

ambenomium chloride (Mytelase) are the drugs most commonly used. They may not prove equally effective for all patients; while they are being tried, the patient is usually hospitalized and observed for his reaction and for any drug side effects. He will be sent home on a very specific regime with drugs to be given at times that will produce the maximum effect when most needed. Some patients must learn to wake themselves up at night for a dose.

The adrenocorticotropic hormone (ACTH) may be used to induce relief of a severe exacerbation. The reason for its usefulness is not entirely understood, although it may be related to the effect of corticoids on the immunologic process. ACTH treatment is administered under medical surveillance, preferably in an intensive care unit. A course of the drug is given over 8 to 10 days. On the third or fourth day the patient's condition usually becomes much worse and assisted mechanical ventilation will probably be necessary. In some centers a tracheostomy is performed before treatment is commenced to prevent the risk of respiratory insufficiency. Improvement usually begins approximately 48 to 72 hours after the ACTH has been discontinued. Hopefully, the patient remains in an improved condition for about 7 months. The treatment may then have to be repeated. Some patients require several courses of treatment during their lifetime.

SURGERY. Thymectomy has proven successful for patients with hyperplasia of the thymus gland. It is a major operative procedure and is recommended only for those who have involvement of parts innervated by bulbar nuclei, as well as jaw, limb and trunk muscles, and who cannot be controlled by drug therapy.

NURSING CARE. It is important for the nurse caring for a patient with myasthenia gravis to know the patient, especially his fears, abilities and response to treatment. Personnel caring for the patient will be responsible for observing and recording the effects of the drugs and for recognizing the times they are most needed, as well as any untoward side effects. It is necessary to be constantly alert for respiratory problems and report any coughing or swallowing difficulties. The patient is taught to restrict his activities to avoid becoming overfatigued. He is advised to rest before meals, since chewing may deplete his muscular potential. The patient and family are also counseled that an

episode may be precipitated by emotional upsets, the ingestion of alcohol, and respiratory infection.

During an exacerbation the patient is confined to bed and requires total nursing care. He is given rest periods while being fed and his food should be soft and easy to manage. Nasogastric feedings may be necessary. If the swallowing muscles are involved, positioning to avoid aspiration of secretion is important. Frequent mouth care is necessary to maintain clearance of secretions. The nurse should be aware that infection will worsen symptoms and should take necessary precautions to protect the patient.

If the patient is to have ACTH therapy, or if surgery is planned, the probable sequence of events is explained to reduce his fear. If mechanical ventilatory assistance is anticipated, care is similar to that cited on p. 426.

When the patient is transferred from an intensive care area he may demonstrate his fear by being very demanding and inventing excuses to have someone in his room. The nurse recognizes the patient's anxiety and explains that staff can be contacted quickly and a nurse will check on him at frequent intervals. The amount of time spent with him is gradually decreased as the patient regains his independence.

MYASTHENIC CRISIS. The patient with myasthenia gravis is predisposed to sudden acute episodes of severe muscular weakness in which respiratory insufficiency and the inability to swallow are manifested. The episode is referred to as a crisis since it is immediately life-threatening. The crisis may be categorized as myasthenic, cholinergic or brittle. The *myasthenic type* is attributed to a temporary resistance to or inadequate dosage of the cholinergic preparation being administered. The *cholinergic crisis* is caused by an excess of anticholinesterase medication. The patient becomes pale and experiences diaphoresis, increased salivation and bronchial secretion, abdominal cramps, diarrhea, nausea, vomiting and blurred vision. In a *brittle crisis,* there is an unpredictable response to drugs; the patient's condition is not improved by increasing or decreasing the anticholinesterase preparation.

To differentiate between the types of crises, the patient may be given an intravenous injection of edrophonium chloride (Tensilon) by the physician. If the crisis is myasthenic, the patient's muscle weakness is reversed and regular dosage of the cholinergic drug is increased. If the muscle weakness is increased, a decrease in the drug administration is indicated. Respiration is supported by intubation and mechanical ventilation with positive pressure. If necessary for more effective removal of respiratory secretions, a tracheostomy is done and deep suctioning used. In the case of a brittle crisis, drug administration is discontinued and the patient supported on a mechanical respirator. Atropine sulfate may be prescribed for the patient to decrease the secretions. Fluids are given intravenously to sustain the patient.

TEACHING. The patient and family require extensive teaching and support when myasthenia gravis is diagnosed. The necessity of the patient adjusting his life style to his symptoms is explained, as is the importance of taking his medication exactly as directed by the physician. They are advised of significant side effects and the appropriate action to take if they occur. The family should be aware of the symptoms of an oncoming crisis and the need to report them immediately so that the patient can be hospitalized and treated promptly. It is advisable to have some family member trained in mouth-to-mouth resuscitation in case artificial respiration is needed before the patient reaches the hospital.

Because many drugs can cause a worsening of myasthenia gravis, the patient is advised not to take any medication that has not been prescribed by his physician. For example, diazepam or barbiturate and opiate preparations depress respirations. Antibiotic therapy is usually only given in the hospital under close supervision.

If the diet requires adjustment because of weakness of the chewing and swallowing muscles, details as to preparation, content and serving times are reviewed.

A patient whose periods of exacerbation are brought under control can, with care, live a fairly normal existence. If the patient's condition is such that he requires assistance with his personal care and requires closer supervision, a referral may be made to a visiting nurse organization. The patient and family are informed of the services of the Myasthenia Gravis Foundation[12] and given copies of the brochures published by this organization.

---

[12]The Myasthenia Gravis Foundation, c/o the Muscular Dystrophy Association of Canada, 74 Victoria St., Toronto, Ontario, Canada.

The Myasthenia Gravis Foundation, Inc., 2 East 103rd St., New York, New York, U.S.A.

NEOPLASMS OF THE NERVOUS SYSTEM

Intracranial Newgrowths

Primary intracranial newgrowths most commonly arise from the neuroglial tissue, meninges, cerebral blood vessels, hypophysis and nerve fibers. They are named according to their tissue origin and may be benign or malignant (see Table 23–4 for the names, origins and most frequent sites of intracranial tumors). The brain is not an infrequent location for metastatic tumors; the most frequent sites of the primary malignancy are the lungs, breast, skin, gastrointestinal tract and the kidneys. Primary malignant neoplasms of the brain differ from those elsewhere in the body in that they rarely metastasize to other parts.

MANIFESTATIONS. Any intracranial newgrowth is a space-occupying lesion which imposes on surrounding tissue and raises the intracranial pressure by increasing the content of the cranium. The signs and symptoms are extremely variable and are classified as general or focal. *Focal symptoms* are the result of the local effects of the neoplasm and reflect its location. The compression or tissue destruction that it causes interferes with the function(s) of that particular area of the brain and may be motor, sensory or psychological. Examples of focal manifestations include weakness or paralysis of a limb, ataxia, convulsions, aphasia, change in personality, disorientation, impaired intellect, impaired vision, loss of hearing, facial paralysis and loss of sensations. They usually develop gradually and may be single or multiple from the onset.

General symptoms occur as a result of increased intracranial pressure and ensuing compression of brain tissue. The increase in the pressure may be due directly to the space-occupying lesion within the rigid cranium or to the associated cerebral edema, venous congestion or an obstruction in the cerebrospinal fluid pathway.

Manifestations of increasing intracranial pressure due to an intracranial tumor may include the following:

Headache, which may also be due to traction on pain-sensitive structures such as blood vessels and cranial nerves, is usually one of the early symptoms and is intensified by activities such as coughing, vomiting, straining at stool and lowering of the head.

TABLE 23-4 INTRACRANIAL TUMORS

Name of Neoplasm	Origin	Most Frequent Sites	Comments
Gliomas	Neuroglial tissue		Commonest type of intracranial neoplasm; rate of growth varies with type of glioma
Astrocytoma	Astrocytes	Adults—cerebrum Children—cerebellum	Most common glioma; grows very slowly; infiltrates surrounding tissue
Glioblastoma	Undifferentiated glial cells	Frontal, parietal and temporal lobes	Highly malignant
Medulloblastoma	Undifferentiated glial cells	Cerebellum	Rapid extension; highly malignant
Ependymoma	Ependymal cells of the lining of the ventricle and aqueducts	Fourth ventricle	Rare; frequently papillomatous; may obstruct flow of CSF
Oligodendroglioma	Oligodendrocytes	Cerebral hemispheres	Rare; grows very slowly; tends to calcify
Meningioma	Meninges	Along the course of the intracranial venous sinuses	Are extracerebral, causing compression of brain tissue; usually encapsulated; grow slowly
Hemangiomas Angioma	Blood vessel wall	Middle cerebral artery	(Not a true neoplasm) Congenital mass of tortuous, enlarged vessels; benign, but may interfere with adjacent tissues
Angioblastoma	Blood vessel wall	Cerebellum	Tendency to form cysts
Pituitary Adenomas Chromophobe adenoma	Adenohypophyseal glandular tissue	Anterior pituitary lobe (adenohypophysis)	Encapsulated; compresses pituitary gland tissue and optic nerves, leading to hypopituitarism and impaired vision
Chromophil adenoma (acidophilic adenoma)	Adenohypophyseal glandular tissue	Anterior pituitary lobe (adenohypophysis	Seen less often than chromophobe adenoma; causes hyperpituitarism (gigantism or acromegaly)
Craniopharyngioma	Embryologic defect in craniopharyngeal duct	Anterior to the pituitary stalk	Produces pressure on surrounding structures, interfering with function
Acoustic Neuroma	Eighth cranial (acoustic) nerve		Encapsulated

Mental disturbances gradually appear and may be mild at the onset, probably taking the form of fatigue, listlessness, a short attention span, restlessness, irritability or emotional instability. They become more marked as the pressure increases and may progress through disorientation and stupor to an eventual loss of consciousness.

Vomiting may occur due to pressure on the vomiting center in the medulla. It may not be preceded by nausea and usually occurs during the night or early morning.

Papilledema and *visual disturbances* may occur.

Changes in vital signs occur as a result of pressure on the brain stem and venous congestion. The blood pressure rises and is accompanied by a slowing of the pulse rate. The respirations tend to become slower, then irregular or Cheyne-Stokes.

Dilation and *failing reaction to light of one or both pupils* may occur due to pressure on the third cranial (oculomotor) nerve.

A *seizure* may be the first presenting symptom.

Progressive loss of function of limbs may occur.

The patient undergoes an extensive neurological examination for motor sensory and intellectual functions.

Various diagnostic procedures are done which may include roentgenograms, an arteriogram, computerized transaxial tomography, ventriculogram, brain scan using a radioisotope, electroencephalogram and biopsy (see p. 830).

TREATMENT AND NURSING CARE. The type of treatment used for the patient with an intracranial neoplasm depends on the location and type of tumor, and his general condition. Surgery or radiation may be used. Whenever possible, surgical excision of the neoplasm is the method of choice but, in many instances, the neoplasm may be inaccessible or may involve vital areas, making removal impossible (e.g., brain stem). Nonencapsulated neoplasms infiltrate surrounding tissue, thus making surgery less effective. Radiation therapy may then be used. The tumors most successfully treated by surgery are meningiomas, acoustic neuromas, pituitary adenomas, and astrocytomas; these tumors, with the exception of the astrocytomas, are extracerebral. In the case of an inoperable neoplasm which is obstructing the cerebrospinal fluid pathway, a tube may be placed between the lateral ventricle and the cisterna magna (subarachnoid space in posterior area below the brain) to bypass the obstruction (Torkildsen operation) or between the ventricle and the peritoneal cavity (ventriculoperitoneal shunt). When the lesion is inaccessible or cannot be removed because of a vital area (such as the midbrain) being involved, a palliative decompression operation may be performed in which a portion of the skull is removed to reduce the intracranial pressure. This retards brain damage and relieves some symptoms.

The nurse carefully notes and records the patient's motor and sensory functions, speech ability, complaints such as headache, dizziness, tingling or numbness of a part, responses and behavior, orientation, ability to carry out usual daily activities, pupillary size and reaction to light, and vital signs. Observation is an ongoing process through successive contacts so that changes and newly developed symptoms may be promptly recognized. The nurse's recognition and accurate recording of deviant physical and behavioral factors may play an important role in the diagnosis and localization of the intracranial newgrowth. Knowing that a space-occupying growth is suspect, the nurse is especially alert for signs of increasing intracranial pressure. Measures such as side rails on the bed are used to prevent possible accidents.

Nursing care is planned according to the patient's needs which are determined mainly by the disturbances, dysfunction and dependencies caused by the intracranial lesion. He is kept ambulatory if his condition permits. If confined to bed, the head of the bed is elevated to promote cerebral venous drainage, which helps to reduce the intracranial pressure and headache. The nurse changes his position at regular, frequent intervals if the patient is lethargic, listless or semiconscious and tends to remain immobile. Particular attention is paid to his nutritional status; an adequate intake is especially important if surgery is anticipated.

The patient may be very upset emotionally and in despair about his future. Acknowledging his fear as understandable, encouraging him to talk about the situation and his feelings, and adequate explanations in preparation for the various diagnostic procedures may reduce his insecurity. The family's anxiety is understandable. Recognition of their concerns, stopping to talk with them and keeping them informed about the patient and what is being done for him instills confidence and helps them to accept the situation. In some instances, it is necessary to suggest that they avoid conveying their emotions to the patient, explaining that he is in need of their support and positive attitude.

A mild analgesic such as acetylsalicylic acid may be used for the relief of headache. Diphenylhydantoin sodium (Dilantin) may be prescribed for oral or intravenous administration to control seizures. To reduce intracranial pressure, osmotic diuresis may be induced by the intravenous injection of mannitol (Osmitrol) or a hypertonic solution of urea and glucose (Urevert). These preparations are not reabsorbed by the renal tubule, and, by their osmotic action, they reduce the amount of water reabsorbed from the glomerular filtrate and increase the urinary output. Dexamethasone (Decadron), an adrenocorticosteroid drug, is frequently prescribed for patients with an intracranial lesion to control intracranial pressure that may be aggravated by the inflammatory process. It may be administered orally or by intramuscular injections.

Immediate preoperative and postoperative care is that cited on p. 864.

Spinal Neoplasms

Newgrowths which arise within or encroach upon the spinal cord may be benign or malignant, primary or secondary (metastatic), and may be classified according to their origin as extradural or intradural. The *extradural neoplasms* occur in the vertebrae or the space between the dura mater and vertebrae and are most commonly metastases. As they enlarge, they encroach on the cord because of the limited space and cause pressure on nerve roots and cord. *Intradural tumors* are extramedullary (outside the spinal cord) or intramedullary (arise within the cord). The intradural-extramedullary type constitutes about 50 per cent of all spinal neoplasms. They may arise from the meninges (meningiomas), nerve roots (neuromas or neurofibromas) or blood vessels (hemangiomas). Gliomas comprise the majority of intramedullary newgrowths.

MANIFESTATIONS. The compression of nerve roots or tracts and neurons within the cord by a neoplasm is manifested by sensory and motor dysfunction. The parts of the body affected depend upon the level of the lesion. In the case of nerve root involvement, the affected areas correspond to those innervated by those particular spinal nerve fibers. Involvement of cord tracts and neurons may interfere with functions in all parts on one or both sides of the body which derive their innervation from the cord below the level of the lesion.

Damage and eventual loss of impulse conduction in the anterior (motor) nerve roots by an extramedullary growth produce progressive muscle weakness, flaccid paralysis, loss of tendon reflexes and muscle wasting comparable to lower motor neuron paralysis (see p. 826). Irritation of the posterior (sensory) nerve roots causes pain and abnormal sensations (e.g., tingling, "pins and needles"). Eventually, as the neoplasm extends, interruption of the impulses results in a loss of sensations.

Newgrowths within the cord or compression by an extramedullary tumor may involve sensory or motor tracts. Pain, pressure and temperature sensations may be dulled or lost, and the patient may be unable to appreciate the position of affected limbs due to interference with proprioception impulse pathways. Damage to the pyramidal tracts (corticospinal motor tracts) produces muscle weakness at first, then spastic paralysis, exaggerated tendon reflexes, and bladder and bowel dysfunction similar to that of an upper motor neuron lesion (see p. 826).

Disturbed motor or sensory function may involve parts of one or both sides of the body, depending on the extent of the compression.

Investigative procedures usually include a lumbar puncture to determine possible obstruction to the cerebrospinal flow, roentgenograms of the spine, and a myelogram (see p. 833).

TREATMENT AND NURSING CARE. Primary extramedullary neoplasms are removed by surgery as soon as diagnosed; unnecessary delay may result in permanent paralysis. Intramedullary growths are more difficult to remove without seriously damaging the spinal cord and interrupting motor and sensory tracts. When the spinal neoplasm is inoperable or metastatic, relief of compression of the cord by laminectomy and probably partial resection of the newgrowth may be done. Radiation therapy of the involved area or chemotherapy may be used as an adjunct to surgery or alone if the lesion is inoperable. For preoperative preparation of the patient for spinal surgery, and postoperative nursing care, see page 878.

The care required by the patient who is inoperable or during investigation depends on the discomfort and disability he experiences. Loss of voluntary muscle power may vary from slight loss of strength in one group of muscles to paraplegia or quadriplegia and complete dependence.

Close observation is made for exaggeration of the patient's symptoms and for the appearance of new ones, indicating compression and damage. Significant factors to be noted are motor abilities (strength, coordination and motion), complaints of pain, abnormal sensations or loss of feeling, bladder dysfunction, which may be manifested by frequency, urgency incontinence or retention, bowel dysfunction (constipation or fecal incontinence), condition of the skin, especially over the vulnerable bony prominences, and the patient's reactions to the illness.

TRAUMA OF THE NERVOUS SYSTEM

Head Injuries

Head injuries have become a major problem because of the present-day mechanization and increasing number of automobile accidents. In areas where wearing seat belts has become mandatory, there appears to be a lessening of the number of severe head injuries due to motor vehicle accidents. An accident may result in laceration of the scalp, skull fracture or brain injury. If there is a wound in the scalp and a fracture of the skull, permitting communication between the air outside and the cranial cavity, the injury is termed open. Conversely, a closed injury is one in which the skull remains intact.

LACERATION OF THE SCALP. The scalp is quite vascular and, when lacerated or torn away from the skull, it bleeds readily. The wound is cleansed thoroughly and sutured. Repair is usually delayed if fracture of the skull and brain injury are suspected or if the patient is in shock. In such cases the wound is cleansed, and a sterile dressing is applied. Efforts are made to determine if the patient has had immunizing tetanus toxoid injections. If he has, a booster dose of the toxoid may be ordered; if there has been no previous immunization, a prophylactic dose of human tetanus immunoglobulin will be prescribed. Before this is given, the patient or his family is questioned as to any history of allergic reactions, eczema and asthma, and a small test dose is administered intracutaneously.

FRACTURE OF THE SKULL. When a patient is known to have received a blow on the head or is unconscious following an accident, roentgenograms are made of the skull and examined for possible fracture. A skull fracture may be classified as linear, comminuted, compound or depressed.

A linear or simple fracture is one in which there are two fragments which remain in apposition or are not displaced.

In a comminuted fracture, multiple linear fractures occur, but the fragments are not displaced. No specific treatment is used for a simple linear or comminuted skull fracture, but the patient is kept at rest and the head of his bed is elevated. He is under close observation because a fracture rarely occurs without injury to blood vessels and the brain. Meningeal blood vessels may have been torn, and this will lead to extradural, subdural or subarachnoid hemorrhage. Concussion or contusion of the brain is a frequent concomitant.

A compound fracture implies that there is communication with the outside because of a scalp wound, predisposing to infection of the bone and cranial contents. The scalp wound is cleansed thoroughly, débrided[13] and repaired as soon as the patient's condition permits to reduce the possibility of infection.

A depressed fracture is one in which the fragments are driven inward, compressing or piercing the meninges and brain. As well as direct injury to the cranial contents at the site of the fracture, there is likely to be a rapid increase in the intracranial pressure, affecting total brain functioning. This type of skull fracture requires early surgical treatment in which the fragments are elevated and any loose pieces or splinters are removed. In some instances, the surgeon may find it necessary to remove a portion of the skull which has been severely fragmented. Later, a cranioplasty may be done in which a "plate" of inert material, such as Vitallium, may be inserted to protect the brain and improve the patient's appearance. The care of the patient following skull decompression is similar to that cited on page 862.

The bone is thinner in some areas of the base of the skull, making it less resistant to force. Basal fractures are more hazardous because they may open into paranasal sinuses or the middle ear, predisposing to infection. In this type of fracture, the drainage of blood and cerebrospinal fluid from the nose and external ear may occur. Cranial nerves emerging through the skull may be injured or, if the fracture is adjacent to the medulla oblongata, vital centers may be seriously damaged.

Rarely, a basal skull fracture results from an indirect blow. The commonest cause is a fall from a height in which the person lands on his feet or buttocks. The impact of the spine against the base of the skull may produce a serious basal fracture.

BRAIN INJURY. Slight or severe brain injury may result from a blow to the head and

---

[13]Débridement is the removal of foreign material and macerated, devitalized tissue.

may or may not be associated with a fracture of the skull. A head injury may cause concussion, contusion, laceration, hemorrhage and/or compression. Injury may occur on the same side of the brain as the site of the impact and/or on the opposite side. If the area of the brain just beneath the site of the skull trauma is injured as a result of its rebound against the cranium, it is referred to as a *coup injury*. The injury on the opposite side is due to the wave of pressure created by the blow, compressing the soft gelatinous-like brain substance against the bony ridges and opposite cranial wall. This is referred to as a *contracoup injury*. For instance, a fall on the back of the head may cause injury to the frontal and temporal cerebral lobes. Superficial and deeper cerebral vessels may be ruptured, meninges may be torn, and the brain tissue may be bruised, lacerated or compressed. The brain injury may be mild and reversible or may be severe and irreversible, leaving residual neurological deficits and disabilities if the patient survives. Cerebral edema and intracranial hemorrhage increase the intracranial pressure which, if severe, may compress the brain stem and its vital centers.

Concussion is characterized by a brief period of unconsciousness due to jarring of the brain and its sudden forceful contact with the rigid skull. Normal brain activity is temporarily interrupted, including the reticular-activating system of the brain stem which normally maintains the conscious state. The period of unconsciousness varies from a few minutes to several hours, depending on the severity of the injury. The patient presents a picture of shock; the face is pale, the pulse rate and respirations are depressed, the skin is cold and clammy and reflexes are diminished. Concussion is usually spontaneously reversible, leaving no permanent damage. When the patient regains consciousness he may be dazed, confused, restless and unable to recall what happened preceding the accident. Pulse and respirations improve and muscle tone and reflexes return. Vomiting is common in this recovery period, and the patient usually complains of headache.

Contusion (bruising) of the brain causes small, diffuse venous hemorrhages (Fig. 23–23). The area in the region of the offending force becomes edematous and swollen, and intracranial pressure increases. The patient may recover from the associated concussion,

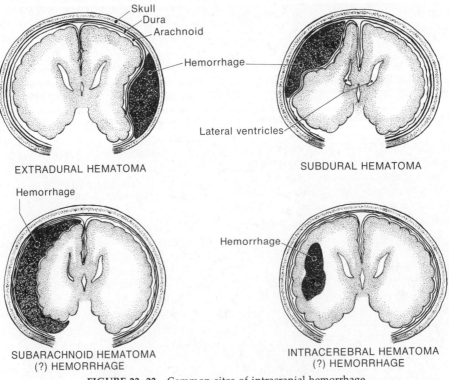

Skull
Dura
Arachnoid

Hemorrhage

Lateral ventricles

EXTRADURAL HEMATOMA

SUBDURAL HEMATOMA

Hemorrhage

SUBARACHNOID HEMATOMA
(?) HEMORRHAGE

Hemorrhage

INTRACEREBRAL HEMATOMA
(?) HEMORRHAGE

FIGURE 23–23   Common sites of intracranial hemorrhage.

but then he progressively regresses as the bleeding continues and intracranial pressure increases. Recovery from contusion may take several weeks. Permanent tissue damage and scarring may result in impaired motor, sensory and/or intellectual functions, or epilepsy.

Cerebral lacerations may occur when the brain is forced against rough and sharp ridges of bone. Meninges and vessels are torn, and intracranial hemorrhage follows, causing pressure. The intracranial bleeding is usually subdural or, rarely, epidural. The latter is between the skull and the dura mater and is frequently caused by the laceration of the middle meningeal artery or dural sinuses. The loss of blood is severe, incurring serious brain compression; emergency surgery is necessary to remove the blood and arrest the bleeding. The blood loss may necessitate a transfusion.

Subdural bleeding is due to a damaged vessel on the surface of the brain. The bleeding and accumulation of blood in the subdural space may occur slowly over several hours or days. The development of symptoms may be delayed and initially may be vague but progressively increase, and eventually the patient may become comatose.

Compression of the brain may result from a depressed fracture, edema and swelling of the brain and intracranial hemorrhage, which may be epidural, subdural, subarachnoid or intracerebral. The patient manifests progressive deepening of unconsciousness and symptoms of increasing intracranial pressure.

Supratentorial herniation is a very critical condition that may be associated with brain trauma. The tentorium is a fold of the dura mater which lies below the cerebrum, separating it from the cerebellum and brain stem. As the brain stem ascends to join the cerebrum it passes through a space referred to as the tentorial hiatus. The rigid skull prevents any outward expansion of the contents of the intracranial cerebral area; as a result a space-occupying lesion, such as a hematoma, may precipitate the herniation of a portion of the cerebrum through the tentorial hiatus. This leads to compression of the brain stem and its vital centers. The patient becomes comatose due to interference with the reticular-activating system and respiratory failure may develop. Drugs are administered to remove fluid from the intracranial cavity and emergency surgery is undertaken to relieve the compression.

To summarize, the signs and symptoms associated with a head injury depend on the nature and severity of the tissue damage. They may appear immediately following the accident or several hours afterward as a result of cerebral edema, swelling of the brain or intracranial bleeding and the ensuing brain compression and elevation in intracranial pressure. The symptoms may include: unconsciousness, which may develop at the time of injury and last for a varying length of time or may occur following a lucid interval and progressive drowsiness and stupor due to intracranial hemorrhage; headache and dizziness; disturbed vision; dilation and failure to react to light of one or both pupils; changes in vital signs, which may be characteristic of shock at first (low blood pressure, weak pulse and shallow respirations), then indicative of increasing intracranial pressure (abnormal elevation in blood pressure, slowing of the pulse); disorientation and confusion; motor and sensory deficits; convulsions; speech impairment; nuchal rigidity (stiffness of the neck) and hyperextension due to meningeal irritation; the escape of blood and cerebrospinal fluid through the nose or external ear; and hyperthermia due to interference with the heat-regulating center in the hypothalamus.

TREATMENT AND NURSING CARE IN HEAD INJURIES

EMERGENCY CARE. As in all emergencies, the first consideration is to insure a clear airway for respiratory exchange. The brain cells are very dependent upon a continuous oxygen supply and, if injured, adequate provision becomes even more imperative. A clear airway is also important because obstruction tends to increase cerebral venous congestion and intracranial pressure. Keeping the spine straight, the patient is carefully turned to a lateral or semiprone position to minimize the danger of aspiration. Flexion or hyperextension of the head is avoided in case there is a cervical vertebral fracture or dislocation that could seriously damage the spinal cord with movement. An open scalp wound is covered with available clean material. The victim is covered and kept quiet and undisturbed while arrangements are made to transport him to the hospital, even if he remains conscious.

On arrival at a hospital, further consideration is given to the airway; suctioning may be used to remove mucus, blood or vomitus and an intratracheal tube may be introduced, or a tracheostomy may be done immediately. A mechanical respirator may be used if there is respiratory depression and insufficiency. The patient receives a quick, complete examination to determine the extent of the total injuries. Intravenous solutions, a blood transfusion and administration of a vasopressor drug such as levarterenol (Levophed) may be necessary for the treatment of shock. If there is an open wound, a reinforcing dose of tetanus toxoid may be ordered or human tetanus immunoglobulin may be given. X-rays of the skull are taken as soon as the initial emergency treatment is completed, and a lumbar puncture may be performed to determine if there is blood in the cerebrospinal fluid. If there is a compressed or compound fracture, or there are indications of a developing hematoma, immediate surgery may be necessary to relieve compression of the brain (see the care of the patient with intracranial surgery, p. 864).

The patient who has what appears to be a minor injury and who did not lose consciousness or recovered it within a few minutes of the accident may be permitted to go home after being examined by the physician. A family member or friend should remain with the patient and *is advised to rouse and observe him hourly*. The physician should be notified or the patient taken to the hospital if he becomes abnormally drowsy or dizzy, vomits or experiences headache of increasing severity, visual disturbance or loss of strength in a limb.

Care of the nonsurgical patient with a head injury includes the following considerations.

OBSERVATIONS. Observation is an extremely important nursing responsibility in the care of the patient with a head injury so that significant changes and complications may be recognized in the early stage and treated promptly. On admission to the hospital, an assessment and recording are made of the patient's vital signs, level of consciousness, comprehension, orientation, responses to stimuli and commands, motor power of the limbs, and pupillary size and reaction. These initial observations serve as a guide in planning nursing care and as a baseline so that even slight changes may be readily recognized. The neurological evaluation is repeated usually at half-hour to hourly intervals for 24 hours. The physician is notified promptly of changes such as an increase in the blood pressure, decrease in pulse rate, change in respirations, dulling or loss of consciousness, inequality of pupils, and loss of strength in one or more limbs. The interval is gradually lengthened to 2, 3 and 4 hours as indicated by the physician on the basis of the patient's progress. The rectal temperature is usually recorded every 2 hours from the onset unless hyperthermia develops, making hourly recordings necessary. Some neurological units have a special form on which the frequent observations are recorded. In some situations, provison may be made for continuous monitoring of the heart action (electrocardiogram), cerebral activity (electroencephalogram), blood pressure and temperature.

When consciousness is regained soon after the injury, the patient is aroused gently and slowly every hour when he goes to sleep to determine his level of consciousness and to examine him for possible changes.

POSITIONING. If the patient is unconscious, he is kept in a lateral or semiprone position to prevent aspiration. Unless contraindicated by his particular injury, he is turned from side to side at least every 2 hours. The uppermost limbs are supported in order to prevent strain on the joints (see positioning, p. 844). The neck is kept straight and is aligned with the spine. When the patient regains consciousness, the head of the bed is usually elevated slightly to promote cerebral venous drainage.

PROTECTION FROM INJURY. Emergence from coma may be accompanied by restlessness and confusion, which may last for a brief period or for several days. Side rails are used on the bed and may need to be padded if the patient is restless; a nurse, nursing aide or relative remains in constant attendance to prevent self-injury. Restraints only tend to agitate the patient further and increase his thrashing about.

MINIMUM OF STIMULI. The patient is kept as quiet as possible, being disturbed only for essential care. The blood pressure cuff is left on the arm between recordings. A semidarkened room and restriction of visitors help to reduce external stimuli.

FLUIDS AND NUTRITION. The patient may have to be supported by intravenous fluids or nasogastric tube feedings for a period of time. When conscious, oral fluids and a soft diet are given and increased to a light diet as soon as tolerated. The 24-hour volume of fluid may be limited if the patient manifests any signs of increased intracranial pressure. The intake and output are measured and recorded, and the balance is noted.

ELIMINATION. Occasionally, retention of urine may be present and may be responsible for the patient's restlessness. More often, incontinence of urine occurs. An indwelling catheter may be passed to prevent incontinence and to protect the skin and insure that an accurate record may be made of the urinary output. A mild laxative or a glycerin or bisacodyl (Dulcolax) rectal suppository may be ordered after 2 to 3 days if the bowels have not moved. Constipation, straining at stool and impaction must be prevented to avoid increasing the intracranial pressure. No enema is given without a physician's order.

SKIN CARE. While the patient is unconscious, and during the period in which he is confined to bed on restricted activity, pressure areas require special attention to prevent decubitus ulcers. The usual measures of frequent change of position, keeping the skin clean and dry, massage and the use of soft resilient material under pressure areas or an air mattress are necessary. If the patient is restless, the elbows, knees and heels may require extra protection by the application of soft pads and bandages to prevent excoriation.

MEDICATIONS. A mild sedative or tranquilizer may be ordered to prevent exhaustion if the patient is extremely restless. Examples of drugs used are chlorpromazine hydrochloride (Thorazine, Largactil), a barbiturate preparation such as phenobarbital, chloral hydrate and paraldehyde. The use of strong sedatives and narcotics is avoided, since they tend to mask neurological symptoms and, as a result, serious changes may not be recognized.

If the patient has received some brain injury, dexamethasone (Decadron) may be ordered to reduce possible cerebral edema by controlling the inflammatory process. Acute increased intracranial pressure may also be treated by inducing osmotic diuresis by the intravenous administration of mannitol (Osmitrol) or a hypertonic solution of urea and glucose (Urevert).

An anticonvulsant drug such as diphenylhydantoin sodium (Dilantin) or phenobarbital (Luminal Sodium) may be ordered parenterally if the patient has a seizure.

OTHER CONSIDERATIONS. If there is intracranial hemorrhage, the patient may develop a convulsion. The pillows are removed and the patient is placed in a lateral or semiprone position. He is restrained only sufficiently to prevent injury. It is important to note the parts of the body involved and which area was involved first, if the head and eyes turned to one side, the duration of the convulsion, and the condition of the patient following the seizure. (See p. 888 for care of the convulsive patient.)

The patient with a head injury and who is conscious commonly experiences a severe headache for several days following the accident. An ice bag may provide some relief and acetylsalicylic acid (aspirin) may be prescribed.

If bleeding and the escape of cerebrospinal fluid from an ear or the nasal cavities occur with a fracture of the base of the skull, a dry sterile dressing is placed over the external orifice(s) and is changed frequently. The amount and color of the drainage is noted and recorded. If conscious, the patient is cautioned against blowing his nose. Under no circumstances should either area be packed tightly, any fluid introduced or any tubes inserted via the nose.

While the patient is unconscious, the eyes are examined frequently for possible dryness of the cornea and failure of the eyelids to close. Brain injury may result in impaired nerve function, causing exposure of the eye and diminished secretion. Regular irrigation of each eye with sterile normal saline, the instillation of an artificial tear solution such as methyl cellulose in saline and a protective eye shield may be necessary. Any sign of irritation is promptly brought to the physician's attention. Occasionally periocular edema, bleeding into the tissue and swelling are associated with a head injury. Iced compresses or a small ice bag may be applied. The fluid is usually absorbed, and the swelling is relieved in 3 or 4 days.

Hyperthermia may develop following an injury and is due to disturbance of the temperature control center in the hypothalamus or infection. If the patient manifests an elevation of 38° C. (100° F.), the patient is covered only with a light cotton sheet, and fans or air conditioning are used to keep the room temperature at 18° to 20° C. (65° to 68° F.), if possible. If the fever continues to rise, alcohol sponges are used or hypothermia may be ordered (see p. 111). Acetylsalicylic acid (aspirin) may be ordered by mouth or may be given by rectum if the patient is unconscious. A progressive elevation of temperature is an unfavorable sign.

THE FAMILY. The family can be expected to be greatly concerned for the patient. The nurse has a responsibility to assist them and provide support by talking with them at intervals, acknowledging their anxiety, keeping them informed as to the patient's treatment and progress, and making suggestions in the interest of their own welfare, as well, of how they can be most helpful to the patient. When the patient is well enough to leave the hospital, at least one member of the family is advised of the prescribed plan for continuity of care and rehabilitation. In some instances, when the accident victim has been the family provider, a referral to a social service or welfare agency may be necessary.

REHABILITATION. Following a head and brain injury, the patient may have some residual disability. He is evaluated, and a rehabilitation program of physical exercises and retraining is planned and started as soon as his condition permits. Progress may be slow, and the patient tends to become easily discouraged. The nurse plays an important role in providing reassuring support and encouraging him to keep trying. It requires patience and judgment to stand by and let the patient proceed, even though it may at times seem like a "cruel struggle." Activities are stopped if the patient manifests fatigue or complains of headache or dizziness. Before discharge from the hospital, the planned regimen of daily activities is outlined and reviewed with the patient and a member of the family.

Nursing Care of the Patient Treated by Intracranial Surgery

OPERATION. Intracranial surgery necessitates an opening in the skull. The size and location of the opening depend upon the nature and site of the lesion and the amount of exposure needed for the anticipated procedure. If the lesion is in the cerebrum, it is referred to as being *supratentorial,*[14] and the incision is usually well above the hairline. If it is in the cerebellar or brain stem regions, it is designated as *infratentorial,* and the incision is usually in the occipital region. The surgery may involve a craniectomy or a craniotomy. A *craniectomy* refers to the excision of a section of the skull and may vary from a small burr hole to a sizeable area of several centimeters. A *craniotomy* provides a relatively large opening and entails the freeing of a portion of the skull referred to as a bone flap. The flap is usually left attached to the muscle tissue and turned back but in some instances may be freed, set aside and replaced at the completion of the operation. When the bone section is replaced, the procedure is referred to as an *osteoplastic craniotomy*. If it is not replaced because of needed decompression, a cranioplasty may be done later in which a plate of an especially prepared material (Vitallium or tantalum) or a bone graft is placed in the opening to provide protection for the brain and for cosmetic reasons.

Intracranial surgery may be done: to obtain a tissue specimen for biopsy; to aspirate fluid; for exploratory purposes; to remove a neoplasm, hematoma, scar tissue which is causing seizures, or a specific area of tissue for the relief of tremors (e.g., pallidectomy or thalamotomy); to correct an aneurysm or vascular anomaly; to treat a decompressed or compound fracture; to drain an abscess; to relieve intracranial pressure; or to remove a foreign body (e.g., bullet).

PREOPERATIVE PREPARATION. If the patient is oriented and aware of his situation, he is likely to be quite apprehensive when advised by a physician of the need for surgery. Any impending surgery causes some anxiety, but that involving the brain is even more threatening. The alert patient is usually very fearful of permanent changes and disability, loss of competence, and death. The nurse conveys understanding of his concern and encourages the patient to talk about his fears and ask questions. Verbal expression of his anxiety and sharing his problems help to reduce his tension. He should not be left alone

---

[14]The *tentorium* is a fold of the dura mater between the cerebellum and the occipital lobes of the cerebrum.

for long periods. Investigative procedures and what is likely to take place at the time of surgery and afterward are explained to the patient and family.

CONSENT FOR OPERATION. Surgery on the brain may carry the risk of a permanent change in appearance or function; this is explained to the competent patient and family by the physician before the consent for operation is signed. It is the policy of most neurosurgeons and hospitals to require the signature of the patient and a close relative on the consent form. If the patient is not conscious or oriented, two relatives sign. The nurse must be familiar with the policy of the institution as to who may witness the signing of the consents.

IMPROVING THE PATIENT'S CONDITION. As with all surgery, the nutritional and hydrational status of the patient receives attention during the preoperative period, and any secondary or concomitant condition (e.g., infection, anemia) is corrected so that he goes to operation in the best possible condition. This includes the need for observing the patient's emotional reactions to the situation and making every effort to reduce his anxiety. As well as causing suffering and distress for the patient, fear may alter vital physiological activities through its effect on the autonomic nervous system and may influence his ability to cope with the stress of surgery. During this period of preparation, the patient is encouraged to remain ambulatory if his condition permits. If his lesion is such that his balance and mobility are impaired, safety precautions are taken to prevent falls.

OBSERVATIONS. The patient is observed for possible changes from day to day which may indicate a worsening of his condition. The nurse follows the vital signs closely, checks the pupils regularly for size, equality and reaction to light, and notes the patient's alertness, level of consciousness, orientation, sensory perception, motor ability and strength of the limbs. The final preoperative summary of these is essential as a baseline for evaluating the patient's condition after the operation.

ELIMINATION. An enema is not usually ordered if the patient's bowels have been moving satisfactorily. If one is necessary, it is given slowly and the patient must be cautioned against straining to guard against increasing intracranial pressure. The bladder must be empty when the patient goes to the operating room. Frequently an indwelling catheter is passed the morning of operation to prevent postoperative incontinence and so that the output volume can be measured accurately.

SKIN PREPARATION. The hair is clipped and the head shampooed with an antiseptic soap solution. Cutting the hair can be quite disturbing to the patient, since it alters his appearance. Before starting the preparation, a careful explanation is made to the patient as to why it is necessary, and suggestions are made to the female patient as to the wearing of colorful turbans or a wig later. In the case of a female, the hair is saved, being carefully placed in a bag and labelled in the event that the patient may wish to have a wig made later, or in case of death the family may request it. Any rash, infection or abrasion of the scalp is brought to the surgeon's attention. Shaving and further cleansing of the operative site are usually done in the operating room. This more immediate preparation lessens the possibility of contamination. If the site necessitates exposure of an ear, a piece of sterile absorbent is placed in the external auditory canal following its cleansing with an antiseptic.

BLOOD TYPING. The blood loss may be considerable because of the vascularity of the scalp and brain. The patient's blood is typed and cross matched for transfusion. An intravenous infusion may be started before the patient goes to the operating room so that blood or a dehydrating preparation, such as dexamethasone (Decadron) or mannitol (Osmitrol), may be readily administered during operation.

FOOD AND FLUIDS. No food is given after the evening meal the night before operation, and no fluids are taken by mouth within the 4- to 6-hour period preceding the scheduled time of surgery.

MEDICATIONS. A mild sedative may be ordered at bedtime the night before operation to insure a good night's rest. Atropine sulfate may be prescribed to control respiratory secretions during inhalation anesthesia, but a narcotic is not usually given because of its depressing effect on respirations. Dexamethasone (Decadron) may be given to counteract subsequent brain edema and swelling.

THE FAMILY. It is natural that intracranial surgery creates a long, anxious period for the family. The physician explains the patient's condition and what will be done at operation, and they are advised of any possibility of residual change in the patient's function, personality and appearance. The nurse acknowledges their concern, talks with them, answers their questions and keeps them informed about the patient's condition, giving them as much support and assistance as possible.

The day of operation, one or two family members are usually permitted to visit the patient briefly before he is taken to the operating room. Knowing they are near is reassuring to the patient. They are advised of the need to control their emotions when with the patient, as he is in need of their support. When he leaves the ward, they are told how long the operation might be (3 to 5 hours, depending on what is done) and are directed to a waiting room. The nurse visits them at intervals and suggests where they may go to have coffee or lunch. Appreciation of their concern increases their confidence in those caring for the patient.

PREPARATION TO RECEIVE THE PATIENT. Preparation of the unit to receive the patient after operation includes the assembling of the following equipment:

The bed should have a low headboard so that the patient's head will be readily accessible, and should have side rails.

The bed is made up with cotton sheets because of the neurosurgical patient's tendency to develop a high body temperature.

Tongue forceps
Suction tubing and catheters
Airway (oropharyngeal and intratracheal) tubes
Tracheotomy tray
Sphygmomanometer and stethoscope
Flashlight
Rectal thermometer
Special recording sheets for frequent neurological assessment
Intravenous pole
Urine drainage receptacle
Mouth care tray

If the temperature of the room is thermostatically controlled it is usually set at 18° to 20° C. (65° to 68° F.). A hypothermic blanket should be available.

POSTOPERATIVE CARE. Care following the operation includes the following considerations (obviously these are modified according to the findings and what was done at operation and the surgeon's orders).

POSITIONING. The patient is placed in a lateral or semiprone position. A small pillow may be necessary under the head to maintain good neck alignment. It is positioned so that the mouth is dependent at the edge of the pillow to allow free drainage of secretions and vomitus. The limbs are positioned and supported as for any unconscious patient (see p. 159). The surgeon's orders will indicate if the head of the bed is to be elevated or kept flat. If the surgery has been on the cerebrum, the head of the bed is usually slightly elevated unless contraindicated by shock. Following infratentorial surgery (cerebellum or brain stem), the bed is generally kept flat for 2 to 3 days.

The patient's position is changed from side to side to back (only if conscious) to side every 2 hours unless contraindicated. If a relatively large space-occupying lesion has been removed, he is usually not permitted to lie on the operative side in order to prevent a shifting of the brain into the remaining space. In the case of surgery in the occipital region, restrictions are usually placed on the dorsal recumbent position for 2 to 4 days, since the brain stem may have been affected, resulting in a dulling of the gag and swallowing reflexes, predisposing to aspiration. Keeping this patient off his back also prevents pressure on the incision as well as possible forward flexion of the head which places a strain on the incision. It is helpful in avoiding mistakes if a notice indicating the restricted position is posted in a prominent place on the head of the bed.

When the patient is repositioned, he is turned slowly and with adequate support for the head so that it and the trunk are turned as if they were one single unit. Sudden movement and jarring are avoided at all times. Particular attention is paid to bony prominences and pressure areas each time the patient is turned to prevent pressure sores. The bedding must be kept dry and free of wrinkles. An air mattress may be used, and pieces of soft, resilient material are placed under vulnerable areas.

OBSERVATIONS. The blood pressure, temperature, pulse and respirations are recorded, and the size, equality and reaction to light of the pupils and the level of consciousness are noted at regular frequent intervals. If the patient is conscious, his alertness and orientations as well as the motion and strength of his limbs are also checked. The required frequency of these observations is indicated by the physician but usually begins with 15-minute intervals which are lengthened to 1/2 hour and then 1 hour if the signs remain stable. Other significant observations include the color, condition of the skin (dry or moist and the temperature) and the fluid balance (fluid intake and output). Careful scrutiny is made of the dressing frequently for moisture and bloodstains.

CLEAR AIRWAY. As well as lateral or semiprone positioning to maintain a patent airway, it may be necessary to remove secretions from the mouth and nose by means of suctioning. The catheter is moistened in normal saline or water before introducing it and is used gently to prevent injury to the mucous membrane lining. The respirations are checked frequently for any manifestations of an obstructed airway or respiratory distress. The lower jaw and tongue must be forward to prevent blocking of the pharynx.

If there are indications of accumulated secretions in the lower respiratory tract or that the patient is having respiratory difficulty, a tracheostomy may be performed to permit deep suctioning of the trachea and bronchi with a sterile endobronchial catheter (see p. 420 for tracheostomy care).

If the patient is capable of responding, he is required to take seven to ten deep breaths every 2 to 3 hours. Coughing is used as a part of the chest routine only if approved by the physician because of the danger of increasing intracranial pressure.

HEAD DRESSING. If the dressing becomes moist or bloodstained, it is promptly reinforced with sterile pads and reported. Depending on the operative procedure, a drain may have been inserted and is usually removed in 24 to 48 hours. Following an infratentorial operation, the head may be slightly hyperextended when the dressing is applied. Long strips of adhesive may extend from the head down to the scapular region. This immobilizes the head and prevents lateral and forward flexion which would place a strain on the incision.

The initial dressing is usually changed in approximately 5 days by the surgeon. The sutures may be removed then or on the sixth or seventh postoperative day. The area may then be left exposed. The scalp may be cleansed with hydrogen peroxide to remove old blood. An application of oil or petroleum jelly will soften any crusts that may have formed and the scalp may then be washed with an antiseptic solution. The incision is inspected once or twice daily and is cleansed with a prescribed antiseptic.

RESTLESSNESS. Restlessness is usually associated with cerebral disturbances, but it should be kept in mind that it might also be caused by head bandages being too tight, retention of urine, or feces in the rectum. To prevent the restless or disoriented patient from dislodging tubes (nasogastric, catheter, tracheotomy, intravenous) or his head dressing, restraint mitts may be applied. Dressing pads are placed between the fingers which are slightly flexed over a roll of dressing placed across the palm of the hand. A large dressing pad is then wrapped over the fingers and the hand bandaged, usually with flannelette bandages for security. A piece of tubular stockinette is then pulled over the bandaged hand and secured with adhesive. Mitts are changed daily; the hands are washed and lightly powdered; the fingers and thumb are massaged and passively moved several times through their range of motion. Ordinary restraints are not used because straining against them only tends to further agitate the patient and may also raise the intracranial pressure.

If the patient is extremely restless, the skin will require additional care. Friction areas may be lightly oiled or powdered at frequent intervals, and the elbows and heels may have to be padded and bandaged for protection. Side rails may have to be padded to prevent injury.

Side rails are kept in position unless someone is at the bedside with the patient. This applies for a considerable period of time even though the patient has regained consciousness and is oriented. Following intracranial surgery, patients frequently are subject to spells of dizziness and lapses of orientation or may be slow in regaining their postural reflexes.

FLUIDS AND NUTRITION. Fluids are generally given intravenously for the first 24 to 48 hours. The amount is specifically limited (usually 1000 to 2000 ml.) and is given slowly to avoid a rapid increase in the intravascular volume and an ensuing rise in blood pressure. If the patient remains unconscious or semicomatose after 3 or 4 days, nasogastric feedings are given every 3 to 4 hours to provide necessary fluid and nutrition. When oral fluids are permitted, only a small amount is given at first through a drinking tube, and the patient is observed closely for any depression of the swallowing reflex. Following certain operations, especially those that are infratentorial, the ability to swallow may be impaired. If there is no difficulty in swallowing and no vomiting, fluids are given freely unless limited to a certain volume per 24 hours because of cerebral edema and increased intracranial pressure. The diet is gradually increased to include soft solid foods and is progressed to a full diet as tolerated. The patient is fed for the first few days to avoid fatigue and to insure an adequate intake.

ELIMINATION. Since these patients may be incontinent or may have retention of urine, an indwelling catheter may be passed previous to surgery or after the patient is returned to the neurosurgical unit. Because a retention catheter predisposes to bladder infection, a continuous drip of an antimicrobial solution may be attached to the catheter which is connected also to a closed drainage system. In the case of a male patient who is incontinent, the physician may prefer the use of an external penile sheath (condom) to the indwelling catheter. The sheath is connected by tubing to a urine receptacle. The urinary output is measured hourly for the first 24 to 36 hours and then every 8 or 12 hours if the patient's condition is satisfactory. The daily fluid intake and output are recorded and the fluid balance noted.

Bowel elimination is usually disregarded for 3 or 4 days postoperatively. A mild laxative such as mineral oil or milk of magnesia may be ordered on the third day. If this is ineffective, a small enema may be prescribed, depending on the patient's condition.

MOUTH AND EYE CARE. Following intracranial surgery, especially during the unconscious period, one or both eyelids may remain open, exposing the conjunctiva and cornea to drying and injury. A special eye shield (not a pad) may be applied for protection. The eyes are bathed with sterile normal saline or water at regular intervals, and the instillation of an artificial tear solution such as methyl cellulose in saline or an ointment may be prescribed. The eyes are carefully inspected for any irritation, blood streaks and discharge which, if present, are brought to the physician's attention.

It is important, especially if the patient is on restricted fluids, that the teeth and mouth receive frequent cleansing to prevent drying and the accumulation of sordes, which predispose to infection (e.g., parotitis).

MEDICATIONS. Sedatives and analgesics are not usually used because they may mask important neurological symptoms and depress respirations. Discomfort and headache may be controlled by acetylsalicylic acid (aspirin) or propoxyphene (Darvon). If the patient is extremely restless or develops a convulsive seizure, sodium phenobarbital or diphenylhydantoin sodium (Dilantin) may be ordered parenterally. Dexamethasone (Decadron) is frequently given to counteract cerebral edema resulting from the inflammatory process incurred by the trauma of surgery.

EXERCISE AND AMBULATION. The limbs are moved passively through a full range of motion two or three times daily to preserve joint mobility. Active limb exercises are begun when indicated by the physician. The patient is assisted out of bed as soon as his condition permits. Before this takes place, the head of the bed is gradually elevated, and the patient is observed for any untoward reactions. When up in a chair, a draw sheet may be secured around the waist and the back of the chair to prevent a possible fall should the patient develop dizziness or sudden weakness. A nurse remains with the patient, closely observing his reactions. If he complains of headache or dizziness or shows signs of fatigue or a fall in blood pressure, he is returned to bed. The time he remains up is gradually increased as tolerated. When he begins to walk, someone must accompany him until he is quite safe on his feet and sure of his balance.

PERSONAL APPEARANCE. The female patient may be very self-conscious about her appearance without her hair. She is encouraged to use colorful scarves as turbans. The suggestion of a wig may also be made.

If the patient is lethargic and disinterested in appearance and dress, he is urged to improve his grooming and to dress when he is well enough to be up most of the day, rather than spend the day in a dressing gown. Gradually this tends to improve the patient's morale.

REHABILITATION. Following intracranial surgery, the patient is quite dependent upon the nurse for complete care for a few days but, as soon as he is well enough, he is encouraged to perform self-care activities. In some instances, there may be loss of movement in one or more limbs or impairment of speech and intellectual ability. A rehabilitation program is planned and instituted as soon as possible with the goal of restoring the patient to independent, useful living within his potential. This may involve the physiotherapist, speech therapist and social worker as well as the physician and nurse. The patient may have to relearn the performance of ordinary daily activities and progress from the simple to the more complex, much as the child learns. It is frequently a slow process, and both the patient and his family are likely to have periods of depression and discouragement. The nurse must maintain an optimistic attitude and patience, providing support and encouragement for both the patient and family, but at the same time appreciate and acknowledge their problems. Emphasis is placed on the positive, and the patient is praised when he accomplishes certain activities. He may not be able to resume his former occupation, and eventual retraining for a different type of work may be undertaken as part of the rehabilitation. The social worker may help the family with the socioeconomic problems resulting from this illness.

Before the patient is discharged from the hospital, he and his family are informed about the exercises and activities that are to be continued. It is helpful if a day's schedule is given to them in writing. A referral is made to the visiting nurse agency so that guidance and support are continued. A referral may also be made to a rehabilitation center, or the patient may remain under the supervision of the hospital rehabilitation department.

COMPLICATIONS. The most common complications that may develop after intracranial surgery include hyperthermia, increased intracranial pressure, respiratory failure and convulsive seizures.

Following intracranial surgery, the patient tends to develop an elevation of temperature due to a disturbance of the temperature-regulating center and mechanisms in the hypothalamus and brain stem. To counteract this tendency, if his temperature is normal, the room temperature is kept at 18° to 20° C. (65° to 68° F.) and only a cotton sheet and spread are used as covers. If the patient's temperature rises above 38°C. (100°F.), it is reported to the physician. The spread is removed from the bed, and the sheet is arranged to cover only the lower half of the body. Acetylsalicylic acid (aspirin) by rectal suppository and an increase in the fluid intake may be ordered. If the temperature continues to rise, especially if it exceeds 38° C. (100° F.), cool sponge baths and an electric fan directed on the patient may be helpful. If these measures are not successful in controlling the hyperthermia, a hypothermia blanket with ice water or alcohol circulating through the coils may be used.

Edema of the brain resulting from the trauma and inflammation incurred by surgery is generally the cause of postoperative increased intracranial pressure, but it may also develop as a result of hemorrhage. The signs and symptoms have been cited previously on page 861. Close observation of the patient and prompt reporting of any significant changes may prevent compression of brain tissue and death of the patient. The head of the bed is elevated to promote cerebral venous drainage, the fluid intake is restricted, and drugs may be given to dehydrate the brain. The drugs administered are principally hypertonic solutions which are given intravenously. They cause the transfer of fluid from the brain tissue into the vascular compartment by osmosis and increase the urinary output. Those most commonly used are mannitol (Osmitrol) and urea and glucose (Urevert). Fifty per cent glucose may also be used. Dexamethasone (Decadron) which is anti-inflammatory may be given postoperatively to reduce the incidence and severity of cerebral edema. A larger dose may be ordered for parenteral administration if the patient manifests increased intracranial pressure.

Respiratory failure may result from compression of the respiratory center in the brain stem (medulla). It is more likely to occur following surgery in the posterior fossa (infratentorial area). The patient's respirations may be rapid and stertorous for a period; then, gradually, they may change and become Cheyne-Stokes or slow and shallow. Any change in the respirations is reported immediately.

The patient may develop convulsive seizures following intracranial surgery as a result of brain irritation, compression or scar tissue. It may be preceded by restlessness and twitching or may occur suddenly without warning. Pillows are removed and the patient is turned on his side as soon as possible to prevent obstruction of the airway and facilitate the drainage of accumulated oropharyngeal secretions. Only sufficient restraint to prevent injury is used. He must not be left alone, but someone is dispatched to notify the physician as soon as possible. The nurse notes the time and nature of the onset, the initial or focal site of involvement, the direction in which the head and eyes are turned, whether the muscle responses are tonic or clonic, the duration of the seizure and the condition of the patient following the convulsion. Sodium phenobarbital or diphenylhydantoin sodium (Dilantin) may be ordered parenterally.

If the seizure occurs when the patient is in a chair, he is gently eased to the floor. A folded towel or whatever is available is placed under his head to prevent injury.

If the family or visitors were present at the onset of the seizure, they are given an explanation of the probable cause and reassured of the patient's condition. If there are other patients in the room, a screen is placed around the patient as soon as possible, since they may become quite disturbed and frightened.

Spinal Cord Injury

Accidental injury to the spinal cord is most commonly associated with a fracture of one or more vertebrae. The fracture may be the result of sudden forceful angulation of the spine (hyperflexion or hyperextension), excessive force applied along the axis of the spine (e.g., landing on the feet or buttocks from a height) or a direct blow. In some instances, rupture and posterior extrusion of the intervertebral disk may also occur. The degree of damage sustained by the cord varies, depending mainly on whether or not the fracture fragments are displaced (fracture dislocation). The cord may be contused, lacerated, or subjected to compression. Bleeding into the tissue and edema may occur, causing swelling and compression of nerve tracts. The damage may be slight and completely reversible, or it may leave a minor degree of residual impairment. A laceration which transects the cord or causes severe compression may result in complete, irreversible interruption of ascending or descending tracts. Interruption of ascending tracts causes loss of sensation below the site of injury. Interruption of descending tracts results in paralysis of the parts deriving their innervation from the cord below the level of the lesion. Autonomic nervous function may also be disturbed.

MANIFESTATIONS. The symptoms of cord injury depend on the level and degree of damage. The patient may complain of pain in the neck or back or in areas supplied by the nerves leaving the injured spinal region. Angulation of the spine may be evident. There is likely to be loss of sensation, motor ability (weakness or paralysis) and reflexes below the level of the lesion. The bladder is atonic, resulting in retention of urine, and vomiting and abdominal distention may develop as a result of paralysis of intestinal peristalsis (paralytic ileus). There may be a lack or excess of perspiration by the skin below the lesion due to disturbed autonomic innervation.

Cervical cord injury may cause paralysis from the neck down (quadriplegia). Respiratory insufficiency or complete failure occurs if there is involvement of the nerve supply to the diaphragm and intercostal muscles. Injury below the cervical region may cause paralysis of the lower limbs, bladder and rectum (paraplegia). Any recovery usually occurs within 1 to 2 weeks; if the loss of function persists beyond this period, the damage is usually irreversible. The cord and its tracts are not capable of regeneration, but regeneration of the nerve roots (outside of the cord) can occur if the neurilemma is not severely damaged (see p. 814). Spasticity of the paralyzed muscles and exaggerated tendon reflexes usually follow the initial flaccidity of the first few days in cord injury. The bladder becomes hypertonic and frequent automatic emptying develops. When paralysis occurs as a result of injury to the cauda equina (lumbar or sacral region), flaccid paralysis and an absence of reflexes persist.

TREATMENT AND NURSING CARE. When a spinal injury is known to have occurred or is suspected, the handling and transportation of the patient is of great importance in the prevention of cord damage or additional impairment.

EMERGENCY CARE. At the scene of the accident, the victim is advised to lie still. To determine if there is cord injury and the level, he may be requested to move his toes and fingers. Loss of sensation may be assessed by gentle pinching at various levels. He is covered and kept flat while other immediate emergencies (respiratory insufficiency and bleeding) are cared for, and movement and transportation are quickly organized. A firm, flat improvised stretcher such as a door or wide plank is provided. Five or six persons are recruited to lift the patient and are instructed that he must be moved as a single rigid unit; even slight flexion and twisting of the spine may cause irreversible cord damage. One person is stationed at the patient's head and one at his feet. All other persons are positioned on one side of the patient so that when he is lifted he may be transferred in one movement. *Slight* traction is applied to the head and lower extremities as he is lifted to the stretcher. Straps or strips of cloth are placed over the patient and around the stretcher to secure the patient and prevent movement. Something firm is placed at either side of his head and someone remains at the head of the stretcher, providing additional support to prevent any movement of the neck in transit.

On arrival at the hospital, the patient usually remains on a stretcher during examination and x-rays and while the treatment bed or frame which is to be used is prepared to insure a minimum of movement.

TREATMENT. The treatment depends on the location of the fracture and whether or not there is dislocation and indications of cord compression. Traction or hyperextension may be used to reduce the fracture.

Cervical spinal injury is usually treated by skeletal traction of 10 to 30 pounds, which is applied by means of tongs (Crutchfield or Barton) that are inserted into the skull at approximately the midlateral line, a short distance above the ears. The sites of insertion of the tongs are inspected daily for signs of inflammation and infection and, following cleansing with a prescribed antiseptic, fresh sterile dressings are applied. If only slight traction is required, a halter-like arrangement may be used in place of the tongs, but prolonged continuous application usually causes considerable discomfort and skin irritation for the patient by the pressure and pull of the straps, especially under the chin.

The patient may be nursed on an ordinary bed with a low headboard that allows clearance for traction equipment. The head of the bed is raised on blocks or shock pins to enable the body to act as countertraction for the weights. This prevents the patient's body from sliding toward the head of the bed. The Foster turning bed may be used in place of an ordinary bed; it provides a pivoting device which permits turning without interference to the appliance or traction. When reduction and sufficient healing are achieved, the patient is fitted with a neck brace or plastic collar to provide cervical immobilization and support, and he is ambulated slowly and progressively.

When there is a *thoracic or lumbar spinal* fracture without dislocation of the fragments, the patient may be placed flat on a firm mattress and fracture board on an ordinary bed or on a turning bed for several weeks. If the ordinary bed is used, specific directions are received as to whether the patient must remain on his back at all times. If turning is permitted, precautions are taken to insure good alignment and avoidance of movement and displacement of the fragments. When the patient must remain on his back continuously, a sponge rubber mattress may be placed on top of the firm mattress. This facilitates the changing of the lower bed linen and the giving of frequent back care. A nurse on each side of the bed, working from the head down, uses one hand to depress the mattress while caring for the skin or changing the linen with the other one. When there is sufficient healing, the patient is gradually ambulated. A brace or firm corset may be necessary for several months to provide support and immobility of the spine.

A fracture dislocation of thoracic or lumbar vertebrae may be treated by hyperextension of the spine which may be achieved by various methods. The patient may be placed on the regular Gatch bed and the Gatch frame raised in line with the fracture. This may necessitate placing the patient's head at the foot of the bed. An alternative method is the placing of a firm roll or sandbag across the bed under the mattress to provide the required angulation. Fracture boards are placed on the springs, and a very firm mattress is used on which a sponge rubber mattress is placed, since the patient must remain in the supine position.

In some instances a plaster cast is used to

immobilize the spine following a fracture in the thoracic or lumbar region. It usually extends from the shoulders to below the hips. An opening may be cut in the cast over the abdomen to prevent pressure and discomfort in that area. The cast edges are bound by the stockinette, which is under the cast, being turned back and secured with adhesive. The skin areas at the borders of the cast are examined daily for possible irritation. The cast is cut back over the buttocks sufficiently to accommodate the use of the bedpan without soiling of the cast. Extra precautions are taken to protect it by the use of pieces of waterproof material such as plastic.

Surgical treatment may be necessary in some spinal injuries to relieve compression of the cord or if the dislocation cannot be reduced by traction or hyperextension. The operation may involve a laminectomy and spinal fusion (see p. 000 for nursing care).

NURSING THE PATIENT WITHOUT CORD INVOLVEMENT. If the spinal cord is intact and undamaged in the case of a spinal fracture, nursing care is directed toward: (1) the maintenance of alignment and stability of the spine to prevent cord and nerve damage and promote healing of the fractured vertebra; (2) the prevention of complications such as decubitus ulcers and respiratory disease; and (3) general supportive care (psychological and physiological).

Observations. The patient is observed closely for signs of cord compression. Any loss of motor strength or ability, loss of sensation, respiratory distress, retention of urine or incontinence, or vomiting and abdominal distention which might be indicative of paralytic ileus must be reported promptly.

Skin Care and Positioning. During the period of immobilization, pressure areas require frequent attention and are inspected two or three times daily for early signs of irritation and breaks in the skin. Usually, the patient is restricted to the supine position if on an ordinary bed; frequent changing of lower sheets is achieved by two nurses working together as cited previously. If there is a possibility of restlessness or of the patient moving, a draw sheet placed over the patient and secured at the sides may deter moving and turning, or long sandbags placed along either side of the patient may be necessary, especially during the night. If the physician sanctions turning, sufficient persons are nec-

essary to maintain alignment and stability of the spine while turning the patient as one immovable unit (log-rolling).

Having the patient on a turning bed (Stryker frame or Foster bed) has several distinct advantages. It facilitates turning the patient from the supine to prone position and vice versa with minimal risk of movement of the vertebrae and reduces the discomfort and strain for the patient in the process. It allows more frequent turning to protect the skin and the use of a bedpan without the patient having to be raised, as well as eliminating the need for more than two nurses to turn the patient (see Fig. 23–24).

The turning bed has two metal frames to which sheets of canvas are firmly attached. The patient's position is changed by turning the whole frame on which he lies. This is possible by pivots at each end of the frame which are locked except during the turning. The frame that is used when he is on his back (posterior frame) has an opening in the canvas in the buttocks and perineal area which permits the use of a bedpan that is placed on a rack beneath the opening when necessary. One end of a piece of waterproof material may be tucked under the buttocks while the other end is placed in the bedpan to direct the flow of excreta and protect the canvas. Following the use of the bedpan, the patient may be turned to thoroughly clean and dry the perineal area and buttocks. A strip of canvas attached to one side of the frame is brought across the opening in the frame and secured when the patient is not using the bedpan.

The sheets used to cover the frames must be free of wrinkles and usually are secured by

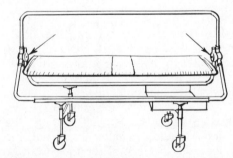

FIGURE 23–24 The Stryker frame, which facilitates the turning of certain patients (e.g., those who have had spinal injury or surgery or who have sustained severe burns). (From Sutton, A. L.: Bedside Nursing Techniques, 2nd ed. Philadelphia, W. B. Saunders Co., 1969, p. 198.)

large safety pins on the undersurface. In the case of the posterior frame, two sheets are used, one above and one below the opening. A narrow strip of sheeting is used over the canvas covering the opening.

In the supine position, a small flat pillow may be permitted under the head. A small bolster of foam rubber or toweling may be placed under the knees to provide support *without flexion.* A footboard attaches to the frame to support the feet in dorsiflexion. The arms are supported on arm rests to which sponge rubber pillows are secured. The patient's gown is usually left open at the back and tucked against his sides to avoid his lying on wrinkles. Sufficient lightweight top covers are used to keep the patient comfortable. If the patient finds the canvas too hard, the doctor may permit the use of a thin layer of sponge rubber on each frame. This is usually enclosed in cotton to which tapes are added for securing the mattress to the frame.

To turn the patient from the supine to prone position, the arm and foot supports and top bedding are removed, and the anterior frame is placed over the patient and secured to the "bed" frame at either end by means of heavy screws. Unnecessary exposure is avoided at all times; the pubic area is covered with a towel or draw sheet that can be easily removed after turning. Two or three straps are then securely placed around the frames and the spring lock released at each end. The frames are then turned quickly and smoothly. The spring locks automatically when the frame bearing the patient is in the correct position but should be tested before the turners' holds are released. The posterior frame is then removed and the arm rests are replaced and, as the frame is narrow, restraining straps are fastened around the patient and the frame, usually at the lower abdomen and thighs and loosely around the chest. The upper border of the canvas on the anterior frame only extends to the neck. The head is supported by a strip of canvas on which the forehead rests. This leaves the patient's face free. A rack placed below the head will hold a book, meal tray or other personal articles which should be readily accessible to the patient. A pillow is used under the ankles, and the feet are suspended over the end of the canvas.

The turning bed is not used when the spinal lesion is treated by hyperextension or, in the case of a cervical injury, without the use of tongs. Rarely, it is not appropriate because of the patient's excessive height or weight or persisting fear of the turning.

Diet and Fluids. During the prolonged period of immobility, a high-protein, high-vitamin diet is recommended to help prevent pressure sores, promote healing, maintain resistance to respiratory complications and prevent a negative nitrogen balance. Prolonged immobilization predisposes to the movement of calcium out of the bones and ensuing hypercalcemia. This favors the formation of renal and bladder calculi. The patient is encouraged to take a minimum of 3000 ml. of fluid daily to prevent concentration and stasis of the urine. The daily calcium intake, mainly in the form of milk and milk products, may have to be restricted to some degree. Swallowing is difficult for the patient who must remain flat on his back or in a position of spinal hyperextension; choking and aspiration may occur readily. Suction should be readily available in the event of aspiration, since he cannot be turned or raised. The patient is fed slowly, and only small amounts of food and fluid taken into the mouth at one time.

Deep Breathing and Exercises. The patient is urged to practice brief periods of deep breathing several times a day. With the physician's permission, a daily exercise regimen may be established. The limbs are gently moved through their full range of motion, and isotonic and isometric active exercises may be gradually introduced. These activities are important in maintaining joint mobility and muscle tone and in stimulating circulation.

Bowel Elimination. Constipation may be a problem because of the inactivity; dietary adjustments such as the inclusion of increased roughage and fruit juices may be necessary. A mild laxative or glycerin or bisacodyl (Dulcolax) suppositories may also be used.

Diversion. Some provision is made for diversion, for the hours and days generally pass slowly for the patient. A mirror attached to the head of the bed may permit him to see what is going on about him. Special prism glasses may be provided for reading, and visitors are encouraged to spend time with him.

Ambulation. When the patient is allowed up after such a prolonged period of immobility, he assumes the upright position slowly and gradually, and someone should be with him in case fainting or dizziness is a problem. The patient may be required to wear a brace or corset for a considerable period of time. A good walking shoe or a firm slipper with a heel should be worn when beginning ambulation. He is instructed how to prevent strain on his spine; lifting and bending are avoided usually for several months and previous activities are resumed gradually.

NURSING THE PATIENT WITH CORD DAMAGE. The most obvious disability in cord injury is paralysis of limbs (paraplegia or quadriplegia), but it is only one of a number of dysfunctions, some of which are a direct result of the cord damage while others are secondary consequences.

Direct neurological effects include loss of voluntary movement, varying degrees of muscle spasm in the paralyzed parts, impairment of sensation which interferes with the patient's adaptation to his environment, and disturbance of some autonomic functions. Interference with autonomic nerve pathways may be manifested by an excess or absence of perspiration which may cause impairment in body temperature regulation. Lack of vascular responses may also occur which may cause postural hypotension, posing a problem later when the patient assumes a sitting or standing position.

The secondary or extraneurological effects of cord injury include bladder and bowel dysfunction, pressure sores which may develop very rapidly due to the immobility, loss of sensation and alterations in local circulation, mobilization of bone calcium, negative nitrogen balance, and emotional reactions to the disabilities and their implications.

The care of the patient with spinal cord involvement is planned according to the amount of damage and the individual patient's reactions and specific needs. The paraplegic patient is nursed on a turning bed, if possible, to facilitate frequent turning. It is easier for the quadriplegic patient if he is nursed on a bed. He usually has breathing difficulty due to paralysis of respiratory muscles and, if turned on his abdomen as he must be on either a Stryker or Foster bed, breathing is even more difficult. Also, if nursed on a bed, he may be positioned on his back and on either side which gives him a more normal outlook on his surroundings. If he is on a turning bed he sees only the ceiling and the floor.

Observations. The paralyzed limbs are tested and observed for signs of any return of sensation and movement. A close check is made of the urinary output, and the amount of perspiration on parts below the level of the lesion is noted. The vulnerable pressure areas are examined frequently for discoloration, edema and broken areas, and the patient's psychological reactions are observed.

Elimination. The bladder generally goes through three stages. It is atonic at first, causing a complete retention of urine without the patient experiencing any discomfort or sensation of needing to void. Then hypotonicity develops, manifested by retention with overflow, and the patient involuntarily voids small amounts frequently. Later, the bladder becomes hypertonic; its capacity is diminished, and frequent reflex voiding develops. Bladder infection leading to pyelonephritis and eventual renal insufficiency is probably the most serious complication of paraplegia and the greatest constant threat to the patient's life. Stasis and residual urine predispose to infection and the formation of calculi. The bladder should be completely emptied at regular intervals, and the patient should have a minimal fluid intake of 3000 ml. daily. Strict aseptic precautions in catheterization and a sterile closed drainage system are extremely important in preventing infection.

An indwelling catheter is introduced soon after admission to prevent bladder damage by overdistention and involuntary voiding with ensuing skin irritation and maceration. Continuous drainage is used at first; then later, either the catheter is clamped for stated intervals to counteract the hypertonicity and diminished bladder capacity or intermittent catheterization is begun. An antiseptic bladder irrigation may be ordered three or four times daily, or a continuous drip may be used as a prophylactic measure. Frequent change of position also helps to prevent residual urine and calculus formation.

The sensation for the need to defecate is lost, and the lower bowel functions reflexly, causing involuntary stools. Because of the immobility and loss of tone, the paralyzed patient is predisposed to constipation and impaction, especially in the early stages of his illness. An enema or suppository may be used daily or every other day to evacuate the bowel at first; then, as the patient's general condition improves and his diet becomes more normal, involuntary stools occur. The diet may be adjusted to the stool consistency and frequency to help in regulation. A regular hour for bowel elimination is established by using a glycerin or bisacodyl (Dulcolax) suppository or by inserting a lubricated gloved finger to initiate defecation.

Following a high cord injury, intestinal peristalsis may be depressed, causing severe abdominal distention and vomiting (paralytic ileus). A Miller-Abbott tube may be passed and gastrointestinal suction established (see p. 500). A peristaltic stimulant such as neostigmine (Prostigmin) and bethanechol chloride (Urecholine Chloride) may be prescribed, and a rectal tube is inserted or an enema given. During this period the patient is sustained by intravenous solutions.

Nutrition. A high-protein, high-vitamin diet is important to combat the tendency toward a negative nitrogen balance due to immobility and to promote tissue resistance and healing power. An adequate intake may be a problem as a result of the patient's emotional reactions and inactivity. Dietary supplements between meals may be given to meet the patient's needs. Food is placed conveniently within reach, and the paraplegic is encouraged to feed himself as soon as his general condition permits. The quadriplegic has to be fed until appropriate assistive devices are available. Food and fluids with a high calcium content (e.g., milk and milk products) may be restricted because of the tendency to renal and bladder calculi formation. If a stone develops, the patient may be placed on an acid-ash or alkaline-ash diet, depending on the composition of the calculus.

Skin Care. To prevent pressure sores to which paraplegic and quadriplegic patients are especially predisposed, frequent skin care must begin within a few hours of the injury. The patient is turned every 1 or 2 hours, day and night. The skin is kept clean and dry, and circulation is stimulated by gentle massage, especially the vulnerable areas such as the sacrum, buttocks, scapulae, heels and ankles. The bedding is kept free of wrinkles, crumbs, tissues, etc. Pieces of resilient material such as sponge rubber and synthetic sheepskin may be used under pressure areas. If the patient is on an ordinary bed, an alternating pressure mattress is helpful. If the skin is dry, oils or lanolin are useful. Talcum powder is used sparingly; an excess may form granules, especially if the patient's skin is moist, and cause irritation. If a decubitus ulcer develops, various methods of treatment are used; examples include compresses of antimicrobial preparations, cleansing with hydrogen peroxide followed by the application of vaseline gauze, and heat lamp therapy. Nursing aims are to keep the wound clean, as dry as possible and free of infection to promote healing. If the area is large and resists healing, débridement and skin grafting may be necessary. With a large open area there is a marked loss of serum and protein. The patient's protein and vitamin C intake is increased to replace the loss, increase resistance to infection and promote healing.

Positioning. Each time the patient is turned, the nurse checks the position of the paralyzed limbs to insure good alignment. Trochanter rolls and supports may be necessary to prevent contractures and deformities that may develop with spasticity in the affected limbs. With the doctor's approval, limbs are moved through their full range of motion two or three times daily. Active exercises of nonparalyzed limbs are introduced when the patient's condition permits and are progressively increased in preparation for rehabilitation. The patient may require mild analgesics — acetylsalicylic acid, propoxyphene (Darvon), codeine — for pain.

Understandably, the disabilities associated with spinal cord injury and their implications are a severe shock to the patient and his family. Each patient will react in his own particular way but will go through the various stages of denial before accepting his disabilities.

THE QUADRIPLEGIC PATIENT. The quadriplegic patient's problems are greater than the paraplegic's; many of the activities of daily living may be impossible for him and he remains greatly dependent on others for the remainder of his life. This patient usually poses the greater challenge to the nurse and should be given constant nursing attention for about a week. He is normally in a state of shock for the first 48 to 72 hours and, because of edema of the injured cord, requires close observation for signs of respiratory distress. Tracheostomy and assisted ventilation may be necessary. About the third or fourth day the patient may become confused and have sensory hallucinations. This appears to happen with greater frequency when the patient is nursed on a turning bed. Perhaps this is due to the fact that not only is he unable to feel any portion of bed but, because of its narrowness, he cannot see what he is lying on. The room will not look normal as he will only be able to see the ceiling and the floor. He will need constant reassurance and support throughout this phase to help him hold on to reality. The nurse, by nonverbal and verbal communication, conveys understanding and appreciation of what the patient is feeling about his situation and is alert for the patient's readiness to talk about his condition and future.

REHABILITATION. As soon as the patient is well enough, an active rehabilitation program is planned and instituted, beginning with simple self-care activities which can be incorporated into the regular plan of care for the patient. The reader is referred to Chapter 2 on rehabilitation.

Ruptured or Herniated Intervertebral Disk

The bodies of the vertebrae are separated by fibrocartilage disks that serve as cushions and shock absorbers. Each disk consists of a tough, firm outer capsule and a central core of resilient pulpy material referred to as the nucleus pulposus. The capsule is attached to the bodies of the adjoining vertebrae and the anterior and posterior longitudinal ligaments. If injury or degenerative change causes tearing or a weakened area in the capsule, the nucleus pulposus extrudes, resulting in a protrusion that may press on a spinal nerve root, giving rise to symptoms.

Heavy lifting and chronic strain on one or more disks bring about degenerative changes. Poor body mechanics, especially lifting with the trunk in acute flexion, are frequent precipitating causes in herniation and rupture. Injury may be the initiating factor in degenerative changes; the immediate symptoms at the time of injury are not usually significant but signs of nerve compression appear months or years later when the disk becomes weaker and less resilient with the tissue changes.

There is a high incidence of herniated and ruptured disks. As a result, many persons suffer a good deal of pain and discomfort and become restricted in their activities. The nurse has the responsibility to practice and teach good body mechanics, which play a significant role in the prevention of disk problems. The following factors are of particular importance in avoiding undue strain on back muscles and ligaments. When picking up objects from the floor, working at a lower level or lifting heavy objects, the knees and thighs should be flexed and the back kept straight so the greater strain is placed on the muscles of the thighs and buttocks. Bending at the waist with the knees straight and twisting of the spine are avoided. Heavy objects are carried close to the body. Pulling taxes the back muscles less than pushing. Objects with which one is working should be kept at a comfortable level and close enough to avoid the strain of reaching. When sitting, the hips should be well back in the chair so that the weight is on the thighs and lower part of the buttocks, and the back is kept straight. Exercising the trunk muscles (especially the abdominal and gluteal) to promote strength and tone contributes to the patient's ability to function with a minimal risk of strain and injury to the disks.

MANIFESTATIONS. The patient with a ruptured or herniated intervertebral disk experiences pain in the back and in the area of distribution of the involved nerve. The pain is usually worse on bending, lifting, straight-leg raising and with sneezing and coughing. The condition may occur at any level of the spine but the lumbar and lumbosacral disks are most frequently affected, causing pressure on the sciatic nerve. The patient complains of pain in the lower back which radiates into one buttock and down the posterolateral aspect of the thigh and leg. Continued pressure may produce degenerative changes in the involved nerve; decreased or absence of tendon reflexes, loss of sensation, weakness of the urethral sphincter resulting in incontinence, and muscular weakness may develop. There is restricted motion of the spine and postural deformity may be evident due to muscle spasm.

Compression of a nerve by a cervical disk causes pain and disturbed sensations in the arm and hand, and limitation of neck movement. The onset of symptoms may be sudden, following severe strain or twisting, or may develop gradually. The distress may be continuous or intermittent.

DIAGNOSTIC PROCEDURES. Investigative procedures to confirm the diagnosis and locate the lesion may include a lumbar puncture to determine if the protrusion is blocking the flow of cerebrospinal fluid in the subarachnoid cavity, an x-ray which may reveal abnormal curvature of the spine and flattening of the intervertebral disks, and a myelogram (see p. 833).

TREATMENT AND NURSING CARE. The patient with a ruptured or herniated disk may be treated conservatively or by surgery. Surgery is usually reserved for those patients who do not respond to conservative therapy and are experiencing continuous pain and increasing signs of nerve or cord compression and disability.

Conservative treatment usually consists of rest, heat, exercises and some form of back support on ambulation. In the acute phase, the patient is placed at rest on a firm mattress and fracture board. The patient may be comfortable absolutely flat or may find that slight elevation of the legs and thighs reduces the tension of the back and thigh muscles. If the patient is flat, a *small* roll or pillow may be used under the knees for support, but it must be small enough to avoid flexion. Intermittent applications of heat may be prescribed, and passive and active exercises are introduced gradually as the acute phase subsides. The exercises which are done in a warm pool may help to reduce the associated muscle spasm and discomfort.

Observations are made from day to day for any motor or sensory changes. Precautions against burning are necessary when using local heat applications, since the patient may have some sensory dulling or loss. The patient is advised of the importance of maintaining good alignment of his spine and is taught to roll like a log onto his side with the uppermost leg flexed when turning. He is also warned to avoid sudden movements and twisting his trunk. A fracture bedpan is used if the patient is not allowed to go to the bathroom or use a commode at the bedside. A rolled towel placed behind the bedpan helps to reduce the strain on his back.

Constipation is a common problem and the patient is cautioned against straining at stool which increases intraspinal pressure and pain. A mild bulk-producing laxative and increased roughage and fluids in the diet are used to promote soft stools and regular elimination. A mild analgesic such as acetylsali-

cylic acid (aspirin) and propoxyphene hydrochloride (Darvon) may be ordered for the relief of pain. In some instances, muscle spasm is responsible for much of the patient's discomfort and a muscle relaxant such as methocarbamol (Robaxin) or diazepam (Valium) may be prescribed.

When ambulated, the patient may be required to wear a brace or therapeutic corset to provide spinal support and immobilization. The principles of body mechanics to be observed in posture and activities are taught and demonstrated. He is also advised to always use a straight chair rather than a large overstuffed one and to avoid quick, jerky or twisting movements. In some instances, the physician may advise the patient against resuming his occupation. This may cause considerable concern for the patient. A social worker may be brought in to advise and assist him in obtaining suitable employment, or his previous employer may be contacted and asked to make some adjustment. The importance of the prescribed exercise regimen in the prevention of recurring attacks is emphasized when preparing the patient for discharge from the hospital.

In the case of a herniated cervical disk, intermittent or continuous traction may be applied by means of a halter. After a period of rest and traction, the patient resumes activities gradually and usually wears a plastic collar or a firm cuff for support and to limit neck movements.

If conservative treatment fails to provide the necessary relief, acute attacks are recurring more frequently, or there are signs of increasing neurological deficit due to compression, *surgical therapy* is undertaken. A laminectomy is done, followed by decompression of nerve roots or the cord by excision of the herniating disk tissue. If more than one disk is involved, the spinous processes of several vertebrae in the region may be fused by bone grafts for stabilization and immobilization of the area. The grafts may be taken from an iliac crest or tibia. If a fusion is done, the patient's movement following the operation is more restricted, and he is usually required to remain in bed for a longer period. A bivalve body cast extending from the axillae to below the sacrum is sometimes applied on completion of the operation or later, before the patient is ambulated. When the cast is removed, he is fitted for a brace or therapeutic corset, which he is required to wear for at least 6 months. For nursing care following spinal surgery, see the section that follows.

Nursing Care Following Spinal Surgery

SPINAL OPERATIONS. Spinal surgery is most often performed for the removal of a neoplasm, a herniated or ruptured intervertebral disk, or bony fragments following injury, the reduction of a fractured vertebra and decompression of the cord following injury, or the relief of intractable pain or spasticity and involuntary movements. In most instances these procedures involve a *laminectomy* (the removal of one lamina or more) to obtain access to the lesion.

A *cordotomy* is the neurosurgical procedure used to interrupt the spinothalamic tract in the anterolateral portion of the cord, which carries pain impulses from the trunk and lower limbs. The tract is usually severed in the high thoracic region of the cord for the relief of severe intractable pain associated with terminal disease, generally cancer. Spinothalamic cordotomy also abolishes the temperature sense and may be unilateral or bilateral, depending on the involvement of the patient's pain. More recently a simpler procedure has been developed that is used in place of open surgery. Interruption of pain impulses is achieved by producing a lesion in the spinal cord. A spinal needle is introduced in the high cervical region and directed, under x-ray, into the appropriate region of the cord. An electrode is passed through the needle, and radiofrequent currents are discharged into the tissue to destroy the tract fibers.

A *rhizotomy* consists of surgical interruption of spinal nerve roots within the spinal canal. Depending on the purpose, it may involve division of the anterior or motor spinal nerve fibers to check involuntary skeletal muscle contractions or spasticity which increase the patient's handicap and pain. Interruption of posterior or sensory spinal nerve fibers may be done for the relief of intractable pain in the areas which the nerves supply.

Diskectomy implies the removal of herniated disk tissue. *Spinal fusion* is the immobilization of vertebrae by the overlay of pieces of bone taken from another bone.

PREOPERATIVE PREPARATION

PSYCHOLOGICAL PREPARATION. The pa-
tient who is advised of the need for spinal surgery generally becomes quite apprehensive; in most cases the patient is fearful about pain and helplessness. The nurse explains in detail what he may expect following the operation, takes time to answer any questions that he and his family may have, and encourages the patient to talk about his concerns. His condition may be such that he may have a prolonged period of bed rest and convalescence before resuming former activities. This may create socioeconomic problems, especially if the patient is the wage earner and chief support of the family. The nurse may be able to have a social service worker visit the patient and assist in arrangements for necessary help. Less apprehension and fewer worries contribute to relaxation and more favorable progress postoperatively.

If there is a risk or anticipation of any permanent changes in functional ability or appearance associated with the planned surgery, these are explained to the family and patient by the surgeon, and the signature of a close relative as well as the patient's may be necessary on the consent for operation.

PHYSICAL PREPARATION. The importance of maintaining spinal alignment following surgery and how it is achieved are explained. Turning as though the body were one unsegmented unit (log rolling) is discussed and practiced. The patient is advised of the deep breathing and graduated exercises (isometric and active) that he will be required to do and of how his various needs will be met (nutrition, elimination, etc.). If a turning bed is to be used, it is described or demonstrated. Other factors, such as nutritional and hydrational status cited in general preoperative care (Chapter 10) are also applicable.

Spinal operations are usually lengthy procedures, producing greater predisposition to shock. The patient's blood is typed and cross matched, and blood is made available. He may be fitted preoperatively for a back brace or therapeutic corset which will be worn when he is ambulated, or a bivalve cast (anterior and posterior shells) may be made which will be used immediately after surgery to facilitate immobilization of the spine and turning. Provision is made for padding its inner surfaces to protect the wound and bony prominences. Straps are provided to hold the cast in position when it is applied.

Local skin preparation entails shaving and

thorough cleansing of the back from the shoulders to the lower border of the buttocks and from side to side. Surgery in the cervical region necessitates higher preparation and may require clipping of the lower hair and shaving of the lower posterior scalp. If a spinal fusion is anticipated, the surgeon may also require similar preparation of the leg or iliac crest region from which the grafts are to be taken. A cleansing enema is given the afternoon or evening before operation, and an indwelling catheter may be passed the morning of operation. Retention is a common problem for a few days following operation, especially if activity is restricted.

A summary is made of the vital signs and of the patient's sensory and motor status to serve as a baseline in assessing the patient postoperatively.

PREPARATION TO RECEIVE THE PATIENT. It should be determined preoperatively from the surgeon whether the patient is to be cared for on a turning bed (Stryker frame or Foster bed) or the ordinary bed so that it will be ready to receive the patient. If the ordinary bed is used, fracture boards and a firm mattress are necessary, and a footboard, cradle, bolsters, extra pillows for placing under the full length of the lower limbs, and long sandbags or firm rolls to prevent outward rotation of the lower limbs are convenient for positioning after the patient is in bed. Suction should be available and, if the surgery is in the cervical region, a respirator, oxygen and tracheostomy tray should be at hand in the event of respiratory failure. A sterile tubing and closed receptacle are assembled to attach to the indwelling catheter for urinary drainage. The remainder of the equipment is the same as that cited in Chapter 10.

POSTOPERATIVE CARE. The care following spinal surgery varies with the particular surgery done, the patient's response to it and the individual surgeon. For example, some patients are immobilized for weeks while others are ambulated a day or two following the surgery. An understanding of what was done and specific directives are necessary in planning care, especially in relation to positioning and movement.

POSITIONING. Unless the patient is on a turning bed, he may be required to remain in the supine or prone position for 8 to 12 hours after operation without being turned. If he is restless, sandbags along either side may be indicated for immobilization. When the surgeon permits turning, it is usually done every 2 hours. The patient is reminded of the instructions received preoperatively regarding turning and is cautioned not to take an active part except to maintain a rigid straight line. *The major principles to be observed are the maintenance of spinal alignment and prevention of strain on the back muscles.* Twisting, jerking and angulation of the spine must be avoided.

The use of a draw sheet under the full length of the spine and buttocks is helpful as a turning sheet. The patient's arms are placed at his sides or folded across his chest. The turning sheet is rolled tightly toward the patient from each side and, with the lifters keeping the sheet taut to provide the necessary support, the patient is eased to one side of the bed. The sheet on that side is then grasped by the nurses on the other side of the bed and steadily pulled to roll the patient toward them. An adequate number of personnel is necessary so that one person may turn the lower limbs and support the uppermost leg to prevent any dragging weight being placed on the back during the process. In the supine position pillows may be permitted under the full length of the lower limbs, without flexion of the knees, to reduce strain. If pillows are not used, a small bolster may be placed under the knees to prevent hyperextension, but it is important to guard against flexion. In the prone position, a pillow is placed under the ankles. When lying on the side is permitted, supports are placed under the uppermost limbs. In the case of high thoracic or cervical spinal surgery, a pillow under the head is not permitted. A small sponge rubber pillow may be allowed under the neck for support, and the head and neck may be immobilized with sandbags. A footboard is used to maintain a dorsiflexion position of the feet, and the heels are protected from pressure. Sandbags or firm rolls extending laterally along the outer surface of the lower limbs from above the hip joint to below the knee may be necessary to prevent outward rotation.

If the patient is placed in the bivalve cast mentioned previously or on a turning bed, turning is facilitated and there is greater assurance of maintaining immobilization. For details for the turning bed, see page 872.

OBSERVATIONS. The patient's vital signs, color and responses are checked at frequent intervals for signs of shock or bleeding. If he is in the lateral or prone position, the dressings are examined for indications of possible bleeding or leakage of cerebrospinal fluid. Edema or bleeding at the site of the surgery may cause cord or nerve compression and interference with sensory and motor functions. Sensation and motor ability of the extremities are tested every 2 to 3 hours during the first 2 to 3 days to detect any change from the preoperative status. Any complaint of tingling or numbness is recorded and reported immediately. The color and temperature of the extremities are also noted in case of circulatory stasis. Pressure areas are examined for irritation and edema whenever the patient is turned. The urinary output is noted; less than 20 to 30 ml. per hour is reported, since it may indicate hypotension, dehydration or renal insufficiency. If an indwelling catheter is not used, the frequency of voiding and the amount of urine are checked. The lower abdomen is examined for possible urinary retention and bladder distention if the output seems inadequate.

When the surgery is in the cervical region, the patient is watched closely for any signs of respiratory distress or failure. Trauma or edema of the cervical cord or nerves may temporarily cause paralysis of the respiratory muscles.

NUTRITION AND FLUIDS. The patient frequently receives blood during the operation and immediately following. The nurse sees that the flow is maintained and observes the patient for early signs of possible reaction (chill, urticaria, dyspnea or complaints of pain in the back). Intravenous fluids may be given for the first day or two or until the patient is taking adequate amounts orally. He should have 2500 to 3000 ml. daily unless contraindicated. Solid food is introduced as soon as it is tolerated, and the patient is encouraged to take sufficient amounts to promote normal intestinal peristalsis. The patient will probably have to be fed for the first 2 or 3 days because of his position and restricted movement. Precautions are necessary to prevent choking and aspiration if the patient is in the supine position. He is fed slowly, and only small amounts are given at a time.

SKIN CARE. Because of the immobilization, the skin requires special attention. Vulnerable areas are gently massaged every 2 hours or each time the patient is turned. If the skin is dry, a small amount of oil or lanolin may be used to prevent cracking. Resilient material may be placed under pressure areas for protection as long as they do not interfere with body alignment. The bottom sheets are kept clean, dry, and free of wrinkles and crumbs. If a bivalve cast is applied, sufficient padding is necesssary to protect bony prominences. A vest or piece of stockinette is worn under a brace or therapeutic corset to protect the skin and also keep the appliance clean.

RELIEF OF PAIN. The patient will probably complain of considerable pain in the operative area and may also experience some pain and spasm in the muscles of the back and lower limbs due to irritation and trauma of spinal nerves at the time of surgery. An analgesic such as morphine or meperidine hydrochloride (Demerol) is given as ordered. If the surgery has been in the cervical region, morphine is not given because of its depressing effect on respirations. After 2 to 3 days, the patient should require less analgesic, and a milder form may be ordered, reducing the danger of addiction. A change of position or gentle exercise of the limbs when permitted may provide the necessary relief. The patient's position should also be rechecked for possible strain and inadequate support.

ELIMINATION. Urine retention is a common problem in patients following spinal surgery because of the possible trauma and edema of the cord or nerves in the operative site. As cited previously, in anticipation of possible retention an indwelling catheter is generally passed before or immediately after operation. Continuous drainage in a closed sterile system is usually permitted for the first 24 to 48 hours; then the surgeon may suggest clamping the catheter for intervals so that normal bladder tone and capacity may be maintained. The volume of the urinary output is measured and recorded every 8 hours. A minimal daily fluid intake of 2500 to 3000 ml. is important to prevent concentration and stasis of urine and bladder infection. If a catheter is not used, a female urinal or emesis basin may be used to collect the urine to avoid having to raise the female patient onto a bedpan.

No laxative or enema is given without the surgeon's order. Straining at defecation must be avoided. If abdominal distention occurs, it is reported. A rectal tube may be inserted and an intramuscular injection of a peristaltic stimulant such as neostigmine (Prostigmin) may be prescribed. A laxative or enema may be ordered after the third or fourth postoperative day. To place the patient on a bedpan, the patient is turned onto his side, a fracture pan is positioned, and a small pillow or padding is placed behind it to support the back. He is then rolled back onto the pan.

WOUND CARE. If the dressing remains dry, it usually remains undisturbed for several days or until the sutures are removed. The first dressing and the removal of the sutures are done by the physician. If the patient develops an elevation of temperature or there is reason to suspect possible wound infection, the dressing may be removed earlier for wound inspection. Protection of the incision by a dressing may be used for a longer period than with other wounds because of the pressure it may be exposed to when the patient is in the supine position or when wearing a cast or brace.

Following a fusion, the donor site of the grafts will also require attention. The area is checked for bleeding in the immediate postoperative period. When the tibia has been used, the leg is handled carefully, avoiding movement of the knee, and it is supported on a pillow. When the patient is allowed up, a crepe or elastic bandage may be applied for support.

EXERCISES AND AMBULATION. Beginning on the day of operation, the patient is encouraged to take five to ten deep breaths every 2 or 3 hours to increase lung expansion and pulmonary exchange. The patient may find this painful because of the strain placed on the operative site. The nurse explains its importance and remains with the patient to provide necessary encouragement and support. When possible, it may be timed with the administration of the prescribed analgesic to reduce discomfort. Coughing is usually contraindicated.

Passive movements of the limbs may be restricted for the first few days. When they are begun they must be done smoothly and gently to prevent any jerking and twisting of the spine. Periodic massage of the limbs during the period of immobilization frequently proves comforting and relaxing to the patient. A specific directive is received as to active exercises. These may be started quite early with some patients, whereas with others, especially fusion patients, active exercises may be prohibited for 2 or more weeks. After the sutures are removed and there is sufficient wound healing, the patient may be lowered into a warm pool for passive and active exercises. This type of therapy is usually quite helpful if the patient is experiencing considerable muscle spasm.

When the patient is ready to be assisted out of bed, a bivalve cast or brace may be applied for support. He is normally advised not to sit for the first few days, although he may stand or walk. To assist him out of bed, the patient is moved to the side of the bed and, without flexing his legs, he is brought to his feet in the erect position. Someone remains with the patient and notes his reactions the first few times he is up. The frequency and length of his time up are gradually increased. Activities and self-care are introduced and increased according to his capacity and responses.

REHABILITATION. The resumption of former activies and the required rehabilitation program must be individualized on the basis of the nature of the patient's surgery, his response and capacity and whether there are residual disabilities. Self-care and independence are encouraged as soon as his condition permits. In many instances, the patient is fearful of "undoing" the surgery by resuming activities and tends to become overdependent. The nurse must be alert for this and provide the necessary reassurance and encouragement as well as the opportunities for him to regain his confidence and independence. What he may and may not do, the therapeutic exercise regimen to be followed, and the continued wearing of a brace or corset are usually outlined by the physician. Detailed explanations of these and assistance in planning necessary adjustments are given to the patient and family by the nurse. The patient is followed closely by regular visits to the clinic or the physician's office for a period of 6 months to a year. If necessary, when the patient is discharged from the hospital, a referral may be made to a visiting nurse agency for guidance and supervision at home. Assistance may be necessary in making arrangements to transport the patient several times weekly to a rehabilitation or physiotherapy center.

NEUROPATHIES

Disorders of the cranial nerves are frequently secondary to other diseases, but a few are primary to specific nerves. These few disorders, include trigeminal neuralgia and Bell's palsy. Peripheral nerve dysfunction may be incurred by direct local trauma (pressure, severance, infection and inflammation) or may be secondary to a variety of general conditions such as malnutrition, alcoholism and chemical poisoning.

Trigeminal Neuralgia (Tic Douloureux)

The trigeminal nerve (fifth cranial) has both sensory and motor fibers. The sensory fibers transmit impulses from the corresponding side of the face and anterior half of the skull. The nerve has three main divisions: the ophthalmic, whose fibers are distributed to the anterior part of the scalp, the forehead, eye and nose; the maxillary, which supplies the skin of the cheek, upper lip, upper jaw and teeth, and palate; and the mandibular, consisting of sensory fibers which carry impulses from the lower lip, chin, lower jaw, teeth, and the tongue, and motor fibers which innervate the muscles of mastication. The sensory fibers of all three divisions pass to the gasserian ganglion which lies in a fold of the dura mater in the temporal region. From the ganglion, the sensory impulses are transmitted along fibers (axons) which terminate in a nucleus in the pons. The motor fibers originate in a small nucleus of neurons also situated in the pons and join the sensory fibers of the mandibular division just beyond the ganglion.

Trigeminal neuralgia[15] is characterized by brief, recurring attacks of agonizing pain along the distribution of one or more divisions of the nerve. The mandibular branch is most often affected. Abnormally hypersensitive areas occur along the pathway of the nerve (trigger zones) which, on very slight stimulation, initiate the paroxysms of pain. The patient may describe the pain as "stabbing," "knife-like," "searing" or "burning." Usually, the attack is very brief, lasting only seconds to 2 to 3 minutes. It may be followed by dull aching and frequent, recurring acute spells over a period of days or weeks after

---

[15]*Neuralgia* is defined as pain in a nerve.

which there may be a remission of varying length (weeks or months). Generally, exacerbations become progressively more frequent in the sixth and seventh decades.

The onset of trigeminal neuralgia may occur spontaneously or may coincide with movement of the face or exposure to a draft. The patient may relate the precipitation of pain to eating, talking, cleaning the teeth, or washing or shaving of the face. As a result, he tends to avoid these activities and becomes withdrawn and occupied with preventing an attack. During the intense pain, twitching, grimacing, frequent blinking and tearing of the eye may be observed.

The cause of the neuralgia is not known; because it usually occurs in later life, it is thought it may be the result of some "aging" change in the sensory nerves but no significant organic factor has been identified. The sinuses, teeth and mouth are usually examined for possible local infection as an aggravating factor. The incidence of the disease is not great. It occurs more often in women, usually appearing between the ages of 40 and 60.

TREATMENT AND NURSING CARE. Various forms of medical treatment are used in the early stages of the condition, but eventually surgical resection of the sensory nerve roots of the affected division(s) usually is necessary to provide relief. Medications which may be used in conservative treatment include analgesics. The drugs most effective in the control of the pain in trigeminal neuralgia are carbamazepine (Tegretol), diphenylhydantoin (Dilantin), codeine, and propoxyphene hydrochloride (Darvon). Cyanocobalamin (vitamin B_{12}) and/or thiamine (vitamin B_1) may also be administered.[12] There is no specific drug for the condition; what may provide relief or shorten an attack for one patient may prove of little or no value to another. Injection of absolute alcohol into the affected nerve branch may be done to interrupt the sensory impulses and usually provides relief for several months. During the period of effectiveness the patient experiences loss of sensation and feelings of numbness, stiffness and heaviness in the areas of distribution of the injected nerve branches.

Surgical therapy involves sectioning the sensory nerve roots of the affected divisions of the nerve between the gasserian ganglion and the brain, which necessitates an intracranial operation. The ophthalmic division is spared whenever possible, since severance of it produces a loss of sensation in the respective cornea, abolishing the corneal reflex and predisposing the patient to drying of the cornea, keratitis (inflammation of the cornea) and ulceration of the eye. If the ophthalmic trigeminal division is also affected, necessitating its section, special protective measures will be necessary afterward.

An alternate form of surgical treatment that may be used is radiofrequency retrogasserian neurotomy. Lesions are produced in the gasserian ganglion and preganglionic fibers destroyed. An electrode is passed through the cheek and advanced to the ganglion.[16] This procedure requires a shorter period of hospitalization.

During an exacerbation of the patient's disease, factors which are likely to precipitate an attack of the severe pain are avoided. He is protected from exposure to cold and drafts. Food and fluids are served lukewarm. Solid foods requiring chewing may be replaced by puréed foods, and concentrates may be added to liquids to increase the patient's caloric intake. He is kept undisturbed and as quiet as possible. Jarring of the bed and unnecessary activity around him are avoided. Because of the fear of aggravating his condition, the patient may neglect the usual care of his face, hair and teeth. Understanding and tact are necessary on the part of the nurse; it may be helpful to provide warm water and a very soft cloth or absorbent cotton and suggest to the patient that he might like to wash his face. The importance of mouth hygiene in preventing complications is explained, and a warm mouthwash is provided. The opportune time for these activities may be following the administration of an analgesic.

If a nerve resection is to be done, the *preparation of the patient* includes an explanation of its possible permanent effects (loss of sensation, numbness, stiffness and heaviness) and the protective measures that he will have to observe. Some surgeons prefer the patient to have had treatment by alcohol injection previously so that he can appreciate what the permanent effects of surgery will be. Specific orders are received as to the preparation of the operative area. The approach is usually in the temporal region in front of the ear. A minimal amount of hair is removed, and the area is cleansed and shaved. In the case of a female, the remainder of the hair is brushed away from the area and secured.

The general principles of *postoperative care* are applicable following the surgery. As soon as the patient responds, the head of the bed is gradually elevated. He is usually ambulated in 24 to 48 hours and progressively increases his activities. Observations are made for signs of difficulty in mastication due to possible interference with the motor fibers of the mandibular nerve and for temporary facial paralysis on the operative side that may result from trauma of the facial (seventh cranial) nerve. It is not uncommon for the patient to develop herpes simplex (cold sores) around the mouth.

A full diet is introduced as soon as the patient can tolerate it. He is advised to place the food in the unaffected side of his mouth and to avoid hot foods because he would be unaware of burning in the desensitized area. Special attention to oral hygiene is necessary because of the possible accumulation of food particles on the insensitive side. The teeth should be cleansed and a mouthwash used after meals and at bedtime. Since dental problems in the desensitized area will not produce the usual warning by pain, the importance of a dental checkup every 6 months is stressed in discussions with the patient. Patients with dentures are encouraged to use them although they may be uncomfortable at first.

If surgery involves resection of the ophthalmic division of the trigeminal nerve, leaving the conjunctiva and cornea insensitive to foreign particles and injury, irrigation of the eye with normal saline two or three times daily is usually ordered. The patient is taught to do this as he will be required to continue the care at home. The importance of examining his eye at least twice daily for redness and irritation and of voluntarily closing his eyelid frequently to keep the surface lubricated is explained. Glasses should be worn for protection.

Bell's Palsy

This condition is due to dysfunction of one of the facial (seventh cranial) nerves which have both motor and sensory components.

---

[16]Lynne Stanton Ostrow: "New Hope for Patients with Trigeminal Neuralgia." Am. J. Nurs., Vol. 76, No. 8 (Aug. 1976), pp. 1301–1303.

The motor fibers of each nerve originate in the pons and innervate the facial muscles and submaxillary and sublingual salivary glands on the corresponding side. The sensory fibers of the facial nerve transmit impulses from taste buds of the tongue to the geniculate ganglion in the temporal bone and then into the brain stem (medulla).

Bell's palsy is manifested by a loss of the ability to move the muscles on one side of the face that occurs independently of other conditions such as stroke, intracranial tumor and injury. The cause is unknown, but it is suggested that it may be due to compression of the nerve fibers by edema associated with inflammation as a result of virus infection, such as that causing herpes zoster.

The patient may complain of pain posterior to the ear for a day or two; then paralysis of one side of the face appears. The affected side of the face becomes flaccid, the mouth is drawn to the unaffected side, drooling occurs, and the patient is unable to wrinkle his brow, whistle, or retract the corner of his mouth. The eyelid on the affected side does not close and, when the patient attempts closure, the eyeball rolls up. The taste sensation is lost over the anterior two-thirds of the tongue on the respective side. Herpes lesions may appear on or in the corresponding ear.

TREATMENT AND CARE. An adrenocorticosteroid preparation such as dexamethasone (Decadron) may be administered to reduce the inflammation and edema and the resulting nerve compression. The head is protected from exposure to cold and drafts which aggravate the symptoms. Massage and electrotherapy of the face are used to stimulate circulation and muscle tone and prevent muscle atrophy. The patient is encouraged to take an adequate diet and is instructed to direct his food into the unaffected side of the mouth for mastication. Oral hygiene is emphasized to prevent the accumulation of residual food in the affected side of the mouth which predisposes to sordes and parotitis. If there is loss of the ability to close the eyelid, measures are used to prevent drying, infection and ulceration of the conjunctiva and cornea. Irrigations of normal saline and the instillation of an artificial tear solution such as methyl cellulose in saline or a protective oil or ointment may be prescribed. Protective glasses or a shield may be worn.

The affected muscles usually begin to regain tone in a few weeks, and movement is generally progressively restored over a period of months. When recovery is evident, the patient is instructed to carry out a regimen of active facial exercises several times a day. Some residual deficit may occur and, rarely, permanent paralysis results from nerve degeneration.

Polyneuritis (Multiple Peripheral Neuritis)

Although neuritis implies inflammation, it is more frequently applied to dysfunction and painful conditions of peripheral nerves that are not inflammatory. Polyneuritis is a condition in which there is pain and impaired function along the distribution of many peripheral nerves. It is usually symmetrical and is manifested by both sensory and motor disturbances in the involved parts. The symptoms generally start in the parts supplied by the distal portions of the nerves and spread proximally. The patient experiences pain, "pins and needles," tingling and weakness occurring first in the hands and feet. There may be a progressive loss of sensation, diminished tendon reflexes and inability to perform finer movements. The areas are tender and sore when subjected to even light pressure.

The condition is most commonly associated with vitamin B deficiency, malnutrition, alcoholism, prolonged gastrointestinal disease or chemical poisoning. It may also occur in uncontrolled diabetes or peripheral vascular disease (arteriosclerosis) or as a result of toxins produced in an infection (e.g., diphtheria).

The cause is determined and treated. Vitamin B complex is administered, and the patient's nutritional status improved. The patient tends to immobilize the affected parts because of the pain and weakness. Limbs are supported in the optimum position, and a cradle is used to protect the feet and legs from the weight of the bedding. The limbs are gently moved through their range of motion three or four times daily to prevent ankylosis of joints. Heat therapy (e.g., infrared lamp) may be prescribed but must be used cautiously because of the danger of burns due to the patient's reduced sensitivity. Gentle massage may be helpful unless the areas are excessively tender. Analgesics are generally necessary to control the pain in the acute stage.

EPILEPSY (SEIZURES)

An epileptic attack (or seizure) is the manifestation of abnormal electrical activity in the brain characterized by sudden temporary disturbances in brain function manifested by sensory, motor and autonomic dysfunction and change in level of consciousness.

It is generally agreed that the term epileptic implies a person who experiences recurring seizures[17] rather than someone who has had only one attack due to some provoking situation. In the normal brain a certain stability exists between excitation and inhibition. When a seizure occurs, the ability to suppress abnormal neural activity may be impaired or lost, or there may be increased excitation within the neurons. The normal seizure level or threshold is lowered, resulting in an uncontrolled discharge of impulses in response to minimal stimuli. The abnormal neural activity may occur in a small group of neurons and remain relatively localized or may spread to involve extensive areas of normal neurons. In some seizures, no focal origin of discharge is identified; large areas of the brain appear to be involved simultaneously.

Etiology and Incidence

Seizures may be caused by almost any intracranial, pathologic condition and by many general systemic disorders. They may be a manifestation of increased intracranial pressure or brain damage associated with a head injury, cerebral edema, or an intracranial space-occupying lesion, hemorrhage or infection. They may be a sequel to brain injury or infection that has caused tissue damage and scar tissue formation.

General systemic conditions in which seizures most commonly occur include hypoglycemia, hypocalcemia (tetany), renal insufficiency (uremia), hypoxia, high fever (especially in children), toxemia of pregnancy and chemical poisoning (e.g., by alcohol,

strychnine, amphetamines, lead, some insecticides). Seizures associated with conditions such as these do not recur when the causative factor is corrected and homeostasis is restored.

If the epileptic seizures are due to a residual structural or physiological defect following a craniocerebral injury or disease, the condition is classified as *symptomatic epilepsy*. In many instances the cause remains obscure, and the epilepsy is referred to as being *idiopathic*. An inherited predisposition is thought to play a role in idiopathic epilepsy. Studies of epilepsy in identical and fraternal twins report a much higher incidence in both identical twins as compared with its occurrence in both fraternal twins. Identical twins have the same genetic pattern, while that of fraternal twins may be quite *dissimilar*.[18] It has also been reported that relatives of an epileptic frequently have an abnormal electroencephalographic tracing although they may not be subject to seizures.

Epilepsy has an incidence of approximately 4 per 1000 of the population.[19] The greater majority of patients develop their recurring seizures before the age of 20. If the onset takes place after the age of 20 to 30, an organic lesion or previous tissue damage is suspected.

Unless the patient's seizures are known to be secondary to an established systemic disease, he undergoes an extensive physical and neurological examination to determine if there is organic disease. The neurological investigation may include skull x-rays, a lumbar puncture and examination of the cerebrospinal fluid, cerebral arteriogram and a ventriculogram. An accurate, detailed description of a seizure and an encephalogram are important in making the diagnosis (see p. 830 for neurological diagnostic procedures).

Types of Seizures

The seizures which characterize epilepsy vary in form and length, depending on the origin of the abnormal neural activity and the extent and course of its spread within the brain. The manifestations may include loss of

---

[17]R. Bannister (Ed.): Brain's Clinical Neurology, 4th ed. London, Oxford University Press, 1973, p. 149.

[18]R. P. Schmidt, and B. J. Wilder: Epilepsy. Philadelphia, F. A. Davis, 1968, p. 48.
[19]Bannister, op. cit., p. 150.

consciousness, changes in behavior, involuntary uncoordinated movements, abnormal sensations and alterations in visceral function. The seizures may vary in length from a brief transitory phase of a few seconds to several minutes.

GRAND MAL OR MAJOR SEIZURE. In many patients, the grand mal seizure is preceded by a momentary warning of the attack (aura) which may take the form of a sensory hallucination, a disturbed mental state or compulsive movement. The sensory aura may be referred to one of the special senses (auditory, visual, gustatory, olfactory), or the patient may experience numbness or tingling in an area of the body or distress in the epigastric region. The aura is specific for each patient and relates to the function of the focal area of involvement. It coincides with the beginning of the abnormal neural activity.

The first objective symptom may be an involuntary cry caused by the sudden contraction of the thoracic and abdominal muscles, forcing air through the spastic glottis. The person loses consciousness and falls. The convulsive phase of the seizure commences with a strong tonic spasm of the muscles, causing rigidity and distortion of the body. The head and eyes may be turned to one side; the deviation is always to the same side with each seizure. Respirations are arrested, and the patient may become cyanosed. After a few seconds, the sustained, rigid contraction of the muscles is replaced by clonic convulsive movements which are irregular and jerky. Breathing is reestablished and is stertorous. There may be foaming at the mouth and some evidence of bleeding due to the tongue being bitten in the clonic phase. The pupils are dilated and do not react to light. Incontinence of urine is common and, rarely, fecal incontinence occurs.

The convulsive movements gradually become less frequent and finally cease. Consciousness is usually regained soon after the cessation of the muscular contractions. The patient may be confused or dazed or may respond normally. He generally drops off into a deep sleep which may last several hours. On waking, he has no memory of the previous conscious interlude. Headache and physical weakness are common after a seizure.

Major seizures vary greatly in frequency from one patient to another. Some experience only a single seizure in a year or two; in others they occur with much greater frequency at irregular intervals.

PETIT MAL OR MINOR SEIZURE. This type of seizure is characterized by a sudden, brief, transitory cessation of awareness and motor activity. The person stares blankly into space, the eyes usually roll upward and he stops what he is doing. Objects he was holding may be dropped. It lasts only 2 or 3 seconds and may pass unnoticed. The patient resumes his activities, often unaware that there has been an interruption. Occasionally, the attack is accompanied by a few involuntary jerky movements and falling. Petit mal seizures are sometimes referred to as absence seizures, which imply loss of awareness unaccompanied by convulsive movements. They start in infancy or early childhood, and either cease during the adolescent period or develop into grand mal seizures.

PSYCHOMOTOR SEIZURES. This category of seizures is characterized by automatisms, psychosensory disturbances, and a clouding of consciousness. The person, in a trance-like state, usually carries out a stereotyped, inappropriate action which may be quite bizarre. Rarely, violent or unlawful acts may be performed. Following the attack, the victim is totally unaware of what took place. He may also experience various psychosensory symptoms. These may include hallucinations of hearing, smell, taste or vision, a disordered sense of reality and a sense of detachment from his surroundings, a feeling that what is happening at the present moment, has been experienced before, or a sense of strangeness with familiar persons, objects or events, or an abnormal sense of well-being or fear. The attack may last from one to several minutes. During the psychomotor disturbances, the patient is unresponsive to any effort on the part of the observer to check his actions. In this type of seizure the temporal lobe is frequently the site of foci of dysfunction. For this reason this type of seizure may be referred to as a temporal lobe seizure.

JACKSONIAN OR FOCAL SEIZURE. Seizures of this type usually have a well-defined focal origin in the cerebral cortex and are generally considered a symptom of an organic brain lesion. The manifestations are usually motor but may be only sensory or both in some instances. Clonic convulsive movements begin in one part of the body, the most common sites being the thumb and index finger, the great toe, and the angle of the mouth on the side of the body opposite to the cerebral focus on onset. It spreads to involve the entire extremity or face and other parts of the same side. In some instances it becomes bilateral, producing a major seizure with loss of consciousness.

STATUS EPILEPTICUS. This is a serious condition characterized by a rapid succession of seizures without any intervening period of consciousness. Unless the seizures can be arrested, hyperpyrexia develops, coma deepens, the patient becomes exhausted and death occurs.

Excitatory Factors

Certain factors tend to precipitate seizures in some persons. These may be external stimuli such as sudden loud noises, intermittent flashing lights, some types of music or prolonged television viewing, especially if the picture is flickering or is particularly exciting. The seizure may consist of rapid, jerky muscular contractions without alteration in consciousness and ceases when the stimulus is interrupted. This type of disturbance may be referred to as reflex epilepsy.

Excitatory factors also include emotional stress, excitement, fatigue, ingestion of alcohol, fever, alkalosis and menstruation.

Precursory Symptoms of Seizures

Some epileptics manifest or experience preseizure symptoms several hours or days before an attack; many have no precursory changes. The symptoms may include irritability, depression and withdrawal, headache, light flashes, dizziness, muscular twitching or isolated jerky contractions in the limbs, or a voracious appetite.

Treatment

When the patient's seizures are a symptom of identifiable organic disease (e.g., uremia or brain tumor), treatment is directed toward eliminating the cause and may include the administration of an anticonvulsant drug. Regular administration of one or more anticonvulsant drugs remains the most effective method of treating patients with epilepsy. This does not cure their disease but, with the majority, seizures are sufficiently con-

trolled to permit them to be self-supporting and live a relatively normal life. The patient's acceptance of his condition and general pattern of living play an important role in successful control. Surgical treatment may be helpful to a smaller number of epileptics whose disease has certain characteristics.

ANTICONVULSANT DRUG THERAPY. There are numerous anticonvulsant drugs presently being used in the management of the patient with seizures. Some of the more common are phenobarbital, diphenylhydantoin (Dilantin) and primaclone (Mysoline, Primadone) for major convulsions, and ethosuximide (Zarontin) and trimethadione (Tridione) for petit mal seizures. In status epilepticus, paraldehyde may be administered intramuscularly or diazepam (Valium) intravenously. If these drugs do not control the seizures in status epilepticus, an anesthetic agent such as sodium thiopental (Pentothal) may be administered intravenously. If this situation arises, equipment for mechanical ventilatory assistance should be available, since these agents may seriously depress respirations.

The patient and family are made aware of the importance of the patient adhering strictly to the prescribed regime of drug therapy, even if he remains seizure-free. He may have to remain on drug therapy for life, although intermittent assessments may be made to determine if his electroencephalogram still shows epileptiform activity. Drug dosage may be adjusted based on the report. The patient is also made aware of the common toxic side effects to the drugs that may occur. Dilantin, if given in large doses over a period of time, may produce hyperplasia of the gums. Phenobarbital may produce skin rashes on some individuals. Dizziness, headache, drowsiness, ataxia and photophobia are also fairly common side effects of the anticonvulsant drugs. Any of these manifestations should be reported to the physician.

SURGICAL TREATMENT. Surgery is employed in the treatment of a small number of patients with seizures. If the symptoms are a result of a cortical tumor or scar tissue, excision of these lesions may stop the seizures. In temporal lobe epilepsy, the focus may be detected with electroencephalography and excised. Part or all of the lobe may be removed, with dramatic results. In selected cases of children with uncontrollable seizures and severe behavior problems hemispherectomy[20] may be performed, leaving the child seizure-free and with only a mild hemiplegia.

Nursing Care

CARE DURING A CONVULSIVE SEIZURE. When a patient has a seizure, the most important functions of the nurse are first, to protect the patient from injury and, second, to make a close observation of exactly what is happening to the patient. An accurate detailed description of the seizure may be important in determining whether the patient has an organic lesion or focal or generalized epilepsy. A convulsion cannot be stopped once it has begun; it is self-limited, and no immediate treatment will shorten it.

If the patient is in bed, the pillow is removed and the top bedding turned back so that the convulsive movements can be observed. If the patient falls to the floor, a folded blanket or thick towel is placed under his head to prevent him banging his head during the clonic phase. If nothing is within reach, his head may be supported on the nurse's thigh. Any restrictive clothing at the neck is loosened, and the immediate area is cleared of anything that might contribute to injury (e.g., furniture, electric fan, lamps). The patient must not be left alone. Only restraint sufficient to prevent the patient from injuring himself is used. For example, the arms may be held loosely to prevent them from striking a hard surface. No attempt should be made to insert a protective device between the teeth; the damage to the tongue has probably already occurred and the effort is likely to result in injury to the gums and teeth.

A seizure can be very frightening and upsetting to those who have never seen one. If there are others in the room, the patient is screened as quickly as possible, and they are reassured later that he has recovered. It is also comforting to the patient when he regains consciousness to find that he has been screened from exposure to others.

The following observations are made and recorded: (1) the time of onset and duration of the convulsion; (2) the mode of onset — did

the patient cry out? Was there deviation of the head and eyes? Did the muscular contractions start in one part of the body and, if so, what course did the spread take? Was there a tonic phase? Did the patient become cyanosed?; (3) symmetrical or asymmetrical movements; (4) dilation and size of both pupils; (5) incontinence; (6) frothing at the mouth; (7) the condition of the patient when the seizure terminated and he regained consciousness — Was he oriented? Was he able to move his extremities and, if so, was the motor power normal? Was there a compulsive act (automatism)? Was his speech normal? Did he fall asleep?

When he has recovered sufficiently, the patient may be asked what he was doing at the time of onset and to describe any warning (aura) he may have had.

After a seizure, the patient is made comfortable and allowed to rest. Fluids containing sugar are encouraged to insure an adequate supply of glucose to the cerebral neurons.

STATUS EPILEPTICUS. A succession of recurring convulsive seizures without the patient regaining consciousness is a critical situation requiring prompt medical treatment and constant nursing observation and attention. External stimuli are reduced to a minimum. The patient is kept flat and in the prone or semiprone position, if possible, to prevent aspiration of the oropharyngeal secretions. Suction is used to clear the mouth and pharynx of mucus between seizures, and the mouth is cleansed with swabs moistened with an antiseptic. A light application of petroleum jelly may be made to the lips. The bed sides are padded to prevent the patient from injuring himself. The vital signs are recorded frequently; fever commonly develops, and respiratory and cardiac failure may occur as a result of extreme exhaustion. Oxygen administration may be necessary. If unconsciousness is prolonged, fluids and nutrients are usually administered by a nasogastric tube. The skin requires special attention because of the friction to which it is subjected. Soft undersheets are used and may be powdered to reduce friction.

PHYSICAL, PSYCHOLOGICAL AND SOCIAL FACTORS. Occasionally, an epileptic receives a physical injury during a seizure. A head injury or fracture of a limb may occur with the sudden fall, or trauma or a burn may result if he falls against a machine in operation or a hot object. Fortunately, such accidents

---

[20]*Hemispherectomy* is the removal of one of the cerebral hemispheres.

have been rare in recent years with the improved anticonvulsant therapy. A few patients may recognize the onset by the aura they experience and have time to move to a safe area and lie down. Some mental deterioration due to organic changes may develop in patients who experience frequent, severe grand mal seizures. This is generally attributed to the brain being repeatedly subjected to hypoxia incurred by the seizures.

In most instances, the most serious problems faced by the epileptic arise from the misconceptions and biases in our society in relation to his condition. Although attitudes have shown considerable improvement in the last two decades, many still equate epilepsy with impaired mentality and ability, and attach a stigma which has been prevalent since ancient times. Mental capacity, talents and abilities are as varied in epileptics as in the general population. Yet, all too often, the person who has epilepsy is an object of pity and rejection, mistrusted and feared, and not given the opportunity to develop and use his potential attributes. It is frequently necessary and often helpful to remind the patient and prejudiced persons, as well as ourselves, that many famous people in history were subject to seizures. A long list of such persons includes Julius Caesar, William Pitt, Lord Byron, Charles Dickens, Martin Luther, Vincent Van Gogh, Ludwig van Beethoven, George Handel, Peter Tchaikovsky and Alfred Nobel.

Abilities vary in epileptics just as they do in nonepileptics; each one's capabilities and liabilities must be assessed on an individual basis. The fact that epilepsy is not synonymous with mental retardation or psychosis requires emphasis. The condition is not incompatible with normal or even superior intellect, independence and a normal satisfying life free of undue limitations. Today it can be successfully controlled in the majority of affected persons just as the diabetic's disease can be controlled. The person should receive the educational opportunities warranted by his actual intelligence and capabilities; he should be considered employable, encouraged to participate in safe recreation with others, and treated as a respected citizen.

Because of the attitudes and rejection with which so many epileptics have met, many tend to conceal their condition and do not seek assistance from available sources of help. The person lives in a constant state of anxiety, fearful of a seizure revealing his secret.

There is no characteristic personality associated with epilepsy. The same range of personality differences exists in persons with epilepsy as in nonepileptics. Personality and behavioral disturbances are more likely to be associated with seizures caused by an organic lesion (e.g., psychomotor epilepsy). However, the person with epilepsy frequently does undergo personality changes and may become resentful, moody, emotionally unstable and suspicious. These traits observed in the so-called epileptic personality are not the direct result of his disease per se, but usually develop because of the injustices, rejection and frustrations to which the person may have been subjected.

On of the most difficult problems experienced by the epileptic is that of employment, even though his seizures are well controlled. Many employers associate impaired ability with epilepsy and are unwilling to accept the fact that the majority of these persons receive successful anticonvulsant therapy. They are fearful of absenteeism and of accidents to the epileptic and others. The regulations of workmen's compensation boards do not preclude the employment of epileptics in industry. As cited previously, each one must be evaluated individually. Selection of an occupation or job depends on the type of seizures and the degree of control which the person has, but a wide range of employment remains open to most epileptics without jeopardizing their safety or that of others. Granted, there is a relatively small group whose seizures cannot be sufficiently controlled to permit employment other than in sheltered workshops.

A great deal remains to be done in educating society about epilepsy. Certainly, considerable progress has been made and much credit is due the epilepsy associations in this respect. As well as counseling and assisting epileptics and their families, they provide information on epilepsy in various ways for the general public, employers, teachers, police and other interested groups.

GENERAL NURSING CONSIDERATIONS. The nurse has an important role in assisting the patient and family to accept the diagnosis of epilepsy and make the necessary adjustments. The aims of care are to prevent seizures and set realistic goals toward a self-supporting, satisfying social life. Both the patient and family are encouraged to talk about the condition. This is likely to bring misconceptions and anxieties out into the open, giving an opportunity for clarification and suggestions for managing the patient's life. They are advised that persons with epilepsy may be found in many fields of occupation; it does not necessarily preclude education, usefulness, employment and socialization. A reasonable amount of activity is actually considered to contribute to the prevention of attacks.

Persons with epilepsy are generally advised to avoid activities and occupations which, in the event of a seizure, could be dangerous for them and others. These include climbing, swimming (unless with someone who knows about the condition and could handle the situation), working at a height or with certain machinery, riding a bicycle or horse, and driving a car. In reference to driving, the law pertaining to a driver's license varies from one province or state to another; the majority now provide a permit for the person if he has been completely free from seizures for 2 or 3 years. The forms of occupation and recreation considered safe for the epileptic are decided by the physician on an individual basis, depending on the type, frequency, and severity of the seizures. Limitations are kept to a minimum so that feelings of being "different," or resentment and undesirable outlets are less likely to develop.

The patient and family are informed about the epilepsy association[21] and its services and are urged to become members of a local branch. Moderation and normality in the general pattern of living for the epileptic are emphasized in discussions. Seizure-provoking factors which should be avoided are reviewed with them. The use of a firm bed pillow is suggested in case a seizure occurs at night. The family and friends are instructed on the care of the epileptic during a seizure and cautioned that overprotection and rejection must be avoided. The nurse explains to the patient the importance of always carrying an identification card which indicates his name and address, the name, address and telephone number of his next of kin, his condition and medication, what to do if he has a seizure, and the physician or clinic to be called for a directive.

In the case of a child, parents are urged to have him continue at school. The teacher should be advised of the possibility of seizures, of what to do if one occurs and of any restrictions made by the physician on sports or physical education. The epilepsy associations have excellent programs and several helpful brochures for teachers which provide an understanding of epilepsy and their role with epileptic children. If frequent attacks preclude the child's attendance at a public school, arrangements may be made for a visiting teacher or enrollment in a special class.

INFECTIONS OF THE NERVOUS SYSTEM

Poliomyelitis (Anterior Poliomyelitis, Infantile Paralysis)

Poliomyelitis is an acute infectious disease caused by a group of related viruses which have a predilection for the motor neurons of the spinal cord and brain stem. The causative virus is found in the nasopharyngeal secretions and feces of infected persons. The main portal of entry is considered to be the mouth, and viral growth begins in the oropharynx and gastrointestinal tract. The infection may be spread by personal contact or by contaminated food, milk or water. The incubation period is 7 to 14 days, and the most communicable period is during the latter part of this period and the first week of the acute illness. Antibody formation may confine the viruses sufficiently to prevent their invasion of the nervous system and the more serious forms of the disease.

INCIDENCE AND PREVENTION. The disease has a higher incidence during the summer and early autumn and among children and young adults. It may occur sporadically or in epidemics. There has been a sharp decline in the incidence of this disease since 1955 as a result of the widespread usage of poliomyelitis vaccine.

Preventive measures include isolation of infected persons during the communicable stage and immunization by means of a series

[21]Epilepsy Foundation of America, Suite 406, 1828 L Street N.W., Washington, D.C. 20036

National Epilepsy League, 116 S. Michigan Ave., Chicago, Illinois 60603

Canadian Epilepsy Association, 1195 West 8th Ave., Vancouver, British Columbia, Canada of doses of a vaccine. Two types of vaccine are available: the Salk vaccine, which is a solution of killed viruses that is given intramuscularly (see immunization program, p. 61); and the Sabin vaccine, which is a preparation of attenuated living viruses that is administered orally.

MANIFESTATIONS AND COURSE. The severity and course of poliomyelitis vary markedly, depending on whether or not the nervous system is invaded and according to the level of involvement and degree of damage to motor neurons.

THE ONSET. Early symptoms are nonspecific and include headache, fever, malaise, sore throat and gastrointestinal disturbances. The infection may go unrecognized at this time or may be suspected only by reason of known contact or epidemic. The disease may not progress beyond this stage and is then classified as abortive poliomyelitis.

NONPARALYTIC PHASE. In this stage of the disease the symptoms cited above usually become more intense. Due to invasion of the nervous system by the viruses, the patient manifests restlessness, limited spinal flexion and tenderness in the muscles and usually complains of pain in the back and limbs. Positive Kernig's and Brudzinski's signs may be demonstrated and are characteristic of meningeal irritation. Kernig's sign consists of resistance to straightening of the knee when the patient's thigh is flexed on the abdomen. Brudzinski's sign is reflex flexion of a thigh when the opposite one is passively flexed and the reflex flexion of both hips and knees in response to passive flexion of the neck. Examination of the cerebrospinal fluid reveals an increase in the number of leukocytes and protein content.

The symptoms may subside within a week or two without further development of the disease, and the patient is said to have had nonparalytic poliomyelitis.

PARALYTIC PHASE. The patient who progresses to this stage develops paralysis of one or more parts of the body as a result of dysfunction or destruction of motor neurons. The parts which become paralyzed vary with the level of the lesions. If the paralysis occurs in muscles innervated by motor neurons in the cord, the condition is referred to as *spinal paralytic poliomyelitis*. When motor neurons in the brain stem are attacked, the disease is classified as *bulbar poliomyelitis*. Involve-ment of neurons in both the brain stem and cord is designated as *bulbospinal poliomyelitis*. Rarely, neurons at a higher level than the brain stem are affected, producing encephalitic poliomyelitis.

Spinal paralytic poliomyelitis is more commonly seen than the other types. The paralytic phase is characterized by pain and tenderness of varying severity, loss of reflexes and the development of weakness or flaccid paralysis in the affected muscles. The site of the paralysis varies; the disease may be patchy and asymmetrical in distribution.

Involvement of the lumbar portion of the cord may cause paralysis of one or both lower limbs and weakness of the lower abdominal and back muscles. The urinary bladder may also be affected. Disease of the thoracic level of the cord may produce weakness of the chest and upper abdominal and back muscles. The affected thoracic muscles may result in reduced respiratory function. Infection of the cervical cord is critical, since it may result in weakness or paralysis of the diaphragm as well as the muscles of the neck and one or both arms and shoulders.

Bulbar poliomyelitis may attack the neurons of various cranial nerve nuclei and regulatory centers of vital functions (respiratory, cardiac, vascular) which are situated in the brain stem. The patient may manifest dysphagia, weakness of the jaws and facial muscles, inability to cough, and respiratory and cardiac arrhythmias and insufficiency.

The paralysis may be temporary or permanent. Neurons may recover as the disease process is arrested, and hyperemia and edema disappear. The return of muscle power may slowly take place over several months. In some instances, maximal recovery requires a year or two. If the neurons are irreversibly damaged and replaced by glial scar formation, the disability is permanent. The affected muscles atrophy; in the case of a limb, its growth is stunted, it remains flail-like and vasomotor disturbances frequently persist, resulting in coldness and mottling.

TREATMENT AND NURSING CARE. There is no specific treatment for poliomyelitis. The care is principally symptomatic and is directed toward minimizing pain, paralysis and deformities and the promotion of maximum rehabilitation if there is permanent disability.

Isolation precautions are necessary for 7 to 14 days after the onset of symptoms, or longer if the temperature remains elevated. The stools are disinfected before disposal, and the bedpan is disinfected after each use. The patient's dishes and cutlery are disinfected after use, and the bed linen is also disinfected before laundering. Precautions are necessary in the handling and disposing of any articles which may be contaminated by nose and mouth secretions or excreta.

During the preparalytic stage, it is important to keep the patient at rest, since the extent and severity of paralysis are thought to be increased by muscular exercise in this period. An analgesic and sedative may be necessary to relieve the pain and reduce restlessness. The patient is observed closely for indications of muscular weakness and paralysis. He is allowed up when he is symptom-free and there is no evidence of paralysis. The physician usually recommends that the patient who has had nonparalytic poliomyelitis be followed for at least 2 or 3 months after recovery for assessment of muscular function.

The patient who progresses to paralytic poliomyelitis requires more intensive, supportive care. The mattress should be firm or a fracture board may be used, and good body alignment is maintained. When the affected limbs are moved, they must be handled very gently to prevent precipitating a spasm and pain, and the joints are supported to prevent overstretching of muscles and tendons. Appropriate supports (footboard, pillows, sandbags and bolsters) are used to maintain a neutral position and relaxation of the paralyzed muscles and to prevent footdrop, outward rotation of the lower limb, hyperextension of the knee, wristdrop and contractures of the involved parts. A cradle may be used to relieve the weight of bedding on the hypersensitive limbs.

Hot moist packs or dry heat may be used to reduce the pain due to muscle spasm. Changes of position may also contribute to relief of pain as well as to the prevention of pressure sores and respiratory and cardiac complications. Splints may be applied to assist in preventing stretching, injury and contracture of the weak or paralyzed muscles.

The patient is observed closely for signs of respiratory difficulty, especially if the arm muscles are weak or paralyzed which indicates involvement of the cervical portion of the cord. Equipment for suctioning the patient and a respirator should be readily available. The nurse must also be alert to the possibility of urinary retention.

In order to keep the muscles in as good condition as possible and preserve range of motion, an exercise program is begun as soon as the acute pain and muscle tenderness subside and the temperature remains normal. Passive movements, assistive and active exercises and exercise against resistance are used in and out of water to strengthen weakened muscles and minimize muscle atrophy and shortening. Residual disabilities such as footdrop may require the use of a brace to facilitate ambulation. Surgical intervention may eventually be considered necessary to correct problems such as a contracture or a foot- or wristdrop which increase the patient's handicap. For example, the footdrop associated with flaccid paralysis of a leg may be corrected by an ankle arthrodesis (surgical ankylosis or fixation of a joint). A tendon transplant may be done so that a functioning muscle may take over the work of the paralyzed muscle. Muscle reeducation and rehabilitation of the patient with paralysis generally requires long-term care. He may be faced with many of the physical, psychological and socioeconomic problems cited in the discussion of rehabilitation of the handicapped in Chapter 2.

In bulbar poliomyelitis, constant nursing attention is necessary. If the patient's swallowing is impaired, secretions collect in the pharynx and may be aspirated. Frequent suctioning and positioning to promote oral drainage are necessary. The foot of the bed may be elevated, and the patient is kept in the semiprone position. A nasogastric tube is passed so that fluids and nutrition may be administered.

The vital signs are recorded frequently so that early signs of involvement of vital centers are recognized. If respiratory insufficiency develops, a mechanical respirator may be necessary (see p. 424). A tracheostomy may be done if the airway is occluded by secretions or laryngeal spasm (see p. 418).

A diagnosis of poliomyelitis creates considerable anxiety for the patient's family; they require the nurse's support and need to be kept informed about the patient's condition. They should be advised that the paralysis may not be permanent but that it may take several months for the return of function. The exercises and physiotherapy program are explained, and suggestions are made as to their role in supporting and assisting the patient. If he is the wage earner, the family may be referred to a service or social welfare organization for assistance with their social and economic problems.

Meningitis

This is an inflammatory disease of the pia and arachnoid meningeal membranes.

ETIOLOGY AND INCIDENCE. Meningitis may be caused by the invasion of any pathogenic organism that gains entrance to the intracranial or intravertebral spaces. The most common offenders are viruses, influenza bacillus, tubercle bacillus, meningococcus, staphylococcus, streptococcus and pneumococcus. When it is caused by one of the last three bacteria, it is usually secondary to infection elsewhere in the body but may be the result of direct invasion through a cranial or spinal wound. The meningococcal type is communicable, being spread by droplet infection. In tuberculous meningitis, the bacilli are transmitted via the blood from a lesion in another part of the body (e.g., lung, bone) to the meninges.

Viral meningitis is now the most common type; incidence of that caused by other organisms has been rare since antibiotics became available. The disease may occur at any age but is seen more commonly in children.

SYMPTOMS. The onset tends to be insidious in viral and tuberculous meningitis and is more sudden and acute in the other types. The patient complains of headache of increasing severity, pain in the back and limbs, and photophobia. The temperature is elevated, and there is marked neck rigidity. Kernig's and Brudzinski's signs, characteristic of meningeal irritation, are present (see p. 828). The patient tends to remain in a lateral position with the back arched and the head retracted. He is drowsy and probably confused, and coma may develop later. Convulsions are common in children. The cerebrospinal fluid is under increased pressure, is cloudy and has a high leukocyte count, high protein content and reduced concentration of glucose. The leukocyte blood count may show an elevation, depending on the causative organism which is identified through examination of the cerebrospinal fluid.

TREATMENT AND NURSING CARE. There is no specific treatment for viral meningitis; the patient is kept at rest and is given supportive care. Tuberculous meningitis is treated with isoniazid (orally), para-amino-salicylic acid (PAS) (orally) and streptomycin (intramuscularly). These medications are continued over a prolonged period. The dosage is usually high for 2 to 4 weeks, depending on the patient's response, and then decreased and continued for as long as 1 to 3 years. In severe cases, a special preparation of isoniazid may be injected into the subarachnoid cavity (intrathecal injection). When the disease is due to other types of organisms, antibiotics may be administered intrathecally as well as parenterally.

Isolation precautions are necessary if the patient has meningococcal (epidemic) meningitis. Those caring for the patient should know that nasal and oral secretions are contaminated. Frequent mouth care is necessary because of the fever and vomiting.

The room is darkened because of the patient's photophobia. An ice bag may help to relieve the headache, and analgesics are usually necessary for the relief of pain. Temperature sponges may be used if the fever is high. The environment is kept quiet and stimuli at a minimum, particularly with children. Sudden noises and movements may precipitate seizures. The fluid intake is increased to a minimum of 3500 ml., and the fluid balance is noted. An adequate fluid and caloric intake may be a problem because of nausea and vomiting or anorexia. Intravenous fluids and nasogastric feedings may be necessary.

Side rails are used on the bed in case of disorientation. Frequent observations are made for changes in vital signs, level of consciousness and neurological deficit such as impaired hearing and vision, or motor weakness.

Tetanus (Lockjaw)

This disease is caused by the effects on the nervous system of the exotoxin released by tetanus bacilli (Clostridium tetani). It is characterized by hypertonicity of the skeletal muscles and recurring attacks of intense tonic spasms. The organism is spore-forming and anaerobic and is found in the fecal discharge of animals and man as well as in soil. The spores or bacilli enter the body via a wound where they germinate and multiply in anaerobic conditions. Wounds contaminated with soil, deep penetrating wounds and those in which there is necrotic tissue and a reduced concentration of oxygen are more prone to develop tetanus. The bacilli remain localized but produce a toxin which is thought to be absorbed into the blood stream. The tetanus exotoxin acts on the neuromuscular junctions and the motor neurons of the spinal cord and brain stem, producing muscular spasm.

The incubation period, which may vary from 2 days to several weeks, usually ranges from 6 to 14 days. The disease is not communicable except by transmission of discharge from the patient's wound to an open wound of another person. It may be prevented by active or passive immunization. Active immunization is conferred by a series of doses of toxoid. It is now usually given to children in combination with other vaccines (see p. 61). If the patient has not had a booster dose of toxoid within the past 5 or 6 years and the wound is heavily contaminated with soil, the patient is given passive immunization with 250 to 500 units of human tetanus antitoxin (HTAT; human tetanus immunoglobulin). This preparation rarely causes a sensitivity reaction.

MANIFESTATIONS. The first symptom is usually hypertonicity of the jaw muscles. The patient complains of difficulty in opening his mouth and in chewing. This progresses to painful spasms (trismus) in which the jaws are rigidly clamped. The spasticity of the facial muscles distorts his expression. The throat and tongue muscles are affected, making swallowing and speech difficult. Eventually, the tonic rigidity spreads to involve all the skeletal muscles. Periodic spasms of increased intensity occur and are extremely painful and exhausting. During these attacks, the head is sharply hyperextended and the back may be arched off the bed (opisthotonus), respirations are arrested because of spasm of the larynx and respiratory muscles, cyanosis develops, and there is danger of asphyxiation.

The patient's temperature is elevated, and he perspires freely with the energy expenditure. The patient remains conscious and oriented unless severe exhaustion, hypoxia or complications such as pneumonia intervene. The paroxysmal muscle spasms gradually decrease in frequency and severity after 7 to 10 days, but it may take several months before normal muscle tone is sustained.

TREATMENT AND NURSING CARE. The patient receives human tetanus immunoglobulin, 3000 to 6000 units, to counteract the tetanus toxin. Penicillin or tetracycline is administered to destroy tetanus bacilli. Sedatives, tranquilizers and muscle relaxants are prescribed to control the convulsive spasms. These include: diazepam (Valium) orally, intramuscularly or intravenously; chlorpromazine (Thorazine, Largactil) orally or intramuscularly; meprobamate (Miltown) orally or intramuscularly; phenobarbital (Luminal) orally or parenterally; and curare (tubocurarine) intravenously. A tracheostomy is usually done immediately because of laryngeal spasm and the accumulation of excessive secretions. It facilitates deep suctioning and respiratory assistance.

The patient requires constant nursing attention in a quiet, darkened room. All external stimuli are kept to a minimum. Disturbances such as a sudden noise, jarring of the bed and quick handling of the patient may precipitate a tonic spasm of the muscles. Everything must be done as gently as possible; a calm, low voice is used when speaking within the patient's hearing, and he is advised when he is going to be moved or touched.

If a tracheostomy is not done, frequent suctioning is necessary to remove oropharyngeal secretions, and the foot of the bed may be elevated to promote postural drainage. Padded side rails are used on the bed to prevent the patient from injuring himself during a spasm. Mouth and skin care are important in preventing sordes, parotitis and pressure sores. Care is given following the administration of a sedative or muscle relaxant to lessen the possibility of precipitating a spasm. A foam rubber mattress helps to protect the skin. Fluids may be given intravenously and, as soon as the convulsive spasms can be sufficiently controlled, nasogastric feedings are introduced. These are of high caloric value because much energy is expended by the muscle contractions. The patient is observed for retention of urine; catheterization may be necessary. Constipation is a common problem, and enemas may have to be used to prevent or correct fecal impaction.

Herpes Zoster (Shingles)

Herpes zoster is an acute infectious disease caused by the same virus that causes chickenpox (varicella). It is thought that in many instances the virus is reactivated after having remained dormant in the body for varying lengths of time. It has an affinity for the sensory neurons of the dorsal root ganglia of the spinal nerves and the ganglia associated with the sensory divisions of the cranial nerves, but can also involve the posterior horn of the gray matter of the spinal cord and peripheral nerves. It rarely occurs in children and increases in incidence and severity in the older age group. Fatigue, illness and malnutrition are predisposing factors.

MANIFESTATIONS. Herpes zoster is characterized by hypersensitivity, pain and a vesicular rash along the course of the sensory nerves emanating from the affected ganglia. The vesicles usually crust and dry up in a few days, but the area may remain painful for much longer. Fever and general malaise may accompany the onset. The lesions are generally unilateral. The gasserian ganglion of the trigeminal (fifth cranial) nerve is not infrequently affected. Lesions along the distribution of its ophthalmic division involve the eye; vesicles develop on the cornea which may lead to ulceration, scarring and permanent impairment of vision. Some patients, especially the elderly, may be left with permanent intractable pain.

TREATMENT AND NURSING CARE. There is no specific treatment for herpes zoster; treatment and care are directed toward the relief of pain and the prevention of secondary infection of the vesicles. Acetylsalicylic acid (aspirin), codeine and, rarely, stronger analgesics are used for the relief of pain. A calamine preparation may be applied to the local skin lesions and, if they are on the trunk, may be protected from clothing by a light, soft cloth or petroleum jelly gauze.

The patient is not usually confined to bed unless the fever is high or the herpes is a complication of another disease. Well-balanced meals high in vitamins, and extra rest are encouraged.

References

Books

American Rehabilitation Foundation: Rehabilitative Nursing Techniques: Minneapolis, American Rehabilitation Foundation. No. 1. Bed Positioning and Transfer Procedures for the Hemiplegic, 1962; No. 2. Selected Equipment Useful in the Hospital, Home or Nursing Home, 1963; No. 3. A Procedure for Passive Range of Motion and Self-Assistive Exercise, 1964.

Bannister, R. (Ed.): Brain's Clinical Neurology, 4th ed. London, Oxford University Press, 1973.

Carini, Esta, and Owens, Guy: Neurological and Neurosurgical Nursing, 6th ed. St. Louis, C. V. Mosby, 1974.

Chusid, Joseph G.: Correlative Neuroanatomy and Functional Neurology, 15th ed. Los Altos, Cal. Lange, 1973.

Clark, R. G. (Ed.): Manter & Gatz's Essentials of Clinical Neuroanatomy and Neurophysiology, 5th ed. Philadelphia, F. A. Davis, 1975.

Elliott, Frank A.: Clinical Neurology, 2nd ed. Philadelphia, W. B. Saunders, 1971.

Ganong, William F.: Review of Medical Physiology, 7th ed. Los Altos, Cal., Lange, 1975. Sections 2 and 3.

Gardner, Ernest: Fundamentals of Neurology:, A Psychophysiological Approach, 6th ed. Philadelphia, W. B. Saunders, 1975.

Gilroy, John, and Meyer, John Stirling: Medical Neurology, 2nd ed. New York, Macmillan, 1975.

Krenzel, J. R., and Rohrer, L. M.: Paraplegic and Quadriplegic Individuals — Handbook of Care for Nurses. Chicago, The Paraplegic Foundation, 1966.

Krupp, Marcus A., and Chatton, Milton, J.: Medical Diagnosis and Treatment. Los Altos, Cal. Lange, 1975. Chapter 16.

Luhan, J. A.: Neurology. Baltimore, Williams and Wilkins, 1968.

Merritt, Houston H.: Neurology, 5th ed. Philadelphia, Lea and Febiger, 1973.

Robertson, D. M., and Dinsdale, H. B.: The Nervous System. Baltimore, Williams and Wilkins, 1972.

Scott, D.: About Epilepsy. London, Duckworth, 1973.

Sorenson, L., et al.: Ambulation — A Manual for Nurses. Minneapolis, American Rehabilitation Foundation, 1966.

Stryker, Ruth P.: Rehabilitative Aspects of Acute and Chronic Nursing Care. Philadelphia, W. B. Saunders, 1972.

Sutherland, J. M., et al.: The Epilepsies — Modern Diagnosis and Treatment, 2nd ed. Edinburgh and London, Churchill Livingstone, 1974.

Sutton, Audrey Latshaw: Bedside Nursing Techniques in Medicine and Surgery, 2nd ed. Philadelphia, W. B. Saunders, 1969. Chapter 17.

Walton, John N.: Brain's Diseases of the Nervous System, 8th ed. New York, Oxford University Press, 1977.

Periodicals

Adolphus, Patricia, et al.: "Stroke." Can. Nurse, Vol. 72, No. 2 (Feb. 1976), pp. 15–25.

Beven, Edwin G.: "Carotid Endarterectomy." Surg. Clin. North Am., Vol. 55, No. 5 (Oct. 1975), pp. 1111–1123.

Blount, Mary, and Kinney, Anna Belle: "Symposium on Neurologic and Neurosurgical Nursing." Nurs. Clin. North Am., Vol. 9, No. 4 (Dec. 1974).

Bruya, Margaret Auld, and Bolin, Rose Homan: "Epilepsy: A Controllable Disease." Am. J. Nurs., Vol. 76, No. 3 (March 1976), pp. 388–397.

Cooper, Clyde R.: "Anticonvulsant Drugs and the Epileptic's Dilemma." Nurs. '76, Vol. 6, No. 1 (Jan. 1976), pp. 45–50.

Erikson, Roberta: "Cranial Check: A Basic Neurological Assessment." Nurs. '76, Vol. 4, No. 8 (Aug. 1974), pp. 67–72.

Fischbach, Frances Talaska: "Easing Adjustment to Parkinson's Disease." Am. J. Nurs., Vol. 78, No. 1 (Jan. 1978), pp. 40–44.

Fowler, Roy S., and Fordyce, Wilbert: "Adapting Care for the Brain-Damaged Patient." Am. J. Nurs., Vol. 72, No. 10 (Oct. 1972), pp. 1832–1835.

————: "Adapting Care for the Brain-Damaged Patient." Am. J. Nurs., Vol. 72, No. 11 (Nov. 1972), pp. 2056–2059.

Fox, Madeline J.: "Patients with Receptive Aphasia: They Really Don't Understand." Am. J. Nurs., Vol. 76, No. 10 (Oct. 1976), pp. 1596–1598.

————: "The Person with a Spinal Cord Injury." Am. J. Nurs., Vol. 77, No. 8 (Aug. 1977), pp. 1319–1329.

Gomez, M. R., Mellinger, J. F., and Reese, F.: "The Use of Computerized Transaxial Tomography in the Diagnosis of Tuberous Sclerosis." Mayo Clin. Proc., Vol. 5, No. 10 (Oct. 1975), pp. 553–556.

Hekmatpanah, Javad: "The Management of Head Trauma." Surg. Clin. North Am., Vol. 53, No. 1 (Feb. 1973), pp. 47–57.

Hinkhouse, Ann: "Craniocerebral Trauma." Am. J. Nurs., Vol. 73, No. 10 (Oct. 1973), pp. 1719–1722.

Jiminez, J., et al.: "Evaluation of Stroke Disability." Can. Med. Assoc. J., Vol. 114, No. 7 (April 1976), pp. 614–616.

Johnson, Marion R.: "Emergency Management of Head and Spinal Injuries." Nurs. Clin. North Am., Vol. 8, No. 3 (Sept. 1973), pp. 389–399.

Jontz, Donna Lynn: "Prescription for Living with MS." Am. J. Nurs., Vol. 73, No. 5 (May 1973), pp. 817–818.

Keller, Margaret R., and Truscott, B. Lionel: "Transient Ischemic Attacks." Am. J. Nurs., Vol. 73, No. 8 (Aug. 1973), pp. 1330–1331.

Kryk, Helena, et al.: "Grand Rounds on Brain Tumor." Can. Nurs., Vol. 71, No. 9 (Sept. 1975), pp. 42–46.

Langan, Rebecca J., and Cotzias, George C.: "Do's and Don'ts for the Patient on Levodopa Therapy." Am. J. Nurs., Vol. 76, No. 6 (June 1976), pp. 917–918.

Liverani, L., and Osserman, R. S.: "Myasthenia Gravis: A Nursing Care Plan." Nurs. Clin. North Am., Vol. 7, No. 1 (March 1972), pp. 185–195.

Lougheed, W. M.: "The Surgical Treatment of Extracranial Arterial Occlusion." Neurol. Med. Chir. (Tokyo), Vol. 14, Part 1 (1974), pp. 1–4.

Meyd, Constance: "Acute Brain Trauma." Am. J. Nurs., Vol. 78, No. 1 (Jan. 1978), pp. 40–44.

Norsworthy, Edith: "Nursing Rehabilitation after Severe Head Trauma." Am. J. Nurs., Vol. 74, No. 7 (July 1974), pp. 1247–1250.

Ostrow, Lynn Stanton: "New Hope for Patients with Trigeminal Neuralgia." Am. J. Nurs., Vol. 76, No. 8 (Aug. 1976), pp. 1301–1303.

Pfaudler, Marjorie: "After Stroke: Motor Skill Rehabilitation for Hemiplegic Patients." Am. J. Nurs., Vol. 73, No. 11 (Nov. 1973), pp. 1892–1896.

Skelly, M.: "Aphasic Patients Talk Back." Am. J. Nurs., Vol. 75, No. 7 (July 1975), pp. 1140–1142.

Sky, Ruth: "Multiple Sclerosis and the Family Physician." Can. Family Physician, Vol. 23, No. 8 (Aug. 1977), pp. 83–86.

Stackhouse, Joan: "Myasthenia Gravis." Am. J. Nurs., Vol. 73, No. 9 (Sept. 1973), pp. 1544–1547.

Swift, Nancy: "Head Injury — Essentials of Excellent Care." Nurs. '74, Vol. 4, No. 9 (Sept. 1974), pp. 26–33.

————: "Helping Patients Live with Seizures." Nurs. '78, Vol. 8, No. 6 (June 1978), pp. 25–31.

Westlund, Drexel: "Tetanus: A Case Study." Can. Nurse, Vol. 70, No. 7 (July 1974), pp. 17–21.

Wheeler, Priscilla: "Care of a Patient with a Cerebellar Tumor." Am. J. Nurs., Vol. 77, No. 2 (Feb. 1977), pp. 263–266.

Wortzman, G.: "Computerized Transaxial Tomography — Its Role in the Postoperative Tumor Case." Can. J. Neurol. Sci., Vol. 3, No. 1 (Feb. 1976), pp. 51–58.

Pamphlets and Associations

Cerebrovascular Accident

Strokes — A Guide for the Family
Strike Back at Stroke
Aphasia and the Family
Stroke: Why Do They Behave That Way?
Diganosis and Management of Stroke
Do It Yourself Again
Up and Around
Distributed by local branches of the American Heart Association and Canadian Heart Foundation.

Epilepsy

Epilepsy Foundation of America, Suite 406, 1828 L Street, N.W., Washington D.C. 20036
National Epilepsy League, 116 South Michigan Ave., Chicago, Illinois 60603
Canadian Epilepsy Association, 1195 West 8th Ave., Vancouver, British Columbia Canada V6H1C5

Multiple Sclerosis

National Multiple Sclerosis Society, 257 Park Ave. South, New York, New York 10010
Multiple Sclerosis Society of Canada, 130 Bloor St. W., Toronto, Ontario, Canada

Myasthenia Gravis

The Myasthenia Gravis Foundation, Inc. 2 East 103rd St., New York, New York
Myasthenia Gravis Foundation, c/o Muscular Dystrophy Association of Canada, 74 Victoria St., Toronto, Ontario Canada
Professional Information Committee of National Medical Advisory Board: "Myasthenia Gravis: A Manual for the Nurse." Myasthenia Gravis Foundation Inc., New York, 1977.

24

Nursing
in
Bone
Disorders

STRUCTURE AND FUNCTION OF BONES

BONE TISSUE

Bone is a rigid connective tissue consisting of bone cells, calcified collagenous intercellular substance and marrow. Each bone, except at joint surfaces, is covered by a tough, supportive membrane called the *periosteum*. It is firmly attached to the underlying bone by penetrating fibers, and its blood vessels give off many branches which enter the tissue to provide the essentials for growth, repair and maintenance. The inner layer of the periosteum gives rise to the osteoblasts, which function in the development and replacement of bone. The shaft of the long bones is hollow and is lined with a comparable membrane referred to as the *endosteum*. Although approximately two-thirds of bone tissue is inorganic mineral substance, which gives it the characteristic hardness and inert appearance, it is viable tissue undergoing constant metabolic processes, just as other tissues.

Bone tissue contains a network of minute anastomosing canals and spaces which contain blood vessels, lymphatics, lymph and bone cells. The rigid intercellular substance is formed in scale-like sheets or layers (la-

mellae) around the canals and spaces. It is composed of a tough collagenous network of fibers which becomes impregnated with mineral salts, principally tricalcium phosphate and calcium carbonate.

There are three types of bone cells — osteoblasts, osteocytes and osteoclasts. The *osteoblasts* are found beneath the periosteum on the surface of growing bones and in developmental or ossification areas within the bones. They are responsible for the formation of the collagenous fibers, the organic bone matrix and the deposition of the mineral salts. The *osteocytes* are matured osteoblasts which become imprisoned in small spaces by the calcification. The *osteoclasts* are considered responsible for the breaking down and reabsorption of bone tissue. Normally, there is a constant turnover of the mineral deposits. This continuous breaking down, reabsorption and new bone formation is necessary, since old bone becomes weak and brittle. The bone cells respond by internal reconstruction according to the forces acting upon the tissue. The mineralization and strength of the bones are influenced by the amount of weight-bearing and muscle pull to which the bones are subjected. Those of the active person and of an athlete are stronger and more resistant to stress than the bones of nonactive persons. One of the complications of prolonged bed rest is the decalcification and weakening of the bones, with ensuing hypercalcemia. In older persons the bones tend to become brittle and less resistant to stress, increasing the possibility of fractures. This is due to the general decline in cell reproduction which results in a slower rate of production of the collagenous matrix and mineralization as well as of reabsorption.

Types of Bone Tissue

Each bone is composed of two types of tissue — compact and cancellous. Outer layers consist of dense, *compact tissue,* and the interior is of a spongy or porous nature *(cancellous).* The numerous larger spaces of cancellous tissue contain *red bone marrow.* The thickness of each type of tissue varies in different bones as well as in parts of the same bone.

In the long bone (e.g., humerus, tibia, femur), the extremities have a thin outer layer of compact tissue enclosing a larger mass of cancellous tissue (Fig. 24–1). The shaft is formed mainly of two thick layers of compact bone separated by a small amount of porous tissue. The central hollow portion of the shaft forms the medullary canal, which is filled with fatty, *yellow marrow.* Flat bones (e.g., skull bones, scapula, ribs) have a thicker layer of cancellous tissue lying between two relatively thinner layers of compact tissue. Short and irregular bones such as those of the wrist and ankle have a thin shell of compact tissue enclosing a fair thickness of cancellous tissue.

Functions of Bones and Contained Marrow

The bones are bound together by ligaments and collectively form the skeleton, which provides a supporting framework for the body and protection for vital structures. They assist in body movement by providing attachment for muscles and leverage for their action. The bones also serve as the body's store of calcium. A constant level in the blood and tissue fluid is necessary for several physiological processes (e.g., blood clotting, normal muscular activity, normal

heart action). If the blood calcium falls below the normal level, the deficit may be met by the withdrawal of calcium from the bones. Conversely, much of the excess in the blood is desposited in bone tissue.

The red bone marrow is a highly vascular hematopoietic tissue contained within the spaces of cancellous tissue. It produces erythrocytes, granular leukocytes and thrombocytes (blood platelets). During childhood, all cancellous tissue contains red marrow. In the adult, much of this is replaced by yellow marrow, and the cancellous tissue of the ribs, sternum, skull bones, vertebrae, pelvic bones and the proximal ends of the long bones play the major role in hematopoiesis. Yellow bone marrow consists mainly of fat cells and blood vessels; the largest amount is found in the medullary canals of long bones.

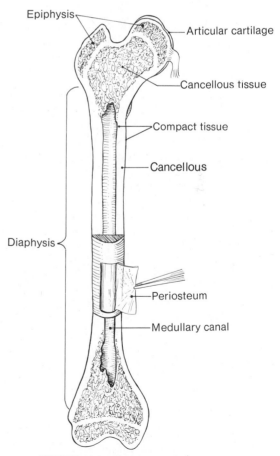

FIGURE 24–1 Diagram of a long bone.

The Development and Growth of Bones

The development of the bones begins early in embryonic life and is not normally completed until the late teens or early twenties. They are preformed of membranous connective tissue or cartilaginous tissue, which is gradually replaced by bone in the process of ossification.

The cranial bones and the mandible (lower jaw) develop by *intramembranous ossification*. There is a marked increase in the vascularity of the membranous tissue. This is followed by the appearance of localized centers of ossification from which bone formation proceeds to the periphery. Radiating bundles of fibers and osteoblasts appear between the blood vessels, followed by the development of the collagenous fibrous matrix which becomes impregnated with calcium salts. The original membrane becomes the periosteum. As the conversion to bone proceeds outward, the edges of the membranous tissue continue to grow. When ossification overtakes the growth of the membranous tissue, the full size of the bone has been reached. The continued growth of the membranous tissue of the cranial bones accounts for the "soft" areas or fontanels in the skull in the infant.

The bones which are preformed of cartilage undergo *intracartilaginous (endochondral) ossification,* which involves destruction of the cartilage and its replacement by bone tissue. Osteoblasts develop at the surface of the cartilage and intiate the formation of surface layers of bone tissue by producing a collagenous fibrous matrix in which mineral salts are deposited. Then osteoblasts, osteoclasts and blood vessels invade internal areas of the cartilage, setting up ossification centers around which cartilage is progressively removed and replaced by bone tissue.

In long bones (Fig. 24–1), an ossification center appears within the shaft *(diaphysis)* and later in each end *(epiphysis)*. As ossification proceeds, growth of the cartilage continues, resulting in a persisting thin strip of cartilaginous tissue between each epiphysis and the diaphysis, which is referred to as the *growth or epiphyseal plate.* The bones continue to grow as long as new cartilage develops to maintain this plate. Cessation of growth occurs when it becomes ossified, and the epiphyses are fused with the diaphysis. Bones grow in circumference by the formation of layers of bone beneath the periosteum.

FACTORS IN BONE DEVELOPMENT, GROWTH AND REPAIR. Several factors influence the development, growth and maintenance of normal bone structure. A diet which is adequate in calcium and phosphorus is essential for ossification and the constant formation of new bone to replace that which is reabsorbed. Vitamin D is necessary for the absorption and utilization of the minerals. A deficiency of any one of these substances in children may lead to *rickets,* which is characterized by soft deformed bones, failure of closure of the fontanels, soft and poorly developed teeth, bleeding tendency and muscle spasms. In adults, a deficiency of calcium and phosphorus or vitamin D may cause a weakening of bone structure referred to as *osteomalacia.* Milk and milk products provide an abundant source of the minerals. Vitamin D may be formed by exposure of the skin to sunlight, which acts on a sterol (7-dehydrocholesterol) that is a component of the skin. To insure an adequate supply of vitamin D, a preparation of a fish liver oil (e.g., cod liver oil) or of ergosterol which has been exposed to ultraviolet rays (calciferol) is usually administered to infants and young children. The nurse must be cognizant of the fact that excessive amounts of vitamin D can cause hypercalcemia, which may be manifested by anorexia, nausea, vomiting, drowsiness, headache, heart irregularity, bladder irritation and renal calculi.

Adequate dietary amounts of protein and vitamin C are necessary to bones for the formation of the collagenous, fibrous, intercellular matrix in which the minerals are deposited. Vitamin A, which is essential to all tissue growth, is also necessary.

Bone growth and ossification are also influenced by certain hormones — namely, the somatotrophic or growth hormone produced by the adenohypophysis (see p. 751), thyroxine (see p. 760) and the parathyroid hormone (see p. 770).

In addition to the above factors, the demand placed on the bones by weight-bearing and muscle pull plays an important role. Inactivity and less than the normal demand weaken the structure; calcium and phosphorus are lost from the bone, and the condition known as *osteoporosis* may develop. Osteoblastic activity is slowed, and bone deposition is depressed. Muscle pull and the degree of stress also influence the shaping of the bone. For example, processes such as the greater and lesser trochanters of the femur, the tibial tuberosity of the tibia, and the deltoid tuberosity of the radius develop as the result of muscle pull when the bones are developing and growing.

NURSING IN BONE DISORDERS

FRACTURES

A fracture is a break in the continuity of a bone, separating it into two or more parts, which are referred to as *fragments*. The soft tissues in the area are also injured.

Causes

The majority of fractures are due to violence incurred by falls, blows or twisting. The force, in excess of the bone's resistance, may be applied directly or indirectly. In direct violence, the fracture occurs at or near the site of the applied force. When indirect violence is the cause, the force is applied at a point remote from the site of the fracture. For example, in a fall on the outstretched hand, the stress may be transmitted to the radius, ulna, humerus or clavicle. A fracture rarely may be due to a sudden, forceful contraction of attached muscles.

Occasionally, a fracture occurs as the result of disease of the bone which has weakened its structure to the point that it cannot withstand the normal degree of stress. Metastases, primary tumors (e.g., sarcoma, osteitis fibrosa cystica due to hyperparathyroidism), osteogenesis imperfecta (a congenital condition affecting the formation of osteoblasts) and osteoporosis are examples of diseased conditions of bone that may lead to spontaneous fracture. Prolonged stress may also cause a fracture in certain bones. For example, a long march may cause a metatarsal fracture.

Types of Fractures [1]

TRAUMATIC OR PATHOLOGIC. The fracture may be designated as traumatic when it is the result of violence or as pathologic or spontaneous if it is due to disease of the bone.

COMPLETE OR INCOMPLETE. A fracture is complete if the bone is separated into two distinct parts or incomplete if the break is not all the way through the bone (Fig. 24–2). The greenstick fracture seen in children is an incomplete fracture in which the bone is broken on one side and bent or crumpled on the opposite side.

SIMPLE OR COMMINUTED. A fracture may be described as simple if it produces only two fragments or as comminuted if it consists of three or more fragments.

OPEN (COMPOUND) OR CLOSED. An open or compound fracture is associated with an open wound in the overlying skin which establishes communication between the fracture site and the outside air. This type of fracture is potentially infected. The skin wound may be produced by the force that inflicted the fracture or by a fragment of the bone. Conversely, in a closed fracture the overlying skin remains intact and there is no communication with the outside.

ACCORDING TO THE DIRECTION OF THE FRACTURE LINE. The break may be described as *transverse, longitudinal, oblique* or *spiral,* according to the direction of the fracture line in relation to the longitudinal axis of the bone. When one fragment is driven into the other one, the fracture is referred to as *impacted.*

COMPRESSION. This is an impacted fracture in which there is a crushing of the bone tissue at the margins of the fragments as they are compressed together.

SPECIAL. A few fractures have been named for physicians associated with studies of fractures in certain areas. The commonest of these are the Colles' and Pott's fractures. In a *Colles' fracture,* a break occurs in the distal portion of the radius and possibly in the styloid process of the ulna. A *Pott's fracture* involves a break

---

[1]*Note:* Injury and fracture of the spine and skull are discussed in Chapter 23 because of the serious associated neurological involvement.

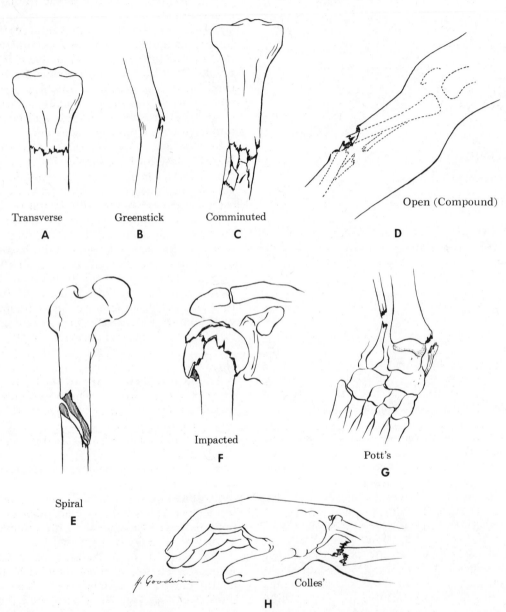

FIGURE 24–2 Types of fractures. *A*, Simple complete transverse. *B*, Incomplete (greenstick). *C*, Comminuted. *D*, Compound (open). *E*, Spiral. *F*, Impacted. *G*, Pott's. *H*, Colles'.

through the distal ends of the tibia and fibula. An *epiphyseal separation* or fracture occurs when the break is through the epiphyseal or growth plate. When a ligament or tendon under excessive stress fractures or tears away its bony attachment, the break in the bone is described as an avulsion fracture.

Effects and Manifestations

LOCAL EFFECTS. A fracture is always accompanied by some degree of damage to the contiguous soft tissues. Blood vessels within the bone, the periosteum and surrounding tissues are torn, resulting in hemorrhage and then the formation of a hematoma. The periosteum at the site may be stripped from the underlying bone tissue, interrupting the blood supply into the area and thus contributing to the death of bone cells. There may also be hemorrhage into adjacent muscles and joints and damage to ligaments, tendons and nerves. Soon after a fracture occurs the muscles in the area go into spasm, causing severe pain and possible displacement of a fragment due to tendon pull.

Depending on the location of the fracture, visceral injuries may occur, actually provoking a threat to the patient's life. Examples of such injuries are rupture of the bladder by a fractured pelvis and rupture of the spleen or perforation of a lung by a fractured rib.

SYSTEMIC EFFECTS. The patient suffers some degree of shock which is influenced by the severity of the injury, the amount of soft tissue damage, associated disorders or multiple injuries, and the patient's age and general condition at the time of injury. (See p. 372 for predisposing factors and manifestations of shock.) Usually a slight elevation of temperature and leukocytosis occur in the first 2 or 3 days.

MANIFESTATIONS. The symptoms of a fracture vary with its location, type, the amount of displacement of the fragments and the degree of damage to soft tissue structures.

The patient or an observer usually relates a history of a fall, blow or sudden forcible movement, and the victim may actually say that he heard the bone break. Sudden severe pain at the site is experienced which may or may not persist. Frequently, because of injury and shock, nerve function is impaired, and pain may be absent for a brief period following the injury. As function returns, muscle spasm in the area, as well as tissue damage, accounts for much of the pain, which becomes worse with any movement. Obvious deformity may be present as a result of displacement of the fragments, and there may be shortening of the affected limb due to contraction of attached muscles. Impaired mobility and loss of mechnical support occur, and, in the case of long bones, there may be obvious movement in a part that is normally rigid. Complete loss of function may result from nerve compression by displaced fragments; this is usually restored when the fracture is reduced and the fragments are placed in normal apposition.

Crepitus (grating sound produced by movement of the ends of the fragments) may be noted if the patient moves the part. Under no circumstances should any attempt be made to elicit the symptom of crepitus because of the possibility of further serious damage to soft tissues (e.g., blood vessels and nerves), unnecessary displacement of fragments and the production of an open fracture. Swelling may develop rapidly over the site of the fracture because of bleeding and the escape of fluid into the tissue. After 2 or 3 days this area frequently becomes discolored (ecchymosis).

In the case of the rupture of viscera by a fragment, symptoms of impaired function of the damaged organ appear. With rupture of the bladder by a fractured pelvis, extravasation of urine gradually becomes evident, and blood appears in the urine. Rarely, perforation of the intestine is associated with pelvic fracture and causes severe shock and peritonitis; the abdomen becomes distended and board-like. A serious complication of a rib fracture may be puncture of a lung. The patient manifests severe shock, respiratory distress, coughing and hemoptysis.

Some fractures, especially those which are incomplete or of short bones, may produce few signs and symptoms. The fracture may be suspected only on the basis of the history of violence, tenderness on pressure over the site or the patient's complaint of pain upon use of the part or weight-bearing on it. Again, no attempt should be made by the person administering first aid or a nurse to elicit symptoms by having the person move or stand. The patient is treated as having a fracture if there is any doubt.

The physician bases his diagnosis of a fracture on the history of the accident, physical examination of the patient and roentgenograms of the affected part.

Fracture Healing

Bone is different from many of the specialized tissues because of its ability to regenerate and bridge a gap to unite broken bones. Many tissues heal by laying down nonspecialized fibrous scar tissue.

Immediately following a fracture, the space between the fragments and around the fracture line is filled with blood and inflammatory exudate. The blood clots and the exudate are invaded by fibroblasts and capillaries from adjacent connective tissue and blood vessels, forming granulation tissue. The fibroblasts differentiate to form fibrous tissue and cartilage. Simultaneously, osteoblasts proliferate, mainly from the inner surface of the periosteum (and endosteum in a long bone), and invade the granulation tissue and cartilage. Calcium salts are deposited, forming a loosely woven, bone-like tissue referred to as a callus. It forms a "collar" around the bone at the fracture site, giving it greater thickness than the original bone. The callus unites and helps to stabilize the fragments but is not strong enough to bear weight or withstand stress. As the bone-forming cells increase, the callus is gradually restructured and remodeled by ossification (production of a collagenous fibrous network which becomes impregnated with mineral salts) to form true bone tissue.

In some instances, a fracture is complicated by malunion, delayed healing or nonunion. *Malunion* implies healing of the fracture in an abnormal position. There may be angulation of the bone or overriding of the fragments which alters the shape and length of the limb. Function may be impaired. The cause is usually ineffective reduction and/or fixation during healing. *Delayed healing* simply implies that the fracture is not healing as rapidly as is normally expected. In *nonunion,* the granulation tissue that formed between the fragments following the fracture is converted to dense fibrous tissue instead of normal callus and bone tissue. Causes of delayed union or nonunion include too wide a gap between the fragments, the interposition of soft tissues or a foreign body between the fragments, inadequate immobilization, poor blood supply to the site, loss of the initial hematoma by the escape of blood through an open wound or surgical intervention, infection of the bone and malnutrition.

General Principles and Methods of Treatment of Fractures

EMERGENCY CARE. The patient's general condition and the extent of his injuries are quickly evaluated, and priorities are set. Respiratory insufficiency, hemorrhage or shock may be evident and take precedence over injured bones.

The first aid treatment that the patient with a fracture receives is very important; movement of the patient or improper handling may cause serious tissue damage and increased pain, hemorrhage and shock. If a fracture is obvious or suspected, care at the site of the accident and during transportation to a hospital is directed toward reducing pain and preventing further tissue damage, visceral injury, and a closed fracture's becoming open. The patient should receive a minimum of handling; unless there is danger of further injury, he is left where he is until lifted onto a stretcher or into a vehicle for transportation to the hospital. The patient is told what is going to be done and why, and that he should remain immobile. Before moving the patient, the fracture site and the joint above and below are immobilized. A splint is made from whatever is available (e.g., a board, two or three thicknesses of cardboard, a folded quilt or blanket, pillows). In the case of a board, the surface applied to the patient must be padded (towels or clothing may be used) to prevent pressure. If the limb is in an abnormal position, it is splinted in that deformed position; no attempt is made to reduce the fracture or restore the limb to a normal position. If splint material is not available, a lower limb may be immobilized by placing a pillow or folded blanket between the legs and tying them together. The uninjured limb serves as a splint. In the case of an arm, it may be secured against the trunk by binders or bandages. If it is an open fracture, the wound is covered with the cleanest material available (e.g., a clean handerchief). If the bone is protruding from the wound, no attempt is made to replace it or reduce the fracture. Nothing is given by mouth in case a general anesthetic will be necessary.

When the patient arrives at the hospital, a quick assessment is made of his general condition, and if there is respiratory insufficiency, bleeding or shock, appropriate treatment is instituted before the fracture receives attention. When the general condition is satisfactory, roentgenograms are made of the fracture area. Clothing is removed from the uninjured side of the body first. When it is necessary to cut the clothing on the injured side, this is done along a seam if possible so the garment may be repaired later.

TREATMENT. The treatment of a fracture usually involves reduction, immobilization of the part while the bone heals, and then a period of physical therapy to restore normal function. Some fractures, such as those of distal phalanges of the fingers and toes, may heal without reduction and immobilization equipment. The patient keeps the part at rest and, in the case of a toe, elevated when sitting. An analgesic is prescribed for relief of pain.

REDUCTION. This is the procedure by which fragments are brought into their preinjury position so that the normal shape and length of the bone are restored and union is promoted. Obviously, reduction is only necessary if there is some displacement of the fragments. It is carried out as soon as possible. A delay makes it more difficult to obtain satisfactory alignment because of the rapid organization of the blood clot and the development of associated muscle spasm. Also, there is likely to be less tissue trauma with early reduction.

A fracture may be reduced by closed manipulative reduction, traction applied distal to the fracture, or open (internal) reduction. In *closed reduction,* the physician manipulates the fragments into position by manual traction, pressure, and/or rotation. In fractures in which one fragment is overriding the other and there is considerable muscle pull, continuous *traction* may be applied to the distal fragment to bring it into apposition and to maintain the alignment. This method of reduction is used most often in fractures of the femur because the pull of the strong thigh muscles tends to displace the fragments and cause overriding. The traction may be applied to the skin (skin traction) or directly to bone (skeletal traction). (See the discussion of traction under Immobilization.) In some fractures, reduction can only be achieved through an *open surgical incision.*

Reduction may necessitate a general anesthetic. The nurse determines from the patient when he last had food and fluid and what was taken. This is reported to the physician. Reduction may have to be delayed a few hours to allow the stomach to empty and reduce the risk of vomiting and aspiration.

IMMOBILIZATION. Various methods are used to maintain reduction and immobilize the fragments. They may be categorized as external fixation, traction or internal fixation. The method used depends upon the particular bone (e.g., location — short, long or flat), the type of fracture and the muscles involved.

External fixation is most commonly achieved by enclosing the part in a plaster cast. A *plaster cast* is made by the application and molding of moist plaster of Paris bandages to the affected part. The bandages are strips of crinoline-like material impregnated with gypsum (anhydrous calcium sulfate). They are immersed in warm water, 21° to 24° C. (70° to 75° F.), for a few seconds and then are lightly compressed by pushing both ends toward the middle to remove excess water before application and to prevent telescoping of the bandage. The addition of water to the bandage causes the gypsum to crystallize. While wet it is possible to mold the soft moist bandage to the affected body part. As it is applied, each layer is rubbed into that below to prevent separation of the case into layers. As the water evaporates from the bandages, the plaster hardens and the application becomes rigid.

Before the cast is applied, the skin is cleansed and examined for any contusions or abrasions. The part is then enclosed in circular stockinette for skin protection.

Extra padding is used over bony prominences or to fill in spaces which might weaken the cast.

When the application of the plaster bandages is completed, the stockinette which extends beyond the cast is turned back over the cast edges and is secured by incorporation into the cast or with adhesive tape. The cast applied to a limb may be referred to as a *circular cast*. A *walking cast* may be applied with simple fractures of the tibia and fibula. A stump or walking iron is incorporated into the cast which encloses the leg and most of the foot. This device permits the patient to be up, walk and bear his weight on the limb. If a stirrup is not used, additional layers of plaster on the sole may be used. A *spica cast* is applied to the trunk and one or both lower or upper limbs (e.g., shoulder spica, hip spica). A cast which is applied to the trunk is called a *jacket or body cast*. A *bivalve cast* is one which has been molded to the limb or trunk, allowed to dry, and then cut down each side so it may be removed for brief periods to allow skin or wound care or other treatment. The sections are held in position by bandages or straps. See the discussion of nursing care of the patient with a cast on page 912.

A *splint* is occasionally used as a means of external fixation and may be of wood, metal, plastic or molded plaster of Paris. It should be long enough to immobilize the joints immediately above and below the fracture and is shaped or molded according to the part to which it is applied. Padding is placed between the skin and the splint to prevent irritation and pressure and to fill in spaces. The splint is secured by straps or firm bandages. Precautions are necessary in order to have the splint held stationary without interfering with circulation. Any swelling, discoloration, coldness or numbness of the distal parts of the limb is reported immediately so the splint may be loosened.

Traction is most commonly used to reduce and maintain reduction in fractures of the limbs by overcoming the effects of gravity and muscle pull.[2] It involves the application of a force along the long axis of the bone distal to the fracture. Countertraction (a force in the opposite direction) is necessary and is provided by elevating the foot of the bed in the case of a lower limb; the weight of the body on the incline supplies the required countertraction. A fracture board is placed under a firm mattress to prevent sagging which could change the direction of the force being applied and interfere with alignment of the fragments. An important use of traction is to overcome the deforming muscle pull that is associated with many fractures. For example, a fracture in the femur is accompanied by marked displacement of the fragments due to the contracture of the very strong muscles of the thigh and hip. The adductor muscles produce a lateral bowing (see Fig. 24–3).

As cited in reduction, traction may be applied to the skin or directly to the bone. *Skin traction* is established by the application of moleskin or adhesive tapes to the medial and lateral surfaces of the limb. These are secured by a firm encircling cotton or elastic bandage. The adhesive strips extend beyond the foot and attach to a plate, bar or block (spreader) wide enough

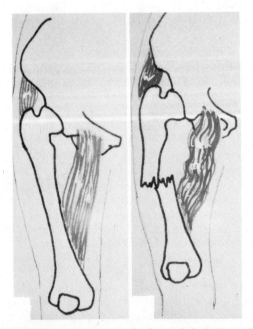

FIGURE 24–3 Fracture in the femoral shaft. The pull by the adductor muscles causes a displacement of the fragments. (From Gartland, John J.: Fundamentals of Orthopaedics, 2nd ed. Philadelphia, W. B. Saunders, 1974, p. 31.)

---

[2]*Note:* Traction may also be employed to correct a deformity, relieve pressure on a spinal nerve or prevent a contracture deformity in cases in which there is muscle spasm.

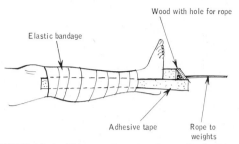

Elastic bandage

Wood with hole for rope

Adhesive tape

Rope to weights

FIGURE 24–4 Skin traction on a lower limb. (From Sutton, A. L.: Bedside Nursing Techniques, 2nd ed. Philadelphia, W. B. Saunders, 1969, p. 190.)

to prevent the tapes from contacting the malleoli. A rope connected to the spreader is carried over a pulley on a crossbar at the foot of the bed and suspends a prescribed weight (usually 6 to 8 pounds for an adult) to exert the traction force (see Fig. 24–4). The disadvantage of skin traction is the limited number of pounds of traction that can be used without damaging the skin. It may be used for a temporary period with an adult, but is used more often with fractures in children.

Skeletal traction is obtained by the insertion of a metal wire (e.g., Kirschner wire) or pin (e.g., Steinmann's pin) through the bone distal to the fracture. A special traction stirrup or bow is fastened to the protruding ends of the wire or pin and is then attached to a rope leading to a pulley and weight system. When skeletal traction is used, the limb is usually suspended on a special splint (see Fig. 24–5).

The appliance used may produce straight traction, balanced suspension traction or vectored traction. *Straight traction* implies a pull along the long axis of the extremity; an example is Buck's extension. The patient may not turn even slightly, since the leg is resting on the bed and the proximal fracture fragment would turn against the distal fragment. In *balanced suspension* traction, the entire limb is suspended or "floats" off the bed surface. The arrangement is such that a single weight suspends the limb and exerts a pull along the long axis of the bone distal to the fracture (e.g., Russell traction). The traction remains constant and the fragments remain stationary when the patient raises up or turns slightly.

Vectored traction implies the application of traction in two or more different directions. The lines of force are at or close to a

right angle to each other. The resultant pull or vectored force is somewhere between the lines of pull which are positioned to produce the traction in the necessary direction for apposition and immobilization of the fragments. Vectored traction is frequently applied in the treatment of a fractured femur, using balanced suspension and skeletal traction. A half- or full-ring Thomas splint with a Pearson attachment is used. See Figure 24–6 for examples of traction.

Various arrangements are used in applying traction to the lower limbs. Those commonly employed are Buck's extension, Bryant's traction (gallows suspension), Russell traction and balanced or suspension traction.

Buck's extension involves simple skin traction by means of adhesive strips applied to the sides of the leg and their attachment to a spreader which in turn attaches to a rope leading to a pulley and suspended weights.

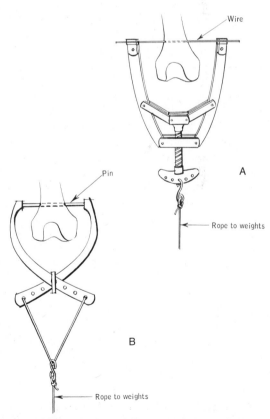

Wire

Pin

A

B

Rope to weights

Rope to weights

FIGURE 24–5 Skeletal traction may be applied by a Kirschner wire and traction stirrup (*A*) or Steinmann pin and traction stirrup (*B*). (From Sutton, A. L.: Bedside Nursing Techniques, 2nd ed. Philadelphia, W. B. Saunders, 1969, p. 191.)

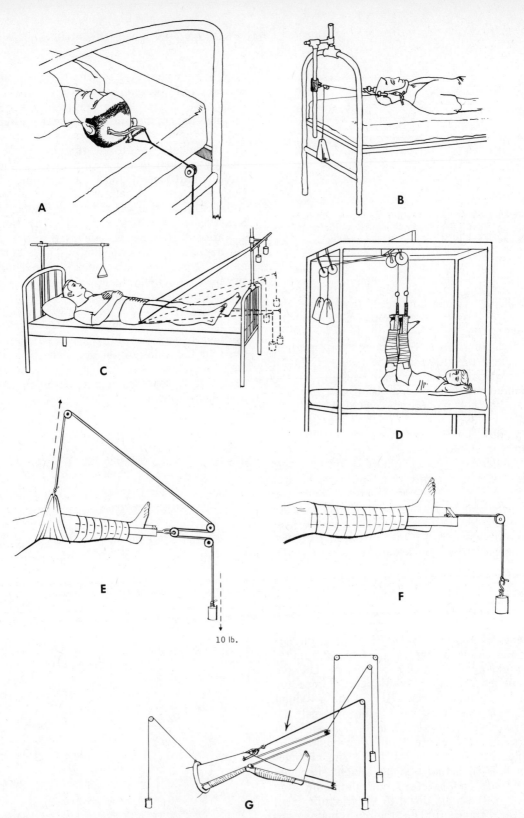

FIGURE 24–6 Types of traction. *A,* Cervical traction using tongs. *B,* Cervical traction using a halter. *C,* Pelvic traction. *D,* Bryant's traction. *E,* Russell traction, which may be used in the treatment of the shaft of the femur. *F,* Buck's extension. *G,* Balanced suspension traction using a Thomas splint with a Pearson attachment. (*A* through *D* from Miller, Benjamin F., and Keane, Claire B.: Encyclopedia and Dictionary of Medicine, Nursing and Allied Health, 2nd ed. Philadelphia, W. B. Saunders, 1978, p. 1015; *E* through *G* from Sutton, A. L.: Bedside Nursing Techniques, 2nd ed. Philadelphia, W. B. Saunders, 1969, pp. 191–192.)

It is usually only used temporarily for reduction of a fracture. The skin should be clean and dry before the traction tapes are applied. The physician may or may not want the leg shaved. Some consider that shaving removes epithelium, leaving the skin more vulnerable to irritation by the adhesive. An application of tincture of benzoin may be ordered to protect the skin and provide better adherence of the tapes. The tapes may be nicked (approximately ¼ inch) every 1 to 1½ inch along the edges; this provides better adherence by allowing the adhesive to follow the contour of the leg closely. The knee is usually held in slight flexion during the application of the adhesive to avoid hyperextension when the weight is attached. The adhesive is not applied over the malleoli or foot but is extended unattached to the spreader beyond the sole of the foot. If the lateral tape is applied over the head of the fibula, precautions are taken to place a pad over the area under the tape to prevent compression of the peroneal nerve which lies close to the surface. Damage to the nerve could result in interference with normal ankle movement. A pillow is usually placed lengthwise under the leg and knee for support, leaving the heel suspended, free of pressure.

Bryant's traction is used in a fracture of the femoral shaft of a young child (under 6 years). Two overhead bars extend the length of the bed. Each has two pulleys, one in line with the child's pelvis and the other just beyond the foot of the bed. Tapes and bandages similar to those used in Buck's extension are applied to both limbs, which are suspended at right angles to the body. Ropes from the spreaders are carried over the pulleys and suspend sufficient weight to lift the buttocks just clear of the bed. A restraining jacket is usually necessary to keep the child in position. The dorsum of the foot and the heel are examined frequently for pressure from the bandage. Any discoloration, edema, loss of motion or sensation, or coldness indicating interference with circulation is reported promptly.

Russell traction is also used in the treatment of a fracture of the shaft of a femur. Vertical traction is applied at the knee at the same time a horizontal force is exerted on the tibia and fibula. The pull on the leg bones is exerted to counteract the contrac-

tion of thigh muscles (quadriceps femoris and hamstring) which insert on the leg bones. Considerable spasm of these strong muscles occurs with a fracture of the femur, causing displacement and overriding of the fragments. The horizontal force is exerted on moleskin or adhesive tapes applied to the medial and lateral surfaces of the leg. The tapes are applied from just below the knee to about 1 inch above the malleoli. They are carried beyond the foot and attached to a spreader. A circular bandage is used to secure the tapes as in Buck's extension. The lateral tapes are terminated just below the head of the fibula to avoid compression of the peroneal nerve. Figure 24–6E illustrates Russell traction.

An overhead bar (Balkan frame) is attached to the bed in line with the affected limb. A crossbar is provided at the foot of the bed to hold the necessary pulleys. One pulley is attached to the overhead bar in line with the tubercle of the tibia, two are secured to the bar at the foot of the bed, one several inches above the other, and a fourth is attached to the spreader plate to which the traction tapes on the leg are attached. A sling or hammock is placed under the knee and attached to a rope that leads vertically to the overhead pulley and then to the uppermost one on the crossbar. From there the rope passes over the pulley on the foot spreader and back to the lower pulley on the crossbar. It then attaches to weights which hang suspended well above the floor. The weight used with an adult patient is usually 8 to 10 pounds. The level of the pulleys on the bar at the foot of the bed is such that the heel is kept clear of the bed to prevent a pressure sore.

The force exerted by the sling is that of the weight at the end of the rope. The horizontal pull on the legs is approximately twice that exerted on the knee by virtue of the pull of the two parallel ropes at the foot. The vertical and horizontal traction are exerted on the same point and together produce a resultant force in line with the femur. A thin pillow is usually placed lengthwise under the thigh; precautions are taken not to increase the slight flexion of the thigh. A second pillow is used under the leg, leaving the heel suspended. A foot support is provided to prevent footdrop. The foot of the bed is elevated to provide countertraction. The popliteal area is padded to protect it from the pressure of the sling, and the color and temperature of the foot are checked frequently, to determine if there is any interference with circulation. The patient is encouraged to flex and extend the toes. The Balkan frame provides a trapeze which the patient uses when he wishes to move.

Balanced suspension traction is also used in an arrangement in which skin or skeletal traction is applied, and the limb is supported on a splint suspended by a system of ropes, pulleys and weights. It is most commonly used in fractures of the shaft of the femur in conjunction with skeletal traction. A half- or full-ring Thomas splint with a Pearson attachment is used (Fig. 26–6G).

Firm cotton slings are secured to the upper part of the Thomas splint to support the thigh and to the Pearson attachment to support the leg. The Thomas splint extends from the groin to beyond the foot in line with the femur. The knee is in a neutral position — that is, slightly flexed to prevent stretching of the posterior knee capsule and ligaments and subsequent joint instability. The heel is suspended beyond the slings to avoid pressure, and some provision is made to support the foot to prevent footdrop. The skeletal traction is usually applied to the proximal area of the tibia. The pull is exerted in line with the femur by means of a rope attached to the bow or stirrup that is fitted to the protruding ends of the wire that passes through the bone. The rope passes over a pulley and suspends a weight. The proximal and distal ends of the splint are suspended by separate cords, pulleys, and weights. When the patient moves up or down in bed the splint moves with him, and traction is maintained. The patient has greater freedom of movement and is usually more comfortable in this system of traction. It also has the advantage of allowing a certain amount of movement in adjacent joints.

See nursing care of the patient in traction on page 914.

Some fractures require *internal surgical reduction and fixation*. Various types of internal fixation devices are used. These include stainless steel or Vitallium wire, screws, plates, rods, and pins, and bone grafts. They may be secured to the sides of the bone, placed through the fragments or passed through the intramedullary cavity of the bone. Internal immobilization is frequently reinforced after the wound is closed by the application of a cast or splint. If a cast is used, a "window" may be made over the wound area to avoid pressure on the incision and promote healing.

Special internal fixation devices are used to immobilize the fragments in a hip fracture or fracture of the femoral neck. Three-flanged nails (Smith-Peters pins or nails), Neufeld nail or a McLaughlin plate and pins may be used (Fig. 24–7). In a few patients, especially the elderly with an intracapsular fracture through the neck of the femur, reduction is not possible and the head of the femur is removed and replaced with a metallic prosthesis. (For further discussion of hip fracture see p. 918.)

See nursing care of patients who have had bone surgery on page 917.

Following any method of reduction and immobilization, roentgenograms are made periodically to determine whether reduction is satisfactory and healing is occurring. In the case of traction, some adjustment in the amount of weight being used may be necessary. For instance, the x-ray may demonstrate too wide a separation of the fragments which would prevent healing and necessitate a reduction in the weight used.

OPEN (COMPOUND) FRACTURES. The patient with an open fracture requires special treatment as soon after the accident as possible. The site is potentially infected, and there is usually a greater amount of soft tissue damage and destruction. Infection and necrosis impede union and may result in serious crippling. As soon as the patient's general condition permits, the physician examines and cleanses the open fracture wound. Gross contaminants and foreign material are removed, and the open wound is covered. The surrounding skin is then cleansed thoroughly with an antiseptic solution. After this initial cleansing, the skin may require shaving, which is then followed by a second cleansing. The open wound may then be irrigated with sterile normal saline. The surgeon explores the wound and a débridement[3] is done, if necessary. The repair of severed or torn ten-

---

[3]*Débridement* is the removal of foreign material and excision of devitalized tissue.

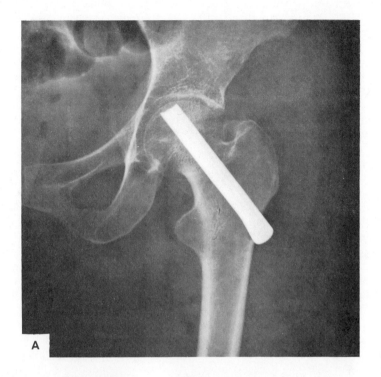

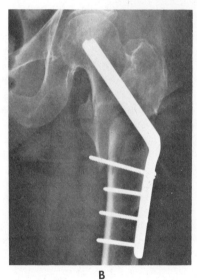

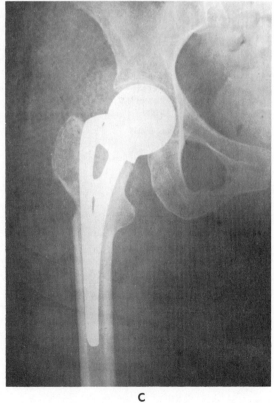

FIGURE 24-7 Roentgenographs showing: *A,* Smith-Peterson nail; *B,* McLaughlin plate and pins; *C,* a femoral head prosthesis. (From Gartland, John J.: Fundamentals of Orthopaedics, 2nd ed. Philadelphia, W. B. Saunders, 1974, pp. 349, 350.)

dons or nerves may be necessary. The fracture is reduced and then immobilized. If there has been gross contamination, the wound may be packed and left open until the danger of infection is past. Antibiotic therapy may be prescribed.

Before the administration of the anesthetic, it is determined if the patient has had previous immunization for tetanus. If he has, a booster dose of tetanus toxoid may be ordered. If he has not been immunized, human tetanus immunoglobulin is given.

Care of the Patient in a Cast

The care of the patient following the application of a cast requires the following considerations.

DRYING OF THE CAST. Complete drying of a cast following its application may take several hours or days, depending on its thickness and the temperature, humidity and circulation of the air. During this period, support of the cast and handling are very important, since the cast is vulnerable to pressure and cracking which could alter its shape, cause indentations that result in undue pressure on an area of the body or make it ineffective. When the part must be lifted, it is supported on the palms of the hands to avoid making indentations by the finger tips. In the case of a body or long leg cast, a fracture board is placed under the mattress to prevent sagging. Pillows with plastic or rubber undercovers are placed under the part encased in plaster so that the cast is not subjected to pressure by the firm mattress. Since it is molded to the contours of the part to which it is applied, support by an extra pillow or folded flannelette sheet may be necessary under such regions as the lumbar or popliteal area.

Drying is promoted by exposure to dry, warm circulating air which evaporates the moisture from the cast. The bedding is arranged so that the cast is left uncovered. A heater with a fan (similar to a hair dryer) may be placed approximately 18 inches from the cast. Unless otherwise indicated by the physician, the patient is turned every 4 to 6 hours to facilitate drying of the complete cast. He is turned toward his uninjured side and, if it is a large or body cast, two or three persons act in unison and pillows are used to avoid strain on any

part of the plaster. A moist cast has a dull gray appearance and produces a dull sound on percussion. When dry, it appears white and shiny and produces a resonant sound on percussion. If a walking cast has been applied, weight-bearing is not permitted for at least 48 hours.

OBSERVATIONS. Following the application of the cast, the patient's general condition is noted at frequent intervals; occasionally, a patient develops delayed shock manifested by sudden weakness, fainting, pallor and weak pulse as a result of the initial injury. During the first 24 to 48 hours, swelling in the area of the fracture may occur, resulting in constriction by the cast. A frequent check is made of the parts distal to the cast (e.g., fingers, toes) for any indication of interference with circulation or pressure on a nerve. Any blanching, discoloration, coldness, swelling, edema, or loss of sensation or motion is reported immediately. Any complaint of pressure of pain at any time must be reported and recorded.

A daily inspection is made of the complete cast for softened areas, and the skin at the cast edges and over pressure areas is examined frequently for any signs of irritation or abrasion. After a few days, if the cast appears to have become loose and less effective, it is drawn to the physician's attention. This may occur as a result of reduced swelling or loss of weight. The nurse is alert for any odor arising from the cast. In some instances, the only indication of a pressure sore having developed under a cast is the offensive, musty odor characteristic of tissue necrosis. If there is a known surgical or accidental wound under the cast, the area is checked frequently for signs of bleeding, infection and drainage. Infection may be detected by an odor or suspected because of an elevation of temperature.

PROTECTION OF THE CAST. Care must be taken during bathing to prevent wetting of the cast. If it approximates the buttocks and perineal area, it requires protection from soiling and wetting when the patient uses the bedpan. Sheets of plastic or other waterproof material may be tucked in well under the edges of the cast, turned back over the outside and secured with adhesive tape. When the patient is placed on the bedpan, pillows are placed under the shoulders and back so that the upper part of the body is level with or slightly higher than the hips and bedpan. The nurse makes sure the patient is thoroughly cleansed and dried following voiding or defecation and that the protective plastic is changed when it becomes soiled. If the cast edges are so close to the perineum that they interfere with adequate care, the physician may permit the cast to be cut to provide greater exposure.

A coat of plastic spray may be applied to the total cast when it is dry to help keep it dry and clean. Superficial soil may be removed with a damp cloth and abrasive powder. If the patient is ambulatory, the cast may be protected by stockinette or a sock or stocking.

SKIN CARE.   If the patient is confined to bed, frequent skin care, especially of pressure areas, is necessary. The bed is kept free of wrinkles and crumbs. If it is a leg that is in a cast it is supported on a pillow to prevent constant pressure on the heel. The crumbling of cast edges can be a source of much discomfort and irritation; the binding may require changing or reinforcing from time to time. The fingers or toes distal to a cast may become irritated by dry, scaly skin; they are bathed, lightly oiled and massaged at least once daily, and frequent active exercise is encouraged.

NUTRITION.   The patient is encouraged to take a regular, well-balanced diet to provide the essentials for tissue healing as well as to maintain normal physiological processes. If activity is restricted, the roughage content may have to be increased to control bowel elimination. If, in the case of a hip spica or jacket cast, intestinal distention becomes troublesome, gas-forming foods may have to be avoided. If the discomfort keeps recurring, the physician may cut a "window" in the cast over the abdominal region.

EXERCISE.   Exercise is important in the care of the fracture patient to stimulate circulation and to prevent muscle atrophy, loss of strength and stiffness of uninvolved joints. Inactivity and immobilization promote the movement of calcium out of the bones, predisposing the person to hypercalcemia and renal calculi. The purpose and details of the exercises are explained to the patient. Uninvolved joints are put through their full range of motion several times daily, and he is encouraged to exercise the unaffected limbs and use them in self-care, turning and raising as much as possible. An overhead trapeze is provided so he can move and lift himself. A schedule of deep breathing and coughing is established for inactive and older persons who are predisposed to pulmonary complications.

The muscles of the immobilized limb are exercised as soon as the physician permits by having the patient contract those muscles immediately above and below the fracture (isometric exercise) frequently, without moving the joint. These exercises may be demonstrated on the unaffected limb so that the patient sees that the muscles can be contracted without moving the limb. For quadriceps setting, the nurse places her hand under the knee and instructs the patient to push down. If it is an arm that is encased in plaster, isometric exercise of the arm muscles is done by having the patient make a fist. The fingers or toes distal to the cast should be exercised several times daily.

DISCHARGED HOME WITH A CAST.   Frequently the patient is allowed to go home as soon as the cast is dry. The patient and his family are advised that the limb should be elevated for the first 24 to 48 hours. Instructions are given to examine the toes and fingers frequently and to report to the physician or the clinic immediately any swelling, blueness, coldness, numbness or inability to move the digits. Persisting pain of the limb or any crack or softening of an area in the cast should also be reported.

The arm with the cast may be supported in a sling when the patient is up. It is important that the sling support the hand to prevent strain and pressure on the wrist. The knot of the sling at the back of the neck is placed lateral to the cervical vertebrae, and a pad may be placed between the sling and the neck to prevent pressure and irritation.

The patient who is discharged with a cast on his leg must know whether or not he may bear any weight on the limb. If he has a walking cast, he is advised as to when he may start to bear weight on it, how to protect the cast, and the necessary precautions to avoid falls. If the patient is to use crutches, they are selected according to the patient's height, and instructions are given in their use (see p. 925).

An appointment is usually made for the patient to have the limb and cast checked in 2 or 3 days and then to return in approximately 10 to 12 days for an x-ray to determine if the callus formation and healing are progressing favorably.

REMOVAL OF THE CAST. When the cast is taken off, the rigid support to joints which have been immobilized for a considerable period of time is removed. The patient is likely to be discouraged by the stiffness, instability and weakness which he encounters and requires reassurance that with exercise and progressive use function will be restored.

The cast is removed by special cast cutters. Soaking the cutting line with dilute acetic acid (vinegar) softens the plaster, making the cutting less difficult. The limb must be handled gently and with support under the joints. The skin is bathed gently, and an application of oil or lanolin is made to soften the accumulation of dry, scaly skin. Vigorous rubbing is discouraged to avoid skin irritation and abrasions.

A regimen of passive and active exercises and massage is established to restore joint and muscle function. Weight-bearing and activities are gradually resumed. When the cast is removed and the limb becomes dependent, edema and swelling are likely to occur. The patient is advised to elevate the limb when sitting and lying, and an elastic or crepe bandage may be applied when he is ambulatory to control the edema which gradually becomes less troublesome as muscle tone improves and there is increasing activity.

Care of the Patient in Traction

It is important that the nurse be familiar with the purpose of the traction and that she understand how the appliances being used are designed and applied to achieve this purpose.

RESPONSIBILITIES IN RELATION TO THE APPLIED TRACTION. Traction must be constant to be effective in the treatment of fractures. The complete traction system is inspected frequently as well as after any movement or treatment of the patient to detect possible interference with the traction or the direction of its pull. Ropes must be taut, ride freely over pulleys and be kept free of the bedding. Knots are examined frequently for security, and the weights, which must never be lifted or changed, are checked for free suspension.

Areas that may be subjected to irritation by adhesive tapes, constriction by circular bandages, or pressure or friction by contact with a part of the appliance are examined several times daily, and any interference with circulation or skin irritation is reported and recorded promptly. Distal portions of the extremity are checked for discoloration, coldness, swelling, edema, and loss of sensation or movement. The nurse is alert for any sign of discharge or a musty odor that might indicate skin necrosis in an area covered by adhesive tapes or bandages. Any change in the alignment of the limb, such as outward rotation, hyperextension or footdrop, is brought to the physician's attention. Every complaint of pain or discomfort deserves investigation and reporting.

Countertraction is maintained by elevation of the bed under the part to which the traction is applied and by preventing a change of position. For example, the patient should not be allowed to slide down so that the foot plate or bar rests against the foot of the bed or a crossbar. The heel, which is so vulnerable to pressure, must remain suspended, and the foot is supported to prevent plantar flexion (footdrop). If the limb is supported in a ring splint (e.g., Thomas' or Thomas-Pearson splint), the ring should not cause undue pressure in the groin. The skin under the ring is bathed frequently, thoroughly dried and lightly powdered. If the patient keeps "sliding into the ring" or if skin irritation occurs, the weights may require adjustment by the physician. When the Pearson attachment is used with a Thomas' splint in suspension traction to support the leg from the knee down, the patient's knee should rest over the point of attachment of the Pearson extension. When traction is applied to the neck with tongs in the head (skeletal traction) or a halter, the head of the bed is elevated to provide countertraction. Some physicians have the patient's head at the foot of the bed to accommodate the traction equipment. This also facilitates care of the patient.

When skeletal traction is used, the wounds are covered with small sterile dressings. The surrounding skin is inspected daily for any redness or discharge that may indicate infection. The protruding ends of the wire or pin are covered with cork or adhesive tape.

POSITIONING, SKIN CARE AND EXERCISES. The patient in traction is required to remain on his back; this becomes tiresome and is a source of discomfort for the patient. An explanation is made to the patient of the reason the dorsal position is necessary, and he is told that turning would prevent immobilization of the fracture area which is essential to healing. A directive is obtained from the physician as to how much movement is permitted and if the patient may or may not use a trapeze. Good body alignment is important; a firm mattress on a fracture board is used. The upper part of the body is kept straight; if the patient lies diagonally, it may alter the desired position of the affected limb and the direction of the pull on it. The patient in leg traction frequently has a tendency to keep his unaffected leg in flexion. He may need to be reminded to extend it for intervals to prevent shortening of the flexor muscles.

Frequent skin care (at least every 2 to 3 hours) of the back, buttocks and the heel of the unaffected leg is very important to prevent pressure sores, especially in elderly persons. Brisk massage helps to stimulate circulation in the areas and increase the resistance of the skin. An occasional light application of lanolin or oil may be necessary to prevent excessive drying and possible cracking of the skin. Squares of synthetic sheepskin or sponge rubber are placed under the vulnerable areas. Thorough cleansing and drying following the use of the bedpan and keeping the bedding clean, dry and free of wrinkles and crumbs are important nursing measures. Vulnerable areas are carefully inspected frequently for any discoloration, mottling, edema or break in the skin. A second person is necessary to assist with the raising of the patient while back care is given and the lower bed linen is changed. If the patient cannot be raised, the person assisting pushes down on the mattress, permitting the nurse to slide her hand in to give the necessary care. The patient may be permitted to raise himself slightly by pulling on a trapeze suspended from the overhead frame. Linen changes are made by working from the unaffected side toward the affected side or from the top of the bed toward the foot. The method which proves easier and least disturbing for the patient is used. The top bedding is arranged to avoid interference with the traction. Small lightweight blankets may be used over the limb in traction for warmth. If suspension traction is used, the patient usually has greater freedom of movement and can be raised with less danger of disturbing the frac-

ture site. *When slight turning of the trunk is permitted for care, the turning is toward the leg in traction.*

The patient is required to practice deep breathing and coughing every 1 to 2 hours to prevent pulmonary complications. To stimulate his circulation and prevent muscle atrophy and joint stiffness, active exercises of uninvolved limbs are carried out several times daily. Self-care activities are encouraged and an explanation of their role in his progress is made to the patient. He is also taught to practice static exercises (isometric contractions or muscle setting) of the abdominal and gluteal muscles.

NUTRITION. A well-balanced diet is provided, and the patient is advised of the need for adequate nutrition to provide the essential materials for healing of the fracture and to maintain resistance. The protein and vitamin C (ascorbic acid) intake receive special attention; a deficiency of these elements predisposes the skin to pressure sores. The reduced activity and subsequent constipation may necessitate increased dietary roughage. Immobilization causes some decalcification of the bones and resultant hypercalcemia, predisposing to the formation of renal and bladder calculi. The patient is encouraged to take 2500 to 3000 ml. of fluid daily (unless contraindicated) to promote elimination of the excessive blood calcium. He may have to be fed at first but should gradually be encouraged to do this for himself. The nurse makes sure that the food is within easy reach of the patient and that he receives the necessary assistance in cutting his meat, buttering bread, pouring coffee, etc.

ELIMINATION. The use of the bedpan by the patient in traction frequently presents some difficulty, mainly because of the elevation of the foot of the bed for countertraction. Unless contraindicated, the patient assists in raising himself onto the fracture pan by using the trapeze and unaffected leg. A pillow may be placed under the back and shoulders so that the patient is more level with the bedpan. For voiding, a female urinal or an emesis basin may be used for female patients. The nurse must see that the patient and bed are left clean and dry.

As cited previously, the enforced inactivity may give rise to constipation and flatulence. If the problem is not corrected, fecal impaction may develop, necessitating digital disimpaction and cleansing enemas, which are distressing and exhausting for the patient. Dietary adjustments and a mild laxative may prevent this problem.

DIVERSION. The fracture patient is usually in traction for several weeks; time passes slowly, and he is likely to be discontented, depressed and unable to sleep. The provision of diversion and some form of occupation is an essential part of the nursing care plan. The patient's need for socialization, interest and occupation may be discussed with his family and friends. It may be suggested that they plan their visits so that he is not alone for several days and then visited by everyone at the same time. The patient's interests should be determined; reading material, a radio or television (if permitted by the hospital) and small handicrafts frequently prove helpful. In the case of a housewife and mother, her family might be encouraged to have her participate in planning and decision making regarding home matters so that she feels that she is still active in family affairs. Similarly, it is psychologically beneficial to the father or businessman to be consulted. Mental and purposeful physical activity help to produce normal fatigue; the patient is likely to sleep and rest better at night and will require less sedation.

CONVALESCENCE AND REHABILITATION. When the traction is removed, the patient will probably be surprised and depressed by the weakness and joint instability in the limb. Before he is allowed up, the head of the bed is elevated so he may adjust to having his head and trunk in an upright position after being flat and in the countertraction position for so long. The elevation is gradual; otherwise he may experience faintness.

Appropriate passive, active and resistive exercises of the affected limb are introduced. These may be planned and supervised by a physiotherapist, but the nurse must be familiar with the plan so that the necessary assistance is provided when the therapist is not at the bedside. In some situations the nurse may have to assume responsibility for teaching the exercises and for helping the patient to resume activity and mobility. In the case of a lower limb, arm and shoulder exercises are continued to strengthen the upper limbs in preparation for the use of a walker or crutches. When the patient is allowed up the casters are removed from the bed; having it lower makes it easier and safer for him to get

in and out. Specific orders are received from the physician as to when weight-bearing and ambulation may begin. Depending on the strength and age of the patient, a walker may be used before crutches or canes are introduced. It is usually used with elderly and debilitated patients because there is less danger of falls and they feel more secure. Firm, low-heeled walking shoes should be worn, preferably an oxford with a rubber heel.

When the patient's ability and confidence increase, he may then progress through crutch walking to a cane. When relearning to walk, he may need prompting to maintain an erect posture (avoid bending forward) and to increase the degree of flexion of his thigh and leg when raising a foot off the floor to take a step in order to overcome the tendency to shuffle. Most patients require a good deal of encouragement and reassurance from the nurse. Physical assistance and support are gradually withdrawn, but the nurse remains with the patient when he is getting in and out of the bed or a chair until it is evident that he can safely manage on his own.

Before the patient is discharged, it is important to know the home situation in order to suggest necessary adjustments. Will he have to use stairs to get to the apartment or to the bathroom? Will there be someone there with him all the time? The necessary information may be obtained from the patient or family, or a visit may be made by a visiting nurse to assess the situation and suggest adjustments in the environment and arrangements for care. It may be necessary for him to spend an interim period in a convalescent home. When he goes home, a referral may be made to the visiting nurse agency so that he receives regular assistance and supervision. Resumption of his former occupation and activities will depend on his progress in relation to mobility and independence. He is seen at frequent intervals in the clinic or by his physician until fully rehabilitated.

Nursing the Patient with Internal (Surgical) Fixation

PREOPERATIVE PREPARATION. How soon the operation for internal fixation is performed after a fracture has occurred depends on the patient's condition and whether there are associated injuries or health problems. It is usually done as soon as possible to minimize soft tissue injury and before any fibroblasts develop, but may have to be delayed because of shock or because the patient has eaten recently and as a result should not have a general anesthetic until the stomach empties. During the preoperative period, some temporary form of immobilization may be applied to the injured part (e.g., sandbags, splint or Buck's extension). It must be handled as little as possible to prevent movement of the fragments and further tissue damage. An analgesic such as morphine, meperidine hydrochloride (Demerol) or codeine may be ordered for relief of pain. Older patients may not tolerate these drugs and, if given, must be observed closely, especially for respiratory depression, shock and disorientation. Side rails are placed on their beds as a precautionary measure, and their condition may necessitate constant attendance at the bedside. The patient's blood is typed and cross matched, and blood is given to counteract shock or hemorrhage. If the patient manifests dehydration, intravenous infusions of electrolyte and glucose solutions are administered. If the patient is elderly, as so many are who have internal fixation, intravenous solutions (including blood) are given slowly to avoid an excessive demand on the heart caused by a rapid increase in the circulating intravascular volume. The urinary output and fluid intake are measured, and the balance is determined so that any renal insufficiency may be detected and reported. The preoperative assessment may include blood tests and an electrocardiogram. If the period between the accident and the operation is more than a few hours, the patient is required to cough and breathe deeply every 1 to 2 hours. Frequent special skin care may also be necessary because of the immobility and constant dorsal position.

Because of bone tissue's susceptibility to infection and the difficulty in bringing it under control if it occurs, meticulous preoperative cleansing of the skin is very important. Specific directions are usually received from the surgeon. A large area is carefully shaved and cleansed with an antiseptic solution. The cleansing may be repeated, depending on the amount of time available. If the surgery is to be performed on a limb, special attention is paid to the skin between digits and to the nails.

POSTOPERATIVE CARE. Following internal reduction and fixation, the general principles of postoperative care are applicable (see p. 178 ff.). The patient is observed closely for any changes in color, blood pressure, pulse and respirations that may reflect shock, hemorrhage or cardiac failure. If the surgery was performed on a limb, the extremity is elevated on pillows to prevent edema. The operative site may be enclosed in a cast, making it difficult to detect early signs of external bleeding. The area is checked for any staining of the cast or oozing from its edges. The initial area of staining may be encircled with a pencil mark so that continued bleeding may be recognized and assessed. As with any plaster application, the part of the limb distal to the cast is examined frequently for any nerve compression or interference with circulation. After the cast is dry, the surgeon may order a "window" to be cut out over the incision. This allows for a change of dressing, if necessary, and permits exposure to air, which helps to keep the wound dry.

The limitations of positioning and activity are indicated by the surgeon. During the period of confinement to bed, exercises of uninvolved parts of the body and self-care activities are usually encouraged to maintain the normal range of joint movement and muscle tone and reduce the mobilization of calcium out of the bones. A trapeze attached to an over-the-bed bar (Balkan frame) allows the patient to move and shift his weight. He is instructed to cough and take eight to ten deep breaths every 2 to 3 hours if activity is restricted. When crutch walking is anticipated, exercises to strengthen the arms and shoulders are introduced. Frequent skin care, especially to susceptible pressure areas (scapular areas, sacrum, heels), is necessary. If turning is permitted, the patient is turned onto the unaffected side; the affected limb is supported during the process and is positioned on pillows to maintain good alignment and prevent strain. A side rail on the side of the bed toward which he turns provides something for him to grasp when turning.

The patient may be allowed out of bed but, in the case of surgery on a lower extremity, he is not usually permitted to bear any weight on it for several weeks. He may be allowed the use of a wheelchair and is gradually introduced to the use of crutches (see p. 925).

When sitting in either a stationary chair or a wheelchair, provision is made for elevation and support of the affected limb. Precautions against pressure sores and slumping posture are necessary when the patient is allowed up in a chair for long periods. He is returned to bed for skin care at regular intervals or may be taught to shift his weight frequently so that no one area is subjected to continuous pressure. Adjustments may also be necessary to avoid prolonged pressure on the popliteal area of the unaffected, dependent leg and to prevent forward sagging of the shoulders.

Exercises of the affected part are started as soon as the physician permits. They may be limited to isometric contractions for a period, followed by the gradual introduction of passive and active movements and resistive exercises. In the case of a lower extremity, weight-bearing is not introduced until roentgenograms indicate satisfactory healing. The overambitious patient is cautioned not to attempt standing or walking without the assistance of a physiotherapist or nurse. He should have a firm, rubber-heeled pair of walking shoes and be assisted first to stand. The nurse stands facing the patient and places her hands to the sides of his lower chest. She encourages him to stand erect, knees extended and head up. When he is sure of his balance in the upright position, he is then assisted with the next step, which may be the use of crutches, a walker or simply walking with only the assistance of the nurse. If the nurse provides the only assistance, support is given to the affected side.

Fracture of the Hip

This refers to a fracture of the proximal extremity of the femur and may be classified as intracapsular or extracapsular. The *intracapsular fracture* occurs through the neck of the femur and is slower in healing because frequently there is an associated interruption of the blood vessels in the medullary canal which are the main blood supply to the head of the bone. The *extracapsular hip fracture* may pass through either the greater or lesser trochanter or the intertrochanteric area. A fracture of the hip is usually treated by internal (surgical) reduction and fixation. A variety of metallic nails, plates and screws are available as fixation devices. The selection depends on the location and angle of the fracture. If the intracapsular fracture is comminuted, if satisfactory reduction cannot be obtained, or if the surgeon suspects that avascular necrosis and nonunion are likely to develop because of injury to blood vessels, the femoral head may be removed and replaced by a metal (Vitallium) prosthesis. It has a ball-shaped head which fits into the hip socket (acetabulum) and a lower intramedullary rod which is fitted into the lower neck and upper part of the shaft of the femur.

The majority of patients who suffer a fracture of the hip are elderly persons. They do not tolerate the prolonged immobilization and bed rest imposed by traction and spica casts; under such treatment they are prone to develop pulmonary and circulatory complications, pressure sores and rapid debilitation. Internal fixation makes it possible to have the patient exercise and be out of bed much earlier than with traction, thus reducing the risk of serious complications.

Following the surgical reduction and fixation, constant nursing attention and close observation of the vital signs are necessary; the older person is more likely to develop shock, respiratory depression and cardiac failure. The patient is placed on a firm mattress on a fracture board to prevent sagging and flexion of the hips. The surgeon may order the affected limb supported on pillows the full length of the extremity. When the patient is in the dorsal position, alignment is maintained by sandbags placed along the lateral aspect. Occasionally, traction is applied for 2 or 3 days to overcome muscle spasm.

Postoperative disorientation and restlessness are common with elderly persons. Side rails are placed on the bed for protection. Analgesic drugs and sedatives are used judiciously; the patient must not be allowed to suffer unnecessarily, but the reduced tolerance of older persons for these drugs, especially opiates and barbiturates, may depress respirations and cause disorientation.

As soon as the patient regains consciousness, a schedule for frequent coughing and deep breathing is established. He is turned frequently as soon as possible to help prevent pulmonary congestion. Change of position may be restricted to turning on the unaffected side for a few days. The affected limb is supported during the process and is positioned on pillows, keeping the hip and knee in the same plane to prevent strain on the operative site.

Retention of urine or incontinence may be experienced in the early postoperative period. An indwelling catheter may be passed as part of the preoperative preparation, or it may be introduced following the operation. Its use should be limited to as brief a period as possible because of the danger of bladder infection. The catheter is usually clamped for stated periods, allowing a normal volume of urine to collect in the bladder to promote tone and normal capacity. A fluid intake of approximately 2500 ml. is encouraged unless contraindicated by circulatory or renal insufficiency. When the catheter is removed, the bedpan is given every 2 hours until normal bladder function and control are established. Constipation is a common problem, and fecal impaction is prone to develop. A mild laxative such as milk of magnesia or psyllium hydrophilic mucilloid (Metamucil) may be ordered, and the diet is adjusted to include increased roughage.

Exercises of the unaffected extremities are started as soon as possible, and the patient is encouraged to flex and extend the toes and ankle of the affected extremity alternately to stimulate circulation. The surgeon may order the application of elastic or crepe compression bandages to the lower extremities to prevent venous stasis, which predisposes the patient to thrombophlebitis. Specific exercises are prescribed for the affected limb; passive movements may be introduced first, followed by active exercises. The patient is assisted or lifted out of bed into a chair on the second or third day. The affected leg is usually extended and supported the first few days unless otherwise indicated by the surgeon, and then lowered and observed for swelling and discoloration. The patient is taught to stand on the unaffected extremity and to transfer to a chair without bearing any weight on the affected limb. He may then be permitted early ambulation with crutches. In most instances, the elderly patient is not taught crutch walking because of the danger of his falling. Weight-bearing on the affected leg is not allowed until there is x-ray evidence of satisfactory healing. When permitted, the older patient is taught to use a walker.

Continued pain or muscle spasm is reported and recorded; it may be due to unsatisfactory reduction or avascular necrosis of the head of the femur. When a prosthesis has been implanted, unless the limb is in traction, a specific directive is received as to the positioning of the patient and the affected extremity. It varies with the location of the operative approach through the joint capsule. If it has been posterior, the patient lies flat, and the leg is abducted and positioned in external rotation; if the approach through the capsule was anterior, the limb is internally rotated, and the patient may be permitted to sit up.

Firm healing of the bone following a hip fracture and the resumption of walking is a long slow process. Periods of discouragement and depression are common. The patient requires a good deal of support. Self-care activities are promoted to reduce his feelings of dependence as well as to maintain muscle tone. Various forms of diversion in which he is interested are provided. The patient may be permitted to go home before weight-bearing is allowed. Adjustments in the home environment and care of the patient are discussed in detail with members of the family. A referral may be made to a visiting nurse agency.

Complications

Complications that may occur with fractures include malunion, delayed healing and nonunion of the fracture (see p. 904). The enforced immobilization associated with the treatment of some fractures predisposes the patient to hypostatic pneumonia, renal calculi and phlebothrombosis. It is important that a regimen of frequent deep breathing and coughing be established from the onset to prevent shallow respirations and the retention of secretions which readily become infected. Circulation and venous return are stimulated by exercising unaffected limbs regularly, encouraging as much movement by the patient as is permitted and promoting self-care. Movement of calcium out of the bones into the blood, which may lead to the formation of kidney or bladder stones, is reduced by patient movement and exercises. The patient is also encouraged to take 2500 to 3000 ml. of fluid daily, unless contraindicated, to promote elimination of calcium by the urine.

Nerve compression and permanent damage may be incurred by prolonged pressure on the nerve by a part of a traction appliance or a plaster cast, or by direct injury to the nerve by a fracture fragment. Frequent observation and prompt reporting of the patient's complaint of pain and pressure may result in an adjustment or correction being made before permanent damage occurs, with consequent loss of function.

The patient with a lower extremity in traction should have the foot supported in the normal position (almost at a right angle to the leg) to prevent prolonged stress on the peroneal nerve which could result in a permanent footdrop.

A fat embolism may occur due to the liberation of fat into the blood from the marrow of the injured bone. The embolus is most often carried to the pulmonary arteries and eventually blocks a vessel, causing a lung infarct. The patient develops sudden severe chest pain, respiratory distress and shock.

Infection of the fracture site develops most often because of the contamination associated with a compound fracture. It may occasionally follow open reduction and fixation.

AMPUTATION OF A LIMB

The incidence of amputation of a part of a limb has been reduced in the last two to three decades. This is attributed to the medical progress made in vascular surgery, the treatment of infection and the control of diabetes mellitus. For those for whom an amputation is a necessity, the loss of the limb has become less obvious and less disabling as a result of improved prostheses and rehabilitation programs. A lower extremity is more frequently involved, and amputation occurs more often in males.

Reasons for Amputation

An amputation is done to preserve the patient's life or may be undertaken to improve function and usefulness. The conditions which necessitate amputation include: (1) insufficient blood supply to the part and resulting gangrene; (2) severe, uncontrollable infection such as gas gangrene (*Clostridium perfringens* infection) or chronic osteomyelitis in which there is marked bone destruction; (3) malignant neoplasm (e.g., osteosarcoma); (4) an injury that has resulted in irreparable crushing of the limb or laceration of arteries and nerves; and (5) a handicapping deformity (e.g., flail limb).

Level and Types of Amputation

Occasionally an amputation is an emergency surgical procedure performed because of irreparable traumatic damage to a part. But, when possible, the level of the amputation is decided before operation so that the patient may be informed of the anticipated extent of the loss. The decision as to the level is based on achieving (1) complete removal of the diseased tissue, (2) viable tissue and an adequate blood supply to the remaining part of the limb, and (3) a stump that will allow for a satisfactory fitting and functional movement of a prosthesis. Adequate soft tissues (skin, subcutaneous tissue and muscle) are preserved so that the end of the bone is well padded and covered. If possible, the stump should be the optimum length for adequate leverage on the prosthesis. Too long a stump may interfere with the function of the prosthesis joint below. In amputation of the lower extremity the knee joint is maintained, if at all possible, since mobility and agility are more readily acquired. The prosthesis for the above knee amputation limits the person, especially if elderly, because of the high energy demands for locomotion.

Two types of operative procedures are used, the closed or flap type of amputation and the guillotine or open amputation.

In the *flap type* of procedure, fascia, probably muscle, and full-thickness skin flaps are brought over the end of the bone. In a lower limb amputation, the anterior flap is usually longer in order to bring the suture line well to the posterior aspect. This arrangement prevents direct pressure on the scar by the prosthesis in weight-bearing. When it is an upper limb that is involved, the anterior and posterior flaps are generally equal in length, producing a terminal scar. The skin flaps are dissected to provide a smooth surface over the end of the stump, free of wrinkles and folds, and the skin edges are sutured in apposition with a minimum of tension.

A *guillotine or open amputation* is reserved for emergency cases in which the limb has been severely traumatized and contaminated or in which an infection such as gas gangrene has already developed. The skin and other soft tissues are severed at the same level as the bone. The wound is left open to promote adequate drainage and closed later when infection is brought under control. Traction may be applied to the skin while it remains open to prevent retraction of the soft tissues.

Traumatic amputation implies the loss of a whole or part of a limb in an accident. This is frequently a life-threatening situation because of the concomitant hemorrhage. A second problem incurred by such circumstances is contamination of the wound. Immediate emergency care is directed toward arrest of the bleeding and getting the person to where blood replacement may be instituted. Precautions are taken to handle and transport the amputated part with the patient carefully, since efforts may be made to reattach the separated unit.

Disarticulation is the term used when the amputation is at the level of a joint.

Preoperative Nursing Care

PSYCHOLOGICAL PREPARATION. When the amputation is an elective procedure, the surgeon advises the patient and family of the need for the operation and the level at which the limb will be removed. The loss may not be very important functionally, or it may prove a serious handicap. For example, an individual can readily adjust to the loss of a second, third or fourth finger but, if it is a thumb, the ability to pick up or grasp an object is seriously impaired. However, when the patient is first advised of the loss of a part of the body, regardless of how functionally insignificant, the information is still likely to be a shock, causing considerable emotional disturbance. The patient's body image and independence are seriously threatened, and he needs the support of an understanding nurse. He is encouraged to verbalize his feelings and, through listening, the nurse identifies his particular fears and concerns. These and the reactions vary among patients, depending on their personality, life situation and ability to handle crises. For example, the wage earner is likely to be greatly distressed about a loss of earning power to support his family. For another, an amputation may mean a complete change in his accustomed activities and occupation.

The patient and family receive explanations of how the problems associated with the loss of a limb may be handled through a planned rehabilitation program. The knowledge that the interest and assistance of specialists in this area are available helps the patient to develop a hopeful and positive attitude toward overcoming the handicap. Opportunities are provided for questions and discussions about what is likely to take place before and after the operation. The patient may derive support from a visit by someone who has had a similar amputation and has been successfully rehabilitated.

The policy relating to the operative consent for an amputation may vary from that used generally. Some institutions and surgeons require the signature of the patient and the closest relative. If the patient is confused and his responsibility questionable, two of his next of kin may be required to sign the consent.

PHYSICAL PREPARATION. During the preoperative period the patient is taught deep breathing and coughing. If his condition permits, exercises are introduced which will facilitate his postoperative mobilization and rehabilitation. These include active exercises of the unaffected limbs to prevent loss of muscular strength. If crutch walking is anticipated, push-ups may be introduced to strengthen the shoulder and arm muscles. Frequent skin care and change of position may be necessary for the patient confined to bed or a wheelchair to prevent pressure sores, since he often tends to remain immobile to reduce pain. Overprotection of an affected lower limb usually results in continuous flexion of the hip and knee joints, leading to contractures. This is discouraged by having the patient assume the prone position several times a day.

Attention is directed toward promoting optimum nutritional and hydrational status. The importance of adequate protein, vitamins and fluids in postoperative progress is explained to the patient. If the patient is overweight, the caloric intake may be moderately reduced, since excess weight may retard postoperative ambulation and rehabilitation. Too restricted a caloric intake (below 1000 to 1200 calories) and a rapid weight loss are avoided because of the danger of causing acidosis, especially postoperatively. Blood typing and cross matching are done, and compatible blood is made available; hemorrhage is always a hazard in an amputation. A transfusion may be given during the preoperative period, as well as during and following the operation, to improve the patient's general condition. The blood pressure and the pulse rate and volume are noted to serve as a base line in postoperative care.

Preoperative preparation of the skin involves the usual shaving and thorough cleansing well above and below the anticipated level of amputation.

Preparation to Receive the Patient After Amputation

In preparing the postoperative bed, a fracture board is placed beneath a firm mattress to assist in maintaining good body alignment, facilitate postoperative exercises and, in the case of a leg amputation, prevent sagging of the bed at hip level which predisposes to flexion contracture. Obviously, amputation necessitates the severing and ligation of large blood vessels. A heavy tourniquet is placed at the bedside and is ready for immediate use in the event of hemorrhage. Provision is also made for elevation of the foot of the bed in case of hemorrhage or shock. Blood, fluids and equipment are made available for prompt intravenous infusion.

Postoperative Nursing Care

OBSERVATIONS. The blood pressure, pulse and respirations are recorded, color noted and the stump examined at frequent, regular intervals for the first 48 hours for early signs of shock and hemorrhage. The patient is observed for general apathy and psychic trauma following the amputation. Even though he was prepared for and consented to the operation, the actual loss of the body part may cause severe depression. The nurse is also alert for any indications of infection such as fever, increased pain, reddened streaks or areas and wound discharge.

CARE OF THE STUMP. The stump may be enclosed in a thick soft dressing and elasticized bandages. If it is a lower extremity and a below-the-knee amputation, it may be enclosed in a plaster cast in which a metal socket is implanted to accommodate a pylon[4] or early training prosthesis when the patient is permitted to bear weight on the stump (Fig. 24–8). Straps may be incorporated into the cast which attach to a belt around the

---

[4]A *pylon* is a peg-like tube to which an artificial foot is attached.

patient's waist while he is in bed to prevent the cast from moving and slipping off. When he is up, the straps are extended over the shoulders. The plaster cast application controls swelling and edema; prevention of edema favors more rapid healing. There is also less danger of hemorrhage with the steady pressure and immobilization. The inclusion of the knee in the cast prevents flexion contracture. The plaster cast permits earlier ambulation which encourages and motivates the patient. The disadvantage with the enclosure of the stump in a rigid plaster dressing is that the condition of the wound cannot be visualized and readily assessed. The cast must be examined frequently and any stain appearing on the cast is reported, outlined with a pencil and the time noted so that continued bleeding or drainage may be recognized. Any complaint of pain in the stump, offensive odor from the area or elevation of temperature must be reported promptly. These symptoms may indicate infection or pressure and tissue necrosis.

When a soft dressing is used, any blood-staining is reported immediately and the tourniquet is applied, if necessary, until the bleeding is brought under control by the surgeon. A tissue drain or Hemovac may be placed in the wound at the time of operation; if serious drainage soaks through the dressing, it is promptly reinforced. The drain is removed in 2 to 3 days and the sutures are left in place for 10 to 12 days.

The surgeon may order the stump elevated on a pillow for the first 24 to 48 hours only or, in the case of a lower limb, the foot of the bed may be elevated for approximately 24 hours. Prolonged use of the pillow under the stump with the patient in the supine position leads to flexion contracture and later difficulty in mobility and the fitting of a prosthesis. With an arm amputation, precautionary measures are used to prevent contracture of the shoulder adductor and inward rotator muscles. Following an amputation above the knee, the nurse must guard against shortening of the hip flexors and abductors. In an amputation below the knee, the patient is encouraged to maintain extension of the knee to avoid contracture of the hamstring muscles. A splint may be necessary with the patient who does not have the rigid plaster dressing to prevent flexion contracture of the knee.

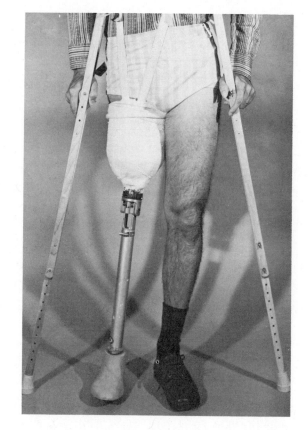

FIGURE 24–8 Plaster cast enclosure of the stump and attachment of a pylon with foot. (From Buck, Barbara, and Lee, Allen D.: Amputation: Two views. Nurs. Clin. North Am., Vol. 11, No. 4 (Dec. 1976), p. 650.)

When a rigid cast is not used and the wound has healed, a compression bandage (elastic or crepe) is applied to the stump to reduce edema and promote firming and molding of the tissue in preparation for a prosthesis. A generous number of long, recurrent, vertical folds are made over the end of the stump and are secured by circular turns. The bandage must be sufficiently firm to compress and shape the soft, flabby tissue, but one must guard against any interference with the blood supply by excessive tightness. The bandage is removed and reapplied three or four times daily. While it is off, gentle massage of the tissue may be prescribed to stimulate circulation and prevent adherence of the scar tissue to the bone. The patient or a member of the family is taught the care of the stump and the correct application of the bandage. The stump is bathed daily with a mild soap and rinsed and dried thoroughly. Nothing is applied to the skin unless it is prescribed by the physician. Certain activities may be ordered which apply pressure to the stump in preparation for the use of a prosthesis and weight-bearing. Contact is first made with something quite soft and, as tolerance is developed, the firmness and resistance of the contact surface and pressure are progressively increased. If the patient complains of muscular spasms and discomfort, heat and massage to the stump may provide relief.

When the plaster cast is used, it remains for approximately 2 weeks unless there is some indication of bleeding or infection. The sutures are removed and a second cast applied which is changed again in 2 weeks.

SAFETY PRECAUTIONS. Side rails on the bed are a necessary precaution, especially with older patients. They may become disoriented or, in turning, may readily lose their balance and fall out of bed.

PAIN AND DEPRESSION. An analgesic is necessary the first 2 or 3 days to control the pain and is then usually tapered off gradually to discourage drug dependency. Some patients experience pain or other sensations which are interpreted as originating in the portion of the limb which has been removed.

This is referred to as *phantom pain* (see p. 118). It may be temporary but, if it persists, the nerve endings in the stump may be injected with alcohol or resected.

The nurse may assist the patient in overcoming despair by conveying an understanding of his feelings and by making positive references to future activity, mobility and rehabilitation.

FLUIDS AND NUTRITION. Intravenous fluids may be necessary during the first 24 to 48 hours to maintain an adequate intake. Oral fluids are given freely, and the patient progresses to a regular diet as soon as it is tolerated. An explanation is made, if necessary, of the importance of adequate nutrition in maintaining and promoting his muscular strength for the exercises that will assist in rehabilitation.

EXERCISES. An hourly routine of coughing and deep breathing and frequent change of position are necessary until the patient is allowed up and becomes sufficiently active to prevent limited ventilation and circulatory stasis.

As soon as he is well enough, a daily regimen of exercises is introduced to maintain and promote the muscular strength and joint mobility that are needed for rehabilitation. The tone of the trunk muscles, as well as that of the limb muscles, receives attention since adjustments and compensation are necessary for the amputee to maintain his balance. If the lower limb has been amputated above the knee, the hip extensors and adductors play an important role in remobilization. To prevent flexion contracture of a thigh stump, the patient lies in the prone position for ½ hour every 3 or 4 hours. A pillow may be placed under the abdomen, stump or ankle of the unaffected limb if the foot is not suspended over the edge of the mattress. While in the prone position, he is encouraged to do push-up exercises to strengthen the shoulder and arm muscles. If the leg is removed below the knee, the quadriceps of that limb is exercised. Following the amputation of an arm, the shoulder muscles of that limb are exercised to prevent adduction and rounding of the shoulder.

REHABILITATION. The patient is allowed out of bed as soon as possible. Assistance must be available until he can maintain his balance and is able to maneuver safely. In the case of a lower limb, the patient first learns to stand, get up from a chair, get in and out of bed and walk with crutches (see below). Attention is paid to posture; any tendency to lean forward or to one side should be corrected.

When an upper limb has been amputated, the patient is assisted and encouraged to begin self-care activities with his one arm as soon as possible. Certain simple adjustments in the serving of food, clothing fasteners, etc. are made to facilitate independence.

When the stump has sufficiently shrunk and is conditioned, measurements are taken, and a permanent prosthesis is made. It usually requires at least 5 to 6 weeks. A special wool stump sock is worn with the prosthesis, and the patient is instructed on the importance of it being well-fitting, free of wrinkles and changed daily. He is also advised to inspect the stump daily for redness, swelling, irritation and calluses. If any symptoms develop, he should avoid weight-bearing on the area and consult his physician.

If a hand has been removed at the wrist or there is a below-the-elbow amputation, a prosthesis can be provided which permits supination and pronation as well as voluntary opening and closing for grasping. The prosthesis used following an elbow disarticulation or mid-upper arm amputation is capable of internal and external rotation, flexion and extension and terminal grasping. The patient who has an arm disarticulation at the shoulder is more handicapped, since the more proximal the amputation, the less efficient is the activity and control of the terminal part of the prosthesis. Prostheses are used that provide units comparable to the upper arm, forearm and hook-hand, but they are more difficult in operation.

Following a below-the-knee amputation, the patient is fitted for a patellar tendon weight-bearing socket which suspends the prosthesis (Fig. 24–9). It is lightweight and held in place by a strap around the thigh, thus eliminating the trunk support previously worn with a below-the-knee prosthesis. This newer model also eliminates the need for knee hinges and provides for greater freedom and agility by the wearer. With an above-the-knee amputation a full-length prosthesis is necessary, and is supported by a pelvic band or corset-like arrangement. The knee is hinged and the upper portion is quadrilateral in shape. Most of the person's weight on the

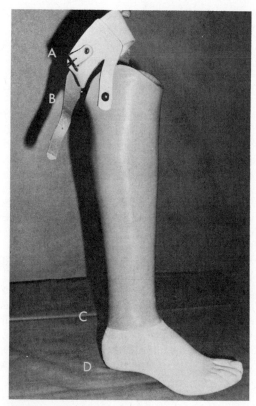

FIGURE 24–9 Patellar tendon-bearing prosthesis. (From Engstrand, Janet: Rehabilitation of the patient with a lower extremity amputation, Nurs. Clin. North Am., Vol. 11, No. 4 (Dec. 1976), p. 666.)

affected side is borne by the ischial tuberosity. The individual with this type of prosthesis uses considerably more energy in getting around than the person with a patellar tendon weight-bearing prosthesis.

When learning to use a lower limb prosthesis, the patient first uses crutches for support, then progresses to canes and, finally, when he achieves a satisfactory stable gait, he is encouraged to discontinue the use of a cane. All of this takes considerable time and perseverance; the amputee will require encouragement and support from his family and those working with him in rehabilitation. If the patient is elderly and adjustment to a prosthesis is too difficult, he is instructed in wheelchair activities.

Crutch Walking

Crutch walking may be a permanent or temporary means of ambulation when one or both lower limbs are disabled. The initial instruction in the use of crutches is usually done by a physiotherapist with support, assistance and reinforcement of instructions provided by the nurse. In some instances, the nurse may have to assume full responsibility. In either situation, she must understand the principles involved and have a knowledge of the various gaits which may be used.

Ambulation through the use of crutches may mean that the patient becomes mobile much faster than would otherwise be possible. Preparation, physical and emotional, begins long before the actual event. Maintenance of good body alignment during the period of bed rest helps to insure good posture and balance when the upright position is resumed. Joints are put through their full range of motion daily, and active exercises are encouraged in order to maintain joint mobility and muscle strength. These activities prevent restricted movement, weakness and deformities, such as footdrop, which could interfere with walking.

It is necessary to strengthen the extensor muscles of the upper arm, namely the triceps, in readiness for crutch walking. Several exercises can be done by the bed patient to achieve this. The patient lies on his abdomen and lifts his chest off the bed using both arms, he lies flat on his back and straightens his elbows several times while holding a weight in each hand or, while sitting on the side of the bed with his foot or feet dangling over the edge, he presses down on the mattress with both hands and lifts his hips off the bed. This last exercise also gets the patient used to bearing his weight on the palms of his hands. Quadriceps muscles may be strengthened while the patient is sitting by isometric contractions or by lifting his stump off the mattress. These exercises may be done two or three times daily but always with sufficient support and not to the point of undue fatigue.

The patient's prognosis, physical condition and emotional make-up will greatly influence his progress in the use of crutches. It may be a slow process which requires considerable physical effort and can quickly lead to feelings of discouragement and hopelessness. A nurse who is sincere in her interest and in giving instruction, encourages the patient to express his feelings, and willingly provides reassurance to him and his family is of great value. Care is taken that both patient and nurse understand the physician's directions regarding weight-bearing. The plans for teaching the skill are adapted to the patient according to future activities, attitude, age, weight and strength. Setting attainable goals for each session, such as walking to the window, will help to combat frustration and perhaps stimulate some interest in what goes on beyond his bed. Enlisting the patient's help in planning and assessing his daily progress helps to maintain his enthusiasm.

Selection of proper crutches is of the utmost importance. There are several ways in which the length is determined. One method is to measure the patient while he is lying flat with his arms at his sides from the axilla to a point 6 inches out from the side of his foot, allowing ¾ of an inch that will be added by the crutch tip. Another is to subtract 16 inches from the patient's height. With children who require prolonged use of crutches, they must be changed periodically to allow for normal growth. The hand bars on which the palms of the hands bear the weight must allow for flexion of the elbow at a 30° angle, or almost complete extension of the arm. A third factor in the selection of crutches is to allow space between the crutch top and the axilla. Undue or prolonged pressure here can cause severe, and occasionally permanent, paralysis of the radial nerve. The axillary bar may be padded with material such as sponge rubber wrapped in soft cloth.

Some minor adjustments may be necessary after the patient becomes more skilled in crutch walking. Good quality rubber tips on the ends of the crutches are imperative for safety. These must be checked frequently. A suction cup tip is available which is particularly helpful for those who are severely disabled and must place their crutches at a wide angle for good balance.

The efforts of all concerned are directed toward assisting the patient to use crutches to walk smoothly and evenly while maintaining good posture. The patient's disability and strength will determine which gait he is to use — the swinging, the four-point, three-point or two-point. Lessons should be given in an environment that avoids crowding, has a smooth floor surface, is free of hazards such as electric cords or rugs, and is equipped with a full-length mirror, if possible.

When only one leg can bear weight, the patient may use the *swinging-to gait*. Both crutches are placed at an equal distance in front while the patient is resting his weight on his good leg. Placing his weight on the hand bars of the crutches, he swings ahead so his legs are in line with the crutches, and then repeats the sequence. Smoothness and speed increase with practice, and emphasis is placed on the maintenance of good balance and a short stride. In using the *swing-through gait,* both crutches are moved forward, the person places his weight on the handbars and, lifting the body, then swings through the crutches to a position ahead of them. This gait is used by paraplegics and those with a fused or immobile hip.

The *four-point alternate gait* is used when both lower limbs are affected but can bear at least part of the patient's weight. One crutch is brought forward, then the opposite leg, then the second crutch and finally the other leg. Having the patient count to 4 may aid in achieving smoothness. This method provides stability since there are always three points of contact with the floor.

If one leg is affected but partial weight-bearing is allowed, the *three-point gait* may be taught. Both crutches and the weak leg are brought forward, and then the good leg is advanced. Emphasis is placed on taking steps of equal length to avoid a limp that may persist even after crutches are discarded. As his strength increases, the patient may progress to the *two-point gait,* which is more rapid and appears closer to the normal. Weight is borne on one crutch and the opposite leg while the other crutch and leg advance; then the weight is shifted to the latter pair, and the process is repeated.

OSTEOMYELITIS

When bone tissue becomes infected the condition is known as osteomyelitis. The pathogenic organisms may be introduced directly through an open fracture or from infected contiguous tissue but are more commonly carried by the blood to the bone from a distant primary focus such as boils (furuncles), an abscessed tooth or infected tonsils. When the infection is bloodborne, the condition is referred to as *hematogenous osteomyelitis*. The most common bacterial offender is the *Staphylococcus aureus,* but the disease may also result from the invasion of streptococci, pneumococci or other strains of staphylococci.

Growing bone is more susceptible to hematogenous osteomyelitis and, as a result, the incidence is highest in children and adolescents. The infection usually develops in long bones at the diaphyseal side of the growth plate. Unless it is checked at the onset, the inflammatory process forms a purulent exudate that collects in the minute canals and spaces of the bone tissue. The pressure of the exudate builds up because of the resistant, rigid bone and compresses the blood vessels, causing thrombosis and occlusion. The accumulation under pressure eventually breaks through the cortex of the bone into the subperiosteal space. The periosteum at that site becomes elevated and stripped from the bone, interrupting the blood vessels that lead into the bone. Interference with the blood supply results in an area of dead bone tissue, which is called a *sequestrum.* The periosteum may rupture, and the infection may then extend into the adjacent soft tissues, forming a sinus tract that discharges onto the skin surface. Small sequestra, separated from the living bone tissue, may escape with the exudate through the sinus. The infection may destroy the growth plate (epiphyseal line), leading to reduced growth of the limb, or it may extend into the adjacent joint with ensuing permanent loss of joint function. The periosteum initiates the formation of new bone tissue around the affected area. The new tissue is called the *involucrum*[5] and may enclose and trap sequestra and infecting organisms. These organisms continue to grow in the confined area and the osteomyelitis becomes chronic, characterized by recurring abscess formation and sequestration.

Signs and Symptoms

The onset of acute osteomyelitis may be manifested by a chill, high fever and rapid pulse. The patient has the appearance of being acutely ill; he perspires freely, is restless and irritable and may be nauseated and

___
[5]*Involucrum* is a membranous covering or envelope.

vomit. Severe pain develops in the limb as a result of the pressure by the accumulating exudate and the destruction of bone. The pain is aggravated by slight movement or jarring of the bed. The patient protects the limb by avoiding weight-bearing and movement and usually holds the adjacent joint in flexion. The local area is very tender on slight pressure and becomes red and swollen when the infective process reaches the subperiosteal area and surrounding soft tissues.

There is a marked increase in the leukocyte count, and the erythrocyte sedimentation rate is elevated. After 1 to 2 weeks, roentgenograms reveal destructive bone changes and periosteal elevation and reaction.

Treatment and Nursing Care

Antimicrobial drug therapy and rest in the early stage of osteomyelitis may bring the infection under control with minimal bone damage and before a sinus is formed. In more advanced cases, surgery may be necessary to provide drainage to relieve the pressure within the bone and periosteum and to remove dead bone tissue.

Efforts are made to identify the infecting organism by making cultures of the blood, nose and throat secretions and discharge from any skin lesions (e.g., boils). If a positive culture is obtained, sensitivity tests may then be made to determine the most effective antibiotic therapy.

Large doses of antibiotic are given, usually by parenteral channels. If the response is favorable and the infective process controlled, antimicrobial therapy is generally continued for several weeks to insure destruction of the organisms.

The patient is placed at rest, and the affected limb is handled very gently. It is positioned and supported to prevent contractures and deformities. A splint may be used to immobilize the adjacent joint. The patient tends to remain in one position because of fear of pain. He must be assisted to turn at frequent intervals to guard against pressure sores and respiratory complications. Fluids are given liberally because of the fever and blood infection. A high-calorie, well-balanced diet is encouraged to increase the patient's resistance. If nausea and vomiting are a problem, intravenous infusions of parenteral fluids and a blood transfusion may be necessary.

If surgical drainage or a sequestrectomy is performed, the wound is packed and allowed to heal by granulation from within toward the surface. Antibiotic or sulfonamide preparations may be introduced locally into the wound. The dressing is changed often enough to keep the wound clean and to prevent the development of an offensive odor that may become very distressing to the patient and those in his environment. Precautions must be taken to observe aseptic technique when dressing or treating the wound to prevent the introduction of secondary infection and to prevent the transmission of the patient's infection to others.

When the patient is allowed up, he must be cautioned against falls and injury to the limb. The loss of bone substance may weaken the bone structure, predisposing it to fracture when subjected to even slight injury or pressure. In the case of a lower extremity, weight-bearing may be contraindicated for many weeks while new bone tissue is being formed. The patient may then have to be taught to use crutches. He may be discharged from the hospital but is likely to require guidance and supervision for a considerable period of time.

As cited earlier, hematogenous osteomyelitis is seen most often in children as a result of infection in some area of the body and, unless treated early, it may lead to a long illness and serious crippling. Nurses (especially those visiting in homes and schools) and parents must be constantly alert to the possible significance of focal and recurring infections, such as boils. Medical treatment should be sought for the child. Any complaint of tenderness or pain in a limb, especially if it is associated with fever or general malaise, requires prompt attention.

OSTEOPOROSIS

Osteoporosis is a metabolic bone disorder characterized by decreased density and atrophy due to a decrease in the formation of bone tissue by the osteoblasts. There is a diminished production of the collagenous matrix in which calcium and phosphorus are deposited; as a result, bone tissue is worn down more rapidly than it is replaced. The trabeculae are fewer, and the tissue is rarefied as compared to normal bone. The calcium and phosphorus levels of the blood are normal or may be elevated if the intake is normal.

The weight-bearing vertebrae (lower thoracic and lumbar) and pelvis are usually the first bones to be involved. As the disease becomes more advanced, the long bones, ribs and skull are affected. Osteoporosis has a higher incidence in females, especially after menopause, and is commonly seen in elderly persons.

Etiology

The cause of osteoporosis in many instances is unknown, and it is termed idiopathic. In some patients, the disorder is attributed to the decreased demand and strain associated with immobilization or sedentary life that reduces the stimulation of osteoblastic activity, a diminished secretion of anabolic sex hormones (e.g., estrogen) as occurs after the climacteric and in senility, a negative calcium balance or a deficient protein intake. The disease may be secondary to some endocrine disturbances such as hyperthyroidism and Cushing's syndrome (adrenocortical hyperfunction) or may be the result of therapeutic doses of corticoids.

Signs and Symptoms

The initial symptom in most patients is usually pain in the back due to a flattening or collapse of vertebrae and resulting pressure on spinal nerves. Muscle spasm and limited movement may also develop. Remissions occur and, frequently, exacerbations are precipitated by lifting or stooping. Kyphosis (forward curvature of spine), loss of the normal lumbar curve and loss of stature may become apparent. The bones fracture more readily and osteoporosis contributes to the high incidence of fracture of the hip in older persons. Spontaneous compression fractures are common in vertebrae of the thoracolumbar region. In many instances, the condition goes unrecognized until the person receives a fracture in a simple fall and the x-rays reveal a loss of density in bone tissue.

Treatment and Nursing Care

During an acute episode, the patient is placed on bed rest and given analgesics such as acetylsalicylic acid (aspirin) or propoxyphene hydrochloride (Darvon) to relieve the pain. A firm mattress on a fracture board is important. As soon as the pain and muscle spasm are reduced the patient is mobilized, for prolonged bed rest only contributes to further weakening of the bone structure and muscles. For comfort and mobility, the patient may require a brace to support the spine.

A diet high in protein, calcium and phosphorus, with vitamin D supplement, is usually recommended. A liberal daily fluid intake is taken to reduce the possibility of hypercalciuria and ensuing renal or bladder calculus formation. The caloric intake is controlled to avoid overweight, which places added strain on the weakened bone structure. Activity is encouraged to stimulate osteoblastic activity, and a daily exercise regimen is frequently prescribed.

Medications that may be prescribed include a preparation of calcium (e.g., calcium gluconate), sodium fluoride and estrogen (e.g., diethylstilbestrol) or androgen (e.g., testosterone propionate). The latter hormone is given for its anabolic effect. In the case of a female receiving estrogen therapy, close observations are made for any sign of vaginal bleeding, which is reported promptly.

The patient is instructed to avoid lifting heavy objects and to keep his spine straight and flex his thighs and knees when he wants to reach something at floor level. Patients, especially older persons, are cautioned against falls. Scatter rugs, footstools or other objects in the environment that might lead to a fall are removed. A firm supportive shoe with a walking heel should be worn.

OSTEOMALACIA

Osteomalacia is an adult disorder comparable to rickets in children and, for this reason, it is occasionally referred to as *adult rickets*. It is characterized by an insufficient plasma concentration of calcium and inorganic phosphate for normal calcification of bone tissue. The bones become soft and weak. The person complains of tenderness and an aching pain in the bones. Some bowing of long bones and deformities may develop. A loss of weight and muscular strength may be manifested and, if the calcium defi-

ciency is marked, tetany may be exhibited (see p. 767).

Osteomalacia may be the result of an insufficient amount of calcium reaching the plasma or an excessive urinary excretion of the mineral. In the first instance, the deficiency of calcium may be due to a lack of calcium-containing foods in the diet, insufficient absorption of the mineral from the intestine (caused by steatorrhea or prolonged diarrhea), or a deficiency of vitamin D, which is necessary for normal absorption of calcium and its deposition in bone tissue. Osteomalacia may also occur during pregnancy if the woman does not receive additional calcium to meet the increased demand incurred by the developing fetus.

The second major cause of the disease — that is, an excessive urinary excretion of calcium — is usually the result of acidosis associated with renal failure or of renal tubular damage and malfunction.

The treatment consists mainly of the administration of calcium and vitamin D. If the serum calcium concentration is markedly low, calcium (e.g., calcium gluconate 10 per cent) may be given intravenously.

PAGET'S DISEASE (OSTEITIS DEFORMANS)

Paget's disease is a chronic bone disease of unknown etiology characterized by structural changes. These are due to accelerated and excessive abnormal bone destruction (osteolysis) and regeneration. The disorder seldom occurs in persons younger than 50 and the incidence increases in the later years.

Symptoms

The patient complains of skeletal pain and headache. Softening of the bones results in deformities; anterior bowing of the tibia and kyphosis become apparent. An x-ray shows thickening of the bones and an irregularity in their contour. There is a marked increase in the vascularity of the affected bones. The changes in bone structure begin at one end of the bone and spread progressively toward the other end. The blood calcium and phosphorus levels are normal, but the alkaline phosphatase concentration is elevated. The disorder seems to be a predisposing factor in the development of osteosarcoma, since some patients with Paget's disease develop this malignancy. Pathologic fractures are a common complication.

Treatment

Treatment and nursing care are supportive and symptomatic; there is no specific or curative treatment. A high-calcium, high-protein diet with vitamin C and D supplements is recommended. Medications that may be prescribed include acetylsalicylic acid (aspirin), parathormone, thyrocalcitonin, mithramycin and sodium fluoride.

BONE NEOPLASMS

Primary and secondary neoplasms may develop in bone tissue. Primary newgrowths may be benign or malignant; secondary bone neoplasms are metastases from malignant disease in another area of the body and have a much higher incidence than primary neoplasms. Primary sites that frequently cause bone metastases are the breast, prostate, lung, thyroid and kidney. The bones that are the most common sites of metastases are the vertebrae, pelvic bones, femora and humeri.

Most primary bone neoplasms develop in children and adults younger than 40 years. They may be classified by the type of cell from which they originate, whether they are benign or malignant, and whether the tissue response is osteolytic or reactive. The newgrowth may cause a breakdown of the bone structure, with loss of calcium from the tissue; this type of reaction is referred to as osteolytic. The response of bone tissue to some types of neoplastic cells is the formation of dense bone tissue around the lesion, which may be referred to as a nidus. This type of reaction is called reactive bone formation.

The more common primary bone neoplasms are listed in Table 24–1.

Manifestations

Neoplasms of bones may be asymptomatic for a period of time and may only be discovered when the person has an x-ray for some other reason (e.g., sustained injury) or has a pathologic fracture. Persisting pain, progressively increasing in severity, and limitation of activity of the affected part are common characteristics. Local tenderness, swelling and warmth may be present. If the newgrowth is malignant, systemic symptoms such as weight loss and anemia develop.

Diagnostic Procedures

Investigation of the patient with the symptoms mentioned may include roentgenograms, bone scan, blood tests (hematocrit, leukocyte count, blood smear, sedimentation rate and serum alkaline phosphatase level) and biopsy.

Bone scanning is very useful in detecting early primary lesions or metastatic lesions. A radioisotope is administered that is normally picked up by bone. Examples of radioactive materials used are technetium-99m-tagged phosphate, fluoride-18, gallium-67 and strontium-85. When technetium, fluoride or gallium is used, the scan is made about 3 hours after its administration; if strontium is administered, a period of 2 to 3 days usually elapses before scanning.

Treatment

Benign bone neoplasms are treated by excision or curettage. The bone structure may have to be reinforced following the removal of the lesion by filling in the space with bone chips or small grafts. Treatment of primary malignant neoplasms involves a combination of surgery and chemotherapy. Radical excision is done if the lesion is accessible or, in the case of an extremity, the limb is amputated. For nursing care of the patient, the reader is referred to Care in Amputation, page 921, and Care of the Patient Receiving Chemotherapy, page 143.

The treatment of the patient with skeletal metastases depends principally on the origin of the primary malignant disease. Chemotherapy, hormones and/or irradiation may be used. Irradiation may be used to reduce the severity of the pain experienced by the patient. Analgesics are prescribed to keep the patient comfortable; a small dose is used at first but usually has to be increased as the condition worsens and the patient develops a tolerance for the drug. Precautions are taken to prevent possible falls or injury because of

TABLE 24-1 COMMON PRIMARY BONE NEOPLASMS

Cell of Origin	Neoplasm	Benign/Malignant	Comments
Osteocyte	Osteoid osteoma	Benign	Small, reactive lesion. Femur and tibia common sites. Especially painful at night.
	Osteochondroma	Benign	Commonest benign bone neoplasm; a hamartoma* consisting of bony outgrowth with a cartilage cap. Distal end of femur, proximal end of tibia and proximal end of humerus are common sites. Symptoms depend upon impingement on surrounding tissues.
	Osteogenic sarcoma (osteosarcoma)	Malignant (rapid spread)	Destroys medullary and cortical bone tissue. Usually develops in end of long bone; almost 50 per cent involve the knee joint. Severe pain and tenderness; area may be hot and swollen. Treatment consists of amputation and chemotherapy.
	Osteoclastoma	Benign—may become malignant	Develops most often in epiphyseal region of femur, tibia or humerus of young adults. Rarefaction of bone occurs. It causes pain, swelling and rarely pathologic fracture. Treated by curettage and bone chips or by resection of the bone and replacement with a bone graft. If malignant, the limb is amputated.
Chondrocyte	Chondroma	Benign	Growth of tumor cells within the bone may cause a pathologic fracture. Treated by curettage and packing of the cavity with bone chips to strengthen the bone.
	Chondroblastoma	Benign	Develops toward end of adolescence. Common sites are femur, tibia and humerus. Highest incidence in males. Causes pain and swelling in epiphyseal area. Treatment is curettage and bone grafts.
	Chondrosarcoma	Malignant (slower spread than osteosarcoma)	Age group most often affected 30 to 60 years. Common sites are scapula, pelvis, humerus and femur. Treatment involves radical excision or amputation.
Fibrocyte	Nonosteogenic fibroma	Benign	Most common site is end of diaphysis of long bone. If asymptomatic, it may be left untreated. If painful, it is excised.
	Fibrosarcoma	Malignant	Rare. Usually in adults. Treated by amputation if in a limb.
Uncertain; reticulocyte suggested	Ewing's tumor or sarcoma	Malignant	May involve ilia, ribs, vertebrae and shafts of long bones. Begins in marrow cavity and gradually erodes the bone tissue. Manifestations include severe pain, swelling, fever and leukocytosis. Treatment is combination of irradiation and surgery.

*A *hamartoma* is a benign tumor formed by an overgrowth of normal mature cells characteristic of the area.

the weakened bone structure; a pathologic fracture is a common complication. The nurse is challenged to provide compassionate care, understanding and comfort measures to support the patient and reduce the suffering. When the condition restricts movement and persisting pain is being experienced many simple nursing measures can mean much to the patient, and indicate understanding and caring. Examples are frequent gentle change of position, placing a support under a part, turning pillows, bathing and providing essential hygienic care, prompt administration of the needed analgesic, provision of fluids and nourishment when the patient feels more comfortable and is able to take it, and merely remaining with the patient frequently for even a few minutes so he is not alone for long periods with the severe pain and fear of the future.

References

Books

Beeson, Paul B., and McDermott, Walsh (Eds.): Textbook of Medicine, 14th ed. Philadelphia, W. B. Saunders, 1975. Part 19, Chapters 878–908.

Bunch, Wilton H., and Keagy, Robert D.: Principles of Orthotic Treatment. St. Louis, C. V. Mosby, 1976.

Gartland, John J.: Fundamentals of Orthopaedics, 2nd ed. Philadelphia, W. B. Saunders, 1974.

Lewis, Royce C., Jr.: Handbook of Traction, Casting and Splinting Techniques. Philadelphia, J. B. Lippincott, 1977.

Pearson, J. R., and Austin, R. T.: Accident Surgery and Orthopaedics. London, Lloyd-Luke, 1973.

Raney, R. Beverly, et al.: Shand's Handbook of Orthopaedic Surgery, 8th ed. St. Louis, C. V. Mosby, 1971.

Ryan, James R.: Orthopedic Surgery. Flushing, Medical Examination Publishing, 1977.

Sabiston, David C., Jr. (Ed.): Davis-Christopher: Textbook of Surgery, 11th ed. Philadelphia, W. B. Saunders, 1977.

Periodicals

Bosanko, Lydia A.: "Immediate Postoperative Prosthesis." Am. J. Nurs., Vol. 71, No. 2 (Feb. 1971), pp. 280–283.

Buck, Barbara (Ed.): "Symposium on Orthopedic Nursing." Nurs. Clin. North Am., Vol. 11, No. 4 (Dec. 1976), pp. 639–724.

Dandy, D. J., and Jackson, R. A.: "The Diagnosis of Problems After Meniscectomy." J. Bone Joint Surg., Vol. 57B, No. 3 (Aug. 1975), pp. 349–352.

Fanalls, John: "Crutches and Walkers." Nurs. '72, Vol. 2, No. 12 (Dec. 1972), pp. 21–24.

Foss, Georgia: "Breaking the Architectural Barrier with Crutches, Wheelchairs and Walkers." Nurs. '73, Vol. 3, No. 10 (Oct. 1973), pp. 17–31.

Haddad, John G., Jr.: "Paget's Disease of Bone: Problems and Management." Orthop. Clin. North Am., Vol. 3, No. 3 (Nov. 1972), pp. 775–785.

Hamey, Ronnie: "The Signs and Treatment of Paget's Disease." Geriatrics, Vol. 32, No. 6 (June 1977), pp. 89–93.

Hogan, Karen, and Sawyer, Janet: "Fracture Dislocation of the Elbow." Am. J. Nurs., Vol. 76, No. 8 (Aug. 1976), pp. 1266–1268.

Jordan, Helen S., and Cypres, Robert M.: "All-Around Care for the Leg Amputee." Nurs. '74, Vol. 4, No. 4 (April 1974), pp. 51–55.

Jowsey, Jenifer: "Osteoporosis: Dealing with a Crippling Bone Disease of the Elderly." Geriatrics, Vol. 32, No. 7 (July 1977), pp. 41–50.

Kurth, Janet Sparks: "Thomas Splint and Pearson Attachment." Nurs. '73, Vol. 3, No. 7 (July 1973), pp. 20–24.

McFarland, Mary Brambilla: "Fat Embolism Syndrome." Am. J. Nurs., Vol. 76, No. 12 (Dec. 1976), pp. 1942–1944.

Ryan, John: "Compression in Bone Healing." Am. J. Nurs., Vol. 74, No. 11 (Nov. 1974), pp. 1998–1999.

Soika, Cynthia Vaughan: "Combatting Osteoporosis." Am. J. Nurs., Vol. 73, No. 7 (July 1973), pp. 1193–1197.

Staudt, Annamay Ricco: "Femur Replacement." Am. J. Nurs., Vol. 75, No. 8 (Aug. 1975), pp. 1346–1348.

Stein, Alice M.: "Multiple Fractures: How to Prevent the Pulmonary Complications." Nurs. '74, Vol. 4, No. 11 (Nov. 1974), pp. 26–34.

Synnestvedt, Norwin: "The Dos and Don'ts of Traction Care." Nurs. '74, Vol. 4, No. 11 (Nov. 1974), pp. 35–41.

Whitehead, Dolores J.: "Emergency Care in Orthopedic Injuries." Nurs. Clin. North Am., Vol. 8, No. 3 (Sept. 1973), pp. 435–440.

Wiley, Loy (Ed.): "Traumatic Amputation." Nurs. '72, Vol. 2, No. 11 (Nov. 1972), p. 4045.

25

Nursing in Joint and Collagen Disease

JOINT STRUCTURE AND FUNCTION

A joint or articulation is formed at the junction of two bones. Joints may be classified according to their structures or the degree of movement they permit. *Synarthroses,* or fibrous joints, are immovable and have a layer of connective tissue which unites the bones. The cranial bones form synarthroses. *Amphiarthroses,* or cartilaginous joints, are slightly movable; the bones are separated by a layer of fibrocartilaginous tissue which allows a limited amount of bending or twisting. The symphysis pubis of the pelvis and the joints between the vertebral bodies form amphiarthroses.

Most of the articulations of the skeleton are *diarthroses* or synovial joints, which are freely movable (Fig. 25–1). The bones are separated by a small cavity enclosed in a tough fibrous capsule which is continuous with the periosteum of the bones. This arrangement serves to stabilize the joint and keep the bones in normal apposition. The joint may be further reinforced by ligaments extending from one bone to the other. The capsule is lined with a synovial membrane (synovium) and the joint surfaces of the bones in diarthroses are covered by a layer of cartilage. The capsule contains synovial fluid which bathes the cartilage, supplying nutrients to it in addition to functioning as a lubricant to promote smooth movement. Most of the fluid is a transudate of plasma which escapes from the vasculature of the synovium. Some constituents of synovial fluid are secreted by the synovial membrane. Some diarthrotic joints have flat, crescent-shaped pieces of cartilage lying in the cavity between the ends of the bones. These and the layer of cartilage on the joint surfaces buffer the impact of the rigid bone and cushion and protect the bone tissue. For example, in the knee joint, between the condyles of the femur and tibia, are semilunar cartilages referred to as menisci (singular — meniscus) (see Fig. 25–2). The medial and lateral menisci are frequent sites of internal joint derangement.

The shapes of the articulating surfaces vary with the particular type(s) of movement required of that area of the skeleton.

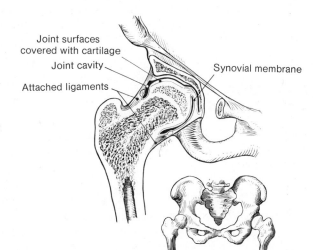

Joint surfaces
covered with cartilage

Joint cavity

Synovial membrane

Attached ligaments

FIGURE 25–1 Diagram of a freely movable joint (diarthrosis).

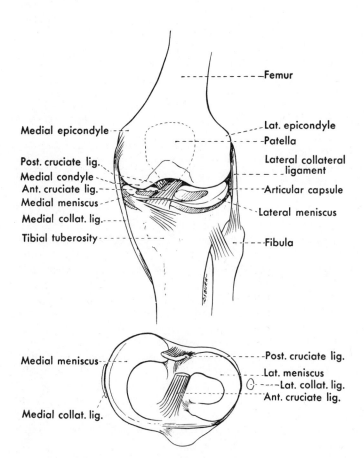

Femur

Medial epicondyle

Lat. epicondyle

Patella

Post. cruciate lig.

Medial condyle

Ant. cruciate lig.

Medial meniscus

Medial collat. lig.

Tibial tuberosity

Lateral collateral ligament

Articular capsule

Lateral meniscus

Fibula

Medial meniscus

Post. cruciate lig.

Lat. meniscus

Lat. collat. lig.

Ant. cruciate lig.

Medial collat. lig.

FIGURE 25–2 Knee joint, showing supporting ligaments and medial and lateral menisci. (From Gartland, John J.: Fundamentals of Orthopaedics, 2nd ed. Philadelphia, W. B. Saunders, 1974, p. 362.)

For instance, the shoulder and hip joints are ball-and-socket in structure to allow all types of movement. The elbow and knee are hinge-like, allowing only flexion and extension.

COMMON JOINT DISORDERS

The more common joint disorders may be traumatic, degenerative, inflammatory or metabolic.

Diagnostic Procedures

Investigation of a joint condition involves a history of why the patient is seeking assistance in addition to the usual record of past health and illness. Physical examination of the patient assesses the body as a whole and the part of which he complains. Posture and alignment of the body and its parts, and anything unusual when the person stands, sits, walks, bends and lies down, are noted. The area in question is *inspected and palpated,* and the *range of motion* and *muscular strength* are assessed. A comparison may be made with the unaffected limb by *measurements* (length and circumference).

Roentgenograms are made of the joint(s) and may include *arthography*. In the latter, a radiopaque substance is injected into the joint cavity to provide a constrast medium so that the soft tissue components may be visualized. This is generally done with investigation of a knee.

Aspiration of synovial fluid may be done to obtain a specimen for laboratory examination for the presence of blood, pus, organisms, sodium urate crystals or malignant cells. A local anesthetic is used and strict asepsis must be observed.

An *arthroscopy* may be done to provide endoscopic examination of a joint. It is used most often in knee disorders. The physician is able to visualize and assess the synovium, articular surfaces, menisci and ligaments, and a biopsy may also be done.

The examination is made in the operating room under strict aseptic conditions. A local or general anesthetic may be administered; the latter is used if surgical intervention is anticipated and is to follow the arthroscopy immediately.

The general and local preparations are the same as for surgery (see p. 164). A large-bore needle is introduced into the joint following anesthesia and normal saline is introduced to "fill out" the cavity. The arthroscope, which is a fiberoptic instrument, is then introduced. Following the examination, if no surgery is performed, the puncture area is sealed and a compressive bandage applied. Activity is usually limited for approximately 3 days.

Laboratory *blood and serum tests* that may be used in joint investigation include: (1) erythrocyte and leukocyte counts; (2) determination of hemoglobin, erythrocyte sedimentation rate (ESR), serum phosphatase, calcium and phosphorus concentrations, and blood uric acid level; and (3) examination for rheumatoid (Rh) factor and human leukocyte antigen B_{27} (HLA B_{27}).

The blood cell counts, hemoglobin and ESR are used to determine the presence of anemia, infection or tissue destruction. The serum phosphatase level is elevated in malignant disease, as is the ESR. The phosphorus and calcium concentrations are significant in bone disease, and the blood uric acid level is increased in gout. The presence of the rheumatoid factor in serum is a characteristic of rheumatoid arthritis.

COMMON JOINT INJURIES

Bursitis

A bursa is a protective structure consisting of a small, flat, fibrous sac lined with synovial membrane. The walls of the sac are separated by a film of synovial fluid. Bursae are located in areas that are subjected to friction or pressure, such as between a bone and overlying tendon or skin. Although inflammation of a bursa is not an internal joint disorder, the affected bursa most frequently is very close to or lies over a joint and results in its impaired function. Bursitis may develop in response to injury or infection. The bursae most commonly encountered clinically in bursitis are those situated between the olecranon process of the ulna and the skin, patella and the skin, shoulder muscles or their tendons and the head of the humerus or scapula, and tendon of Achilles and the calcaneus (heel bone). Excess fluid accumulates within the bursa in response to injury or irritation. There are swelling, pain, tenderness and impaired function.

Treatment may involve aspiration of the fluid and instillation of a corticosteroid preparation, local heat application and, if accessible, as in prepatellar, olecranon and Achilles tendon bursitis, a pressure dressing may be applied. Chronic recurrence of bursitis may necessitate surgical removal of the affected bursa.

Sprain

A sprain is the tearing of ligaments of a joint and overstretching of the joint capsule by twisting or wrenching. The injury may also involve damage to blood vessels, tendons and/or nerves in or around the joint. The person experiences pain, which worsens on movement or weight-bearing, and loss of joint movement. Swelling develops and, if blood vessels are ruptured, extravasation of blood into the tissues causes discoloration. An x-ray of the injured part is usually recommended to rule out a fracture. The ankle is the most frequent site of this type of injury.

Treatment includes rest of the part and the application of cold for 12 to 24 hours to control edema, bleeding and swelling; heat may then be used for comfort. The joint is immobilized and supported by adhesive strapping; rarely, a plaster cast or splint may be necessary. Weight-bearing may be restricted for a considerable period of time, necessitating the use of crutches for mobility.

Dislocation

In a dislocation the bones of a joint are displaced and are no longer in normal anatomic apposition. An incomplete or partial dislocation is referred to as a *subluxation*. The dislocation may be caused by a fall, blow or an unusual effort or movement. Some injury is sustained by the soft tissues of the joint (joint capsule, ligaments, semilunar cartilages, nerves and/or blood vessels).

Manifestations of a traumatic dislocation include pain, deformity, loss of motion of the involved part, and swelling. The joints most commonly affected are the shoulder, finger, thumb, knee and mandible. Dislocation of a hip in an infant or child is usually due to congenital failure of normal joint development. Most often the problem is a shallow acetabulum that will not accommodate the head of the femur, or laxity of the ligaments and joint capsule.

The patient with a dislocation should receive prompt treatment which involves closed or open reduction and immobilization. The area is x-rayed to assess the extent of the injury and the dislocation reduced as soon as possible. The patient is usually given a general anesthetic; reduction involves manual traction and possibly abduction and/or rotation. The joint is then immobilized by the application of adhesive strapping, splint or plaster cast. The immobilization period varies from 2 to 6 weeks, depending upon the extent of damage to the joint capsule and ligamentous structures. Severe tearing and stretching of soft tissues may necessitate surgical repair in order to restore joint stability.

Internal Derangement of a Joint

Injury to a joint may incur tearing of the joint capsule, supporting ligaments and/or semilunar cartilages, resulting in a painful and weak joint with impaired function. The knee is the most common site of internal joint derangement.

The medial meniscus is very vulnerable to injury when the knee is subjected to rotation while flexed and then quickly extended. Tears do not heal; cartilage is less vascular than other tissues and does not regenerate readily. The patient experiences pain which is worse when the limb is used. Displacement of a torn part of the cartilage may cause locking of the joint. The knee is x-rayed and an arthroscopy may be done to assess the damage. Injury to the lateral meniscus occurs much less often than tearing of the medial cartilage.

Rest of the joint, heat application and the administration of acetylsalicylic acid (aspirin) may provide relief for the patient. Surgical excision of the meniscus is done (meniscectomy) if pain and disability persist.

Preoperative preparation is the same as for any bone surgery; local preparation includes the whole limb.

Postoperatively, the leg is elevated on pillows in slight flexion for 12 to 18 hours.

The patient is taught to contract the quadriceps muscles several times at intervals throughout the day while confined to bed. Ambulation with crutches is usually commenced on the second postoperative day; weight-bearing on the operative limb may be gradually increased after 1 week. Exercises are introduced to attain satisfactory range of joint motion. Full activity is usually resumed in about 5 to 6 weeks.

DEGENERATIVE JOINT DISEASE

Osteoarthrosis (Osteoarthritis)

Osteoarthrosis is a common chronic joint disorder which is also known as osteoarthritis, hypertrophic arthritis, degenerative arthritis or senescent arthritis. The term osteoarthrosis or degenerative joint disease is a more accurate designation; arthritis is a misnomer, since inflammation is not a part of the pathologic process. The disorder is characterized by degenerative changes in articular cartilage and marginal bony overgrowth.

MANIFESTATIONS AND ETIOLOGY. Early symptoms appear in the middle or later years of life. It may develop in both males and females, but has a higher incidence in women. The cartilage on the articular ends of the bones becomes thin and worn and gradually breaks down, leaving the underlying bone exposed. The reaction of the denuded bone is manifested in outgrowths of bone from the joint margins, resulting in thickening of the ends of the bones and protruding ridges and spurs (osteophytes) which impair joint movement. Spurs may break off and become loose in the joint, causing further impairment of movement and more pain.

The weight-bearing joints, such as the spinal, hip and knee, and the interphalangeal joints are most frequently the site of degenerative joint disease. It may occur in a single joint or may involve several. The principal cause is thought to be the cumulative strain and wear on the joints through the preceding years, and the aging process. Trauma of the joint, overweight, and malalignment, probably due to poor posture, may be causative factors.

The patient complains of stiffness, soreness and pain in the affected joint(s), and crepitus may be felt or heard on movement. The range of motion becomes increasingly limited because of pain, muscle spasm and the bony outgrowths. Joint enlargement and instability develop. The joints feel hard and irregular. Bony outgrowths on the dorsal surface of affected interphalangeal joints give the knuckles a knobby or gnarled appearance; these knobby protrusions are referred to as *Heberden's nodes*.

CARE OF THE PATIENT. Most patients are treated conservatively but, if the pain becomes intractable and the disability severe, partial or total replacement arthroplasty may be used in selected instances.

In conservative treatment, strain on the affected joints is kept to a minimum. A full explanation of the nature of the disorder should be made to the patient in terms he can understand. This may be supplemented by providing the patient with a booklet provided by a national arthritis organization that describes the disorder and care.[1] Reduced use of the joints and living within the tolerance of the involved parts are stressed. The use of a cane or crutches is encouraged, if necessary, to reduce weight-bearing and keep the patient ambulatory. The patient may have to change his occupation and give up any strenuous sport or other form of recreation. If overweight, the patient is urged to lose weight. During periods of acute pain, a brief period of bed rest, heat applications and medication may be necessary.

Medications used in treating the patient with osteoarthrosis are prescribed primarily to control pain. They include acetylsalicylic acid (aspirin), indomethacin (Indocid), phenylbutazone (Butazolidin, Phenbutazol) and propoxyphene hydrochloride (Darvon). A course of phenylbutazone is usually given over a period of 3 to 4 weeks, or it may be given for 2 weeks and then gradually decreased to a maintenance dose that keeps the patient comfortable and mobile. The drug may be more readily tolerated when taken with meals or a glass of milk. The patient is followed closely and erythrocyte and leukocyte counts are done every 1

---

[1]Arthritis Society: Osteoarthritis, A Handbook for Patients. Arthritis Society, Toronto, Canada.

or 2 weeks, since agranulocytosis and aplastic anemia are possible side effects. Some patients develop gastrointestinal irritation, nausea or a skin rash.

Indomethacin may not be tolerated by the patient, since it may cause gastrointestinal irritation or nausea as well as light-headedness and a feeling of detachment.

Appropriate exercises may be prescribed to maintain muscle tone and movement and promote good alignment and joint stability. The patient is encouraged to be posture-conscious and to review his regular daily activities and posture. Work should be interspersed with short intervals of rest, and unnecessary walking, climbing stairs, lifting and bending should be eliminated. A fitted brace may be helpful to immobilize and provide support in the case of degenerative changes in the spine. A firm mattress with a "fracture" board between it and the bedsprings is recommended to promote good alignment and support for the affected joints.

The application of heat usually contributes to the relief of pain. It promotes circulation through the part and relaxation of the muscles. Precautions are observed to prevent burns.

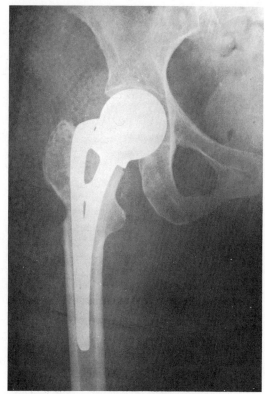

FIGURE 25–3 A partial hip arthroplasty prosthesis. (From Gartland, John J.: Fundamentals of Orthopaedics, 2nd ed. Philadelphia, W. B. Saunders, 1974, p. 350.)

Surgical Therapy in Osteoarthrosis

When an arthritic or deformed joint causes intractable pain and severe disability, surgical intervention may be undertaken. The operative procedures used are osteotomy, arthrodesis, partial replacement arthroplasty or total replacement arthroplasty.

Osteotomy is the reshaping of the bone by cutting or curettement to correct deformity and promote normal joint motion.

Arthrodesis is the surgical fusion of a joint, which results in loss of joint movement. It is done to provide relief from pain or to correct joint instability. In this surgery, the articular cartilage is removed and bone grafts are implanted across the joint surface.

An *arthroplasty* is a reconstructive procedure that may entail replacement of part of the joint or of the whole joint with a prosthesis. It is done to relieve pain and permit patient mobility.

Partial Hip Replacement. The head of the femur is frequently the part of the hip joint degenerated or damaged and that requires replacement. The prosthesis consists of a spherical head and stem of Vitallium or stainless steel; these are inert substances (Fig. 25–3). The head and neck of the femur are removed and the stem of the prosthesis is cemented[2] into the medullary portion of the proximal part of the femoral shaft. The head of the prosthesis fits into the acetabulum.

Total Hip Replacement. Total hip arthroplasty is being used frequently with patients with degenerative joint disease and involves surgical replacement of both sides of the joint. The femoral head and neck are removed. The cartilage is removed from the acetabulum and a polyethylene cup is fitted into the socket. Surgical bone cement is used to secure the plastic cup to the sur-

---

[2]The surgical bone cement that is used in securing prostheses is methyl methacrylate.

face of the acetabulum. The head and neck of the femur are then replaced by a metal prosthesis consisting of a spherical head and stem (Fig. 25–4). The latter is implanted and cemented into the proximal portion of the femoral shaft. The ball part of the prosthesis is fitted into the acetabulum and tested for a range of motions to make sure it does not dislocate on movement. When the wound is closed Hemovac drainage is established. The extremity is placed in a position of abduction which must be maintained until the surgeon indicates that adduction may be resumed gradually.

PREOPERATIVE PREPARATION. In preparing the patient for a replacement arthroplasty, 2 or 3 days are required to advise him of what to expect postoperatively and his role in self-care. A complete physical investigation is made during this period and includes an electrocardiogram, chest x-ray and blood examination (e.g., blood cell counts and determination of hemoglobin, serum electrolyte levels and prothrombin time). The patient's blood is typed and cross-matched and blood is made available for blood replacement during the surgery, and postoperatively if necessary.

An overhead bed frame with a trapeze bar is used to demonstrate how the patient may help with raising himself off the bed after the operation. Instruction is given in deep breathing, coughing and the exercises that will be required. The importance of these is explained while they are being taught. The exercises include isometric quadriceps and gluteal contractions, flexion and extension of toes and ankles and of the nonoperative leg at the knee. The patient is advised that when he is permitted to be turned in bed he will require the assistance of at least two nurses; one will handle the affected limb and maintain its position of abduction. While in the lateral position on the nonoperative side, abduction of the limb is maintained by several pillows.

During the preoperative period, an anticoagulant and antibiotic may be prescribed. The anticoagulant is administered to reduce the risk of thrombophlebitis and ensuing embolism, and to promote microcirculation in the operative site. The drug used may be acetylsalicylic acid, a warfarin preparation, heparin, or a solution of dextran. The latter reduces thrombocyte cohesiveness. Because infection is a very serious postoperative complication the physician may commence antibiotic therapy before the surgery as a prophylactic measure.

Local preparation involves shaving and thorough cleansing of the extremity to mid-calf, the complete hip and the trunk as high as the lower rib with a prescribed antiseptic solution. A cleansing enema is given the day before surgery. Other general preoperative measures (as cited in Chapter 10) are applicable.

POSTOPERATIVE CARE. The postoperative regimen following a hip replacement varies with surgeons and with individual patients. For example, an elderly, weak and debilitated patient may require a different plan of care than that used for a 60-year-old. Following the operation, directives are received from the physician as to the exact position in which the leg is to be maintained and the desired degree of ab-

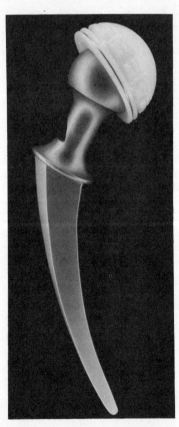

FIGURE 25–4 A total hip arthroplasty prosthesis. (From Burton, David S.: The current status of hip replacement. Primary Care, Vol. 2, No. 1 (March 1975), p. 49.)

duction and rotation, the extent to which the patient may be moved, and the exercises to be done and when they are to commence.

As with all postoperative patients, the plan of care includes the concerns cited in Chapter 10 (vital signs, ventilation, coughing, fluid balance, diet, elimination, hygienic care and comfort) as well as the following specific considerations.

Positioning. The patient's bed is prepared and taken to the operating room so that the patient is moved only once. The surgeon positions the operative limb in abduction. The desired position may be maintained by placing a special hard, triangular pillow between the legs, which are secured to the pillow by straps. The skin surface in contact with the pillow is protected by thick padding to prevent pressure on nerves and on the skin.

In some instances, Russell traction is applied to the operative limb to reduce muscle spasm and maintain abduction. An overhead frame is attached to the bed in both instances, and a trapeze bar is provided so that the patient can assist with raising himself off the bed for skin care and for using the bedpan. The latter should be a small, flat fracture pan to minimize the extent of elevation of the hips.

The patient with the abduction splint remains in the supine position until the surgeon indicates he may be turned. The legs remain attached to the pillow and a minimum of two nurses are required for the procedure. One nurse supports the limb, maintaining the abduction position, while the second person turns the patient almost completely over onto his nonoperative side. Pillows are placed anteriorly and posteriorly to provide support in the tilted position. The period of bed rest required when the abduction splint is used is variable. If traction is used, it is usually maintained for 1 week. Following the removal of the splint or traction, the patient must be cautioned against lying on the operative side and against putting weight on it to "push up in bed" until advised that he may do so.

Observations. The position, circulation and nerve function of the operative limb are monitored hourly for the first 24 hours then 2 hourly. The amount and characteristics of the Hemovac drainage are noted; if it contains bright blood it is reported promptly.

The temperature, pulse and respirations are recorded three times daily even though they remain normal; it is important that any elevation which might indicate infection of the wound or chest be recognized immediately. Patient complaints of pain and/or discomfort are recorded. If the patient complains of sudden severe pain in the hip, or if numbness or a tingling or burning sensation develops, dislocation should be suspected. A firm palpable mass may be felt in the operative area.

Exercises and Ambulation. Active foot and ankle exercises and gentle flexion and extension of the good knee are started the first or second postoperative day, if approved. The patient is reminded to do the isometric exercises that were taught preoperatively several times a day after the order has been given to start them. A limited range and slow flexion of the operative hip are introduced by the surgeon and then gradually increased in range and frequency under the supervision of the nurse or physiotherapist. The patient is usually assisted out of bed on the fourth to seventh postoperative day unless in traction; the surgeon will indicate if the patient is to bear weight at this time or if crutches or a walker should be used for weight support. Walking is commenced after 1 week using crutches or a walker. The patient usually remains in hospital for 2 to 3 weeks.

Wound Care. A Hemovac drainage system is established at the time of operation. The length of time the tubes are left in the wound depends upon the amount of drainage; they are usually removed the first or second day after operation. The surgeon may replace the large pressure dressing on the second day with a smaller, lighter one so that the wound is kept dryer. Strict asepsis is very important in wound care; infection is disastrous in arthroplasty. Good healing is essential for a successful functioning prosthesis.

Pain. The patient usually requires an analgesic for pain relief during the first day or two. Frequently, the hip replacement patient is an older person and narcotics may cause respiratory depression. Precautions are necessary to check the respirations before repeating a dose and again at intervals following administration. On the other hand, the analgesic should not be withheld unnecessarily when the patient is in pain because the suffering and loss of rest predispose to shock.

Skin Care. Since the patient must remain in the supine position, dorsal pressure areas (sacral areas, buttocks, shoulders) require attention every 2 hours. A square of sheepskin is placed under the sacral region and the areas are massaged frequently. One nurse helps the patient raise himself with the trapeze bar while a second gives back care. The lower bedding is changed, working from the top of the bed towards the foot.

Prevention of Complications. The administration of a prophylactic antibiotic which was commenced 1 or 2 days before operation may be continued for several days. Close observations are made for early signs of infection (elevation of temperature, elevation of white blood cell count, complaints of pain and pressure in the affected hip, headache and general malaise).

The immobility of the lower limbs and probably the patient's age predispose to thrombus formation. Preventive measures include the application of elasticized bandages or stockings to both legs after the surgery, the administration of an anticoagulant and approved exercises.

The required position and restricted movement also predispose the patient to hypoventilation and pneumonia. Frequent deep breathing and coughing are very important with this patient. The chest is auscultated twice daily to determine if the segments are being adequately ventilated and if there is any retained secretion.

Psychological Support. When activity and ambulation are commenced, the nurse should be aware of the patient's need for considerable support. Having experienced so much pain and instability before the operation when he walked, the patient is likely to require repeated reassurance that he can now walk comfortably — that he can depend on the new joint. Early attempts with the walker or crutches are anxiety-producing experiences; the patient needs someone close by. The support is very gradually withdrawn so that when he has sufficient control to be safe, he will have gained confidence and independence.

Discharge Preparation. To prepare for going home and becoming as independent as possible, the patient gradually takes over self-care and is instructed in "getting around" and walking up and down stairs. The patient is advised that he should continue to avoid lying on the affected side for at least 2 months, as well as avoid sitting in low chairs. A firm, straight-backed chair and a raised toilet seat are recommended. The importance of continuing the exercises and walking is stressed; crutch-walking distance should be increased gradually.

A referral is made to a visiting nurse or rehabilitation agency. A visit is made to the home before the patient is discharged to assess the situation and suggest, if necessary, any adaptations that would facilitate the person's independence, progress and safety. When the patient goes home regular visits are usually made to the home to supervise the care and exercises and to assess progress. Assistance may be necessary in arranging a visit to the clinic or physician.

KNEE REPLACEMENT. Surgical implantation of a knee prosthesis may be done for the patient whose degenerative disease (e.g., osteoarthrosis) is causing intractable pain and severe incapacity. Various types of prostheses have been introduced but many were discarded because they did not provide sufficient joint stability. The device currently in use consists of a metal femoral condylar unit and a polyethylene tibial plateau unit. The components of the prosthesis are secured by bone cement (methyl methacrylate). This model of prosthesis is proving to provide greater joint stability than those used previously, and to be more functional.

As with hip replacement, the postoperative plan of care varies with different surgeons. The leg is extended and may be immobilized by the application of a splint for several days. Some surgeons have the leg supported on a pillow placed under the lower part of the limb, but not under the knee, and encourage earlier gentle movement of the knee. The nurse requires specific information about the position of the limb, whether support is required, if flexion is permitted, the exercises to be done, and when weight-bearing is to commence. Assessment and nursing considerations are similar to most of the factors cited above for hip replacement. Ambulation begins with the use of the walker and the gradual introduction of partial weight-bearing on the operative knee. The patient progresses to crutches, and eventually uses only a cane for support.

INFLAMMATORY JOINT DISEASES

Rheumatoid Arthritis

Rheumatoid or atrophic arthritis is a chronic inflammatory disease of connective tissues; the dominant site is the joints.

The disease is a major health problem, being responsible for much of the existing chronic illness and crippling incapacity of adults. The incidence is three times higher in women than in men. It may have its onset at any age but most commonly begins between the ages of 30 and 60.

The cause of rheumatoid arthritis remains obscure. Several etiologic factors, such as heredity, infection and nutritional deficiencies, have been suspected from time to time but none have been substantiated. In recent years, attention has been focused on the possibility of an autoimmune reaction being the causative factor. Currently, this theory receives considerable support because of the presence of the *rheumatoid factor* in the blood of 70 to 80 per cent of persons with rheumatoid arthritis. This is a large antibody-like protein molecule which is thought to be produced in response to an altered gamma globulin in the connective tissues and the antigen-antibody reaction that occurs in the various connective tissues but is greatest within the synovium.

CLINICAL COURSE AND FEATURES. The onset is usually insidious; the person experiences a period of general fatigue, nonspecific illness, and morning stiffness and tenderness in some joints. The small joints of the hands or feet or of the wrists, elbows or knees are generally the first to be involved. The disease develops symmetrically and, as it progresses, the affected joints become swollen, painful, red and increasingly difficult to move. Their range of motion is reduced. The overlying skin may take on a stretched, smooth glossy appearance.

The severity of the disease varies in different persons, and remissions and exacerbations may occur. Physical or psychological stress may be a precipitating factor or may aggravate the disease.

Muscle weakness and spasm are common in the early stages and are frequently followed by marked muscular atrophy. Unless early treatment is instituted, progressive joint tissue destruction and deformities develop, leading to permanent disability. Partial dislocation (subluxation) and flexion contractures occur. Deformities commonly seen include hyperextension of the distal phalanges, flexion contracture or ulnar deviation of the fingers due to metacarpal-phalangeal joint involvement, and flexion contraction of the wrists, knees and hips. Subcutaneous nodules (*rheumatoid nodules*) appear principally on extensor surfaces or areas subjected to pressure. These are composed mainly of fibrinoid material (degenerative tissue cells) and granulation tissue.

The initial pathologic, changes within the joints are inflammation, effusion and swelling of the synovial membrane and joint capsule. The process is reversible in the early stage, and the joint may be left undamaged and functional. As the inflammation continues the synovium proliferates and, with the fibrin of the inflammatory exudate, forms a thick spreading membrane of granulation tissue known as a *pannus*. It spreads over the joint surfaces, gradually eroding the cartilage, and may even destroy the denuded bone surfaces. An x-ray may show rarefaction of the ends of the involved bones. Instability and irritation of the joint may cause muscle contraction with a resulting flexion or extension deformity or subluxation of the joint. Fibrous scar tissue and adhesions develop between the opposing joint surfaces, leading to fibrous ankylosis of the joint. The exposed, roughened ends of bone tissue may eventually proliferate bone cells into the joint cavity, resulting in calcification and bony ankylosis.

The patient with rheumatoid arthritis may also have diffuse involvement of nonarticular connective tissue. Degenerative lesions of the collagen component of the connective tissue may develop in muscles, tendons, blood vessels, pleura, heart or lungs.

General constitutional disturbances are manifested; the patient is pale and looks ill. He experiences anorexia, loss of weight and energy, and mental depression. Low-grade fever, tachycardia, anemia and a mild leukocytosis may be present. Later, leukopenia may develop. The erythrocyte sedimentation rate is usually elevated (normal: Westergren, 15 mm. per hour; Wintrobe, 0 to 9 mm. per hour for males and 0 to 20 mm. per hour for females) and, later in the disease, a blood examination may reveal the presence of the rheumatoid factor. When rheumatoid arthritis develops in children, it may be referred to as *Still's disease*. In addition to the symptoms mentioned for adults, they usually have some enlargement of the lymph nodes (lymphadenopathy).

ASSESSMENT AND CLASSIFICATION. In assessing the patient, the physician may classify the disorder according to the pathologic changes (clinical stages) and the loss of functional capacity (functional classification). (See Table 25–1.)

TREATMENT AND NURSING CARE. The care of the patient with rheumatoid arthritis is directed toward the suppression of the inflammatory process, the prevention of deformities, and the maintenance and promotion of joint function. The earlier treatment

is instituted, the less advanced and less crippling the disease is likely to be.

The patient may be hospitalized during the initial investigative and therapeutic periods and is then followed at home by a visiting nurse or at the clinic. Bed rest may be prescribed for a brief period when many joints are acutely inflamed and when systemic disturbances such as fever, anemia and severe fatigue are manifested.

DRUG THERAPY. Various drugs are used in the treatment of rheumatoid arthritis, including salicylates, ibuprofen, indomethacin, gold salts, antimalarial preparations, corticosteroids, phenylbutazone, cytotoxins and immunosuppressive preparations.

The *salicylate preparation* most commonly used is acetylsalicylic acid (aspirin). It is prescribed in relatively large doses and must be taken regularly at the intervals stated in order to maintain effective plasma salicylate levels. Salicylates may produce some adverse effects for which the nurse must be alert. The patient may complain of gastrointestinal disturbances, tinnitus (a ringing or roaring in the ears) and loss of auditory acuity. Since they frequently cause gastrointestinal irritation, the prescribed salicylate is likely to be tolerated better if taken with or soon after meals or with milk or some bland food between meals. Enteric-coated tablets may be used if the

TABLE 25–1 CLASSIFICATION OF RHEUMATOID ARTHRITIS

	By Clinical Stages		By Functional Classification	
Stage	*Manifestations*	*Class*	*Manifestations*	
1 (Early)	No evidence of joint destruction or osteoporosis.	1	No loss of functional capacity.	
2 (Moderate)	Evidence of some destruction of cartilage and probably of subchondral bone. No deformity but full range of motion may be limited. Adjacent muscle atrophy present.	2	Able to carry out usual activities despite some discomfort and limited joint mobility.	
3 (Severe)	Cartilage and bone destruction quite evident. Muscle atrophy and joint deformities such as hyperextension, flexion contracture, ulnar deviation and subluxation present.	3	Functional capacity impaired; occupational and self-care activities quite limited.	
4 (Terminal)	Criteria of Stage 3 plus fibrous or bony ankylosis present.	4	Confined to a wheelchair or bed; not able to carry out self-care. Dependent.	

patient cannot tolerate the plain forms. Gastric or intestinal bleeding is not an uncommon side effect, and patients with any history of peptic ulcer do not usually receive salicylate therapy.

Ibuprofen (Motrin) is an anti-inflammatory, analgesic drug that has recently been used in the treatment of arthritis. The principal side effects that develop with some patients are nausea, vomiting, diarrhea and dizziness.

Indomethacin (Indocid) may be prescribed for its anti-inflammatory and analgesic effects. Some patients cannot tolerate it because of side effects, which may be gastrointestinal irritation and ulceration, nausea, headache, depression, dizziness and a sense of detachment.

When a preparation of *gold salts* such as gold sodium thiomalate (Myochrysine) or gold thioglucose (Solganal) is given, the patient is observed closely for signs of toxic reactions. The initial dose is small to test the patient for adverse reactions. Such reactions may be seen as stomatitis (inflammation of the oral mucous membrane), dermatitis, renal damage and bone marrow depression leading to severe anemia, leukopenia (agranulocytosis) and thrombocytopenia. Gold therapy usually involves an intramuscular injection given two or three times each week for a period of 4 to 6 months. Urine analysis and blood cell counts are done weekly, and the patient is checked for possible signs or symptoms of adverse side effects.

The *antimalarial drugs* such as chloroquine (Nivaquine B or Aralen) and hydroxychloroquine sulfate (Plaquenil Sulfate) may be prescribed over a period of several months for some patients. Toxic effects that may develop include skin eruptions, headache, anorexia, nausea, vomiting and auditory or visual disturbances. Frequent blood cell counts are done because occasionally bone marrow depression occurs.

Adrenal corticosteroids are now usually reserved for patients whose rheumatoid arthritis is rapidly progressing, is very painful and has not responded to therapeutic courses of other antirheumatic drugs. Examples of oral preparations used are prednisone, prednisolone and hydrocortisone. The dosage is individualized and kept to a minimum because of the unfavorable side effects which may develop. It is important that the patient

understand that the drug will be given only for a limited period. The dosage is gradually reduced and then completely withdrawn. Adverse side effects which are likely to develop with overdosage or prolonged therapy include reduced lymphocyte and antibody production, leading to increased susceptibility to infection, sodium and water retention, excessive potassium excretion, mood swings or euphoria, restlessness or overactivity, hyperglycemia and glucosuria, fullness or rounding of the face (moon face), and growth of hair on the face in the case of a female. The patient who has experienced increased appetite, a marked sense of well-being and some remission of the disease while receiving a corticosteroid may feel quite depressed and let down when the drug is withdrawn, and will require considerable emotional support from the nurse.

When only one or two joints are affected, intra-articular injections of a corticosteroid may be made to arrest the inflammatory process.

Phenylbutazone (Butazolidin) is occasionally prescribed, and unfavorable effects may be reflected in skin eruptions, bone marrow depression or gastrointestinal irritation. Blood cell counts are monitored frequently.

The *immunosuppressive drug* azathioprine (Imuran) has been used in treating the patient with rheumatoid arthritis, using the rationale that the cause is an antigen-antibody reaction. It is prescribed for patients who are unresponsive to any of the drugs mentioned previously in this section. The suppression of leukocyte and antibody formation makes the patient very susceptible to infection. The rheumatoid arthritic patient is frequently debilitated and already has a lowered resistance. Precautions are necessary to protect him from exposure to infection; recognition of early symptoms is reported promptly so an antibiotic may be prescribed. Side effects that may be experienced by the patient receiving azathioprine include gastrointestinal intolerance and liver dysfunction.

The *cytotoxic drug* cyclophosphamide (Cytoxan) is being used occasionally with severe rheumatoid arthritis that is unresponsive to more conventional drug therapy (for side effects, see p. 144).

D-*Penicillamine* has been introduced recently as an anti-rheumatoid drug. It is considered effective through its action of altering collagen metabolism, but toxic side effects are common. The patient may experience anorexia, nausea and vomiting, skin eruption, thrombocytopenia and nephritis.

The last three drugs cited (cyclophosphamide, azathioprine, D-penicillamine) may produce life-threatening, toxic side effects; their use is limited to patients with severe rheumatoid disease who have shown no improvement with other drugs. The physician explains the risk associated with them to the patient and family and may require a signed consent for administration.

POSITIONING AND THE APPLICATION OF SPLINTS. During the acute inflammatory stage, the affected joints are especially painful on movement. The involved part usually assumes the flexed position because of spasm of the dominant flexor muscles, and contracture deformity is likely to develop. Limb joints may be placed at rest and immobilized in a neutral position by the application of padded splints to reduce the severity of pain and prevent contractures and deformities. At first, these may only be removed during the daily passive exercise or heat therapy periods. Later, as the muscle spasm lessens, the splints are left off for most of the day and may only be necessary during the night.

To prevent hip and spinal flexion, a fracture board is placed under the mattress and the patient is encouraged to use only a small pillow to maintain good cervical alignment. If the patient is confined to bed for a period longer than 24 hours, he is advised to change his position frequently. Two or three periods of ½ hour or more should be spent in the prone position to prevent flexure contraction at the hips. A footboard is provided to keep the feet at almost right angles while in the dorsal position. When positioning or assisting the patient, the affected parts must be handled very gently, and support is given to the joints. Jarring and quick, jerky movements are avoided. Independence and active movements are encouraged as acute inflammation subsides; the patient moves slowly and the nurse and family must learn to be patient and allow him the necessary time.

When the arthritic is up, attention is paid to posture. He is encouraged to stand erect and "sit straight" to avoid forward flexion of the trunk and drooping of the shoulders.

HEAT APPLICATIONS. Various forms of heat applications are used to help reduce muscle spasm, pain, joint stiffness and swelling. Soaks in water at 38° to 39° C. (100° to 102° F.) or the application of dry heat (hot water bottle, electric heating pad or infrared heat lamp) may be prescribed. Hot paraffin immersion is also used. Paraffin mixed with mineral oil (3½ pounds of paraffin to 1 cup of mineral oil) is heated to 51.4° to 54° C. (125° to 130° F.). The affected limb is repeatedly dipped in the solution until six to eight coats are applied and then wrapped in paper and a thick bath towel. If the affected joint cannot be immersed in the paraffin, several layers may be applied to it quickly with a paint brush. The wax coating is left for approximately 1 hour and then is peeled off and reused.

Whatever form of heat is used, precautions must be used against burning; the skin over acutely inflamed joints is more sensitive and is readily burned. Heat is not used if there is any break in the skin.

EXERCISES AND ACTIVITY. As soon as possible, a daily exercise schedule is introduced to achieve and preserve the most complete range of motion possible, as well as to maintain muscle strength. Exercises are planned and prescribed on an individual basis and are carefully supervised by a physical therapist or nurse until they are understood and are familiar to the patient. Indiscriminate movements or overstretching may cause a dislocation or torn tendons.

When acute inflammation, swelling and severe pain preclude joint movements, isometric exercises are recommended. Joint exercises may be passive or active-assisted to start with and are gradually progressed to active and resistive exercises within the limits set by the physician. The exercises are only of value if carried out at regular intervals. The patient's reaction to the exercises is noted; excessive fatigue or increased pain necessitates some modification in the exercise program. A balance must be struck between rest and exercise. An explanation is made to the patient and family of the purpose and importance of the exercise regimen. The exercises may be performed with less difficulty if preceded by some form of heat application which promotes muscle relaxation. Special shoes, canes, a walker or braces may be recommended to assist with weight bearing and mobility.

Self-care and the activities of daily living are encouraged. If the range of motion is limited because of joint destruction or ankylosis, self-help devices may be provided to promote maximum independence in such activities as dressing, grooming and feeding. Good grooming and taking pride in appearance are encouraged by providing the essentials and commending the patient.

SURGICAL TREATMENT. Surgery is playing an increasing role in the treatment of rheumatoid arthritis. The thickened inflamed synovium is removed (*synovectomy*) from the affected joint(s) early in the disease, prior to cartilage and bone destruction or the formation of fibrous adhesions and ankylosis.

In more advanced disease in which there has been irreversible joint damage that has led to deformity and loss of function, various surgical procedures may be undertaken to reduce the handicap. Arthrodesis (fixation of the joint) to provide joint stability or arthroplasty (reconstructive procedure) with the use of prosthetic devices may be done. A rigid exercise program following surgery is usually very necessary to insure functional improvement for the patient.

GENERAL SUPPORTIVE MEASURES. In planning care for the arthritic, the nurse also gives consideration to the *psychological support, rest* and *nutrition* needed by the patient.

The diagnosis of rheumatoid arthritis is likely to produce considerable emotional response in the patient because of the chronic nature of the disease and because the possible crippling effects are common knowledge to most persons. The patient may become resentful, depressed and uncooperative. The nurse, recognizing the patient's reactions as normal responses to threatening situations, accepts them and watches for opportune situations to convey her understanding of his feelings and to encourage him to talk about his problems, at which time she may offer explanations as to the available assistance and suggestions as to how he may adjust. He is advised of the variability in the severity and rate of progress and should be reminded that many patients lead a normal, useful life with only slight modifications in their pattern of living.

Some activities which previously seemed very simple and were taken for granted may become quite a chore and time-consuming. Adjustments in the daily routine may be made to allow more time for such tasks. Many of the patients afflicted with rheumatoid arthritis are in what are referred to as the most productive years. Restricted employment, reduced earning capacity and limited social and recreational activities add considerable stress to the situation and are frequently a source of great concern for the patient and his family. A social worker's assistance, a chaplain's counsel and the assurance that there is a planned therapeutic and rehabilitation program available may help with emotionally disturbing factors. Successful adjustment in the initial stage of the disease is important. If the patient accepts and follows the prescribed modifications and treatment regimen at the onset, he is usually less distressed and more likely to respect the necessary adjustments during an acute recurrence.

The person with rheumatoid arthritis generally requires extra rest. The amount depends on the severity of his disease. The daily schedule may require modification to allow rest periods through the day and more hours in bed at night. The arthritic must appreciate that rest alone or exercise alone is not good, but rather that both are essential. Controlled activity and exercise must be balanced with an appropriate amount of rest. The amount of each is recommended by the physician but is an individual factor, frequently requiring modification from time to time.

A well-balanced diet, similar to that essential to the health of all persons, is recommended for the arthritic. The total caloric intake may require some adjustment with a view to achieving or maintaining the person's normal weight. Overweight is avoided for it increases the strain on joints and may also reduce motivation in exercise.

INSTRUCTION AND REHABILITATION. The long-term goal in planning and implementing care for the person with rheumatoid arthritis is to have him be as independent and as useful as possible, gainfully employed and living as normal a social and family life as possible.

It is important for the patient and family to understand the nature of rheumatoid arthritis and that much of the disability and deformity commonly associated with the disease can be prevented if early treatment is instituted and the prescribed regimen followed. The nurse's explanation can be reinforced by providing booklets especially prepared for patients and the public by national arthritis societies.[3]

---

[3]The Canadian Arthritis Society, Toronto, Ontario, Canada. The Arthritis Foundation, New York, N. Y., U.S.A.

Rehabilitation depends largely on the severity of the patient's disease and whether or not the pathologic process in the joints is arrested. Obviously, if the disease is severe and more and more joints are progressively involved, the patient is less likely to be well enough to return to his former occupation and will require a more active and closely supervised care program. Many patients are well enough to go to work and adjust their daily life to provide for extra rest as well as continuance of a daily physical exercise regimen. Some find it necessary after the onset of arthritis to change their former type of work. This may necessitate assistance in finding suitable employment or in interpreting the patient's condition to the employer, who may be persuaded to employ him in another type of job. A period of vocational training may be necessary before the arthritic can be reemployed.

Before leaving the hospital or clinic, the patient is given a written outline of his exercises. These are reviewed and discussed with him and a family member. If there is some restriction in the range of motion of some joints which interferes with self-care activities, arrangements are made for the provision of self-help devices. The family members are made aware of the importance of encouraging the patient to do things for himself. They are advised that he may be very slow in achieving various activities which seem very simple to them. They should appreciate the need for additional patience and for planning that will provide the required extra time.

If drug or heat therapy is to be continued as well as the exercises, or if the patient is sufficiently handicapped to require physical care, a referral may be made to the visiting nurse or rehabilitation agency. The visiting nurse frequently is of assistance in assessing the home situation and making recommendations for adjustments that will simplify the care of the patient and will increase mobility and independence. For example, suggestions may be made for reorganizing the kitchen in order to make equipment more readily available and lessen the demands on the worker. Such recommendations for simplification of household chores may enable a woman with arthritis to carry on the care of her home.

The importance of maintaining good body alignment is stressed; in addition to fracture boards and footboards for the bed, a comfortable straight chair of appropriate height and good walking shoes are needed.

The patient and his family are acquainted with the services of the Arthritis Society and its publications which may be helpful. Transportation is frequently a problem for the arthritic. If he is required to go regularly to a physical therapy clinic or rehabilitation unit, the society will usually provide transportation, if requested.

In discussing the necessary care, emphasis is placed on the avoidance of becoming overtired, emotionally upset about things that cannot be corrected and exposure to cold. The patient is also reminded to minimize as much as possible the strain and pressure normally placed on the affected joints. He and his family are cautioned against quack and folk remedies and the taking of unprescribed drugs. Regular attendance at a clinic or the physician's office is essential for repeated ongoing evaluation and appropriate adjustments in treatment.

The nurse is alert for economic problems that may be imposed by the illness, and a referral is made, when necessary, to a welfare or service agency for assistance.

Ankylosing Spondylitis

This is a chronic disorder characterized by inflammation and ensuing ankylosis of the sacroiliac joints and spinal articulations. It may also be designated as Marie-Strümpell arthritis or rheumatoid spondylitis. The pathologic process is similar to that seen in rheumatoid arthritis, but there is a greater tendency toward calcification. In most instances the disease remains confined to the joints cited above but occasionally does spread to peripheral joints.

The highest incidence is in young men, the onset occurring most often in the late teens or the twenties. The cause is unknown, but heredity is suspected of having a role, since a large majority of those afflicted have a family history of some form of inflammatory arthritis.

CLINICAL FEATURES. The onset of this disease is usually insidious; the patient first complains of stiffness of the back in the morning or following a period of inactivity. Progressively, this becomes more noticeable; limitation in the range of spinal flexion develops, chest expansion is reduced and there is low back pain radiating to the buttocks and thighs along the sciatic nerve pathways. General systemic symptoms are usually absent or are limited to unusual fatigue and probably some weight loss.

Laboratory examinations indicate an increase in the erythrocyte sedimentation rate but in most cases the rheumatoid factor is absent. Recently it has been recognized that the histocompatibility antigen HL-A$_{27}$ is present in these patients; this has become a confirming diagnostic factor of ankylosing spondylitis. Leukocytosis and anemia may be present and the protein concentration of the cerebrospinal fluid is frequently increased.

Remissions and exacerbations of the acute disease are common. In more advanced stages, some patients develop some peripheral rheumatoid arthritis. A few develop circulatory complications due to aortitis and aortic valvular insufficiency. Uveitis[4] is also seen in about 25 per cent of the patients.

Progressive involvement of spinal segments may continue over a period of years and eventually leave the patient with practically the whole spine firmly ankylosed, producing what may be referred to as a poker back or poker spine. Rarely, rheumatoid spondylitis has an abrupt, acute onset and spreads rapidly through the lumbar, thoracic and cervical segments, leaving the patient with a poker spine in a relatively short period.

TREATMENT AND NURSING CARE. Care of the patient with ankylosing spondylitis is directed toward the relief of pain, maintenance of good spinal alignment and preservation of maximum spinal function.

During acute phases, the patient usually receives acetylsalicylic acid (aspirin), phenylbutazone (Butazolidin) or indomethacin (Indocid) (see p. 945 for side effects).

Good body alignment at rest and good posture at all times are extremely important so that ankylosis of the affected joints occurs while they are in the normal neutral position, thus preventing deformity and handicap. The patient is advised of the need for constant attention to good posture when he is up, with emphasis on contraction of the buttock and lower abdominal muscles and keeping the chest up, shoulders back and head erect. In some instances, he is fitted with a back brace to maintain optimum alignment of the affected joints. A fracture board and a firm mattress are placed on his bed, and it is suggested that he not use a pillow or, if necessary, only a very small one. The small of the back may be supported by a small pillow, but hyperextension is avoided. The patient is advised to sleep straight and flat on the back or in the prone position to discourage possible flexion of the spine.

A daily physical exercise program is prescribed with the objective of strengthening the muscles which help to support the spine, maintain good alignment and promote the patient's functional capacity. Since ankylosis of the costovertebral joints may occur and reduce the ventilatory capacity, breathing exercises are also included in the suggested exercise regimen.

Heavy lifting and activities which place strain upon the back are restricted. The patient assists in determining his level of tolerance of physical activity; that which produces pain should be avoided. The disease may necessitate a change of occupation and vocational retraining before suitable employment can be found.

If hip and spinal deformities develop, surgical correction may be undertaken to facilitate the patient's mobility and rehabilitation. The commonest deformity is fixed flexion of the spine (kyphosis).

METABOLIC JOINT DISEASE

Gout

Gout is a disorder of uric acid metabolism, characterized by recurring episodes of acute inflammation, pain and swelling in a joint. Any joint may be affected, but those of the foot are more susceptible; the condition usually develops first in the great toe. Gout occurs more commonly in men over 40 years of age and is rarely seen in females.

The disorder is thought to occur as the result of a genetic defect in the metabolism of purine. It causes an excessive concentration of uric acid in the plasma (hyperuricemia) which may be brought about by an overproduction or faulty disposal by the kidneys. Urate crystals may be precipitated and deposited within joint tissues, setting up irritation

---

[4]*Uveitis* is inflammation of the iris, ciliary body and choroid of the eye.

and a local inflammatory response. The small masses of crystals, which are called *tophi,* may also form in cartilage, the kidneys or soft tissues in other areas of the body.

Secondary gout may develop in disorders such as blood dyscrasias in which there is a marked breakdown of cellular nucleic acid. When the urate crystals are deposited in joints and produce inflammation, the condition may be referred to as *gouty arthritis.*

SIGNS AND SYMPTOMS. Acute episodes are characterized by the sudden onset of excruciating pain in the affected joint. It becomes very tender, red, hot and swollen. Veins in the area stand out because of congestion and distention. The patient may also experience anorexia, headache, fever and constipation. The blood uric acid concentration is elevated (normal: 2.5 to 5 mg. per cent). Subcutaneous tophi are frequently apparent in the ears or over joints or knuckles. Precipitations of urates may occur in kidney tissue, leading to impaired renal function. In some patients, the excessive concentration of uric acid results in the formation of kidney stones.

The acute attack usually subsides in a few days, and in the early stages of the disease the joint returns to normal. Remissions may gradually become shorter, and the disease may become chronic. More joints become involved, and there are irreversible changes, leading to deformity and loss of function.

TREATMENT AND NURSING CARE. During an acute attack of gout, the patient is placed on bed rest, and drug therapy is promptly instituted. The preparation that has proved most effective to date and is most commonly used is colchicine. It may be administered orally or intravenously. If it is given intravenously, precautions are taken to avoid any of the drug being deposited in the subcutaneous or extravascular tissues because of its local irritating effect. Side effects include nausea, vomiting, abdominal discomfort and diarrhea. The drug generally relieves the pain fairly quickly but does not lower the hyperuricemia. If the patient cannot tolerate or does not respond to colchicine, phenylbutazone (Butazolidin), indomethacin (Indocid) or an adrenocorticosteroid preparation such as prednisone may be prescribed. For possible side effects of these, see page 945.

Probenecid (Benemid) or sulfinpyrazone (Anturan) may also be administered to increase the pH of the urine and the renal excretion of uric acid to avoid the formation of renal calculi.

Hot or cold applications to the affected joint(s) may provide some relief, but frequently the patient cannot tolerate either. Discomfort is usually less when the part is protected as much as possible from any direct contact with applications and bedding.

A fluid intake of 2500 to 3000 ml. is encouraged to promote dilution and renal elimination of the uric acid. The urinary output is recorded, and the fluid balance is determined.

The diet is generally restricted to fluids for the first day or two; then it is gradually increased as tolerated to include mainly soft carbohydrate foods. The protein and fat contents are kept low and then are added in specified, limited amounts. The patient then progresses to a well-balanced diet that is low in fat and has a controlled protein content; he is advised to follow this diet during remissions. The prescribed diet prohibits foods high in purines such as organ meats (liver, kidneys, heart, sweetbreads), shellfish, sardines and meat extracts. If the patient is overweight, the caloric intake is adjusted to promote a gradual reduction to the optimum weight. Some physicians recommend that the patient subject to acute attacks of gout should abstain from drinking alcohol. Others permit their patients to have a limited amount. The importance of a high fluid intake is explained to the patient, and a minimal daily intake of 2000 to 2500 ml. is continued during remissions.

Patients who are having frequent and severe attacks may receive a uricosuric drug routinely. This type of preparation promotes the urinary excretion of uric acid and lowers the serum uric acid level by inhibiting renal tubular reabsorption. The patient must have a high fluid intake, and an effort is made to keep the urine alkaline. The patient is taught to take alkaline-producing foods and fluids or sodium bicarbonate tablets and to test the pH of the urine. If the urine reaction is acid while he is receiving the drug, it is reported to the physician. The uricosuric drug that may be prescribed for the patient with chronic gout is allopurinol (Zyloprim, Bloxanth) or probenecid (Benemid). Salicylate, thiazide and furosemide preparations are not administered when the patient is receiving a uricosuric agent, since they counteract the desired effect.

COLLAGEN DISEASE

Systemic Lupus Erythematosus (Disseminated Lupus Erythematosus)

This disorder is a multisystem disease which is characterized by diffuse inflammation and biochemical and structural changes in the collagen fibers of connective tissues in organs and tissues throughout the body. Originally, lupus erythematosus, dermatomyositis and scleroderma comprised the collagen diseases. In recent years, some references include rheumatoid arthritis, rheumatic fever and polyarteritis nodosa in the classification of collagen disease.

Systemic lupus erythematosus (SLE) is poorly understood. It usually runs a chronic, irregular course and may prove fatal. The cause is not known, but the presence of certain immunoglobulins (antibodies) in the blood supports the theory that an autoimmune mechanism is responsible. Several factors are suspected of having a role in precipitating the onset or an acute exacerbation of the disease; these include exposure to the sun's rays, emotional stress, infection and drugs (e.g., sulfonamide, penicillin, procainamide, isoniazid).

SIGNS AND SYMPTOMS. The disease may begin at any age in either sex, but is seen most often in young women. The signs and symptoms, especially at the onset, vary greatly from one person to another, depending upon the systems and organs involved. Those most commonly seen include fever, general malaise, excessive fatigue, weakness, anorexia, weight loss and joint pain. An erythematous rash may be evident on the face, neck and/or extremities. If the disorder is confined to the skin it is referred to as *discoid lupus erythematosus*. The lesions on the face typically spread over the nose and cheeks to form a butterfly pattern. Angioneurotic edema[5] with burning or itchy sensations, patchy vitiligo or areas of hyperpigmentation, mucosal ulceration and alopecia may develop.

---

[5]*Angioneurotic edema* is the temporary appearance of large edematous areas in the skin or mucous membrane due to a disturbance in the innervation of the vasomotor system.

In the systemic type of lupus erythematosus, generalized lymphadenopathy occurs. The patient may complain of impaired vision as a result of corneal involvement and retinopathy. Raynaud's phenomenon may be troublesome, especially if the patient is exposed to even slight cold. As the disease progresses, serious visceral involvement and ensuing dysfunction are likely to develop. Impaired pulmonary, cardiovascular and kidney function are common. Renal failure is the most frequent cause of death of the patient with SLE. Central nervous system involvement is also common.

The erythrocyte sedimentation rate is elevated (normal: Westergren, < 15 mm. per hour; Wintrobe, 0 to 9 mm. per hour for males and 0 to 20 mm. per hour for females), and anemia is a frequent development. The presence of the LE cell or factor in the serum facilitates diagnosis. LE cells are polymorphonuclear leukocytes which are enlarged as the result of "ingested" nucleoprotein that has been released by damaged leukocytes in an antigen-antibody reaction. Recently, antinuclear antibodies have been identified in the serum of most patients with SLE. The hematocrit falls and thrombocytopenia may be manifested in petechiae and purpura.

TREATMENT. The care of the patient is mainly supportive and symptomatic; at present, no therapy is considered curative. In remissions, the patient is advised against exposure to sunlight, infection and excessive fatigue which are thought to predispose or precipitate an exacerbation of the disease process. Lotions may be recommended by the physician that will screen out the ultraviolet sun rays when the person has to be exposed. Cold should be avoided because of the vascular reaction (Raynaud's).

Medications which may be prescribed include acetylsalicylic acid (aspirin) to control fever and joint involvement, an antimalarial drug such as hydroxychloroquine (Plaquenil) for the patient with skin and joint involvement if the condition is unresponsive to salicylates, and an adrenocorticosteroid preparation. The latter is used for the more severe stage of SLE when there is renal, central nervous system, cardiovascular and hemopoietic involvement. The steroid drug is given in relatively large doses during an acute exacerbation, and then gradually reduced to a maintenance dose or withdrawn completely. If hydroxychloroquine is given, frequent ophthalmologic examinations are necessary since the drug may precipitate retinopathy. A cytotoxic immunosuppressive drug such as cyclophospamide (Cytoxan) or azathioprine (Imuran) may be used when the patient with severe disease is unresponsive to the more conservative drugs.

Blood transfusions may be necessary because of the anemia and thrombocytopenia; packed cells may be administered if cardiac and respiratory embarrassment have been manifested. Hemodialysis may be necessary when the disease attacks the kidneys.

Dermatomyositis

In this form of collagen disease the skin and voluntary muscles are the principal focal sites of the pathologic inflammatory process. The incidence is higher in females. The onset is insidious and may be manifested by an erythematous skin rash, subacute fever, and tenderness, edema and weakness of the muscles. Contracture of the skin and muscles due to the fibrous scar tissue may lead to tightly drawn skin in the affected areas, muscle contracture and loss of function. Involvement of the respiratory muscles may cause respiratory insufficiency and frequently is the cause of death. In some instances the condition is confined to muscle tissue and is referred to as *chronic polymyositis;* the skin is not involved. Diagnosis includes an electromyogram, muscle and/or skin biopsy and blood determination of enzyme levels. The serum glutamic-oxaloacetic transaminase (SGOT) is elevated in dermatomyositis.

This collagen disease may be treated with an adrenocorticosteroid preparation, but the outlook is generally unfavorable.

Scleroderma (Progressive Systemic Sclerosis)

This is a chronic disorder in which the collagen component of the skin undergoes degenerative changes and becomes sclerotic. The dermal changes and contraction produce deformities and restricted movement. The pathologic sclerosing process may spread to viscera, causing systemic disturbances and organ dysfunction similar to those that may occur in systemic lupus erythematosus. The rate of progress varies with patients; some survive many years, while the disease may prove fatal to others in a few months.

Polyarteritis Nodosa

This disorder is characterized by diffuse inflammatory and necrotizing lesions in the walls of smaller arteries with resultant fibrosis of vascular walls, thrombosis and infarction. The vessel wall is weakened at the site of the lesion and an aneurysm may develop. In other instances, thrombosis within the lumen of the vessel may lead to occlusion.

The incidence of polyarteritis nodosa is greater in males. Vague and varying signs and symptoms occur, as with other collagen diseases, and are referable to multiple systems and organs. Although any organ may be affected, those most commonly involved are the kidneys, muscles, heart, lungs, liver and gastrointestinal tract. If the arteries in vital organs such as the kidneys and heart are attacked, essential life-supporting functions may be threatened.

As with other collagen diseases, there is no specific treatment; adrenocorticosteroids may be administered and may provide a temporary remission. Care is symptomatic and supportive.

References

Books

Beeson, Paul B., and McDermott, Walsh (Eds.): Textbook of Medicine, 14th ed. Philadelphia, W. B. Saunders, 1975. Parts V and VI.

Ehrlich, George E. (Ed.): Total Management of the Arthritic Patient. Philadelphia, J. B. Lippincott, 1973.

Gartland, John J.: Fundamentals of Orthopaedics, 2nd ed. Philadelphia, W. B. Saunders, 1974.

Herman, Jerome H., et al.: Rheumatoid Arthritis: Theoretical and Clinical Aspects. New York, MSS Information, 1973.

Marmor, Leonard: Surgery of Rheumatoid Arthritis. Philadelphia, Lea and Febiger, 1967.
Macleod, John (Ed.): Davidson's Principles and Practice of Medicine, 11th ed. Edinburgh, Churchill Livingstone, 1974, pp. 768–792.
Pearson, J. R., and Austin, R. T.: Accident Surgery and Orthopaedics. London, Lloyd-Luke, 1973.
Raney, R. Beverly, et al.: Shand's Handbook of Orthopaedic Surgery, 8th ed. St. Louis, C. V. Mosby, 1971.
Scott, J. T. (Ed.): Textbook of the Rheumatic Diseases, 5th ed. Edinburgh, Churchill Livingstone, 1978.
Wintrobe, Maxwell M., et al. (Eds.): Principles of Internal Medicine, 7th ed. New York, McGraw-Hill, 1974. Section 14.

Periodicals

Ball, Barbara (Ed.): "Helping Patients Adjust to Rheumatoid Arthritis." Nurs. '72, Vol. 2, No. 10 (Oct. 1972), pp. 11–17.
Beurgin, Pat: "Ravages of Rheumatoid Arthritis." Nurs. '75, Vol. 5, No. 6 (June 1975), pp. 44–47.
Bowden, Susan Ackerman: "New Surgery for Arthritic Hands." Nurs. '76, Vol. 6, No. 8 (Aug. 1976), pp. 46–48.
Burton, David S.: "The Current Status of Hip Replacement." Primary Care, Vol. 2, No. 1 (March 1975), pp. 47–55.
Calabro, John J.: "Arthritis of the Spine: Management of Ankylosing Spondylitis." Med. Times/Contents, Vol. 105, No. 11 (Nov. 1977), pp. 80–96.
Calin, Andrei: "Rheumatoid Arthritis." Am. Fam. Physician, Vol. 18, No. 1 (July 1978), pp. 89–94.
Decker, John L.: "From Willow Bark to Cytoxids: The Management of Rheumatoid Arthritis." Med. Times/Contents, Vol. 105, No. 11 (Nov. 1977), pp. 28–34.
Denman, A. M.: "Viruses, Poisons and Arthritis." Rheumatol. Rehabil., Vol. 16, No. 4 (Nov. 1977), pp. 205–214.
Drain, Cecil B.: "The Athletic Knee Injury." Am. J. Nurs., Vol. 71, No. 3 (March 1971), pp. 536–537.
Driscoll, Pamela Webb: "Rheumatoid Arthritis: Understanding It More Fully." Nurs '75, Vol. 5, No. 12 (Dec. 1975), pp. 26–32.
Eyre, Mary K.: "Total Hip Replacement." Am. J. Nurs., Vol. 71, No. 7 (July 1971), pp. 1384–1387.
Feeley, R. H.: "Systemic Lupus Erythematosus: A Review." Rheumatol. Rehabil., Vol. 17, No. 2 (May 1978), pp. 79–82.
Gwilliam, Suzanne: "Total Knee Arthroplasty." Can. Nurse, Vol. 70, No. 9 (Sept. 1974), pp. 33–36.
Hartley, Bonnie: "Systemic Lupus — A Patient Perspective." Can. Nurse, Vol. 74, No. 2 (Feb. 1978), pp. 16–20.
Hunt, T. E.: "The Rheumatoid Arthritic at Home." Can. Fam. Physician, Vol. 23, No. 1 (Jan. 1977), pp. 50–54.
Janecki, Chet J., et al.: "Arthroscopy of the Knee." Am. Fam. Physician, Vol. 17, No. 3 (March 1978), pp. 109–116.
Janul, Linda C.: "Dermatomyositis-Polymyositis: A Perplexing Disorder." Am. J. Nurs., Vol. 77, No. 7 (July 1977), pp. 1184–1186.
Jennings, Kate: "The Cheerful Operation: Total Hip Replacement." Nurs. '76, Vol. 6, No. 7 (July 1976), pp. 32–37.
Johnson, Kenneth: "When Total Knee Arthroplasty is Indicated." Geriatrics, Vol. 31, No. 3 (March 1976), pp. 71–75.
Kealey, Louis A.: "Treatment of Gout and Hyperuricemia." Med. Times/Contents, Vol. 105, No. 11 (Nov. 1977), pp. 28–34.
Loxley, Alice Keating: "The Emotional Toll of Crippling Deformity." Am. J. Nurs., Vol. 72, No. 10 (Oct. 1972), pp. 1839–1840.
Millender, Lewis H., and Sledge, Clement (Eds.): "Symposium on Rheumatoid Arthritis." Orthop. Clin. North Am., Vol. 6, No. 3 (July 1975).
O'Dell, Ardis J.: "Hot Packs for Morning Joint Stiffness." Am. J. Nurs., Vol. 75, No. 6 (June 1975), pp. 986–987.
Pigg, Janice: "50 Helpful Hints for Active Arthritis Patients." Nurs '74, Vol. 4, No. 7 (July 1974), pp. 39–41.
Pitorak, Elizabeth Ford: "Rheumatoid Arthritis: Living With It More Comfortably." Nurs. '75, Vol. 5, No. 12 (Dec. 1975), pp. 33–35.
Rhodes, Mitchell L., and Smith, Jan D.: "The Lung in Autoimmune Collagen Vascular Disease (A-CVD)." Heart Lung, Vol. 6, No. 4 (July-Aug. 1977), pp. 653–659.
Roe, Robert L.: "The Anti-Inflammatory Agents Used in Rheumatic Disorders." Primary Care, Vol. 2, No. 2 (June 1975), pp. 259–273.
Schaller, Jane G.: "Diagnosis and Treatment of Arthritis in Children." Med. Times/Contents, Vol. 105, No. 11 (Nov. 1977), pp. 65–74.

Sculco, Cynthia D., and Sculco, Thomas P.: "Management of the Patient with an Infected Total Hip Arthroplasty." J. Nurs., Vol. 76, No. 4 (Apr. 1978), pp. 584–587.

Shearn, Martin (Ed.): "Symposium on Rheumatic Diseases." Med. Clin. North Am., Vol. 61, No. 2 (March 1977).

Simmons, E. H., and Brown, M. E.: "Surgery for Kyphosis in Ankylosing Spondylitis." Can. Nurse, Vol. 68, No. 5 (May 1972), pp. 24–29.

Resource Organizations

The Arthritis Foundation, 1212 Avenue of the Americas, New York, N.Y.

The Arthritis Society, 920 Yonge St., Toronto, Ontario, Canada M4W3J7

26
Nursing in Skin Disorders and Burns

STRUCTURE AND FUNCTIONS OF THE SKIN

The skin (integument) is composed of two layers — a thin, avascular, epithelial layer called the epidermis, and a supporting layer of connective tissue on which the epidermis rests, called the dermis, or corium (Fig. 26–1). The *epidermis* has several layers of cells which differ in shape and composition from layer to layer. The cells are produced in the basal (germinating) layer and then gradually move through the other layers to the surface. As they ascend, they progressively undergo degenerative changes. The nuclei disintegrate, the cell substance changes to a water-repellent, waxy, protein-like substance called *keratin,* and the cells become flat. They are continuously reproduced in the basal layer and cast off from the surface. It is thought that normally they reach the surface in approximately 27 to 30 days. The cells that are shed disintegrate, leaving their keratin on the surface; this keratin helps to protect the skin. The germinating layer is supported by the diffusion of nutrients from capillaries in the dermis.

The thickness of the epidermis varies in different areas of the body, being thickest on the soles of the feet and palms of the hands and thinnest on the lips and eyelids. It is thinner than the dermis.

The *dermis,* consisting of fibrous and elastic connective tissue, contains many blood vessels, lymphatics, nerves and their end-organs, sebaceous and sweat glands, ducts and hair follicles. The undersurface merges with the loose, *fatty subcutaneous tissue.*

Lying between the epidermal, germinating layer and the dermis are the melanocytes, which produce the pigment melanin and deliver it to the epidermal cells. The amount of pigment is mainly determined by the person's genetic inheritance. The activity of the pigment-producing cells may also be influenced by the melanin-stimulating hormone (MSH), which is released by the pituitary gland, and by exposure to sunlight and friction.

The *sebaceous glands* secrete an oily substance (sebum) which reaches the skin surface via the hair follicles. The secretion prevents drying of the hair and skin and helps to keep the skin soft and pliable. Blackheads (comedones; sing.: comedo) are discolored accumulations of sebum in hair

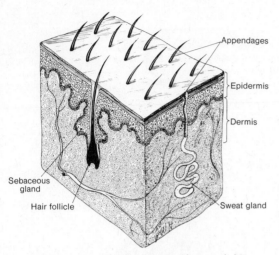

FIGURE 26–1 Section showing layers of skin.

follicles and frequently provide a medium for organisms, causing pimples or the condition *acne*. Sebaceous gland activity increases at puberty and decreases in later life due to the influence of gonadal hormones on the output of sebum. The growth of hair on certain areas of skin is also stimulated by gonadal hormones, principally the androgens.

The skin has five important functions — protection, sensation, heat regulation, absorption and storage.

The skin protects the internal structures from injury, drying and the invasion of organisms by its continuity, the water-repellent, waxy nature of the surface cells, desquamation (separation of the superficial cells), and the acid pH (4.5 to 6.5) of the secretion on the surface; this secretion has a bactericidal effect on many organisms.

The abundance of sensory receptors and nerves in the skin function in the sensations of touch, pressure, pain and temperature. These sensations serve as an important protective mechanism for the body and also convey impulses that contribute information about the external environment. For example, through touch we can appreciate shape, composition and texture.

The skin plays an important role in regulating body temperature by varying the caliber of its blood vessels and the activity of the sweat glands. These controlled mechanisms may promote the dissipation of the body heat or conserve it according to the need indicated by the heat-regulating center in the hypothalamus. For further details of temperature regulation, see Chapter 6.

The absorptive function of the skin is mainly limited to the absorption of ultraviolet rays from the sun or special lamps; it then converts sterol substances in the skin to vitamin D. A few drugs which may be included in ointments or lotions may be absorbed in small amounts.

The dermis and subcutaneous tissue may act as a storage area for water and fat. For instance, when an excess of water is retained in the body, the accumulation in these tissues becomes evident as edema. The subcutaneous tissue serves as one of the main fat depots.

With advancing years, the sebaceous and sweat glands become less active as a result of the decreased production of hormones, and the skin becomes dry. Degenerative changes occur in the elastic tissue and collagenous component of fibrous tissue, and the skin becomes wrinkled. Frequently, areas of melanocytes produce more pigment, and "brown spots" characteristic of aging skin appear.

DISORDERS OF THE SKIN

Skin disorders may be primary or may be secondary to a systemic disease or reaction. It is not the author's intention to present an all-inclusive discussion of many specific skin disorders but, rather, to offer a brief description of common manifestations, general principles of nursing care of patients with skin disorders, and a discussion of a few conditions that are encountered frequently.

For more detailed information relating to skin diseases, the reader is referred to dermatology texts; several are listed in the references at the end of this chapter.

Manifestations of Skin Disorders

LESIONS. Various changes in areas of the skin may occur, and the exact nature of these is important in diagnosis and treatment. Characteristic *primary lesions* in which the skin is usually intact include the following:

Erythema — an area in which the blood vessels become dilated, causing redness, warmth and increased firmness of the skin.

Macule — a circumscribed, smooth, flat, discolored area up to 1 cm. in size.

Papule — a small circumscribed elevated area that may or may not be discolored and is not more than 1 cm. in diameter.

Vesicle — an elevated area that contains clear fluid.

Pustule — a small elevation of the skin that contains pus.

Nodule — a solid elevation larger than a papule, usually involving both the skin and subcutaneous layers.

Wheal — a localized, elevated, edematous area that is red at the margins with a blanched center.

Bulla — an elevation larger than 1 cm. of superficial skin layers containing serous or purulent fluid.

Comedo (blackhead) — a plug of sebum and keratin within a hair follicle.

Telangiectasia — a lesion composed of a group of small blood vessels that are abnormally dilated.

Secondary lesions are those that develop as a result of a break in the skin and destruction of cells. These include:

Crust — a rough, dry area formed by the coagulation and drying of plasma and exudate over a primary lesion.

Scales — thin, flat, minute plates of dried epidermal cells which have not completely undergone the normal keratinization process before being separated. Desquamation is the term which refers to the separation of scales or patches of cells.

Fissure — a split or crack in the surface, extending through the epidermal layers and possibly into the dermis. If it extends into the dermis, bleeding occurs. This type of lesion is most likely to occur in a natural skin or surface crease such as those located over knuckles, at the angles of the mouth, in the groins, between the buttocks and behind the ears.

Excoriation — an abrasion in which the epidermis is removed.

Ulcer — a denuded area of irregular size and shape extending into the dermis due to necrosis of superficial tissue.

Lichenification — the thickening and hardening of skin as a result of continued irritation.

Leukoplakia — a white plaque which is seen most commonly in the mucous membrane of the oral cavity or tongue but may occur on the lips and, rarely, on other atrophied skin areas.

Cicatrix (scar) — an area of fibrous tissue replacing tissue destroyed by trauma or disease.

Keloid — an irregularly shaped, elevated scar resulting from excessive formation of collagen during the healing process.

Hyperkeratotic plaque (corn, callus) —an excessive thickness of the epidermis caused by chronic pressure and/or friction. In the case of a corn, the hyperkeratosis is sharply circumscribed.

PRURITUS. Generalized or localized itching is a common complaint in skin disorders. The sensory nerve endings or end-organs are irritated, giving rise to the desire to scratch. The patient is hard-pressed to refrain from scratching which further irritates the area and is frequently responsible for fissures, abrasions and subsequent secondary infection. Itching does not occur if the skin has been removed, as in a severe burn.

PAIN. The pain associated with skin lesions may be described as prickly or burning. It may be caused by chemical, mechanical or pressure irritation of the cutaneous sensory nerves, actual cellular damage or exposure of the nerve endings due to tissue destruction and erosion.

REDNESS. Erythema or redness of the skin indicates vasodilation and hyperemia in the area. Erythematous lesions are initially macular but frequently become papular because of the edema or developing exudate in the affected tissues.

SWELLING. A puffy swollen area of the skin is usually due to localized edema, resulting from increased permeability of the capillaries, or to localized inflammatory reaction.

SYSTEMIC DISTURBANCES. The skin reflects the individual's general physical and emotional status. Skin lesions are frequently manifestations of a systemic disorder (e.g., measles, systemic lupus erythematosus) or a systemic or emotional disturbance may be secondary to primary skin lesions. An elevated temperature is likely to be present if the skin disorder involves infection.

Assessing the Patient with a Skin Disorder

A skin disorder cannot be examined "in isolation"; information about the patient's total health can reveal very significant diagnostic factors and influence the therapeutic plan. The social and occupational history as well as the health history are significant.

In taking the patient's history, particular attention is given to eliciting information about:

1. Any previous skin disorders, their nature, the patient's age and the season of the year at which they occurred and the treatment.
2. Any known allergy or drug reactions.
3. Drugs that are being taken, and for what reason.
4. Known food(s), fluid(s) or contact substances (e.g., soap, certain material) that worsen the condition.
5. Substances that are brought in contact with the skin throughout daily activities (e.g., cosmetics, chemicals at work).
6. Dietary habits.
7. Recreational customs or hobbies.
8. Family history, especially in relation to skin disorders, allergy and systemic disease; for example, a history of asthma may lead the physician to suspect that heredity may have a role in the patient's disorder.

In questioning the patient about the present skin condition, it is necessary to determine:

9. When it was first observed.
10. Whether the lesion(s) persist or come and go, or change in appearance.
11. The extent to which it has spread.
12. Whether it itches or pains.
13. Whether the lesions are dry, moist or discharging.

The history-taking is followed by an examination of the skin. This involves inspection and palpation. A good light is essential and the skin must be clean; if cleansing is necessary it must be done gently to avoid injury and change in skin color. Vigorous rubbing could cause temporary erythema.

The lesions are inspected and palpated; the nature of the lesion (e.g., macule, papule, ulcer, etc.) is established and its characteristics recorded according to size, shape, color and whether it has a dry or wet surface. The entire skin surface of the body is examined to determine the general condition of the total skin in addition to the distribution of the affected areas. The latter is of assistance in diagnosis since certain disorders are known to develop more frequently in certain areas. For example, acne, impetigo, contact dermatitis, herpes simplex and discoid lupus erythematosus develop most commonly on the face. The oral mucosa is usually included in an examination of the entire skin.

If the lesions are moist or discharging, a swab of the exudate may be obtained for culture. If the affected areas are dry or scaly, scrapings may be taken for examination and/or culture. It should also be noted if an odor is associated with the affected areas. Other laboratory tests may be done, such as leukocyte and thrombocyte counts, examination for the lupus erythematosus (LE) cell, and erythrocyte sedimentation rate determination. A biopsy of a lesion may be done if malignancy is suspected. If the condition is dermatitis, patch, intracutaneous or scratch tests may be done during a remission to identify the allergen or substance to which the person is sensitive. The substances are administered intracutaneously or applied to the back by the physician and observed at intervals over 48 hours. If positive, the reaction is manifested by inflammation and papules or vesicles.

Although the skin lesions prompted the patient to seek medical assistance, the disorder may have internal or systemic components. This may necessitate other investigative procedures, such as urinalysis, x-rays, pulmonary function tests or further blood work.

General Principles in Nursing Patients with Skin Disorders

The nursing care varies greatly with these patients. The extent of the skin involvement as well as the nature of the condition determines whether or not the patient continues activities, is ambulatory and is treated at home. The patient's reaction to the disease also influences the plan of care and progress. The following are general considerations which will require adaptation and modification according to the individual; this, of course, is true of all nursing.

PSYCHOLOGICAL SUPPORT. The patient with skin lesions is likely to be quite sensitive and become emotionally disturbed over the condition. Many are self-conscious about their appearance, worry constantly and tend to withdraw, believing that a skin disease carries a stigma. The disease may be such that it persists over a long period, interfering with the patient's ability to work or go out socially. The understanding nurse guards against showing any reluctance to care for the patient and any expression of displeasure or revulsion because of his appearance. The patient is advised that the disorder is not contagious, and there should be no hesitation on the part of the nurse to touch the affected parts when giving care. An effort is made to convey to the patient an appreciation of his feelings, to have him aware that he is accepted and to provide the necessary support and care which will help to reduce the patient's anxiety.

LOCAL CARE

CLEANSING. A specific directive is received from the physician regarding the cleansing of the skin or affected areas(s). In some instances the application of soap and water may be contraindicated, and an alternative method of cleansing is necessary. For example, it may be necessary to cleanse the skin with a vegetable oil. If soap is permitted, it should be mildly alkaline and used very sparingly. A soft washcloth is preferable, and the surface is washed lightly and gently to avoid injury and erythema. If there are open, discharging lesions, sterile absorbent may be used in place of a washcloth.

Special local or general therapeutic baths may be prescribed. These may be used to relieve itching, remove scales or crusts, or apply medications as well as for cleansing purposes. Caution is used against having the water or solution hot; a temperature higher than 35° to 38° C. (95° to 100° F.) is likely to be too hot for the sensitive areas. Also, higher temperatures are likely to promote hyperemia and itching. Various preparations may be added to the bath according to its purpose. The patient is usually encouraged to remain in the prescribed bath for 10 to 20 minutes, and an attendant remains with the patient or close by, depending on his condition and age. Assistance is provided while he gets into and out of the tub. Measures are taken to prevent the patient from slipping, since many of the preparations used (e.g., oatmeal, bran, an emollient such as Alpha-Keri) make the surface of the tub especially slippery.

MOIST COMPRESSES. Wet dressings may be applied over lesions, especially if they are open and discharging. The compresses are generally left uncovered and dry out very quickly, necessitating frequent changing. The prescribed solution is usually used at room temperature. Wet dressings are not usually applied to dry or scaly lesions; an ointment or creamy lotion is more appropriate.

TOPICAL APPLICATIONS. Many different drug preparations are used in treating skin diseases. Topical applications may be in powder, lotion, oil, cream, paste or ointment form. They may be classified according to their effect.

Antipruritic preparations are applied to relieve itching. Examples are calamine lotion and corticosteroid cream or ointment.

Keratolytic agents soften and remove scales and the horny layer. An example is salicylic acid ointment.

Antieczematous agents are applied to relieve itching and remove the vesicular drainage. Examples are corticosteroid lotion or spray and coal tar solution.

Keratoplastic preparations stimulate the epidermis, increasing its thickness. An example is a weak salicylic (1 to 2 per cent) acid ointment.

Antimicrobial agents destroy or inhibit the reproduction of bacteria and fungi. Examples are antibiotic ointments such as neomycin (Neosporin) and gentamicin (Garamycin).

Zinc undecylenate (Desenex) is a common *antifungal* agent.

Antiparasitic preparations destroy or inhibit parasites. Examples are benzyl benzoate lotion (Acabiol) and gamma benzene hexachloride (Kwell).

Emollients are used to soften the skin. Examples commonly used are lanolin, petroleum jelly and Nivea oil.

Frequently, topical preparations are a combination of two or more agents which have been selected for their specific effect.

OBSERVATION. Following each cleansing and before each local therapeutic application, the lesions are examined carefully. Any increase or spread, or change in size, color or appearance is noted and reported. The nurse is constantly alert for factors in the patient's environment (e.g., contacts, diet, drugs) with which exacerbations of the condition may be associated. The patient's reaction to the disease and progress are noted.

PHYSICAL AGENTS. Ultraviolet rays may be prescribed in the treatment of psoriasis, acne and seborrheic dermatitis. Irradiation is used if the lesion is malignant. Electrosurgery or cautery may be employed in the removal of warts, leukoplakia and seborrheic or senile keratoses (areas of horny thickening of epidermis).

SYSTEMIC THERAPY. If the skin disorder is secondary to a systemic disease, treatment is directed principally toward curing the primary condition.

SYSTEMIC DRUGS. The treatment of primary skin disorders may include the administration of systemic drugs. The drug will depend upon the nature of the disorder and the patient's general health and response to his condition. An oral corticosteroid (e.g., prednisone) is frequently prescribed in dermatitis, urticaria and pemphigus. If the skin lesions are infected, an antibiotic (e.g., tetracycline) may be ordered to be given orally. An antihistamine such as chlorpheniramine maleate (Chlor-Tripolon, Novo-Pheniran) may be used in urticaria. Vitamins may be given to improve the patient's appetite, general condition and resistance.

Concern about the condition and fear of disfigurement and rejection as well as itching may result in a considerable loss of sleep for the patient. A sedative may be necessary to provide rest which plays an important part in the patient's recovery.

NUTRITION. Attention is paid to the patient's nutritional status and to whether he is taking sufficient food. Frequently severe anorexia is a problem with the dermatological patient because of the skin irritation he experiences as well as the emotional disturbance. Dressings, ointments, lotions or similar applications on the hands may preclude his feeding himself.

INSTRUCTION. In the clinic or during preparation for discharge from the hospital, the patient and a family member are advised of the day-to-day care required and precautionary measures applicable to the prevention of an exacerbation of the skin disorder. Verbal and written directions are given about the local applications and taking of medicinal preparations. For example, adrenocorticosteroid preparations in the form of an ointment or cream are used topically to suppress inflammation and reduce sensitivity of the tissues. The patient must be cautioned to apply the corticoid preparation sparingly. If compresses or therapeutic baths are to be continued, specific details of the preparation, temperature and application are outlined and demonstrated if necessary. In the case of contact dermatitis, the patient may not be able to return to his former occupation. A referral to the social service may be helpful in finding a suitable job.

Pruritus (Itching)

Pruritus is the sensation that arouses a desire to scratch. It is a symptom of many common skin disorders and may be generalized or localized. It may be associated with an internal disorder or excessive dryness as occurs with overbathing, dry atmosphere due to warm environs in winter and the aging process. Physiologically, it is considered to be a modified form of pain; the impulses are carried on slow-transmitting sensory nerve fibers.

Pruritus is extremely irritating and difficult to tolerate. Local treatment varies with the cause and specific lesions if present, and also depends on whether the skin is dry or moist. Measures that may contribute to the relief of pruritus include:

1. The application of lotions, ointments, or creams which contain an antipruritic drug (e.g., calamine, corticosteroid).
2. The application of moist drying agents (wet compresses) or powders if the skin is moist.
3. A *lukewarm* bath (15 minutes, two or three times daily) if the pruritus is generalized. After bathing excessive rubbing to dry the skin is avoided; the moisture is simply blotted gently with a towel.
4. The suggestion that fewer baths be taken. For elderly persons, and if the

skin is dry, a bath only once or twice weekly is recommended. Excessively hot water should be avoided.

5. The avoidance of soaps and detergents.
6. A simple, adequate diet without rich and spicy foods.

The patient is advised to refrain from scratching because of the danger of infection as well as the damage to the skin. The fingernails are kept short and clean. A systemic antipruritic drug may be prescribed (e.g., an antihistamine preparation, such as chlorpheniramine maleate) and, if the patient is very distressed and agitated, a sedative may be necessary.

Urticaria

Urticaria is a skin disorder which is characterized by itching wheals of varying size which may develop very rapidly and become widespread. The lesions are a reaction to an external agent or to an irritating substance reaching the skin via the blood stream. The reaction consists of dilatation and increased permeability of the capillaries and arteriolar dilatation. The combination of these is referred to as the triple response. The patient may experience general malaise and fever, especially if the urticaria is over an extensive area. The lesions usually disappear in a few hours when the blood vessels return to normal. The condition is commonly referred to as *hives*.

CAUSES. Urticaria may be a manifestation of an allergic reaction to a food, drug, vaccine or serum, or it may be caused by insect bites, contact with certain plants or chemicals or prolonged exposure to heat, cold, physical pressure or sunlight. It may also be associated with a systemic infection or internal disorder such as hepatitis.

TREATMENT. Urticaria is treated by the administration of an antihistamine preparation or, if it is widespread and causing considerable irritation, epinephrine (Adrenalin) 1:1000 may be ordered subcutaneously and usually provides immediate relief. The application of calamine lotion or a cream of calamine, diphenhydramine and camphor (Caladryl) may be useful in reducing the itching and local response. Unless the cause is definitely known, an investigation is made to identify the offending substance.

Intracutaneous, patch or scratch sensitivity tests may be done (see p. 958).

A severe and possibly life-threatening form of this disorder is known as *angioneurotic edema* or *giant hives*. Very large wheals develop rapidly on the skin and mucous membranes. The commonest cause is a severe allergic reaction to a drug, food or insect bite. The patient is observed closely for respiratory distress due to laryngeal obstruction. Prompt action is necessary. A corticosteroid preparation such as hydrocortisone (Sulu-Cortef) is given intravenously; this usually reverses the reaction.

Acne Vulgaris

This is a disorder of the sebaceous glands in which there is an increase in the secretion of sebum. The accumulation becomes lodged in the follicle, forming a comedo (blackhead) which becomes infected. The lesions, which appear commonly on the face, progressively form comedones, papules and pustules or cysts.

The incidence is greatest in adolescents after puberty. The increased sebaceous gland activity is associated with the increased production of sex hormones.

Treatment is directed toward preventing obstruction of the follicles by which the sebum escapes onto the skin surface and avoiding those factors, such as certain foods, which aggravate the condition; these foods include fatty foods, chocolate, and pork. Thorough washing of the face three or four times daily with soap and warm water is recommended. The hair should be shampooed twice weekly. The comedones should be removed with a comedo expressor and young persons should be discouraged from squeezing the lesions and using unprescribed medicated preparations.

Contact Dermatitis

Contact dermatitis is a very common inflammatory disease of the skin and, according to the cause, may be referred to as *primary-irritant dermatitis* or *allergic contact dermatitis*.

CAUSES. The former type is caused by contact of the skin with a substance (primary irritant) that results in inflammation upon initial contact. Examples of primary irritants are strong soaps and some acids or alkalies. Allergic contact dermatitis is the result of an inflammatory reaction to a substance by a hypersensitive or allergic skin. The causative agent does not irritate the skin of a nonallergic or nonsensitized person. The person may not develop dermatitis with the first several contacts but repeated skin exposures sensitize him. The number of contacts with the substance before sensitization occurs varies with individuals. Examples of allergens which cause contact dermatitis are poison ivy, cosmetics, hair dye, soaps, and certain types of clothing material and dyes, plastic and insecticides. Dyes, flour, mineral dust, metal and industrial chemicals are examples of sensitizers.

Any causative agent can affect any area of the body but, because certain substances are commonly in contact with only certain areas, they become suspect. For example, lesions on the head, neck and face may be caused by cosmetics, soap, hair dye, or nickel (earrings). If the lesions are confined to the trunk, soaps, dusting powder and clothing may be suspect. Knowledge of the distribution of the dermatitis caused by different agents facilitates identification of the cause.

MANIFESTATIONS. The lesions in contact dermatitis usually progress through various forms, beginning with an erythematous area on which small papules develop and rapidly progress to vesicles. The vesicles may rupture and discharge their contents. Those vesicles which do not rupture dry and form crusts or scales. The affected areas may become denuded, leaving a red glazed surface which probably oozes a serous discharge, giving rise to what is referred to as *"weeping eczema."* As the denuded areas are recovered by regenerated epidermis, more lesions may develop so that various stages (papular, vesicular, scaly, weeping, healing) exist at one time unless the reaction is corrected in the early stages. The patient experiences itching and burning, and scratching may result in infected lesions. The affected areas may remain localized to certain parts of the body or become disseminated.

TREATMENT. Local applications such as wet compresses, lotions, creams and ointments are used to reduce the itching and tissue response and provide protection. If lesions are extensive, involving large areas of the body, therapeutic baths are used. An antibiotic ointment may be prescribed if there is infection.

A systemic drug may also be ordered for the relief of itching (e.g., diphenhydramine), and an adrenocorticosteroid (e.g., prednisone) may be administered to reduce the tissue response and inflammation. The patient is advised of the importance of avoiding scratching and the fingernails are kept short and clean. The application of arm splints or mittens may be necessary to control scratching in children.

The patient undergoes an investigation to determine the precipitating factor or allergen when the episode is controlled (see p. 958). When the causative agent is identified, contact must be avoided. It should be remembered that dermatitis may be aggravated by emotional disturbances. Kind, sincere attention by the nurse may reduce the patient's tension or lead to discussions that reveal his concerns and disturbances.

Dermatitis is sometimes classified as drug dermatitis, because of the obvious cause; exfoliative dermatitis, characterized by extensive scaling and thickening of the skin; infantile dermatitis, or eczema; or infective dermatitis because infection has been superimposed.

Psoriasis

Psoriasis is a relatively common, chronic inflammatory skin disorder characterized by remissions and exacerbations and dry, scaly lesions. The lesions develop initially as dull, red papules on which silvery white, waxy scales accumulate in layers due to rapid, uncontrolled cell proliferation of the epidermis. Normally, the epidermis is replaced in 28 days; in psoriasis, it is reproduced in 4 days.[1] The lesions gradually increase in size, and several may coalesce, forming large, prominent, scaly plaques. Removal of the scale produces small, pinpoint bleeding areas.

The patient may or may not experience itching. Any skin area, including the nails, may be involved, but common sites are the

[1]Carolyn North and Gerald D. Weinstein: "Treatment of Psoriasis." Am. J. Nurs., Vol. 76, No. 3 (March 1976), p. 410.

extensor surfaces of the arms and legs (especially pressure areas such as the knees and elbows), the scalp, and the lumbar and sacral regions. The amount of involvement varies from one attack to another, and chronic patch areas vary in individuals; that is, it may always appear first on the fronts of the knees, on the elbows or on the back. If the nails become affected, they usually manifest pitting, discoloration and separation from the underlying tissue, which tends to become thick, dry and hard (keratosis).

The onset may be gradual or sudden. The lesions may persist for weeks or months and then may disappear spontaneously.

ETIOLOGY. The cause of psoriasis is not known, but there is general agreement that heredity plays a role. Males and females are equally affected, and the incidence is much higher in temperate climates. The onset of the disease may be at any age but most commonly begins in adolescence. Psoriasis is occasionally seen in persons with rheumatoid arthritis. Exacerbations are more prevalent in winter months. Patients who move from a cold, wintery climate to a warm, sunny climate have found that their psoriasis usually clears spontaneously and quickly. Many persons with the disease indicate knowing of someone in their family who is or was affected. The disorder is frequently precipitated by trauma, infections and psychological stress.

TREATMENT. The treatment consists principally of local applications, baths and exposure to ultraviolet rays. One preparation may prove effective for one patient and not for another. The treatment is individualized —this must be impressed on the patient. Various preparations in the form of ointments, creams or pastes are used and include anthralin, derivatives of coal tar and adrenocorticosteroids.

The patient has a daily therapeutic bath, remaining in it for 20 to 30 minutes to soften and promote separation of the scales. The lesions may be scrubbed, gently using a soft brush or rough terry cloth. If the scalp is affected, daily shampooing is also necessary. Following the bath, the patient is exposed to ultraviolet light. Colored glasses are worn during the ultraviolet ray therapy. The period of exposure is very brief at first (1 minute) and then is increased very gradually. An application of the prescribed ointment or cream is applied. A coal tar preparation is generally used for the patient receiving ultraviolet therapy; it is considered to increase the effectiveness of the ultraviolet rays.

Anthralin paste is used less often than coal tar and corticosteroid preparations and only for severe psoriasis. It is an irritant, and precautions are taken to avoid getting it on unaffected skin. A protective substance such as petroleum jelly is applied around the lesions. The affected areas to which the anthralin is applied are left uncovered.

Methotrexate given orally may be used rarely for severe psoriasis that is not improving with local treatment. It is a chemotherapeutic antimetabolite (a folic acid antagonist) and has proved effective with some patients.

A more recent plan of care involves the oral administration of methoxsalen tablets 2 hours before exposure to a high intensity ultraviolet light of a long wavelength (UVA). The treatment is given 3 or 4 days weekly over a 1-month period on an outpatient basis.

The psychological impact of psoriasis for the patient and family is very great. Although it is noninfectious and not contagious, the appearance of the lesions frequently results in associates and even family members avoiding the person, especially personal skin contact. The patient experiences rejection and isolation, withdraws, and may seek undesirable emotional outlets and undergo personality changes. The nurse uses every opportunity available to provide support, especially understanding and willingness to help foster acceptance and encourage the person to face his problems. A full explanation of the disorder is made to the family (and employer, if necessary). Suggestions are made as to how they may help the person with his problems.

Scabies

Scabies is a contagious parasitic infestation caused by *Acarus scabiei* (itch mite). The disease is associated with overcrowding and uncleanliness; it is transmitted by personal contact or occasionally by contact with the clothing or bedding of an infected person.

The parasite burrows under the skin and lays eggs which hatch in 3 to 4 days. On the skin surface grayish-white, slightly elevated, zigzag lines appear and the patient experiences severe itching which is worse at night, resulting in loss of rest and sleep. Secondary lesions in the form of vesicles, papules, pustules and encrustations develop. Common infestation sites are the flexor surfaces of the wrist, palms, between the fingers and toes, groins and the areolae of the breasts.

TREATMENT. The patient takes a hot bath, vigorously scrubbing the affected areas to open the infested burrows. Following the bath, a benzyl benzoate preparation (Benzoped) or gamma benzene hexachloride (Kwell) is applied over the entire skin surface. All clothing and bed linen are changed following each bath. Linen and clothing are washed in boiling water or pressed with a very hot iron. All close contacts of the patient are also treated.

Tinea (Ringworm)

Ringworm is a contagious, fungal infection of the skin which may develop on any part of the body. Common forms are designated according to the location; for example, ringworm of the feet (athlete's foot), ringworm of the scalp (tinea capitis), ringworm of the nails (tinea unguium), and ringworm of the body (tinea corporis).

The lesions vary with the area of the body infected. For example, ringworm of the scalp is manifested by round, gray scaly patches. In athlete's foot, the primary lesions appear on the soles and between the toes in the form of itching, burning vesicles which lead to secondary moist lesions and then to scaly areas. The lesions in tinea corporis may have an advancing peripheral ring of vesicles and a pustular or scaly center. The area heals from the center. The diagnosis of tinea is made by the microscopic examination of scrapings from the lesions. The specimen is placed in 10 per cent potassium hydroxide.

The drug commonly used in the treatment of tinea is griseofulvin, an antibiotic, and is administered orally. Toxic reactions include headache, dizziness, drowsiness, urticaria and gastrointestinal distress. It is least effective with ringworm of the hands and athlete's foot.

Cancer of the Skin

Carcinoma of the skin has a high incidence and occurs more often in males. The prognosis in skin cancer is usually more favorable than when the disease is located in other tissues and organs. Malignant skin lesions are readily discovered, which results in early treatment, and they generally progress quite slowly.

The symptom that most frequently prompts the patient to seek medical advice is a discolored lesion which persists and progressively increases in size or an open sore (ulcer) which does not heal and progressively becomes deeper. The nurse should be alert for lesions that frequently precede malignant changes. Most significant of these are soft black moles that tend to increase in size, leukoplakia (white patches) and a sore which does not heal.

Epithelioma is the type of skin cancer most commonly seen. The primary nodular lesion most often develops on the face, slowly enlarges and ulcerates, and is referred to as a *rodent ulcer*. The lesion may be treated by excision and/or radiation. The neoplastic cells rarely metastasize, and the disease remains controlled.

Squamous cell carcinoma develops in the skin occasionally and is more serious than the epithelioma type because it tends to invade surrounding tissues and metastasize more readily. The primary lesion ulcerates and enlarges. The common sites are similar to those of epitheliomas — namely, the face, lips, nose, forehead and arms. The treatment is also similar, and the patient is followed closely for possible metastases.

Malignant melanoma arises from a pigmented nevus or preexisting mole and is a rapidly spreading cancer that readily metastasizes and presents a grave prognosis. Wide excision of the primary lesion is done, and the regional lymph nodes may also be removed. The surgery may be followed by radiation therapy if involvement of the lymph nodes is suspected.

NURSING THE BURNED PATIENT

Burns continue to be a major cause of suffering, disfigurement, disability and death, and a large proportion of those that occur are due to carelessness and could be prevented. More emphasis on safety measures, especially in the home, seems necessary. Through increased public education by the use of such aids as mass media and printed pamphlets, we have been able to alert the public to the danger signals of cancer and the importance of early treatment. A comparable program relating to burn statistics, causes of fire and safety measures might produce greater caution in the home and elsewhere.

Causes of Burns

A burn may be inflicted by dry or moist heat, irradiation, electrical current or chemicals. The burn that is caused by dry or moist heat may be referred to as a thermal burn and is the type of greatest incidence. The discussion that follows pertains to the burn incurred by heat.

Classification and Assessment of Burns

Burns may be classified according to cause (thermal, electrical, chemical or irra-

diation), the extent of the body surface burned, and the depth of tissue damaged or destroyed. The assessment of the severity of a burn is made principally on the last two factors. The seriousness is also influenced by the patient's age, health at the time of the accident and whether or not any other injury was incurred at the same time.

The most accurate estimation of the percentage of body surface burned may be based on the Lund and Browder chart (see Fig. 26–2). The chart assigns a certain percentage to various parts of the body and includes a table indicating the adjustments necessary for different ages, since the head and trunk represent relatively larger proportions of body surface in the early stages of development. Copies of these charts may be kept available in the emergency department or intensive care unit so that the burned areas can be mapped out when the patient is examined and the percentage estimated.

If the Lund and Browder chart is not available, a quick approximate estimate of the percentage of body surface burned may

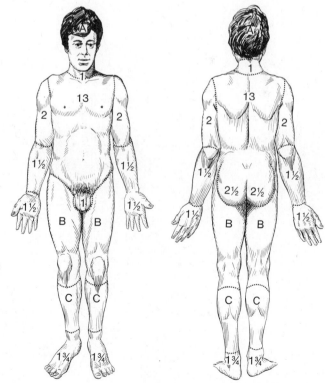

FIGURE 26–2 The Lund and Browder burn chart.

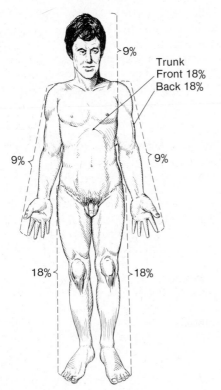

9%

Trunk
Front 18%
Back 18%

9%

9%

18%

18%

FIGURE 26–3 Rule of Nines; used for estimating the percentage of body surface burned.

be made on the Rule of Nines (see Fig. 26–3). The body is divided into areas, each of which represents 9 per cent. The apportionment is as follows: an arm is 9 per cent, a thigh 9 per cent, a leg (below the knee) 9 per cent, the anterior chest 9 per cent, the posterior chest 9 per cent, the abdomen 9 per cent, the lower half of the back (lumbar and sacral regions) 9 per cent, the head and neck 9 per cent, and the perineum 1 per cent. It should be remembered that in infants and children the head represents a relatively large percentage, but the extremities compose a smaller portion of the body surface.

If approximately *10 per cent or more of the body surface of a child or 15 per cent or more of that of an adult is burned, the injury is considered to be a major burn.* The patient requires hospitalization and fluid replacement.

The depth of tissue damage and destruction in a burn is indicated by the classification as first, second, or third degree, or as full-thickness or partial-thickness burns (Fig. 26–4). A *first-degree burn* is characterized by erythema with destruction of only superficial layers of the epidermis. It may be quite painful for a short time but

FIGURE 26–4 Classification of burns according to depth.

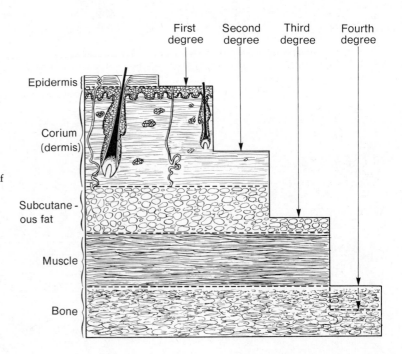

First degree

Second degree

Third degree

Fourth degree

Epidermis

Corium (dermis)

Subcutaneous fat

Muscle

Bone

heals quickly without residual evidence of tissue injury. Systemic effects may accompany a first-degree burn if a large percentage of the body surface is involved. First-degree burns are considered minor unless more than 10 per cent of the body surface of an infant, young child, or elderly person is involved.

Second-degree burns involve the destruction of several layers of the skin, but sufficient viable dermal tissue remains to promote regeneration of the cells to replace those burned. This type of burn is very painful. Separation of epidermal layers occurs by the collection of fluid in the tissues, forming blisters which are characteristic of second-degree burns.

The term *partial-thickness* may also be used to describe the depth of tissue and severity of damage. It indicates a combination of both first- and second-degree burns.

A *third-degree burn* or a *full-thickness* burn is characterized by the destruction of the full thickness of the skin and its appendages. Underlying tissues such as the subcutaneous fat, muscles, tendons and bone may also be burned. The sensitivity of the area is reduced because of the destruction of sensory nerve endings. However, the patient usually experiences pain because the burn is mixed — third-degree with second-degree burns that may be marginal to the major tissue damage. The injured area may be charred or have an opaque white appearance. Because the burn is of full-thickness depth, spontaneous regeneration and replacement of the skin is not possible. The area may be slowly filled in with granulation tissue and then fibrous scar tissue, proliferated from marginal or underlying connective tissue, or it is recovered by skin grafting.

The age of the patient is an important factor in the seriousness of a burn. The severity of the burn increases with age when the patient is over 55 to 60 years. The person of 40 withstands a burn much better than the patient of 60, even though the percentage of body surface burned and the degree are the same in both. Infants and young children also tolerate burns less well than those who are more mature.

Pathophysiological Effects of Burns

The patient who suffers a major burn manifests shock which, in some cases, may be irreversible. Immediately following the injury, the pain and fear which may be experienced by the injured person are considered to be responsible for widespread vasodilation and subsequent hypotension and impaired circulation. This phase may be referred to as *primary or neurogenic shock*. The duration varies; it may be brief or may persist to become a part of the *hypovolemic (oligemic) shock* that develops rapidly as a result of the loss of fluid from the circulating blood volume. Increased permeability and dilation of the capillaries in the burn area result in a shift of protein-rich fluid out of the vascular compartment into the interstitial spaces, causing the formation of blisters and edema. Large volumes of the fluid, which is similar in composition to plasma, may seep into the tissues. Some is carried away via the lymphatics, but an amount in excess of what can be drained into the lymphatic system accumulates. The edema is also promoted by the loss of blood proteins with the fluid and the ensuing reduction of the intravascular colloidal osmotic pressure. In a third-degree burn, the fluid loss is extensive and, in areas of greater vascularization, such as the face, the edema and swelling may be very severe.

The intravascular volume diminishes, the blood pressure falls, the cardiac output is reduced, and the blood flow through the tissues is reduced. *Hypovolemic shock* develops unless there is adequate fluid replacement. The reduction in the intravascular volume produces a corresponding hemoconcentration, evidenced by an increase in the hematocrit and hemoglobin levels (normal hematocrit: 40 to 50 per cent; normal hemoglobin: 12 to 16 Gm. per cent). The greater concentration of cellular elements in the blood increases the demand on the heart and predisposes to thrombosis and circulatory insufficiency.

An actual decrease in the number of red blood cells occurs especially in deep burns, due to trapping and heat injury of those in the skin capillaries at the time of the injury. Normal red blood cell production may also be reduced because of depression of the bone marrow.

Inhalation of smoke and chemical fumes can seriously impair ventilatory function; irritation of the mucosa may cause laryngeal edema and airway obstruction or pulmonary edema and severe respiratory insufficiency.

The urinary output is decreased as a result of the decreased intravascular volume and subsequent hypotension. If considerable muscle cell destruction occurs, the subsequent release of free hemoglobin and myoglobin into the blood is reflected in the appearance of brownish-black urine. The filtration of these globins may result in plugging of the renal tubules, with ensuing renal failure. If the blood supply is markedly reduced in the shock phase, renal tubular damage may also result. Diuresis and increased sodium excretion occur in 3 to 5 days and are favorable signs.

In severe burns gastrointestinal peristalsis is depressed; nausea, vomiting and abdominal distention may occur.

Toxemia may develop in 3 to 5 days, especially with a large surface area burn. This is attributed to absorption of the decomposition products of dead tissue.

Electrolyte imbalances develop because of the burn edema, loss of fluid through the open wound, impaired renal function in the associated shock, and excessive release of potassium by the damaged tissue cells and erythrocytes. The disturbances are also influenced by the adrenocortical response (increased secretions) to the stress which results in sodium retention and increased potassium excretion by the kidneys if they are functioning satisfactorily. The adrenocortical hyperactivity also accelerates protein catabolism, resulting in a negative nitrogen balance.

The effects of the heat at the site of the burn depend on the intensity of the heat. The layer of burned tissues may form a dry, charred, coagulated surface, called an *eschar*, or a soft, moist noncoagulated area. Inflammation and edema develop at the wound margins and below the layers of dead tissue. Many small blood vessels below the devitalized tissue may be thrombosed, promoting further cellular destruction. The decomposition of dead tissue and sloughing produce a favorable culture medium for organisms and the development of serious infection. Most major burns are mixed in depth; some areas will have partial-thickness skin loss while other areas suffer full-thickness destruction.

Treatment and Nursing Care

Treatment and care are directed toward the following: (1) the prevention of shock, or its reversal should it occur; (2) the prevention of wound contamination and the treatment of infection; (3) the alleviation of pain; (4) the prevention of contractures and deformities; and (5) maximum rehabilitation of the patient.

Care of the patient who is severely burned can be divided into that necessary throughout the initial *emergent period,* the *acute phase* and the *rehabilitation period*.

Care during the emergent period includes first aid at the site of the injury and the initial medical and nursing care. This initial care is directed toward establishing and maintaining an airway if necessary, reversing hypovolemic shock and cleansing and assessing the severity of the burned areas. The emergent period may last for 2 to 7 days and the patient requires constant nursing care throughout this period.

The acute phase of burn care involves wound care to promote healing and recovery of skin, physical and psychological support, the prevention of complications and the treatment of complications, if they occur.

The rehabilitation period is the phase of regaining function and resuming a normal active and useful pattern of life.

FIRST AID. The initial move in the case of burning due to flames is to smother the fire if possible or remove the victim from exposure to it. If his clothes are on fire, he should remain stationary because movement fans the flames, and lie down on the floor or ground. This position may prevent the igniting of his hair and the inhalation of flames, with subsequent respiratory damage. He is quickly rolled in a rug, blanket or something comparable to smother the flames or is doused freely with water. If nothing is quickly available, the flames may be extinguished if he rolls on the ground.

The immediate application of cold either by holding the part under cold running water, immersion, or the application of cold, moist towels or compresses is recommended as a valuable first aid measure. The cold reduces pain and may decrease the effect of the heat on the tissues.

Oils, ointments, lotions and other preparations *should not* be applied, and no attempt is made to remove clothing that is adherent. The burn area is covered with the cleanest material available to exclude air, which stimulates pain, and to reduce contamination. While awaiting transportation, the patient is kept at rest. A minimal amount of movement and handling is important, but any constricting shoes, clothing and jewelry are loosened or removed.

In the case of chemical burns, the area is washed with generous amounts of water. The patient's clothing is removed, since it is most likely holding some of the offending substances.

Most first- and second-degree burns involving approximately *less than 10 per cent* of body surface are treated at home or in the clinic. Systemic effects in such cases are minimal and are not considered sufficiently significant to require hospitalization. However, it should be remembered that there are variables; concomitant disease or injuries, if the patient is under 18 months of age or over 60 years, the patient's reactions and the availability of home care are a few factors which may influence the decision as to whether hospitalization is required.

PREPARATION TO RECEIVE THE BURNED PATIENT. If notified of the imminent admission of a severely burned patient, preparations include assembling the following equipment for prompt use:

Tray and tubes for an intubation or tracheostomy

Oxygen, and mechanical respirator

Intravenous infusion and blood transfusion sets

Colloidal and electrolyte intravenous solutions

Equipment for taking blood specimens for typing and cross matching and determination of hematocrit, hemoglobin, creatinine and electrolyte levels

Sphygmomanometer, stethoscope and a central venous pressure set

Catheterization tray with indwelling catheter (Foley catheter), sterile closed system with a urimeter for determining hourly output, tubing and drainage bag

Sterile gowns, masks and gloves for physicians and nurses

Appropriate instruments, sterile towels, burn dressings and bandages for cleansing, débridement and dressing of the burn areas.

Solutions for cleansing the area (e.g., sterile water, normal saline, mild surgical soap)

Burn applications (antimicrobial topical preparations such as Sulfamylon, gentamicin and silver sulfadiazine

Tetanus toxoid, human tetanus immuno-globulin, analgesics such as morphine and meperidine hydrochloride (Demerol), and injection equipment

Bed made with sterile sheets, cradle and extra sterile sheets

If the victim is known to have received major trunk or circumferential burns, a Stryker frame or CircOlectric bed is prepared to receive the patient following the initial assessment and treatments.

CARE ON ADMISSION. An immediate *assessment* of the patient's general condition is made by the physician before attention is directed to the burn wound. A history as to how the burn was sustained is obtained from the patient or the person who accompanied him; this may indicate the need to search for other injuries. The burn patient is usually sufficiently alert to provide information; if drowsy, confused or comatose, other disorders or injuries are suspected (e.g., hypoxia, head injury, cerebral aneurysm or stroke).

RESPIRATORY FUNCTION. Damage to the respiratory tract and respiratory insufficiency demand prompt attention. Respiratory impairment is frequently associated with burns of the face or neck and may be the result of the inhalation of smoke, a gaseous chemical or flames. To assess ventilatory function, observe respiratory efforts and listen for inspiratory wheezes, check odor of breath (a smoky or chemical odor may be detected which indicates inhalation of smoke or fumes), listen for hoarseness, and examine any sputum for blood and carbon particles. Humidified oxygen is administered, if necessary, and suctioning may be helpful to clear the airway of secretions. Intubation or a tracheostomy may be done if respiratory embarrassment increases. If there is marked insufficiency, a mechanical ventilator may be used in conjunction with the tracheostomy tube. Frequent estimations of the blood gases and expiratory or tidal volume may be done. See Chapter 15 for the care required in respiratory insufficiency and tracheostomy.

Respiratory insufficiency may develop later in circumferential or severe chest burns due to restricted respiratory excursion as a result of the firm unyielding coagulum or eschar. The physician may have to make several incisions in the eschar to relieve the thoracic restriction. Following the initial assessment and treatment, the patient is required to breathe deeply and cough hourly if intubation or a tracheostomy is not necessary.

When satisfactory ventilation is established, attention is directed toward fluid therapy and assessment of the extent and severity of the burn and any other injuries.

FLUID REPLACEMENT. The control of shock resulting from the loss of intravascular volume in a severe burn is dependent upon prompt, adequate fluid replacement. A reliable intravenous route is established by the insertion of a polyethylene cannula or catheter immediately on admission. The intravascular fluid shift commences immediately after burning but signs of shock may not appear for a few hours. Solutions that may be administered include colloidal solutions[2] such as plasma, whole blood and a plasma expander (e.g., dextran), or a solution of electrolytes (e.g., lactated Ringer's solution) and glucose 5 per cent in distilled water. The volume, composition and rate of flow of the intravenous fluids are based on the hourly urinary output, arterial blood pressure and central venous pressure, the patient's daily weight, hematocrit and hemoglobin and serum electrolyte concentrations, especially potassium and sodium. Hematocrit determinations are usually done every 4 to 6 hours.

Fluid is given orally, when tolerated, and may be restricted to the following formula: sodium chloride 4 Gm. (1 level tablespoonful) and sodium bicarbonate 1.5 Gm. (1 level teaspoonful) dissolved in 1 liter of water. The solution is chilled and may be flavored with fruit juice. Generally, after the first 24 to 36 hours, fluid extravasation into the tissues lessens and the intravascular volume tends to stabilize gradually. The intravenous fluid therapy is gradually reduced and may be discontinued when laboratory studies indicate satisfactory concentrations and the patient is able to take adequate amounts of fluid orally. He is observed closely for signs of circulatory overload, since much of the fluid in the interstitial spaces is reabsorbed into the intravascular compartment as capillary integrity is reestablished. Overloading of the circulatory system may be manifested by a urinary output greater than 100 ml. per hour within the first 48 hours, pulmonary edema, a

central venous pressure in excess of 13 cm. of water and a weak pulse. If renal function is normal, the excessive amount is controlled by diuresis. A blood transfusion may be necessary later if the hematocrit or red blood cell count indicates anemia.

INDWELLING URINARY CATHETER. An indwelling (Foley) catheter is passed as soon as the patient is admitted so that the hourly urinary output may be noted. This serves as a guide in determining intravenous fluid requirement and also provides information about the patient's general circulatory status and renal function. The urinary output should be at least 25 to 30 ml. per hour for an adult, 20 to 25 ml. per hour for a child and 10 to 20 ml. per hour for an infant. A volume below the normal minimum is reported promptly. Urine specimens are sent once or twice daily for determination of specific gravity and sugar, acetone and creatinine levels. Dark urine, indicating the presence of hemoglobin and myoglobin, is brought to the physician's attention promptly. The intravenous fluid volume is increased, and a diuretic such as mannitol or furosemide (Lasix) may be prescribed to dilute the globins and produce diuresis.

The catheter is removed as soon as the patient's condition is stable and shock is reversed, since the indwelling catheter predisposes to bladder infection and loss of bladder tone.

OBSERVATIONS. The patient is observed closely during the early postburn period for symptoms of shock. The blood pressure, pulse and level of consciousness are noted every 15 to 30 minutes and the urinary output per hour is recorded. A diminishing intravascular volume and subsequent circulatory failure may be reflected by a fall in blood pressure, weak pulse, abnormal drowsiness, disorientation and a urinary output of less than 30 ml. per hour. A long venous catheter may be passed via the cephalic vein into the vena cava so that the central venous pressure may be monitored hourly (see p. 297); this provides information about the intravascular volume and is a guide to the volume and rate of intravenous fluid administered. If it is significantly elevated, intravenous infusion is reduced (normal central venous pressure: 10 to 15 cm. of water).

Frequent hemoglobin and hematocrit determinations are made; abnormal elevations indicate hemoconcentration due to loss of intravascular fluid into the tissues. After 2 or 3

---

[2] A *colloidal solution* contains large nondiffusible particles of solutes which will not leak out of the capillaries.

days a deficiency of erythrocytes and hemoglobin may indicate the need for a blood transfusion. Serum protein and electrolyte concentrations are also determined frequently; these help in selecting the type of intravenous solutions required. An accurate record of the fluid intake (oral and intravenous) and the output is necessary. The patient is weighed daily as soon as the condition permits. A gain is manifested at first because of the increased extracellular fluid and the intravascular infusion. Then a marked weight loss accompanies the diuresis that corresponds with the recovery from shock. During this period the patient is observed closely for any sign of overhydration. Much of the fluid which escaped into the interstitial spaces is reabsorbed into the vascular compartment. If the intravenous infusion is continued at the previous rate of administration at this time the vascular system may become overloaded, placing an excessive demand on the heart and causing pulmonary edema. The reabsorption of the tissue fluid can usually be recognized by a marked increase in the urinary output.

After the emergent period the nurse is alert for an elevation of temperature, rapid pulse, leukocytosis and odor and discharge from the burned area which may indicate infection.

The patient's position, especially that of the burned parts of the body, is checked frequently during the day and night for optimum alignment. Flexion contracture may develop very quickly and preclude restoration of function.

RELIEF OF PAIN. Unless contraindicated by respiratory impairment or depression, the patient is usually given an analgesic on admission to relieve pain and reduce anxiety, since both contribute to shock. A small dose of morphine, codeine or meperidine hydrochloride (Demerol) may be given by the physician. The intravenous route is used because the circulatory disturbance, shock and edema reduce absorption of subcutaneous injections.

An analgesic may be necessary three or four times in 24 hours for 2 to 3 days to keep the patient reasonably comfortable. Some patients require the administration of the prescribed narcotic only before the burn areas are dressed. The nurse must be alert for signs of addiction; generally, the drug order is changed to a milder sedative after 3 to 4 days.

PSYCHOLOGICAL SUPPORT. Following a severe burn, the patient and family experience considerable emotional disturbance. As with any psychological concern, the reactions and adaptive mechanisms may vary markedly from one person to another, depending mainly on the particular situation and past experiences of each person. Factors which generate fear and anxiety in both the patient and family include the actual threat to life, permanent incapacity and disfigurement, the prolonged period of treatment necessitating dependence as well as separation, and the uncertain future. An understanding of the problems of the patient and family should be appreciated by the nurse in order to convey understanding support and to help the patient work through to acceptance and a more positive outlook. He may have guilt feelings about the accident, especially at first. Withdrawal, depression and resentment are commonly manifested. Long periods of the patient being alone are avoided; the visitors permitted are encouraged to visit regularly. Reading material and a radio or television usually help and, as he improves, constructive activities in which he may be interested are gradually introduced by the occupational therapist.

It is important that the patient be given honest, realistic explanations of progress and of the plans for treatment (e.g., skin grafting) and rehabilitation. It is more supportive when the patient and family can relate to one or two key persons in the therapeutic team throughout the entire course of the illness. Constant change of personnel can be very disconcerting and may undermine the patient's confidence.

WOUND CARE. Infection is a serious hazard in severe burns and is a major cause of death of burned patients. The skin, which is damaged or destroyed, is the normal protective barrier against environmental organisms as well as those commonly found on the skin, in hair follicles and in sweat and sebaceous ducts. Thrombosis and damage of local vessels and stasis of circulation in the burn area frequently prevent antibodies and systemic antimicrobial medications from reaching the wound to destroy organisms. At the same time the patient's ability to produce antibodies may be reduced.

Various forms of local treatment are used to prevent further wound contamination and tissue destruction, suppress the growth of bacteria in the area, and promote separation of the devitalized tissue and its replacement with skin. Sterile sheets are used under and over the patient, and staff members providing direct care wear sterile gowns, caps, mask and gloves. Placement of the patient receives consideration; if there is no special burn care unit the patient is placed in a single room where reverse isolation technique can be used to reduce the risk of infection. If there is a burn care ward the patient is transferred there from the emergency room for wound care, since it will have a hydrotherapy tub which facilitates cleansing.

Initially, the burn is cleansed of dirt, foreign substances and detached epithelium, using gauze and a mild soapy solution, water or normal saline. The temperature of the burn bath solution is kept at 37° to 38° C. (99° F.) to approximate body temperature. If a hydrotherapy bath is not available, the cleansing is done on the transfer carriage or in the patient's bed. Loose, sloughing skin and debris are removed with sterile forceps and the physician removes the skin from blisters. The cleansing must be *very gentle* to avoid damage of exposed viable tissue and the area is rinsed with generous amounts of water or saline. If the skin on the periphery of the burn is hairy, it is shaved during the initial cleansing and then at intervals until healing occurs. Hair tends to harbor infectious agents.

Following the cleansing, the patient is placed on a fresh sterile sheet and an estimate made of the extent and depth of the burns.

First-degree burns may be left exposed or may recieve an application of an ointment. The ointment frequently contains a local anesthetic for the relief of pain; an example is dibucaine hydrochloride ointment (Nupercain Hydrochloride). Cold, moist applications for the first few hours will also provide relief of the pain of first-degree burns.

In *second-degree burns,* opinion differs as to whether blisters are better left intact or should be opened and the overlying devitalized tissue removed. It is suggested that the dead tissue and the fluid encourage the development of infection. There is a consensus, however, that blisters on the palms of the hands, where the skin is thick and not easily ruptured, should be left intact.

The more common, current methods of local treatment of *major* and *third-degree burns* include exposure treatment, closed treatment methods and skin grafting.

EXPOSURE TREATMENT. In this method of treatment the wound (with or without topical application) is exposed to the air; no dressings are applied. The exposure results in drying and the formation of a protective coagulum of serum. A cradle is used over the patient to support a sterile sheet and blanket to reduce body heat loss. Exposure is the preferred form of treatment for facial, neck, head and perineal burns. If infection develops under the coagulum, it is removed and baths and topical antimicrobials used. This method of treatment is useful when care is necessary for a large number of casualties.

CLOSED TREATMENT. In the closed method the burned areas may be covered with a topical antimicrobial preparation and gauze. The topical applications commonly used include silver sulfadiazine, mafenide (Sulfamylon) and gentamicin sulfate (Garamycin cream). The cream or ointment is applied to sterile gauze which is then placed over the wounds and covered with gauze. The dressings are changed at least once daily and the wound cleansed, preferably in a bath. Contraindications to using the hydrotherapeutic bath include a fall below normal of the patient's blood pressure, or a sudden elevation in the blood pressure or pulse, fever of 39.4° C. (103° F.), electrolyte imbalance, extensive edema, endotracheal intubation or tracheostomy, other injuries and if skin grafting has been done.

A second closed form of treatment is the occlusive dressing, in which a single layer of petroleum jelly gauze or gauze impregnated with an antimicrobial water-soluble preparation is applied directly to the burns. In the case of a hand or foot, the digits are separated and each is completely covered with gauze to prevent any direct surface contact between them. The initial layer of gauze is then covered with a thick layer of fluffed absorbent gauze and dressing pads. The dressing is secured in place by stockinette or an elasticized bandage and left undisturbed for several days.

The purposes of this form of treatment are to protect the area from contamination, immobilize the area and provide slight compression to reduce vascular and lymphatic stasis. The dressing is applied firmly enough to eliminate dead space and prevent irritation of viable tissue by its movement but not firmly enough to interfere with the blood supply to the part.

Disadvantages of this form of wound treatment are that changes in the wound(s) are not observed and the closure and unevaporated moisture foster infection. The dressings are examined frequently by the nurse; if moisture soaks through to the outer surface or there is an odor or other signs of infection, the physician is notified.

HEALING. In a second-degree burn, healing (i.e., reepithelialization) occurs under the coagulum, which gradually separates. When a third-degree (full-thickness) burn is sustained, the nonviable tissue changes in 3 to 5 days to a hard, tough black layer called the *eschar,* providing a protective surface which organisms cannot penetrate as long as it remains dry and intact. The underlying dead tissue eventually sloughs off, liquefies and detaches the eschar from the viable tissue. There may be considerable drainage before there is complete separation. If a patient has a circumferential burn on a limb, close observations are made for signs of interference with the circulation as a result of the constricting effect of the dry, shrinking eschar. In the case of a circumferential eschar of the trunk, the constriction may restrict chest excursion and embarrass respiratory function. If signs of constriction appear, an escharotomy is done immediately under aseptic conditions.

Infection may develop under the eschar as a result of organisms that were present deep in ducts or on adjacent areas which were not destroyed at the time of the burn. As the eschar is removed by slough or débridement, granulation tissue consisting of fibroblasts and capillaries is gradually formed. If the granulation tissue is allowed to mature to fibrous scar tissue, the natural shortening of the collagenous fibers results in contracture of the area and possible deformity or loss of function, depending upon the location. Some marginal growth of epithelium may take place but, unless the burn is very small, this is usually insignificant.

The usual procedure is to apply split-thickness skin grafts to the area as soon as it is reasonably clean and some granulation tissue has formed. Frequent dressings may be ordered for a period following the removal of the eschar to promote drainage and bring any infection under control in preparation for grafting.

The patient's general condition and the size of the burn area determine whether the grafting will require several stages. Priority is given to areas where scarring and contraction produce loss of movement and marked deformity. The grafts are usually laid on (not sutured) and covered with petroleum jelly-impregnated gauze, pads and an elastic or crepe bandage. If the grafts are around or over a joint surface, a splint or plaster cast may be applied to immobilize the part. Unless necrosis and infection are suspected from the patient's symptoms, the dressing usually is not changed for 5 to 6 days. Further information is offered about skin grafts at the end of this discussion on the care of the burned patient.

PRECAUTIONS AGAINST INFECTION. If the patient with a deep burn has been immunized within the preceding 5 years for tetanus, a booster dose of toxoid is given. The patient with no tetanus immunization is given a prophylactic dose of human tetanus immunoglobulin. This necessitates questioning the patient or family as to whether he has ever had asthma, eczema or any known drug reaction or allergy.

Infection of the burn area may originate with bacteria that were present in the area before the burn and survived the heat. Special protective measures are used to minimize the possibility of contamination from outside sources. Reverse isolation technique and sterile bed linen are used. Strict aseptic technique is observed in providing wound care and changing dressings. Masks, caps and sterile gowns and gloves are worn by those participating in direct care. The patient may be moved to a special burn dressing room or to a small operating room for dressing changes. Obviously, personnel with infection (e.g., cold, sore throat, skin infection) are not allowed to care for the patient. Visitors are restricted in number and are given an explanation of their role in protecting the patient. They are required to wear caps, gown and masks while with him.

When changing the dressing, the inner layers of gauze are removed very gently to minimize tissue bleeding and damage. Moistening of the gauze with a sterile solution or in a bath may be necessary to prevent trauma. The dressing procedure is likely to be painful and anxiety-producing for the patient, especially in the early stages; an analgesic such as meperidine hydrochloride (Demerol) or codeine may be ordered for administration 15 to 30 minutes before the burn is dressed.

One of the most serious complications in third-degree burns is septicemia; this generally develops during the second or third week. It may have a sudden onset, ushered in by chills and a rapid elevation of temperature, or it may develop gradually over 2 to 3 days. It is characterized by high fever which may fluctuate, rapid pulse, drowsiness and disorientation. Paralytic ileus is a common concomitant, and petechiae, ecchymoses and oozing from the burn areas frequently appear, since a bleeding tendency develops. Blood cultures are made to identify the organism(s) which have invaded the blood stream. Common offenders are *Staphylococcus aureus,* hemolytic streptococcus, and *Pseudomonas aeruginosa.*

Treatment of septicemia includes massive doses of antibiotics intravenously, promotion of the separation of the eschar to permit drainage and the application of a topical antimicrobial preparation, and supportive therapy. Intravenous fluids are given to sustain the patient. Gastrointestinal decompression suction is established if there are vomiting and abdominal distention. Blood transfusions may be given and, if the patient's condition deteriorates, which may be manifested by a subnormal temperature and shock, a corticosteroid preparation such as Solu-Cortef may be given intravenously.

POSITIONING AND EXERCISES. The patient is turned every 2 to 3 hours to prevent respiratory congestion and circulatory stasis. If the back is burned or the involvement is circumferential, care is facilitated if the patient is nursed on a Stryker frame or CircOlectric bed. Because of the edema, burned extremities are elevated on pillows or another form of support during the initial phase. Frequent attention is paid to body alignment; flexion contractures, outward rotation of thighs and foot drop must be prevented.

Splints may be applied to limbs after the emergent period if the closed wound care procedure is used. They may be used for immobilization to promote healing and to prevent contracture and deformity. The splint used must be nonsupportive to bacterial growth, fit the contour of the part to which it is applied and be secured well enough to provide stability but not cause pressure or interfere with circulation.

Burned parts which involve joints are moved through their range of motion as soon as possible and as indicated by the physician.

If the patient is placed in a bath, he is encouraged to exercise while soaking. As healing occurs, the activity program is progressively increased to preserve normal range of motion and function.

NUTRITION. In addition to fluid therapy, nutrition plays an important role in the recovery of the burned patient. In the initial shock period in severe burns the patient is sustained mainly by intravenous fluids. If oral fluids are tolerated, they may be given freely. Following recovery from shock, if there is no vomiting or abdominal distention, the intake is progressively increased from fluids, through soft foods, to a full normal diet.

The patient develops a negative nitrogen balance as a result of tissue catabolism and the reduced intake, which increases susceptibility to infection and debilitation and delays healing. A high-calorie, high-protein (150 to 200 Gm. per day for an adult) and high-vitamin diet is recommended to provide the essentials for tissue repair and the production of antibodies and blood cells. Vitamin C is essential in the synthesis of corticosteroids and in tissue repair, and the vitamin B complex is needed in the many cellular enzyme systems essential to normal cellular responses.

Ingenuity and resourcefulness are necessary on the part of the nurse to have the patient take the essential food. He should be advised of the important role of nutrients in his diet, and small frequent feedings of high-calorie foods are offered. Supplements of protein concentrates may be added to fluids. Likes and dislikes are determined and respected, and the family is encouraged to bring in occasional "treats" in the form of favorite foods. Adequate assistance is provided so that taking meals does not require too great an effort. A close check is made of the patient's daily intake, and the weight is also recorded daily.

REHABILITATION. Rehabilitation of the burned patient is fostered throughout the acute stages by conscientious attention to good body alignment, the prevention of infection and contractures, and the maintenance of joint and limb mobility as much as possible. Following recovery from the burn, the patient may require considerable reconstructive surgery and retraining before he can resume independent and self-supportive functioning. Rehabilitation is a lengthy process for many, and they and their families may require social guidance and financial assistance as well as psychological support throughout. Retraining for a different occupation may be necessary. In some instances the patient finds it very difficult to resume social contacts and to take his place in society because of scarring and gross disfigurement.

GRAFTS

A graft implies the placement of body tissue or other material in an area of the body where it becomes a part of the local structure, substituting for absent or damaged tissue.

Types of Grafts

Various terms are used to describe grafts and are defined as follows:

AUTOGRAFT OR AUTOGENOUS GRAFT. The autograft is obtained from the recipient's own body and may be skin, vein, artery, fascia, tendon or bone, depending on the particular recipient site and correction to be made. No tissue rejection is involved.

ISOGRAFT OR ISOLOGOUS GRAFT. This is a graft between identical twins. Because of the same germ cell origin, the graft is biologically compatible with the recipient's tissue, and there is no tissue rejection.

HOMOGRAFT (HOMOLOGOUS GRAFT OR ALLOGRAFT). The donor and recipient of the graft are of the same species. It may be obtained from a living person or taken from a body shortly after death. Homografts commonly used include skin, cornea, bone and blood vessel. Homografts do not survive indefinitely because the tissue is recognized as "unlike self" and rejected. The rejection phenomenon is an immunologic reaction in which the graft is an antigen and antibodies are formed by the host in response to it (see Rejection Process, Chapter 19). The tissue is attacked, and an inflammatory process ensues, ending in a breakdown of the graft. The graft must receive nutrients and oxygen from a blood supply; therefore, donor tissue which normally requires a lesser blood supply, such as the cornea, withstands rejection for a longer period. The transplanted cornea functions for a period during which it is rejected very slowly while at the same time repair slowly replaces it. Rarely, homografting of skin may be used in extensive third-degree burns as a temporary means of providing a

covering to protect the patient against massive infection and excessive loss of fluid. In donor selection, the person most closely related to the patient is selected if possible. The survival period for the graft varies, but it is usually 1 to 3 weeks. By this time, the patient's condition may have improved sufficiently that a series of autogenous grafting may be done.

Arterial and venous homografts are rejected slowly and, during the process, new host tissue replaces the graft wall. These grafts are frequently complicated by thromboses and closure of the vessels.

Bone homografts seem to be one of the more successful of homologous tissue transplants.

Organ transplant from one person to another is currently receiving a great deal of attention. Renal homotransplants appear to have had the most gratifying results; many persons with renal insufficiency that was incompatible with life have received a kidney transplant and, with the aid of immunosuppressive drugs, are living extended, useful lives.

HOMOSTATIC GRAFT. The tissue in the homograft may or may not be viable when placed in the recipient. It serves temporarily as a framework for new host tissue that forms or provides materials for new host tissue when it disintegrates. Bone tissue grafts are an example.

SUBSTITUTE GRAFT. This graft is made of inert material to which there is a minimum of tissue reaction. It may serve as a replacement for weak or destroyed tissues or as a framework for the formation of host tissues. An example of the latter is a porous Teflon tube which is placed in the aorta during the correction of a coarctation. The Teflon is eventually incorporated into the host tissue as the tissue grows through the pores. Other examples of substitute grafts are patches of inert material used to strengthen or correct an area (e.g., defect in the cardiac wall).

HETEROGRAFT. This implies the transfer of tissue between species and results in rapid rejection.

Skin Grafting

A large proportion of reconstructive surgery and the correction of cutaneous defects involves skin autografts. As indicated in the preceding discussion on the care of the burned patient, skin grafting is necessary in many third-degree burns to prevent handicapping and disfiguring contractures.

A skin graft may be classified as a *free graft* when it is completely separated from the donor site and is transferred to another area of the body. If the graft remains attached at one end to the donor site in order to maintain a blood supply, it may be referred to as a *pedicle graft or a flap.* The detached end is moved to the recipient area and, when sufficient blood vessels form to establish an adequate circulation between the graft and the surrounding tissue, the pedicle or flap is then separated from the donor area. The thickness of skin grafts varies. The graft may be of *split thickness,* which consists of the epidermis and a portion of the dermis. A *full-thickness* graft includes the epidermis and complete dermis.

Types of free grafts include the Ollier-Thiersch grafts, which are thin strips or sheets of partial thickness; pinch or Reverdin grafts, which are very small pieces (approximately 0.5 cm. in diameter) of full thickness; and Wolfe's grafts, which are full-thickness pieces of skin that are larger than pinch grafts. The donor sites most commonly used for free autografts are the thighs and trunk. The donor site for a flap or pedicle graft must be within reach of the recipient site, since one end is attached to each site. When grafts are placed in position, they may be held in place by dressings or may be sutured and left exposed.

Nursing Care

The donor area is shaved and cleansed as for any other surgery. The recipient site may receive frequent moist antiseptic dressings or the application of a topical antimicrobial preparation to render it as free of organisms as possible. If a thick layer of granulation tissue has developed, it may be pared down by the surgeon before the application of a graft.

The patient's blood is typed and cross matched, and blood is made available for transfusion. Débridement (the removal of granulation tissue and oozing from the donor area) may result in a considerable loss of blood, which could interfere with the growth of the graft.

Following the operation, unless the graft is sutured, the area is covered with fine mesh, petroleum jelly gauze, dressing pads and elastic or crepe bandages. If the recipient site involves or is adjacent to a joint, a splint or plaster cast is applied to immobilize the part. The dressing remains undisturbed for 4 to 6 days unless infection is suspected because of fever, leukocytosis, or an offensive odor and discharge from the area.

The donor site may be covered with petroleum jelly gauze for 24 to 48 hours and then exposed. This area may be painful and, in some instances is a greater source of discomfort than the recipient area.

References

Books

Archambeault-Jones, Claudella, and Feller, Irving: Procedures for Nursing the Burned Patient. Ann Arbor, Michigan, National Institute for Burn Medicine, 1975.

Harmon, Vera M., and Steele, Shirley M.: Nursing Care of the Skin: A Developmental Approach. New York, Appleton-Century-Crofts, 1975.

Huckbody, Eileen: Nursing Procedures for Skin Diseases. Edinburgh, Churchill Livingstone, 1977.

Jacoby, Florence Greenhouse: Nursing Care of the Patient with Burns, 2nd ed. St. Louis, C. V. Mosby, 1976.

Krupp, Marcus A., and Chatton, Milton J.: Medical Diagnosis and Treatment. Los Altos, Cal., Lange, 1975. Chapter 3.

Lynch, J. B., and Lewis, Stephen R. (Eds.): Symposium on the Treatment of Burns, Vol. 5. St. Louis, C. V. Mosby, 1973.

Moschella, Samuel L., et al.: Dermatology, Vol. 2. Philadelphia, W. B. Saunders, 1975.

Muir, I. F. K., and Barclay, T. F.: Burns and Their Treatment, 2nd ed. London, Lloyd-Luke, 1974.

Polk, Hiram, C., and Stone, H. Harlan (Eds.): Contemporary Burn Managment. Boston, Little, Brown, 1971.

Rudowski, Wittold, et al.: Burn Therapy and Research. Baltimore, Johns Hopkins Press, 1976.

Sauer, Gordon C.: Manual of Skin Diseases, 3rd ed. Philadelphia, J. B. Lippincott, 1973.

Sneddon, I. B., and Church, R. D.: Practical Dermatology, 3rd ed. London, E. A. Arnold, 1976.

Solomons, Bethel: Lecture Notes on Dermatology, 4th ed. Oxford, Blackwell, 1977.

Sutton, Richard L., Jr., and Waisman, Morris: The Practitioner's Dermatology. New York, Dun-Donnelley, 1975.
Von Prince, Kilulu M. P., and Yeakel, Mary H.: The Splinting of Burn Patients. Springfield, Ill., Charles C Thomas, 1974.

Periodicals

Boswick, John A., and Pandya, Narendra J.: "Emergency Care of the Burned Patient." Surg. Clin. North Am., Vol. 52, No. 1 (Feb. 1972), pp. 115–123.
Brown, Marie Scott, and Alexander, Mary M.: "Examining the Skin." Nurs. '73, Vol. 3, No. 9 (Sept. 1973), pp. 39–43.
Burton, J. L., and Thompson, Lorna: "What Do Dermatology Patients Believe?" J. Adv. Nurs., Vol. 1, No. 4 (July 1976), pp. 293–302.
Chaney, Patricia (Ed.): "Burns: Breaking the Anger-Despair Cycle." Nurs. '75, Vol. 5, No. 5 (May 1975), pp. 44–49.
Corliss, Sylvia: "Improving Care of Severe Burn Wounds." Nurs. '72, Vol. 2, No. 4 (April 1972), pp. 6–12.
Derbes, Vincent J.: "Rashes: Recognition and Management." Nurs. '78, Vol. 8, No. 3 (March 1978), pp. 54–59.
Fortier, Rosemarie Repa: "Nutrition and the Burn Patient." Can. Nurse, Vol. 73, No. 8 (Aug. 1977), pp. 30–31.
Hawkins, Kathy: "Wet Dressings: Putting the Damper on Dermatitis." Nurs. '78, Vol. 8, No. 2 (Feb. 1978), pp. 64–67.
Huntley, Carolyn Coker: "Atopic Dermatitis and Contact Dermatitis in Children." Am. Fam. Physician, Vol. 16, No. 2 (Aug. 1977), pp. 111–118.
Jacoby, Florence Greenhouse: "Individualized Burn Wound Dressings." Nurs. '77, Vol. 7, No. 6 (June 1977), pp. 62–63.
Jepsen, Lois: "Malignant Melanoma." Nurs. '77, Vol. 7, No. 12 (Dec. 1977), pp. 38–43.
Johnson, Hugh A. (Ed.): "Symposium on Plastic Surgery for General Surgeons." Surg. Clin. North Am., Vol. 57, No. 5 (Oct. 1977).
Johnson, Sture A. M. (Ed.): "Symposium: Coping with Common Skin Conditions. Part 1 and Part 2." Geriatrics, Vol. 30, No. 2 (Feb. and Mar. 1975), p. 50.
Jones, Claudella A., and Feller, Irving: "Burns: What To Do During the First Crucial Hours." Nurs. '77, Vol. 7, No. 3 (March 1977), pp. 22–31.
———: "Burns: Avoiding and Coping with Complications Before and After Grafting." Nurs. '77, Vol. 7, No. 11 (Nov. 1977), pp. 72–81.
LaPerriere, Robert J.: "Acne Vulgaris." Primary Care., Vol. 1, No. 3 (Sept. 1974), pp. 417–448.
LeFort, Sandra: "Burn Update." Can. Nurse, Vol. 73, No. 8, (Aug. 1977), pp. 16–26.
Minckley, Barbara A.: "Expert Nursing Care for Burned Patients." Am. J. Nurs., Vol. 70, No. 9 (Sept. 1970), pp. 1888–1893.
North, Carolyn, and Weinstein, Gerald D.: "Treatment of Psoriasis." Am. J. Nurs., Vol. 76, No. 3 (March 1976), pp. 410–412.
Parks, Donald H., et al.: "Management of Burns." Surg. Clin. North Am., Vol. 57, No. 5 (Oct. 1977), pp. 875–894.
Rice, Alice K.: "Common Skin Infections in School Children." Am. J. Nurs., Vol. 73, No. 11 (Nov. 1973), pp. 1905–1909.
Roach, Lora B.: "Color Changes in Dark Skins." Nurs. '72, Vol. 2, No. 11 (Nov. 1972), pp. 19–22.
———: "Assessing Skin Changes: The Subtle and the Obvious." Nurs. '74, Vol. 3, No. 3 (March 1974), pp. 64–67.
Rogenes, Paula R., and Moylan, Joseph A.: "Restoring Fluid Balance in the Patient with Severe Burns." Am. J. Nurs., Vol. 76, No. 12 (Dec. 1976), pp. 1952–1957.
Savedra, Marilyn: "Coping with Pain." Can. Nurse, Vol. 73, No. 8 (Aug. 1977), pp. 28–29.
Shoss, Robert G., and Lumpkin, Lee: "Current Therapy of Psoriasis." Am. Fam. Physician, Vol. 5, No. 1, (Jan. 1977), pp. 114–116.
Stinson, Velda: "Porcine Skin Dressings for Burns." Am. J. Nurs., Vol. 74, No. 1 (Jan. 1974), pp. 111–112.
Stone, Stephen P.: "Scabies." Am. Fam. Physician, Vol. 15, No. 5, (May 1977), pp. 152–153.
Talabere, Laurel, and Graves, Patricia: "A Tool for Assessing Families of Burned Children." Am. J. Nurs., Vol. 76, No. 2 (Feb. 1976), pp. 225–227.
Vistnes, Lars M.: "Grafting of Skin." Surg. Clin. North Am., Vol. 57, No. 5 (Oct. 1977), pp. 939–960.
Wagner, Mary M.: "Emergency Care of the Burned Patient." Am. J. Nurs., Vol. 77, No. 11 (Nov. 1977), pp. 1788–1791.
Wiley, Loy (Ed.): "Burn Care." Nurs. '72, Vol. 2, No. 7 (July 1972), pp. 32–37.
———: "Psoriasis." Nurs. '76, Vol. 6, No. 11 (Nov. 1976), pp. 35–38.
Wright, Edwin T.: "Identifying and Treating Common Benign Skin Tumors." Geriatrics, Vol. 33, No. 6 (June 1978), pp. 37–44.

27

Nursing in Disorders of the Eye

STRUCTURE AND FUNCTION OF THE EYES

Vision, like all other sensory mechanisms, requires receptors, an afferent pathway to carry the impulses into the central nervous system and an interpretive center. The eyes serve as receptors which are sensitive to light rays, the pathway is formed by the optic nerves and tracts within the brain, and the interpretive centers are composed of groups of neurons localized in the cortex of the cerebral occipital lobes (visual centers). In addition, the visual apparatus includes intrinsic and extrinsic muscles which play an important role in vision. There are also several accessory structures which function to protect the eyes.

Location of the Eye

Each eyeball rests in a cone-shaped cavity (the orbit) in the skull. The orbit is covered posteriorly by a fibrous sac lined with a smooth moist membrane which promotes smooth movement of the eye in its socket.

Accessory External Structures

The accessory structures include the eyelids, lacrimal system and extrinsic ocular muscles.

EYELIDS (PALPEBRAE). The upper and lower eyelids are curtain-like structures lying in front of the eyeball. They serve as protective coverings by shutting out intense light, dust and foreign bodies. The space between them is referred to as the palpebral fissure; the angles or corners where the lids meet are known as the inner (medial) and outer (lateral) canthi. Each eyelid has an outer layer of skin, a layer of firm fibrous tissue (tarsal plate), sebaceous-like glands (meibomian glands) which secrete an oily substance onto the free margins of the lids, and a mucous membrane lining called the conjunctiva. The conjunctiva is reflected over the anterior of the eyeball. The secretion of the meibomian glands prevents adherence of the lids when the eyes are closed and also prevents the overflow of normal amounts of lacrimal secretion. The eyelashes emerge from the free borders of

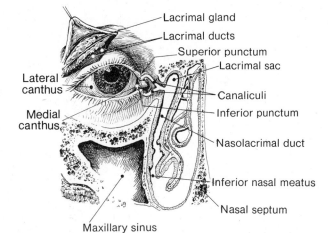

FIGURE 27–1 The lacrimal system.

the eyelids to protect the eye from dust and perspiration.

LACRIMAL SYSTEM. The lacrimal apparatus protects the eye by continuously secreting a fluid that "washes" over the anterior surface of the eyeball, keeping it moistened and cleansed. The system of each eye consists of a gland, ducts and a drainage system (Fig. 27–1).

The lacrimal gland lies in a slight depression in the outer superior portion of the orbit. Several ducts carry the secretion of the gland onto the inner surface of the upper eyelid. The secreted fluid is distributed over the anterior surface of the eye and then drains through two small openings (puncta) in the medial canthus into two short canals (lacrimal canaliculi). The canals drain into a small sacular structure, the lacrimal sac, which narrows to form the nasolacrimal duct, which carries the secretion into the nasal cavity.

A volume of lacrimal secretion in excess of what the drainage system can handle results in fluid overflowing the eyelids and forming tears. Increased lacrimal secretion occurs in response to irritation of the conjunctiva or to certain emotions.

EXTRINSIC OCULAR MUSCLES. Several external muscles have their origin in orbital structures and insert on the eyeball to provide movement of the eye within its socket. There are four straight muscles (*recti muscles*); each is named for the direction in which it moves the eye. The superior rectus turns the eye up, the inferior rectus turns it downward, the medial rectus turns it in, and the lateral moves it in the reverse direction. In addition to the recti muscles, two *oblique muscles* (a superior and an inferior) provide rotation and modification of straight movements. For most movements, more than one external ocular muscle generally operate; various combinations of recti and oblique muscle action are necessary (Fig. 27–2).

The external ocular muscles include the levator palpebrae superioris muscle which inserts in the upper eyelid. It is responsible for raising the upper eyelid (opening the eye).

Eyeball

The eyeball is spherical with a slight anterior bulge. It is composed of three layers of tissue which enclose the iris and special

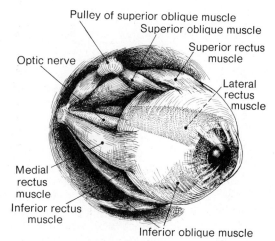

FIGURE 27–2 Extraocular muscles of the left eye.

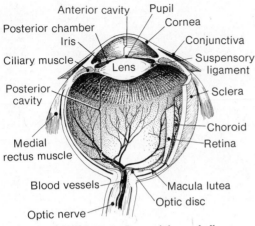

Anterior cavity · Pupil
Posterior chamber · Cornea
Iris · Conjunctiva
Ciliary muscle · Suspensory ligament
Lens
Posterior cavity · Sclera
Medial rectus muscle · Choroid
Retina
Blood vessels · Macula lutea
Optic disc
Optic nerve

FIGURE 27–3 Parts of the eyeball.

transparent, refracting structures (Fig. 27–3). The tough, outer coat forms the sclera and cornea. The *sclera,* which covers the posterior five-sixths of the eyeball, is white, opaque fibrous tissue. The *cornea* is a continuation of the sclera over the anterior portion of the eye. It consists of transparent, special connective tissue that is devoid of blood vessels. The corneoscleral junction is referred to as the *limbus.*

Underlying and attached to the sclera is a thin, heavily pigmented, vascular coat, the *choroid,* which extends forward to what is referred to as the ciliary body. The pigmentation prevents the reflection of the light rays.

The *ciliary body* consists mainly of muscle tissue which takes its origin at the corneoscleral junction and inserts in the suspensory ligaments that are attached to the lens, holding it suspended in position. The action of the ciliary muscle influences the curvature, and thus the refractive power, of the lens.

The second layer of the eyeball continues forward and inward beyond the ciliary muscle to form the iris. The *iris* is composed of circular and radial muscles and pigmented cells and is perforated centrally, creating the opening referred to as the *pupil.* Contraction of the circular muscle fibers (sphincter pupillae) constricts the pupil; dilation is controlled by the radial fibers.

The *retina* is the innermost and nervous coat of the posterior two-thirds of the eyeball. It consists of several strata of cells through which light rays pass before reaching the outer layer of cells, which are light-sensitive receptors that convert luminous energy into nerve impulses. There are two types of receptor cells — the rods and cones. The rods have a lower response threshold, making them more sensitive to lower levels of illumination. The cones have a higher response threshold and, as a result, function in bright light and provide color and detailed vision.

In the center of the retina, a small area occurs in which the inner layers of cells are absent and only cones are concentrated. Light rays falling on this site strike the cones directly and produce the greatest visual acuity. This area is referred to as the *fovea centralis* and occurs as a slight depression in a small, elevated, yellowish area called the macula lutea, or yellow spot. Slightly medial to the macula there is a pale papillary area called the *optic disk,* or *fundus oculi.* It is at this point that the optic nerve and ophthalmic blood vessels leave and enter the eyeball. The disk is a blind spot, since the area is devoid of rods and cones.

The eyeball is "filled out" by contents composed of fluids (aqueous humor), a biconvex disk (lens) and a jelly-like mass (vitreous humor).

The *lens* is elastic and crystal-clear and is suspended just behind the iris by ligaments which attach to the ciliary body. Its shape varies with age; it is spherical in infancy, gradually flattening to a disk shape with age. In the elderly, the lens tends to flatten and become less elastic.

DIVISIONS OF THE INTERIOR OF THE EYEBALL. The interior of the eyeball is divided into the anterior and posterior cavities. The *anterior cavity* is the space between the cornea and lens and is subdivided into the *anterior and posterior chambers,* which are areas frequently referred to in clinical work. The anterior chamber lies posterior to the cornea and in front of the iris. The posterior chamber is situated posterior to the iris and anterior to the lens. The content of the two chambers is *aqueous humor.*

The posterior cavity lies posterior to the lens and is the remainder of the interior of the eyeball. It is filled with the *vitreous humor,* or *vitreous body.*

FLUID SYSTEM OF THE EYE AND INTRAOCULAR PRESSURE. The interior of the eyeball is filled by the aqueous and vitreous humors and the crystalline lens. The *vitreous humor* is a clear, jelly-like mass enclosed in a hyaloid membrane which anteriorly is continuous with the capsule of the lens. The vitreous humor fills out the larger and posterior portion of the eyeball that lies behind the lens.

The anterior and posterior chambers are filled with a clear fluid, the *aqueous humor*. There is a continuous flow into and out of the eye. The fluid originates from capillaries contained in processes of the ciliary body. Some fluid diffuses into the vitreous body from the posterior chamber; the greater proportion flows through the pupil into the anterior chamber. From here, a small amount of the aqueous humor continuously drains into the canal of Schlemm, from which it is carried into the venous circulation. The *canal of Schlemm* is a channel that circles the eye in the region of the corneoscleral junction. Small spaces (spaces of Fontana) leading to the canal occur in the tissues at the angle formed by the junction of the cornea with the anterior surface of the iris. This may be referred to as the *filtration angle*. The production of aqueous humor and its drainage are constant in order to maintain a *normal intraocular pressure,* which is 15 to 25 mm. Hg. Any interference with normal drainage of the fluid from the anterior chamber raises the pressure, leading to decreased blood supply, pain and impaired vision.

Visual Impulse Pathway

Impulses generated by the rods and cones synapse through several neurons to ganglionic cells whose axons course toward the site of the optic disk where they unite to form the optic nerve. This nerve differs from most nerves in that it has no neurilemma; thus, it is incapable of regeneration if damaged or destroyed. At the base of the brain, the nerve fibers from the medial half of the retina of each eye cross, going to the opposite side of the brain. The fibers from the lateral halves of the retinae do not cross but continue on to the corresponding side of the brain. This arrangement forms the optic chiasma (see Fig. 27–4). Within the brain, the fibers from the lateral half of the right eye and those from the medial half of the left eye continue on as the right optic tract. The fibers of each tract synapse

with the lateral geniculate in the thalamus on the corresponding side. From there, the impulses are transmitted along the postsynaptic fibers (optic radiations) to the visual center in the occipital cerebral cortex of the same side, where they are interpreted as sensations of light, color and form. Other cerebral areas are necessary for normal vision; correlation with information stored as memory in association areas has to occur in order to give meaning to what is seen. For example, a written word or an object may be seen but, unless the person has heard or experienced its meaning, he is unable to interpret it.

Visual Fields

The retinae of both eyes receive light rays at the same time from an object within the field of vision (binocular vision). Light rays from an object in the left outer visual field are received on the medial, or nasal, side of the left retina and on the lateral, or temporal, side of the right retina. The ensuing impulses are carried over fibers of the left and right optic nerves but, with the crossing of fibers in the chiasma, the impulses will travel along the right optic tract

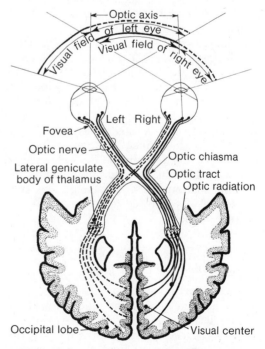

FIGURE 27–4 Left and right visual fields and the visual impulse pathway.

to the visual center in the right occipital lobe for interpretation. Conversely, rays from objects in the right visual field will fall on the lateral area of the left retina and nasal area of the right retina, with the resulting impulses ending up in the visual center of the left occipital lobe. There is some overlapping between the two halves of each retina and, as a result, the central half of each is represented in each hemisphere.

If the optic nerve of one eye is destroyed blindness occurs in that eye, but destruction of fibers of the optic tract (i.e., beyond the optic chiasma) causes blindness to occur in half of each retina, limiting the field of vision. The term for this blindness is *hemianopia.*

Eye Reflexes

The eye reflexes are used frequently in assessing the patient's condition. Some fibers of each optic tract terminate in a group of neurons referred to as the superior colliculus (superior colliculus quadrigeminae) in the midbrain. From here, efferent impulses originate, resulting in blinking of the eyelids, movement of the head, or dilation or constriction of the pupil.

The conjunctival and corneal reflex of blinking is a protective response elicited by touching the conjunctival surface.

Pupillary reaction is observed by flashing a light into the eye; this normally results in constriction of the pupil. A second reflex that may be noted is the accommodation reflex. The pupils are observed while the person shifts his gaze from a distant to a near object. The normal response is constriction of the pupils. In some pathologic conditions (e.g., syphilis), the response of the pupil to light may be absent while the accommodation reflex is present. This type of response is referred to as an Argyll Robertson pupil.

Refraction, Accommodation, Pupillary Modification and Convergence

Several processes may be necessary to focus the light rays on the retina in order to form a clear image.

REFRACTION. When light rays pass obliquely from one medium to another of a different density their velocity is altered, and they are bent or deflected. The process is referred to as refraction (Fig. 27–5). If the rays pass into a medium of greater density, they are deflected toward the perpendicular; conversely, in a medium of lesser density the rays are bent away from the perpendicular. Parallel rays striking a surface at right angles are not refracted. Parallel light rays striking the center of the cornea and lens pass through unrefracted. At either side of the center of the convex surfaces of the cornea and lens, light rays enter at an angle to the surface and are refracted toward the perpendicular. The greater the curvature or convexity of the surface, the greater is the degree of refraction.

The cornea and lens are the principal refractive media in the eye; the lens is particularly significant in that its curvature and degree of refraction can be varied by the ciliary body, according to the amount required to focus the light rays on the retina. The aqueous and vitreous humors also contribute to refraction but the degree, as with the cornea, remains the same. Without strain or modification, the normal eye will refract light rays from an object 20 or more feet away sufficiently to focus them on the retina. For objects that are near, refraction must be increased, and for distant objects, the eye must decrease its refraction. When greater refraction is necessary, the ciliary muscles contract and the suspensory ligaments, which are attached to the lens and the ciliary body, move forward, reducing their pull on the lens. As a result, the lens increases its convexity and thickness and, thus, its refractive power. When light rays reflected by distant objects enter the eye, the ciliary muscles relax, and the suspensory ligaments exert greater tension on the lens. This reduces convexity, thickness and refractive power of the lens, and focus of the light rays on the retina is achieved.

Various errors of refraction occur which interfere with the ability of the eye to focus light rays on the retina, resulting in impaired vision.

Emmetropia implies normal refraction.

Nearsightedness, called *myopia,* is the result of light rays from an object at 20 feet or more being focused at a point in front of the retina. Close objects can be seen, but distant objects are blurred. Correction may be made by use of a concave lens, since a

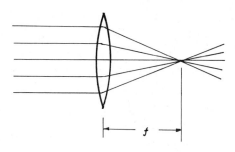

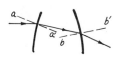

a. A double convex lens focuses light.

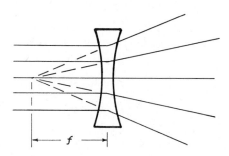

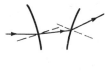

b. A double concave lens causes light to diverge.

FIGURE 27–5 Diagram showing refraction. *A,* Refraction of light rays by a double convex lens (convergence). *B,* Refraction of light rays by a double concave lens (divergence). (From Nave, Carl R., and Nave, Brenda C.: Physics for the Health Sciences. Philadelphia, W. B. Saunders, 1975, p. 231.)

concave lens produces divergence of light rays (see Fig. 27–6A).

Farsightedness (*hypermetropia*) is due to insufficient refraction and, as a result, light rays from an object at 20 feet or less are focused at a point behind the retina. The person sees distant objects more clearly than close ones. Correction may be made by use of a convex lens, since a convex lens focuses light rays by convergence (see Fig. 27–6B). In the later years of life, as part of the aging process, the lens loses its elasticity and becomes thinner and flatter. This lessens the normal degree of refraction and the person becomes farsighted, a refractive error referred to as *presbyopia*.

In some persons, the horizontal and vertical curvatures of the cornea are uneven, producing differences in the degree of refraction. This results in different focal points; some light rays may be focused on the retina, but others may fall short or be carried to a point beyond the retina. This type of refractive error is known as *astigmatism*.

ACCOMMODATION. This is the process by which the degree of refraction by the lens is changed in order to focus rays from objects at various distances. This is made possible by the elastic nature of the lens and the action of the ciliary muscles on the suspensory ligaments, as explained under refraction (Fig. 27–7).

PUPILLARY MODIFICATION. The pupillary aperture is varied to control the amount of light entering the eye. For clear vision of near objects, the iris constricts the pupil of each eye to prevent divergent rays from entering. The opening is also reduced to restrict the entrance of excessively bright light, which may harm the retina. The iris constricts the pupil through parasympathetic innervation; sympathetic nervous stimulation produces dilation of the pupil. In dim light and when focusing on a distant, wider visual field, the iris dilates the pupil to admit more light rays.

CONVERGENCE. Although light rays from the same object(s) fall on both retinae, only single vision is experienced. This is due to light rays from the object falling on corresponding points of the two retinae. This is brought about by convergence, which involves the extrinsic muscles (recti

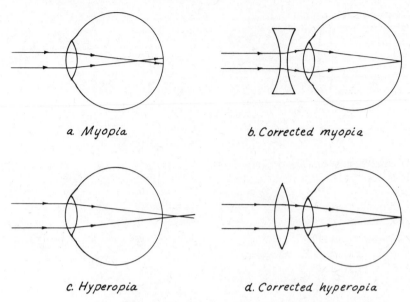

a. *Myopia*

b. *Corrected myopia*

c. *Hyperopia*

d. *Corrected hyperopia*

The use of lenses to correct common eye defects.

FIGURE 27–6 Diagram showing: *A,* Myopia and correction by concave lens. *B,* Hypermetropia and correction by convex lens. (From Nave, Carl R., and Nave, Brenda C.: Physics for the Health Sciences. Philadelphia, W. B. Saunders, 1975, p. 236.)

and oblique). The movements of the two eyes must be coordinated accurately. As an object is brought closer to the eyes, convergence of their axes occurs as they turn inward. For distant objects convergence is not necessary; the eyes remain parallel. *Strabismus* is a defect which interferes with coordination of the eye movements, and the light rays do not fall on corresponding points of the two retinae. It is usually due to an abnormal extrinsic muscle. Two images result and the person "sees double"; this is termed *diplopia*.

Light and Dark Adaptation

LIGHT ADAPTATION. When exposed to intense light, adaptation takes place by constriction of the pupils and lowering of the eyebrows, eyelids and head; the visual purple (rhodopsin) within the rods is bleached which reduces their sensitivity and responses.

DARK ADAPTATION. When a person goes from a light to a dark area, he cannot see immediately; then gradually he sees outlines of objects. This vision in dim light

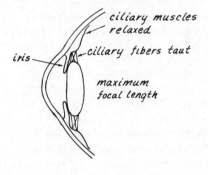

ciliary muscles relaxed

iris

ciliary fibers taut

maximum focal length

a. *Distant vision*

ciliary muscles contracted

ciliary fibers loosened

lens becomes more rounded, focal length shorter

b. *Close vision*

FIGURE 27–7 Diagram showing the ciliary body, suspensory ligaments and lens and the changes in accommodation. (From Nave, Carl R., and Nave, Brenda C.: Physics for the Health Sciences. Philadelphia, W. B. Saunders, 1975, p. 234.)

is due to an increased sensitivity of the rods as they produce a chemical pigment, visual purple or rhodopsin. Vitamin A is essential for the formation of the chemical; if it is deficient, the person experiences night blindness. At the same time that the rods increase their sensitivity, the pupils dilate to admit more light.

IMPAIRED VISION

Man is very dependent upon his sense of vision, since most of his knowledge of his environment is obtained through his eyes. The eyes are also used in expressing emotions. Any impairment or loss of vision is a serious threat. In many instances the ability to freely move about safely and the privilege of enjoying color, form, depth, beauty and distance are lost. Loss of vision results in reduced sensory input and stimulation; this may lead to boredom and reduced responsiveness on the part of the person unless stimuli by other channels (e.g., hearing) are increased and the person's interest maintained.

Nursing is concerned with the prevention of visual impairment, curative aspects when a disorder exists, and the rehabilitation of the patient with a loss of vision. The nurse should appreciate the incalculable value of sight and the natural anxiety and concern of the patient when it is threatened. Reduced vision affects his whole way of life socially, physically, economically and emotionally.

Factors in the Preservation of Sight

GOOD GENERAL HEALTH. There is a tendency to consider the eyes as being independent of general health. The vision remains good in some serious bodily disorders, while others may have a serious effect on visual acuity. Occasionally, general body disease is discovered because of changes in the eyes and vision (e.g., hypertension, diabetes).

OPTIMUM DIET. A well-balanced diet contributes to good eye health as well as to good general health. Vitamins A and B complex are considered important; a deficiency of vitamin A may cause drying and changes of the cornea and conjunctiva and a decreased production of the retinal pigment, rhodopsin, leading to night blindness. A deficiency in the vitamin B complex may predispose to retinal changes.

PROTECTION OF CHILDREN'S EYES. There is a legal requirement that a silver nitrate preparation be instilled in the eyes of every newborn infant in order to prevent possible infection, especially gonorrhea, which leads to corneal scarring and blindness. A child's eyes are not fully grown until he is at least 7 years of age. The infant's eyes require protection from prolonged exposure to direct sun and artificial light. Toys and playthings should be selected to avoid broken, sharp and pointed parts that predispose to injury. Children are taught to keep dirty fingers and other objects away from their eyes and are also instructed in the necessary precautions when old enough to play with such things as arrows, catapults and peashooters.

AVOIDANCE OF EYESTRAIN. Good lighting for reading and on close work is important to prevent eyestrain. Unshaded lights, glare and working with a light directly in front of the eyes are to be avoided. The rays should come from the back and one side onto the work area, which is kept free of shadows. Reading material or close work is held 14 to 16 inches from the eyes. Immobility is maintained when reading or doing close work; this precludes reading in moving vehicles.

When doing detailed and exacting work, the person should take frequent rests and look off into the distance. Close work should be avoided when fatigued.

REGULAR PERIODIC EYE EXAMINATION. Some eye diseases and changes develop insidiously without markedly reducing vision or causing pain until they are well advanced. Regular eye examination may reveal early signs, and a serious disease may be checked before it progresses to loss of vision and blindness. If glasses are necessary, only those which have been properly prescribed should be used. Lenses are individually ground for each eye according to the testing and examination findings. (See Table 27–1 for a list of terms which relate to eye examinations and errors of refraction.)

PROMPT TREATMENT. No "eyedrops" or solutions should be instilled in the eyes unless prescribed by a physician. In the event of a persisting foreign body which

TABLE 27–1 TERMINOLOGY AND ABBREVIATIONS

Term	Meaning
Ocular dexter (O.D.)	Right eye
Ocular sinister (O.S.)	Left eye
Ocular unitas (O.U.)	Both eyes
Emmetropia	Normal vision (normal refraction)
Myopia (M.)	Shortsightedness
Hypermetropia (hyperopia; H.)	Farsightedness
Presbyopia	Reduced accommodation associated with the aging process
Astigmatism	Uneven curvature of the cornea; results in different focal points
Diplopia	Perception of two images of a single object (double vision)
Entropion	Turning in of the eyelid
Ectropion	Turning out of the eyelid
Ptosis	Drooping of the upper eyelid
Photophobia	Hypersensitivity to light
Ophthamologist (oculist)	A physician who specializes in the treatment of eye disorders
Optometrist	A person who examines the eyes to assess vision and prescribes corrective eyeglasses or lenses
Optician	A specialist who prepares eyeglasses or lenses according to prescription

cannot be gently washed or wiped away, inflammation or any other disturbance in an eye, early treatment by a physician or oculist (ophthalmologist) should be secured.

USE OF PROTECTIVE DEVICES. To avoid injury by chemicals, dust, mechanical objects, wind, sun rays, and the like, appropriate safety goggles, shields or glasses should be worn.

Manifestations of Visual Disorders

The development of signs and symptoms of impaired vision varies greatly; as cited previously, the onset of changes may be very insidious; the person may continue to see well, but may actually be experiencing acute eyestrain. In others, the onset of a disorder and its manifestations may occur suddenly. One or both eyes may be involved. The symptoms may be principally objective, with changes being noted only by an observer.

The person may be seen holding reading material or an object nearer than 12 inches to the face or beyond the distance of 16 to 18 inches. He may scowl or have a strained expression when making an effort to see. A child may fail to develop at a normal rate or make normal progress at school.

Errors may be observed because of misread information or directive. The person may complain of difficulty in seeing or, that persons and objects are blurred or foggy. The field of vision may be limited, the outline and size of objects may be distorted, or diplopia may be experienced. Colored halos around lights may be seen if the intraocular pressure is increased.

With some conditions, the patient may complain of flashes of light or stars, increased sensitivity to ordinary light (photophobia), spots before the eyes, itching, burning, or pain and irritation. There may be redness of the eye or lids, excessive lacrimal secretion and tearing, or serous or purulent discharge.

Eye Examinations

Tests for evaluation of eye function include the following:

MEASUREMENT OF VISUAL ACUITY. Visual acuity implies the ability to distinguish details of objects and is measured as a means of evaluating ocular function. Each eye is tested separately; the eye not being examined is completely covered. A wall chart (Snellen chart) with rows of letters of decreasing size is used and placed 20 feet from the patient. The person is required to read the chart through to the line of smallest letters that he can see. The distance from which the normal eye can read each line is known. The top line of the Snellen chart is perceived by the normal eye at 200 feet, the second line at 100 feet, the third at 70 feet, the fourth at

50 feet, the fifth at 40 feet, the sixth at 30 feet, the seventh at 20 feet, the eighth line at 15 feet and the ninth line at 10 feet. Visual acuity is expressed as a fraction; the numerator represents the distance between the chart and the patient, and the denominator is the distance from which a person with normal vision could read the same line. Visual acuity recorded as 20/20 means normal vision. If the patient 20 feet from the chart can only read the line that the normal eye could read at 60 feet, the visual acuity is expressed as 20/60 and his vision is one-third of normal. The larger the denominator recorded, the poorer is the vision. In a person with severe impairment who can only see a hand moving in front of his face, the visual acuity may be recorded as H.M. (hand movements). If the person can only distinguish between light and dark, the recording is L. P. (light perception).

REFRACTION. The testing of the eyes' ability to focus the light rays on the retina is done by using a series of trial lenses as well as by assessing the person's visual acuity. In doing a refraction test, the physician may require the instillation of a cycloplegic drug, such as atropine 0.5 to 2 per cent or hyoscine 0.2 to 0.5 per cent, which temporarily inhibits ciliary muscle action and dilates the pupil.

VISUAL FIELD MEASUREMENT (PERIMETRY). A special semicircular instrument, called a perimeter, which is marked in degrees, is used to determine if the patient's visual fields are normal or restricted. Defects in the visual fields are frequently associated with intracranial lesions or damage to an optic nerve.

OPHTHALMOSCOPIC EXAMINATION. With an ophthalmoscope, the posterior, internal surface of each eye is magnified and observed. The blood vessels, retina, optic nerve and disk are examined. In order to get a wider view, the pupil is frequently dilated by the instillation of a mydriatic such as atropine 0.5 to 2 per cent.

MEASUREMENT OF INTRAOCULAR PRESSURE. The detection of increased intraocular pressure is important; an excessive pressure is very painful and progressively causes permanent damage within the eye, leading to loss of vision. The pressure is measured by an instrument called a tonometer. A few drops of a local anesthetic (e.g., cocaine 0.5 to 5 per cent) are instilled in each eye. The tonometer is then placed on the corneal surface, causing indentation; the extent of the indentation reflects the intraocular pressure. If the pressure is high, the cornea resists indentation. The calibrated scale of the tonometer records the pressure in mm. of Hg. The normal intraocular pressure is approximately 15 to 25 mm. Hg.

A second instrument that is now generally employed to measure the ocular tension is the applanometer. This is an electronic device which is considered to provide a more accurate measurement of the intraocular pressure.

ASSESSMENT OF THE RETINA. An electroretinogram may be done to record the extent of the electrical response made by the retina to light stimulation.

GONIOSCOPY. This involves the examination of the angle of the anterior chamber by means of an optical instrument (gonioscope) with an intense light.

COMMON EYE DISORDERS

Conjunctivitis

Inflammation of the conjunctiva may be caused by bacteria, viruses, chemicals or an allergic reaction. Sources of eye infection include foreign bodies, dust, hands, infected neighboring structures (nose, face, sinus) or contaminated equipment or solutions used in treatment. Infection by the Koch-Weeks bacillus causes a very contagious form of conjunctivitis called pinkeye. Prompt isolation precautions and therapeutic measures are necessary to prevent its rapid spread to others.

The infection may begin or be confined to the conjunctival lining of the eyelids. Involvement of the lids is referred to as *blepharitis*.

MANIFESTATIONS. The inflammation is manifested by irritation, pain, redness, encrustations and excessive lacrimation or serous and purulent discharge. The patient may complain of photophobia. When infection is present a culture may be made from a swab of the discharge for identification of the invading organism.

TREATMENT. Hot wet compresses or irrigations may be prescribed. Frequent gentle cleansing of the lid margins is necessary to prevent encrustations. Precautions must be observed to treat each eye separately so that infection is not transferred from one to the other. A specific antimicrobial ointment or solution may be prescribed for instillation. In severe infection, an antibiotic may be prescribed for systemic administration. In an allergic reaction, an antihistamine preparation may be prescribed to relieve the irritation. The patient is advised to keep the hands away from the eyes and, if responsible for instilling medications or applying compresses, the patient must be cautioned to wash the hands thoroughly under running water before starting. The affected eye is left uncovered.

Hordeolum

A hordeolum, or stye, is a small abscess that develops within a marginal gland or hair follicle of an eyelash. A small, red, swollen tender area appears. Spontaneous drainage of pus may be hastened by the application of hot moist compresses. Rarely, a small incision is necessary to drain the abscess. The patient with a stye is cautioned not to squeeze the area, as this may "break down" the localization and lead to cellulitis.

Chalazion

A chalazion is a cyst that forms in a meibomian gland. It may remain as a small, firm, painless swelling in the lid for a long period. Eventually it may become infected, frequently necessitating a small incision in the eyelid for drainage and curettage.

Glaucoma

This disorder is characterized by an increase in the intraocular pressure above the normal. Normal pressure is generally maintained by a balance between the production of aqueous humor by the ciliary body and its drainage from the anterior chamber. If an imbalance occurs between production and drainage, the pressure increases, compressing the retina and the blood vessels within the eye (Fig. 27–8). Permanent optic nerve damage leading to blindness results unless there is early recognition and treatment of the disease.

Glaucoma usually develops gradually

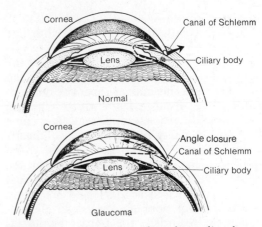

FIGURE 27–8 This diagram shows how a disturbance in the balance of fluid within the eyeball increases pressure in the eye and can result in glaucoma.

but, in some instances, may have a sudden onset. It may be chronic or acute; the latter form may be referred to as *acute angle-closure glaucoma* and the chronic form, with an insidious onset, may be classified as *open-angle glaucoma*.

The disorder may be primary or secondary and is due to some interference with the outflow of aqueous humor from the anterior chamber into the canal of Schlemm. Secondary glaucoma may be associated with inflammation, trauma, infection or a tumor within the eye. The cause of primary glaucoma is not understood, but the tendency to familial incidence points to an inherited predisposition. It has a high incidence in persons over the age of 35 or 40; surveys have indicated that one in every 50 persons over 40 years of age has glaucoma.

In *acute glaucoma,* the intraocular pressure increases rapidly as a result of a complete block in the outflow of the aqueous humor. The iris appears to have been pushed forward, narrowing the peripheral angle between it and the cornea (see Fig. 27–8) and, with dilation of the pupil and the concomitant thickening of the iris, the openings in the angle which lead into the canal of Schlemm become occluded. Rapid compression of the retinal blood vessels develops, and destruction of the optic nerve cells and fibers occurs.

MANIFESTATIONS AND TREATMENT. The patient with acute glaucoma experiences severe pain, nausea and vomiting, halos or rainbows around artificial lights and blurring of vision. On examination, the pupil is seen to be dilated, and there is evidence of congestion and a marked increase in intraocular pressure. The cornea becomes edematous and may eventually lose its luster and transparency.

Prompt treatment is necessary to prevent blindness. A miotic preparation such as pilocarpine hydrochloride, isofluorphate (Floropryl) or echothiopate iodide (Phospholine Iodide) is instilled to constrict the pupil; this effects an increase in the peripheral angle by moving the iris away from the cornea. A drug such as acetazolamide (Diamox) or dichlorphenamide (Oratrol) may be administered orally to reduce the formation of aqueous humor, or an osmotic agent such as urea or mannitol may be given intravenously to increase the urinary output, which reduces fluid volume and thus, intraocular pressure.

The patient is kept on complete bed rest with the head and shoulders elevated. An analgesic is prescribed to relieve the pain.

If an immediate, satisfactory response to drug therapy does not occur, surgical intervention is undertaken. A small section of the iris is removed (*iridectomy*) to prevent it from being imposed on the drainage system. Alternative surgical procedures which may be used are iridencleisis and cyclodialysis. These promote drainage of the aqeous humor from the anterior chamber. *Iridencleisis* creates an opening between the anterior chamber and subconjunctival space; aqueous fluid is absorbed into the conjunctival tissues. *Cyclodialysis* involves the establishment of a communication between the anterior chamber and the suprachoroidal space.

Chronic glaucoma, which is the more common form, has an insidious onset and is frequently well advanced before the person seeks assistance. The visual field progressively diminishes, and the individual may become aware that something is wrong when he learns of objects on either side of him that he "missed" or if he persistently sees halos around artificial lights. The condition may be discovered during a routine examination. As the condition progresses, the person may complain of some pain in the eye(s), especially in the morning on awakening. If chronic glaucoma is not recognized and treated in the earlier stages, the person eventually experiences symptoms similar to those cited for acute glaucoma.

Treatment of chronic glaucoma in the early stages usually consists of daily instillation of a miotic. Preparations are available now which have a more prolonged effect, requiring instillation only once in 24 hours. An example of such a preparation is echothiopate iodide (Phospholine Iodide). Surgical treatment may become necessary. As in acute glaucoma, an iridectomy, iridencleisis or cyclodialysis may be done.

Following surgery for glaucoma, the patient may be kept flat for 12 to 24 hours and then is gradually elevated and allowed to move.

Because glaucoma accounts for such a large proportion of blindness, more effort has been directed toward informing the general public about the disease and the significance of early recognition. Clinics have been organized so that mass surveys may be made in order to identify persons in the early stages of the disorder.

Glaucoma cannot be cured, but blindness can be prevented by continuous use of a miotic as prescribed and by medical supervision, if it is begun early in the disease.

An important nursing responsibility is to alert the patient to activities and situations that predispose to a rise in intraocular pressure. The condition is explained to the patient and family, and emphasis is placed upon the need for some precautions to prevent visual damage. Emotional and stressful situations are avoided as much as possible; the patient must learn to accept calmly what cannot be changed. Limitations are placed on the length of periods for reading, watching television and close work. Tight clothing around the neck is avoided. Constipation is dangerous, since it leads to straining at stool which causes an elevation of intraocular pressure.

The patient and family must appreciate the importance of regularly scheduled visits to the physician for measurement of the intraocular pressure and visual field and acuity testing. They are taught the correct method of instilling the prescribed miotic, and cautioned against the use of any solution or medication that is not prescribed by the physician. An identification card or Medic Alert pendant indicating that the person suffers from glaucoma is recommended. He is encouraged to continue his former occupation unless it requires prolonged periods of close visual concentration. If it does require such concentration, some job modification or change may be made if the employer is approached and is given an explanation of the employee's condition. Patients with advanced glaucoma and loss of vision are referred to the National Association for the Blind.

Cataract

A cataract is a clouding of the crystalline lens, resulting in opacity. It develops most commonly in persons over 50 years of age and is then classified as *senile cataract*. In a few instances it is present at birth and is then termed *congenital cataract*. It may develop secondary to trauma, exposure to radiation or extreme heat, or disease at any age. The cause of senile cataract is not known; it is suggested that an inherited predisposition to develop the characteristic lens changes plays a role. Some deficiencies in nutrients, such as vitamins C and B, or a metabolic change in the lens protein have also been suggested as possible etiologic factors. Cataract is frequently associated with diabetes mellitus. Congenital cataract occurs most often in infants whose mothers have a history of a viral infection (e.g., German measles) during the first trimester of pregnancy.

SYMPTOMS. The opacity develops very gradually and may be localized to the center of the lens, incurring early impairment of vision, or it may start in the periphery. A cataract, even in its early stage, is readily recognized through the pupil, using an ophthalmoscope. As it matures, the examiner is not able to visualize the fundus or optic disk.

The loss of the normal refractive ability of the lens prevents light rays from being focused on the retina. Vision becomes blurred and objects may appear distorted. Visual loss is very gradual and is directly proportional to the degree of opacity of the lens.

TREATMENT. The patient with a cataract is treated by surgical removal of the lens. The procedure of choice is the *intracapsular extraction* in which the lens is removed, complete with its capsule. An *extracapsular extraction* is used principally with traumatic cataracts and those in younger persons. The anterior portion of the capsule and the lens content are removed, leaving the posterior part of the capsule because of its adherence to the vitreous body. A third procedure that is used rarely is discission or "needling," in which a small opening is made in the anterior surface of the lens capsule to permit the flow of aqueous humor in and out of the lens, washing away the opaque content. The meth-

od of intracapsular extraction now commonly employed is *cryoextraction*. A probe-like instrument is introduced so that it lies against the lens and is cooled to −30° C. to −35° C. The lens and its capsule freeze to the probe and are removed when the probe is withdrawn. This procedure is less traumatizing than lens excision with forceps. A recent extraction procedure that may be used is *phacoemulsification*. It employs high-frequency ultrasonic vibrations, irrigation and aspiration. The lens is broken up and removed by suction.

Cataract extraction is done on only one eye at a time. If both eyes are involved they are treated in separate operations; these may be done during the same hospital stay.

PREOPERATIVE CARE. The preoperative preparation of the patient includes orientation to the environment, an explanation of what may be expected during and after the operation, and an opportunity for the patient and family to ask questions about the procedure and care. If it is anticipated that certain postoperative positions and activities will be restricted, the patient is advised of them and their significance.

Preoperative medication usually includes a sedative so that the patient is less apprehensive. Local anesthesia is used in cataract extraction. The surgeon may request that a mydriatic drug (e.g., atropine solution) be instilled before the patient is taken to the operating room.

POSTOPERATIVE CARE. Following the operation the patient may be kept at complete rest for at least 24 hours. The head of the bed is usually elevated 30 to 45 degrees and the patient is permitted a low pillow. Positioning when in bed is restricted to lying on the back and unoperative side for at least a week or two. The patient is usually allowed out of bed the day after surgery. Activity and ambulation may be limited at first, and the patient is cautioned not to bend over because of the risk of increasing intraocular pressure and hemorrhage. He is also advised to control coughing or sneezing, avoid straining at stool and move slowly.

A dressing and perforated metal shield are applied to the affected eye for protection. Rarely, the unoperated eye may also be covered for 1 or 2 days. Pain is not usually a problem following cataract extraction. If the patient does complain of severe pain, it is brought to the surgeon's attention immediately since it may indicate intraocular hemorrhage. The dressing is usually kept on the eye for 7 to 10 days. When the dressing has been taken off colored glasses are worn because the patient may experience discomfort with full exposure to the light, and some adaptation is necessary. Temporary glasses with thick convex lenses are used for approximately 2 months; the patient is then provided with permanent glasses or contact lenses. Most patients have some difficulty in adapting to the convex glasses; their depth and distance perception may not be accurate at first. Objects are magnified and appear closer than they really are; this may lead to errors and accidents. Precautions are necessary when using stairs or crossing a road. A patient has to learn to turn the head so that objects are brought into the central line of vision. If the patient receives contact lenses instead of glasses, the problem of objects having to be brought into the direct central line of vision is eliminated. Also, depth, distance and size perception are more accurate and less of a problem. Contact lenses are used principally with younger persons; in most instances older persons are not able to insert and remove them.

The patient's diet postoperatively starts with fluids and then, if tolerated, increased progressively from soft foods to a light diet. Vomiting should be avoided because of the associated strain.

Detachment of the Retina

Retinal detachment is separation of the retina from the choroid as a result of tears or holes in the retina. These openings permit fluid from within the eye to leak through and accumulate behind the retina, separating it from the choroid.

The cause may be degenerative retinal changes associated with the aging process, trauma or tumor. The damaged areas are usually toward the periphery of the retina.

SYMPTOMS. The manifestations appear suddenly and include flashes of light, blurred vision, floating particles in the line of vision, the sensation of a curtain coming in front of a part of the eye, restricted visual field and eventual loss of vision.

TREATMENT. The patient is placed on complete bed rest, and both eyes are covered. A mydriatic and cycloplegic drug such as cyclopentolate hydrochloride (Cyclogyl,

Mydplegic) may be prescribed for instillation to dilate the pupils and arrest accommodation by depressing ciliary action. He is positioned so that the detached area of the retina will approximate the underlying choroid. A sedative or tranquilizer is usually prescribed to reduce the patient's fear and apprehension and promote immobility.

Surgical intervention is usually undertaken fairly early. Various procedures are used, but the underlying principle is scarring of the area. As the scar tissue forms, it fills in the retinal hole and provides attachment to the underlying sclera. The surgical procedures include *electrodiathermy, cryosurgery, photocoagulation* which involves the application of heat by means of directing a very intense light into the eye (laser beam), and *scleral buckling*. In scleral buckling, the accumulated fluid is removed, the area is treated to produce scar tissue, and a fold is then made in the underlying sclera, which buckles the overlying choroid and retina, bringing them in contact.

After the operation, the patient is kept in bed at complete rest with both eyes bandaged for several days. Elevation, self-care, movement and ambulation are resumed very gradually. The patient must be cautioned against bumping the head, rapid eye movements, reading and close work.

Uveitis

Inflammation due to injury or infection may develop in the uveal tract, which includes the choroid, iris and ciliary body. It may also be associated with collagen disease (e.g., rheumatoid arthritis, sarcoidosis). The patient complains of pain, photophobia, and impaired vision in the affected eye. The pupil usually remains constricted.

Treatment may include rest of the eyes and the administration of an antimicrobial drug if infection is suspected as being the cause. A mydriatic (e.g., atropine, epinephrine) is instilled to dilate the pupil and prevent adhesions from developing between the iris and the lens. A corticoid preparation may be given systemically to arrest the inflammatory process and scar formation, since scar formation is likely to cause loss of vision.

Keratitis

This term is used for inflammation of the cornea and is a serious condition. It may be due to infection or trauma and is likely to lead to ulceration and scarring. The affected areas lose their transparency, diminishing the light rays entering the eye. Keratitis is manifested by irritation, discharge if the cause is infection, redness of the eye due to injection of the peripheral areas of the cornea by blood vessels, photophobia and tearing.

Prompt medical treatment is necessary to prevent visual damage. Keratitis frequently may be prevented by early removal of foreign bodies as well as early treatment of injuries and infection.

Treatment includes rest, the use of antimicrobial drugs, warm moist compresses, the instillation of a mydriatic and a local anesthetic solution to relieve pain. The eyes are covered to protect them from light and to keep them at rest.

Keratoconus

This is a degenerative disorder of the cornea that is seen rarely in young persons. There is a degenerative thinning and protrusion of the central cornea, usually of both eyes. Irregular astigmatism develops, causing visual impairment.

An excessive amount of fluid collects posterior to the protruding cornea and scar tissue develops as a result of the damage to tissue by stretching and rupture. The person experiences blurring of vision in the early stages but progressive changes may eventually lead to complete loss of vision. The patient may be helped at first by the wearing of hard contact lenses but may finally require keratoplasty.

Keratoplasty (Cornea Transplantation)

Loss of vision due to destruction of the cornea, keratoconus or loss of transparency may be corrected by a cornea transplantation. The central portion of the affected cornea is removed and replaced with a cornea obtained from a cadaver. The period between death and removal of the graft should not exceed 6 to 8 hours, and the transplant must be performed within 24 to 48 hours. During the interval following enucleation the donor eye is refrigerated at 4° C. to minimize degenerative changes. Rejection is less of a problem with corneal transplantation than with other types of organ transplantation. It is suggested that this is due to the avascularity of the cornea. In the absence of blood vessels,

donor tissue antigens do not get into the recipient's blood to initiate the formation of antibodies and sensitized lymphocytes. However, "10 to 15 per cent of corneal transplants are rejected."[1]

PREOPERATIVE PREPARATION. A detailed discussion of all that is involved in a keratoplasty occurs between the surgeon and the patient and family. The patient is informed that several weeks will elapse following the transplant before the results can be evaluated. If the patient elects to have the transplant, he is placed on a waiting list and should be prepared to go to the hospital on very short notice when a donor cornea becomes available.

The immediate preoperative period is as brief as possible. Blood specimens are collected for the usual preoperative blood studies, the face is thoroughly cleansed with surgical soap and the physician usually prescribes the instillation of pilocarpine 2 per cent in the affected eye to constrict the pupil so that the lens is protected during surgery. Acetazolamide (Diamox) or mannitol may be prescribed to reduce the intraocular fluid volume and tension. Local anesthesia is generally used.

TYPES OF KEROPLASTY. The operative procedure may be a penetrating keroplasty or a lamellar transplant. The *penetrating transplant* involves a full-thickness removal of the central portion of the affected cornea and replacement with an equivalent full-thickness section of the donor cornea. In a *lamellar keratoplasty,* a partial-thickness piece of the donor cornea replaces superficial layers of the recipient's cornea.

POSTOPERATIVE CARE. Both eyes may be covered for a few days; during this period the patient may require a good deal of support and assistance. The nurse observes him closely and anticipates his needs since he may be somewhat confused and unable to express his needs and feeling of distress. The patient experiences some pain, not severe, and a mild analgesic or sedative may be prescribed.

Bathroom privileges may be permitted the first postoperative day and, by the second or third day, he is allowed up as much as he wishes.

The eye is protected by a dressing and metal eye shield. The patient is cautioned not

---

[1]Linda Levenson and Jeremy Levenson: "Corneal Transplantation." Am. J. Nurs., Vol. 77, No. 7 (July 1977), pp. 1160–1163.

to stoop and to move slowly, to lie on his back or unaffected side, keep the hands away from the eye and always wear a shield or protective glasses until otherwise advised by the surgeon.

Topical medications prescribed for daily instillation for a period of time may include, in addition to a mydriatic (e.g., atropine), a corticosteroid preparation to suppress inflammation which would reduce the clearness and transparency of the cornea. A prophylactic topical antibiotic may also be used for a few days. When instilling ointments or drops, as always, precautions are observed to avoid any pressure on the eye and having the dropper or the tube applicator touch the eye.

During the weeks and months following the transplantation, the patient has alternating periods of optimism and discouragement. It is important for the patient to be informed before leaving the hospital that healing will be slow because a transparent cornea does not have blood vessels.

A family member and the patient receive demonstrations and instruction in the care of the eye and the instilling of medications in preparation for leaving the hospital. If a family member or the patient is not able to undertake the care safely, a referral may be made to a visiting nurse agency. The patient is followed closely by frequent visits to the clinic or surgeon.

Injury to the Eye

An eye may be traumatized by a foreign body, laceration or chemical. Persisting pain, loss of vision and bleeding usually manifest a serious injury.

A *foreign body* may lodge on the conjunctiva or may be embedded in the conjunctival or corneal tissue, causing inflammation and possible ulceration. In some accidents, the injury may penetrate the lens or even the retina. If a foreign body is not easily and lightly wiped off or washed out, the patient is promptly referred to a clinic or oculist. Deep metal foreign bodies may be removed by the use of a strong electric magnet.

Lacerations of the eyeball seriously threaten vision because of the formation of scar tissue in healing and by predisposing the eye to infection. Prompt treatment and strict asepsis are very important.

Various *chemicals,* acids and alkalies may cause serious irritation or burns of the conjunctiva and cornea. Emergency treatment consists of washing the eye with copious amounts of water or saline. The lids must be wide open and assistance may have to be provided in order to keep the eye open during the flushing. The person is referred to a physician as quickly as possible.

Strabismus (Squint)

Normally, both eyes perform an equal range of movement and assume corresponding lines of position when focusing on an object. Strabismus ("cross eyes") is characterized by the deviation of one eye from the position of the other. One eye (the normal or fixing eye) focuses directly on the object, but the other one (the deviating eye) appears to be focused on a different object or area.

The inequality in the movement of the eyes is due to an imbalance in the function of one or more extrinsic ocular muscles. The defect may result in the eye being turned medially, producing a convergent strabismus (*esotropia*). If the eye is turned laterally, the condition is referred to as divergent strabismus (*exotropia*). The result of the unequal movement and two points of focus is double vision (*diplopia*). Two images are formed on the retinae and the visual centers in the brain receive two sets of impulses, each producing a separate picture.

Strabismus may also be classified as being nonparalytic or paralytic and monocular or alternating. Nonparalytic strabismus (the more common) is the result of a congenital abnormality. The defect is in the central nervous system mechanism which coordinates the movements of the eyes in order to bring them into the positions that will focus the light rays from an object on corresponding areas of the two retinae. The person may be able to focus the right eye on an object of attention but the left deviates, presenting a second image. If the person has alternating strabismus, he may be able to focus first with one eye on the object, then with the other. The eye that is in the correct position is referred to as the fixing eye; the other is called the deviating eye. If it is always the same eye, the strabismus is said to be monocular.

The person with strabismus develops single vision, seeing only what the fixing or nondeviating eye perceives by involuntarily suppressing the confusing image presented by the deviating eye. Nonparalytic strabismus is generally recognized in early childhood.

Paralytic strabismus is due to the inability of the extraocular muscles to move the eye into the position corresponding to that of the other eye. As a result the person experiences diplopia. The cause of paralytic strabismus may be a defect in the muscle itself or a disturbance in the muscle innervation. The condition may be a manifestation of a disorder within the brain or orbit that interferes with the transmission of impulses by the third (oculomotor), fourth (trochlear) or sixth (abducens) cranial nerve.

TREATMENT. Strabismus requires medical treatment; unfortunately, in some instances parents think it will correct itself as the child becomes older. A delay may result in permanent damage; constant suppression of the image presented by the deviating eye may lead to loss of vision in that eye. The form of treatment will depend on the cause and severity of the strabismus. Obviously, if it is secondary to a lesion that is interrupting nerve impulses, the primary condition is surgically treated, if possible. Strabismus in the child may be corrected by the wearing of prescribed glasses. The good eye may be covered for periods to enforce the use of the deviating eye. Special eye exercises may be ordered (*orthoptics*).

If the condition does not respond to these conservative forms of treatment, surgical correction may then be undertaken. The procedure may involve shortening or lengthening of one or more extrinsic eye muscles. Following the surgery, exercise and the wearing of glasses may still be necessary for a period of time. The patient requires continued medical supervision.

Enucleation

Enculeation is the removal of an eyeball and may be necessary because of a malignant newgrowth, deep infection, severe trauma or persisting pain in a blind eye. Rarely, an enucleation is done to remove a disfiguring blind eye. When an eyeball is removed, the extrinsic muscles are severed close to their insertion, and the Tenon's capsule is retained. These may be arranged around a plastic ball to provide support and movement for an artificial eye.

Occasionally, the operation performed is an evisceration in which the contents of the eyeball are removed, leaving the sclera.

A more radical procedure may be necessary in malignancy or severe trauma. The operation performed is called *exenteration* and involves the removal of the eyeball and the surrounding structures.

Sympathetic Ophthalmia

Following an eye injury, especially a deep penetrating one, the patient may develop uveitis (inflammation of the ciliary body, choroid and iris) in the uninjured eye. This response is not understood; it has been suggested that it may be an allergic reaction to the pigment released by the damaged eye. Any redness or tearing of the uninjured eye and any complaint of photophobia, pain or loss of vision must be reported promptly. The condition may develop soon after the injury or several months or years later. Unless the inflammatory reaction is checked promptly, loss of vision results. Corticoid preparations are used locally and generally. Rarely, the injured eye is removed to prevent the sympathetic ophthalmitis from developing.

General Considerations in Nursing the Patient with an Eye Disorder

FEAR AND INSECURITY. Impairment and threatened loss of vision arouse considerable fear, insecurity and emotional reactions. All the implications which impaired vision may have in the present and future crowd in on the patient. Fears and worry may be greatly exaggerated, and the patient becomes panicky and loses control. The understanding of the nurse as to what the patient may be experiencing and the provision of emotional support contribute greatly to the care of this patient.

Factors which help to reduce the patient's anxiety include the following suggestions. The patient is carefully oriented to any new environment; if confined to bed, the orientation is by a verbal description. If he is allowed up, the verbal description is combined with helping him to explore it. An explanation is made of how the usual daily needs will be met.

The patient is given the opportunity and encouragement to express concerns and to ask questions. The person who cannot see is spoken to as he is approached and is advised who it is. If the nurse is working in the room but not with the patient, he is told. Anything that is going to be done for him is outlined (e.g., treatment, investigative procedure). It means a great deal to the patient to always have the call button within reach; it reassures him that help is always at hand. He should not be left alone for long periods; he may not require a lot of physical care but still requires support and contacts. The nurse takes time to converse with the patient; the flowers and cards which he receives and details of the environment are described vividly. He has visual memory from which he can recall sufficiently to form a mental picture of that being described. Some appropriate form of diversion, such as a radio, visitors to chat with the patient or read to him, and records, is provided. Noisy, confusing situations are avoided; if in darkness, the patient becomes more alert and is more sensitive to sounds and voice inflections. An effort is made to anticipate the patient's needs.

PREVENTION OF INJURY. Adequate orientation and frequent observations are important to prevent accidents when the patient's vision is seriously impaired. Side rails are placed on the bed until he is accustomed to the situation. If the patient is disoriented, it may be necessary to have someone remain with him to insure his safety. The environment must be checked carefully for any hazards for the unseeing, ambulatory person. He should be escorted around the area until he becomes familiar with it. Stools, rugs or other such articles over which he might trip are removed. Furniture is not moved from its original position, and doors are kept closed or wide open. The person is cautioned about nearby stairs and radiators.

OBSERVATIONS. The nurse is required to be familiar with any specific observations that are important in certain eye disorders. Generally, significant factors that should be brought promptly to the physician's attention include elevation of temperature, discharge, unrelieved pain, headache, retraction of the eyelid, any evidence of disturbance in the unaffected eye, drying of the cornea, and signs of bleeding in the anterior chamber.

POSITIONING AND ACTIVITY. The position which the patient with an acute eye disorder is to assume varies with different conditions and is usually indicated by the physician. For instance, if increased intraocular pressure is a concern, as in glaucoma, the head of the bed is elevated; if detachment of the retina occurs, the patient is kept flat; following a cataract extraction, some surgeons require the patient to lie flat for a stated period of time and others permit the

head of the bed to be elevated 30 to 45 degrees. Usually, if the patient with an eye disorder is permitted to turn, he lies on the side of the unaffected eye only. Prolonged restriction of activity is rare; patients worry less and have fewer complications when allowed up as soon as possible. If the patient is required to remain in bed, lying flat with the head immobilized, the arms and lower limbs are moved through a range of motion, and active exercises of the legs are begun as soon as the physician permits.

INFECTION. Infection within the eye can be very serious and may lead to loss of vision. Strict asepsis is observed in all eye treatments. Clean dressings are done before infected ones. If both eyes are infected, separate equipment is used for each one. If only one eye is infected, precautions are taken to protect the unaffected eye. For instance, when irrigating or cleaning the affected eye, the nurse works from the inner canthus toward the outer corner, making sure no fluid escapes over the bridge of the nose into the other eye. In conjunctivitis, the eyes are left exposed; frequent cleansing may be necessary to remove the discharge and crustations.

DRESSINGS AND INSTILLATIONS. In order to keep the affected eye at rest, the unaffected eye may be covered. Adaptation to light is resumed gradually; the unaffected eye may first be exposed by wearing a shield with a small central opening. This minimizes eye movement. A similar shield may also be used later on the affected eye. Extreme gentleness is used when changing a dressing or doing any treatment; caution is used to avoid pressure on the eyeball.

Preparations of drugs used for instillations should be fresh; the labels carry the date of expiration. A fresh sterile dropper is used for each solution. Drops are placed on the inside of the lower lid and not directly on the eyeball to avoid reflex squeezing of the eye.

NUTRITION. The patient frequently experiences anorexia due to anxiety and because of the difficulty with taking food when he cannot see. The necessary assistance is provided and, when feeding him, the food is described; only small amounts are offered to avoid choking and coughing, since coughing raises the intraocular pressure. As soon as the patient is well enough, he is encouraged to start feeding himself and to become independent. Assistance is withdrawn gradually, not all at once.

ELIMINATION. Constipation and straining at stool are avoided, since they tend to cause an elevation in the intraocular pressure. A mild laxative may be administered and the diet modified to encourage normal bowel evacuation.

PREOPERATIVE PREPARATION. The surgeon advises the patient and family of the anticipated surgery, but the nurse is prepared to clarify the explanation and answer their questions. Many eye operations are performed under local anesthesia; the patient is told what to expect and is cautioned against squeezing the eye during operation. Any anticipated postoperative restrictions in activities and positioning and their significance are explained. A cleansing enema is usually given the night before operation unless the intraocular pressure is elevated above normal. Food and fluid are withheld the morning of operation if a general anesthetic is to be used. If the patient is to have local anesthesia, a fluid or soft diet may be given at breakfast.

A specific directive is received as to the local preparation required. The area around the eye is thoroughly cleansed but not shaved, and drops (e.g., mydriatic, miotic, prophylactic antibiotic and local anesthetic preparations) are generally instilled 1 or 2 hours before the scheduled time.

REHABILITATION OF THE BLIND. The patient with marked visual impairment or with total loss of vision needs a great deal of assistance in adjusting to the situation. He must be persuaded that life still holds something for him. Emphasis is placed on what he can do. He still has visual memory of form, color, and space and can learn that other senses can be put to greater use.

The development of independence is started as soon as possible, beginning with self-care (feeding, bathing, dressing and hair). He is assisted with moving about the room and then from room to room, locating furniture and necessary articles by touch. The environment is organized to provide safety. Furniture is left in the same place unless he is advised and oriented to its new position; rugs, footstools and other such hazardous objects are removed. Doors are kept wide open or closed.

Anyone walking with a blind person allows him to take an arm rather than grasping his and pushing. Writing is practiced, beginning with the signing of his name. Differentiation by touch is also tested and practiced. The person learns to tell the time by opening the crystal of a watch.

Various forms of diversion and recreation are introduced (records of books and music, radio, games). The patient is referred to the national associations for the blind,[2] which provide vocational training, assistance in learning Braille and in finding a job, recreation, transportation, and financial assistance when necessary. The use of the white cane is introduced and the necessary guidance given on excursions beyond the house until the person is capable of safely getting around alone.

The patient and family are advised of the financial assistance available for the blind and are assisted in making application for it. The family may require help in accepting the blind patient and in organizing the home environment in the interest of his safety and independence.

---

[2]The Canadian National Institute for the Blind, 1929 Bayview Avenue, Toronto, Ontario, Canada.

The American Foundation for the Blind, 15 W. 16th Street, New York, New York, U.S.A.

References

Books

Keeney, Arthur H.: Ocular Examination, 2nd. ed. St. Louis, C. V. Mosby, 1976.

Krupp, Marcus A., and Chatton, Milton, J.: Current Medical Diagnosis and Treatment. Los Altos, Cal., Lange, 1975. Chapter 4.

Martin-Doyle, J. C., and Kemp, Martin, H.: A Synopsis of Ophthalmology, 5th. ed. Bristol, England, J. Wright, 1975.

Meredith, Travis A.: The Eye: Disease, Diagnosis, Treatment. Englewood Cliffs, N.J., Prentice-Hall, 1975.

Nave, Carl R., and Nave, Brenda C.: Physics for the Health Sciences. Philadelphia, W. B. Saunders, 1975. Chapter 19.

Scheie, Harold G., and Albert, Daniel M.: Textbook of Ophthamology, 9th ed. Philadelphia, W. B. Saunders, 1977.

Vaughn, Daniel, and Asbury, Taylor: General Ophthamology, 8th. ed. Los Altos, Cal., Lange, 1977.

Periodicals

Allen, Henry Freeman (Ed.): "Symposium: Insight into the Aging Eye." Geriatrics, Part 1, Vol. 30, No. 4 (April 1975); Part 2, Vol. 30, No. 5 (May 1975).

Ammon, Lillian Louise: "Surviving Enucleation." Am. J. Nurs., Vol. 72, No. 10 (Oct. 1972), pp. 1817–1821.

Boyd-Monk, Heather: "Helping the Corneal Transplant Patient to See Again." Nurs. '78, Vol. 8, No. 2 (Feb. 1978), pp. 47–51.

Chodil, J., and Williams, B.: "The Concept of Sensory Deprivation." Nurs. Clin. North Am., Vol. 5, No. 3 (Sept. 1970), pp. 453–465.

Dupont, Jeanne: "What To Do For Common Eye Emergencies." Nurs. '76, Vol. 6, No. 5 (May 1976), pp. 17–19.

Fernsebner, Wilhelmina: "Early Diagnosis of Acute Angle-Closure Glaucoma." Am. J. Nrus., Vol. 75, No. 7 (July 1975), pp. 1154–1155.

French, Eileen: "Glaucoma: Awareness Prevents Blindness." Can. Nurse, Vol. 73, No. 10 (Oct. 1977), pp. 20–25.

Gould, Herman: "How To Remove Contact Lenses from Comatose Patients." Am. J. Nurs., Vol. 76, No. 9 (Sept. 1976), pp. 1483–1485.

Hiles, David A.: "Strabismus." Am. J. Nurs., Vol. 74, No. 6 (June 1974), pp. 1082–1089.

Kahn, Howard: "Visual Dysfunctions." Nurs. '74, Vol. 4, No. 10 (Oct. 1974), pp. 26–27.

Kwitko, Marvin L.: "New Lenses for Old: A Promising Method of Treating Cataracts." Can. Nurse, Vol. 71, No. 11 (Nov. 1975), pp. 34–38.

Levenson, Linda, and Levenson, Jeremy: "Corneal Transplantation." Am. J. Nurs., Vol. 77, No. 7 (July 1977), pp. 1160–1163.

Marmor, Michael F.: "The Eye and Vision in the Elderly." Geriatrics, Vol. 32, No. 8 (Aug. 1977), pp. 63–67.

Mechner, Francis: "Examination of the Eye." Am. J. Nurs., Vol. 74, No. 11 (Nov. 1974), pp. 2039–2062.

Ohno, Mary I.: "The Eye-Patched Patient." Am. J. Nurs., Vol. 71, No. 2 (Feb. 1971), pp. 271–274.

Rooney, Maureen: "Children With Strabismus." Can. Nurse, Vol. 74, No. 1 (Jan. 1978), pp. 24–27.

Smith, Joan F., and Nachazel, Delbert: "Retinal Detachment." Am. J. Nurs., Vol. 73, No. 9 (Sept. 1973), pp. 1530–1535.

Steenburg, Yvonne, et al.: "Eye Enucleation." Nurs. '74, Vol. 4, No. 8 (Aug. 1974), p. 14.

Weinstock, Frank J.: "Emergency Treatment of Eye Injuries." Am. J. Nurs., Vol. 71, No. 10 (Oct. 1971), pp. 1928–1931.

28

Nursing in Disorders of the Ear

STRUCTURE AND FUNCTIONS OF THE EAR

The ear is concerned with the special sense of hearing as well as with the maintenance of equilibrium. It has three divisions: the external and middle ears for the collection and conduction of sound waves and the internal ear, which actually serves as the receptor. The eighth cranial (auditory or acoustic) nerve provides the afferent impulse pathway of the sensory unit. Part of its fibers carry impulses to the interpretive centers for sound in the temporal lobes, and the others transmit impulses to areas of the brain stem and cerebellum associated with control of body posture.

Ear Structure (Fig. 28–1)

EXTERNAL EAR. The outer ear consists of the *auricle (pinna)* and the external auditory meatus. The auricle is an immobile cartilaginous framework covered with skin and may contribute slightly to the collection of sound waves. The external auditory meatus is an S-shaped tube approximately 1 inch long. The tube ends at the tympanic membrane (eardrum), which separates the

external and middle ears. The skin lining the canal is covered with fine hairs near the opening and has special glands which produce a yellow waxy secretion called *cerumen* for protection against insects and dust particles. The *tympanic membrane* is a thin, semitransparent membrane covered externally with skin and internally with mucous membrane which is continuous with that which lines the middle ear cavity. The middle layer is composed of thin elastic and fibrous tissue. A white streak is normally seen extending from the periphery towards the center; this is the handle of the malleus in the middle ear (Fig. 28–2).

MIDDLE EAR. This portion of the ear is contained within a small cavity in the temporal bone. The cavity communicates with the nasopharynx by means of the *eustachian or auditory tube* and with the mastoid cells. The eustachian tube permits the entrance of air into the middle ear; this equalizes the pressure on the internal surface of the eardrum with atmospheric pressure (that which is exerted on the external surface of the drum). The cavity is lined with mucous membrane which is continuous with that of the eustachian tube and mastoid cells. The *mastoid cells* are small air spaces within the posterior portion of the

998

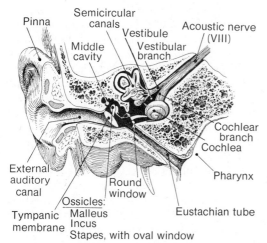

FIGURE 28–1 The parts of the ear.

temporal bone, just behind the middle ear. Obviously, the continuity of the lining membrane provides a ready means for the spread of infection from the throat to the middle ear and from the middle ear to the mastoid.

The middle ear cavity contains three small bones called the auditory ossicles, which are movable for the purpose of transmitting sound vibrations. The first ossicle, the *malleus,* is attached to the eardrum and articulates with the second ossicle, the *incus.* The incus articulates with the third ossicle, the *stapes,* which is attached to the membranous oval window (fenestra ovalis) that leads into the internal ear. The middle ear also has two small muscles; one, the tensor tympani, is inserted on the malleus and the other, the stapedius, is inserted on the foot plate of the stapes. Contraction of these muscles re-

duces the amplitude of the sound waves entering the middle ear and cochlea.

INTERNAL EAR (LABYRINTH). The inner ear consists of a system of irregularly shaped cavities which contain fluid and complex membranous structures which initiate nerve impulses as a result of sound waves or change of position. The *bony (osseous) labyrinth* is divided into a series of channels — the cochlea, vestibule and semicircular canals. Within the bony labyrinth is a membranous labyrinth which conforms fairly closely to the shape of the bony-walled cavities (Fig. 28–3). The fluid contained within the osseous cavities is called *perilymph,* and that within the membranous cavities is known as *endolymph.*

The complex snail-shaped structure, the *cochlea,* consists of three tubes wound two to three times around a central column called the modiolus. The channels formed by the tubes are called the scala vestibuli, scala media (cochlear duct) and scala tympani (Fig. 28–4). The scala vestibuli is closed at one end by the membrane of the oval window. As a result, vibrations transmitted to the membrane by the stapes set up waves in the fluid within the scala vestibuli. The scala vestibuli communicates with the scala tympani at the apex of the cochlea so that when the fluid within the scala vestibuli is set in motion, the fluid in the scala tympani is similarly affected. The base of the scala tympani is closed off by the membrane covering an opening into the middle ear which is known as the *round window (fenestra rotunda).*

The scala media is walled off from the scala vestibuli by Reissner's membrane and from the scala tympani by the basilar mem-

FIGURE 28–2 Diagram of tympanic membrane (ear drum). (From Sabiston, David C., Jr. (Ed.): Davis-Christopher Textbook of Surgery, 11th ed. Philadelphia, W. B. Saunders, 1977, p. 1398.)

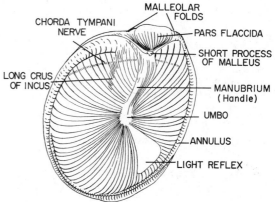

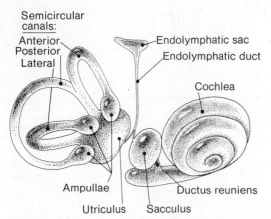

Semicircular canals:
Anterior
Posterior
Lateral

Endolymphatic sac
Endolymphatic duct

Cochlea

Ampullae

Ductus reuniens

Utriculus   Sacculus

FIGURE 28–3   The membranous labyrinth in the ear.

sists of three *semicircular canals* hollowed out of the temporal bone at right angles to each other. They communicate with the osseous vestibule and contain perilymph. Three semicircular membranous ducts suspended within the osseous canals contain endolymph and communicate with the utricle. Each membranous semicircular canal has a dilated portion at one end, called the ampulla, which contains special sensory hair cells, forming the *crista acustica,* or crista ampullaris. The crista is sensitive to movement of the endolymph within the ampulla and initiates neural impulses that are transmitted by the vestibular portion of the acoustic (eighth cranial) nerve to the central nervous system.

brane. On the surface of the basilar membrane are special cells with hair-like projections which collectively are known as the organ of Corti. Contained within the organ of Corti are receptor cells which produce auditory nerve impulses when stimulated by vibrations of the basilar membrane (see Fig. 28–5).

The *vestibule* lies between the cochlea and the semicircular canals. The bony-walled cavity contains perilymph. The suspended membranous portion is divided into two sacs, called the utricle and the saccule, which contain endolymph. Within these cavities are hair-like projections and calcium carbonate concretions (otoliths) which respond to movements of the head by giving rise to neural impulses concerned with the maintenance of equilibrium.

The third division of the inner ear con-

Auditory Pathway

Sound waves passing into the external ear strike the tympanic membrane, causing it to vibrate with the same frequency as the sound waves. This in turn results in vibrations of the ossicles in the middle ear. The stapes, being attached to the oval window, causes its membrane to move in and out. The ossicles serve as amplifiers but, if the amplitude of the waves is excessive, producing excessive loudness, the vibrations may be modified by contraction of the tensor tympani and the stapedius. The tensor tympani decreases tympanic membrane contractions and the stapedius pulls the stapes away from the oval window, reducing the force of the vibrations which strike the oval window. The vibrations are transferred into the perilymph of the scala ves-

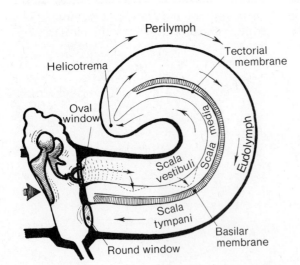

Perilymph

Tectorial membrane

Helicotrema

Oval window

Scala media

Endolymph

Scala vestibuli

Scala tympani

Basilar membrane

Round window

FIGURE 28–4   Schematic drawing of the cochlea.

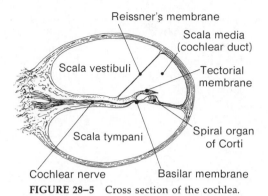

FIGURE 28–5   Cross section of the cochlea.

tibuli of the inner ear and in turn through the Reissner's membrane and through the endolymph in the scala media to the basilar membrane. Movements of the endolymph and basilar membrane stimulate the receptor cells of the organ of Corti, initiating neural impulses which are transmitted via nerve fibers to a ganglion in the central core (the modiolus) of the cochlea. The axons of the ganglionic neurons form the cochlear branch of the acoustic (eighth cranial) nerve. The cochlear branch synapses with a group of neurons in the medulla (cochlear nucleus). The impulses are then transmitted to the inferior colliculi which are the centers for auditory startle reflexes, through the thalami and eventually reach a cortical area of the temporal lobe (auditory center) where they are interpreted as sound. Each ear delivers impulses to both auditory centers.

The movements of the perilymph, initiated by the vibrations of the oval window, are transmitted through the helicotrema (communicating channel between the scalae at the apex of the cochlea) to the scala tympani and subsequently to the membrane of the fenestra rotunda (round window).

Pitch and Intensity of Sound

The pitch of a sound depends upon the frequency of the vibrations (number per second). The number of vibrations or cycles per second (CPS) are expressed as a unit of frequency referred to as a hertz (Hz) which is used in measuring the pitch of sound. The fibers of the basilar membrane vary in length. It is thought that different frequencies stimulate selective areas of fibers and cells of the membrane — that is, each place on the basilar membrane is sensitive to sound waves of a certain frequency.

The intensity, or loudness, of a sound depends upon the amplitude or force of movement of the vibrations. The louder the sound, the greater is the displacement back and forth.

Physical Equilibrium

When the head moves, neural impulses originate in the crista acustica of the semicircular canals and the maculae acusticae of the utricle and saccula and are transmitted by nerve fibers which form the vestibular branch of the acoustic nerve. The vestibular nerve fibers pass to groups of neurons (vestibular nuclei) in the brain stem from which impulses may be delivered to the cerebellum, reticular formation, down the vestibulospinal tracts to motor neurons which innervate skeletal muscle, the oculomotor center and the thalami. The principal purpose of these impulses is to orient the person in space, and reflexly stimulate muscles so that he may assume an upright position or maintain the position that has been assumed against gravity.

AUDITORY DISORDERS

LOSS OF HEARING

The incidence of loss of hearing in varying degrees is very high and, in many instances, the person is unaware of it until it is well advanced. Hearing limitations interfere with the ability to communicate with others, which is extremely important. It may also result in the individual not being alerted to a threatening object or situation. Obviously, the effects and problems vary with the degree of loss and the age at which it developed. In the child, it retards development, affecting the learning of speech and normal adjustment within society. It creates physical, emotional and socioeconomic problems for both the person and family.

The degree of loss of hearing may be indicated by classifying those affected as "hard of hearing" or "deaf." The hearing is defective in those who are hard of hearing but is not totally absent. They have sufficient hearing, either with or without the use of a hearing aid, to cope with ordinary activities. Persons who are described as deaf have a marked or total loss of hearing that makes it very difficult, if not impossible, to function normally.

Manifestations of Impaired Hearing

Indications of a hearing deficit may include failure to respond when addressed, frequent requests for repetition, and misinterpretation of what was said, especially of words that sound alike. A short attention span or lack of attention, lack of interest, a strained confused expression, turning of the head to direct the "good" ear to the source of sound, irritability because of the strain and withdrawal from the group may be manifested. Changes in speech, such as a lack of inflections, and a low or excessive volume, may also develop. A person with conductive deafness tends to speak softly; the person with nerve deafness usually speaks loudly.

In the case of a child, impaired hearing may be suspected if there is a failure in the development of speech, a lack of normal progress in school, no response to voice or sound, or no interest in noisemaking toys. The severity of the speech defect depends on when the hearing deficit developed and the degree of loss. If the person is partially deaf with loss for high frequency (high pitched) sounds, he may hear vowels but not consonants. The deaf child responds more readily to movements than to sound and, when in need of comfort and reassurance, responds to cuddling or touch rather than to verbal expressions. He may develop and persistently use gestures to indicate needs or wishes rather than producing vocal expressions.

Classification and Causes of Loss of Hearing

A hearing deficit may be congenital or acquired and may be classified as conductive, sensorineural, central or combined.

In a *conductive hearing loss,* sound waves fail to reach the internal ear as a result of some disturbance in the external ear, middle ear or the oval window (fenestra ovalis).

In *sensorineural deafness,* which may also be called *nerve or perceptive deafness,* the disorder is located in the organ of Corti, cochlear division of the acoustic nerve, or auditory impulse pathway or center within the brain.

Central hearing loss denotes a hearing deficit resulting from disturbances within the brain, principally the auditory center in the temporal lobe.

Combined hearing loss occurs because of impairment within both the conductive and neural auditory mechanisms.

Congenital loss of hearing may be due to a prenatal malformation or lack of development of a part of the auditory apparatus. Heredity may play a role, or it may be the result of a viral infection in the mother during the first trimester of the pregnancy, the effect of a toxic drug taken by the mother during pregnancy, hypoxia or a birth injury.

Acquired impairment of hearing may be caused by obstruction of the external auditory canal by a foreign body or impacted cerumen, infection (e.g., otitis media, labyrinthitis, meningitis), a newgrowth (e.g., acoustic neuroma), an ototoxic drug (e.g., streptomycin, quinine), trauma associated with a skull fracture or excessively loud noise, obstruction of the eustachian tube, or degenerative changes in the auditory pathway frequently associated with the aging process (presbycusis).

Assessment and Investigation of the Ear

Assessment of the ear may include inspection of the external ear, tests for eustachian tube patency, evaluation of hearing, labyrinth tests, a roentgenogram of the mastoid region, blood tests, and cultures. Obviously, the selection of investigational procedures depends upon the presenting signs and symptoms.

INSPECTION OF THE EXTERNAL EAR. The ear is inspected inside and outside. The pinna (auricle) is examined for lesions and the mastoid process is palpated, especially if infection of the middle ear is suspected. The inside of the auditory canal is inspected with an otoscope which has a magnifying lens in addition to providing a light. The canal is inspected for lesions, foreign bodies and the amount and characteristics of the cerumen (wax). The tympanic membrane is viewed and the color (normal:light pearl-gray) and tension noted. It is examined for retraction or bulging, increased vascularity and perforation(s). During examination of the tympanic membrane, the patient is asked to take a breath and then to try to exhale forcibly through the nose with it tightly pinched and the lips closed. The normal eustachian tube opens to admit air into the middle ear and the tympanic membrane may be seen to move outward. This latter procedure is referred to as the Valsalva method of testing the patency of the eustachian tube.

HEARING EVALUATION. In hearing evaluation, the examiner assesses the degree of hearing loss and establishes whether it is due to conductive or sensorineural impairment.

TUNING FORK TESTS. These are used to differentiate the type of deafness. The tuning fork may produce a frequency of 512 or 1024 cycles per second (cps). The tests should be made in a room free of noise.

Rinne Test. The fork is set in vibration and the stem is held alternately against the mastoid process and 1 to 2 inches in front of the entrance to the external auditory canal, to determine whether the loss of hearing is conductive or sensorineural. In each instance, the patient is asked whether he hears the sounds and to indicate when they become inaudible. He also indicates whether the sound, if heard, is greater in one position than in the other. (In the normal ear, air is a better conductor than bone.) If the patient responds negatively when the fork is held in front of the ear, or if he hears the sound longer by bone conduction, a conduction loss is indicated and the Rinne test is reported as negative.

The procedure may be carried out by placing the prongs of the vibratory fork in front of the external auditory meatus. When the patient indicates that the sounds are inaudible, the stem is transferred to the mastoid process; if sound is heard, conduction impairment is indicated.

Weber's Test. This test is used to compare the degree of impaired hearing in the two ears. The fork is set in vibration, the stem is held against the middle of the forehead or the vortex and the patient is asked if he hears the sound better in one ear than the other. If the sound is heard better in one ear than the other, conductive deafness

is present in that ear or in greater degree than in the other ear. If the sound is heard equally well in both ears, the hearing loss is the same in both ears.

In neural loss of hearing, if the middle ear is normal, the sound will be louder in the ear with conductive loss of hearing than in the ear with the normal conductive system and sensorineural impairment.

Thus, if the sound is louder in one ear there may be conductive loss of hearing in that ear or there may be a sensorineural deafness in the other ear.

Schwabach Test. This test compares the patient's bone conduction with that of the examiner, whose hearing is normal. The tuning fork is set in vibration and the stem is placed against the patient's mastoid process. The patient is instructed to indicate when the sound becomes inaudible. The stem of the tuning fork is then transferred to the mastoid bone of the examiner. If the sound is still audible to the latter, the patient has some sensorineural loss of hearing.

VOICE TEST. The patient's ability to hear the normal speaking voice and then the whispered voice is tested in a room free of sounds. The ear opposite to the one being tested is covered. The normal ear can hear the spoken word at 20 feet and the whisper at 15 feet.

AUDIOMETRIC TESTS. These tests provide information as to the degree of hearing loss. The unit used to express the intensity (or loudness) of sound is the *decibel*. The audiometer is operated to produce sounds of known intensity and frequency (cps). Hearing is evaluated by recording the minimum intensity of sounds of various frequencies that are just audible to the patient.

Audiometric tests are conducted in a soundproof room and the patient wears earphones. The audiometric methods of assessing hearing that are commonly used are the pure-tone and speech tests.

Pure-Tone Audiometry. The audiometer produces a range of pure tones of varying frequencies (cps or Hz). The intensity is adjusted in 5-decibel steps. The procedure is explained to the patient before the earphones are put on, and he is instructed as to when and how to signal. The test commences with a sound of high intensity which is gradually reduced to below the patient's threshold of hearing sound. The patient signals when the sound disappears. The intensity then is increased very slowly until the patient signals that the tone is just discernible. A range of frequencies is used, and the threshold intensity for each frequency is recorded on a chart called an audiogram. This indicates any hearing loss and the range of tones most affected. The test may be made of bone or air conduction. The greater the number of decibels recorded at which sound is perceived, the greater is the degree of defective hearing. The symbol O on the graph represents the right ear in air conduction, X the left ear in air conduction, [the right ear in bone conduction and] the left ear in bone conduction.

Speech Audiometry. In this test, a recording of lists of words representing normal vocabulary sounds is played at varying volumes. The patient indicates the words he hears. The percentage of words correctly heard for each intensity is recorded.

Speech audiometry plays an important role in diagnosing the type of deafness and is especially helpful in the selection of a hearing aid.

LABYRINTH TESTS.[1] Tests used to assess the function of the labyrinth of the internal ear involve observing responses to certain stimuli. Strong stimulation normally produces vertigo or the falling to one side, nystagmus (involuntary, rhythmic eye movement) and nausea.

ROTATION TEST. The patient is seated in a chair that can be rotated, with the head tilted forward and the eyes closed. The chair is rotated quickly for ten full turns and stopped suddenly. The patient is asked to look at the physician's finger which is held in front of the patient. Nystagmus is a normal response and its duration is timed. It should continue for about 25 to 40 seconds.

CALORIC TEST. This test is also used in neurological investigation of the vestibular portion of the acoustic (VIII) nerve (see p. 835). The nystagmus is timed, and past-pointing and testing for swaying to one side may be done. The test is carried out in each ear. Pathologic disturbances in the

---

[1]*Note:* Since the labyrinth tests may cause vertigo, nausea and vomiting, the nurse remains with the patient, prepared to provide the necessary support and assistance. Precautions are taken to prevent possible falls when the patient moves or attempts to walk.

labyrinth may result in an absence of responses or excessive reaction.

ELECTRONYSTAGMOGRAPHY. This is an electroencephalographic recording of the eye movements in nystagmus. A study is made of the frequency, speed and amplitude of the eye movements. The recording is carried out in darkness or with the eyes closed to prevent fixation which suppresses nystagmus.

ROENTGENOGRAM. An x-ray examination of the temporal bone may be done to determine if mastoiditis has developed.

BLOOD EXAMINATIONS. Leukocyte and differential cell counts may be ordered if acute infection of the middle ear or labyrinthitis is suspected. In the case of acute infection and inflammation, the leukocyte count is usually above normal, the increase being principally in neutrophils.

CULTURE. Any discharge from the ear is usually cultured as soon as observed in order to identify the causative organism. Sensitivity tests to antibiotics may also be done.

PRESERVATION OF HEARING

Nurses, especially those working with industrial workers and schoolchildren, have an important role in the prevention of hearing loss. The public requires education about the causes and early signs of impaired hearing and significant preventive measures.

Good prenatal care and the avoidance of contact with persons with measles or other viral infections are important in preventing congenital deafness. Prompt treatment of respiratory infection and infectious diseases may allay the complication of otitis media. Prompt medical treatment and follow-up are urged for persons with an ear disorder.

The danger of introducing foreign objects into the external ear canal should be emphasized; for example, cleansing the ear with applicators, matches and hairpins is dangerous. If the wax (cerumen) becomes dry and impacted or an insect or foreign body becomes lodged in the canal, a few drops of warm oil or glycerin may be instilled and followed by a warm water or normal saline irrigation in a few minutes. If this does not remove the foreign object or impacted wax, the person is advised to seek medical attention promptly.

Routine tests of schoolchildren's hearing are important so that early recognition may be made of any impairment. Teachers and school nurses must be familiar with manifestations of a hearing deficit.

The nurse caring for a patient receiving a preparation of streptomycin or quinine must be alert for early signs of damage to the hearing.

The occupational health nurse, especially in an industry in which there is prolonged, intense noise in the work environment, must be cognizant of the possibility of noise-induced hearing loss. Frequently the employees tend to accept noise simply as a necessary part of the occupation and do not realize that hearing damage may be insidiously developing. Gradual loss of hearing usually involves, first, failure of response to high frequency sounds. Later, areas of the cochlea which respond to lower frequencies become damaged. In order to protect persons exposed to noise that endangers hearing, protective devices in the form of earmuffs, ear plugs or a special helmet should be provided. Employees should receive regular hearing tests and be exposed to an active educational program.

SUGGESTIONS TO THOSE SPEAKING TO A PERSON WHO IS HARD OF HEARING

Do not speak until you have the person's attention. The speaker's face should be in full view of the listener so that he has the opportunity to observe lip movement.

Determine which is the better ear and go to that side if possible. Look directly at the listener.

Speak slowly, enunciate clearly and avoid raising the pitch of voice. The volume is increased, but actual shouting is avoided. Guard against running words together. The natural form of conversation is used rather than broken statements and incomplete sentences.

Exaggerated lip movement only confuses the listener.

If repetition is necessary, rephrasing the communication may be helpful; remember that vowels are heard more readily than consonants.

Patience, tact and understanding are needed. Avoid any irritation or annoyance; such reactions on the part of the speaker only discourage the listener.

Do not prolong a conversation unnecessarily, since the listener tires under the strain.

If a hearing aid is used, give the person time to adjust it. Do not get within 4 to 5 feet of the aid and use natural volume and tone.

A misinterpretation must not be ridiculed or treated as a joke.

When a deaf person enters a room, an effort is made to draw him into the group. He is advised of the topic of conversation and is encouraged and given the opportunity to participate. Otherwise, he tends to withdraw and become isolated.

If it is not possible to communicate verbally, write the message.

If a patient is totally deaf and does not lip-read, pictures or symbols that represent objects may be helpful to orient the patient and for use during hospitalization.

SUGGESTIONS TO THOSE WHO ARE HARD OF HEARING

Look directly at the speaker, since observation of lip movements proves helpful.

Concentrate on the speaker.

Observe the total situation, since this may give a lead to the topic of conversation.

Acknowledge your hearing deficit; do not guess at things rather than ask for repetition.

ASSISTANCE AND HEARING AIDS

Some persons with a hearing deficit may be helped by using a hearing aid, which is a small, battery-operated instrument which amplifies sounds. Aids are helpful to persons who have reduced conduction of sound waves into the inner ear. Few of those with sensorineural loss of hearing receive help from hearing aids; amplification of sound does not assist with the distortion and impaired discrimination resulting from impairment of the neural elements of the auditory apparatus. Before purchasing a hearing aid, the person with a hearing deficit should be examined by a physician for evaluation of the residual hearing and identification of the type of hearing loss. *The selection of the aid is based on the patient's particular type of hearing loss.* If an aid is recommended, it should be worn for a trial period to determine if it does help.

Those who are deaf or hard of hearing and their families should be familiar with the American or Canadian Hearing Association and its local branches.[2] Assistance may be provided in the form of procuring medical examination and treatment, counseling as to the type of hearing aid that would be helpful, obtaining vocational training and employment, arranging for special classes (e.g., speech) and obtaining printed advice in pamphlets.

COMMON DISORDERS OF THE EAR

Impacted Cerumen

The normal secretion of the external auditory canal (cerumen) may accumulate and become hard and dry. The retention may be due to abnormal narrowness of the canal, dryness of the skin or excess hair in the canal, or it may be associated with the person's occupation. It is a common problem for those working in a dusty environment.

Symptoms develop with the obstruction of the canal; the person may experience a sense of fullness, noises, loss of hearing or, rarely, a cough. The latter is a reflex response to stimulation of the vagus nerve. Examination of the ear with an otoscope reveals a firm yellow or dark mass.

Removal of the mass may be by the instillation of a warm solution of oil to soften it, followed by irrigation with warm water. It is important that any solution introduced into the ear be warmed to approximately 40° C. (104° F.); cold or hot solutions may stimulate the labyrinth and cause nystagmus, vertigo and nausea. If the mass cannot be removed by irrigation, the physician may remove it with a dull-ring curette.

External Otitis

This is a generalized inflammation of the external ear that may vary in severity from a mild dermatitis to cellulitis. The tympanic membrane may be affected. The causative factor is usually bacteria but, in some instances may be a fungus. A predisposing factor is moisture in the ear. The infection is more likely to develop in a warm moist atmosphere or if the person swims frequently. It may be secondary to trauma inflicted by efforts to remove wax. External otitis may also be due to allergic dermatitis.

SYMPTOMS. The patient may complain of pruritus if the disorder is dermatitis, and the skin may be dry and scaly at first. If the cause is infection, the ear is painful and examination may reveal redness, swelling, edema and purulent lesions. An elevation of temperature and increased leukocyte count indicate a serious infection.

TREATMENT. Ear irrigations and the topical application of an antibiotic preparation are prescribed in the case of infection of the canal. If allergic dermatitis is the cause a corticosteroid ointment or solution may be prescribed. Inflammation of the auricle (pinna) may be treated by warm compresses.

The patient with severe infectious otitis that has extended beyond the skin receives an oral or parenteral antimicrobial preparation as well as local treatment. An analgesic may also be necessary to provide relief from the pain.

Acute Otitis Media

This is an inflammation of the middle ear and is most often due to infection that has gained access through the eustachian tube. Rarely, the organisms may have entered through a perforation in the tympanic membrane. It is frequently a complication of a respiratory infection or an infectious disease such as measles. The disorder is usually acute but may become chronic.

The initial inflammatory response causes congestion and swelling of the mucous membrane lining of the middle ear, and the cavity fills with exudate. The tympanic membrane bulges externally and, unless the infection is checked, the exudate generally becomes purulent. If the cavity is not surgically drained, the tympanic membrane may rupture spontaneously.

MANIFESTATIONS. The patient with otitis media experiences a sensation of fullness in the ear and dullness of hearing at

---

[2]The Canadian Hearing Society, 60 Bedford Road, Toronto, Ontario, Canada.

The National Association of Hearing and Speech Agencies, 18th St. N.W., Washington, D.C.

first, then severe pain, and increasing loss of hearing because of failure of the conduction of sound waves through the middle ear. The temperature and leukocyte count are elevated, and the patient feels generally ill. Examination of the eardrum by means of an otoscope reveals redness, hyperemia and external bulging due to the pressure of the collection of exudate in the middle ear, or rupture and drainage of the advanced stage.

TREATMENT. The patient is given an antibiotic and, if the infection has progressed to the suppurative stage, the eardrum is surgically opened to permit drainage. The operative procedure is referred to as a *myringotomy*. Incision and drainage is preferable to leaving the condition until there is spontaneous rupture of the tympanic membrane. Such delay predisposes to mastoiditis, chronic otitis media and permanent hearing loss.

The patient having a myringotomy receives a local anesthetic or a brief-acting general anesthetic. Fluid is aspirated from the middle ear cavity through the incision, and a culture is taken. Absorbent cotton is placed loosely in the outer ear to absorb the drainage. The patient is encouraged to lie on the affected side to promote drainage. A persistent elevation of temperature, pain and deep tenderness in the region of the mastoid, headache, drowsiness or disorientation is reported to the physician. These may indicate the onset of a serious complication such as mastoiditis, meningitis or brain abscess.

Serous Otitis Media

Serous otitis media is characterized by an accumulation of fluid in the middle ear. The effusion is usually caused by obstruction of the eustachian tube incurred by enlarged adenoids, severe nasopharyngitis or an allergic reaction. It may also develop following acute otitis media that has not been completely resolved. Rarely, the condition may be associated with a benign or malignant neoplasm of the pharynx which blocks the eustachian tube.

The fluid is a thin and watery transudate. Blockage of the eustachian tube results in a negative pressure in the middle ear cavity which promotes movement of fluid out of the mucous membrane capillaries.

MANIFESTATIONS. The patient experiences loss of hearing and uncomfortable sensations in the affected ear. Examination of the eardrum reveals its immobility and the amber fluid level in the middle ear. The nasopharyngeal area is investigated for disease that is the likely primary cause.

TREATMENT. Any nasopharyngeal disorder is corrected; for example, if hypertrophied adenoids are found to be the cause, an adenoidectomy is performed. The allergic reaction is treated if it is found to be the problem. If nasopharyngitis due to infection is obstructing the eustachian tube, the patient receives antibiotic therapy.

A myringotomy is done and the fluid aspirated. This may be followed by repeated Valsalva maneuvers to clear the eustachian tube (see p. 1003) and ventilate the middle ear. Following the myringotomy, a plastic, indwelling tympanostomy tube may have to be inserted via the external auditory canal. This permits continuous ventilation and drainage of the middle ear (see Fig. 28–6). The tube is left in position until patency of the eustachian tube is reestablished; this may be a period of several weeks or months. The patient is closely supervised following the surgery. Usually he is seen in the clinic or physician's office every 2 or 3 weeks, and the tube and the patient's hearing are checked.

When the tube is inserted the nurse instructs the patient, and the parents if the patient is a child, about the care of the affected ear and the restrictions on activities. Daily, or more often if necessary, an absor-

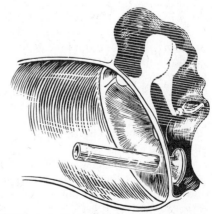

FIGURE 28–6 Tympanostomy tube. (From Sabiston, David C., Jr. (Ed.): Davis-Christopher Textbook of Surgery, 11th ed. Philadelphia, W. B. Saunders, 1977, p. 1404.)

bent ear dressing is placed *loosely* in the external auditory meatus. If the physician prescribes the instillation of drops, an explanation and demonstration are given to the parents, and an opportunity provided for one of them to carry out the procedure under supervision. They are cautioned that if the medication causes pain following the instillation, the procedure is discontinued and the physician contacted promptly. The physician is also notified immediately of any increase or change in the fluid drainage, increasing deafness or pain. The patient must guard against getting water into the ear. During a bath or shower, a cotton ball coated with petroleum jelly is placed in the entrance to the ear canal. Swimming is contraindicated unless the physician has indicated that the patient may do so, and then only if tightly fitting ear plugs and a swimming cap are used. If swimming is approved, the patient is cautioned against diving.

Chronic Otitis Media

This chronic inflammatory disorder of the ear is associated with a permanent perforation of the tympanic membrane. It usually is a sequela of repeated episodes of acute otitis media that were not treated or were caused by virulent or antibiotic-resistant organisms. The perforation may also be the result of mechanical trauma or blast injury.

The location of the perforation is an important factor in the seriousness of the disease. If it is central or at least does not involve the margin of the eardrum, the perforation is less serious and can be treated more effectively. This type of perforation is categorized as *tubotympanic*. If the perforation involves the tympanic margin in the posterior-superior area, the disorder is a more serious and life-threatening problem. There are usually several perforations and, because of their location, may be referred to as *attic perforations*.

MANIFESTATIONS. The otitis media associated with a central perforation is manifested by purulent discharge with an offensive odor. The discharge may be greatly increased during periods of acute upper respiratory infections or if water gets into the ear during bathing or swimming. Over a period of time, middle ear structures are damaged by the infection and necrosis.

There is usually some impairment of hearing which worsens during exacerbations.

TREATMENT. The initial treatment of the patient with a *tubotympanic perforation* is directed towards eliminating any upper respiratory tract infection as well as that in the ear. An antibiotic is administered orally or parenterally. The ear is cleansed by syringing which is followed by the instillation of an antimicrobial solution. If the exudate is excessive, it may be removed by daily aspiration by the physician. When the infection is cleared up, the perforated area very occasionally fills in with scar tissue. If the perforation persists, a tympanoplasty may be done to improve the patient's hearing and reduce the risk of reinfection by establishing a barrier between external and middle ears. The type of surgical procedure used depends upon whether there is damage to the middle ear structures or not and, if so, the extent of the involvement. Tympanoplastic surgery is only undertaken if infection is controlled.

Tympanoplasty Type I indicates a myringoplasty in which a graft is used to repair the perforated eardrum when the middle ear structures are intact and functional. Epithelium from the ear canal, skin from the postauricular area, fascia stripped from the temporal muscle or a section of a vein may be used as a graft. Tympanoplasty Types II, III, IV, and V operative procedures involve plastic correction of the perforated eardrum and repair of damaged middle ear structures. The operations progressively increase in complexity, involving more extensive surgery and structural replacement. The reparative and/or reconstructive procedures are directed toward reestablishing a conductive system from the eardrum through the ossicles and the oval window and providing sound protection for the round window. Reestablishing ossicular continuity may necessitate the replacement of ossicles by a graft or a prosthesis.

Postoperatively, the dressing is left undisturbed for 3 to 4 days; if necessary, the outer part may be reinforced. Dressings are changed and the packing is removed by the surgeon. Precautions are taken to avoid wetting the dressing during bathing. The patient is asked not to blow his nose and to avoid coughing and sneezing to prevent air being forced through the eustachian tube into the middle ear. When he is allowed up, a nurse assists and remains with him for a while since he may experience dizziness and nausea.

In *marginal (attic) perforations,* the disease involves the bony rim of the tympanic membrane and the mastoid cells as well as the middle ear structures. An invasive *cholesteatoma* may develop; this is a mass that forms in the middle ear as a result of the growth of epithelial tissue implanted in the middle ear from the collapsed and invaginated parts of the eardrum when it perforates. The inflammation causes hyperactivity of the basal layer of the epidermis. The epidermal tissue encloses sebum and desquamated epidermal cells; these serve as a good culture medium for organisms. The mass compresses middle ear structures and mastoid cells, causing necrosis and bone erosion. The presence of the cholesteatoma predisposes to the serious complications of labrynthitis and brain abscess. Marginal perforation and the development of a cholesteatoma are treated by radical surgery. A mastoidectomy is done, the cholesteatoma and middle ear debris are removed and reconstruction undertaken to provide a conductive channel. The surgery is done in two stages; the first operation removes the cholesteatoma and clears out the infected and necrotic tissue. The patient receives antibiotic therapy and, when the area is free of infection and there is no drainage, the reconstructive plastic surgery is undertaken.

Mastoiditis

The small spaces (air cells) in the mastoid communicate with the middle ear cavity and are lined with mucous membrane which is continuous with that of the middle ear. As a result, infection may spread readily to the mastoid in acute or chronic otitis media. The patient experiences tenderness over the mastoid process, headache and fever. A roentgenogram of the temporal bone shows a cloudiness in the mastoid cells.

TREATMENT AND NURSING CARE. Generally, early treatment with antibiotics checks the infection and no residual damage to hearing occurs. Rarely, if the infection is neglected or is virulent and unresponsive to the antibiotic given, bone tissue of the mastoid becomes infected, necessi-

tating surgery. A myringotomy and a simple mastoidectomy are done. A simple mastoidectomy involves an incision behind the auricle and the removal of the diseased bone by curettage.

If the patient develops chronic otitis media and chronic mastoiditis, more extensive surgery may be undertaken. A radical mastoidectomy involves the removal of the diseased mastoid tissue and the incus, malleus and remainder of the tympanic membrane, leaving the mastoid and middle ear as one large cavity. This surgery on the middle ear results in loss of hearing.

Preoperative preparation for a mastoidectomy is the same as that for any patient who is to have a general anesthetic (see Chapter 10). The scalp is shaved 1 to 2 inches around the affected ear, and the long hair is combed toward the opposite side and secured.

Postoperatively, the dressing remains undisturbed for 3 to 4 days. Packing is placed in the wound to promote drainage and remains in place until the first dressing change by the physician. The bulky dressing and trauma make it difficult for the patient to move or raise his head. The nurse provides assistance at first, but gradually the patient learns to support his head with the hands when moving.

The patient is observed closely for nystagmus or any sign of facial paralysis. Facial paralysis is a threat in mastoidectomy because of the facial (seventh cranial) nerve's proximity to the operative site. Persisting headache, stiffness of the neck, elevation of temperature or disorientation is brought to the physician's attention, since it may indicate a complicating brain abscess or meningitis. Fluids are given freely and a regular diet is served as soon as it is tolerated.

The patient is generally allowed up on the second day; someone remains with him at first in case of dizziness and nausea that may develop as a result of labyrinth disturbance, especially following a radical mastoidectomy.

If the patient suffers some hearing loss, he is reassured that assistance is available. The nurse advises him how he may help himself in trying to communicate with others and may also refer him to the National Hearing Society.

A radical mastoidectomy may be followed by a tympanoplasty. This is a surgical procedure done to improve conduction through the middle ear (see p. 1008).

Otosclerosis

This is a chronic ear disease in which the stapes becomes immobilized because of progressive growth of bone tissue over the oval window and fixation of the stapes, interfering with the transmission of vibrations into the inner ear. Both ears are affected.

The disease appears to be hereditary and has a higher incidence in females. The ability of the stapes to vibrate progressively decreases, and the loss of hearing usually becomes apparent in the teens or twenties. The person may complain of tinnitus as the deafness becomes more marked. The testing of hearing with a tuning fork reveals that the person has good bone conduction of sound but none by air.

TREATMENT. A hearing aid may be of some help for a period of time, but a stapedectomy has proved to be the treatment of choice at present. By means of a surgical microscope, the surgeon works through the external auditory canal and the middle ear. The stapes is removed, and a prosthesis introduced to transfer the vibrations of the incus through the oval window into the inner ear. Various forms of prostheses have been used and include a wire or polyethylene tube with a section of vein, a "pad" of fat, or Gelfoam. The wire or polyethylene tube is attached to the incus while the vein, fat or Gelfoam is fitted into the oval window. Only one ear is done at a time.

Postoperatively, dizziness and nausea may be troublesome because of the disturbance of the labyrinth. A specific directive is received from the surgeon about the position in which the head is to be maintained. A close check is made for any sign of infection (elevation of temperature and leukocyte count, discharge and pain); if it is suspected, an antimicrobial drug is prescribed. The patient is instructed not to blow his nose to prevent air from being forced through the eustachian tube to the middle ear. The patient is allowed out of bed in 2 or 3 days and is cautioned to move slowly and not to stoop over. If vertigo is experienced, ambulation may have to be delayed. The patient requires assurance that the dizziness is temporary.

Packing is placed in the ear upon completion of the surgery; this is removed by the surgeon in approximately 7 to 9 days. When the packing is removed, the patient may find the noise in the environment very confusing and disturbing. A nurse or family member should accompany him to provide support and reassurance.

Meniere's Disease or Syndrome

This is a disorder of the internal ear characterized by recurrent attacks of severe vertigo, nausea, vomiting, tinnitus and a progressive loss of hearing. The cause is not known but an excess of endolymph (endolymphatic hydrops) resulting in increased pressure and dilation of the canals develops. Vascular spasm and allergic reaction have been suggested as possible etiologic factors. The disorder usually makes its appearance between the ages of 40 and 60 years, and occurs more often in males.

The episodes have a sudden onset, and the patient is generally prostrated by the dizziness and nausea. The duration of an attack varies from hours to days.

During an attack the patient remains in bed in a quiet environment. Siderails may be necessary for safety because of the vertigo. An antiemetic such as dimenhydrinate (Dramamine) and a sedative may provide some relief. Diphenhydramine hydrochloride (Benadryl) given intravenously may arrest an acute attack. In an effort to offset episodes, the patient is placed on a low-sodium diet and receives ammonium chloride; a diuretic such as hydrochlorothiazide (Hydro-Diuril) may also be prescribed to reduce the formation of endolymph. A vasodilator (e.g., nicotinic acid) to discourage vasospasm may be helpful. Although the acute attacks are episodic, the hearing loss tends to be permanent.

The condition can be very incapacitating and may necessitate surgery. The procedure entails the destruction of the membranous labyrinth. More recently, ultrasonic waves have been used. This form of treatment requires a mastoidectomy to permit the application of the probe. If the patient still has considerable hearing in the affected ear, ultrasonic treatment is used because it is thought to be less hazardous for the hearing.

References

Books

Ballantyne, John: Deafness, Edinburgh, Churchill Livingstone, 1977.

Davis, Hallowell, and Silverman, S. Richard: Hearing and Deafness, 4th ed. New York, Holt, Rinehart and Winston, 1978.

DeWeese, David D., and Saunders, William H.: Otolaryngology, 4th ed. St Louis, C. V. Mosby, 1973. Chapters 18–26.

Ganong, W. F.: Review of Medical Physiology, 7th ed. Los Altos, Cal., Lange, 1975. Chapter 9.

Hall, I. Simson, and Coleman, Bernard H.: Diseases of the Nose, Throat and Ear, 11th ed. Edinburgh, Churchill Livingstone, 1975. Chapters 28–42.

Krupp, Marcus A., and Chatton, Milton J.: Current Medical Diagnosis and Treatment. Los Altos, Cal., Lange, 1975, pp. 88–95.

Nave, Carl R., and Nave, Brenda C.: Physics for the Health Sciences. Philadelphia, W. B. Saunders, 1975. Chapter 18.

Periodicals

Blancher, Gertrude C.: "My Trip Through the Semicircular Canals." Am. J. Nurs., Vol. 74, No. 10 (Oct. 1974), pp. 1842–1843.

Brown, Marie Scott, and Alexander, Mary M.: "Examining the Ear." Nurs. '74, Vol. 4, No. 2 (Feb. 1974), pp. 48–51.

————: "Hearing Acuity." Nurs. '74, Vol. 4, No. 4 (Apr., 1974), pp. 61–65.

Conover, Mary, and Cober, Joyce: "Understanding and Caring for the Hearing-Impaired." Nurs. Clin. North Am., Vol. 5, No. 3 (Sept. 1970), pp. 497–506.

Huber, Helen L.: "Draining the Fluid Ear with Myringotomy and Tube Insertion." Nurs. '78, Vol. 8, No. 7 (July 1978), pp. 28–30.

Kearns, J. R.: "Presbycusis." Can. Family Physician, Vol. 23, No. 9 (Sept. 1977), pp. 96–100.

Keim, Robert J.: "How Aging Affects the Ear." Geriatrics, Vol. 32, No. 6 (June 1977), pp. 97–99.

————: "Problem Ear Infections." Med. Times, Vol. 106, No. 2 (Feb. 1978), pp. 68–73.

Lesser, Stanley R., and Easser, B. Ruth: "Psychiatric Management of the Deaf Child." Can. Nurse, Vol. 71, No. 10 (Oct. 1975), pp. 23–25.

Mamaril, Aurora Pizana: "Sudden Deafness." Am. J. Nurs., Vol. 67, No. 12 (Dec. 1976), pp. 1992–1994.

McNamee, Christine: "Communicating with the Hard-of-Hearing." Can. Nurse, Vol. 74, No. 3 (March 1978), pp. 27–29.

Mechner, Francis: "Examination of the Ear." Am. J. Nurs., Vol. 75, No. 3 (March 1975), pp. 1–24 (programmed instruction).

Meyerhoff, William L., and Paparella, Michael M.: "Diagnosing the Cause of Hearing Loss." Geriatrics, Vol. 33, No. 2 (Feb. 1978), p. 95.

Payne, Peter D., and Payne, Regina L.: "Behavior Manifestations of Children with Hearing Loss." Am. J. Nurs., Vol. 70, No. 8 (Aug. 1970), pp. 1718–1719.

Perron, Denise M.: "Deprived of Sound." Am. J. Nurs., Vol. 74, No. 6 (June 1974), pp. 1057–1059.

INDEX

Note: Page numbers in *italic* indicate illustrations; folios followed by t refer to tabular material.